WEIGHT

Metric		Approximate apothecary equivalents		Metric		Approximate apothecary equivalents
30	g	1	ounce	30	mg	$^1/_2$ grain
15	g	4	drams	25	mg	$^3/_8$ grain
10	g	$2^1/_2$	drams	20	mg	$^1/_3$ grain
7.5	g	2	drams	15	mg	$^1/_4$ grain
6	g	90	grains	12	mg	$^1/_5$ grain
5	g	75	grains	10	mg	$^1/_6$ grain
4	g	60	grains (1 dram)	8	mg	$^1/_8$ grain
3	g	45	grains	6	mg	$^1/_{10}$ grain
2	g	30	grains ($^1/_2$ dram)	5	mg	$^1/_{12}$ grain
1.5	g	22	grains	4	mg	$^1/_{15}$ grain
1	g	15	grains	3	mg	$^1/_{20}$ grain
0.75	g	12	grains	2	mg	$^1/_{30}$ grain
0.6	g	10	grains	1.5	mg	$^1/_{40}$ grain
0.5	g	$7^1/_2$	grains	1.2	mg	$^1/_{50}$ grain
0.4	g	6	grains	1	mg	$^1/_{60}$ grain
0.3	g	5	grains	0.8	mg	$^1/_{80}$ grain
0.25	g	4	grains	0.6	mg	$^1/_{100}$ grain
0.2	g	3	grains	0.5	mg	$^1/_{120}$ grain
0.15	g	$2^1/_2$	grains	0.4	mg	$^1/_{150}$ grain
0.125	g	2	grains	0.3	mg	$^1/_{200}$ grain
0.1	g	$1^1/_2$	grains	0.25	mg	$^1/_{250}$ grain
75	mg	$1^1/_4$	grains	0.2	mg	$^1/_{300}$ grain
60	mg	1	grain	0.15	mg	$^1/_{400}$ grain
50	mg	$^3/_4$	grain	0.12	mg	$^1/_{500}$ grain
40	mg	$^2/_3$	grain	0.1	mg	$^1/_{600}$ grain

Pharmacology
in nursing

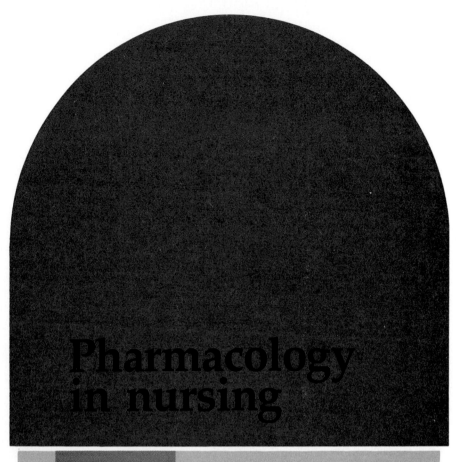

Pharmacology in nursing

Thirteenth edition

BETTY S. BERGERSEN, R.N., M.S., Ed.D.

Formerly Professor of Nursing
and Chairman of Graduate
Medical-Surgical Nursing,
University of Colorado School
of Nursing, Medical Center,
Denver, Colorado

in consultation with

Andres Goth, M.D.

Professor of Pharmacology
and Chairman of the Department,
The University of Texas
Southwestern Medical School,
Dallas, Texas

with 100 illustrations

The C. V. Mosby Company

Saint Louis   1976

Thirteenth edition

Copyright © 1976 by The C. V. Mosby Company

All rights reserved. No part of this book may be reproduced in any manner without written permission of the publisher.

Previous editions copyrighted 1936, 1940, 1942, 1945, 1948, 1951, 1955, 1960, 1963, 1966, 1969, 1973

Printed in the United States of America

International Standard Book Number 0-8016-0631-4

Library of Congress Catalog Card Number 66-10935

Distributed in Great Britain by Henry Kimpton, London

TS/K/B   9   8   7   6   5   4   3   2   1

Preface

Drugs can be beneficial when used with wisdom but harmful when used with inadequate knowledge. This edition of *Pharmacology in Nursing* outlines current concepts of pharmacology and their relationship to clinical patient care. Included in the text are basic mechanisms of drug action, indications and contraindications for drug therapy, toxicity and side effects, and safe therapeutic dosage range. This information should provide the nurse practitioner or student with the means for ensuring rational and optimal drug therapy.

In this edition the following changes have been incorporated: (1) major revision of the chapters on drug legislation, respiratory system drugs, skeletal muscle relaxants, fluids and electrolytes, antimicrobial and antineoplastic drugs, endocrine hormones, and ophthalmic drugs; (2) dosage for children for many drugs approved for use in pediatrics; (3) inclusion of D.E.S.I. ratings (drug efficacy study by the Food and Drug Administration); and (4) expanded coverage of information on drug interactions, pharmacologic effects, and nursing care aspects.

Concern for prevention of teratogenic effects and more extensive research on the effects of drugs has led to the inclusion of a new chapter titled "Effects of Drugs on Human Sexuality, Fetal Development, and Nursing Infant." I wish to thank Eleanor A. Schuster, R.N., D.N.S., Associate Professor of Nursing and Director of the Graduate Program, Department of Nursing, Wichita State University, Wichita, Kansas, for this timely contribution.

I also wish to thank my friend and colleague, Jurate Sakalys, Assistant Professor of Nursing, University of Colorado School of Nursing, for updating the chapter on drug abuse, which she originally wrote, as well as for revising the chapters on antimicrobial and antineoplastic drugs and pharmacodynamics. In addition, I wish to thank Patsy A. Perry, R.N., M.S., Assistant Professor of Medical-Surgical Nursing, University of Colorado School of Nursing, for the much needed revision on respiratory system drugs.

As in the previous edition, each chapter has been critically reviewed by Andres Goth, Professor of Pharmacology and Chairman of the Department, The University of Texas Southwestern Medical School, Dallas, Texas.

I also wish to express my deep gratitude and affection to Elsie Krug, from whom I inherited this textbook, and I extend my appreciation to the many students and educators of nurses who have used this book and contributed to its success.

Betty S. Bergersen

v

Contents

List of tables

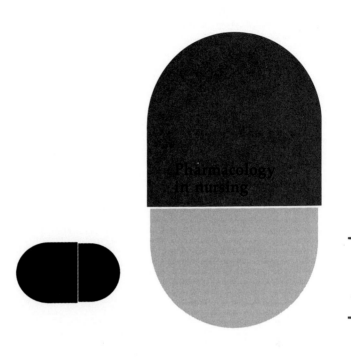

Pharmacology
in nursing

CHAPTER 1

Orientation to pharmacology

Orientation to pharmacology
Drug information sources

ORIENTATION TO PHARMACOLOGY

Medications are an essential part of patient care, and safe administration of drugs requires *sound* and *current* knowledge of their: (1) mode of action, (2) side effects, (3) toxicity, (4) range of dosage, (5) rate and route of excretion, (6) individual differences in response, such as idiosyncratic or allergic reactions, and (7) interactions with other drugs. This knowledge can be obtained from textbooks and periodicals for health professionals, classroom lectures and discussions, and materials available in teaching laboratories. However, actual administration of drugs with careful observation of their effects in individuals and groups of patients will richly supplement and complement a student's knowledge of specific drugs.

Drugs have the power to help or to harm. Nurses, along with physicians and clinical pharmacists, are held legally responsible for safe and therapeutically effective drug administration. Nurses are liable for their actions and omissions and for those duties they delegate to others. The nurse is not exonerated from responsibility when drugs are administered by medication technicians, pharmacy technicians, practical nurses, or even physicians. Indeed, all members of a health team may be held liable for a single injury to a patient. The continued increase in litigation against nurses and physicians indicates that society tolerates only a minimal margin of error in

relation to human life. Claims have been brought against health professionals for drug errors that caused loss of life (Norton v. Argonaut Insurance Co., the Somera case) and permanent injury (Honeywell v. Rogers).* When claims against health professionals are supported with evidence that the conduct of one or more health professionals helped to bring about the loss or injury, those parties are held liable. The law, a legal and social norm, requires health professionals to be safe and competent practitioners and permits compensation to those harmed or injured.

However, the law is a protective force for the knowledgeable, competent, and skilled nurse. The nurse who is knowledgeable about the drugs patients are receiving, who uses proper technique and precautions, who observes for and charts explicitly the drug effects, who keeps up to date by referring to authoritative sources (pharmacist, pharmacologist, professional literature), who questions a drug order that is unclear or that appears to contain an error, and who even refuses to administer a drug and intervenes to prevent others from administering a drug if there is reason to believe harm may come to the patient is safeguarding and protecting patients from drug-induced harm. The law in turn will protect the nurse from unfair litigation.

Drugs deserve the respect of the nurse, but

---

*Murchison, I. A., and Nichols, T. S.: Legal foundations of nursing practice, New York, 1970, The Macmillan Company, pp. 189, 338, and 116.

that respect must be mingled with skepticism. Much remains to be learned about the actual mode of action as well as effects from prolonged use of many commonly prescribed drugs. Furthermore, there is increasing concern about drug-induced disease. Fortunately, drug therapy for most illnesses or for illness prevention is temporary. However, there are those diseases that require life-long use of drugs to sustain life (such as insulin for diabetes mellitus) or prolonged use to maintain relatively normal physiologic or psychologic functioning.

Nurses are entrusted with potent and habit-forming drugs, and they must not abuse or misuse this trust. Used respectfully and intelligently, drugs are comforting and lifesaving. Used unwisely or with undue dependence, they can lead to irreparable tragedy. The nurse who combines diligent and intelligent observation with moral integrity and factual knowledge will be a safe and competent practitioner and a credit to the nursing profession.

Pharmacology is a challenging and interesting subject to study. It requires integrating knowledge from many different disciplines including anatomy and physiology, pathology, microbiology, organic chemistry and biochemistry, psychology, and sociology; thus, clinical drug therapy can be considered to be an applied science. The hundreds of drugs available would make the study of pharmacology formidable if they had to be studied as individual agents. Fortunately, drugs can be classified into a reasonable number of drug groups based on their chemical, pharmacologic, or therapeutic relatedness. Understanding the characteristic effects of a particular group of drugs at the subcellular, tissue, organ, or functional system level permits a student or practitioner to know a variety of facts about many drugs. An individual drug can then be studied according to those characteristics that differentiate it from other drugs within the same classification.

The doses of drugs and indications for use must not be regarded by the student as therapeutic dogma. New knowledge about drugs will be forthcoming from laboratory research and more scientific methods of clinical drug evaluation.

The constant advances in the field of drug therapy, the almost daily appearance of new drugs or new preparations of old drugs on the market and in the hospital, are a challenge to both the student and the graduate nurse to be students always. An examination passed and an R.N. acquired are no lasting guarantees of sufficient knowledge in the field of drugs to make a nurse helpful to the doctor or even safe for the patient. Drugs change and will continue to change. Pharmacology books should become a permanent section of the nurse's library, and year by year as new editions or new books appear the library must be brought up to date. In addition, the official current literature on drugs must be followed carefully, since new drugs are slow in making their way into more permanent literature. For the nurse working in a hospital or health service, doctors, instructors, supervisors, and pharmacists will be on hand to help. In a more isolated practice, greater personal effort will be required to keep abreast of current practices. In any case, a sustained interest in pharmacology will help to keep the nurse well informed about drugs.

Of primary importance is the understanding that learning is an active process and that learning does not take place without activity. Thus, clinical experience with drugs is invaluable for it enables the student to:

1 Note those drugs most commonly used to treat certain diseases or specific signs and symptoms
2 Note the frequency with which certain drugs are administered
3 Observe the degree of effectiveness between specific drugs for relieving particular signs and symptoms
4 Witness the individual differences in patients' reactions to a specific drug
5 Relate knowledge obtained from authoritative sources with real-life situations

Regardless of what subject matter is to be learned, reasoning and the ability to analyze and synthesize information are prerequisites to understanding. These cognitive skills, along with perceptual skills, permit an individual to see meaningful relationships, make comparisons, and determine significance, all of which are essential for sound decision making. The development of cognitive, perceptual, and manual skills is the foundation for professional competence.

DRUG INFORMATION SOURCES

Nurses will find the following sources of drug information very useful in the study of pharmacology and in the practice of nursing involving drug therapy.

THE UNITED STATES DISPENSATORY

The twenty-seventh edition of the United States Dispensatory was edited by Arthur Osol, Robertson Pratt, and Alfonso R. Gennaro and published by J. B. Lippincott Co. (Philadelphia, 1973).

The Dispensatory is an encyclopedia containing comprehensive monographs on individual drugs and general survey articles on pharmacologic classes of drugs alphabetically arranged. The monographs contain descriptions, histories, actions, uses, and facts on toxicology and dosage for adults and children; they are documented by references to medical literature. Official, generic, trade, and chemical names are given in the monographs. The monographs contain drugs listed in *The Pharmacopeia of the United States of America, The National Formulary,* and the *British Pharmaceutical Codex* and drugs not listed in these official compendia. Official, generic (or nonproprietary), and trade (or proprietary) names are included in the general alphabetic index.

AMERICAN HOSPITAL FORMULARY SERVICE

The *American Hospital Formulary Service* is a drug monograph subscription service for the calendar year published by the American Society of Hospital Pharmacists, Washington, D.C. The monograph of each drug is entered under the generic name, giving common synonyms and trade names. Monographs are full and descriptive and emphasize rational therapeutic procedures. Classification is according to the pharmacologic ac-

tions of the individual agents. Each monograph includes a list of the dosage forms most commonly used in hospitals.

MODERN DRUG ENCYCLOPEDIA AND THERAPEUTIC INDEX

The *Modern Drug Encyclopedia,* thirteenth edition edited by Arthur J. Lewis and published by the Dun-Donnelley Corporation (New York, 1975), describes widely used prescription medications. Individual monographs are arranged alphabetically according to generic names. Information for each includes its manufacturer, pharmacologic classification, description, chemical name, trade name, action and uses, method of administration and dosage, cautions and contraindications, and forms and sizes supplied. The general alphabetic index includes both generic and trade names.

A.M.A. DRUG EVALUATIONS

The *A.M.A. Drug Evaluations* contains drug monographs organized according to therapeutic classifications. Each chapter begins with an overall discussion of the therapeutic category followed by brief evaluative monographs of individual drugs. Drugs evaluated include those listed in the official compendia, those that are dispensed exclusively or principally by prescription, those commonly administered, and those judged to be of particular importance to a therapeutic category. Evaluations are based on available and current evidence from scientific literature, unpublished data, and consultants and review committees. The monographs also contain uses, routes of administration, and dosages that may or may not be included in package inserts. Although the drug evaluations are compiled by the A.M.A. Department of Drugs this does not imply endorsement by the American Medical Association. Evaluations may be favorable, unfavorable, or a combination of both.

PHYSICIANS' DESK REFERENCE TO PHARMACEUTICAL SPECIALTIES AND BIOLOGICALS (P.D.R.)

P.D.R., published by Medical Economics, Inc. (Oradell, N.J.), contains an annual listing of drugs arranged in five sections. The pink section is a comprehensive alphabetic listing of brand name products and a list of manufacturers with their products. The blue section is a therapeutic index. The yellow section is a drug, chemical, and pharmacologic index to drugs. The white section is a list of the major products of manufacturers, with information on composition, action, uses, administration, dosage, precautions, contraindications, and supply of each drug. A product identification section shows full-size color photographs of more than 1000 capsules and tablets.

UNLISTED DRUGS

Unlisted Drugs, published by Special Libraries Association (New York), lists new drugs found in literature or advertising when no entries are located for them in *Modern Drug Encyclopedia* or other standard sources. Entries are made for experimental compounds under their research numbers as well as for marketed products. Each entry includes a brief statement of composition, manufacturer, action, dosage, and source of information. This is a monthly publication with a cumulative index for volumes.

COMPENDIUM OF PHARMACEUTICALS AND SPECIALTIES (CANADA)

Compendium of Pharmaceuticals and Specialties (Canada), edited by G. N. Rotenberg and published by Canadian Pharmaceutical Association (Toronto), contains information on the most frequently used drugs available to Canadian pharmacists. The book contains monographs (entered under trade names) that provide descriptions, manufacturers' information, indication, instructions for administration, and dosage, as well as forms and sizes in which drugs are available. A product recognition section is included as an aid for quick visual identification of drug dosage forms. A list of manufacturers

with their products and a therapeutic index are included as well as a cross-reference index for nonproprietary names and chemical names of drugs. Drug schedules of the Food and Drugs Act and regulations issued by the Health Protection Branch, Ottawa, and the location of poison control centers in Canada are also included. This publication consists of three semiannual supplements, which are cumulative.

PACKAGE BROCHURES

Before marketing a new drug product, the manufacturer develops a concise description of the product, indications and precautions in clinical use, guidance for dosage, known adverse actions, and other pertinent pharmacologic information. Federal law requires that a brochure accompany each package of the product, and because this is construed as labeling, the brochure must be approved by the Food and Drug Administration.

THE MEDICAL LETTER

The Medical Letter, a semimonthly periodical published by Drug and Therapeutic Information, Inc. (New York), contains independent brief comments on newly released drug products and related topics by a board of competent authorities who call freely upon specialists in various fields. The letters contain data on drug action and comparative clinical efficacy. They have the advantage of presenting a timely and critical summation of current status in the early phase of promotion of a drug. However, these drug appraisals are tentative.

CLINICAL PHARMACOLOGY AND THERAPEUTICS

Clinical Pharmacology and Therapeutics, a bimonthly periodical published by The C. V. Mosby Co. (St. Louis), contains reports of studies of new drugs, reviews of present knowledge of classes of drugs or advances in therapy of various disorders, and abstracts of reports of adverse reactions to drugs appearing in the world literature. It also contains a section on drug-induced diseases.

DRUGS OF CHOICE 1976-1977

Drugs of Choice 1976-1977, edited by Walter Modell and published by The C. V. Mosby Co. (St. Louis, 1976), is revised every 2 years and contains contributions from outstanding specialists who express their opinions of the drugs in current use in their own fields of specialization. The book is designed to provide clear, concise, and practical answers to questions of drugs of choice for actual therapeutic problems. An alphabetically arranged index of drugs in common use is also included.

JOURNALS

Other important sources of drug information are the various nursing, pharmacy, medical, and allied health journals. In addition to the *American Journal of Nursing, Nursing '76, Nursing Digest,* and *RN* the following prominent periodicals are usually available in medical and health reference libraries:

Pharmacy journals

Journal of the American Pharmaceutical Association
American Journal of Hospital Pharmacy
American Druggist
Pharmacy Times
Drug Topics

Medical journals

Journal of the American Medical Association
New England Journal of Medicine
Postgraduate Medicine
British Medical Journal

CHAPTER 2

History of materia medica

Ancient period
Medieval period
Sixteenth century
Seventeenth century
Eighteenth century
Nineteenth century
Twentieth century

The story of materia medica is as old as the story of man, for sickness has been man's heritage from the beginning of time and the search for ways and means to combat disease has been one of his earliest and most persistent activities. Early man's first experiments in dealing with disease were suggested by the belief common to all primitive people that the world in which they lived teemed with invisible spirits, some of whom were good and some bad. Whatever puzzled man in nature was attributed to these supernatural agencies, and it followed that disease was at first thought to be an evil spirit or the work of such a spirit. If this supposition were true, the logical treatment was to placate the invader by burnt offerings or to frighten it away by resorting to hideous noises or by administering foul-tasting substances. These measures were designed to make the body an uncomfortable habitat for the spirit. The search for obnoxious materials led man to experiment with herbs of the field and the forest, and as the knowledge gained from experience increased, the rudiments of materia medica were assembled. These intuitive efforts of man led to some valuable discoveries. Primitive peoples in separate countries knew the properties of the most fatal arrow poisons, such as curare, veratrine, and ouabain, as well as the virtues of drugs like opium. Centuries ago the Indians of Peru discovered the value of cinchona bark for the treatment and prevention of malaria, and the natives of Brazil knew the worth of ipecac for amebic dysentery. The victims of leprosy in the Far East believed that they received relief by rubbing their wounds with chaulmoogra oil, and for some time chaulmoogra oil was used in the treatment of this disease. The Indians of America used arbutus for rheumatism; lobelia for coughs and colds; wild sage tea, goldenseal, and flowering dogwood for fevers; elders, wild cherry, and sumac for colds and quinsies; inhalations of pennyroyal for headache; sassafras leaves for wounds and felons; and the roots of sassafras for cooling and purifying the blood.

As medical lore accumulated, there appeared individuals who demonstrated a special talent for herb-doctoring, bone-setting, and crude surgery and who employed it as a means of earning a livelihood. They were either the wisewomen who sought by their art to lessen the hardships and dangers of childbirth or certain men of superior intelligence and cunning who, appreciating the credulity of the rank and file, made use of incantations and charms in their therapeutics and established themselves in the community in the role of priest and physician. These nature healers soon perceived not only what substances were good and what were harmful but that a number of poisons were also remedies under certain conditions. This drug and poison lore was the beginning of materia medica and medicine.

ANCIENT PERIOD

EGYPT

The oldest phase of medicine is the Egyptian. The main sources of data are the medical papyri, the most important of which is the Ebers papyrus, written in the sixteenth century B.C. It is a scroll 22 yards long and about 12 inches wide that contains a collection of prescriptions and formulas covering a wide range of uses. Included among them are many invocations and conjuring forms for driving away disease, as well as specific recipes, calling in many instances for drugs that are in common use today, for example, aloes, castor oil, figs, vinegar, turpentine, opium, wormwood, peppermint, and squill.

As the inclusion of invocations and charms in the prescriptions would imply, medicine was closely allied with religion, as it was to remain for many centuries. The doctors were all priests paid out of the royal treasury, but they were allowed to take fees also.

GREECE

The pharmaceutical history of Greece begins with legends regarding gods and goddesses. The reputed activities of these mythical characters are so inextricably woven with the authentic doings of real men and women that it is often hard to determine where legend ends and history begins. The story goes, however, that Chiron, the centaur, originated the pharmaceutical art and imparted his valuable knowledge to Asclepius, son of Apollo. Asclepius, with the aid of his daughters Hygeia and Panacea, in turn taught mortals the art of healing, but he became so successful in combating disease that he incurred the wrath of the god of the underworld, because he was diminishing too greatly the number of shades received in Hades. Zeus destroyed Asclepius with a thunderbolt, but upon the intercession of Apollo, Zeus deified him as

the god of healing. His mortal followers in time made up the organized guild of physicians called Asclepiades. They built temples in his honor in which they practiced their art and increased their knowledge of healing. These temples were situated in hills or mountains, usually near mineral springs, and were managed by trained priests. Hence they were virtually sanatoriums or hospitals for the sick. The patient was received by the physician priests and, after spiritual purification by prayers and sacrifice, was further cleansed by a bath from the mineral springs, catharsis, massage, and inunction and encouraged with medicated wines and soft music to sleep and to dream. The priest then interpreted the dream as a message from Morpheus and offered medical advice accordingly. If the treatment was a success and the patient recovered, a votive tablet giving the history of the case and the treatment was hung in the temple where anyone who wished might consult it. In this way, a considerable body of empirical knowledge was assembled and these Temples of Health took on some of the characteristics of a medical school. The most celebrated ones were at Cnidus and Cos.

The most famous representative of the Asclepiades was Hippocrates, who was born in the Island of Cos, 460 B.C., of a long line of priest physicians and who was reputed by popular tradition to be the seventeenth in direct descent from Asclepius. Hippocrates pursued his early studies at Cos and Cnidus but later came under the influence of the great thinkers and philosophers of the period and soon began to apply their scientific and ethical ideas to medicine. He denounced the belief in the supernatural origin of disease and the use of charms, incantations, and other superstitious devices of priestcraft. He substituted the doctrine that disease resulted from natural causes and that knowledge of it would be gained only through the study of the natural laws. He taught the use of the senses in collecting data for diagnosis and the use of inductive reasoning in arriving at diagnostic conclusions.

His therapeutic measures were decidedly modern. He believed that the body has great power to recuperate and that the role of the physician should be simply to aid Nature in her work. His treatment consisted usually of fresh air, good food, purgation, bloodletting, massage, and hydrotherapy. Although he mentioned over 400 drugs in his writings, he used only a few of the important ones, among them opium. His preparations included foments, poultices, gargles, suppositories, pills, lozenges, ointments, cerates, and inhalations.

Hippocrates is called the Father of Medicine because his influence has extended through the ages and his teachings have established the sound principles that control the practice of medicine to the present day.

Another early Greek physician was Dioscorides, who was an authority on materia medica. He described 600 plants and plant principles of which no fewer than seventy-four are in use today. His work was the chief source of pharmaceutical knowledge of antiquity.

ROME

After the Roman conquest of Greece, Greek medicine migrated to Rome. The most famous Greek physician of this period was Galen (A.D. 131-201). He based his teachings and practice largely upon the work of Hippocrates and established a system of medicine and pharmacy that made him the supreme authority for several hundred years. He originated many preparations of vegetable drugs, which even now are spoken of as galenicals, and was the first to prepare rosewater ointment or cold cream.

MEDIEVAL PERIOD (A.D. 400 to 1500)
EARLY PERIOD—THE DARK AGES
(A.D. 400-1100)

The term *Middle Ages* is given to that period of European history that lies between what are known as ancient and modern times, extending from about the middle of the fifth to the middle of the fifteenth century. The historical event that marked the close of ancient times was the decline and fall of the Roman Empire. This process extended over three or four centuries, during which period successive hordes of Germanic barbarians poured in from the north and east and overran Western Europe. They gradually succeeded in wresting the territory piecemeal from the Romans and in setting up their own tribal organizations. This process of dismemberment of the Roman Empire was completed in the fifth century and was followed by a period of about 600 years known as the Dark Ages, because during this time the old civilization was largely destroyed and there was little progress in learning. The German tribes were slowly learning to combine their primitive institutions with those of Rome and were assimilating the first rudiments of culture through their contact with the Latins. Wars between the tribes were frequent and served to stifle all effort along constructive lines. Their medicine was folklore and tradition, the employment of wonder-cures and temple-sleeps similar to those of the Greeks before the advent of Hippocrates.

Another important movement at the same time was the spread of Christianity. After three centuries of struggle and persecution the Christian church triumphed in 311 through a decree of the emperor, who made it the official church of Rome. Thereupon, religious orders arose whose members scattered throughout Europe preaching the new doctrine and building monasteries, where they could withdraw from the world and devote their lives to the work of the Church. The monasteries, particularly those of the Benedictines, soon became the repositories of all the learning of the period. The Venerable Bede was a Benedictine. The monks collected all available manuscripts and copied and preserved them. Among other things, they preserved the works on pharmacy and medicine. Since it was part of their religious duty to give aid to the sick and needy, they controlled most of the practice of medicine and disseminated much knowledge of healing. Their treatment was usually good food, quiet, rest, and the administration of decoctions of medicinal plants from their gardens. Monastery gardens were an important factor in the development of herbals and books of plant lore, the oldest of which dates 500 years before the invention of printing. Mistletoe was a great panacea. Lycopodium, clover, primrose, henbane, and verbena were common remedies, as were wormwood, belladonna, hellebore, and mandragora.

The first records of the use of some of the remedies now in modern practice are from this period. In the sixth century Alexander of Tralles used colchicum for gout, iron for anemia, cantharides as a blister, and rhubarb for dysentery and liver complaints.

ARABIAN INFLUENCE

In the eighth century the Arabs spread over the Holy Land, Egypt, North Africa, and Spain and began a supremacy that lasted over 500 years. They were especially interested in medicine, pharmacy, and chemistry and built hospitals and schools for the pursuit of their study. They carried forward the knowledge obtained from Greece and Rome and preserved the pharmaceutical art from the sixth to the sixteenth centuries. Their medicine was a blend of the practice of the Greeks and Jews and of the astrology and occult lore of Egypt and India. The teachings of Hippocrates and Galen, which had been translated into Arabic in the seventh century, furnished much of their material.

The Arabs contributed many new drugs. Medicine is indebted to them for the use of senna, camphor, musk, myrrh, cassia, tamarind, nutmeg, cloves, cubeb, aconite, ambergris, canabis, and sandalwood. They were the originators of syrups, juleps, alcohol, and aromatic water. They introduced into Europe the decimal notation, acquired by them from a now forgotten race in India.

The first great Mohammedan author was Geber, who wrote exclusively on chemistry. He is the reputed discoverer of sulfuric acid, nitric acid, nitrohydrochloric acid, corrosive sublimate, and lunar caustic.

Avicenna was an accomplished physician of the tenth century. He wrote the *Canon*, a miscellaneous collection of past medical lore with his interpretations. His works were considered authoritative in universities as late as 1650.

During this period, pharmacy was practiced somewhat as a profession separate from medicine. The first apothecary shops were established and the first pharmaceutical formulary or set of drug standards was produced. This served as a model for the first London pharmacopeia. The Arabian pharmacists were called sandalini. Their stocks were regularly inspected and punishment was meted out to those found guilty of selling spurious or deteriorated drugs.

RISE OF UNIVERSITIES

The word *university* means an association, and the principal universities of Europe had their origin in the voluntary association of guilds of students banded together for mutual protection and established at some place favorable to the pursuit of their studies. Salerno, which was founded in the eighth century, was the first of the educational institutions of the university type. Others founded later were the University of Paris, 1110; Bologna, 1113; Oxford, 1167; Cambridge, 1209; Padua, 1222; and Naples, 1224. They exerted a great influence upon the development of all science, and especially of medicine and pharmacy. Pharmacy was taught in all as part of the medical course. One of the most eminent pharmaceutical authorities of this period was Nicholas of Salerno, Director of the Medical School. He wrote the *Antidotarium*, which was the standard for pharmaceutical preparations for centuries. It contained the basic units of the present apothecaries' system, the grain, scruple, and dram, just as they are used today. At Salerno, the study of anatomy was resumed under a decree that permitted the dissection of a human body every 5 years. Didactic instruction here was based upon Hippocrates, Galen, Avicenna, and the antidotary of Nicholas Praepositus. A famous woman physician, Trotula of Salerno, first used mercury in the treatment of syphilis.

LATE MEDIEVAL PERIOD

In 1095 occurred the first of the Crusades. They extended over a period of nearly 200 years and exerted a profound influence on pharmacy by bringing about a fusion of Arabian science and learning with the primitive practices based upon folklore and tradition in Central and Northwest Europe. Records of the customhouse of the port of Acri in Italy in the early thirteenth century show large traffic in the various spices, opium, and rhubarb. Venetians brought the first sugar to Europe during the time of the Crusades. It was costly and was used exclusively as medicine, as were most of the spices.

Pharmacies as separate places for compounding and dispensing medicines spread through Europe with great rapidity during the thirteenth century. The fourteenth and fifteenth centuries witnessed a great awakening of interest in medicine and pharmacy throughout Europe. The Moors of Spain, who had a great reputation for knowledge and skill in these branches of science and who had been driven out of Granada by Ferdinand in 1492, scattered over Europe, practicing and teaching. Moreover, during this period, epidemic diseases were very prevalent, especially leprosy, ergotism, and the Black Death. The Black Death (bubonic plague) killed 25% of the human race (60 million people) during this period.

In the fifteenth century alchemy, brought in by the Arabs, swept over Europe like a conflagration. Alchemy was the search for means of transmuting base metals into gold. The mere desire to discover such a substance gave rise to a universal belief that one existed, and the so-called philosopher's stone was as much a reality to the alchemist as the actual substances with which he worked. Gradually belief spread that the philosopher's stone could not only transmute all metals into gold but could also cure all diseases, restore youth, and indefinitely prolong life. It thus also became the elixir of life. While the alchemists were carrying on the search for the stone, they made important inventions and discoveries that laid the foundations of the modern science of chemistry. In 1438 printing was invented and the world was flooded with books. One of the earliest printed works extant contains an illustration of a fifteenth-century pharmacy.

SIXTEENTH CENTURY

In the sixteenth century pharmacy came into its own. Drugs were rare and costly, prescriptions were complex, and special art was required in preparing and keeping the drugs. Formularies appeared in such numbers that a need was felt for an authoritative standard. This was furnished by Valerius Cordus, son of a professor of medicine at Marburg. Cordus collected formulas during 12 years of teaching at Wittenberg and compiled these in manuscript form. The physicians of Nuremberg wanted a copy for the local druggists and secured the consent of the senate in 1546 to have it printed. This work of Cordus was the first pharmacopeia to be printed and authorized for use in a community for the sake of uniformity. It drew its material from Greek, Roman, and Arabian sources and quoted freely from Galen, Dioscorides, Avicenna, and Nicholas Praepositus. It contained comparatively few types of preparations, namely, aromatics, opiates, confections, conserves, purges, pills, syrups, plasters, cerates, troches, salves, and oils. Editions were published in Paris, Lyons, Venice, and Antwerp. It held its place till 1666 and was revised five times.

The outstanding figure of the sixteenth century was Paracelsus, the son of a German physician and chemist. At the age of 16 years he began the study of medicine at the University of Basel, but he soon gave it up to experiment with chemistry and alchemy. He traveled widely, gathering a vast amount of knowledge, especially of folk medicine, from barbers, gypsies, and others with whom he associated. He served some time as a military surgeon in the Low Countries and worked in mines in the Tyrol. Here he investigated processes of preparing metals and made experiments as to their medicinal virtues. His cures gained wide publicity and he was called upon to prescribe for many of the great men of his day. In 1526 he was appointed professor of physics and surgery at Basel. Here he inaugurated his career as a teacher by publicly burning the works of Galen and denouncing the Arabian masters whose doctrines were then generally followed. He also flouted tradition by lecturing in German instead of Latin. His defiance of tradition and his arrogant manner aroused the enmity of the other members of the faculty, and he was compelled to leave the university in 1528 and resume his wanderings. At Salzburg he gave offense to a prominent physician, was thrown from a window by the man's servants, and died from the fall.

In spite of his objectionable methods, Paracelsus exerted a profound influence upon the medical beliefs of his time and of succeeding centuries. He attacked the weak points of the prevailing system of medicine; he destroyed the "humoral pathology" that taught that diseases were caused by an excess or deficiency of the "humors" bile, phlegm, or blood and substituted the doctrine that diseases were actual entities to be combated with specific remedies. He improved pharmacy and therapeutics, introduced some new remedies such as calomel and sulfur, made some new chemical compounds, and strove to reduce the overdosing then practiced.

SEVENTEENTH CENTURY

In 1618 the first London pharmacopeia appeared. It was chiefly a compilation of older authorities. It was sponsored by the London College of Physicians, and its use was made obligatory throughout the British realm by a decree of King James. It was very large compared with the modern pharmacopeia, containing 1028 simple drugs and 932 preparations and compounds. The most complex preparation contained 130 ingredients. One substance listed was usnea. This was moss from the skull of a man who had died a violent death. It was not hard to obtain in England in those days, because the bodies of criminals who had been executed were suspended in chains in public places as a warning to other criminals, and the exposure was conducive to growth of moss on the skull.

Great interest was displayed in chemistry and pharmacy in this century, and many preparations that originated then are still in use. Among them are senna or black draught, the alcoholic tincture of opium or laudanum, the compound tincture of benzoin, the balsams of Peru and Tolu, guaiacum, sarsaparilla, and jalap. In 1638 cinchona was imported by the Countess Ana del Chinchon, wife of the Viceroy of Peru, who had been cured of a severe intermittent fever by its use. Coca was likewise introduced from Peru, and ipecac found its way into Europe and was used with such skill by a quack named Helvetius that Louis XIV paid him $4000 for his secret.

EIGHTEENTH CENTURY

The eighteenth century likewise witnessed great progress in pharmacy. A German practi-

tioner by the name of Hoffmann originated the elixir of orange and Hoffmann's anodyne. A Berlin apothecary identified magnesia, the alums, the potassa, and soda and discovered beet sugar. A French pharmacist published an essay entitled "The Superstitions Concerning the Philosopher's Stone" and thereby helped divert alchemy into more profitable channels. In 1775 Louis XVI paid nearly $5000 to a certain Madame Nouffer for a celebrated cure for tapeworm. She inherited the secret from her husband, a Swiss physician. The drug proved to be male fern, commonly known since Galen.

Inoculation against smallpox was introduced in the latter part of the eighteenth century by Edward Jenner, an English physician. For years he had been studying smallpox, swinepox, and cowpox and the development of the two latter diseases when communicated to man. He noticed that milkmaids who were frequently infected with cowpox were immune to smallpox. He made his first public inoculation with vaccine on May 14, 1796, and within a year had won the confidence of the physicians in his theory of immunization.

In 1785 the infusion of digitalis was introduced by William Withering of England for the treatment of heart disease. The foxglove is carved on Withering's monument.

Dover's powder had its origin about this time. Thomas Dover administered the drug in doses of 60 grains and claimed to have given as much as 100 grains. This was equivalent to 10 grains of opium and 10 grains of ipecac. The pharmacists filling his prescriptions usually advised patients first to make their wills.

NINETEENTH CENTURY

During the nineteenth century, chemistry gradually took its place as a highly specialized science, with pharmaceutical chemistry as an important subdivision. The first great pharmaceutical discovery was that of the alkaloid morphine, obtained from opium by a German apothecary, Serturner, in 1815. This was the first active principle to be isolated and it led to enthusiastic research on many vegetable drugs. The result was the discovery of quinine, strychnine, and veratrine by Pelletier and Caventou; of emetine by Pelletier and Magendie; of atropine by Brandes; and of codeine by Robiquet. All of these men were pharmacists. Their discoveries made it possible to administer drugs in an attractive and palatable form. The accurate study of dosage was also possible.

In 1842 Dr. Crawford W. Long of Georgia first used ether as a general anesthetic, and in 1847 Sir J. T. Simpson used chloroform for the same purpose.

About 1856 appeared the first of the numerous coal-tar products. Perkin, in a vain attempt to produce synthetic quinine, discovered instead the first coal-tar dye, called "Perkin's purple" or mauve. This led to the preparation in the laboratory of a great family of remedial agents, some of which, such as salicylic and benzoic acids, duplicated products previously obtained from natural sources, and others of which were new to science, for example, acetanilid and antipyrine.

The discovery of so many new drugs and the invention of new and convenient dosage forms led to the establishment of large-scale manufacturing plants that took over much of the work formerly done by the pharmacist with his mortar and pestle.

This century also witnessed the initial appearance of the important national pharmacopeias. The French *Codex* was first to be produced. It was issued in 1818 and contained one remarkable item, a formula for an extract of opium in which the preparation was to be boiled incessantly for 6 months and the water lost by evaporation to be constantly replaced. The first pharmacopeia for the United States appeared in 1820, the national standard for Great Britain in 1864 to replace those of London, Edinburgh, and Dublin, and that for Germany in 1872, superseding nearly a score of local volumes.

Fewer drugs were prescribed, and the prescriptions given were accompanied with greater knowledge of their expected action. In other words, rational medicine began to replace empiricism. During this period purging and bloodletting became less popular and definite action toward exposing harmful patent medicines and nostrums was taken.

TWENTIETH CENTURY

Great progress has been made in pharmacy and medicine since the beginning of the twentieth century. In pharmacy, growth has been chiefly along the lines of strengthening and improving the work of the professional organizations such as the American Pharmaceutical Association and the National Association of Retail Druggists and with the promotion of legislation controlling the manufacture and sale of drugs. The most important acts were the Food and Drug Acts of 1906 and 1938, the Harrison Narcotic Act of 1914, and the Controlled Substances Act of 1970.

It is said that more progress has probably been made during the past 50 years than in all the years prior to that time. As far as therapeutics is concerned this is largely the result of changes in the concept of the cause of disease. When it was believed that evil spirits caused disease, the treatment given was highly varied and used in the hope that one of the measures would be the right one. Since the acceptance of the germ theory there has been rapid advancement in scientific methods of research. Such methods have been greatly aided by animal experimentation, appropriation of money for research work, and efforts of public health organizations to educate the public and to collect valuable vital statistics.

Of interest to both pharmacy and medicine are the many biologic preparations such as the vaccines, antitoxins, and serums now in common use and the valuable group of anesthetics, which is constantly growing through the isolation and duplication in the laboratory of more and more of the potent vegetable substances found in nature. The introduction into medicine by the German physician Ehrlich in 1907 of salvarsan, the great specific for syphilis, and the discovery by Banting in 1922 of insulin for the treatment of diabetes constitute two epoch-making events.

With the increased knowledge of drugs has grown an increasing awareness of implications in their misuse and abuse. Among other trends in modern medicine is the use of other therapeutic agents either to supplement drug therapy or to replace it. Such therapies include vitamin therapy, diet therapy, and various kinds of physical therapy.

To discover chemotherapeutic agents that will be effective in every infectious disease is one of the goals of research workers in medicine. However, for years there were only a few chemicals that acted as specifics. Among the most important were quinine for malaria and the arsenicals for syphilis. In the last few decades several remarkable chemotherapeutic agents have changed chemical therapy tremendously. Infections that a few decades ago took a tremendous toll in sickness and deaths are now well controlled by the sulfonamides, penicillin, and other antibiotics. In 1908 sulfanilamide was first prepared by Gelmo, a German organic chemist, who was investigating azo dyes. It was not until 1932, however, that its possible therapeutic value was realized. In 1932 Prontosil was patented in Germany by Klarer and Mietzsch. A German worker, Domagk, is credited with the discovery of the therapeutic value of Prontosil. In 1932 Domagk observed that mice with streptococcal septicemia could be protected by Prontosil. It was later shown that Prontosil breaks down into para-aminobenzenesulfonamide, which is the effective substance. In the next few years more and more interest was aroused in these drugs, and today they have a rightful place as some of the most important drugs. Para-aminobenzenesulfonamide was accepted by the Council on Pharmacy and Chemistry of the American Medical Association for inclusion in New and Non-official Remedies in 1937, at which time the name of sulfanilamide was suggested for it. Since then many new sulfonamide derivatives have been tried, and a few of them have become well established in drug therapy.

The story of the development of antibacterial agents of biologic origin, or antibiotics, is one of the most interesting developments in pharmacy. In 1929 Dr. Alexander Fleming at the University of London noted that a mold contaminating a plate of staphylococci produced a zone of inhibition around it in which the staphylococci did not grow. Fleming found that the mold, *Penicillium notatum*, secreted into its medium an antibiotic agent, which he named penicillin. He found it was not toxic to animals, did not hurt white blood cells, and inhibited the growth of certain gram-positive pathogens. He used broth containing penicillin clinically on several cases of skin infections with favorable results. However, little was done clinically about it for the next 10 years.

In 1939 Rene J. Dubos of the Rockefeller Institute for Medical Research published the results of experiments done on certain bacteria found in the soil. Dubos acted on the assumption that all organic matter added to the soil would eventually undergo decomposition by microorganisms. Samples of soil were incubated for a few weeks to bring about decomposition of most of the organic matter present. Then cultures of staphylococci, Group A hemolytic streptococci, and pneumococci were added to the soil at intervals.

After 2 years, a gram-positive, spore-bearing aerobic bacillus capable of lysing the living cells of many gram-positive bacteria was isolated from the soil. The soil bacillus, called *Bacillus brevis*, produced a substance destructive to certain gram-positive bacteria. The destructive substance could be extracted from the bacteria. It was named tyrothricin and was later shown to be composed of two substances, gramicidin and tyrocidine. Gramicidin is much more effective than tyrocidine therapeutically. Unfortunately, gramicidin is hemolytic and can be used only for local infections, never where it can get in contact with the blood.

This story now turns back to penicillin. In 1938 Dr. Howard Florey at Oxford University began to study penicillin and other naturally occurring antibacterial agents. Dr. Florey and his associates are responsible for the isolation of penicillin, its assay and dosage, and proof of its clinical usefulness. The first patient was treated with penicillin early in 1941. Because of World War II it was impossible to start large-scale production in England. Dr. Florey came to the United States in 1941 and asked for the help of the National Research Council in studying penicillin. Production was soon started in the United States, and the first patient in this country was treated with penicillin in March, 1942. Since that time a number of other antibiotics— streptomycin, dihydrostreptomycin, chloramphenicol, chlortetracycline, oxytetracycline, tetracycline, and many others—have been added to the physician's armamentarium.

It should be noted that obtaining antibacterial agents from natural sources is not a new procedure. There are many such substances throughout the plant and animal kingdoms. Quinine, which is produced by a plant, has been used for many years.

In 1935 a series of events occurred that were to have far-reaching significance. Dr. E. C. Kendall and associates of the Mayo Foundation, Dr. Wintersteiner and Dr. Pfiffner of Columbia University, and Professor Reichstein of Switzerland independently isolated a group of crystalline substances from the cortex of the adrenal gland. Continued effort resulted in the discovery of the chemical structure of these compounds. Among these new products was one that proved to be 17-hydroxy-11-dehydrocorticosterone. The name of this compound was shortened to cortisone. It was first used in medicine in 1948. It opened a new era in medical science. Later (1950) hydrocortisone and (1954) aldosterone were isolated and identified.

In 1955 and later in 1961 the announcement of new poliomyelitis vaccines focused the attention of the world upon another achievement that provided mankind with relief from the dreaded disease of poliomyelitis.

During the 1950's and early 1960's many new drugs were introduced, bringing great benefits but also creating many problems. Since the passage of the 1962 Kefauver-Harris Drug Amendments requiring proof of efficacy as well as safety, the introduction of new medicinal agents has become much less frequent. In addition, the number of preparations available is actually decreasing as many older, ineffective drugs are being removed from the market.

Despite the slowdown in the introduction of new drugs, many valuable agents continue to be made available, such as newer anti-infectives, hormonal agents, and antineoplastic agents, to mention a few. Real breakthroughs in therapy continue to occur, such as the discovery of the beneficial effect of allopurinol (Zyloprim) in gout or the dramatic effects of L-dopa in Parkinson's disease. The future of drug therapy continues to be bright.

REFERENCES

Elliott, J. S.: Outline of Greek and Roman medicine, Boston, 1971, Milford House.

Krantz, J. C.: Historical medical classics involving new drugs, Baltimore, 1974, The Williams & Wilkins Co.

Poynter, N.: Medicine and man, London, 1971, C. A. Watts & Co. Ltd.

Rogers, F. B.: A syllabus of medical history, Boston, 1972, Little, Brown & Co.

Scarborough, J.: Roman medicine, London, 1969, The Camelot Press Ltd.

CHAPTER 3

Drug standards and legislation

Drug standards
Drug legislation

DRUG STANDARDS

Drugs have been known to vary considerably in strength and activity. Drugs obtained from plants, such as opium and digitalis, have been known to vary in strength from plant to plant and from year to year, depending on where the plants are grown, the age at which they are harvested, and how they are preserved. Occasionally, one finds on the market drugs of low concentration or drugs that have been adulterated. Since accurate dosage and reliability of effect of a drug depend on uniformity of strength and purity, it has been necessary to find ways by which drugs can be standardized. The technique by which the strength or potency of a drug is measured is known as *assay*. The two general types of assay method used are chemical and biologic. Chemical assay really means chemical analysis to determine the ingredients present and their amount. A simple example would be the determination of the concentration of hydrochloric acid in a solution to be used medically. Thus the acid content of a solution might be measured by titration and then adjusted, for example, to a standardized tenth-normal solution.

Opium is known to contain certain alkaloids (*active principles* was the older term), and these may vary greatly in different preparations. The United States official standard demands that opium must contain not less than 9.5% and not more than 10.5% of anhydrous morphine. Opium of a higher morphine content may be reduced to the official standard by admixture with opium of a lower percentage or with certain other pharmacologically inactive diluents such as sucrose, lactose, glycyrrhiza, or magnesium carbonate.

In the case of some drugs either the active ingredients are not known or there are no available methods of analyzing and standardizing them. These drugs may be standardized by biologic methods—bioassay. Bioassay is performed by determining the amount of a preparation required to produce a definite effect on a suitable laboratory animal under certain standard conditions. For example, the potency of a certain sample of insulin is measured by its ability to lower the blood sugar of rabbits. The strength of a drug that is assayed biologically is usually expressed in units. For example, insulin injection, U.S.P., possesses a potency of not less than 95% and not more than 105% of the potency stated on the label, expressed in U.S.P. insulin units. Both the unit and the method of assay are defined, so that national and sometimes international standards exist.

DRUG STANDARDS IN THE UNITED STATES

In the United States an official drug is one that is included in *The Pharmacopeia of the United States of America, The National Formulary,* or the *Homeopathic Pharmacopoeia of the United States.* Drugs listed in these publications are official because they are so designated by the *Federal Food, Drug, and Cosmetic Act.*

15

The Pharmacopeia of the United States of America (usually referred to as the U.S.P. or *The Pharmacopeia)* is a book in which approved medicinal agents used in present-day medical practice are defined as to source, physical and chemical properties, tests for purity and identity, assay, method of storage, category (general type of drug), and dosage (range of dosage as well as the usual therapeutic dosage).

In most instances, preparations included in the U.S.P. are single drugs. They are listed under their official names. The purpose of the U.S.P. is to provide standards for the identification and purity of drugs and to ensure uniformity of strength. When a drug is prescribed by a physician anywhere in the United States, the pharmacist must fill the prescription with a preparation that meets pharmacopeial standards if the drug is listed in the U.S.P. This assures physicians of uniform potency and purity of all official drugs that they prescribe for their patients.

The first pharmacopeia in the United States was published in 1820. The current edition, U.S.P. XIX, became official in 1975. At one time it was customary to revise the U.S.P. every 10 years, but it is now revised every 5 years. Supplements to the U.S.P. are published between revisions to keep abreast of the rapid changes in this field.

The U.S.P. is revised by a special pharmacopeial committee headed by a full-time director. The committee is made up of outstanding pharmacologists, physicians, and pharmacists who donate their services to this important task. The main committee is assisted by many subcommittees and advisory boards. Drugs included in the U.S.P. are selected on the basis of their therapeutic usefulness and low toxicity. When drugs listed in the U.S.P. have been supplanted in practice by better drugs, the older ones are deleted and the newer or better drugs are added. Sometimes a drug is deleted from the U.S.P. when after extensive use the incidence of toxic reactions is shown to be too high.

Drugs whose content or method of preparation is secret are not admitted to the U.S.P. Trademarked or patented preparations of therapeutic merit may be included; when included they are listed under their official names, not the popular trade names by which they may be commonly known.

The National Formulary (N.F.) serves as a supplement to the U.S.P. It is sponsored by the American Pharmaceutical Association and is usually revised the same year as the U.S.P. Originally *The National Formulary* contained only formulas for drug mixtures. It now contains single drugs as well as formulas for drug mixtures. It contains monographs on therapeutic agents, pharmaceutic aids, and tests for purity and potency. *The National Formulary* establishes standards and specifications for the agents and procedures used therein. *The Pharmacopeia* represents a more critical selection of drugs since they are more carefully screened as to their therapeutic value and toxic qualities. Drugs included in *The National Formulary* XIV are selected solely on the basis of their therapeutic value. Preparations deleted from *The Pharmacopeia* are often transferred to *The National Formulary*. It provides standards for many of the older remedies that the pharmacist is still called upon to dispense. As is true of *The Pharmacopeia,* drugs are listed in *The National Formulary* under their official names only.

The *National Code Directory* contains codes and information on more than 12,000 drugs. It establishes a standard identification system for computer processing of drug information, inventory control, billing, accumulation of drug utilization data, drug recalls, and automated drug ordering. It is expected to have wide application by governmental agencies, hospitals, insurance companies, manufacturers, and distributors.

DRUG STANDARDS IN GREAT BRITAIN AND CANADA

British Pharmacopoeia (B.P.) is similar to the U.S.P. in its scope and purpose. Drugs listed in it are considered official and subject to legal control in the United Kingdom and those parts of the British Commonwealth in which the *British Pharmacopoeia* has statutory force. It is published by the British Pharmacopoeia Commission under the direction of the General Medical Council. Dosage is expressed in metric system, although in some cases dosage is indicated in both metric and imperial systems.

The Pharmacopeia of the United States of America is used a great deal in Canada, and some preparations used in Canada conform to the U.S.P. instead of the B.P. because many of the drugs used in Canada are obtained from the United States.

British Pharmaceutical Codex (B.P.C.) is published by the Pharmaceutical Society of Great Britain. In general, it resembles *The National Formulary*.

The Canadian Formulary contains formulas for preparations used extensively in Canada. It also contains standards for new drugs prescribed in Canada but not included in the *British Pharmacopoeia*. The publication has been given official status by the *Canadian Food and Drug Act*.

The Physician's Formulary contains formulas for preparations that are representative of the needs of medical practice in Canada. It is published by the Canadian Medical Association.

INTERNATIONAL STANDARDS

Various national pharmacopeias have been developed to meet the needs of medical practice in different countries. *The Pharmacopeia of the United States* has been translated into Spanish for the Spanish-speaking parts of the Americas. In addition, an international pharmacopeia has been published.

Pharmacopoea Internationalis (Ph.I.) was first published in 1951. It was published by a committee of the World Health Organization and represents an important contribution to the development of international standards in drugs and unification of national pharmacopeias. The work done on this publication has resulted in better understanding of terms and in uniformity of strengths and composition of drugs throughout the world. It has also demonstrated that members of different nations can sit down together and come to agreement about matters that concern many people of the world.

The *Pharmacopoea Internationalis* is published in English, Spanish, and French. The nomenclature is in Latin, and the system of measurement is metric. It is not intended to convey official status in any country unless it is adopted by the appropriate authority of that country.

DRUG DEVELOPMENT AND EVALUATION

In the United States, when a new drug is discovered the pharmaceutical company must obtain an *Investigational New Drug Exemption* (I.N.D.) from the Food and Drug Administration before any clinical tests can be conducted in man. The pharmaceutical company must submit to the F.D.A. all available information on the drug, including a specific description of the drug, its active ingredients, and results of toxicity tests in animals. The drug must be tested in at least two different mammalian species using male and female animals. Routes of administration must be the same as those proposed for man, and magnitude of dose related to that intended for human use.

Drug development is dependent upon the assumption that a high degree of correlation exists between the effects of drugs in animals and man. It is generally accepted that the principal physiologic and biochemical mechanisms in animals and man are identical although variations exist in size, concentration, and activity in individual systems in different species. However, no amount of experimentation in animals will ensure absolute safety and complete predictability in man. Certain pathologic conditions in humans, such as psychiatric disorders, myocardial infarction, and bone marrow diseases have no satisfactory equivalent in common laboratory animals. A major problem in correlation is that the pharmacodynamic data of healthy animals have to be adapted to the sick man. Attempts are now being made to reduce this source of error by "modeling" the disease in animals. Drug studies today are more intensive and extensive than was true in the past. For example, drug researchers are now trying to determine the following:

1 Toxicity reversibility (Recovery after a reaction to the drug)
2 Tumorigenicity (Is the drug tumor or cancer producing?)
3 Reproductive toxicity (Is the drug teratogenic [causing malformed fetuses] or mutagenic [causing chromosomal changes]? Does it cause changes in fertility and general reproductive performance? Are there undesirable effects during the peri- and postnatal periods? Observations are made for delayed or prolonged labor, abnormalities in lactation and

maternal care, and the drug's direct toxic action on the offspring.)

Throughout the animal studies, detailed biochemical and hematologic measurements are made to determine drug absorption by different routes of administration, drug distribution throughout the body, and drug metabolism. These studies are often linked to pharmaceutical studies in which the drug's physical and physicochemical characteristics are altered to determine how this affects absorption of the drug. The animals' behavior is also closely observed during the study. To further assess the drug's effects on various body tissues, the animals are sacrificed and histopathologic examination of all body tissues is performed.

Clinical studies are divided into three phases by the F.D.A.:

Phase I: Very limited investigations in man to determine toxicity, metabolism, pharmacology, preferred route of administration, and safe dosage range

Phase II: Initial clinical trials on a limited number of patients for treatment or prevention of specific diseases

Phase III: Extensive clinical trials to establish the most effective therapeutic regimens for treating specific diseases, determining the therapeutic effect likely to be achieved, possible side effects, and safety of the drug

There should also be a follow-up phase after the drug is in general use, because the extent and severity of side effects often cannot be determined solely during the experimental stages.

Normal subjects are usually used for phase I testing to permit assessment of the drug's effects in a normal person. These can then be compared with those effects occurring in diseased subjects to determine the extent to which disease modifies the drug's effects. In phase I testing all aspects of drug testing are fully known to both investigator and subject.

If the new drug appears to have a therapeutic effect the following questions need to be answered:

1 Does the drug have significant therapeutic effects when compared with placebo effects?
2 Is the new drug as good as, or superior to, the best drugs presently available for treatment?

There is little value in marketing an inferior product. Controlled studies in phases II and III are designed to answer these questions.

To minimize bias in drug evaluation various safeguards are used. These include:

1 Double-blind administration. Neither the subject nor investigator is aware of which substance is administered: the new drug, a standard drug with which it is to be compared, or an inactive placebo. All are prepared in such a way that they appear identical.
2 Randomization of drug administration
   a. Within-subject trials. All subjects receive each substance included in the study and their responses to each are compared.
   b. Between-subjects trials. Subjects are divided into groups; each group receives only one of the substances in the study. Comparison is made between the responses of each group.
3 Exclusion of placebo reactors from within-subject trials
4 Use of homogeneous subjects, such as all postoperative hysterectomy patients, and matching patients according to sex, age, weight, etc.
5 Formulation of criteria for measurement of effects, and surveillance by trained observers for desired and undesired effects
6 Correlation of therapeutic and toxic effects with blood, tissue, or body fluid levels of drug
7 Comparison of the drug's effects to a standard drug such as morphine or aspirin
8 Proper statistical evaluation

All subjects in experimental drug studies should be true volunteers and not subjected to any coercion. Informed consent should be obtained from them only after they have been given careful explanation of the purpose of the study, procedures to be used, and the risks involved. New drug studies in children and psychiatric patients require special consideration.

The nurse and clinical drug testing. Nurses involved in clinical drug studies should be fully informed about the study and the drug under investigation. All information available to the physician, researcher, or pharmacist should also be available to the nurse. Ethical and legal responsibilities mandate that a nurse's actions be based on adequate knowledge and skill and that the patients be protected from foreseeable harm. This necessitates that the nurse know the recommended dosage range and route of administration, the desired therapeutic effect, and the undesired and toxic effects. Throughout the entire investigation the nurse must strictly adhere to the protocols of the study. Recordings of all observations should be as precise as possible for they will have a direct influence on the study outcome.

The law imposes strict limitations on human experimentation, and the prevailing legal view is that no experimentation of any kind is proper without full disclosure to the patient of all risks and all aspects of the experiment. The nurse as guardian of the patient's rights should take steps to ensure that those rights are not violated. To protect themselves and their patients nurses should become familiar with the Nuremberg Code. This code states the principles for using human subjects in medical research, and it conceivably could be used during litigation of a case involving human experimentation.

The Nuremberg Code was formulated by American physicians and came as a result of the trials at Nuremberg of Nazi physicians and scientists who had conducted experiments on political prisoners. That Code is:

1 The voluntary consent of the human subject is absolutely essential.
2 The experiment should be such as to yield fruitful results for the good of society, unprocurable by other methods or means of study, and not random and unnecessary in nature.
3 The experiment should be so designed and based on the results of animal experimentation and a knowledge of the natural history of the disease or other problem under study that the anticipated results will justify the performance of the experiment.
4 The experiment should be so conducted as to avoid all unnecessary physical and mental suffering and injury.
5 No experiment should be conducted where there is an *a priori* reason to believe that death or disabling injury will occur; except, perhaps, in those experiments where the experimental physicians also serve as subjects.
6 The degree of risk to be taken should never exceed that determined by the humanitarian importance of the problem to be solved by the experiment.
7 Proper preparations should be made and adequate facilities provided to protect the experimental subject against even remote possibilities of injury, disability, or death.
8 The experiment should be conducted only by scientifically qualified persons. The highest degree of skill and care should be required through all stages of the experiment of those who conduct or engage in the experiment.
9 During the course of the experiment the human subject should be at liberty to bring the experiment to an end if he has reached the physical or mental state where continuation of the experiment seems to him to be impossible.
10 During the course of the experiment the scientist in charge must be prepared to terminate the experiment at any stage, if he has probable cause to believe, in the exercise of good faith, superior skill and careful judgment required of him that a continuation of the experiment is likely to result in injury, disability, or death to the experimental subject.

DRUG LEGISLATION

Important though pharmacopeias, formularies, and other publications are to the maintenance of standards for drugs, unless provision is made to enforce the standards the public can be defrauded, drugs adulterated, and the market flooded with unreliable and unsafe preparations. Enforcement of standards is partly a responsibility of individual states, but federal legislation is needed to cover interstate commerce in drugs as well as in other items.

The twentieth century ushered in an era of rapidly expanding scientific knowledge. At the beginning of the century federal laws controlling drug distribution were nonexistent. Illness was treated primarily with well-known botanicals or time-honored products of nature, and many preparations of secret composition were sold to the public for all known diseases.

During the first decade of the twentieth century organic chemicals used in medicine increased in number, and it soon became evident that federal legislation was needed to protect the public in a complex area where individuals were unable to protect themselves. The result was enactment of the first federal drug law in 1906.

UNITED STATES DRUG LEGISLATION

Federal Food, Drug, and Cosmetic Act. In 1906 the Food and Drug Act designated *The Pharmacopeia of the United States of America* and *The National Formulary* as official standards and empowered the federal government to enforce these standards. It was "an act for preventing the manufacture of adulterated or misbranded or poisonous or deleterious foods, drugs, medicines, and liquors, and for regulating traffic therein, and for other purposes." The federal drug law required that drugs comply with the standards of strength and purity professed for them, and it also required that labels on drugs and patent medicines containing morphine or other narcotic ingredients indicate the kind and amount of such substances.

Enforcement of the 1906 law focused primarily on food and patent medicine abuses, with prescription drugs receiving a low priority in the enforcement effort. The number of prescription and known curative drugs was not extensive at this time. Until the mid-twenties drug control efforts were sporadic and unsystematic, primarily because of the paucity of analytical knowledge, inadequate application of available scientific knowledge, and lack of refinement of technologic processes. During the early 1930's drug control was aimed at protecting the public against quacks and drugs dangerous to health when used in the dosage provided or according to the instructions on the label.

In the second decade of the twentieth century the number of chemicals used in medicine continued to increase, and in 1912 Congress passed the Sherley Amendment prohibiting use of fraudulent therapeutic claims. Drug research continued to accelerate during the next two decades. Synthetic organic chemicals made their appearance, and the chemotherapeutic age began.

The Food and Drug Act of 1906 was updated by the Federal Food, Drug, and Cosmetic Act of 1938. Impetus to revise the 1906 drug act was provided by more than 100 deaths in 1937 resulting from ingestion of a diethylene glycol solution of sulfanilamide. The sulfanilamide preparation had been marketed as an "elixir of sulfanilamide" without benefit of investigation of the toxicity of the solvent. The only charge that could be made against the drug was that it was misbranded since it was labeled an "elixir" and the drug failed to meet the definition of an elixir as an alcoholic solution. The Federal Food, Drug, and Cosmetic Act of 1938 contained a provision to prevent premature marketing of new drugs not properly tested for safety by requiring the manufacturer to submit a new drug application to the government for review of safety studies before the product could be sold.

The Federal Food, Drug, and Cosmetic Act of 1938 conferred status on the drugs listed in the *Homeopathic Pharmacopoeia of the United States* as well as those in *The Pharmacopeia of the United States of America* and *The National Formulary*.

Provisions of the Federal Food, Drug, and Cosmetic Act. The provisions include many features designed to prevent misbranding and to ensure careful and accurate labeling. Labeling refers not only to the labels on the immediate container but also to circulars, pamphlets, and brochures that may accompany the preparations or in some manner reach the hands of the consumer. The Act prohibits certain statements from appearing on the label and insists upon certain others:

1 Statements on the label must not be false or misleading in any particular.
2 Drugs must not be dangerous to health when used in the dosage or with the frequency prescribed, recommended, or suggested on the label.
3 The label must indicate the name and the business address of the manufacturer, packer, or distributor as well as an accurate statement of the contents.
4 The label must indicate quantitatively the presence of all habit-forming drugs, such as narcotics, hypnotics, or other habit-forming drugs or their derivatives. The label must also bear the statement: "Warning—May Be Habit Forming."
5 Labels must designate the presence of official drugs by their official names, and if nonofficial they must bear the usual name of the drug or drugs, whether active or not.
6 The Act requires that official drugs be packaged and labeled as specified by *The Pharmacopeia of the United States*, *The National Formulary*, or the *Homeopathic Pharmacopoeia of the United States*. Deviations in strength, quality, and purity are permitted, provided such deviations are clearly indicated on the label.

7 Labels must indicate the quantity, kind, and proportion of certain specified ingredients, including alcohol, bromides, atropine, hyoscine, digitalis, and a number of other drugs, the presence of which needs to be known for the safety of those for whom it is prescribed.

8 The label must bear adequate directions for use and adequate warnings against unsafe use (a) by children and (b) in pathologic conditions.

9 The label must bear adequate warning against unsafe dosage or methods or duration of administration or application in such manner and form as are necessary for the protection of the users.

10 New drugs may not be introduced into interstate commerce unless an application has been filed with the Food and Drug Administration and the application has been permitted to become effective. Adequate scientific evidence must be presented to show that the drug is safe for use under the conditions proposed for its use. The applicant does not have to prove the efficacy of the drug in order to obtain an effective application. During the time that the drug is under investigation by experts, the label of the drug must bear the statement: "Caution: New Drug—Limited by Federal Law to Investigational Use."

NOTE: When tests indicate that the requirements of the Food and Drug Administration have been met, the law permits a period of clinical testing by approved clinicians and clinical groups. Pertinent data are collected and submitted to the Food and Drug Administration for further evaluation. If the Administration is satisfied that the drug has therapeutic merit and is not unduly toxic, distribution and sale of the new drug are permitted.

In 1945 the following amendment was passed and attached to the law:

Certain drugs must be obtained from a batch that has been certified by the Food and Drug Administration. This applies to insulin and the antibiotics. Samples of each batch of these drugs are examined, and if samples conform to standards set forth by the Food and Drug Administration, the batches are referred to as "Certified Drugs."

The Durham-Humphrey Amendment of 1952 further changed the 1938 drug act. This amendment restricts the dispensing of so-called "legend" drugs by the pharmacist to dispensing on prescription only. It also prohibits the refilling of such prescriptions without authorization of the doctor. In addition, it provides for oral or telephone prescriptions of certain legend drugs. Finally, it provides for oral or telephone authorization of refills, subject to certain limitations. This provision modifies a previous provision that recognized only written prescriptions. Legend drugs are those that must bear the legend, "Caution: Federal law prohibits dispensing without prescription." These include all drugs given by injection as well as:

1 Hypnotic, narcotic, or habit-forming drugs or derivatives thereof as specified in the law.

2 Drugs that because of their toxicity or method of use are not safe unless they are administered under the supervision of a licensed practitioner (physician or dentist).

3 New drugs that are limited to investigational use or new drugs that are not considered safe for indiscriminate use by lay persons.

This amendment also recognized a second class of drugs, over-the-counter drugs (OTC's), for which prescriptions are not required.

In 1958, Senator Estes Kefauver of Tennessee began a senate investigation into the drug industry when it became known that the drug companies were making huge profits, and that some drug promotion was false, misleading, and avalanche-like. This investigation received little support until given impetus by the thalidomide tragedy, although for the United States it was more a might-have-been catastrophe than a real one. Thalidomide, a hypnotic marketed in Europe, was found to be responsible for severe deformities in babies whose mothers had taken the drug during the early stage of pregnancy. These events led to passage of the Kefauver-Harris Amendment in 1962.

Fundamentally, there were two objectives advanced by the Kefauver-Harris Amendment: (1) assurance of both the safety and effectiveness of drugs, and (2) improvement of the communication of necessary information concerning these drugs, their side effects and contraindications, as well as their advantages. Specifically, these two related objectives are advanced by provisions that require the following:

1 Substantial evidence of the effectiveness of new drugs before marketing.

2 Manufacture of all drugs under adequate control and good manufacturing practices.

3 Government certification of both the safety and effectiveness of all antibiotics for human use.

4 Prompt reporting by manufacturers to the government of adverse reactions attributed to new drugs and antibiotics.

5 Truthful statements in prescription drug advertisement concerning the effectiveness, side effects, and contraindications of the advertised drugs.

6 Annual registration with the Food and Drug Administration of all persons and firms engaged in the manufacturing, reporting, and labeling of drug products.

7 Inspection of every registered establishment at least once every 2 years.

The law further authorizes the Food and Drug Administration to do the following:

1 Establish official names for drugs in the interest of usefulness and simplicity.

2 Withdraw approval of drugs when substantial doubt arises as to their safety or in the absence of substantial evidence of effectiveness.

3 Have access during inspection of prescription drug manufacturing establishments to all things that have a bearing on violations of the law with respect to such drugs, including records, files, papers, processes, controls, and facilities.

4 Exercise greater controls over shipment and clinical testing of investigational drugs and ensure that adequate preclinical studies are done on the drug before the investigator is asked to do human studies.

From 1938 to 1962 approval of a new drug application was based solely on proof of its safety for use in humans. Since passage of the Kefauver-Harris Amendment, proof of both safety and efficacy is required. To facilitate the enormous task of evaluating all drugs introduced between 1938 and 1962, the F.D.A. signed a contract with the National Academy of Sciences and its research arm, the National Research Council (N.A.S.-N.R.C.) in 1966 to independently study all supporting data for all therapeutic claims. This program of study was called the Drug Efficacy Study Implementation (D.E.S.I.). Early in the study it was agreed that each drug would be rated for effectiveness in each of its stated indications according to the following categories:

Effective: substantial evidence of effectiveness.

Probably effective: additional evidence required to rate the drug effective.

Possibly effective: effectiveness might be shown eventually, but at the present time there is little evidence of efficacy.

Ineffective: no substantial evidence of effectiveness.

Two other ratings were also formulated:

Ineffective as a fixed combination: even though one or more components might be effective if used alone, the product is not acceptable in fixed dosage combination for reasons of safety or because there is no evidence of contribution of each component to claimed effect.

Effective but: although effective there is an appropriate qualification or restriction imposed on the drug, which is still under consideration by the N.A.S.-N.R.C. and the F.D.A.; the drug is effective for some recommended uses but not for all, requiring labeling changes.

Thousands of drugs and therapeutic claims have been evaluated and the "ineffective" drugs are being withdrawn from the market. Those rated as "possibly effective" or "probably effective" are being withdrawn or reformulated; however, the drug may remain on the market while claims are being modified and scientific data collected to substantiate the claims. Drugs in the "probably effective" and "possibly effective" categories must be upgraded to the "effective" category within time limits set by the F.D.A. or the claims and drug withdrawn. The drug rating must be prominently displayed on the label.

"Substantial" evidence is that derived from adequate, well controlled, scientific and clinical investigations by experts qualified by training and experience to evaluate the drug. This evidence validates the actions claimed for the drug under the conditions of use prescribed. Uncontrolled observations and testimonial-type endorsements are not accepted as scientific evidence.

It is important for nurses and other health professionals to familiarize themselves with the D.E.S.I. ratings, particularly for those drugs commonly administered to patients under their care. It is hoped that eventually only drugs in the "effective" category will be available for prescribing, dispensing, and administering.

Narcotic and drug abuse laws. The Harrison Narcotic Act passed in 1914 was the first federal law aimed at curbing drug addiction or dependence. This was the first narcotic act passed by any nation. It established the word "narcotic" as a legal term. This act regulated the importation, manufacture, sale, and use of opium and cocaine and all their compounds and derivatives. Marihuana and its derivatives were also subject to this Act, as were many synthetic analgesic drugs that proved to produce or sustain either physical or psychologic dependence.

This Act and other drug abuse amendments now have only historical import, since they have been superseded by the *Comprehensive Drug Abuse Prevention and Control Act of 1970,* * also called the *Controlled Substances Act.* It became effective May 1, 1971. This law was designed to provide: "increased research into, and prevention of, drug abuse and drug dependence; to provide for treatment and rehabilitation of drug abusers and drug dependent persons; and to strengthen existing law enforcement authority in the field of drug abuse." This law is also designed to improve the administration and regulation of the manufacturing, distributing, and dispensing of controlled substances by legitimate handlers of these drugs to help reduce their widespread dispersion into illicit markets.

Specifically, it does the following:

1 Provides funding for the collection, preparation, and dissemination of drug education material on use and abuse of drugs and prevention of abuse.
2 Provides funding for development and evaluation of programs of drug abuse education directed at the general public, school-age children, and special high-risk groups.
3 Provides funding for the development of treatment, detoxification, and rehabilitation programs for drug-dependent persons.
4 Directs the Secretary of Health, Education, and Welfare to work with professional groups to develop guidelines for treating narcotic addicts.
5 Establishes a "Commission of Marihuana and Drug Abuse" to study and report on:

*Current regulations can be obtained from the nearest Regional Director, Drug Enforcement Administration, or from the Drug Enforcement Administration, Department of Justice, Post Office Box 28083, Central Station, Washington, D.C. 20005.

a. the extent of marihuana use in the United States, type of user, nature of use, and source
b. the efficacy of existing marihuana laws
c. the pharmacology of marihuana; physiologic and psychologic immediate and long-term effects
d. the relationship of marihuana to aggressive behavior and crime and use of other drugs
e. the international control of marihuana
6 Defines a *"drug-dependent person"* as "a person who is using a controlled substance (as defined in the Controlled Substances Act) and who is in a state of psychic or physical dependence, or both, arising from the use of that substance on a continuous basis. Drug dependence is characterized by behavioral and other responses which include a strong compulsion to take the substance on a continuous basis in order to experience its psychic effects or to avoid the discomfort caused by its absence."
7 Defines a *"drug addict"* as "any individual who habitually uses any narcotic drug so as to endanger the public morals, health, safety, or welfare, or who is so far addicted to the use of narcotic drugs as to have lost the power of self-control with reference to his addiction."
8 Resolves some basic philosophical, ethical, and legal issues by:
a. centering the enforcement authority of drug control in the Department of Justice rather than in the Treasury Department
b. making the Attorney General responsible for the enforcement of the drug control law and the Secretary of Health, Education, and Welfare responsible for final decisions on which drugs should be controlled; this separates drug law enforcement from scientific evaluation of drugs for control
9 Schedules or classifies drugs according to medical usefulness and "potential for abuse":
Schedule I. Drugs that currently do not have accepted medical use, have a high potential for abuse, and lack accepted safety measures for use (e.g., heroin, marihuana, LSD, peyote)
Schedule II. Drugs that have medical use and a high abuse potential; abuse may lead to severe psychologic or physical dependence (e.g., morphine, methadone, secobarbital [Seconal], amobarbital [Tuinal], amphetamines; many were formerly known as class A narcotic drugs)
Schedule III. Drugs used in medical practice that have less potential for abuse than those in schedule II; abuse may lead to moderate or low physical dependence or high psychologic dependence

(e.g., barbiturates, nalorphine, drugs combined with codeine or other narcotics, paregoric; these were formerly class B narcotic drugs)

Schedule IV. Drugs that have medical use, lower potential for abuse than those in schedule III; abuse may lead to limited physical or psychologic dependence (e.g., certain tranquilizers such as meprobamate, chlordiazepoxide [Librium], diazepam [Valium], phenobarbital, chloral hydrate)

Schedule V. Drugs that have medical use, lower potential for abuse, and cause less physical or psychologic dependence than drugs in schedule IV; mixtures of limited quantities of narcotics (e.g., over-the-counter drugs such as cough syrup with codeine)

10 Determines the regulation of drug use in research and criminal penalties for illegal possession, use, sale, and manufacture according to drug classification.

11 Requires all persons who manufacture, distribute, or dispense any controlled drug to (a) obtain an annual registration unless exempted, (b) provide effective controls and procedures to guard against theft and diversion of controlled substances, (c) keep inventories and maintain complete and accurate records of all drugs manufactured, dispensed, obtained, or disposed of.

12 Requires researchers using narcotic drugs in their analytical work to register with the Bureau of Narcotics and Dangerous Drugs.

13 Requires that the label of commercial containers of controlled drugs state the schedule to which the drug belongs in letters twice as large as the largest letter printed on the label.

This law does not eliminate state regulations.

Regulations concerning prescriptions include the following:

1 All prescriptions for controlled substances must be dated and signed when issued and bear the patient's full name and address and the name, address, and registration number of the practitioner.

2 Prescriptions must be labeled with the date of filling, pharmacy name and address, serial number of the prescription, patient's name, physician's name, directions for use, and cautionary statements. This labeling is not required for hospitalized patients.

3 Refilling a prescription for a controlled drug listed in schedule II is prohibited; a new prescription is required. For hospitalized patients, not more than a 7 day supply of a schedule II drug is to be dispensed at one time and must not be in the possession of the patient prior to administration.

4 Prescriptions for drugs listed in schedules III and IV cannot be filled or refilled more than 6 months after the date issued and cannot be refilled more than 5 times. For hospitalized patients, not more than a 34 day supply or 100 dosage units, whichever is less, of schedule III or IV drugs is to be dispensed at one time and must not be in the patient's possession prior to administration.

5 A prescription for a controlled substance listed in schedule V can be refilled as authorized by the physician on the prescription. These drugs can be dispensed by a pharmacist without a prescription if the purchaser is at least 18 years old, known to the pharmacist, and a record made of the purchase (e.g., name and address of purchaser, date of purchase, etc.).

6 Pharmacists must keep a record of the receipt and dispensing of controlled drugs for a period of at least 2 years and must make the records available to authorized persons.

In July of 1973, the Drug Enforcement Administration (D.E.A.) in the Department of Justice became the nation's sole law and enforcement agency; it replaced the Bureau of Narcotics and Dangerous Drugs.

Possession of narcotics. It is, of course, unlawful for any person to possess a controlled substance unless obtained by a valid prescription or order, or unless its possession is pursuant to actions in the course of professional practice. A nurse administering special controlled drugs, such as narcotics, from stock supplies must record the date, time of administration, patient's name, physician's name, and his or her own name. Stock supplies of narcotics must be accounted for, and nurses are responsible for maintaining accurate accounting of all narcotics dispensed to their hospital unit or clinic. Nurses need to know that it is a crime to transfer a drug listed in schedule II, III, or IV to any person other than the patient for whom the drug was ordered.

Nurses give narcotics only under the direction of a physician or dentist licensed to prescribe or dispense narcotics. Narcotics ordered but not used for patients must be returned to the source from which they were obtained (e.g., hospital pharmacy). Violation of the Controlled Substances Act is punishable by fine, imprisonment, or both. In addition, a nurse who violates this Act is subject to revocation of his or her license to practice nursing.

Food and Drug Administration. The Food and Drug Administration is charged with the enforcement of the Federal Food, Drug, and Cosmetic Act. Seizure of offending goods and criminal prosecution of responsible persons or firms in federal courts are among the methods used to enforce the Act.

In addition, pharmaceutical firms must report at regular intervals to the F.D.A. all adverse effects associated with their new drugs. The F.D.A. also has an adverse-reaction reporting program with approximately 450 cooperating reporting sources. The purpose of this program is to detect reactions not revealed by previous clinical or pharmaceutical studies.

Public Health Service. The Public Health Service is an agency that is also part of the U.S. Department of Health, Education, and Welfare. One of its many functions is the regulation of biologic products. This refers to ''any virus, therapeutic serum, antitoxin, or analogous product applicable to the prevention, treatment, or cure of diseases or injuries of man.'' The control exercised by the Public Health Service over these products is done by inspecting and licensing the establishments that manufacture the products and by examining and licensing the products as well.

Federal Trade Commission. The Federal Trade Commission is an agency of the federal government that is directly responsible to the President. Its principal control with respect to drugs lies in its power to suppress false or misleading advertising to the general public.

Product liability. In a majority of the states the rule of strict manufacturer's liability has been adopted. This doctrine holds manufacturers liable for injuries caused by defects in their products. Liability exists (1) if a product is defective or not fit for its reasonably foreseeable uses, (2) if the defect arose before the product left the control of the manufacturer, and (3) if the defect caused some person harm. If these three legal requirements are met, the manufacturer must pay money damages for the harm unless he can shift the liability to some other party. Anyone

harmed by a defective product has the right to sue the manufacturer for compensation.

Harm may be caused if a drug contains an ingredient whose danger is not commonly known, or if it contains an ingredient known to be harmful that one would not reasonably expect to find in such a product. Drugs containing potentially harmful ingredients must so state on the label warnings concerning its use; otherwise, the product will be considered defective and the manufacturer liable for resulting harm to unusually susceptible persons who unknowingly use it. Whether or not a product is defective depends on its compliance with current reasonable standards of safety. Manufacturers are legally responsible for knowing the effects of their products; if an unknown risk could have been discovered through a reasonable amount of research, the manufacturer will be held liable for any resulting harm.

The following are examples of drug liability awards:

A 43-year-old woman who sustained retinal damage as the result of taking Aralen, a prescription drug, was awarded $180,000 to be paid by the manufacturer. *Krug v. Sterling Drug, Inc.* (Mo S Ct 1967) ¶ 5789, 416 SW2d

The manufacturer of the drug Chloromycetin was liable for the death of a 7-year-old girl of aplastic anemia. The parents were awarded $215,000. *Incollingo v. Ewing* (Pa Ct Com Pls 1969) ¶ 6388, 48 D&C. (Aff'd Pa S Ct 1971) ¶ 6941.

A 43-year-old male who developed cataracts as the result of taking MER/29, a prescription drug, was awarded $500,000 to be paid by the manufacturer. *Toole v. Richardson-Merrell, Inc.* (Cal Ct App 1967) ¶ 5814, 60 Cal Rptr 398.

The parents of a 3-month-old infant, who developed a permanent brain disorder as the result of injections of Quadrigen, a quadruple antigen, recovered $643,000 from the drug company. *Tinnerholm v. Parke-Davis & Co.* (Ca-2 NY 1969) 6178, 411 F2d 48.

Nurses should be alert to defects in the drugs they administer. Although detection of chemical defects is beyond the nurse's province, detection of observable physical defects is not. Nurses should be keenly aware of the proper physical characteristics of drugs they administer. Discoloration or improper consistency of tablets, pills, or liquids, or precipitates or foreign bodies in parenteral fluids, should be considered suspect. These should be referred to the pharmacist. It might mean that an entire stock supply or batch is defective. Recall of defective drugs will prevent unnecessary harm.

Problems in drug legislation. In addition to the federal laws discussed in the preceding pages, it should be mentioned that many states have laws applicable to the sale and manufacture of drugs within the state. This refers to laws other than those applying to the sale of small amounts of narcotics. Outstanding among them are the regulations for the sale of barbiturates.

It is well to remember that the effectiveness of legislation will depend on the appropriation of adequate funds to enforce the laws, the vigor with which enforcement is pushed by proper authorities, and the interest and cooperation of professional and lay groups.

There are still many problems resulting from indiscriminate and unwise use of drugs, misunderstandings about vitamins, drugs for obesity, and cancer "cures." Although the consumer is often led astray by attractive advertising, clever suggestion, and adroit mishandling of information, there are reliable sources of information concerning drugs. Organizations such as the American Medical Association, American Dental Association, American Cancer Society, American Heart Association, and local, state, and county health departments will supply accurate information free of charge or for a very small fee.

CANADIAN DRUG LEGISLATION

In Canada, the Health Protection Branch (H.P.D.), of the Department of National Health and Welfare is responsible for administration and enforcement of the Food and Drugs Act, as well as the Proprietary or Patent Medicine Act and the Narcotics Control Act. These acts are designed to protect the consumer from health hazards and fraud or deception in the sale and use of foods, drugs, cosmetics, and medical devices. Canadian drug legislation began in 1874 when the Parliament of Canada passed an act to prevent the sale of adulterated food, drink,

and drugs. Since that time there has been food and drug control on a national basis.

Canadian Food and Drugs Act. In 1953 the present Canadian Food and Drugs Act was passed by the Senate and House of Commons of Canada. Since then the law has been amended several times; the most recent amendments occurred in 1974. The law states that no food, drug, cosmetic, or device is to be advertised or sold as a treatment, preventative, or cure for certain diseases listed in schedule A of the Act. Among the diseases included in the list are alcoholism, arteriosclerosis, and cancer. When it is necessary to provide adequate directions for the safe use of a schedule G drug used to treat or prevent diseases mentioned in schedule A, that disease or disorder may be mentioned on the labels and inserts accompanying the drug. In addition, the Act prohibits the sale of drugs that are contaminated, adulterated, or unsafe for use and those whose labels are false, misleading, or deceptive. According to the Act, drugs must comply with prescribed standards as stated in recognized pharmacopeias and formularies listed in schedule B of the Act, or according to the professed standards under which the drug is sold. These include the following:

Pharmacopoeia Internationalis
The British Pharmacopoeia
The Pharmacopeia of the United States of America
Codex Français
The Canadian Formulary
The British Pharmaceutical Codex
The National Formulary

C.S.D. means Canadian Standard Drug. This legend, or abbreviation, must appear on the inner and outer labels of a drug to signify that it meets the standards prescribed for it.

Sale of certain drugs is prohibited unless the premises where the drug was manufactured and the process and conditions of manufacture have been approved by the Minister of National Health and Welfare. These drugs are listed in schedules C and D and include injectable liver extracts, all insulin preparations, anterior pituitary extracts, radioactive isotopes, antibiotics for parenteral use, serums and drugs other than antibiotics prepared from microorganisms or viruses, and live vaccines. For some drugs the batch from which the drug was taken must meet safety approval, and these are listed in schedule E. Among the drugs listed are various arsphenamines and sensitivity disks and tablets. Distribution of samples of drugs is also prohibited, with the exception of distribution of samples of drugs to duly licensed individuals such as physicians, dentists, or pharmacists. Schedule F (Section 15) states that no person can sell any drug described in schedule F. Thalidomide, a hypnotic known to be a teratogenic substance, is the only drug presently listed. However, thalidomide may be sold in powdered form to qualified investigators for experimental and investigational use in animals upon approval by the Minister of National Health and Welfare. Schedule F of the Act contains a list of drugs that can be sold only on prescription, and such prescriptions shall not be refilled, unless the prescriber has so directed. Refills may be permitted at specified intervals but cannot exceed 6 months. Drugs listed in schedule F include the antibiotics, sulfonamides, and phenothiazine derivatives. They must always be properly and clearly labeled and include directions for use. Labels on containers of schedule F drugs should be marked with the symbol Pr (prescription required). These drugs cannot be advertised to the general public.

Controlled drugs are those listed in schedule G and include amphetamines, barbituric acid and its derivatives (barbiturates), methaqualone, pentazocine, and phenmetrazine. Controlled drugs must be marked with the symbol ⟨C⟩ in a clear and conspicuous color and size on the upper left quarter of the label. The proper name of the drug must appear on the labels either immediately preceding or following the proprietary or trade name. Controlled drugs can be dispensed only on prescription.

When dispensed by prescription the labels of a controlled drug must carry the following:

1 Name and address of the pharmacy or pharmacist
2 Date and number of the prescription
3 Name of the person for whom the controlled drug is dispensed
4 Name of the practitioner
5 Directions for use

6 Any other information that the prescription requires be shown on the label

Prescriptions for controlled drugs cannot be refilled unless at the time the prescription was issued, the practitioner so directed in writing and specified the number of times it could be refilled and the dates for, or intervals between, refilling. All information on the labels must be clearly and prominently displayed and readily discernible. Controlled drugs cannot be advertised to the general public.

Designated drugs are the following controlled drugs: (1) amphetamines, (2) phenmetrazine, and (3) phendimetrazine. Physicians may prescribe a designated drug for the following conditions: (1) narcolepsy, (2) hyperkinetic disorders in children, (3) mental retardation (minimal brain dysfunction), (4) epilepsy, (5) parkinsonism, and (6) hypotensive states associated with anesthesia.

Controls were relaxed on the amphetamines in 1973. Physicians are no longer required to notify the federal government when they prescribe amphetamines, phenmetrazine, or phendimetrazine, nor are they required to obtain confirmation of their diagnosis when amphetamine treatment is to exceed 30 days. Permission can be obtained to prescribe amphetamines for patients with diagnoses other than those listed.

Restricted drugs are those listed in schedule H and include the hallucinogenic drugs lysergic acid diethylamide (LSD), diethyltryptamine (DET), dimethyltryptamine (DMT), and dimethoxyamphetamine (STP; DOM). Sale of these drugs is prohibited. These drugs may be obtained for research by a qualified investigator if authorized by the Minister of National Health and Welfare. Precautions must be taken to ensure against loss or theft of a restricted drug.

The following are additional requirements to be found in the Food and Drugs Act:

1 Labels of drugs must show:
   a. Proper name of the drug immediately preceding or following the proprietary or brand name.
   b. Name and address of the manufacturer or distributor.
   c. Lot number of the drug.
   d. Adequate directions for use.
   e. Quantitative list of medicinal ingredients and their proper or common names.

f. Net amount of drug.

g. Common or proper name and proportion of any preservatives used in parenteral drugs.

h. Expiration date if the drug does not maintain its potency, purity, and physical characteristics for at least 3 years from the date of manufacture.

i. Recommended single and daily adult dose; if the drug is for children the label must state: "Children: As directed by physician" or:

Age in years	Proportion of adult dose
10-14	One-half
5-9	One-fourth
2-4	One-sixth
Under 2	As directed by physician

j. A warning that the drug be kept out of the reach of children and any precautions to be taken (e.g., "*Caution:* May be injurious if taken in large doses for a long time. Do not exceed the recommended dose without consulting a physician." Warning is to be preceded by a symbol—octagonal in shape, red in color, and on a white background).

k. Contraindications and side effects of nonprescription drugs.

l. On and after July 1, 1974, the drug identification number assigned to the drug, preceded by the words "Drug Identification Number" or the abbreviation "D.I.N."; to be shown on the main labels of a drug sold in dosage form (i.e., one ready for use by the consumer).

2 Other specific regulations such as:

a. Manufacturers must be able to demonstrate that a drug in oral dosage form represented as releasing the drug at time intervals actually is released and available as represented.

b. Oral tablets must disintegrate within 60 minutes. Enteric-coated tablets must not disintegrate for 60 minutes when exposed to gastric juice but must disintegrate within an additional 60 minutes when exposed to intestinal juice.

c. Drugs containing boric acid or sodium borate as a medicinal ingredient must carry a statement that the drug should not be administered to infants or children under 3 years of age.

d. No manufacturer or importer shall sell a drug containing phenacetin in combination with any salt or derivative of salicylic acid.

The regulations allow the government to withdraw from the market drugs found to be unduly toxic. New drugs introduced to the market must have shown effectiveness and safety in human clinical studies to the satisfaction of the manufacturer and the government.

For more specific information, the nurse can obtain a copy of *The Food and Drugs Act and Regulations*, issued by Department of National Health and Welfare, from the Queen's Printer and Controller of Stationery, Ottawa, Canada.

Canadian Narcotic Control Act. The regulations of the Canadian Narcotic Control Act govern the possession, sale, manufacture, production, and distribution of narcotics. The Canadian Narcotic Control Act was enacted in 1961. This act revoked the Canadian Opium and Narcotic Act of 1952. The 1961 Act has been amended a number of times.

Only authorized persons can be in possession of a narcotic. Authorized persons include a licensed dealer, pharmacist, practitioner, person in charge of a hospital, or a person acting as an agent for a practitioner. A licensed dealer is one who has been given permission to manufacture, produce, import, export, or distribute a narcotic. Practitioners include persons registered under the laws of a province to practice the profession of medicine, dentistry, or veterinary medicine. However, persons other than these may be licensed by the Minister of National Health and Welfare to cultivate and produce opium poppy or marihuana or to purchase and possess a narcotic for scientific purposes. Members of the Royal Canadian Mounted Police and members of technical or scientific departments of the government of Canada or of a province or university may possess narcotics for the purpose of, and in connection with, their employment. A person who is undergoing treatment by a medical practitioner and who requires a narcotic may possess a narcotic obtained on prescription. This person may not knowingly obtain a narcotic from any other medical practitioner without notifying that practitioner that he is already undergoing treatment and obtaining a narcotic on prescription.

All persons authorized to be in possession of narcotics must keep a record of the name and quantity of all narcotics received, from whom narcotics were obtained, and to whom narcotics were supplied (including quantity, form, and dates of all transactions). In addition, they must ensure the safekeeping of all narcotics, keep full and complete records on all narcotics for at least 2 years, and report any loss or theft within 10 days of discovery.

The schedule of the Act lists those drugs, their preparations, derivatives, alkaloids, and salts that are subject to the Canadian Narcotic Control Act. Included in the schedule are opium, coca, and marihuana. Before a pharmacist legally may dispense a drug included in the schedule or medication containing such a drug, he must receive a prescription from a physician. A signed and dated prescription issued by a duly authorized physician is essential in the case of all narcotic medication prescribed as such or any preparation containing a narcotic in a form intended for parenteral administration. Oral medication containing a narcotic may be dispensed by a pharmacist on the strength of a verbal prescription received from a physician who is known to the pharmacist or whose identity is established. Prescriptions of any description calling for a narcotic may not be refilled.

There is one exception to the prescription requirement. Certain codeine compounds with a small codeine content may be sold to the public by a pharmacist without a prescription. In such instances the narcotic content cannot exceed $1/8$ grain per unit in tablet, capsule, or other solid form and $1/3$ grain per fluidounce in liquid form. In products of this kind, codeine must be in combination with two or more nonnarcotic substances and in recognized therapeutic doses.

Additionally, items of this nature are required to be labeled in such a fashion as to show the true formula of the medicinal ingredients and a caution to the following effect: "This preparation contains codeine and should not be administered to children except on the advice of a physician." These preparations cannot be advertised or displayed in a pharmacy. It is also unlawful to publish any narcotic advertisement for the general public.

Labels of containers of narcotics must legibly and conspicuously bear the proprietary and proper or common name of the narcotic, name of the manufacturer and distributor, the symbol "*N*" in the upper left-hand quarter, and net contents of the container and of each tablet, capsule, or ampule.

It should be pointed out that local or provincial laws modify to a certain extent regulations governing the sale and administration of narcotics.

Although the administration of the Canadian Narcotic Control Act is legally the responsibility of the Department of National Health and Welfare, the enforcement of the law has been made largely the responsibility of the Royal Canadian Mounted Police. Prosecution of offenses under the Act is handled through the Department of National Health and Welfare by legal agents specially appointed by the Department of Justice.

The Narcotic Control Act defines a narcotic addict as "a person who through the use of narcotics, has developed a desire or need to continue to take a narcotic, or has developed a psychological or physical dependence upon the effect of a narcotic." A person brought into court for a narcotic offense may be placed in custody by the court for observation and examination. If the person is convicted of the offense and found to be a narcotic addict, the court can sentence him to custody for treatment for an indefinite period.

Amendments to this Act place special restrictions on methadone. No practitioner can administer, prescribe, give, sell, or furnish methadone to any person unless the practitioner has been issued an authorization by the Minister of National Health and Welfare.

Application to nursing. A nurse may be in violation of the Canadian Narcotic Control Act if he or she is guilty of illegal possession of narcotics. Ignorance of the content of a drug in the nurse's possession is not considered a justifiable excuse. Proof of possession is sufficient to constitute an offense. Legal possession of narcotics by a nurse is limited to times when a drug is administered to a patient on the order of a physician, when the nurse is acting as the official custodian of narcotics in a department of the hospital or clinic, or when the nurse is a patient for whom a physician has prescribed narcotics. A nurse engaged in illegal distribution or transportation of narcotic drugs may be held liable, and heavy penalties are imposed in violation of the Canadian Narcotic Control Act.

Proprietary or Patent Medicine Act. The Proprietary or Patent Medicine Act, first passed in 1908, was designed to ensure to the Canadian public safe and effective home medication with proprietary or patent medicines (P.P.M.). The word "patent" in medicine originated in England in the early eighteenth century when a royal patent, or exclusive right, could be obtained for a drug formula based on claims that it would help the sick. Unlike official drugs, the composition of which was available to medical science, the formulas of patent medicines were usually secret.

The Proprietary or Patent Medicine Act regulates the sale and manufacture of patent medicines. It was enacted when it was found that some of the cure-all mixtures were worthless, fraudulent, and even harmful to health since they contained substances such as cocaine, arsenic, strychnine, and high levels of alcohol. For example, "Mrs. Winslow's Soothing Syrup" contained morphine with claims that it was a source of comfort to both teething baby and fretful mother. "Hotstetter's Bitters," sold as a tonic for the entire body, contained the equivalent of one ounce of whisky per four tablespoons of medicine!

Passage of the Act in 1908 prohibited inclusion of cocaine in patent internal medicine, limited the amount of alcohol, controlled the use of hazardous drugs, and required the manufacturer to be registered.

In 1919, the Proprietary and Patent Medicine Act was amended to do the following:

1 Require registration and annual licensing for each formula
2 Forbid patent medicines to be represented as curing disease
3 Ban all false, misleading, or exaggerated advertising
4 Require declaration on the label of all patent drugs in the formula
5 Require that the drug be effective for the claims advanced
6 Forbid distribution of samples to the public
7 Establish an advisory board to determine dosage of drug and alcohol content

P.P.M. drugs registered by the Health Protection Branch have been evaluated and found acceptable for sale to the public. These products are checked for dosage, efficacy, compatibility of ingredients, action, proper directions for use, and for false and misleading claims.

Labels of P.P.M. drugs must show:

1 Name of drug
2 Name and address of manufacturer
3 Net contents
4 Directions for use and special instructions, such as "shake well" or "for external use only"
5 A caution or warning statement, if applicable
6 Expiration date
7 Registration number, the words "Proprietary or Patent Medicine Act," and any drugs listed in the P.P.M. schedule

Registered preparations have a number assigned to them; any change in the formula or name requires a new registration application. To advertise a patent medicine on radio or television, the manufacturer must have the commercial or script previewed by the Health Protection Branch. Newspapers and periodicals are checked regularly for noncompliance with drug advertising legislation. If advertisements are found contrary to the law, they must be altered or withdrawn or the offenders are subject to legal action.

Distribution of P.P.M. preparations is under the jurisdiction of the provincial governments. These preparations may be sold in registered pharmacies or other retail outlet such as grocery stores. Nurses should be aware of the home remedies or patent medicines commonly used by patients.

INTERNATIONAL DRUG CONTROL

International control of drugs legally began in 1912 when the first "Opium Conference" was held at The Hague. International treaties were drawn up legally obligating governments to: (1) limit to medical and scientific needs the manufacturing of and trade in medicinal opium; (2) control the production and distribution of raw opium; and (3) establish a system of governmental licensing to control the manufacture of and trade in drugs covered by the convention.

In 1961 government representatives formulated the "Single Convention on Narcotic Drugs," which became effective in 1964. This Act consolidated all existing treaties into one document for the control of all narcotic substances by:

1 Outlawing their production, manufacturing, trade, and use of nonmedicinal purposes
2 Limiting possession of all narcotic substances to authorized persons for medical and scientific purposes
3 Providing for international control of all opium transactions by the national monopolies (countries designated to produce opium, e.g., Turkey) and authorizing production only by licensed farmers in areas and on plots designated by these monopolies
4 Requiring import certificates and export authorizations

An International Narcotics Control Board was established to enforce this law. Since this is an immense task it is impossible to prevent illicit trafficking of drugs. For example, during a 1 year period it was estimated that 1,200 tons of opium were circulated in the illicit market when 800 tons were considered sufficient for world medical needs. This law needs to be updated and stricter control enforced.

QUESTIONS

For study and review

1 State the purpose of the Federal Food, Drug, and Cosmetic Act.
2 Explain the need for drug standards.
3 State the purpose of the National Code Directory.
4 Explain the reason for testing new drugs in at least two different animal species.
5 Why are normal subjects often used for phase I clinical testing of a new drug?
6 Discuss the various safeguards used to minimize bias in clinical drug studies.
7 Why would the effects of a new narcotic analysis be compared with those of a standard narcotic such as morphine or codeine?
8 What responsibilities does a nurse have when participating in new drug studies?
9 Why did the Drug Efficacy Implementation Study (D.E.S.I.) come into being?
10 Formulate criteria for measuring the effectiveness of a new narcotic analgesic.
11 What is the purpose of using homogeneous subjects in clinical drug studies?

12 State the purpose of the Controlled Substances Act.
13 How does the Controlled Substances Act define a "drug-dependent person"? A "drug addict"?
14 Interview various hospital or clinic personnel to determine ways in which narcotics can be "pilfered" from hospital units or clinics.
15 Discuss the nurse's responsibility when a physician orders a narcotic for a patient by telephone.

Objective questions

Select the correct combination answer.

Controlled Substances Act (U.S.)

16 Schedule I drugs are those that:
  a. have high potential for abuse.
  b. do not have an acceptable medical use.
  c. include the hallucinogenics.
  d. lack accepted safety measures for use.
17 Schedule II drugs are those that:
  a. have an accepted medical use.
  b. have high abuse potential.
  c. may cause severe dependence.
  d. include the barbiturates.
18 Schedule III drugs are those that:
  a. may cause moderate or low physical dependence.
  b. have low abuse potential.
  c. may cause high psychologic dependence.
  d. include the barbiturates
19 Schedule IV drugs:
  a. include major tranquilizers.
  b. may cause minimal dependence.
  c. include phenobarbital.
  d. have moderate potential for abuse.
20 Schedule V drugs:
  a. include over-the-counter drugs containing limited amounts of narcotics.
  b. lack potential for abuse.
  c. do not cause physical dependence.
  d. may cause psychologic dependence.

Canadian Food and Drugs Act

21 Match the following:
  _____ **1.** Designated drugs   **a.** Sale of these drugs is prohibited
  _____ **2.** Restricted drugs
  _____ **3.** Controlled drugs   **b.** Prescription drugs
           c. These drugs to be prescribed only for specific listed conditions

22 Which of the following statements are correct?
  a. Hallucinogenics are restricted drugs.
  b. Obesity is one of the listed conditions for which amphetamines may be prescribed.
  c. The legend "C.S.D." on a drug label indicates that the drug meets the standards prescribed for it.
  d. Amphetamines and barbiturates cannot be advertised to the general public.

REFERENCES

Aviado, D. M.: Krantz and Carr's pharmacologic principles of medical practice, ed. 8, Baltimore, 1972, The Williams & Wilkins Co.

Blackwell, B.: For the first time in man, Clin. Pharmacol. Ther. **13**:812, 1971.

Black, J. B., editor: Safeguarding the public—historical aspects of medicinal drug control, Baltimore, 1970, The Johns Hopkins Press.

Blissett, C. W., Webb, O. L., and Stanaszek, W. F.: Clinical pharmacy practice, Philadelphia, 1972, Lea & Febiger.

Di Palma, J. R.: DESI ratings, a revolution in the making, R.N. **36**:51, 1973.

Nichols, T. S.: Human experimentation in clinical nursing research. In Anderson, E. H., and others, editors: Current concepts in clinical nursing, Vol. IV, St. Louis, 1973, The C. V. Mosby Co.

Palmer, R. F.: Controversies in clinical pharmacology and drug development, Mount Kisco, N.Y., 1972, Futura Publishing Company, Inc.

Palmer, R. F.: Products liability—minimizing the hazard, New York, 1971, Commerce Clearing House, Inc.

Silverman, A., and Lee, P. R.: Pills, profits and politics, Los Angeles, 1974, University of California Press, Ltd.

Turner, P., and Richens, A.: Clinical pharmacology, London, 1973, Churchill Livingstone.

Uehleke, H.: Animal data in perspective, Int. J. Clin. Pharm. **8**:239, 1973.

Official publications

Code of Federal Regulations, #21 Food and Drugs, Washington, D.C., 1973, U.S. Government Printing Office.

Public Law 91-513, 91st Congress, H.R. 18583, Washington, D.C., 1972, U.S. Government Printing Office.

The Food and Drugs Act and Regulations, 1972, with Amendments to March 26, 1974, Roger Duhamel, F.R.S.C. Ottawa, Ontario, Queen's Printer and Controller of Stationery.

Narcotic Control Act and the Narcotic Control Regulations, Roger Duhamel, F.R.S.C. Ottawa, Ontario, Queen's Printer and Controller of Stationery.

Patent Medicines, #14. Educational Services, 1971, Food and Drug Directorate, Ottawa, Ontario, Department of National Health and Welfare.

CHAPTER 4

Names, sources, active constituents, and pharmaceutical preparations of drugs

Names of drugs
Sources of drugs
Pharmaceutical preparations

NAMES OF DRUGS

The present-day use of a variety of names for the same drug is cause for confusion for all health professionals. One name under which a drug may appear is its official name, another is the generic name, another is its chemical name, and a fourth by which it may be known is its trade name.

The *official name* is the name under which it is listed in one of the official publications. The official name may also have one or more synonyms by which it is known. Before a new drug becomes official it will have assigned to it a *generic name.* This name is simpler than the chemical name, although it may reflect the chemical family to which the drug belongs. The generic name is never changed and can be used in all countries. It is not protected by law. It is usually initiated or proposed by the company that develops the drug. When it is selected careful investigation is made to make certain that it does not conflict with already existing names. Then it is usually processed by way of the American Medical Association Council on Drugs and through the World Health Organization, which has a Committee on International Non-Proprietary Names. In that way the name may be adopted on a worldwide basis.

The *chemical name* is meaningful principally to the chemist, who sees in the name a very precise description of the chemical constitution of the drug and the exact placement of atoms or atomic groupings. For example, the chemical name of one of the antibiotics is 4-dimethylamino-1,4,4a,5,5a,6,11,12a-octahydro-3,6,10,12,12a-pentahydroxy-6-methyl-1,11 dioxo-2-napthacenecarboxamide. Its generic name is tetracycline, and it is known under a number of trade names—Achromycin, Panmycin, Tetracyn, and Steclin.

A *trademark name* or a *brand name* frequently appears in the literature with the sign® at the upper right of the name to indicate that the name is registered and that its use is restricted to the manufacturer who is the legal owner of the name. The first letter of the trade name is capitalized but the generic name is not capitalized. Many times the generic name is stated and the trade name is given in parentheses.

The name of a drug is not patented but a patent may be issued by the U.S. Patent Office to cover the drug as a chemical entity, the method of manufacture, the method of use, or any combination of these. Patents expire after 17 years; then other manufacturers may make the drug under its generic name but they must select a different trade name. Two or more drug companies may make the same drug under different

33

trade or trademark names. Sometimes a single drug may be sold under ten or twenty different brand names, which results in a great deal of undesirable confusion.

In order to promote sales under the trademark name, extensive advertising is usually necessary. This involves considerable expense, which is borne mainly by the consumer. On the other hand, much of the research in new drugs is done in laboratories of reputable drug firms, and in order to realize a legitimate return for the cost of research, they need to patent their product and have exclusive rights of its manufacture and sale.

There is a real need to give more attention to generic and official names. Some hospital pharmacies in the United States label medications with their official or generic names and place the trade name or trademark name at the bottom of the label. This would appear to place the emphasis properly.

Further confusion is fostered when mixtures or combinations of otherwise well-known drugs are sold under a name that does not reflect the content. For example, combinations of phenacetin, aspirin, and caffeine are sold under a variety of names such as Empirin compound, APC, and PAC, as well as aspirin compound.

The word *proprietary* is also used in referring to drugs. This means that the drug is protected from competition in some manner. In other words, the drug or its name belongs to someone.

SOURCES OF DRUGS

Drugs are derived from four main sources: (1) plants, examples of which are digitalis, opium, and belladonna; (2) animals, from which drugs such as epinephrine, insulin, and ACTH are obtained; (3) minerals or mineral products, such as iron, iodine, and Epsom salt; and (4) chemical substances made in the laboratory. The drugs made of chemical substances are pure drugs, and some of them are simple substances, such as sodium bicarbonate and magnesium hydroxide, whereas others are products of complex synthesis, such as the sulfonamides and the adrenocorticosteroids.

ACTIVE CONSTITUENTS OF PLANT DRUGS

The leaves, roots, seeds, and other parts of plants may be dried or otherwise processed for use as medicine and, as such, are known as crude drugs. Their therapeutic effect is caused by chemical substances contained in the crude preparation. When the pharmacologically active constituents are separated from the crude preparation, the resulting substances are more potent and usually produce effects more reliable than those of the crude drug. As might be expected, these active principles are also more poisonous, and the dosage must be smaller. Some of the types of pharmacologically active compounds found in plants, grouped according to their physical and chemical properties, are alkaloids, glycosides, gums, resins and balsams, and oils.

Alkaloids. Alkaloids (alkali-like) are compounds composed of carbon, hydrogen, nitrogen, and oxygen. Alkaloids have a bitter taste; they are often poisonous and hence preparations of them are administered in small doses. They are, for the most part, white crystalline solids. The name of an alkaloid ends in "ine," for example, caffeine, atropine, and morphine. Alkaloids will combine with an acid to form a salt. The salts of alkaloids are used in medicine in preference to pure alkaloids because they are more soluble; for example, morphine sulfate is preferred to morphine since it is much more soluble in water. Increased solubility may make possible administration by injection. A number of alkaloids have been chemically synthesized in the laboratory.

Both alkaloids and their salts are precipitated by tannic acid and oxidized by potassium permanganate. Hence these substances can be used under certain circumstances as antidotes for poisoning from alkaloids.

Glycosides. Glycosides are active principles that upon hydrolysis yield a carbohydrate (a sugar) and some other chemical grouping such as an aldehyde, acid, or alcohol. The carbohydrate may be glucose, in which case the compound may be called a glucoside, but carbohydrates other than glucose may occur in the molecule, hence the use of the more general term *glycoside*. The carbohydrate molecule is usually not necessary for the action of the glycosides, and in the body it may be removed to liberate the active aglycone or genin. The presence of a sugar in the molecule of the glycoside is thought to modify activity by increasing solubility, absorption, permeability, and cellular distribution. An important glycoside used in medicine is digitoxin.

Gums. Gums are exudates from plants. They are polysaccharides that vary in the degree of their solubility in water. Upon the addition of water some of them will swell and form gelatinous or mucilaginous masses. Some remain unchanged in the gastrointestinal tract, where they act as hydrophilic (water-loving) colloids; that is, they absorb water, form watery bulk, and exert a laxative effect. Agar and psyllium seeds are examples of natural laxative gums. Synthetic hydrophilic colloids such as methylcellulose and sodium carboxymethyl cellulose may eventually replace the natural gums as laxatives. Gums are also used to soothe irritated skin and mucous membranes. Tragacanth gum, upon the addition of water, forms an emulsion used as a base for a greaseless catheter lubricant or for chapped skin. Acacia (gum arabic), U.S.P., B.P., is used as a suspending agent in making emulsions and mixtures.

Resins. Resins are crude drugs or an extraction from a crude drug. The rosin used by violinists is an example of a solid resin. A few are devoid of color, and some give off an aromatic fragrance as a result of admixture of a volatile oil. Resins form the sap of certain trees. They are insoluble in water but soluble in alcohol, ether, and various oils. Resins are local irritants and some have been used in medicine as cathartics. Podophyllum resin is a constituent of aloin, belladonna, cascara, and podophyllum pills (Hinkle's Pills) and is a rather irritating cathartic.

Balsams also contain resins in addition to benzoic or cinnamic acids. Benzoin, U.S.P., B.P., Peruvian balsam, and tolu balsam, U.S.P., B.P., are examples.

Oils. The term *oil* is applied to a large number of liquids characterized by being insoluble in water and highly viscous. Their greasy feel is the result of these properties. Oils are of two kinds, volatile and fixed.

Volatile oils are liquids that impart an aroma to a plant. They evaporate easily and leave no greasy stain. Because of their pleasant odor and taste they are frequently used as flavoring agents. Because of their volatility and consequent power of penetration they may be irritating, mildly stimulating, and antiseptic in effect. Peppermint oil and clove oil are listed in the U.S.P. and the B.P. and are occasionally used in medicine.

Fixed oils are those that feel greasy and do not evaporate readily. They hydrolyze to form fatty acids and glycerin. Some fixed oils are used as food, for example, olive oil. Others are used in medicine, such as castor oil, and some as vehicles in which to dissolve other drugs, such as sesame oil.

PHARMACEUTICAL PREPARATIONS

Pharmaceutical preparations are the preparations that make a drug suited to various methods of administration. They may be made by the pharmacist or by the pharmaceutical company from which they are purchased. The nurse who has some knowledge of these preparations is likely to bring more understanding to the task of administering drugs.

SOLUTIONS AND SUSPENSIONS

Aqueous solutions. Aqueous solutions have one or more substances dissolved in water. *Waters* are saturated (unless otherwise stated) solutions of volatile oils or other aromatic substances in distilled water. Peppermint water and concentrated peppermint water, B.P., are examples. Other aqueous solutions, sometimes referred to as *true solutions*, are made by dissolving a nonvolatile substance in water. Examples are strong iodine solution (Lugol's Solution), U.S.P., epinephrine nasal solution, U.S.P., and aluminum acetate solution, U.S.P.

Syrups are sometimes used for their demulcent (soothing) effect on irritated membranes of the throat. Syrup, U.S.P., is an aqueous solution of sucrose (85%). Syrups may be flavored and used as a vehicle in which to disguise unpleasant-tasting medicines and also as a preservative. Examples listed in the *National Formulary* are orange and cherry syrups. Promethazine hydrochloride syrup, U.S.P., is an example of a syrup that reflects medicinal content, an antihistaminic.

Aqueous suspensions. Aqueous suspensions are defined in U.S.P. XIX as preparations of finely divided drugs either intended for suspension or already in suspension in some suitable liquid vehicle. Sterile suspensions are prepared by adding sterile, distilled water for injection to the preparation, for example, sterile chloramphenicol for suspension. A sterile suspension ready for use is sterile penicillin procaine G suspension, U.S.P. Sterile suspensions are intended for intramuscular or subcutaneous injection, but they cannot be given intravenously or intrathecally. Oral suspensions may be prepared in much the same way, but they are not sterile and must not be injected. Suspensions for ophthalmic use are sterile and contain a bacteriostatic agent. Hydrocortisone acetate ophthalmic suspension, U.S.P., is a good example. Suspensions tend to settle slowly and should be shaken well before use to provide uniform distribution of the drug in the aqueous medium.

Mixtures. Mixtures are any solid material suspended in a liquid. No mixtures are listed in the U.S.P. The B.P. records a mixture of magnesium hydroxide. The term *mixture* is also used to mean any preparation of several drugs, such as a cough mixture. However, the term is usually restricted to mean only preparations for internal use.

Emulsions. Emulsions are suspensions of fats or oils in water with the aid of an emulsifying agent, which lowers the interfacial tension between the two substances, masking its oily feel. These oils are more easily digested than undispersed oils. Emulsions are stabilized by agents such as acacia and gelatin, which coat the tiny droplets of oil and prevent them from coming in direct contact with water. An example is cod liver oil emulsion.

Magmas. Magmas are sometimes called milks because they are white and resemble milk. They are bulky suspensions of insoluble preparations in water. Milk of magnesia, U.S.P., or magnesium hydroxide mixture, B.P., is an example.

Magmas tend to settle or separate upon standing and should be shaken well before they are poured.

Gels. Gels are aqueous suspensions of insoluble drugs in hydrated form. The particles suspended are approximately the size seen in colloidal dispersions. Magmas and gels are similar except that the particles suspended in a magma are larger; aluminum hydroxide gel, U.S.P., is an example.

Spirits. Spirits are concentrated alcoholic solutions of volatile substances. They are also known as essences. The dissolved substance may be solid, liquid, or gaseous. Most spirits contain from 5% to 20% of the active drug. The alcohol serves as a preservative as well as a solvent. Peppermint spirit, N.F., is sometimes used as a carminative and also a flavoring agent.

Elixirs. Elixirs are aromatic, sweetened, alcoholic preparations, frequently used as flavored vehicles, such as aromatic elixir, U.S.P., or as active medicinal agents if they are medicated elixirs, such as phenobarbital elixir, U.S.P., or cascara elixir, B.P.

Tinctures. Tinctures are alcoholic or hydroalcoholic solutions usually prepared from plant drugs or from chemical substances. Tinctures of potent drugs contain 10 Gm. of drug in 100 ml. of tincture. Most other tinctures contain 20 Gm. of drug in 100 ml. of tincture. Tinctures are prepared by extracting the drug from its crude source or by making an alcoholic solution of the drug. Iodine tincture, U.S.P., is made by dissolving iodine in an alcoholic solution of sodium iodide. The alcoholic content of tinctures improves their stability and facilitates solution of drugs that are poorly soluble in water. Tinctures listed in the B.P. are preparations extracted from crude drugs, not simple solutions. The usual dose of a potent tincture is about 1 ml. (0.3 to 1 ml.) or 5 to 15 minims.

Fluidextracts. Fluidextracts are alcoholic liquid extracts of vegetable drugs made so that 1 ml. of the fluidextract contains 1 Gm. of the drug. They are the most concentrated of any of the fluid preparations, being of 100% strength and ten times stronger than potent tinctures. Since many of them precipitate in light, they should be kept in dark bottles and not used if precipitate has formed. Glycyrrhiza fluidextract is used as a flavoring agent, whereas aromatic cascara sagrada fluidextract, U.S.P., and cascara liquid extract, B.P., are used as cathartics.

NOTE: Spirits, medicated elixirs, tinctures, and fluidextracts are preparations that tend to be potent and therefore the dosage is likely to be small. A nurse would never expect to administer as much as 30 ml. (a fluidounce) of any of them. A fraction of a milliliter (a few minims) up to as much as 2 to 4 ml. (1 to 2 fluidrams) is likely to be the range of dosage. Furthermore, these preparations are never injected, one reason being that they all contain alcohol. Most tinctures contain resins that make them incompatible with water.

Extracts. Extracts are concentrated preparations of vegetable or animal drugs obtained by removing the active ingredients of the drugs with suitable solvents and then evaporating all or part of the solvents. Extracts are made in three forms: semiliquids or liquids of syrupy consistency, plastic masses or pillular extracts, and dry powders known as powdered extracts. Extracts are intended to preserve the useful constituents of a drug in a form suitable for medication or for the making of other dosage forms such as tablets or pills. Liver extract is a dry extract. Cascara dry extract, B.P., is used to make cascara tablets, B.P.

DOSAGE FORMS

Capsules, sustained-release capsules, tablets, pills, and troches are used to divide a drug or mixture of drugs into definite doses and avoid the inconvenience of preparing the dose from dry powders. They are therefore referred to as dosage forms. Capsules and coated tablets are a convenient way of giving drugs that have an unpleasant taste. It has been true in the past and to some extent continues to be true that some patients are more impressed with a vile-tasting medicine than a pleasant-tasting or tasteless preparation. However, most patients appreciate preparations that are not unpleasant to take.

Capsules. Capsules are one of the most popular dosage forms for the oral administration of powders, oils, and liquids. They dissolve readily in the stomach and make the contents available for absorption only slightly less quickly than a liquid medicament. New drugs for oral use are often introduced in capsules in order to avoid problems of disintegration, stability, or taste. When these problems have been solved, tablet forms of the drug are generally used because they are less costly to produce. Capsules are usually made of gelatin and may be hard or soft, depending on the amount of glycerin in the gelatin. Gelatin capsules may be coated with a substance that resists the action of gastric juice and so will not disintegrate until they reach the alkaline secretions of the intestine. Such capsules are said to be *enteric coated*. Sizes of capsules range from 5 to 000 (see Figure 4-1). Capsules are often of a distinctive color or shape to identify the manufacturer.

Dosage forms providing for gradual but continued release of drug are sold under a number of different names, such as Spansules, Gradumets, and Timespans. Sustained-release dosage forms contain small particles of the drug coated with materials that require a varying amount of time to dissolve. This provides for a long contin-

Figure 4-1
Various sizes and numbers of gelatin capsules, actual size.

000   00   0   1   2   3   4   5

uous period of absorption and effect. Some particles dissolve and are absorbed almost immediately, others require 2 or 3 hours, and some do not dissolve for 10 or 12 hours. An increasing number of drugs are available in sustained release form; prochlorperazine edisylate, U.S.P. (Compazine Edisylate), is available in this dosage form.

Tablets. Tablets are preparations of powdered drug that are compressed or molded into small disks. They may be made with or without a diluent (dextrose, lactose, starch), and they may differ greatly in size, weight, and shape. *Compressed tablets* are made with heavy machinery. The granulated form of the preparation is formed, under great mechanical pressure, into tablets. Compressed tablets usually contain in addition to the drug a diluent, a binder, a disintegrator, and a lubricant. Binders are substances that give adhesiveness to the powdered drug. Diluents are used when the amount of active ingredient is small, and lubricants keep the tablet from sticking to the machines. A disintegrator, such as starch, helps the tablet to dissolve readily when it is placed in water, because the starch expands when it gets wet. Tablets are sometimes scored (marked with an indented line across the surface) so that they can be broken easily if half a tablet is the dose required. Tablets may be coated with sugar or chocolate to enhance their palatability. They may be covered with a colored coating to make them more attractive to patients, easier to swallow, or identifiable by the use of distinctive colors and legible imprinting. Both tablets and capsules may be enteric coated, either to protect the drug from the effect of the gastric secretions or to prevent drug irritation of the gastric mucosa.

Enteric coatings should never render the drug ingredient less available, but this problem may occur. When enteric-coated medication seems to fail or proves less effective than expected, the patient may be excreting the tablets intact.

The absorption of drugs from tablets and capsules is receiving much attention these days. It was discovered that the absorption may vary greatly depending on the manufacturing practices of different firms. For this reason the Food and Drug Administration is paying more and more attention to "bioavailability" in the approval of different medicinal preparations. This concept takes into consideration not only the amount of active drug in a preparation but also the percentage of its absorption. A tablet may be so poorly made that its dissolution and absorption are defective. It has been shown, for example, that digoxin tablets made by different manufacturers may produce quite different blood levels although the amount of the active drug in the tablets is the same. There is every reason to believe that eventually bioavailability data will be available on virtually all drugs.

Compressed tablets are usually administered orally. *Molded tablets* or *tablet triturates* are made by mixing the moistened powdered drug with dextrose or lactose and powdered sucrose, so as to make a plastic mass suited for manual pressure into small molds. Later the tablets are ejected and dried. They disintegrate readily when placed in water. Molded tablets are administered orally, sublingually, or sometimes by inserting them in the buccal pouch (between the cheek and the teeth), depending on the type of medication they contain and the purpose for which they are given. Hypodermic tablets are compressed or molded tablets that dissolve completely in water, making a solution suitable for injection. They must be prepared under aseptic conditions and dissolved suitably before administration.

Tablets may "case harden" on storage, which would interfere with absorption, or deteriorate when exposed for long periods of time to high humidity, thereby reducing the availability of the drug. Tablets so affected should be discarded.

Numerous sustained-release products are also available as tablets that may (1) disintegrate into discrete particles in the gastrointestinal tract, (2) gradually erode but retain their original shape while getting smaller, and (3) retain their original shape but give up active drug by leaching.

Troches. Troches or lozenges are flat, round, or rectangular preparations that are held in the mouth until they dissolve, liberating the drug or drugs involved. They usually contain water, sugar, and a mucilage in addition to the drug and are dried in hot air. They temporarily produce a high concentration of the drug in the oral cav-

Figure 4-2 How to use Tubex-sterile needle units. *(Courtesy Wyeth Laboratories, Philadelphia, Pa.)*

How to use
Tubex®-sterile needle units

To load the syringe

1

Grasp barrel of syringe with one hand. With the other hand, pull back firmly on the plunger and swing the entire handle section downward so that it locks at right angle to the barrel.

2

Insert Tubex-sterile needle unit, needle end first, into the barrel. Engage needle ferrule by rotating it clockwise in the threads at front end of syringe.

To administer

Method of administration is the same as with conventional syringe. Remove rubber sheath, introduce needle into patient, aspirate, and inject.

3

Swing plunger back into place and attach end to the threaded shaft of the piston. Hold the syringe barrel with one hand and rotate plunger until both ends of Tubex are fully but lightly engaged. To maintain sterility, leave the rubber sheath in place until just before use. To aspirate before injecting, pull back slightly on the plunger.

To remove the empty Tubex

4

Disengage plunger from piston by rotating counterclockwise and open syringe as in step 1. Do not pull plunger back before disengaging or syringe will jam. Rotate Tubex-sterile needle unit counterclockwise to disengage at front end of syringe, remove from syringe, and discard.

TO ADAPT 2 CC. SYRINGE
TO 1 CC. TUBEX

The 2 cc. syringe can be used for a 1 cc. Tubex. Engage both ends of Tubex and push the slide through so the number "1" appears. After use, the syringe automatically resets itself for 2 cc. Tubex.

ity. They are held in the mouth until entirely dissolved. That which is swallowed may produce systemic effects.

Pills. Pills are mixtures of a drug or drugs with some cohesive material. The mass is molded into globular, oval, or flattened bodies convenient for swallowing. Pills are not suitable for injection. They have been replaced to a great extent by capsules and tablets. Although *pill* is a popular, general term for tablets or capsules, this is a misuse of the term. In fact, very few true pills are on the market today.

Powders. Powders are finely divided solid drugs or mixtures of drugs for internal or external use.

Ampules and vials. Ampules and vials contain powdered or liquid drugs usually intended for injection. *Ampules* are sealed glass containers and usually contain one dose of the drug. *Vials* are glass containers with rubber stoppers and usually contain a number of doses of the drug. The powdered drug must be dissolved in sterile distilled water or in isotonic saline solution before administration.

Disposable syringes. Disposable syringes containing doses of drug preparations have become popular. Various antibiotic preparations are commonly given this way. Another dosage form employs the cartridge type of container, which is fitted into a metal framework and a needle attached, such as Tubex. The cartridge contains the drug that is given by injection and the whole resembles a hypodermic (Figure 4-2).

ADDITIONAL PREPARATIONS

Liniments. Liniments are liquid suspensions or dispersions intended for external application. They are applied to the skin by rubbing. In addition to one or more active ingredients they may contain oil, soap, water, or alcohol. The oil and the soap of liniments adhere to the skin and serve as lubricants while the preparation is being rubbed on. Liniments usually contain an anodyne (to relieve pain) or a rubefacient (to redden the skin). Liniments may temporarily relieve pain and swelling by counterirritation and by improving circulation of blood to the part.

Lotions. Lotions are liquid suspensions or dispersions intended for external application. Lotions usually should be patted on the skin and not applied by rubbing. This is particularly true if the skin is irritated or inflamed. Lotions can be protective, emollient, cooling, cleansing, astringent, or antipruritic, depending on their content. Calamine lotion, U.S.P., B.P., is an example of a lotion that has a soothing effect.

Ointments. Ointments are semisolid preparations of medicinal substances in some type of base such as petrolatum and lanolin that are intended for external application to the skin or mucous membranes. The base helps to keep the medicinal substance in prolonged contact with the skin. Ointments do not wash off readily unless surfactants have been added. A number of other bases can be used in ointments, some of which are miscible with water. Ointments are used for their soothing, astringent, or bacteriostatic effects, depending on the drug or drugs contained in the preparation. Sulfur ointment, U.S.P., B.P., rose water ointment, N.F., and zinc oxide ointment, U.S.P. (zinc ointment, B.P.), are examples.

Ophthalmic ointments are sterile, specially prepared ointments for use in the eye. The ointment base selected must be nonirritating to the eye, must permit free diffusion of the drug throughout the secretions of the eye, and must not alter or destroy the drug that it incorporates. Chloramphenicol ophthalmic ointment, U.S.P., is an example.

Pastes. Pastes are ointment-like preparations suited only for external application. Many of them consist of thick stiff ointments that do not melt at body temperature. They tend to absorb secretions and they soften and penetrate the skin to a lesser extent than do ointments. Zinc oxide paste, U.S.P., and compound zinc paste, B.P., are examples.

Plasters. Plasters are solid preparations that serve as either simple adhesives or counterirritants. When applied to the body the heat softens them and makes them adhere. The base is usually a rubber mixture called rubber plaster. Adhesive tape, U.S.P., and salicylic acid plaster, U.S.P., are two examples.

Suppositories. Suppositories are mixtures of drugs with a firm base that can be molded into

Figure 4-3
Various forms of suppositories: rectal, vaginal, and urethral.

shapes suitable for insertion into a body cavity or orifice. The base may be glycerinated gelatin, a hard soap, cacao butter (cocoa butter), or carbowax (a polymer of ethylene glycol). These substances melt at body temperature and dissolve in the secretions of mucous membranes to produce local or systemic effects. The shapes and sizes are suitable for insertion into the rectum, vagina, or urethra. Urethral suppositories are called *bougies*. Aminophylline suppositories and aspirin suppositories are listed in the U.S.P.

Poultices. Poultices are soft moist preparations, the purpose of which is to supply moist heat to a skin area. If applied too long they cause maceration of the skin. They tend to be regarded as home remedies. There are no poultices listed in the U.S.P.

PHARMACEUTICAL ACCESSORIES

Coloring substances. Coloring substances may be added to medicines to make them more acceptable to patients. Red and green colors seem to be favorites. The coloring agent must be either an official agent or one that has been certified under the Federal Food, Drug, and Cosmetic Act. Amaranth solution, U.S.P., imparts a vivid red color to a preparation such as phenobarbital elixir, U.S.P. Compound amaranth solution is listed in the N.F.

QUESTIONS

For study and review

1 What is meant by the generic name of a drug? How does it differ from a trade name?
2 What is the advantage of labeling drugs with both their generic and trade names?
3 How can you recognize a trademark name when it is used in medical literature?
4 From what source do most of our new drugs come? What advantages do they have from the standpoint of dosage and reliability of effect?
5 Define an active principle and name several.
6 What is meant by a crude drug? Why were so many of the early drugs used in this country as well as in other countries preparations of crude drugs?
7 What are the main differences between alkaloids and glycosides?
8 What seems to be the main role or function of a carbohydrate in the molecular makeup of a glycoside?
9 Name four medicinal preparations that contain alcohol. How would you expect to administer them to patients and why? What general statement could you make about their dosage?
10 What differences exist between compressed and molded tablets that are of significance to a nurse?
11 What is meant by an enteric-coated tablet? What is the purpose of the enteric coating?
12 What purpose is served by sustained-release dosage forms of drugs?

REFERENCES

Campbell, J. A., and Morrison, A. B.: Oral prolonged medication, J.A.M.A. **181**:102, 1962.

Crossland, J.: Lewis's pharmacology, Baltimore, 1970, The Williams & Wilkins Co.

DiPalma, J. R., editor: Drill's pharmacology in medicine, ed. 4, New York, 1971, McGraw-Hill Book Company.

Friend, D. G.: One drug—one name, Clin. Pharmacol. Therap. **6:**689, 1965.

Grollman, A., and Grollman, E. F.: Pharmacology and therapeutics, ed. 7, Philadelphia, 1970, Lea & Febiger.

Hallister, L. E.: Studies of delayed action medication, New Eng. J. Med. **266:**281, 1962.

Jerome, J. B.: Selecting generic names for drugs, J. New Drugs **2:**276, 1962.

Martin, E., editor: Remington's pharmaceutical sciences, ed. 14, Easton, Pa., 1970, Mack Printing Company.

Official drug compendia

British Pharmacopoeia, ed. 10, London, 1968, The Pharmaceutical Press.

The National Formulary, ed. 14, Easton, Pa., 1975, Mack Printing Company.

The Pharmacopeia of the United States of America, ed. 18, Easton, Pa., 1970, Mack Printing Company.

CHAPTER 5

Weights and measures

Brief history of weights and measures
Metric system
Apothecaries' system
Conversion from one system to another
Household measures
The preparation of solutions and doses

BRIEF HISTORY OF WEIGHTS AND MEASURES

The several systems of weights and measures used today have developed over a long period of time and in different cultures. Many measures used by English-speaking nations grew out of Egyptian, Roman, and Greek measures based on the human hand, finger, or foot. The Egyptian cubit was the distance from the elbow to the tip of the middle finger. The Roman mile was 1000 paces, a pace being 5 Roman feet. King Henry I of England is said to have made the yard (cloth yard) the distance from his nose to his outstretched thumb. The drachma (dram) is from the Greek and meant a handful.* The hand meant the breadth of the palm. These were early attempts to define a symbol to represent a definite quantity of a substance.

Measures based on common objects or parts of the body were highly variable although useful to meet the simple needs of people at one time. The ruling monarch of a country frequently decided on the amount of a measure in order that some conformity could prevail in his country.

The King of England adopted the avoirdupois pound as an outgrowth of trade relations with France where the pound was 16 ounces. This resulted in two weights for pounds in England and later in the United States, the apothecaries' pound (12 ounces) and the avoirdupois pound (16 ounces).

Britons and Americans are not referring to the same measurement when they speak of gallons or quarts. Both the British gallon and the American gallon contain 4 quarts. However, the American quart contains 32 ounces and the British quart contains 40 ounces. Today there are various standards established by state or national authority as a rule for the measure of quantity. Late in the nineteenth century the International Bureau of Weights and Measures was founded and prepared international standards in the metric system.

The metric system is the system prescribed by law in most European countries, and Canada is now converting to the metric system. Several legislative attempts have been made to render its use obligatory in the United States also. It is now used in the sciences, in weighing foreign mail, in weighing at the mints, and in other government departments, particularly the medical departments of the Army and Navy.

---

* This ancient Greek unit of measurement had several values.

43

There are two systems of weighing and measuring drugs in the United States—the metric system and the apothecaries' system. There is a growing tendency to use the metric system entirely, but until such time that change to the metric system is complete, nurses will need to know something about both. Moreover, since these systems are often used interchangeably, nurses need to be able to convert from one system to the other. In the home, patients or nurses may use teaspoons or other common household containers to measure drugs. Therefore, nurses also need to know the approximate equivalents for the household system.

METRIC SYSTEM

The metric system of weights and measures was invented by the French in the latter part of the eighteenth century. For this purpose a committee of the Academy of Sciences, consisting of five men, was appointed under authority of the government. They had two preconceived ideas regarding the proposed system: (1) that the standards should be based upon some unalterable object in nature, so that the correctness of the measures accepted as models might be redetermined, if necessary, and (2) that the system should employ the decimal scale. Of the three natural linear bases proposed—namely, the length of a second's pendulum, a fourth of the earth's circumference measured along the equator, and a fourth of the earth's circumference measured across the poles—the committee recommended the last, ten-millionth of which should be the standard unit of linear measure. They calculated the distance from the equator to the North Pole from surveys made along the meridian that passes through Paris, and this distance, divided by 10 million, was chosen as the unit of length, the meter. The meter is the fundamental unit of the metric system. A bar of platinum of this length was constructed and deposited in the French Archives to serve as a model for the meter measures intended for actual use. There was also constructed and deposited in the Archives a weight of platinum of such size as to counterpoise in vacuo 1 cubic decimeter of water at its greatest density. This weight constituted the fundamental standard of mass and was to serve as the model for the kilogram weights (and indirectly for the other weights) intended for actual use.

The metric standards were adopted in France in 1799. In 1875 the International Metric Convention met in Paris. Seventeen countries including the United States participated. This convention resulted in the foundation of the International Bureau of Weights and Measures, whose first work was the preparation of an international standard meter bar and an international standard kilogram weight with duplicates for each of the countries that had contributed to the support of the bureau. For the international standard meter, a bar of platinum iridium was selected and two lines were drawn on its surface at a distance from each other equal to 1 meter measured when the bar was at the temperature of melting ice (0° C.). The distance between these lines is the official unit of the metric system. The international standards were placed in the custody of the International Bureau of Weights and Measures near Paris. The duplicates were distributed by lot, the United States drawing meters No. 21 and No. 27 and kilograms No. 4 and No. 20. Meter No. 27 and kilogram No. 20 were selected as our national standards and are carefully preserved in the United States Bureau of Standards at Washington, D.C. Meter No. 21 and kilogram No. 4 are used as working standards.

METRIC UNITS OF MEASUREMENT

Metric units of measurement are the meter, the liter, and the gram. The *meter* is the unit for linear measurement, the *liter* for capacity or volume, and the *gram* for weight.

The metric system is a decimal system; the basic unit can be divided into 10, 100, or 1000 parts, or the basic unit may be multiplied by 10, 100, or 1000 to form secondary units that differ from each other by 10 or some multiple of 10. The names of the secondary units are formed by joining Greek and Latin prefixes to the names of the primary unit. Subdivisions of the basic unit can be made by moving the decimal point to the left, and multiples of the basic unit are indicated by moving the decimal point to the right.

The prefixes used to designate subdivisions of the unit are deci- (0.1), centi- (0.01), and milli- (0.001) and are from the Latin; those used to designate multiples are deka- (10), hecto- (100), and kilo- (1000) and are from the Greek. The subdivisions of a meter are known as decimeters, centimeters, and millimeters; and the multiples of the meter are known as dekameters, hecto- meters, and kilometers. The following diagram compares the subdivisions or denominations of the metric system with the scheme of the decimal system.

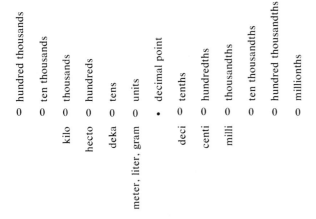

Meter. The meter is the unit from which the other metric units were derived (Table 5-1). The meter is comparable to the yard although it is several inches longer (39.37 inches).

The first part of Table 5-1 is most frequently used and is similar to the system of money used in the United States: one dollar = 10 dimes, or 100 cents, or 1000 mills.

Centimeters and millimeters are the chief lin- ear measures used in hospital work. Measure- ment of the size of body organs is made in centi- meters and millimeters, and students will recall that the sphygmomanometer used in measuring blood pressure is calibrated in millimeters. Mi- crons, which are one millionth of a meter, are used in measuring minute distances, such as the length or size of bacteria. There are approxi- mately 2.5 centimeters (25 millimeters) in 1 inch.

Liter. The liter is the unit of capacity. The con- tents of a cube whose sides measure 1 decimeter (10 centimeters) constitute the unit of capacity. It was originally intended that the liter and the cubic decimeter should be exactly the same. Be- cause of the difficulty of measurement, however, the liter is found to be 1.000028 cubic deci- meters.

The liter, therefore, is 28 parts per 1,000,000 larger than intended. The difference is so small that it is of no importance except in determi- nations of great precision. The weight of a liter of water at 4° C. is 1 kilogram.

If the liter contained exactly 1000 cc., the cubic centimeter and the milliliter would be ex- actly the same volume and each the one thou- sandth part of the liter. However, since the liter in common use is 1000.028 cc., the cubic centi- meter is less than the milliliter by 0.000028 cc. *In practice the cubic centimeter and the milliliter are considered equal.*

Fractional parts of a liter are usually ex- pressed in milliliters or cubic centimeters. For example, 0.6 L. would be expressed as 600 ml. or 600 cc. Multiples of a liter are similarly ex- pressed: 2.4 L. would be 2400 ml. or cc.

Gram. The gram is the metric unit of weight that is used in weighing drugs and various phar- maceutical preparations. Originally, the unit of

Table 5-1 Metric linear measurement

1 meter =	10 decimeters (dm.)
=	100 centimeters (cm.)
=	1000 millimeters (mm.)
10 meters =	1 dekameter (Dm.) — *microns i millionth of meter*
100 meters =	1 hectometer (Hm.)
1000 meters =	1 kilometer (Km.)
	(approx. ⅝ mile)

Table 5-2 Weight

1 gram = (Gm.)	10 decigrams (dg.)
=	100 centigrams (cg.)
=	1000 milligrams (mg.)
=	1,000,000 micrograms (μg.)
10 grams =	1 dekagram (Dg.)
100 grams =	1 hectogram (Hg.)
1000 grams =	1 kilogram (Kg.)

Figure 5-1

Metric measures suited to the measurement of volume. Both containers are marked in milliliters. The cylindrical graduate on the left is marked so that small amounts can be measured more accurately than with the graduate on the right.

measurement of weight was the kilogram, but this proved too large to meet the practical needs of the pharmacist. The gram is the weight of 1 milliliter of distilled water at 4° C. Either Gm. or g. is an acceptable abbreviation for gram.*

In studying Table 5-2 it becomes apparent that 1 decigram is 10 times greater than a centigram and 100 times greater than a milligram. To change decigrams to centigrams one would therefore multiply by 10; to change decigrams to milligrams one would multiply by 100. To change milligrams to centigrams one would divide by 10; to change milligrams to decigrams one would divide by 100; and to change milligrams to grams one would divide by 1000.

In reading a whole number expressing a metric quantity only one unit is used, however large the number, such as 2750 Gm. is read twenty-seven hundred fifty grams, not two kilograms, seven hectograms, five dekagrams; 7500 ml. is read seven thousand five hundred or seventy-five hundred milliliters.

In expressing a fraction of a gram, the terms *decigram* and *centigram* are seldom used. The quantity is expressed in its equivalent grams or milligrams; for example, 6 decigrams, written 0.6 Gm., is called six-tenths gram; 5 centigrams, written 0.05 Gm., is called preferably fifty milligrams. The thousandth part of a gram and multiples or fractions of it are commonly expressed as milligrams; for example, 0.001 Gm. may be expressed as 1 mg.; 0.003 Gm. as 3 mg.; and 0.0005 Gm. as 0.5 mg.; 0.001 mg. is 1 microgram.

*This book uses a capital G (Gm.) to avoid confusion with gr. for grain.

The kilogram is the only multiple of the gram used in medical work. Nurses will observe that this measure is used in weighing patients and in calculation of dosage in terms of kilograms of body weight (1 kilogram = 2.2 pounds avoirdupois weight).

To ensure accuracy in reading, a zero always should be used before the decimal point in writing a fractional part of a metric unit—0.5 Gm., 0.6 ml., or 0.001 L. The misplacement of the period or point may be the cause of serious error. When the abbreviations for gram, milliliter, and cubic centimeter are omitted, it is taken for granted that 1.0 means 1 Gm. when expressing weight or 1 ml. when expressing liquid quantity. When metric abbreviations are used, the numerals are always expressed in Arabic (rather than Roman) numerals and precede the abbreviation—for example, 20 Gm., 50 ml., 250 mg.

The metric system has many advantages, chief of which are as follows: all the standard units of weight and measure bear a simple relation to the fundamental unit, the meter; the prefixes deci-, centi-, milli-, deka-, hecto-, and kilo- have a numerical significance and have other applications in our language that make them readily understood; the uniform decimal scale of relation between the successive units makes the use of the decimal notation possible; and the system is universal.

The early Greeks had an advantage when they described the quantity of a substance as a handful. The person hearing these words could look at his hand and imagine how much it would hold. To use the metric system to accomplish the same purpose today, it is necessary to obtain a mental picture of the quantity represented by the denominations that are a part of the system. The laboratory suggestions in this chapter are designed to help the student develop these concepts.

LABORATORY SUGGESTIONS

1 Gather the following materials for use: glass measures marked in milliliters, gram scales, salt, water, and colored solution of alcohol.
2 Study the gram scale. Balance it and note how the scale is marked to indicate the subdivisions of the gram.

3 Study the various metric measures that can be used to measure liquids. Note the amount of water contained in 4 ml., 30 ml., 180 ml., and 500 ml. Try to build a mental concept of these quantities.
4 Weigh out 3 Gm. of salt and add it to 30 ml. of water; notice how much constitutes each of these amounts. Is the volume of the liquid noticeably changed? Why? How much salt is there in each milliliter of solution?
5 Normal (physiologic) salt solution is made by adding 9 Gm. of sodium chloride to 1000 ml. of water; weigh out the amount of salt needed for 0.5 liter of normal (physiologic) salt solution.
6 Add 15 ml. of alcohol to 30 ml. of water. Is the volume of the liquid increased? How much? Why? What is the ratio strength of the finished solution? How much alcohol would be needed to make 1 liter of solution of the same strength?
7 Add 10 ml. of alcohol to 60 ml. of water. How much alcohol is there in each milliliter of solution?

Before undertaking any arithmetic operations using the metric system of measure, it is necessary to recall a few basic rules and definitions.

A number such as 2 or 7 taken by itself, without reference to anything concrete, is called an *abstract* or *pure* number. A number that designates a quantity of objects or units of measure, such as 2 grams or 7 milligrams, is called a *concrete* or *denominate* number.

Four basic rules govern the arithmetic operations used here.

1 Numbers of different denominations have no numerical connection with each other and cannot be used together in any arithmetic operation.
2 A denominate number may be added or subtracted from any other number of the same denomination.

> Example: 2 grams + 7 grams = 9 grams

3 A denominate number may be multiplied or divided only by a pure number.

> Example: 2 × 7 = 14

NOTE: The result of any of these operations is always a number of the same denomination.

4 When both sides of an equation are multiplied or divided by the same pure number, the resulting products or quotients are equal.

> Example: 1 gram = 1000 milligrams
> 10 × 1 gram = 1000 milligrams × 10
> 10 grams = 10,000 milligrams

Conversion is the process that enables one to describe the same quantity of a substance in different terms. Tables have been developed to show relationships among subdivisions within a system or between systems. Entries from these tables provide the starting point for the conversion process. The arithmetic operation is multiplication or division of both sides of the equation by the same pure or abstract number:

1 To express 4.75 Gm. in terms of milligrams: 1 Gm. = 1000 mg. (Table 5-2, p. 45)
The pure number selected is 4.75; the operation selected is multiplication.

$$4.75 \times 1 \text{ Gm.} = 1000 \text{ mg.} \times 4.75$$
$$4.75 \text{ Gm.} = 4750 \text{ mg.}$$

2 To express 568 cm. in terms of meters: 1 meter = 100 centimeters (Table 5-1, p. 45)
a. The pure number selected is 100; the operation selected is division.

$$1 \text{ M.} \div 100 = 100 \text{ cm.} \div 100$$
$$0.01 \text{ M.} = 1 \text{ cm.}$$

b. The pure number selected is 568; the operation selected is multiplication.

$$568 \times 0.01 \text{ M.} = 1 \text{ cm.} \times 568$$
$$5.68 \text{ M.} = 568 \text{ cm.}$$

EXERCISES

Metric system

1 a. What part of a gram is a decigram?
b. What part of a gram is a milligram?
c. What part of a gram is a centigram?
2 a. How many dekagrams are there in a kilogram?
b. How many centigrams are there in a kilogram?
c. How many centigrams are there in a hectogram?
3 In the calculation of the following problems, state the process of reasoning:
a. Convert the following to milligrams: 3 Gm., 7 dg., 4 cg., 0.5 Gm.
b. Add this series of measurements and express the sum in grams: 200 mg., 40 cg., 15 dg., 2 Gm.
c. Add this series of measurements and express the sum in centigrams: 250 mg., 1.3 Gm., 12 dg., 0.7 cg.
d. Add this series of measurements and express the sum in milligrams: 0.02 Gm., 0.13 cg., 0.125 Gm., 0.08 dg.
4 A preparation of medicine is made by dissolving 30 mg. of drug in 200 ml. of water. If 3 mg. is the dose of drug desired, how many milliliters must be given for each dose?
5 If the dose of cascara sagrada is 4 ml., how many doses will there be in 0.2 liter?

6 If 0.2 Gm. of drug is added to 200 ml. of water, how many milligrams of drug are there in each milliliter of solution?
7 If 20 ml. of alcohol is added to 80 ml. of water to make a certain desired strength of solution, how much alcohol would be required to make a liter of solution?

APOTHECARIES' SYSTEM

The apothecaries' system of weights and measures was a part of the system used in England at the time of colonization in the United States. It has now been superseded by the imperial system, which is official in Great Britain.*

The basic unit of weight in the apothecaries' system is the grain, which originally meant a grain of wheat. The other units of weight are the scruple, the dram, the ounce, and the pound. The scruple is seldom used and therefore is not included in Table 5-3. Quantities less than 1 dram are usually expressed in grains. The abbreviation lb. is for libra, the Latin word meaning pound.

The unit of fluid measure is a minim (Table 5-4), which is approximately the quantity of water that would weigh a grain. The symbol O is the abbreviation of the Latin word *octarius* meaning an eighth (eighth of a gallon), and the letter C is the abbreviation for the Latin word *congius*, meaning a vessel holding a gallon.

When symbols are used, the quantity is usually expressed in Roman numerals, which are placed after the symbols: three grains is written gr. iii; five drams, ℨ v; ten ounces, ℥ x. Fractions are usually expressed in Arabic numerals; gr. $\frac{1}{4}$, gr. $\frac{1}{8}$, gr. $\frac{1}{2}$; the symbol "ss" may be used for $\frac{1}{2}$ (ss = *semis*, Latin for one-half); thus, two and one-half grains, gr. iiss. † However, it is ac-

---

* The imperial system of weights and measures as well as the metric system is used in the *British Pharmacopoeia* and the *Canadian Formulary*. The imperial system is being replaced by the metric system.

1 pound (lb.)	= 16 ounces = 7000 grains
1 ounce (℥)	= 437½ grains
1 dram (ℨ)	= 60 grains (unofficial)—officially 1 grain is 1/7000 part of a pound
1 pint (O)	= 20 fluidounces (f℥)
1 fluidounce (f℥)	= 8 fluidrams (fℨ)
1 fluidram (fℨ)	= 60 minims (min.)

† When the numeral for "one" is used, a dot is frequently placed over it to avoid confusion with the Roman numeral L, meaning 50, which is sometimes written as a small letter.

Figure 5-2
Disposable medicine glasses made of plastic material. Household, apothecaries', and metric measures are indicated.

Table 5-3 Weight

60 grains	= 1 dram (ℨ)
480 grains or 8 drams	= 1 ounce (℥)
12 ounces	= 1 pound (lb.)

Table 5-4 Fluid measure

60 minims (♏)	= 1 fluidram (fℨ)
8 fluidrams or 480 minims	= 1 fluidounce (f℥)
16 fluidounces	= 1 pint (pt. or O)
2 pints	= 1 quart (qt.)
4 quarts	= 1 gallon (C)

ceptable to use either Roman or Arabic numerals with the sign for minim and with the abbreviations for grains and grams (for example, gr. viiss or $7^{1}/_{2}$ gr.).

The minim (♏) is often assumed to be identical with the drop (gtt. from the Latin word *gutta*), but such measurement is inaccurate. A minim of water or of an aqueous solution is approximately equal to a drop; a minim of an alcoholic solution, such as digitalis tincture, equals approximately 2 drops; a minim of ether contains 3 drops; and a minim of chloroform equals approximately 4 drops. A minim of a gummy substance is less than a drop. Minims should always be measured when minims are ordered, and a minim glass or minim pipet should be used to measure accurately. When drops are ordered, they may be measured by means of a medicine dropper.

EXERCISES

Apothecaries' system

1 Read the following:
  a. ℨ iiss
  b. gr. xiii
  c. ℥ ss
  d. ℨ xviii
  e. ♏ viii
  f. gr. xxx
  g. ℨ iv
  h. ℥ vi
  i. ♏ xxiv
  j. O v

2 Write the following expressions as they should be written in a prescription: 15 minims, 3 fluidrams, 7 fluidounces, 1 pint, $2^{1}/_{2}$ drams, 20 grains, 12 minims, 5 ounces, $^{1}/_{2}$ ounce.

3 How many grains are there in:
  a. ℨ vi
  b. ℥ iss
  c. ℨ ii
  d. ℥ vi
  e. lb. i
  f. ℥ ss
  g. ℨ iii
  h. ℨ ix

4 How many minims are there in:
  a. f℥ ss
  b. fℨ ss
  c. fℨ iv
  d. f℥ ii
  e. O ss
  f. f℥ viii
  g. f℥ i
  h. f℥ iiss

5 a. What part of a dram is gr. xl, gr. xiii, gr. xv, gr. xx, gr. i?
  b. What part of an ounce is gr. xxx, ℨ ss, ℨ iv, ℨ vi, gr. lx?
  c. What part of a fluidram is ♏ x, ♏ xv, ♏ xlv, ♏ xxx, ♏ i?
  d. What part of a fluidounce is fℨ vi, fℨ iv, fℨ ii, fℨ ss?

6 Add the following amounts and express the sum in fluidounces: O ss, ♏ 160, f℥ x, ♏ 200.

7 A physician's prescription calls for gr. xxiv of a drug. This would be what part of an ounce?

8 One dose contains gr. xv of a drug; how many drams of this drug would be required to make up sixty doses?

9 How much morphine sulfate would be required to make up 2 fluidounces of solution if every 20 minims of the solution is to contain gr. $^{1}/_{4}$?

10 If a pint of solution contains ℨ ii of drug, how many grains in each fluidounce of solution?

LABORATORY SUGGESTIONS

1 Gather the following materials for use: apothecaries' scales and measures, colored solution of alcohol, and salt.
2 With a minim measure determine the number of minims in:
   a. 1 fluidram
   b. 2 fluidounces
   c. 1 fluidounce
      Why would a minim glass be unsuitable to measure out several fluidounces of a solution?
   d. Observe the various apothecaries' measures set out for your use. Note the amount of their content. Measure out 1 fluidram, 1 fluidounce, 60 minims, 1 pint, and so on. Try to form a mental picture of various quantities and how they compare with each other; for example, compare the amount of water in 15 minims with the amount in 1 fluidram or 1 fluidounce. Compare the weight of 1 grain with 15 grains, with 1 ounce, and with 1 pound.
3 With a fluidram measure determine how many fluidrams there are in 1 fluidounce; in 1 pint. What kind of an apothecaries' measure would you select to measure out ½ pint of a solution if you had the following to choose from: minim glass, fluidram measure, fluidounce measure? Why?
4 Weigh out 60 grains of salt on an apothecaries' scale. This corresponds with how many drams?
5 Dissolve ʒ i of salt in fʒ iv of water. How many grains of salt are there in each fluidounce of solution? In each fluidram?
6 Dissolve gr. xxx of salt in fʒ iiss of water. How many grains of salt would there be in ♏ 40 of the solution?
7 Using the colored solution of alcohol, add 1 fluidram of alcohol to 4 fluidrams of water. What part of the solution will be alcohol? How many minims of alcohol would there be in ♏ 60 of the solution?
8 Add fʒ ii of alcohol to fʒ iv of water. What part of the solution is alcohol? How many minims of alcohol in each fluidram of solution?

CONVERSION FROM ONE SYSTEM TO ANOTHER

The metric system and the apothecaries' system have different size units and subdivisions. The denominations of one system are incompatible with the denominations of the other. Thus, the tables that list the measurement of a denomination of one system in terms of another system are clearly labeled approximate equivalents and should be interpreted in that way.

Since nurses have occasion to use both the apothecaries' and the metric systems in computing dosage of drugs to be given orally or parenterally as well as in preparing solutions for external use, it is essential that they know how to use these systems interchangeably.

Although these systems are used interchangeably, greater emphasis is being placed on the metric system as its convenience is increasingly appreciated. Nevertheless, it is advisable for nurses to learn the tables of weights and measurements and at least some of the approximate equivalents as thoroughly as they learned the multiplication tables. However, the nurse should rely neither on memory alone nor on tables alone. Conversion tables should be available in every medication locker as a means of checking, not as a substitute for the nurse's calculations.

Although it is well to know how to calculate the change from one system to the other, often the accepted equivalent is not the same as the

Table 5-5 Commonly used approximate equivalents

Weight		Volume	
1 Gm.	= 15 grains	1 ml.	= 15 minims
0.06 Gm.	= 1 grain	1 cc.	= 15 minims
4 Gm.	= 1 dram	0.06 ml.	= 1 minim
30 Gm.	= 1 ounce	4 ml.	= 1 fluidram
1 Kg.*	= 2.2 pounds (imperial or avoirdupois)	30 ml.	= 1 fluidounce
		500 ml.	= 1 pint
		1000 ml. (1 L.) =	1 quart

* 1 Kg. is equivalent to 2.6 apothecaries' pounds; however, the nurse has little or no occasion to use the apothecaries' pound.

Figure 5-3
Apothecaries' measures.

Dram — Minim

Ounce — Dram

Minim glass

Fluidounce measure

Table 5-6 Additional approximate equivalents (weight)

gr. xv	= 1.0	Gm.	=	1000	mg.
gr. x	= 0.6	Gm.	=	600	mg.
gr. viiss	= 0.5	Gm.	=	500	mg.
gr. v	= 0.3	Gm.	=	300	mg.
gr. iii	= 0.2	Gm.	=	200	mg.
gr. $1^{1}/_{2}$	= 0.1	Gm.	=	100	mg.
gr. 1	= 0.06	Gm.	=	60	mg.
gr. $^{3}/_{4}$	= 0.05	Gm.	=	50	mg.
gr. $^{1}/_{2}$	= 0.03	Gm.	=	30	mg.
gr. $^{1}/_{4}$	= 0.015	Gm.	=	15	mg.
gr. $^{1}/_{6}$	= 0.010	Gm.	=	10	mg.
gr. $^{1}/_{8}$	= 0.008	Gm.	=	8	mg.
gr. $^{1}/_{12}$	= 0.005	Gm.	=	5	mg.
gr. $^{1}/_{15}$	= 0.004	Gm.	=	4	mg.
gr. $^{1}/_{20}$	= 0.0032	Gm.	=	3	mg.
gr. $^{1}/_{30}$	= 0.0022	Gm.	=	2	mg.
gr. $^{1}/_{40}$	= 0.0015	Gm.	=	1.5	mg.
gr. $^{1}/_{50}$	= 0.0012	Gm.	=	1.2	mg.
gr. $^{1}/_{60}$	= 0.001	Gm.	=	1	mg.
gr. $^{1}/_{100}$	= 0.0006	Gm.	=	0.6	mg.
gr. $^{1}/_{120}$	= 0.0005	Gm.	=	0.5	mg.
gr. $^{1}/_{150}$	= 0.0004	Gm.	=	0.4	mg.
gr. $^{1}/_{200}$	= 0.0003	Gm.	=	0.3	mg.
gr. $^{1}/_{300}$	= 0.0002	Gm.	=	0.2	mg.
gr. $^{1}/_{600}$	= 0.0001	Gm.	=	0.1	mg.

exact amount in the other system, and confusion results. For the most part, exact equivalents are used only by the pharmacist in compounding prescriptions or in converting a pharmaceutical formula from one system to the other. When dosage forms such as tablets and capsules are prescribed in the metric system, the nurse may administer the approximate apothecaries' equivalent and vice versa. If the nurse knows that 1 mg. = gr. $^{1}/_{60}$, the desired equivalent, can be easily calculated.

To express 0.2 mg. in terms of grains: gr. $^{1}/_{60}$ = 1 mg. (Table 5-6). The pure or abstract number selected is 0.2; the operation selected is multiplication.

$$0.2 \text{ (or } ^{2}/_{10}) \times \text{gr. } ^{1}/_{60} = 1 \text{ mg.} \times 0.2$$
$$\text{gr. } ^{1}/_{300} = 0.2 \text{ mg.}$$

The approximate equivalents (Table 5-5) are used in *The Pharmacopeia of the United States of America* and *The National Formulary*, and they have the approval of the F.D.A.

It is important to know how to change from one system to the other in the event that one forgets the corresponding equivalent or that no table with the desired equivalent is available. It must be remembered, of course, that 1 gram is the equivalent of 15 grains and that 1 milliliter is the equivalent of 15 minims. One gram (1 Gm.) divided by 15 is 0.06 Gm., the equivalent of 1 grain, and 0.06 milliliter is the equivalent of 1 minim.

EXERCISES

Conversion from one system to another

Indicate the process whereby you arrive at an answer.

1 Convert the following to their apothecary equivalents:

a. 30 Gm.	**h.** 0.1 Gm.	**o.** 15 ml.
b. 4 Gm.	**i.** 0.03 Gm.	**p.** 15 mg.
c. 4 ml.	**j.** 0.010 Gm.	**q.** 10 mg.
d. 1 ml.	**k.** 500 ml.	**r.** 100 mg.
e. 45 Gm.	**l.** 1000 ml.	**s.** 0.1 mg.
f. 0.6 ml.	**m.** 250 ml.	**t.** 30 mg.
g. 0.6 Gm.	**n.** 120 ml.	

2 Change to metric equivalents:

a. ʒ i	**h.** gr. iss	**o.** gr. $^1/_8$
b. ʒ iv	**i.** gr. $^1/_6$	**p.** gr. v
c. ℥ ii	**j.** gr. $^1/_4$	**q.** fʒ i
d. O ss	**k.** 6 lb.	**r.** ℳ lx
e. C i	**l.** 3 lb.	**s.** f℥ iv
f. ℳ xv	**m.** 35 lb.	**t.** qt. i
g. gr. viiss	**n.** gr. $^1/_{600}$	

3 Without consulting the text, practice giving metric equivalents for:

a. gr. xv	**g.** ℳ x	**m.** gr. $^1/_2$
b. gr. x	**h.** gr. $^1/_6$	**n.** qt. ss
c. v	**i.** qt. i	**o.** O i
d. 11 lb.	**j.** ℳ xv	**p.** gr. viiss
e. gr. iss	**k.** gr. $^1/_{60}$	**q.** gr. $^1/_8$
f. 1 lb.	**l.** ʒ i	**r.** gr. $^1/_{150}$

4 In the same way, give apothecaries' equivalents for:

a. 1.0 Gm.	**j.** 0.1 Gm.
b. 0.3 Gm.	**k.** 500.0 ml.
c. 1 Kg.	**l.** 0.0006 Gm.
d. 1.0 ml.	**m.** 30.0 ml.
e. 1$^1/_2$ ml.	**n.** 0.015 Gm.
f. 0.03 Gm.	**o.** 10 Kg.
g. 4.0 ml.	**p.** 0.065 Gm.
h. 1000 ml.	**q.** 0.008 Gm.
i. 0.5 Gm.	**r.** 250.0 Gm.

5 Change:

a. 3 fluidounces to minims	**g.** 1 liter to fluidounces
b. 1 liter to pints	**h.** 36 drams to grams
c. 6.0 ml. to fluidrams	**i.** 5.0 ml. to minims
d. 75 grains to grams	**j.** 3 pints to milliliters
e. 7.0 Gm. to grains	**k.** 75.0 ml. to fluidounces
f. 40 lb. to Kg.	

6 If the dose of milk of magnesia is 15 ml., how many fluidounces would be necessary to give ten doses?

7 If there are 7$^1/_2$ grains of drug in each 5-ml. ampule of the preparation, how many grams of the drug are there in four ampules?

8 If the dose of a certain medication is 0.5 Gm. and the tablets are marked 7$^1/_2$ gr., how many tablets will be given for each dose? How many tablets will be required for ten doses?

9 If the dose of a medication is 4 ml., how many fluid-ounces would you order from the pharmacy in order to have sixty doses?

10 If a physician orders 15 mg. of a drug and the preparation comes marked "Tablets gr. $^1/_8$," how many tablets or what part of a tablet will you give?

HOUSEHOLD MEASURES

When nursing is done in the home, a graduate for accurate measurement may not be available and some household article may be used to measure, approximately, the amount required. Household measures include glasses, cups, tablespoons, teaspoons, and drops. Pints and quarts are usually found in the home, but they are defined as apothecaries' measures. Household measures are not accurate and their use should be avoided in the administration of medicines. A teaspoon is said to hold a dram, but the average present-day teaspoon often holds 5 ml. or more.* Drops and minims are also said

* An American standard teaspoon has been established by the American Standards Institute as containing approximately 5 ml. and is accepted as such in U.S.P. XIX.

Table 5-7 Approximate equivalents

60 drops (gtt.)	= 1 teaspoonful (t.)
3 teaspoonfuls	= 1 tablespoonful (T.)
2 tablespoonfuls	= 1 fluidounce
6 fluidounces	= 1 teacupful
8 fluidounces	= 1 glassful

Household	Apothecaries'	Metric	
1 drop	1 minim	0.06	ml.
1 teaspoonful	1 fluidram	5 (4)	ml.*
1 tablespoonful	4 fluidrams	15	ml.
2 tablespoonfuls	1 fluidounce	30	ml.
1 teacupful	6 fluidounces	180	ml.
1 glassful	8 fluidounces	240	ml.

*A scant teaspoonful is generally accepted as an equivalent of 4 ml. (cc.) or fʒ i.

to be equivalent, but when the physician orders a certain number of minims of a drug, the dose should be measured in minims. If he orders drops, the dose should be measured with a medicine dropper. The volume of a drop varies with the viscosity of the liquid to be dropped, the diameter of the dropper used, the angle at which the dropper is held, and sometimes the temperature of the solution. Approximate equivalents (Table 5-7) are not absolutely accurate, but they are sufficiently accurate for practical purposes.

EXERCISES

Approximate equivalents

Choose approximate and appropriate equivalents.

1 Using household measures, how would you measure:

a. ℥ i	**f.** ℳ xxx	**k.** 120 ml.
b. f℥ i	**g.** qt. ss	**l.** C ss
c. f℥ iii	**h.** 0.3 ml.	**m.** f℥ iv
d. 30 ml.	**i.** 4 ml.	
e. 1000 ml.	**j.** ℥ ss	

2 Change to the approximate apothecary equivalents:

a. 1 T.	**e.** 1 teacupful	**i.** ½ glassful
b. 2 t.	**f.** 1 glassful	**j.** ½ teacupful
c. ½ t.	**g.** 60 drops	**k.** ½ T.
d. 2 T.	**h.** 4 glassfuls	**l.** 15 drops

3 Give the approximate metric equivalents:

a. 1 teacupful	**g.** 2 T.
b. 1 glassful	**h.** ¼ t.
c. 1 T.	**i.** 20 gtt.
d. 1 t.	**j.** ½ T.
e. 60 gtt.	**k.** 2 teacupfuls
f. ½ t.	**l.** 2 glassfuls

LABORATORY SUGGESTIONS

1 Gather the following materials for use: apothecaries' measures, metric measures, household measures of various sizes and shapes, medicine droppers, water, and oil.

2 Determine the capacity of the household measures provided for you, using apothecaries' and metric measures. Compare the sizes of three or four cups, glasses, teaspoons, and tablespoons. Do you find any discrepancy? What can you say about the reliability of household measures?

3 With a medicine dropper, drop 20 drops of water into a minim glass. How many minims are there? Do the same with a water faucet instead of a medicine dropper. How many minims are there? Under what circumstances would a medicine dropper measure minims accurately?

4 Drop 20 drops of oil into a minim glass. How many minims are there? What factors determine the size of a drop?

THE PREPARATION OF SOLUTIONS AND DOSES
METHODS OF MAKING SOLUTIONS

There are three methods of making solutions. One is on the weight-to-weight basis, commonly designated as W/W. This means that a given part by weight of solute is dissolved in a given number of parts by weight of solvent. This method is used chiefly where a high degree of accuracy is essential, such as in highly technical work.

A second method is the weight-to-volume method, designated W/V, in which a given part by weight of drug (solute) is placed in a graduate and a sufficient amount of solvent is added to make the required amount of solution. This method is commonly used in medicine and pharmacy. Many of the intravenous fluids given to patients, such as the glucose and saline solutions, are prepared on a weight-to-volume basis and are so indicated on the label.

The third method is the volume-to-volume method, in which a liquid solute is added to the liquid solvent and is designated V/V.

The difference in expressing the strength of a solution on a W/V basis or on a V/V basis is very apparent when one considers the difference in weight of two liquids such as alcohol and water. Alcohol weighs considerably less than water so the amount of alcohol in a 50% solution prepared on a weight-to-volume basis would be quite different from that prepared on a volume-to-volume basis.

The strength of solutions is frequently spoken of in terms of molarity or normality. A *normal solution* is one that contains 1 Gm. equivalent weight of solute in each 1000 ml. of solution. An equivalent combining weight is the weight of an element in grams that will combine with 1.008 Gm. of hydrogen or 8 Gm. of oxygen. It is obtained by dividing the atomic weight by the valence. Normal solution of sodium chloride contains 58.454 Gm. of sodium chloride per liter of solution. The atomic weight of sodium is 22.997, and the atomic weight of chlorine is 35.457, making a total of 58.454. Since the valence of both sodium and chlorine is 1, the atomic weight and the equivalent weight of each are the same.

Normal solution of sodium chloride should not be confused with physiologic saline solution, particularly since the physiologic saline solution is sometimes referred to as normal saline. Normal solution of sodium chloride is a 5.8% solution of sodium chloride, whereas physiologic or normal saline is approximately 0.9% strength.

Solutions may be designated as normal (1N), half-normal (0.5N), tenth-normal (0.1N), etc.

A *molar solution* is one that contains a mole (gram molecular weight) of the solute in 1000 ml. of solution. Thus each liter of molar solution of sulfuric acid contains 98.08 Gm. of hydrogen sulfate (H_2SO_4). Since the equivalent weight would be half this amount, a normal solution of sulfuric acid would contain 49.04 Gm. of solute. Solutions containing one tenth of a gram molecular weight of solute in 1 liter of solution are designated as (0.1 M) or M/10.

Solutions are made from pure drugs, tablets, or stock solutions. *Pure drugs* are unadulterated substances in solid or liquid form. They are 100% pure unless otherwise stated. Powders and crystalline substances, such as boric acid, magnesium sulfate, sodium chloride, sodium bicarbonate, and a few liquids, such as cresol, alcohol, and glycerin, are pure drugs.

Tablets containing a definite known quantity of drugs may be used in making solutions. They also save the inconvenience of weighing the pure drug. The tablet is essentially a preparation of pure drug.

Stock solutions are relatively strong solutions from which weaker solutions may be made. It is customary to have stock solutions on hand so that dilution of various strengths may be made without the inconvenience and delay of weighing the pure drug. Examples of stock solutions commonly used are phenol, potassium permanganate, and magnesium sulfate.

Solutions from pure drugs. To prepare a solution of a given strength of a pure drug it is necessary to determine the amount of drug to use to make a given quantity of solution. If ratio and proportion is the method of calculation, the proportion may be expressed as follows: The amount of drug is to the finished solution as the strength in percent* (or equivalent ratio expression):

$$\begin{array}{cccc} \text{(a)} & \text{(b)} & \text{(c)} & \text{(d)} \end{array}$$
Amount of drug : finished solution :: % : 100

In this proportion terms *a* and *b* are concrete or denominate numbers; terms *c* and *d* are abstract or pure numbers. To construct a true proportion terms *a* and *b* must be of the same (or equal) denomination.

Right way

(X) Gm. of drug are to ml. of solution
(X) ml. of drug are to ml. of solution
(X) gr. of drug are to ♏ of solution
(X) f℥ of drug are to f℥ of solution

Wrong way

(X) gr. of drug are to ml. of solution
(X) ♏ of drug are to ml. of solution
(X) ml. of drug are to ♏ of solution
(X) f℥ of drug are to f℥ of solution

In a true proportion the product of the means (terms *b* and *c*) equals the product of the extremes (terms *a* and *d*).

Examples (using the above rule):

1 Prepare 500 ml. of a 5% solution of boric acid. Since no strength of solute is indicated, boric acid crystals or powder are considered 100% pure drug.

X (Gm. of drug) :
500 ml. finished solutions :: 5 : 100
100 X = 2500
X = 25

In any proportion the product of the means equals the product of the extremes.

Proof: 25 × 100 = 2500
5 × 500 = 2500

Substitute the number 25 for X in the original proportion and it reads:

25 Gm. of drug :
500 ml. finished solution :: 5 : 100

---

*The term *percent* and its corresponding sign, %, mean "by the hundred" or "in a hundred." Percent is simply a fraction of such frequent use that its numerator is expressed but its denominator is left understood, for example, 4% or $^4/_{100}$.

Another method that can be used to solve this problem or to prove the answer is as follows:

Five percent means that $^5/_{100}$ of the solution is boric acid. 500 ml. weigh 500 Gm. Hence $^5/_{100}$ × 500 (Gm.) = 25 Gm. It is necessary to use 25 Gm. of pure drug. To prepare the solution, place 25 Gm. of boric acid in a graduate, add enough water to dissolve it, and then add water up to 500 ml.

2 How much drug is needed to make 1 fluidounce of a 1:25 sodium chloride solution?

Amount of drug: finished solution :: specified ratio. Since so small an amount is to be made, it is well to change the fluidounce to minims.

$$X \text{ grains (amount of drugs) :}$$
$$480 \text{ minims finished solution :: } 1 : 25$$
$$25 X = 480$$
$$X = 19.2$$
$$19.2 \text{ grains of drug :}$$
$$480 \text{ minims finished solution :: } 1 : 25$$

Another method of solving the problem is similar to that mentioned under example 1: the ratio 1:25 means that $^1/_{25}$ of the solution is sodium chloride. One fluidounce weighs 480 grains.

$$^1/_{25} \times 480 = 19.2 \text{ gr.}$$

Dissolve 19.2 grains of sodium chloride in a quantity of water so that the total amount of solution measures 1 fluidounce.

3 Prepare a gallon of 1:1000 bichloride of mercury from tablets of $7^1/_2$ gr.

$$X \text{ (Gm.)} : 4000 \text{ (ml.)} :: 1 : 1000$$
$$1000 X = 4000$$
$$X = 4$$
$$4 \text{ Gm.} : 4000 \text{ ml.} :: 1 : 1000$$

Each tablet contains $7^1/_2$ gr. Entry from Table 5-6, p. 51. $7^1/_2$ gr. = 0.5 Gm.

$$1 \text{ tablet} = \text{gr. } 7^1/_2 = 0.5 \text{ Gm.}$$
$$4 \div 0.5 = 8$$
$$8 \times 0.5 \text{ Gm.} = 1 \text{ tablet} \times 8$$
$$4 \text{ Gm.} = 8 \text{ tablets}$$

4 If f℥ 2 of alcohol are added to f℥ 4 of water, what is the percentage strength of the resulting solution? State the strength also as a ratio.

$$\text{Amount of drug : finished solution :: \% : 100}$$
$$2 \text{ (f℥)} : 6 \text{ f℥} :: X : 100$$
$$6 X = 200$$
$$X = 33^1/_2$$

When a liquid drug is added to a given amount of water, the finished solution is the sum of the two. Addition of a dry drug to the water of a solution will not increase the volume appreciably since it will be soluble.

$$33^1/_3\% \text{ means } 33^1/_3 \text{ parts in 100 parts}$$
$$\text{or 1:3 ratio}$$

5 How much water would you add to a pint of pure alcohol to make it an 80% solution?

$$500 \text{ ml. drug: } X \text{ ml.}$$
$$\text{finished solution :: } 80 : 100$$
$$80 X = 50,000$$
$$X = 625$$
$$500 \text{ ml. drug} : 625 \text{ ml.}$$
$$\text{finished solution :: } 80 : 100$$
$$625 \text{ ml.} - 500 \text{ ml.} = 125 \text{ ml. of water}$$

Since the alcohol is a liquid, to determine the amount of water needed the liquid drug must be subtracted from the finished solution.

6 How much potassium permanganate solution 1:100 could you make from fifteen 5-gr. tablets?

Since it is convenient and customary to measure solutions of this type in milliliters, it will be necessary to convert the known available drug to grams.

Entry from Table 5-5, p. 50.

$$1 \text{ Gm.} = 15 \text{ gr.}$$
$$15 \times 5 \text{ gr.} = 75 \text{ gr.}$$
$$5 \times 1 \text{ Gm.} = 15 \text{ gr.} \times 5$$
$$5 \text{ Gm.} = 75 \text{ gr.}$$

$$\text{Amount of drug : finished solution ::}$$
$$\% : 100 \text{ (or ratio of strength)}$$
$$5 \text{ (Gm.)} : X \text{ (ml.)} :: 1 : 100$$
$$X = 500; \text{ therefore 500 ml.}$$
$$\text{of finished solution}$$

EXERCISES

Solutions from pure drugs

1 How much salt would be required to make the following?
   a. 1 gallon of a 0.9% solution
   b. 250 ml. of a 1% solution
   c. O ss of a $^1/_2$% solution
   d. 1 liter of 1:20 solution
2 How much drug would be required to make up the following?
   a. 4 fluidounces of a 2% Lysol solution
   b. 1000 ml. of a 4% vinegar solution
   c. 2 liters of $^1/_5$% soda bicarbonate solution
   d. 1 liter of 5% glucose solution
3 Express the strength of the following in percent:
   a. 200 ml. of solution containing gr. xv of mercuric cyanide
   b. 1 pint of solution containing 50 ml. of glycerin
   c. 1000 ml. of solution containing 4 fluidounces of alcohol
   d. 500 ml. of alcohol added to a liter of water

4 Express the strength of the following in ratio:
  a. 500 ml. of solution containing 20 Gm. of boric acid
  b. 4 fluidounces of solution containing 60 gr. of a drug
  c. 120 ml. of solution containing $1\frac{1}{2}$ fluidrams of a drug
  d. O ss containing 1 ounce of a drug
5 How many tablets would you need for each of the following?
  a. 1 liter of 1:1000 mercuric cyanide, using gr. $7\frac{1}{2}$ tablets
  b. 2 quarts of 1:100 potassium permanganate solution, using gr. 5 tablets
  c. 1 fluidounce of 2% ammonium chloride solution, using gr. 3 tablets
  d. 1 gallon of bichloride of mercury 1:5000, using 0.5 Gm. tablets.
6 How much water would be required:
  a. to prepare a $\frac{1}{2}$% solution from gr. x of soda bicarbonate
  b. to prepare a 40% solution from 200 ml. of pure alcohol
  c. to prepare a 1:10 solution from f℥ iii of glycerin
  d. to prepare a 2% solution from 1 level teaspoon of soda bicarbonate

Solutions from stock solutions. Stock solutions are relatively concentrated solutions that are kept on hand and from which weaker solutions can be made. The problem is always how much stock solution of a given strength is needed to make a certain amount of solution of a lesser strength. The rule is much the same as the one used in the previous lesson. *The amount of drug (stock solution) : the finished solution :: the ratio of strength of the two solutions (lesser to the greater)*

The following are some examples:

1 How would you prepare a quart of a 2% solution of formaldehyde from a stock solution labeled 40%?

$$X \text{ (ml. of stock sol.)} : 1000 \text{ (ml.)} ::$$
$$2 \text{ (\%)} : 40 \text{ (\%)}$$
$$40 X = 2000$$
$$X = 50$$

50 ml. of stock solution : 1000 ml. finished solution :: 2% : 40%

Fifty milliliters of stock solution would be measured in a graduated container and to this amount would be added 950 ml. of water.
2 How would you prepare 2 liters of a 1:2000 potassium permanganate solution from a 1% stock solution?
  In this case, the strength of the stock solution is expressed in percent and the strength of the solution to be made is in terms of a ratio. In

order to be able to compare the strengths, both must be ratios or both must be in percentage.

$$X \text{ (ml. of stock sol.)} : 2000 \text{ (ml.)} ::$$
$$\frac{1}{20} \text{ (\%)} : 1 \text{ (\%)}$$
$$X = 100 \text{ ml. of stock solution}$$

The balance of the 2 liters would be water (1900 ml. water).

EXERCISES

Solutions from stock solutions

1 How much of a 5% solution would be needed to prepare 1 L. of a 2% solution?
2 How much of a 1:5 solution would be needed to prepare 1 pint of a 10% solution?
3 How much water would be needed to prepare 1 gallon of a 3% solution from a 10% solution?
4 How many milliliters of a 20% stock solution would be needed to prepare f℥ ii of a 4% solution?
5 How much water should be added to 50 ml. of a 10% solution to make it a 1:20 solution?
6 How much of a 1:5 stock solution would be needed to prepare 1 gallon of a 1:20 solution?
7 How much of a 25% stock solution would be needed to prepare 10 fluidounces of a 1:25 solution?
8 How much of a $\frac{1}{2}$% solution would be needed to make 20 minims of a $\frac{1}{5}$% solution?
9 How much stock solution 1:10 would be needed to prepare f℥ ivss of a 1:80 solution?
10 How many milliliters would be needed to prepare 5 fluidrams of a 15% solution from a 1:4 solution?
11 How many fluidounces of a 5% glucose solution could be prepared from 2 fluidrams of a 1:4 solution?
12 How many minims of a 1% solution would be needed to prepare f℥ ss of a $\frac{1}{10}$% solution?
13 How much of a 1:2000 solution would be needed to prepare 1 gallon of a 1:10,000 solution?
14 How much of a 12% solution could be made from a fluidounce of a 20% solution?
15 How much stock solution 1:3 would be needed to prepare f℥ v of a 1:5 solution?

Doses from stock solutions. In some hospitals, drugs for parenteral use are kept in solutions of various strengths. The strength is expressed either by percentage or as the number of minims that contain a certain dose, as ♏ x = gr. $\frac{1}{8}$. The problem for the nurse is to determine how many minims or milliliters of the stock solution contain the required dose:

1 How would you give morphine sulfate gr. $\frac{1}{4}$ from a stock solution labeled ♏ 15 contains gr. $\frac{1}{6}$? One half of the proportion describes the relationship between the drug and the solution as it is stated on the label; the other half indicates the relationship between the desired amount of drug and the solution.

gr. $^1/_6$: 15 minims :: gr. $^1/_4$ (desired
dosage) : X minims
$^1/_6$ X = $3^3/_4$
X = $22^1/_2$
gr. $^1/_6$: 15 minims :: gr. $^1/_4$ (desired
dosage) : $22^1/_2$ minims

If the nurse is expected to determine the amount in milliliters (or cubic centimeters), the equation would read:

15 (mg.) : X ml. :: 10 (mg.) : 1 (ml.)
10 X = 15
X = 1.5

2 How would you give atropine sulfate gr. $^1/_{300}$ from a solution containing gr. $^1/_{150}$ per ml.?

gr. $^1/_{150}$: ℥ 15 :: gr. $^1/_{300}$: X (℥)
$^1/_{150}$ X = $^1/_{20}$
X = ℥ $7^1/_2$

EXERCISES

Doses from stock solutions

1 If the bottle of morphine sulfate is labeled 15 mg. = 1 ml., how would you give the following (how many milliliters or what part of a milliliter would you need to give)?
a. gr. $^1/_6$ **c.** gr. $^1/_{12}$
b. gr. $^1/_8$ **d.** gr. $^1/_4$

2 If the solution of Demerol Hydrochloride is labeled 50 mg. = 1 ml., how many milliliters would be required to give the following?
a. 100 mg.   **c.** gr. ss
b. gr. i   **d.** 37.5 mg.

3 If the solution of codeine phosphate is labeled gr. i = 1 ml., how many minims would be required to give the following?
a. 0.03 Gm.   **c.** 60 mg.
b. 0.015 Gm.   **d.** 8 mg.

4 If a solution of atropine sulfate is labeled gr. $^1/_{150}$ = 1 ml., how many milliliters or what part of a milliliter would be needed to give the following?
a. gr. $^1/_{200}$ **c.** gr. $^1/_{100}$
b. gr. $^1/_{300}$ **d.** gr. $^1/_{75}$

5 How would you obtain gr. $^1/_{200}$ of atropine sulfate from bottle of atropine solution marked 0.5 mg. per ml.?

6 How would you obtain 65 mg. of Phenergan from a stock bottle of solution marked 25 mg./cc. Phenergan?

7 How would you obtain gr. $^1/_4$ of morphine sulfate from a solution labeled 1:50?

8 What amount of solution would be necessary if you wished to give gr. $^1/_{150}$ of atropine sulfate and the bottle of atropine solution is marked 0.3 mg./cc.?

Doses from tablets. Potent drugs such as alkaloids and glycosides usually come in tablets containing definite doses. If the dose that the nurse is called upon to give is not the same as that of the tablet, it is necessary to calculate how many tablets or what part of a tablet will contain the required dose.

The drug is found in a solid state called a tablet instead of in solution. For these problems the statement of proportion is adjusted to read: *Amount of drug specified on label : one tablet :: desired amount of drug : tablets required.*

Example:

The physician orders atropine sulfate gr. $^1/_{300}$ to be given hypodermically, the tablets in the medicine cupboard are labeled gr. $^1/_{150}$.

gr. $^1/_{150}$ (drug specified on label) : 1
tablet :: gr. $^1/_{300}$: X tablets
$^1/_{150}$ X = $^1/_{300}$
X = $^1/_2$
gr. $^1/_{150}$: 1 tablet :: gr. $^1/_{300}$: $^1/_2$ tablet

It is important to label the answer of this part of the calculation in terms of a tablet or tablets. But in this instance and in most others in which drugs are given hypodermically, the nurse does not cut the tablet. Since the drug is to be given hypodermically, the tablet gr. $^1/_{150}$ will be dissolved in a suitable number of minims of water and half of the solution will be administered to the patient. The volume of solution given hypodermically is usually between 10 and 20 minims. More than this can make the patient uncomfortable, and less than this increases the margin of error should some of the solution be lost. In this example, 30 would be a good choice of minims in which to dissolve the stock tablet, gr. $^1/_{150}$, because half of 30 minims is 15 minims and the patient will get half of gr. $^1/_{150}$ or gr. $^1/_{300}$. The remaining 15 minims would be discarded.

EXERCISES

Dosage from tablets

1 How would you calculate and prepare the following doses for hypodermic administration?
a. atropine sulfate gr. $^1/_{200}$ from tablets gr. $^1/_{100}$
b. atropine sulfate gr. $^1/_{350}$ from tablets gr. $^1/_{150}$
c. morphine sulfate gr. $^1/_{16}$ from tablets gr. $^1/_6$
d. codeine sulfate gr. $^1/_4$ from tablets gr. $^1/_2$

2 How would you calculate and prepare the following for hypodermic administration?
  a. Dilaudid hydrochloride gr. $^1/_{60}$ from tablets gr. $^1/_{30}$
  b. morphine sulfate 15 mg. from tablets gr. $^1/_6$
  c. codeine sulfate 60 mg. from tablets gr. $^1/_4$
  d. morphine sulfate 0.01 Gm. from tablets gr. $^1/_8$

3 How would you prepare gr. 3 of a drug from a gr. 5 tablet? How would you expect to administer it?

Weights and measures

1 Change to appropriate metric equivalents:
  a. f℥ iv   **e.** C ii   **i.** gr. $7^1/_2$
  b. ℥ ii   **f.** 2.2 lb.   **j.** f℥ ii
  c. ℳ xv   **g.** gr. $^1/_8$
  d. $^1/_2$ cup   **h.** gr. $^1/_{120}$

2 Change to appropriate apothecaries' equivalents:
  a. 30 Gm.   **e.** 0.2 mg.   **i.** 15 gtt.
  b. 0.5 Gm.   **f.** 1 cup   **j.** 500 ml.
  c. 1 L.   **g.** 1 T.
  d. 30 mg.   **h.** 1 t.

3 Change to appropriate household equivalents:
  a. 4 Gm.   **e.** f℥ i   **i.** O ii
  b. 30 ml.   **f.** ℳ xxx   **j.** 1 L.
  c. 1 quart   **g.** ℥ iv
  d. f℥ i   **h.** gr. LX

For the following problems, state the rule by which you solve the problem, indicate the equation you use, and label all answers. Additional information may be indicated in some instances.

4 The bottle of streptomycin is labeled 1 Gm. = 2.5 ml. How much solution will contain 350 mg.?

5 How many gr. $7^1/_2$ tablets of salt would you need to make 2 L. of 1:100 solution?

6 A vial of powdered polymyxin B is labeled 50 mg. or 500,000 units. How would you prepare a solution so that you could administer doses of 300,000 units?

7 How would you prepare a gallon of 1:2000 solution from a stock solution labeled $^1/_{10}$%?

8 If sodium pentothal solution is made by adding 400 ml. of distilled water to 10 Gm. of drug, what is the percentage strength of the solution? The ratio of strength?

9 If 4 fluidrams of drug are added to 4 fluidounces of water, what is the strength of the resulting solution? Express the strength also as a ratio.

10 How much water would you add to a pint of 95% alcohol to make a 70% solution?

11 How much salt (sodium chloride) would be required to make a quart of physiologic saline solution (0.9%)?

12 If you have on hand tablets of morphine gr. $^1/_6$ and the doctor orders gr. $^1/_8$, how would you prepare the dose?

13 The vial of kanamycin is labeled 0.25 Gm./ml. You are to give 15 mg. of drug for each kilogram the patient weighs. The patient weighs 11 lb. How large a dose is required?

14 Change to appropriate metric equivalents:
  a. f℥ i   **e.** 2 T.   **j.** $^3/_4$ cup
  b. 12 lb.   **f.** gr. $^1/_{600}$ **j.** 1 t.
  c. C ss   **g.** gr. x
  d. O ii   **h.** 30 lb.

15 Change to appropriate apothecaries' equivalents:
  a. 250 ml.   **e.** 8.4 Kg.   **i.** 54.5 Kg.
  b. 1 mg.   **f.** 300 mg.   **j.** 0.3 Gm.
  c. 10 mg.   **g.** 10 gtt.
  d. 30 ml.   **h.** 8 mg.

16 Change to appropriate household equivalents:
  a. 80 ml.   **e.** ℳ xxx   **i.** 0.5 L.
  b. 45 ml.   **f.** 120 ml.   **j.** O i
  c. f℥ iv   **g.** 6 ml.
  d. f℥ vi   **h.** 45 Gm.

For the following problems, state the rule by which you plan to solve each problem, state the equation, and label all answers.

1 How would you prepare a gallon of 1:2000 solution from a stock solution labeled $^1/_5$%?

2 How would you make 2 L. of 1:2000 solution from tablets containing gr. $7^1/_2$ of drug in each tablet?

3 How much water is needed to make a 70% solution from a pint of pure alcohol?

4 How much soda bicarbonate is needed to make $1^1/_2$ L. of 2% solution?

5 If a physician ordered 2 Gm. of drug to be given in four equally divided doses and the drug is available in 250-mg. capsules, how many capsules would you give per dose?

6 How much water would you add to a pint of 95% alcohol to make a 50% solution?

7 If the container of Demerol Hydrochloride solution reads 50 mg. per milliliter (cubic centimeter), how many minims would be required to give gr. iss?

8 If a bottle of codeine sulfate solution is labeled 60 mg. per milliliter (cubic centimeter), how many minims would you need to give gr. $^1/_4$?

9 How would you prepare 2 quarts of a 2% vinegar douche for a patient?

10 If a fluidounce of glycerin is added to 120 ml. of water, what is the strength of the solution?

11 How would you prepare $1^1/_2$ quarts of a physiologic saline solution to be used for a throat irrigation?

12 How much water is needed to make a $^1/_{10}$% solution from gr. 2 of a drug?

QUESTIONS

For study and review

1 Explain how you would prepare 1 L. of a 5% solution from a stock solution labeled 12%.

2 Explain how you would prepare 1 L. of 1:1000 solution of Zephiran Chloride using the 17% concentrate solution.

3 How much water would you need to add to 120 ml. of 17% Zephiran Chloride to obtain a 1:5000 solution?

4 How would you give gr. i of sodium phenobarbital from a tablet containing 0.12 Gm.?

5 A 2-ml. ampule of caffeine with sodium benzoate contains gr. $7\frac{1}{2}$ of drug; how much would be necessary to give gr. 5?

6 Explain how you would give morphine sulfate gr. $\frac{1}{64}$ from tablet gr. $\frac{1}{4}$.

7 What is the ratio of strength of a solution in which 10 fluidounces contain 2 drams of drug? What is the percentage strength?

8 How much salt is needed to make 2 quarts of physiologic saline solution?

9 If ♏ xx of solution contain gr. $\frac{1}{4}$ of a drug, how much of the solution would you use to give gr. $\frac{1}{6}$?

10 How would you prepare 1500 ml. of a 7% solution, using gr. 5 tablets?

11 How would you give atropine gr. $\frac{1}{200}$ from a bottle marked 0.5 mg. per ml.?

12 If 2 fluidounces of alcohol are added to a liter of water, what is the percentage strength of solution? What part of the total solution is alcohol?

13 How would you prepare a dosage of 0.02 mg. of digoxin to be given intramuscularly to a child, if the ampule of digoxin (Lanoxin) is labeled 0.5 mg. in 2 ml.?

14 If a physician orders 10 mg. of morphine sulfate and the bottle is labeled gr. $\frac{1}{4}$ ml., how many minims will you give?

15 How would you prepare 750 ml. of half-strength magnesium and sodium citrate solution (Suby-Albright solution) from full-strength stock solution?

16 How much 1:1000 solution could be made from ten gr. $7\frac{1}{2}$ tablets of a drug?

CHAPTER 6

Administration of medicines

Major channels of administration
Orders for medications
Nursing responsibilities relative to medicines and their administration
Administration of medicines on the psychiatric ward
Administration of medicines to geriatric patients
Administration of medicines to infants and children

MAJOR CHANNELS OF ADMINISTRATION

Route of administration of a given drug is determined by its physical and chemical properties, the site of desired action, and the rapidity of response desired. As a rule, drugs are administered for one of two effects: local, in which the effects are confined to the site of application, or systemic, in which the results are realized after the drug is absorbed into the blood and diffuses into one or more tissues of the body. Some drugs given locally may produce both local and systemic effects if they are partly or entirely absorbed. A drug may be injected into a joint cavity and have little or no effect beyond the tissues of that structure.

ADMINISTRATION FOR LOCAL EFFECT

Application to the skin. Medications are applied to the skin primarily for the following effects:

1 *astringent:* resulting in vasoconstriction, tissue contraction, and decreased secretions and sensitivity, thereby counteracting inflammatory effects
2 *antiseptic* or *bacteriostatic:* to inhibit growth and development of microorganisms

3 *emollient:* for a soothing and softening effect to overcome dryness and hardness
4 *cleansing:* for the removal of dirt, debris, secretions, or crusts

These medications may be applied in the form of a lotion, tincture, ointment or cream, wet dressing, baths, or soaks. Effectiveness of medicinals applied to the skin is limited by the fact that the highly specialized layers of skin resist penetration of foreign substances to protect the internal body environment. However, absorption is increased when the skin is thin or macerated, when there is increased drug concentration, or when there is prolonged contact of the drug with the skin.

Application to mucous membranes. Drugs are well absorbed across mucosal surfaces and therapeutic effects are easily obtained. However, mucous membranes are highly selective in their absorptive action and differ in sensitivity. A drug applied to oral mucosa may be twice as concentrated as that applied to nasal mucosa, while its concentration may be reduced one fourth to one half for delicate membranes of the eye or urethra. Aqueous solutions are quickly absorbed from mucous membrane while oily liquids are not. Oily preparations should not be applied to nasal or respiratory mucosa using sprays or nebulae since the droplets of oil may be carried to terminal portions of the respiratory tract and retained there, causing lipoid pneumonia.

Respiratory mucosa may be medicated by means of inhalation or insufflation. The *inhalation* method utilizes *sprays* or *nebulae,* whereby the drug is sprayed into the throat using a nebulizer, or *aerosols,* whereby a flow of air or oxygen under pressure disperses the drug throughout the respiratory tract. In the *insufflation* method a fine powder is blown or sprayed onto nasal mucosa. Drugs so administered tend to have both a respiratory and a systemic effect. The respiratory mucosa offers an enormous surface of absorbing epithelium. If the drug is volatile and capable of being absorbed and if there is more in the inspired air than in the blood, the drug is instantaneously absorbed. This fact is of significance in situations of emergency. Amyl nitrite, ether, oxygen, and carbon dioxide are examples of volatile and gaseous agents that are given by inhalation.

Drugs in suppository form can be used for their local effects on the mucous membranes of the vagina, urethra, or rectum. Packs and tampons may be impregnated with a drug and placed in a body cavity. They are used particularly in the nose, ears, and vagina. Drugs may also be painted or swabbed on a mucosal surface, instilled, or administered by way of a douche or irrigation.

ADMINISTRATION FOR SYSTEMIC EFFECTS

Drugs that produce a systemic effect must be absorbed and carried to the cells or tissues capable of responding to them. The channel of administration used depends upon the nature and amount of drug to be given, desired rapidity of effect, and general condition of the patient. Channels selected for systemic effect include the following: oral, sublingual, rectal, and parenteral (injection)—intradermal, subcutaneous, intramuscular, intravenous, intraspinal, and sometimes intracardiac, intrapericardial, and intraosseous.

Oral. The oral channel of administration is the safest, most economical, and most convenient way of giving medicines. Therefore, medications should be given orally unless some distinct advantage is to be gained by giving them another way. Most drugs are absorbed from the small intestine; a few are absorbed from the stomach and colon.

Following oral administration, drug action has a slower onset and *more prolonged* but *less potent effect* than when drugs are given parenterally. This may result from: (1) *variation in absorption* as a result of drug composition, gastric or intestinal pH and motility, food content, and pathology within the gastrointestinal tract; or (2) *alteration of the drug* resulting from its retention, inactivation, or partial destruction by the liver if the drug traverses the hepatic circulation before entering the general circulation.

Disadvantages of oral administration of certain drugs are: (1) they may have an objectionable odor or taste; (2) they may harm or discolor the teeth; (3) they may irritate the gastric mucosa, causing nausea and vomiting; (4) they may be aspirated by a seriously ill or uncooperative patient; and (5) they may be destroyed by digestive enzymes.

Sublingual. Drugs given sublingually are placed under the patient's tongue, where they must be retained until dissolved and absorbed. The thin epithelium and rich network of capillaries on the underside of the tongue permit both rapid absorption and rapid drug action. In addition, there is greater potency since the drug gains access to the general circulation without traversing the liver or being affected by gastric and intestinal enzymes.

The number of drugs that can be given sublingually is limited. The drug must dissolve readily, and the patient must be able to cooperate; the patient must understand that the drug is not to be swallowed and that he must not take a drink until the drug has been absorbed. Tablets of nitroglycerin are usually administered sublingually.

A drug may be applied against the mucosa of the cheek for *buccal absorption.*

Rectal. Rectal administration can be used advantageously when the stomach is nonretentive, when the medicine has an objectionable taste or odor, or when it can be changed by digestive enzymes. It is a reasonably convenient and safe

Figure 6-1

Withdrawing medication from an ampule. The ampule on the left will break easily when pressure is exerted at the constricted portion. An ampule may be made so that a metal file must be used at the neck to secure a clean break.

Figure 6-2

Inserting hypodermic needle into a stoppered vial. When a hypodermic needle is inserted into a vial of this type, it is important that air be injected first to facilitate withdrawal of the liquid medication. Note that the plunger has been withdrawn and is supported by the index finger. After the plunger has been pushed down to the end of the barrel, the vial can be inverted. The desired amount is then drawn into the syringe.

method of giving drugs when the oral method is unsuitable, as when the patient is unconscious.

Use of this route avoids irritation of the upper gastrointestinal tract and may promote higher bloodstream drug titers because venous blood from the lower part of the rectum does not traverse the liver. The suppository vehicle is far superior to the retention enema because the drug is released at a slow but steady rate to ensure a protracted effect. One disadvantage of the retention enema is unpredictable retention of the drug; another is that much of the fluid passes above the lower rectum and then is absorbed into the portal circulation. An evacuant enema prior to the administration of the medication is usually advisable. The amount of solution that can be given rectally is usually small.

Parenteral. Parenteral administration of drugs includes all forms of drug injection into body tissues or fluids using a syringe and needle or catheter and flask. Drugs given parenterally must be sterile, readily soluble and absorbable, and nonirritating. Since parenteral administration of drugs can be hazardous, precautions are required: (1) sterile aseptic technique must be used to avoid infection, and (2) accurate drug dosage, proper rate of injection, and proper site of injection are essential to avoid harm such as tissue injury and severe or permanent nerve damage. *An injected drug is irretrievable,* and an error in dosage or method or site of injection is not easily corrected.

Given parenterally rather than orally: (1) onset of drug action is more rapid but of shorter duration; (2) dosage is often smaller since drug potency tends not to be altered; and (3) the cost of drug therapy may be greater. Parenteral administration of drugs requires specialized knowledge and manual skill to ensure safety and therapeutic effectiveness. Various methods of parenteral administration may be performed by the nurse, but some are done only by a physician.

Intradermal. Intradermal or intracutaneous injection means that the injection is made into the upper layers of the skin. The amount of drug given is small and absorption is slow. This method is used to advantage when testing for allergic reactions of the patient. Minute amounts

Figure 6-3 Intradermal injection.

Needle penetrates epidermis into the dermis.

Figure 6-4

These syringes are used to accurately measure varying amounts of liquids and liquid medications. The uppermost syringe is known as a tuberculin syringe and is graduated in 0.01 cc. (ml.). It is a syringe of choice for administration of very small amounts. The 2-cc. syringe is the one commonly used to give a drug subcutaneously. It is graduated in 0.1 cc. The larger syringes are used when a larger volume of drug is to be administered.

of the solution to be tested are injected just under the outer layers of the skin. The medial surface of the forearm and the skin of the back are the sites frequently used. These injections are best made with a fine, short needle (26 gauge) and a small barrel syringe (such as a tuberculin syringe) (Figure 6-4). A physician or professional nurse is usually responsible for this procedure.

Subcutaneous. Small amounts of drug in solution are given subcutaneously (hypodermically) by means of a hypodermic syringe and needle, usually a fine 25-gauge needle. The needle is inserted through the skin with a quick movement, but the injection is made slowly and steadily. The piston of the syringe should be withdrawn slightly before injecting the drug to make sure that a blood vessel has not been entered. The angle of insertion should be 45 to 60 degrees and should be made on the outer surface of the upper arm or on the anterior surface of the thigh. In these locations there are fewer large blood vessels, and sensation is less keen than on the medial surfaces of the extremities. Movement of the part after injection tends to increase the rate of absorption. Disposable syringes and needles contribute to accuracy and safety of the procedure. Hypodermically injected medicines are limited to the administration of drugs that are highly soluble and nonirritating and to solutions of limited volume (0.5 to 2 ml.).

Irritating drugs given subcutaneously can result in the formation of sterile abscesses and necrotic tissue. Infection can also occur more easily after subcutaneous administration than when drugs are given intravenously. Care should be exercised to avoid contamination. Subcutaneous injections are not satisfactory in individuals with sluggish peripheral circulation.

The introduction of large amounts of solution (500 to 1000 ml. in adults) into subcutaneous tissues is known as *hypodermoclysis*. Isotonic solutions of sodium chloride or glucose are administered this way. The needle is longer than that used for a hypodermic injection and it is inserted into areas of loose connective tissue such as that under the breasts, in the upper surfaces of the thighs, and into the subscapular region of the back. Fluids must be given slowly to avoid overdistention of the tissues. Hyaluronidase is sometimes added to the solution to facilitate the spread and absorption of fluid by decreasing the viscosity of the ground substance in connective tissues. Some physicians prefer intravenous infusion of fluids to hypodermoclysis because the

Figure 6-5 Subcutaneous injection.

The skin surface has been cleansed and the hypodermic syringe is held at the angle at which the needle will penetrate the tissue. The left hand is used to pinch the arm gently but firmly. When the needle has been inserted into the subcutaneous tissue, the tissue of the arm is released and the solution is steadily injected.

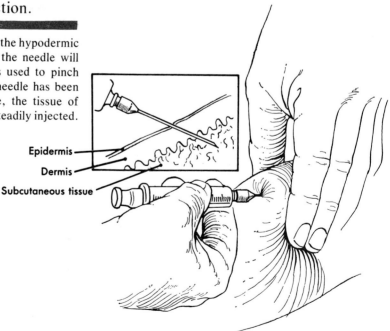

Epidermis
Dermis
Subcutaneous tissue

amount of absorption is more readily determined.

Intramuscular. Injections are made through the skin and subcutaneous tissue into muscular tissue when prompt absorption is desirable and the drug is too irritating to be given subcutaneously. Irritation may not be obvious following intramuscular injection. Larger doses can be given intramuscularly than can be given subcutaneously (1 to 10 ml.). Muscles into which injection can usually be made conveniently are those of the buttock, the lateral side of the thigh, and the deltoid region of the arm. The gluteal muscles are usually thick and well suited to the injection of the larger intramuscular doses. The drug spreads along the muscle fibers and along the fasciae. This affords a large absorbing surface with relatively few sensory nerves.

A drug may be given intramuscularly in an aqueous solution, an aqueous suspension, or a solution or suspension of oil. Suspensions form a depot of drug in the tissue, and slow gradual absorption usually results. Two disadvantages are sometimes encountered when preparations in oil are used: the patient may be sensitive to the oil or the oil may not be absorbed. In the latter case, incision and drainage of the oil may be necessary.

The type of needle used for intramuscular injection depends upon the site of the injection, the condition of the tissues, and the nature of the drug to be injected. Needles from 1 to 3 inches in length may be used. The usual gauge is 19 to 22 (the larger the number, the finer the needle). Fine needles can be used for thin solutions and heavier needles for suspensions and oils. Needles for injection into the deltoid area should be 1 to $1^1/_2$ inches in length, the gauge again depending on the material to be injected. The deltoid can readily absorb up to 2 ml. of drug. For many intramuscular injections the preferable site of injection is the buttock. The needle must be long enough to avoid depositing the solution of drug into the subcutaneous or fatty tissue. The depth of insertion depends upon the amount of subcutaneous tissue and will vary with the weight of the patient. The buttock should be divided into four parts and the injection made into the upper outer quadrant. The crest of the ileum serves as a good landmark and should be palpated to confirm the location of the upper outer quadrant, and then the needle should be inserted straight in, with a firm bold pressure, about 2 to 3 inches below the iliac crest. In this region the muscle is thick and the nerve supply is less profuse than in an area near the middle of the buttock or in the region closer to the rectum. Nurses sometimes make the mistake of giving intramuscular injections too near the rectum or too near the middle of the buttock, where it is possible to cause the patient unnecessary discomfort or actually to injure the sciatic nerve and cause paralysis of the lower extremity. To avoid this injury, von Hochstetter has described the V method of locating the ventral gluteal muscle. Using the left hand, the index finger is placed on the right iliac spine of the patient and the middle finger stretched back to form a V with the index finger. The middle finger is slipped to a point just below the crest of the ilium. The palm of the hand rests on the patient's hip. The triangle between the index and middle fingers is the injection site. The positions of the middle and index fingers are reversed in finding the site on the patient's left side. In case the needle is inserted all the way to the hub, it should be withdrawn just enough to have something to grasp should the needle break.

After the needle is inserted the plunger should be slightly withdrawn to make certain that the needle is not in a blood vessel. Although this problem seldom occurs when the injection is made in the sites mentioned, it is not justifiable to take a chance of injecting a drug into a blood vessel when this is not the route of administration selected for the drug. In certain instances injection of oily or particulate medicines or killed bacteria by inadvertent intravenous administration could result in a serious emergency.

When giving an intramuscular injection, it is usually preferable to have the patient in a prone position, with his head turned to one side and with a pillow under the legs just below the knees. He should be instructed to toe inward; this will help to promote relaxation of the gluteal muscles. If this is not a convenient position for the patient to take, he may be placed on his side with the leg flexed at the knee.

Figure 6-6 Intramuscular injection.

A

Posterior gluteal site. In determining the location of the upper outer quadrant it is important to locate the crest of the ilium above and the inferior gluteal fold below before marking the buttocks into fourths. The X's indicate two of a number of sites that may be used in the upper outer quadrant, although it is well to keep about 2 inches below the iliac crest. An injection near the middle of the buttocks may result in an injury to the sciatic nerve. It is, of course, important to vary the sites of injection, preferably using alternate buttocks. The needle is inserted in with a quick firm movement. After aspirating to make certain the needle is not in a blood vessel, the solution is injected slowly and steadily.

B

Ventrogluteal intramuscular injection site. The V fans out from the greater trochanter. The injection site (X) is centered at the bottom of the triangle.

C

Midlateral thigh intramuscular injection site a handsbreadth below the greater trochanter and a handsbreadth above the knee.

D

Mid-deltoid intramuscular injection site—below the acromion and lateral to the axilla.

To prevent excessive scar formation or tissue irritation, no two injections should be made in the same spot during a course of treatment. When injection is made into the buttocks, it should be given first on one side and then on the other. The technique in which the tissue is pinched between the fingers, rather than spread, may be desirable for patients with very little subcutaneous tissue but is contraindicated for patients who are bruised as a result of repeated injections.

Intravenous. When an immediate effect is desired, or when for any reason the drug cannot be injected into other tissues, or when absorption may be inhibited by poor circulation, it may be given directly into a vein as an *injection* or *infusion.* The technique of this method requires skill and sterile asepsis, and the drug must be highly soluble and capable of withstanding sterilization. This method is of great value in emergencies. The dose and amount of absorption can be determined with accuracy, although the rapidity of absorption and the fact that there is no recall once the drug has been given constitute dangers worthy of consideration. From this standpoint it is one of the least safe methods of administration. Precautions must be taken to prevent extravasation of drug or fluids into surrounding tissue.

INJECTION. In intravenous injection a comparatively small amount of solution (also referred to as a *bolus*) is given by means of a syringe. The drug is dissolved in a suitable amount of normal (physiologic) saline solution or some other isotonic solution. The injection is usually made into the median basilic or median cephalic vein at the bend of the elbow (Figure 6-7). However, any accessible vein may be used. Factors that determine the choice of a vein are related to the thickness of the skin over the vein, the closeness of the vein to the surface, and the presence of a firm support (bone) under the vein. The veins in the antecubital fossa, though readily accessible, are uncomfortable sites for the patient requiring long-term intravenous therapy. For this reason they are frequently reserved for obtaining samples of blood. A vein that is normally distended with blood is much easier to enter than a partially collapsed vein. If a vein of the arm has been chosen, a tourniquet is drawn tightly around the middle of the arm to distend the vein, the air is expelled from the sy-

Figure 6-7 Intravenous injection.

Epidermis
Subcutaneous tissue
Vein

The skin has been cleansed with a solution of alcohol. Thumb of right hand holds the skin taut. Withdrawal of blood indicates needle is in the vein. Solution is injected slowly and steadily.

ringe, and the needle should be introduced quickly and forcefully pointing upward toward the heart. A few drops of blood aspirated into the syringe indicates the needle is in the vein; the tourniquet is then removed; and the solution is injected very slowly. The needle, syringe, and solution must be sterile, and the hands of the doctor and nurse and the skin of the patient at the point of insertion of the needle must be clean.

INFUSION. In intravenous infusion a larger amount of fluid is usually given, varying from 1 to 5 pints, and the method differs somewhat. The solution flows by gravity from a graduated glass flask or plastic bag through tubing, connecting tip, and needle or catheter into a vein.

Infusions are most commonly given to relieve tissue dehydration, to restore depleted blood volume, to dilute toxic substances in the blood and tissue fluids, and to supply electrolytes, drugs, and foods.

The fluid is usually given slowly to prevent reaction or fluid overload, which may impair cardiac and pulmonary function. Ordinarily 3 to 4 hours are required for every 1000 ml. of fluid, depending on the condition of the patient, the nature of the solution, and the reasons for giving it. For children the rate will be slower and is determined by age, weight, and urinary output.

Sodium chloride (0.9%) solution, commonly known as physiologic or isotonic salt solution, is the fluid of choice for intravenous infusion to relieve dehydration not complicated by acidosis.

Five percent dextrose solution is frequently administered and is of value because it provides a means of administering water and a sugar, which is a food. A concentration of 5.5% is approximately isotonic with normal body fluids. Dextrose in physiologic saline solution is sometimes given.

A dextran solution may be given intravenously as an infusion colloid to support blood volume in the management of various types of shock.

A number of commercial solutions are used in intravenous replacement therapy. Some contain not only salts of sodium and potassium but also salts of calcium and magnesium. Vitamins are also added to intravenous fluids when their need is indicated.

Whole blood and blood plasma are likewise given intravenously to restore depleted blood volume as well as constituents of the blood.

Intraspinal. Intraspinal injection is also known as intrathecal (into a sheath), subdural, subarachnoid, or lumbar injection. The technique is the same as that required for a lumbar puncture. Nurses do not administer drugs intraspinally.

In addition, drugs are occasionally administered by intracardiac, intrapericardial, and intraosseous injections; however, nurses do not administer drugs by these routes.

ORDERS FOR MEDICATIONS

The procedure used for ordering medicines for a patient depends on whether the patient is in the hospital, at home, in the doctor's office, or in some institution other than a hospital. On the ward of the hospital there is usually a book or file in which the physician writes the orders. Sometimes orders are written on the patient's chart. In an emergency there may be no time to write an order and it is given verbally. Sometimes the physician gives an order over the telephone. It is customary for the nurse to write the order that has been given verbally indicating the name of the physician who gave the order and how it was given (in person or by telephone). The physician later confirms the order by signing his or her name or initials.

Written orders are a form of protection to everyone concerned with medicines—the patient, physician, pharmacist, and the nurse. They constitute permanent legal records that can be referred to as often as necessary or submitted as evidence in case of litigation. No nurse may modify or in any way alter a physician's order. If there is reason to think that an error has been made, the nurse should ask the physician about it. If inquiry is made courteously, the physician is usually pleased that the nurse is alert and conscientious. The nurse in charge, if available, will appreciate being asked regarding an order about which there is question and may be able to explain something about the order that will clarify matters. *The nurse should not go ahead and give a medicine if there is doubt about an error.* On the other hand, the order cannot be disregarded; the nurse is obligated to seek clarification.

PRESCRIPTIONS

Outside the hospital physicians will write a prescription when they wish to order a drug. Only persons legally licensed to prescribe—physicians, dentists, and veterinarians—may write prescriptions. In some states changes in the law, nurse practice acts, and medical practice acts have extended prescription writing to nurse practitioners and physicians' assistants. However strict limitations are placed on the type of prescription that can be written by nurses and physicians' assistants; they are not usually permitted to prescribe narcotics or drugs with a high abuse or dependence potential. Medicines should be labeled by a pharmacist.

A number of medicinal agents may be purchased over the counter without a prescription, but an amendment to the Federal Food, Drug,

and Cosmetic Act (as mentioned in Chapter 3) requires that all drugs that can be used safely and effectively only under the supervision of a physician must have a prescription. Such prescriptions can be refilled only if authorization is granted by the prescriber. Authorization may be made in writing by indicating on the written prescription the number of times or the frequency with which the prescription may be refilled, or the physician may authorize the pharmacist by telephone. Sometimes the pharmacist telephones the physician if a patient requests that a prescription be refilled and no previous authorization has been given. Prescriptions for narcotics cannot be refilled; they must be rewritten.

A typical prescription is a written formula given by a physician to a pharmacist for dispensing medicine to a patient. It consists of four parts:

1. The *superscription,* which includes the patient's name, address, the date and the symbol

Table 6-1 Abbreviations for orders, prescriptions, and labels

Abbreviation	Derivation	Meaning	Abbreviation	Derivation	Meaning
a͞a	ana	of each	o.h.	omni hora	every hour
a.c.	ante cibum	before meals	o.m.	omni mane	every morning
ad	ad	to, up to	o.n.	omni nocte	every night
ad lib.	ad libitum	freely as desired	os	os	mouth
aq.	aqua	water	oz.	uncia	ounce
aq. dest.	aqua destillata	distilled water	p.c.	post cibum	after meals
b.i.d.	bis in die	two times a day	per	per	through or by
b.i.n.	bis in noctis	two times a night	pil.	pilula	pill
c.	cum	with	p.r.n.	pro re nata	when required
caps.	capsula	capsule	q.h.	quaque hora	every hour
comp.	compositus	compound	q. 2 h.		every two hours
dil.	dilutus	dilute	q. 3 h.		every three hours
elix.	elixir	elixir	q. 4 h.		every four hours
ext.	extractum	extract	q.i.d.	quater in die	four times a day
fld.	fluidus	fluid	q.s.	quantum sufficit	as much as is required
Ft.	fiat	make	℞	recipe	take thou
Gm.	gramme	gram	s	sine	without
gr.	granum	grain	Sig. or S.	signa	write on label
gtt.	gutta	a drop	s.o.s.	si opus sit	if necessary
h.	hora	hour	sp.	spiritus	spirits
h.s.	hora somni	hour of sleep (bedtime)	ss	semis	a half
M.	misce	mix	stat.	statim	immediately
m.	minimum	a minim	syr.	syrupus	syrup
mist.	mistura	mixture	t.i.d.	ter in die	three times a day
non rep.	non repetatur	not to be repeated	t.i.n.	ter in nocte	three times a night
noct.	nocte	in the night	tr. or tinct.	tinctura	tincture
O	octarius	pint	ung.	unguentum	ointment
ol.	oleum	oil	vin.	vini	wine
o.d.	omni die	every day			

Superscription	Mr. James Wiley 210 Elmwood Pl. Minneapolis, Minn.	Age	Date	2/4/76
Inscription	Ampicillin	250 mg.		
Subscription	Dispense #20			
Signature	Sig.: Caps. ī q.i.d.			
Reg. No._____ (DEA No.)			J. B. Tanner, M.D. (address) (phone number)	

℞, an abbreviation for "Recipe" meaning "Take thou." The age of an infant or young child should be included to permit the pharmacist to check the correctness of the dose.

2. The *inscription,* which states the name of the drug, dose form, and amount per dose.

3. The *subscription,* which contains the directions to the pharmacist, which are now usually limited to the number of doses to be dispensed.

4. The *signature,* which is abbreviated "S." or "Sig." and means "Write on the label." This indicates the directions for the patient who is to take the medicine and should include that the name of the drug be placed on the label. This permits identification of the drug if toxicity occurs or the patient changes physicians. Instructions for refilling the prescription should also be included.

The physician's name is also indicated. The physician's name, address, and telephone number are frequently printed on prescription blanks. If the prescription is for a narcotic or any other drug listed in the Controlled Substances Act, the physician's registry number, obtained from the Drug Enforcement Administration, and address must appear on the prescription form. Quantities are expressed in either the apothecaries' or metric system. An example of a prescription is shown above.

The abbreviations in Table 6-1 are used in written orders, prescriptions, and labels on medicines, and it is necessary for the nurse to know what they mean. A difference exists between the abbreviations s.o.s. and p.r.n. The former, when used in connection with medicines, means "if necessary" and refers to one dose only. The latter means "when required," "as often as necessary," or "according to circumstances." The nurse is expected to use judgment about repeating the dose. For example, a physician may leave an order for a patient that reads:

> For Mrs. Smith, Room 210, elixir terpin hydrate dram i q. 3 h. p.r.n. for cough.
>
> John Doe, M.D.

The order means that the patient may have a dose of cough medicine every 3 hours. However, if the patient is not coughing and has no need for the medicine, the nurse may allow longer intervals to elapse between doses.

"Morphine sulfate 10 mg. q. 4 h. p.r.n." means that the dose of morphine sulfate may be given every 4 hours if the patient has need of it. If the nurse thinks that the patient has no need for it—the patient seems to have no pain, is resting comfortably, is asleep most of the time—an interval longer than 4 hours will be allowed to elapse before the dose is repeated. If, however, the order reads "Morphine sulfate 10 mg. s.o.s.," the nurse would give one dose of the drug if the patient seemed to need it and then would give no more. If one dose of the drug is to be given immediately, it would read "Morphine sulfate 10 mg. stat."

NURSING RESPONSIBILITIES RELATIVE TO MEDICINES AND THEIR ADMINISTRATION
CARE OF MEDICINES

Regulations vary in different hospitals, but, regardless of the place, certain principles of organization should be observed in the care of drugs and associated equipment.

1 All medicines should be kept in a special place, which may be a cupboard, closet, or room. It should not be freely accessible to the public.
2 Narcotic drugs and those dispensed under special legal regulations must be kept in a locked box or compartment.
3 In some hospitals each patient's medicines are kept in a designated place on a shelf or compartment of the medicine cupboard or room. Such an arrangement means that the nurse must be careful to keep the patient's medicines in the right area and to make certain that when the patient leaves the hospital his medicines are returned to the pharmacy, unless he is taking them with him. Many hospitals require that medicines be returned to the pharmacy for relabeling if they are to be taken home at the time of dismissal. It is imperative that the medicines have the patient's full name on the label of the container. In some hospitals the medicines are dispensed wholly or in part from a stock supply kept on the ward. Misplaced medicines and equipment can contribute to errors in administration.
4 If stock supplies are maintained they should be arranged in an orderly manner. Preparations for internal use should be kept separate from those used externally.
5 Some preparations, such as serums, vaccines, cer-tain suppositories, certain antibiotics, and insulin, need to be kept in a refrigerator.
6 Labels of all medicines should be clean and legible. If they are not, they should be sent to the pharmacist for relabeling. *Nurses should not label or relabel medicines.*
7 Bottles of medicines should always be stoppered and protected from light.

THE ADMINISTRATION OF MEDICINES

Experience has demonstrated that it is wise to abide by established policies and regulations pertaining to the administration of medicines. Such regulations vary from hospital to hospital, but principles of safety do not vary appreciably. They have been established to protect patients and to save nurses from the traumatizing effects of errors that other nurses have had the misfortune to experience. This does not mean that deviation from the rule or regulation under special circumstances is always bad judgment. The nurse must consider the situation carefully before departing from established policy and, if possible, should consult with a more experienced person, such as the instructor or the nurse in charge. Policies and regulations are protective guides to live by, not to be followed so blindly that thinking and good sense do not enter into decision-making.

Figure 6-8 Read the label carefully.

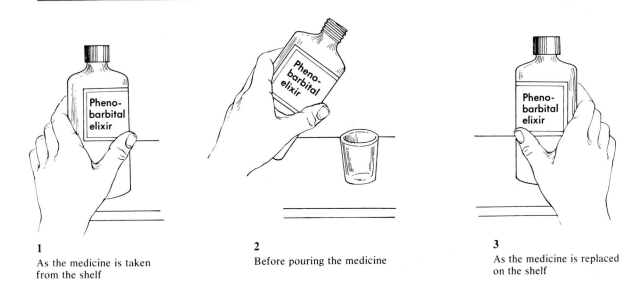

1
As the medicine is taken from the shelf

2
Before pouring the medicine

3
As the medicine is replaced on the shelf

Safety regulations are effective only when they are understood and readily interpreted by the nursing staff as being necessary for the patient's protection. The following are policies or regulations that have been found to be sound relative to the administration of medicines. They are not listed in order of importance.

1 When preparing or giving medicines, concentrate your whole attention on what you are doing. Do not permit yourself to be distracted while working with medicines.
2 Make certain that you have a written order for every medication for which you assume the responsibility of administration. (Verbal orders should be written out as soon as possible.)
3 Develop the habit of reading the label of the medicine carefully before removing the dose from the container.
4 Make certain that the data on the medicine card corresponds exactly with the doctor's written order and with the label on the patient's medicine. A medicine card should accompany each medicine (Figure 6-9). Sometimes skipping a dose of medi-

Figure 6-9

Samples of medicine cards used to accompany medications. Cards should bear the following information: name and room of patient; name of medicine; dosage; time of administration; route of administration if there is any question about how it might be given; and special precautions.

Mrs. Melvin Nigon	Michael Morris
(Name)	(Name)
2 - 190	3 - 160
(Room no.)	(Room no.)
Digitoxin	Compazine
0.2 mg. bid.	Syrup
(orally)	℥ ī T.i.d.
8⁻	8⁻
4⁻	1⁻
Count Pulse	5⁻

cine may be as dangerous as an overdose. It is important that for every drug listed in the Kardex there be a corresponding medicine card.
5 Never give a medicine from an unlabeled container or from one on which the label is not legible.
6 Do not administer medicines that have been prepared by some other person unless that person is a clinical pharmacist.
7 If you must in some way calculate the dosage for a patient from the preparation on hand and you are uncertain of your calculation, verify your work by checking with some responsible person—an instructor, nurse in charge, or pharmacist.
8 Measure quantities as ordered, using the proper apparatus, graduated containers for milliliters, fluidounces, or fluidrams, minim glasses, or calibrated pipets for minims and droppers for drops. When measuring liquids, hold the container so that the line indicating the desired quantity is on a level with the eye. The quantity is read when the lowest part of the concave surface of the fluid is on this line (Figure 6-11).
9 Even though you have cared for a particular patient all morning or for several days, you should have developed the habit of checking his identification each time you give him a medication. If the patient wears an identification band, the name on it must correspond with the name on the medicine card. The problem of identification presents an even greater hazard to the nurse who is responsible for the administration of medications to a group of patients, perhaps an entire unit. For this nurse a 10:00 A.M. injection may be the initial or only contact with the patient. It is important that each patient be called by name. If there is the least doubt of his identity, ask him to state his name. Patients have been known to answer to names other than their own, but they are not likely to give the wrong name when asked to speak it.
10 Remain with the patient until the medicine has been taken. Most patients are very cooperative about taking medicines at the time that the nurse brings them. However, sometimes patients are more ill than they appear and have been known to hoard medicines until they have accumulated a lethal amount and then have taken the entire amount, with fatal results.
11 Never return an unused dose of medicine to a stock bottle.
12 Never chart a medicine as having been given until it has been administered. Sometimes it may be necessary to check the chart before giving the medication. All medications are recorded, but the

Figure 6-10

Two medicine trays with cards. The small tray at the left may be used for a number of patients, as in a double room or a small ward. Souffle cups instead of medicine glasses may be used for capsules or tablets. The large tray is arranged for the administration of medications to a group of patients.

Figure 6-11

When pouring liquid medicine, the thumbnail is placed at the mark on the medicine glass and the medicine is poured on a level with the eye. The bottle should be held so that the medication is not poured over the label.

manner of recording may vary from hospital to hospital. The name of the drug, the dosage, the time of administration, and the channel of administration as well as the patient's reaction to the medication should be recorded.

Additional suggestions relative to the giving of medicines. The following suggestions constitute habits of thought and behavior developed by experienced professional nurses that the nursing student will also be expected to develop.

1 Dosage forms such as tablets, capsules, and pills should be handled in such a way that the fingers will not come in contact with the medicine. Use the cap of the container or a clean medicine card to guide or lift the medicine into the medicine glass or container you will be taking to the bedside of the patient.
2 When pouring liquid medicines, hold the bottle so that the liquid does not run over the side and obscure the label. Wipe the rim of the bottle with a clean piece of paper tissue before replacing the stopper or cover.
3 Assist weak or helpless patients in taking their medications.
4 Most liquid medicines should be diluted with water or other liquid. This is especially desirable when medicines have a bad taste. Exceptions to this rule include oils and cough medicines that are given for a local effect in the throat. The patient should be supplied with an ample amount of fresh water after swallowing solid dosage forms, such as tablets or capsules, unless for some reason the patient is allowed only limited amounts of fluid.
5 Medicine glasses should be thoroughly washed with hot soapy water and scalded with hot water. Glasses used for oils should be washed separately. Disposable medicine containers provide a more sanitary means of dispensing medicines.
6 The nurse should avoid waste of medicines. Medicines tend to be expensive; in some instances a single capsule may cost the patient several dollars. Dropping medicine on the floor is one way of wasting it.
7 If a patient expresses doubt or concern about a medication or the dosage of a medication, the nurse should do everything possible to make sure that no mistake has occurred. Occasionally, the patient is right. Reassure the patient as well as yourself by rechecking to make certain that there is no error. You may need to recheck the order, the label on the medicine container, or the patient's chart.
8 Do not leave a tray of medicines unattended. If you are in a patient's room and must leave, take the tray of medicines with you.
9 As a rule nurses should not prepare mixtures of drugs. They should be prepared by the pharmacist.

Nurse's approach. The reaction of a patient to medicine may be an expression of fear, frustration, or hostility. The nurse who has been caring for a patient can appreciate the many incidents that may disturb him. A physician calls upon a patient to discuss the possibility of serious surgery that will benefit the patient. The proposition leaves the patient rather shaken. He also knows that sometime during the day he must make financial arrangements for continued hospitalization. The nurse who understands this patient is not content to simply chart that the patient refused his 10:00 A.M. medication. The nurse may encourage him to talk about the things that are concerning him so deeply and thus make him feel that his reaction is accepted whatever it may be. The nurse who realizes that a particular medication is an essential part of the patient's care will provide him with other opportunities to refuse less essential care. Recognition of the patient's right to express feelings can lead to greater security for the patient and deeper insight for the nurse.

The medicine containers from which the patient is served his medicine should be scrupulously clean, and water supplied immediately after the medicine should be fresh. Carelessly prepared medicines and lack of consideration in the way a medicine is handed to a patient can disgust him in the same way that poor food, cracked dishes, and inefficient service affect him in a restaurant.

When giving a medicine with an unpleasant taste it is better to admit that it is unpleasant and thereby agree with the patient than to make him feel that his reaction is grossly exaggerated or silly. The nurse can attempt to improve the taste by diluting the medicine (if possible) or by offering chewing gum or a Life Saver immediately after the medicine.

DRUG ORDERING AND DISTRIBUTION

Safer and more expedient methods of drug distribution to hospitalized patients has received much interest during the past decade. However, in many hospitals nurses still transcribe drug orders, make out medicine cards, keep a Kardex containing the patient's medicine orders, and count, pour, and request medicines from the pharmacy. In one study it was found that in more than 300 hospitals located throughout the United States, 89% of all drug orders were still being written on the patients' charts in the nurses' station and that 60% of the time nurses assumed major responsibility for transcribing all drug orders and requisitioning medicines from the pharmacy. There is no doubt that most methods of drug ordering and drug distribution in the hospital now in use are serious usurpers of the nurses' valuable time.

Unit dose package. A number of hospitals have converted to unit dose packages, and it is safe to predict that in the future the use of unit dose packages will be commonplace in all hospitals. A unit dose package contains the ordered amount of a drug for a single administration in the proper form for administration by the prescribed route. All unit dose packages are labeled with the drug's generic name, trade name, strength of dose, warning terms or precautions, expiration date (if this is appropriate), and recommendations for storing (such as the need to store in a cool place or away from direct light). Tablets, capsules, and liquids can be prepared in single unit packages or vials.

Disadvantages of using unit dose packages are primarily those of space for storage and increased cost. In addition, it is practical at this time for pharmaceutical companies to manufacture unit dose packages or single unit packages for only the most widely and commonly used drugs. It has been estimated that 30% to 50% of all drugs commonly used are available in single unit packages. However, small and inexpensive single unit package machines are available for purchase that permit hospital pharmacists to make up unit dose packages from their own stock supplies for medications ordered for patients in their hospital.

The advantages of using unit dose packages far outweigh their disadvantages. The most important advantage is medication safety and a decrease in error, since drug computations are eliminated. The drug is already properly labeled and does not have to be poured. All the nurse needs to do is deliver the package to the patient where it is opened at the bedside and administered. This permits the patient to check on his own drug and be assured of proper medication and dosage, particularly when the drugs are distributed by nonprofessional personnel. Packaging also decreases chance of deterioration and permits giving financial credit to the patient for drugs not used. Often because of fear of contamination, bottles of unused drugs must be discarded and not relabeled for any other patient. Because of this the patient for whom the drug was originally ordered does not get financial credit for drugs he did not receive.

Strip packages permit ease of narcotic counting since all packages in the strip are numbered and only the number needs to be checked. This also prevents contamination caused by pouring narcotic tablets into the hands for ease of counting.

Unit dose dispensing systems in hospitals may be centralized, decentralized, or a combination of both. In the centralized system the pharmacist and pharmacy are located in a central area from which doses for all patients are prepared and distributed to patient care areas. In the decentralized system, clinical pharmacists and satellite pharmacies are located in patient care areas and doses are prepared and distributed to patients in those particular areas. In the combined system, patient medications are prepared in a central area with clinical pharmacists assigned to various patient care areas to oversee drug therapy thus providing safer and more controlled drug ordering and drug distribution.

Medication carts are used in some hospitals for distributing unit doses to the nursing unit and to the patients' bedside. Each patient has a drawer or tray for his medications, which are stocked by the pharmacy staff.

Prefilled disposable syringes. Prefilled disposable syringes for medications to be given subcutaneously, intramuscularly, and even intravenously are available. Advantages of prefilled and disposable syringes are the following:

1 Accuracy of dosage
2 Sterile product
3 Sharp needle
4 Elimination of suspected source of serum hepatitis

5 Less danger of allergic sensitization of personnel handling the drugs
6 Immediate availability of drug for use
7 Charge only for medicine used
8 Reduced likelihood of pilferage of narcotics
9 Less waste by breakage or incomplete use
10 Safer use of practical nurses permitted to administer subcutaneous or intramuscular drugs

Clinical pharmacists. The present trend is toward more extensive use of clinical pharmacists who are stationed in nursing areas to work closely with physicians, nurses, and dietitians. They are drug clinicians responsible for holding pharmacology conferences to discuss not only drug action but also whether or not a particular drug is compatible with other drugs and foods the patient is receiving. In addition these clinical pharmacists may:

1 Obtain a drug history on all patients, including what medicines (prescription or nonprescription) the patient took prior to hospitalization
2 Interpret the physician's medication orders to the nurse and to the patient
3 Recommend drug therapy for particular patients to the physician
4 Work with the nurse in observing patients for drug reactions and keep logs or records of suspected reactions to particular drugs
5 Advise patients about the medications they are to take home with them

Since pharmacists are well educated in the compounding, dispensing, and control of drugs, it is only natural they become more involved in drug therapy for the hospitalized patient. They should not be isolated from the clinical areas where much of the actual compounding and dispensing of drugs in the hospital really takes place.

There are also hospital pharmacies with special "clean rooms" and specially filtered air for compounding various parenteral solutions. The pharmacist may be responsible for putting all additives into intravenous solutions and checking all such solutions for compatibility reactions.

The emergence of clinical pharmacists was long overdue, and nurses have found them to be valuable and irreplaceable members of the health team. In some hospitals clinical pharmacists or clinical pharmacy technicians may actually distribute and administer drugs to patients. It goes almost without saying that whoever is responsible for drug administration is also responsible for being highly knowledgeable about each and every drug administered.

Role of the nurse. Regardless of the changes that may come about in the ordering, distribution, or administration of drugs, nurses are still responsible for their patients and their care 24 hours a day. Automation, clinical pharmacists, and unit package doses do not simplify the task of the nurse but serve to increase the complexity of patient care and responsibility of the nurse. As a result of these changes nurses should be better informed about drugs and their actions. Nurses still need to make their observations of patients, determine whether p.r.n. orders are to be given, and consult with physicians about withholding, discontinuing, or changing the drug dosage. They will continue to assist the physician and pharmacist in teaching patients about drugs and their effects and help patients plan their drug therapy upon returning home. The nurse should become more involved in taking drug histories and in working more closely with the pharmacist.

ADMINISTRATION OF MEDICINES ON THE PSYCHIATRIC WARD

The giving of medicines on a psychiatric unit automatically assumes symbolic meanings present in lesser degree on any hospital ward. All individuals need and seek meaningful interpersonal relationships; most individuals find such relationships outside medical situations. Psychiatric patients, however, are often starved for affection and yearn for some person to whom they may look for security and interest. Frequently, their emotional deprivation is concealed by an appearance of hostility or disdain.

In addition, the immediate personal needs of the patient and the current symptoms against which the patient is fighting must be considered. Overwhelming anxiety, depression to the point of suicide, pain of an uncanny nature, or distortions of thought that constantly separate the patient from his fellow men demand of the nurse much care in any contact, particularly that of medication. To the patient in a state of psychologic disequilibrium, that which is taken by mouth or given by injection may hold threats and symbolic meanings rarely felt by the medical or surgical patient. The fear of poisons or supernatural effects of capsules or the suggestions of witchcraft inherent in a needle often reach the degree of catastrophe unless the nurses are able to interrelate their actions and the thought processes of the patients. The psychiatric patient's tendency toward impulsiveness and his increased emotional sensitivity must constantly be kept in mind.

No practical suggestions can ever take the place of the techniques practiced by the psychiatrically oriented nurse, but the following factors should be considered in the general handling of medications for the psychiatric patient:

1 Drugs used in emergencies must be anticipated and such drugs must be made available.
2 Medicines should be given in paper, not glass, containers. The psychiatric patient is often so impulsive that all possible precautions must be taken to avoid accidents, and glass is always a potential weapon for suicide.
3 Precautions should be used whenever drugs are administered.
4 *The nurse must remain with the patient until oral medications have been swallowed.* This principle is basic in the giving of all medications but one of particular importance to the depressed and suicidal patient; such patients may conceal capsules in the mouth for long periods, only to hoard them until a lethal supply has been accumulated. Frequently, measures such as the piercing of the capsule case and staying with the patient until the drug is dissolved or the practice of using liquid preparations will enforce the actual ingestion of the drug.
5 It is often necessary not only to urge the psychiatric patient to take medication but also to insist upon its acceptance. The psychiatric patient is frequently an indecisive, emotionally confused individual who tends to doubt everything. He often presses the nurse for detailed information about the drug prescribed and frequently rebels because of minor discrepancies in information. Paradoxically, however, he complies quickly if a positive yet interested attitude is presented without undue explanation.
6 It is of utmost importance to report all drug refusals

to the physician in charge. But in the meantime it is frequently also of importance to persuade the patient to take the medicine. Omission of doses may cause the blood level of psychotropic drugs to be lowered so that larger doses than usual may eventually be needed. Intramuscular administration of psychotropic drugs assists in calming the patient within a relatively short period of time, so that oral preparations may then be given. The oral route of administration is preferred and should be instituted as soon as possible.

ADMINISTRATION OF MEDICINES TO GERIATRIC PATIENTS

Elderly patients may pose special problems in relation to their drug therapy. Passive resistance to drug therapy is not uncommon in the elderly; although they will not aggressively refuse drugs, some patients will not take them. It is frequently necessary to observe the patient swallow the drug and to make sure that the patient has not surreptitiously hidden the drug under the tongue, in the buccal cavity, in the hand, or in bed linen. The patient may refuse to take medications because of fear that drugs are harmful or mistrust of nursing and medical personnel.

Older persons should be treated like mature adults capable of being reasoned with; they are entitled to adequate explanations about their drug therapy.

Nurses must remember that effects of certain drugs may be increased or decreased in the elderly. For example, sedatives and other central nervous system depressants have an intensified effect in the elderly and only small doses of these drugs should be given. In addition, the elderly may exhibit bizarre behavior when given a sedative or hypnotic; confusion, disorientation, irritability, and incontinence commonly occur. On the other hand, stimulants are often less effective in the elderly and large doses are usually necessary.

Decreased circulation, impaired liver and kidney function, and constipation can result in cumulative drug effects and toxicity. Since these conditions are common in the elderly, precautions must be taken to prevent toxic accumulation of drugs in the body.

The number of drugs given to an older person should be as few as possible, since a direct relationship exists between the number of drugs taken and drug error as well as drug interactions.

Since visual acuity is diminished in the elderly, all labels should be as legible as possible and preferably in large bold type. If drugs are to be administered intramuscularly and the patient is quite thin or emaciated, it is usually advisable to use a subcutaneous needle rather than an intramuscular needle.

ADMINISTRATION OF MEDICINES TO INFANTS AND CHILDREN

CALCULATION OF DRUG DOSAGES

The responsibility of drug administration to patients on pediatric services requires of nurses a specific knowledge and technique. Physicians prescribe the dosage of medication, but it is the nurse's responsibility to know the safe dosage range of any medication administered to children. A standard dosage of medication is nonexistent in pediatrics; medications are ordered according to the weight or body surface area of the child. Pharmaceutical companies continue to supply most medications in a standard adult dosage strength, and the nurse must calculate the correct dosage before administering the medication.

Since many pharmacology textbooks or drug reference books are geared to standard adult dosages, the nurse must have other resources for estimating safe dosages for children. The methods used to calculate a safe dosage for an individual child are based on the weight or body surface area of the child. Following are some formulas for calculating estimated safe dosages. The formula based on weight is preferred whenever possible since it is considered most accurate.

1 $\dfrac{\text{Average adult dose} \times \text{Weight of child in pounds}}{150} = \text{Estimated safe dose}$

Example: How much aspirin should a 1-year-old child weighing 21 pounds receive if the average adult dose is 10 grains?

$$\dfrac{\overset{10}{(\text{grains})} \times \overset{21}{(\text{weight in pounds})}}{150} = \text{gr. } 1^2/_5$$

*2 $\dfrac{\text{Average adult dose} \times \text{Age of child in years}}{\text{Age} + 12} = \text{Estimated safe dose}$

Example: How much atropine sulfate should an 8-year-old child receive if the adult dose is gr. $^1/_{150}$?

$$\dfrac{8}{8 + 12} \times \text{gr. } ^1/_{150} = \text{gr. } ^1/_{375} = \dfrac{\text{Estimated}}{\text{safe dose}}$$

*3 $\dfrac{\text{Average adult dose} \times \text{Age in months}}{150} = \text{Estimated safe dose}$

Example: The adult dose of atropine is 0.6 mg. How much should a 2-month-old infant receive?

$$\dfrac{0.6 \times 2}{150} = \dfrac{1.2}{150} = .008 \text{ mg.}$$

A nurse preparing calculated dosages of digitalis, insulin, barbiturates, and narcotics should have the calculations as well as the prepared medication dosage checked by another nurse before the drug is administered. Pediatric dosages are often minute, and a slight mistake in calculating the amount of medication to be administered results in greater proportional error.

Body surface area as a basis. More than 100 years ago, Hufeland suggested that drug doses should be calculated on size or a proportional amount of body surface area (BSA) to weight. Many physicians continue to use weight as the basis for calculating drug doses and body surface area for calculating fluid requirements. Most clinicians advocate using body surface area for determining drug dosage for adults as well as children. Physicians usually carry a simple slide rule or nomogram such as the West nomogram

---

*Age alone does not provide a good basis for calculating estimated safe doses. A 1-month-old infant could weigh 3 pounds, 7 pounds, or 16 pounds.

Figure 6-12

BSA is indicated where straight line that connects height and weight levels intersects BSA column or, if patient is about average size, from weight alone (enclosed area). (Modified from data of E. Boyd by C. D. West. From Shirkey and Barba.)

(Figure 6-12) to make rapid conversions from weight alone.

Although the previously stated rules have been devised for relating adult doses to infants and children, it must be emphasized that there are *no* rules or charts that are adequate to guarantee safety of dosage at any age, particularly in the neonate. None of these methods takes into account all variables, particularly individual tolerance differences. Astute, accurate nursing observations of the reactions of individual children to drugs can be of great assistance as the physician chooses drugs and regulates their dosage.

SOME VARIABLES AFFECTING DRUG RESPONSES IN NEONATES, INFANTS, AND CHILDREN

The pharmacologic effects of a drug are determined by the drug's action and the individual receiving the drug. Since the biochemical makeup of individuals may be markedly different, the wide variety of responses to drugs is not surprising, even among adults. The introduction of other variables such as maturation processes and maturity accentuate physiologic and biochemical differences in infants and children. Many articles have appeared on the subject of iatrogenic damage caused by drugs in the fetus, premature infant, and full-term newborn infant. The precautions and dangers of giving drugs to an immature organism can be readily summed up by saying that *most* drugs can be harmful to the immature neonate and *very few* drugs are indicated in his care.

Other variables that add to the problems of drug responses in children are absorption, distribution, biotransformation, excretion, developmental effects, difficulty in evaluating drug response, and actual administration of drug. Add to these variables the influence of disease on an easily disturbed acid-base equilibrium, and there exists a situation that frequently calls for constant observation of a child by physicians and nurses.

Immaturity and maturation process. Pharmaceutical researchers have done few studies on the reactions of drugs in very young animals. Thus there is little basis for knowledge of drug action and toxicity in children except as they may have been delineated in mature animal studies. Immaturity may alter drug actions and toxicities because of inability to excrete medications as rapidly as necessary for the prescribed dosage. Hopefully, future research will give a sounder basis for choice of drugs in immature organisms. The need for this type of research as well as the need for pediatric pharmacologists is evident.

During the neonatal period, there is rapid physical growth and daily changes in organ functions produced by biochemical fluctuations within the cells. If enzyme systems responsible for metabolizing drugs are not fully developed, drugs may have profound effects on the developmental processes occurring in the child. Histologic and laboratory studies have demonstrated that in early infancy normal kidney function is significantly different from that of an adult. The newborn infant has fewer glomeruli than the adult, and there is diminished or immature reserve capacity. This is of critical importance when administering drugs excreted via the renal system.

Drug administration routes. Even assuming that nurses have some knowledge of medications and some experience and skill in giving medications to adult patients, they will find the administration of medications to infants and children challenging, as well as frustrating at times. The ability to give injections skillfully will enhance their security and help to successfully gain a child's cooperation when giving injections. A sound knowledge of growth and development will also provide the nurse with information as to how a child at a certain age might be approached, whether trying to reason with him will help or hinder the process, and also whether as-

sistance will be needed in holding the child securely. Many of the principles of safe administration of medications apply to all age groups, but children are different from adults, and the nurse has certain added responsibilities.

Ideally, a nurse who has established a positive relationship with a child will find it easier to secure his cooperation when administering medications. The child may also find it easier to accept the discomforts associated with injections and some oral medications from the nurse he associates with daily hygiene, feeding, holding, play, and happy times. In addition, the nurse will experience fewer feelings of guilt when it is realized that the child sees the nurse as someone who brings him pleasure and comfort most of the time, as well as some discomfort necessary to his getting well.

Regardless of what kinds of external stimuli produce fear or anxiety in a child, his natural response will be to strike out at the frustration or avoid it. By accepting this behavior as a natural response to some type of frustration or discomfort, the nurse will be able to deal with it and will be able to be honest with the child by telling him when a medication or procedure will be unpleasant or painful.

Many children are courageous, or like to be considered so, and appealing to their courage is sometimes effective. A child 4 years old or over may choose to hold his own medicine cup, to drink unassisted, and to take his pills from the container without any assistance from the nurse. Because of the sense of achievement that follows, he may want to save the medicine cups to show his mother and father.

Honest explanations to children are essential, and the timing and type of explanation should be geared to his ability to perceive and understand. Each child has a right to some explanation of any procedure that concerns him. For the child 2 years of age or younger very simple explanations such as "I have some medicine for you to drink" or "I have an injection to give you, and it will hurt a little" will be sufficient. Long explanations to children up through 5 years of age do little more than delay his anticipated pain and increase his anxiety or his fear. Telling a child of 4 to stop (when he has responded to being told that he is to receive a medication with kicking, hitting, or other avoidance behavior) only conveys to the child that he is not understood and that he will receive little or no help with his feelings of frustration.

Oral medications. Success in administering oral medications usually requires a kind but firm approach with a positive attitude. There should be no evidence of doubt in the nurse's choice of words or tone of voice that the child will take his medicines. The nurse might say: "Jimmy, it's time to take your yellow medicine." This is an indication that he is expected to cooperate and to do it willingly. An unwise approach that reveals doubt on the part of the nurse might be: "I have your yellow pill, Jimmy. Will you take it for me, please?"

Nurses should by all means be aware of the taste of medicines they are giving to anyone, adult or child, so that they can answer such questions as: "Does it taste bad? Will it burn my mouth?" The nurse who knows what a medication tastes like might then reply: "It tastes like cherry to me. Tell me what it tastes like to you." Often the child will accept the suggestion to taste and find out. However, if the medication is bad tasting, attempting deceit or lying to the child is pointless.

Disagreeable tasting medications should be disguised if at all possible. Small amounts of honey, syrup, jam, fruit, and some fruit juices are suitable sweet substances that might provide a vehicle for less palatable drugs. Pills can be crushed and suspended in small amounts of any of these. Many liquid medications are more readily swallowed by infants and children if they are mixed with any of the suggested sweet substances or diluted with a small amount of water. If large amounts of water or other substances are used and the child refuses to take all of the mixture, it is difficult to estimate the amount of medication the child received. Fortunately, many drugs are available in the form of syrups or suspensions that are palatable and well suited for administration to infants and children. The following suggestions may be helpful:

1 Parents are frequently good sources of information about successful methods or vehicles for giving medications to their children.

2 Try to avoid the use of essential foods such as milk, cereal, or orange juice, since the child may become conditioned against future acceptance of that food in his diet.

3 Never underestimate the reaction of a child. He may not require that the taste of his medication be disguised.

4 A sip of fruit juice, a popsicle, or a mint-flavored substance before and after the administration of an unpalatable medicine may effectively dull its taste.

5 Sugarless vehicles such as those sweetened by saccharin should be used to disguise the taste of medications given to diabetic children or those on a ketogenic diet.

6 Honey and syrup are ideal for suspending drugs that do not dissolve easily in water.

7 Since fruit syrups are usually acid in reaction, they should not be used for medicines that react in an acid medium (for example, sodium bicarbonate, soluble barbiturates, and salicylates).

8 Elixirs have an alcohol base that, when undiluted, may cause the child to cough and choke. Small amounts of water added to elixirs of phenobarbital, chloral hydrate, and the like will make them easier to swallow.

9 Much nursing time will be saved if the child's care plan is utilized to communicate the most successful method of administering medications.

It is relatively easy to give oral medications to neonates and young infants, but caution must be exercised to prevent aspiration. It is important to give the medications slowly and in small amounts to avoid causing the infant to choke. Liquid medications may be administered via nipple, plastic medicine cup, plastic dropper, or a plastic syringe without the needle. Glass cups, droppers or syringes should be avoided at all costs because of the obvious danger of breakage in the child's mouth. A dropper or syringe is best suited for placing a liquid medication along one side of the infant's tongue. Older infants and toddlers seem to prefer to take their medications from a plastic medicine cup. If the child is held or placed in a sitting position, he will be less likely to aspirate the medication than if he is lying on his back. When administering a medication with a dropper or syringe, the nurse may purse the infant's lips with one hand to keep the medicine from running out of his mouth.

If the child is still refusing to cooperate after

explanations and encouragement, the nurse may have to ask the child whether he is going to take the medication himself or whether he would like the nurse to give it to him. Physical coercion is seldom necessary, but if and when it is, it should be a mild form used with dispatch and firmness, since there is danger of aspiration. It is important, however, not to combine force with anger, nor should force be resorted to because one nurse has been unable to administer the medication. Careful consideration should be given to such factors as: Why does the child resist? Does he disapprove only of this one nurse? Have his past experiences with medications given at home or in the hospital frightened him? Will forcing a medication cause a struggle that will counteract the effects of the drug if the medication is intended to sedate the child? The use of mild force, when necessary, should be explained to the child in such a way that he gets the idea that this form of treatment is necessary to his well-being. The cooperation of the child cannot be gained if he feels that force was used as punishment for his inability to cooperate, and often his confidence in all personnel will be lost.

Intramuscular injections. The principles and techniques of the administration of injections are the same for children as they are for adults. There has been considerable concern, however, about the advisability of using the buttocks as a site for intramuscular injections for infants and children. Many authorities believe that the risk of sciatic nerve injury is too great to warrant the use of this site of administration. The sciatic nerve is the largest nerve in the body, and its normal pathway is the hollow midway between the ischial tuberosity and the greater trochanter, covered by the gluteus maximus muscle. This, however, varies a great deal from individual to individual. In addition, the small size of the gluteal mass in the infant or neonate and the potential neurotoxicity of many drugs enhance the possibility of iatrogenic trauma secondary to intramuscular injections. According to some authorities, iatrogenic trauma of this kind is the leading cause of sciatic neuropathy in infancy. A lesion at this height of the sciatic nerve is usually tragically associated with marked permanent disability. The gluteal musculature develops

more fully after the child begins to walk, so it is inadvisable to use this site for injection until he has at least reached the toddler stage.

The quadriceps muscle of the midanterolateral aspect of the thigh is the site of choice for injections in infants, children, and adults. Injection sites should be rotated frequently, and if multiple injections over a long period of time necessitate the use of the buttocks in older children, the nurse must be extremely cautious. A method that is relatively safe and adaptable for older children is to establish landmarks by placing the thumb on the trochanter and the middle finger on the iliac crest. The index finger is placed midway between the thumb and middle finger and above them to form a triangle. The index finger indicates the safe area for the injection site. Anatomic landmarks must always be felt, not arrived at by looking at the child, because of individual differences in body structure. Other sites that can be utilized are the deltoid area and the soft flesh inferior to the crest of the ilium.

As stated previously, injections should be given as rapidly as possible to avoid prolonging a fear-provoking experience. The child must be adequately restrained before attempting to give an injection. Children will often tell the nurse that they will "hold still" for an injection, but a wise pediatric nurse will be sure to have another person there to hold the patient so that the injection can be administered safely. Stabilizing a child over 4 years of age in order to give an injection in the thigh may require more than two persons.

Rectal administration. When oral administration is difficult or contraindicated, the rectal route is often advised. A number of drugs are available in suppository form, for example, sedatives, aspirin, and antiemetics. Suppositories made with a cocoa butter base will melt rapidly at normal body temperature, releasing the drug for absorption. After a suppository is inserted in an infant, the buttocks should be held or taped together for 5 to 10 minutes to relieve pressure on the anal sphincter and thereby help to ensure retention and absorption of the medication. Infants and children with diarrhea, however, may easily expel suppositories with their explosive stools. Likewise, a suppository inserted into a child with a constipation problem or a rectum full of stool will be surrounded with stool with little chance for absorption of its contents.

Pharmacists and nurses often have to cut suppositories to obtain correct doses. This is a dangerous practice, since all of the medication might be contained in one area of the suppository. If divided doses must be administered, the pharmacist should be the one to divide the suppository; they should be cut lengthwise and weighed in order to ensure as accurate a dosage as possible.

Nose drops, ear drops, and eye drops. Aqueous preparations of nose drops are the only safe preparations to use, if it is deemed necessary to use them at all, because of the danger of aspiration. Many nose drop preparations act as vasoconstrictors and prolonged or excessive use may be harmful. Infants are nose breathers, and nasal congestion will inhibit their sucking. For this reason, nose drops should be instilled 20 minutes to 1 half hour before feedings.

To instill nose drops:

1 Hold the infant in your arm, allowing his head to fall back over the edge of your arm, or place a small pillow under the shoulders and allow his head to fall back over the edge of the pillow.
2 Place your free arm so that the forearm is around the far side of the child's head, stabilizing his head between your forearm and your body. Use your hand to stabilize his arms and hands.
3 With your free hand you can then instill the prescribed drops with minimum struggle and maximum accuracy.

The instillation of ear drops requires a knowledge of anatomic structure, since the shape of the auditory canal of a young child is different from that of an adult. In children 3 years of age or younger the nurse must gently pull the pinna of the ear slightly down and straight back to properly instill ear drops. In older children and adults, the pinna should be held up and back. Gentle massage of the area immediately anterior to the ear will facilitate the entry of the drops into the ear canal.

Eye drop instillation is done in the same way on children as with adults. The lower lid of the eye is gently pulled down and out so that it has a cup effect into which the correct number of drops is instilled. Many eyedrops cause a burning sensation in the eye for a few seconds, so if both eyes are to be medicated it is wise to do the second instillation quickly before the patient begins to blink and tear as a reaction to the burning sensation occurring in the first eye medicated.

Aqueous preparations of nose, ear, and eye drops may support the growth of bacteria and fungi. For this reason small volumes of such medications are ordered and should be used for only *one* individual (not shared by family members). Examination of these types of drops for clearness of fluid (hold the dropper up to the light) is a good method of checking for contamination. Contaminated fluid will appear cloudy when held up to the light.

Eye and ear drops are more comfortably tolerated if they are warmed before instillation. This can be achieved by running warm water over the side of the bottle without the label or immersing the bottle in some warm water in a medicine cup. Even carrying the bottle in your pocket for half an hour or so will take the chill off of the drops.

Intravenous medications. The use of intravenous drug therapy is widespread on most pediatric services for several reasons. In children with vomiting and diarrhea, medications given by mouth may be vomited so that precious time is lost in drug management of disease processes. These same children may have poor absorption of drugs and fluids as a result of dehydration or peripheral vascular collapse, so that drugs administered via the intramuscular route may be ineffective. Prior to the now widespread use of the midanterolateral thigh muscle for intramuscular injections, there was a great danger of sciatic neuropathy and other neurologic sequelae associated with injections in the gluteal area. For these reasons, as well as the advantages associated with administering long-term drug therapy more accurately via a relatively simple vehicle, the use of intravenous therapy has increased greatly. Considering the dangers and contraindications of intravenous drug therapy, however, its use must be justifiable.

The pediatric nurse responsible for the *administration* of intravenous drugs may find the following suggestions helpful.

1 Intravenous drug therapy should only be utilized when other channels of drug administration have failed. Pediatric nurses skilled in the administration of medications to children via other routes may greatly influence the physician's decisions regarding channels of drug administration.

2 Too rapid intravenous injection causes "speed shock": rapid fall in blood pressure, respiratory irregularity, incoagulability of the blood, and even death.

3 Once a drug is injected intravenously, it is impossible to exert further control except by specific antidote.

4 Drugs must be properly diluted. Too much emphasis cannot be placed on the caution: give the smallest possible dose at the slowest possible rate.

Most older children may be given fluids or drugs intravenously following the same principles and techniques utilized for adults. The younger and smaller the child, the greater the difficulty of administration and the greater the dangers associated with it.

Neonates, infants, and children must be adequately restrained so as not to dislodge or pull out an infusion needle once it is in place. Some of the following may be helpful hints to the nurse *caring* for a patient receiving intravenous therapy.

1 The needle should be fixed with plastic tape.

2 When a loop of tubing directly above the needle is secured to the tape, it relieves some of the pressure on the needle.

3 Since most children move about or are restless, it will be necessary to support the limb and immobilize the site of intravenous therapy.

4 Support should extend to the joints above and below the site (with arm boards or intravenous boards).

5 Tape backed with gauze can be used to secure the limb to the support.

6 If the infusion bottle is too high, it will increase the pressure in the vein and cause fluid seepage into the surrounding tissues.

Other conditions influencing the dosage of drugs in infants and children. Laboratory studies have shown that the same individual under almost identical situations at different time intervals will exhibit variations in measured drug responses. For example, frequent altering of drug dosage is often necessary in relation to insulin administration, digitalis administration, and oral enzyme therapy.

Some of the variables that influence drug dosage were mentioned briefly at the beginning of this section (for example, age, size, weight, and immaturity of the child, and routes and time of administration). A few other variables will be considered here with some specific examples.

Tolerance to drugs exists in infants and children just as it does in adults, and the same principles are followed to handle such a problem. Either a larger dose of the drug is administered or a different drug is selected, preferably one without cross tolerance.

As previously discussed, the dosage of most agents is roughly proportional to the age, weight, and size of the child. According to Barnett, opiates, for example, can be given in dosages proportional to body weight, 0.15 to 0.2 mg. of morphine sulfate per kilogram of body weight being a safe level. On the other hand, infants are more sensitive than adults to a few drugs, so that smaller dosages than those proportional to weight and size are recommended. Atropine sulfate is one of these drugs. For many years atropine was used in the medical treatment of pyloric stenosis as an antispasmodic to relax the pylorospasm. The reason for sensitivity to atropine in infants is not well known, but it may be contingent on the immaturity of the central nervous system. Products less toxic than atropine itself (atropine methylnitrate or Eumydrin) are being utilized with much greater success in the treatment of pylorospasm.

Among the drugs to which older infants and children are more tolerant are epinephrine, barbiturates, and many of the other biologic preparations. Pentobarbital (Nembutal) is such an example. Roughly half of an adult dose will be easily tolerated by a child 2 to 4 years of age and one fourth of the adult dose by an infant of 6 months. Long-term experience with adult doses of pentobarbital given to children ages 3 to 6 in preparation for heart catheterizations has greatly influenced clinical opinions of its tolerance levels in children.

Infants and children have been shown to be more resistant to the effects of digitalis preparations than are adults. At any age, however, digitalis preparations should be administered based on individual tolerance, and suggested safe dosages should be used only as a guide.

Presence of disease. The presence of disease or any basic abnormality in a child may alter his response to drugs. For example, in children with any of the metabolic diseases such as diabetes mellitus, melituria, galactosemia, or phenylketonuria, one can expect altered drug responses. Since the liver, kidneys, intestines, and lungs are the chief channels of drug elimination, the presence of disease in any one of these organs will require that medications be administered with much knowledge and deliberation. It remains the nurse's responsibility in pediatrics to administer medications, to recognize and interpret the child's response to drug therapy, and to teach parents about the drugs their children are receiving. All ethical opportunities for learning about the pharmacodynamics of drugs should be maximally exploited by physicians and nurses alike so that children can benefit sooner from advances in medicine.

Pediatric nurses have a legal, moral, and ethical responsibility associated with drug administration to children. In addition to that, the responsibility of teaching children and parents about the drugs they are receiving, using sound knowledge of pharmacodynamics, has further expanded the nurse's role in relation to drug therapy. These factors, along with a knowledge of principles and techniques of drug administration to children and the application of knowledge of growth and development, will greatly enhance the pediatric nurse's ability to be the decision maker in rapidly changing health care delivery systems.

QUESTIONS

For study and review

1 What are some of the habits that you think would help you to develop safety and accuracy in the administration of drugs?
2 Make a list of precautions that should be observed in a home to prevent accidents in the care and handling of medicines.
3 Write out a plan of instruction for one of your patients who expects to go home and will continue to take several of the medicines that he has been taking while in the hospital. What explanation does the patient need to help him understand what to do, how to do it, and when to do it?

4 How would you interpret the following orders?
Sherry wine $\bar{3}$ ii t.i.d. a.c.
Nitroglycerin gr. $^1/_{100}$ stat. and p.r.n.
Mineral oil and milk of magnesia $\bar{3}$ ss āā b.i.d. and p.r.n.
Phenobarbital gr. ss q.i.d.
5 What advantages does oral administration of drugs have over parenteral administration (subcutaneous, intramuscular, or intravenous)?
6 What is meant by buccal administration of a drug? When is this form of administration used?
7 When are drugs most likely to be administered intravenously?
8 What would you do if one of your patients refused to take the oral medications prescribed for him by his physicians?
9 What precautions should be taken and what are the responsibilities of the nurse for narcotics stored in the clinical area?
10 What length and guage of needle are usually recommended for the administration of drugs to adults by the following routes?
  a. intramuscular
  b. subcutaneous
  c. intravenous
  d. intradermal
11 What is meant by the following?
  a. Store in a tight container.
  b. Keep in a cool place.
  c. Do not expose to direct light.
  d. Do not use if solution is cloudy.
12 Write a paper on the predictions for the future in relation to drug administration in hospitals. Information can be obtained from nursing and pharmacy journals.
13 Briefly explain the relationship of weight and drug dosage in children.
14 Explain why the variable of age alone is not a good basis for calculating safe drug doses for children or adults.
15 Identify and describe four conditions or variables that influence or alter drug dosage in children.
16 Identify and describe four factors that might influence a nurse's ability to administer oral medications to a 4-year-old child.
17 Using the formula based on the weight of the child in pounds, calculate the estimated safe dose of Benadryl for a 1-year-old child weighing 21 pounds if the average adult dose is 50 mg.
18 Identify and explain five factors that will enable a nurse to give an injection most effectively.
19 Identify and explain the responsibilities of a nurse administering drug therapy.

Objective questions

Select the answer that in your opinion is the one best answer.
20 If a drug is injected into the cavity of a joint where its

effect is limited to the tissue of the joint, its action is said to be:

 a. general   c. systemic
 b. local   d. selective

21 Which of the following channels of administration is likely to afford least dependable absorption?

 a. oral   c. intravenous
 b. intraspinal   d. rectal

22 Which of the following must be characteristic of a drug if it is to be administered by inhalation?

 a. volatile   c. nontoxic
 b. sterile   d. water soluble

23 Which of the following routes of administration will afford the most rapid rate of absorption and action?

 a. intramuscular   c. rectal suppository
 b. sublingual   d. subcutaneous

24 Which of the following routes of administration is least likely to cause a systemic reaction?

 a. rectal suppository
 b. application of ointment to the skin
 c. inhalation
 d. spraying of a drug onto mucous membrane

REFERENCES

Ballard, B. E., and Nelson, E.: Physicochemical properties of drugs that control absorption rate after subcutaneous implantation, J. Pharmacol. Exp. Ther. **135:**120, 1972.

Budd, R.: We changed to unit dose system, Nurs. Outlook, **19:**116, 1971.

DiPalma, J. R.: Clinical pharmacist: New member of the health team, R.N. **32:**57, 1969.

DiPalma, J. R.: Drill's pharmacology in medicine, ed. 4, New York, 1971, McGraw-Hill Book Co.

Donn, R.: Intravenous admixture incompatibility, Am. J. Nurs. **71:**325, 1971.

Flack, H. L., et al.: The current status of parenteral hyperalimentation, Am. J. Hosp. Pharm. **28:**326, 1971.

Frazier, W. M.: Administration routes of parenteral injections, Drug Intell. **3:**42, 1968.

Goodman, L. S., and Gilman, A.: The pharmacological basis of therapeutics, ed. 4, New York, 1970, The Macmillan Co.

Levine, M. E.: Breaking through the medication mystique, Am. J. Nurs. **70:**799, 1970.

Lowenthal, W.: Factors affecting drug absorption, Am. J. Nurs. **73:**1391, 1973.

McDonald, D. E.: Prefilling syringes in the hospital pharmacy, Am. J. Hosp. Pharm. **29:**223, 1972.

Modell, W.: Drugs of choice 1976-1977, St. Louis, 1976, The C. V. Mosby Co.

Monahan, J. J., and Webb, J. W.: Intravenous infusion pumps—an added dimension to parenteral therapy, Am. J. Hosp. Pharm. **29:**54, 1972.

Pitel, M.: The subcutaneous injection, Am. J. Nurs. **71:**76, 1971.

Ryan, P. B., et al.: In line filtration—a method of minimizing contamination in intravenous therapy, Bull. Parent. Drug Assoc. **27:**1, 1973.

Shirkey, H. C., editor: Pediatric therapy, ed. 5, St. Louis, 1975, The C. V. Mosby Co.

Stuart, D. M.: Unit dose medication, Pharmindex, April 1973.

Turco, S., and King, R. E.: Sterile dosage forms: Their preparation and clinical application, Philadelphia, 1974, Lea & Febiger.

Turco, S., and Davis, N.: Clinical significance of particulate matter: A review of the literature, Hosp. Pharm. **8:**137, 1973.

CHAPTER 7

Pharmacodynamics

Empiric versus scientific medicine
Theories of drug action
Physiologic processes mediating drug action
Adverse responses to drugs

Because of the constantly increasing number of drugs utilized in medical therapeutics and the nurse's expanded responsibility in this area, it is essential that the nurse have a coherent, rational, and scientifically accurate understanding of the principles underlying pharmacology. The time is long past when anyone can expect to acquire complete knowledge about all drugs. Thousands of drugs exist, requiring that health professionals have some fundamental theoretical framework through which to approach their study and understanding of drug therapy.

Historically, the administration of drugs has been a prominent nursing task. This task, however, is changing in nature and prominence. A shift in responsibility is occurring away from the actual administration of drugs to greater responsibility in relation to other aspects of drug therapy. The nurse's expanded role currently includes a variety of functions, all of which are predicated upon a sound understanding of drug action. In many health care delivery settings, for example, the nurse is no longer the primary administrator and dispenser of drugs. In such settings, the nurse's responsibility has shifted to assuring safe administration of drugs by a variety of specially educated health workers and to observing and interpreting the patient's response to drug therapy. However, the moral, ethical, and legal responsibility of drug administration remains the nurse's. In addition, other nursing roles in relation to drug therapy have been devel-

oped and expanded. Today, more than before, nurses have the responsibility of *teaching* patients about the drugs they are receiving. They have a *data-gathering role* in relation to the patient's previous drug therapy and present and past responses to drug therapy, as exemplified in the function of obtaining a drug history from the patient. They are *decision-makers* regarding p.r.n. medications. By virtue of their interpersonal skills, they may also function as *potentiators* of drug effects. Nurses are *communicators* of knowledge and observations to other health care professionals, notably to the physician who prescribes drug therapy. There is also a change in nurses' roles in relation to drug prescriptions. In some states, nurse practice acts have been changed to give nurse practitioners limited authority in the prescribing of drugs.

These responsibilities require more than memorization of specific drugs, their actions, and their dosages. Rather, their effective implementation is predicated upon a sound comprehension of the theories of drug action, knowledge the nurse can transfer to the individual patient with a specific diagnosis and definable, individualistic needs. Such a background necessitates knowledge of theories of drug action, physiologic processes mediating drug action, variables affecting drug action, and unusual and adverse responses to drug therapy.

The field of pharmacodynamics encompasses such theoretical knowledge. It is defined as the **87** study of biochemical and physiologic effects of drugs and their mechanisms of action. As such, it is concerned with the response of tissues to specific chemical agents and with the absorption, distribution, biotransformation, and excretion of that chemical agent in the body.

EMPIRIC VERSUS SCIENTIFIC MEDICINE

Early medicines could be described as empiric remedies—that is, experience with them revealed that they were sometimes useful in certain conditions, but very little was actually known about the reasons for their therapeutic effectiveness. This type of remedy has been replaced by drugs whose effects are often highly predictable and whose action in the body has, to a great extent, been substantiated through scientific research.

Once a chemical agent is found to be biologically active, pharmacologists perform a variety of tests. The major studies performed include: (1) investigation of the drug's site and mechanism of action; (2) determinations of the drug's metabolic fate in the body; (3) determination of dose-response relationships—that is, how much of the agent is required to produce various effects; and (4) investigation of structure-activity relationships—that is, exploration of the extent to which the agent's effects resemble those of other compounds that have similar chemical structures. A principal method of this scientific research in pharmacology is *biologic assay*, or *bioassay*, the study of the effect of a certain kind and certain amount of a drug upon living organisms.

In utilizing the method of bioassay, it is assumed that a definite quantity of a drug will always produce a certain response in the same animal or in animals of the same species. Methods of bioassay require rigorous statistical control in order to account for biologic variations (such as sex, age, and genetic background) that can exert a major influence on sensitivity to drugs and also in order to account for inevitable variations in laboratory conditions. In order to overcome such variables, reference standards

and international standards have been established, as mentioned in Chapter 3. Consequently, contemporary knowledge about drug effects is predicated upon knowledge of chemical structures of drugs, which enable the scientists to predict to some extent the effects of a drug in the body. It has been found, for example, that drugs containing a certain molecular structure have a tendency to produce allergic responses in patients. Hence, any new drug with this general type of molecular structure may have a tendency to produce hypersensitivity in some patients.

It must be said that scientists still do not have a definite theoretical scheme that allows them to predict accurately which chemical groupings will have specific desired physiologic effects. The advances made in knowledge regarding the chemistry of proteins, the nature and behavior of enzymes, and the metabolism of microbes have contributed greatly to understanding the responses that living systems make to drugs.

THEORIES OF DRUG ACTION

The effects of drugs can be recognized only by alterations of a known physiologic function or process. That is, drugs may increase or diminish the normal functions of tissues or organs, but they cannot confer any new functions on them. For example, drugs may decrease or increase the normal rate of evacuation of the large intestine, or they may decrease the production of saliva. In exerting their effects, drugs can either return a function or process to a normal level or change it to be abnormal. For example, drugs used to treat anemia can restore the adequate production of red blood cells. On the other hand, drugs can decrease the rate of salivation in preoperative patients, which is an essentially abnormal state but a necessary one to decrease the surgical risk of aspiration.

When a drug enters a living system, one can think of its molecules immediately beginning to react with the molecules of the cells and tissues with which it comes in contact. The effects a drug produces must be regarded as ultimate consequences of complex physical and chemical interactions between the drug and molecules in the living organism. Therefore, in order to understand drug action, drug and tissue interactions at the molecular level must be studied.

The means by which drugs exert their effects is known as their mechanism of action. The mechanism of action of most drugs is believed to involve a chemical interaction between the drug and a functionally important component of the living system. Most drugs are believed to produce their effects by combining with cell membranes, enzymes, or other specialized components of cells. The interaction between the drug and the cell is presumed to change the function of the cell, thereby initiating biochemical and physiologic changes. According to some authorities, pharmacologically active compounds can be conceptually divided into two groups: those that are structurally specific and those that are not. Structural specificity refers to the ability of a drug to produce its effects by combining with a specific receptor. Structurally nonspecific drugs, on the other hand, do not combine with specific receptors and may instead penetrate into cells or accumulate in cell membranes.

STRUCTURALLY SPECIFIC DRUGS

Receptor theory of drug action. Structural specificity is an essential postulate of the receptor theory of drug action. Receptor theory hypothesizes that drugs are selectively active substances that have a special affinity for certain chemical groups or parts of cells and not for others. That is, drugs act at some sites to produce their characteristic biologic effects whereas their presence at other cells, tissues, or organs leads to no measurable biologic response. Therefore, receptor theory states, drugs exert their action by becoming attached to specialized regions of a cell. The cellular components with which drugs interact to produce their characteristic biologic effects are called *receptors*. The relationship of a drug to its receptor has often been likened to the fit of a key into a lock. That is, some sort of reciprocal, or complementary, relationship exists between the chemical structure of the drug molecule and the drug receptor. The drug must interact by combining or binding with the

macromolecular tissue element at the site of action in order to produce its characteristic biologic effects. Therefore, there must be some forces that not only attract the drug to its receptors but also hold it in combination with the receptor long enough to initiate the chain of biochemical reactions leading to the drug effect. It is believed that drug receptor binding may result from the formation of hydrogen, covalent, or ionic bonds or from weak binding forces that operate when any atoms are brought together.

The term *affinity* is used to describe the propensity of a drug to be found at a given receptor site and the term *efficacy* is used to describe the drug's ability to initiate biologic activity as a result of such binding. A drug that combines with receptors and initiates a sequence of biochemical and physiologic changes is said to possess both properties and is termed an *agonist*. Drugs that are agonists improve the action of a cell component by modifying the molecule in order to localize or intensify its action. However, most drugs are *antagonists*, designed to inhibit or counteract effects caused by other drugs or undesired effects caused by cellular components during illness. A *competitive antagonist* has an affinity for the same receptor site as an agonist; the competition with the agonist for the site inhibits the action of the agonist; increasing the concentration of the agonist tends to overcome the inhibition. Competitive inhibition responses are usually reversible. A *noncompetitive antagonist* combines with different parts of the receptor mechanism and inactivates the receptor so that the agonist cannot be effective regardless of its concentration. Noncompetitive antagonist effects are considered to be irreversible or nearly so. *Partial agonists* have affinity and some efficacy but may antagonize the action of other drugs that have greater efficacy. Not infrequently, antagonists share some structural common denominators with their agonists.

Because of some basic similarities between the receptor theory and theories of enzymatic action, many drugs are thought to produce their effects by combining with enzymes. Those drugs that are believed to combine with enzymes are thought to do so by virtue of their structural resemblance to an enzyme's substrate molecule (the substance acted upon by an enzyme). A drug may resemble an enzyme's substrate so closely that it may combine with the enzyme instead of with the normal substrate. Drugs resembling enzyme substrates are termed *antimetabolites* and can either block normal enzymatic action or result in the production of other substances with unique biochemical properties. The enzyme, then, becomes the receptor for the drug. However, while enzymes may be receptors, not all receptors are enzymes.

Rate theory of drug action. The rate theory assumes that the most important factor determining drug action is the rate at which drug-receptor combinations take place. It postulates that if a drug-receptor complex dissociates rapidly, it has high efficacy. Conversely, if there is slow dissociation, there is firm binding, prolonged occupancy, and low efficacy. Therefore, drug antagonism is associated with slow kinetics and drug agonism with fast kinetics.

The validity of rate theory is controversial at this time, although it does explain drug phenomena in quantitative as well as qualitative terms.

STRUCTURALLY NONSPECIFIC DRUGS

It is not to be concluded from the previous discussion that all drugs operate through receptor mechanisms. Some drugs demonstrate no structural specificity and presumably act by more general effects on cell membranes and cellular processes. These drugs may penetrate into cells or accumulate in cellular membranes where they interfere, by physical or chemical means, with some cell function or some fundamental metabolic processes. Cell membranes are complex lipoprotein structures that regulate the flow of ions and metabolites in a highly selective manner, thereby maintaining an electrochemical gradient between the interior and exterior surfaces of the cell. Structurally nonspecific drugs are exemplified by the general anesthetics, which are lipid-soluble compounds of unrelated chemical structure but having similar properties. It is believed that general anesthetics alter the properties of lipids in cell membranes of nerves rather than acting on specific receptors.

Other structurally nonspecific drugs may act by biophysical means that do not affect cellular or enzymatic functions. Drugs acting as a result of their obvious physical properties include the ointments and emollients. Hydrophilic indigestible substances exert a cathartic action because of their physical action on the bowel. The interaction of a molecule like lead with an antidotal drug is a true chemical reaction that produces biologic effects. It is not considered a receptor interaction because there are no macromolecular tissue elements involved. Detergents, alcohol, oxidizing agents such as hydrogen peroxide, and phenol derivatives such as Lysol are also structurally nonspecific and act by irreversibly destroying the functional integrity of the living cell.

PHYSIOLOGIC PROCESSES MEDIATING DRUG ACTION

As previously mentioned, pharmacodynamics deals not only with mechanisms of drug action but also with the study of a drug's process through the body. The fate of drugs in the body includes everything that happens to a drug from the time the foreign chemical enters the biologic system until it and all of its products have been eliminated from the body.

In order to produce its effects, a drug must reach appropriate concentrations at its sites of action. That is, the molecules of the chemical must proceed from their point of entry into the body to the vicinity of the tissues with which they react. The concentration the drug attains at its site of action is influenced by a number of factors, the primary ones being: (1) the rate and extent to which the drug is *absorbed* into body fluids; (2) the rate and extent to which the drug is transported or *distributed* to sites of action or storage in the body; (3) the rate and extent to which the drug is *biologically transformed* in the body to breakdown products; and (4) the rate and extent to which the drug is *excreted* from the body via various routes.

Drug molecules free to move to sites of action, biotransformation, excretion, and tissue storage must cross membranes since these sites are all enclosed by membranes. A drug's passage across cell membranes is influenced by (1) the size and shape of the drug's molecules, (2) the degree of ionization of drug molecules, that is, the extent to which a drug's molecules have dissociated or separated into ions, or electrically charged particles, (3) the drug's solubility in lipids and water, or its lipoid (oil)/water coefficient, and (4) the pH of the medium.

Drugs may act at the outer membrane surface or inside the cell. Cell membrane, which consists of lipids and proteins, is penetrated at intervals by aqueous channels or pores through which small water-soluble molecules (dimensions smaller than those of the pores) and ions (e.g., K^+, Cl^-) pass; this process is called *filtration*. Lipid-soluble molecules, like those in anesthetic gases, diffuse readily through cell membranes, a process called *passive diffusion*. The higher the lipid/water coefficient, the greater its lipid solubility and the greater the ease with which the drug moves from the fluids outside the cells into the lipid material in the cell membrane. Moderate sized water-soluble molecules as well as moderate sized ions, including the ionic form of most drugs, do not readily enter cells but require some means of transport. *Active transport* is believed to be conducted by "carriers" which form complexes with drug molecules on one surface of the membrane, carry them through the membrane, and then dissociate from them. Active transport requires an energy source and involves the movement of drug molecules against the concentration gradient (i.e., from areas of low concentration to areas of high concentration) or, in the case of ions, against the electrochemical potential gradient such as occurs with the "sodium pump." Active transport is usually more rapid than passive diffusion. *Facilitated diffusion* refers to the movement of drugs from areas of high concentration to areas of low concentration; an energy source is not required. All of the physiologic processes mediating drug action —absorption, distribution, biotransformation, and excretion—are predicated upon these transfer processes.

ABSORPTION

Absorption refers to the process by which a drug is transferred from its site of entry into the body to the circulating fluids of the body, i.e., the bloodstream and the lymphatic system. With the exception of locally acting drugs, all drugs must reach the bloodstream in order to be carried to their sites of action. Absorption of the drug from its site of administration is largely influenced by the following factors.

Routes of drug administration. A drug may enter the circulatory system either by being injected there directly—for example, intravenously—or by absorption from depots in which it has been placed. The routes of drug entry into the body can be classified into three categories: the enteral (drugs administered via any portion of the gastrointestinal tract); the parenteral (drugs administered by routes that bypass the gastrointestinal tract and that are generally given by injection, thereby avoiding the necessity for absorption across a mucosal barrier); and the percutaneous (drugs absorbed from mucous membranes, either through sublingual administration or by inhalation).

Generally, the oral route of drug administration is the safest, most convenient, and most economical method of drug administration. However, the frequent changes of the gastrointestinal environment produced by food, emotion, and physical activity make it the most unreliable and slowest of the commonly used routes in terms of both the amount and the rate of drug absorption. Generally, slowing the gastric emptying rate will decrease drug absorption and vice versa. This is why so many drugs are administered on an empty stomach with sufficient water to ensure their rapid passage into the small intestine where drug absorption is usually increased because of the larger surface area available to the dissolving drug. An additional limitation of the oral route of administration is that this route cannot be used for drugs that are susceptible to alteration by the biochemical processes involved in digestion. Insulin, for example, is destroyed by the digestive enzymes and must be administered by parenteral routes if it is to be absorbed. Drugs administered sublingually or rectally are not changed by the digestive processes, but sublingual drugs must be readily soluble and depend on the patient's ability to cooperate, while drug retention is frequently unpredictable with rectal administration. Parenteral administration affords relatively rapid drug absorption since the drugs bypass the epithelial barrier and absorption from these sites is more reliable than from enteral routes. The intravenous route of administration completely bypasses the process of absorption and this route represents the most rapid means of introducing drugs into the body. Inhalation drugs, such as gaseous or aerosal drugs, are also extremely rapidly absorbed from the respiratory tract or alveolar surfaces.

Drug solubility. In order to be absorbed, a drug must be in solution. The more soluble the drug, the more rapidly it will be absorbed. Therefore, oral drugs given in solution form are generally absorbed more quickly than drugs administered in capsule or tablet form. Moreover, because cell membranes contain a fatty acid layer, lipid solubility is a valuable attribute of a drug that is to be absorbed from the alimentary tract; this attribute is also necessary for drugs to cross the placental barrier. Because the skin has a lipid barrier, topically applied drugs are poorly absorbed, if at all. However, if this lipid barrier of the skin is altered, for example, by cuts, abrasions, or burns, toxic drug dosage may result. Chemicals and minerals that form insoluble precipitates in the gastrointestinal tract, such as barium salts, or drugs that are not soluble in water or lipids cannot be absorbed. Parenterally administered drugs prepared in oily vehicles, such as streptomycin, will be absorbed more slowly than drugs dissolved in water or isotonic sodium chloride.

Influence of pH. When in solution, drugs are a mixture of ionized and nonionized forms. Nonionized drug is lipid soluble and diffusible (referred to as *nonionic diffusion*); ionized drug is lipid insoluble and nondiffusible. The proportion of drug in the nonionized form depends on the dissociation constant of the drug (pK_a) and on the pH of the medium in which it is dissolved. Most drugs are weak acids or bases. In aqueous solutions drugs that are acid produce hydrogen ions (H^+); drugs that are bases produce hydroxyl ions (OH^-). A drug that is acidic tends to dissociate less in an acid medium while a drug that is a base will dissociate to a greater extent in an acid medium. The reverse occurs when the drugs are in a base medium.

In the stomach the pH is low (about 1.4), and drugs such as the barbiturates which are slightly acidic tend to remain in a nonionized state and thus are readily absorbed from this area. Morphine and quinine are slightly basic; they tend to ionize in the stomach and thus are poorly absorbed from this area. The neutralization of the stomach contents by giving sodium bicarbonate may facilitate the absorption of basic drugs in the stomach.

In the intestines the pH is higher (6 to 8). Nonionized basic drugs will tend to remain nonionized and be readily absorbed in this area while the reverse is true for acidic drugs. Plasma pH is about 7.4, and only drugs that are substantially nonionized in this pH will be widely distributed.

Urinary pH varies between 4.6 and 8.2 and affects the amount of drug reabsorbed in the renal tubule by passive diffusion. Weak acids are excreted more readily in alkaline urine and more slowly in acidic urine; the reverse is true for weak bases. In cases of poisoning by aspirin or phenobarbital, alkalinizing the urine can result in increased urinary drug excretion. However, acidifying or alkalinizing urine to promote drug excretion is seldom of great importance.

Local conditions at the site of administration. These local conditions include circulation to the site and the area of the absorbing surface. Generally, the more extensive the absorbing surface, the greater the absorption of the drug and the more rapid its effects. For example, anesthetics are very rapidly absorbed from the pulmonary epithelium because of its vast surface area and its vascularity. Circulation to the site of administration is also a significant factor in the absorption of parenteral drugs. A patient in shock, for example, may not respond to intramuscularly administered drugs because of poor peripheral circulation. Drugs injected intravenously, on the other hand, are placed directly into the circulatory system and are totally absorbed. This route of administration is desirable when speedy drug effects are necessary, but it carries the potential danger of achieving temporarily toxic effects in vital organs such as the heart or the brain.

Circulation to the site of administration can be externally manipulated in order to hasten or retard the rate of drug absorption. Local cooling of the site will hinder absorption, as will the application of a tourniquet proximally to the injection site. On the other hand, applying heat or friction to the site of administration will hasten absorption.

Drug concentration or dosage. Drugs administered in high concentrations or dosages are more rapidly absorbed than drugs administered in low concentrations. In certain situations, a drug may be initially administered in large doses that temporarily exceed the body's capacity for excretion of the drug. In this way, active drug levels are rapidly reached at the receptor site. Once an active drug level is established by such cumulation of effects, smaller daily doses of the drug can be administered to replace only the amount of the drug excreted since the previous dose. The initial and temporary overloading doses of the drug are *priming doses*, while the smaller daily doses are *maintenance doses*. Such manipulation of drug dosage is frequently used, for example, with digitalis and steroid preparations in acute situations.

Another way in which drug concentration can be manipulated is by pharmaceutical processing. It is possible to combine an active drug with a resin or another substance from which it is only slowly released or to prepare a drug in a vehicle that offers relative resistance to the digestive action of stomach contents (enteric coating). Enteric coatings on drugs are used for the following reasons: (1) to prevent decomposition of chemically sensitive drugs, (2) to prevent dilution of the drug before it reaches the intestine, (3) to prevent nausea and vomiting, and (4) to provide delayed action of the drug. Capsule forms of drugs are absorbed more rapidly than tablets because the powder inside capsules affords a larger surface area than the compressed tablet. Repository dosage forms are produced by suspension of a drug in a substance from which it is slowly released, producing uniform drug absorption for at least 8 hours or longer. For example, protamine zinc insulin is suspended in protamine for slow, sustained release so that its duration of action is 24 to 36 hours. Drug "Spansules" are gelatin capsules containing drug pellets having different coatings designed for timed release of the drug contained within. Advantages of this dosage form include decreased frequency of administration and prolonged maintenance of therapeutic effects. Disadvantages are related to possible failure of the sustained release mechanism, which could result in release of unexpectedly high and toxic levels of the drug or in therapeutically inadequate levels.

DISTRIBUTION

After a drug is absorbed or injected into the bloodstream, it is distributed throughout the body by means of the circulation. Drug distribution is the transport of a drug across cell membranes, resulting in accumulations of the drug in certain tissues. The rate of entry of a drug into the various tissues of the body depends upon the relative rate of perfusion and the permeability of the capillaries for the particular drug molecules. The distribution may be general or restricted. Some drugs cannot pass particular cell membranes and are restricted in their distribution, while other drugs, such as ethyl alcohol, can eventually be found in solution in all body fluids.

Differential distribution of drugs may result from the binding of a drug to plasma proteins and from the unequal passage of a drug across biologic membranes, most notably into the central nervous system and the placenta. The same kinds of bonds that are formed when a drug interacts with its receptor can be formed between drug molecules and other macromolecular tissue components. The difference in these bonds is that the drug-receptor combination leads to drug action, while binding with a nonreceptor substance does not. Binding of drugs can occur at sites of absorption, in plasma, or at extravascular sites, but the proteins of plasma appear to be the most common site of drug binding. Albumin is the protein with which the greatest variety of drugs combine. The binding of drugs decreases the concentration of free drug in circulation and prevents the drug from reaching its site of action in full concentrations. As the free drug is eliminated from the body more drug can be dissociated from the protein to replace what is lost. Other tissues of the body can also act as such reservoirs, or depots, for drugs. Some drugs have preferential sites of accumulation in certain tissues. For example, body fat has a high affinity for some drugs, such as thiopentone. Another common site of drug accumulation is muscle, which may be considered as a storage depot for a drug. The stored drug is in equilibrium with the amount of drug contained in plasma and is released as plasma levels are reduced. Consequently, plasma levels of the drug are maintained for longer periods and, therefore, pharmacologic effects are predicated upon the administration of initially adequate priming doses in order to saturate the storage depots or binding sites.

In relation to the passage of drugs into the central nervous system, it has long been noted that many drugs fail to penetrate into those tissues as readily as into other tissues. This phenomenon has led to the conceptualization of a "blood-brain barrier." Currently, this concept is undergoing scrutiny, and recent research indicates that what has been termed the "blood-brain barrier" is not an absolute barrier. It has been postulated that it is a quantitative rather than a qualitative difference in capillary permeability as compared with other tissues. Still, the fact remains that the distribution of some drugs will be more readily achieved into other parts of the body than into the central nervous system. There is a very slow rate of entry of water-soluble and ionized drugs, such as penicillin, into the brain and spinal cord. Lipid-soluble compounds, on the other hand, enter the brain easily and rapidly. Moreover, some drugs that have no effects on the central nervous system when administered systemically have striking effects when injected directly into the cerebrospinal fluid.

Passage of drugs across the placenta to the fetus is a well-established fact. Again, lipid-soluble substances diffuse across the placenta readily and other substances are assisted by energy-coupled specific transport systems. Some drugs that are easily transported across the placenta include steroids, narcotics, anesthetics, various teratogenic agents, and some antibiotics. The rate of maternal blood flow to the placenta limits the availability of the drug to the fetus. This explains why an alert infant can be delivered to an anesthetized mother, provided that delivery occurs within 10 to 15 minutes after the drug is administered to the mother. Long-term administration of drugs to the mother, however, may produce adverse effects on the fetus. For example, infants born to mothers dependent on narcotics will manifest withdrawal symptoms when the infants are no longer supplied with these drugs after delivery. Teratogenic effects of drugs also occur after exposure of the pregnant woman to certain toxic agents, especially if this occurs during early stages of fetal development.

BIOTRANSFORMATION

Most drugs, once absorbed and distributed, undergo metabolic changes, or biotransformation. This process, which usually takes place in the liver, converts the drug into products which are generally less active and more easily excreted than the original form. For example, most drugs are fat soluble, but the kidney excretes water-soluble compounds; therefore, one function of metabolism is to convert lipid-soluble drugs to water-soluble products.

The term *detoxication* has often been used to describe the metabolism of drugs, but it is not an optimally accurate conceptualization of the process. The term implies that all drugs are toxic to the body and that all are metabolized to less toxic products which is not always the case. Although most types of biotransformation result in inactivation of a drug, occasionally the result of this metabolic process is a more active compound that requires further biotransformation before being excreted. For example, the active ingredient of chloral hydrate is its metabolite, which must then undergo a second reaction to facilitate its excretion. In addition, drugs may be changed to other chemical forms or inactivated before excretion. In other instances, drugs may be excreted from the body unchanged, as is the case with ether, for example.

The chemical alterations of biotransformation are produced by enzyme systems in the blood and in all body cells, but particularly those of the liver. The hepatic enzyme systems responsible for the biotransformation of many drugs seem to be located in the hepatic endoplasmic reticulum and are generally called microsomes, because they are located in the microsomal fraction of the liver. These hepatic microsomal enzymes effect the process of biotransformation through two general classes of chemical reactions: the synthetic and the nonsynthetic. The synthetic chemical reactions, also called *coupling* or *conjugation*, involve the union of the drug (or its metabolite) with another substance. This chemical reaction generally produces a soluble, inactive product that is readily excreted. Nonsynthetic chemical reactions of drug metabolism include oxidation, hydrolysis, or reduction, which can result in activation, a change in activity, or inactivation of a drug.

Research indicates that drug metabolism can be depressed or stimulated. Depression of the microsomal drug-metabolizing system can be produced by conditions that have a deleterious effect on hepatic function, such as starvation and obstructive jaundice. Individuals with any type of hepatic disease, severe cardiovascular disease, or renal disease may be expected to have prolonged drug metabolism. Immaturity of drug-metabolizing enzymes in infants and degeneration of these enzymes in the aged also produce depression of biotransformation. In addition, some drugs are known to inhibit the metabolism of other drugs when they are administered simultaneously. If metabolism of drugs is delayed, cumulative drug effects may be expected and may be manifested as excessive or prolonged responses to ordinary doses of drugs. Stimulation of drug metabolism, on the other hand, may produce a state of apparent drug tolerance. A number of substances are also known to cause an increase in the activity of hepatic microsomal drug-metabolizing enzymes. These include CNS depressants, xanthines, pesticides, food preservatives, and dyes. It is possible that repeated administration of some drugs stimulates the formation of new microsomal enzymes. This is thought to be the case with some hypnotic drugs, whose effect diminishes with prolonged administration.

Biotransformation of drugs does not occur exclusively in the liver. The plasma, the kidneys, and the intestinal mucosa also contain microsomes and function to metabolize drugs, although to a lesser degree.

EXCRETION

A drug continues to act in the body until it is changed or excreted. Drug molecules, intact, changed, or inactivated, ultimately must be removed from their sites of action by the physiologic channels and mechanisms of excretion. The lungs are the major organs of excretion for gaseous substances such as some alcohols and anesthetics. The most important route of excretion for nonvolatile substances, however, is the kidney. Some drug metabolites are also excreted through the intestines via the feces, but the liver, through its secretion of bile into the small intestine, contributes to the major portion of material excreted in this manner. Many of these drug metabolites are also reabsorbed into the blood and excreted in the urine.

Some drugs are excreted almost unchanged in the urine, while other drugs are so extensively metabolized that only a small fraction of the original chemical substance is excreted in intact form. Other routes of drug elimination include the nursing mother's milk, perspiration, tears, and saliva, although the latter three constitute relatively unimportant routes.

Drugs may also be eliminated through the use of extracorporeal dialysis, which was originally designed to substitute for renal function in cases of severe but temporary renal shutdown. Overdosage of drugs may lead to just such a situation. By an artificial process resembling glomerular filtration, dialysis can achieve rapid reduction of high plasma levels of the drugs. As a general rule, substances that are completely or almost completely excreted by the normal kidney can be removed by hemodialysis. Such substances include some CNS stimulants and depressants, some nonnarcotic analgesics, and some metals.

Excretion via the kidneys remains by far the most important route of drug elimination. It accomplishes this process through passive glomerular filtration, active tubular secretion, and reabsorption. The availability of a drug for glomerular filtration depends on its concentration in unbound form in plasma. Some drugs are cleared by tubular secretion and all of the drug, bound and free, becomes available for active secretion. When free drug is eliminated by tubular cells, the bound drug dissociates its bond rapidly in order to maintain a level of equilibrium with plasma water. The renal excretory mechanisms, then, have the net effect of removing the amount of free drug that is brought to the kidneys by the renal arterial blood.

There are several factors that influence the rate

of drug excretion. Prerequisite to successful excretion is the maintenance of effective physiologic mechanisms of distribution (the circulatory system) and excretion (kidney and bowel function, respiratory function, and sweating). Immaturity or deterioration of the renal system, for example, will influence the rate of drug excretion. In newborn infants, whose renal tubular secretory mechanisms are incompletely developed, and in individuals with renal dysfunction, drug elimination is severely hampered and drug toxicity may result. The rate at which the drug is presented to the kidney and the rate of glomerular filtration also influence the rate of excretion. The biologic half-life of a drug is also essential to determining the rate of its excretion. (The half-life of a drug is the amount of time required for the plasma level concentration of the drug to decrease to 50% of the original concentration.) This half-life will not change with the drug dose, i.e., it will always take the same amount of time to eliminate one-half of the drug present in the body. If, for example, 10,000 units of a drug is administered and that drug has a half-life of 4 hours, then 5,000 units of the drug will be excreted in 4 hours. In the next 4 hours, 2,500 units will be excreted, with an additional 1,250 units excreted in the third 4-hour period.

VARIABLES PREDICTABLY INFLUENCING DRUG ACTION

There are some factors that will alter an individual's response to drug therapy. Deviant drug reactions can frequently be traced to the predictable influence of such variables. It is important for the nurse to be cognizant of factors that modify cell conditions and, therefore, modify the activity of a drug. Some of these factors include the following.

Age. It is generally recognized that children and elderly persons are highly responsive to drugs. Infants often have immature hepatic and renal systems and, therefore, incomplete excretory and metabolic mechanisms. Aged individuals may demonstrate different responses to drug therapy because of deterioration of hepatic and renal function, which is often accompanied by concurrent disease processes, such as cardiovascular disease. Modifications of dosage for children may be calculated as a fraction of the adult dose on the basis of body weight or surface area.

Body mass. The relationship between body mass and amount of drug administered influences the distribution and concentration of a drug. In order to maintain a desired drug concentration in individuals of various sizes, drug dosage must be adjusted in proportion to body mass. For a given dose of drug, the greater the volume of distribution, the lower the concentration of drug reached in various body compartments. Since the volume of interstitial and intracellular water is related to body mass, weight has a marked influence on the quantitative effects produced by drugs. The average adult drug dose is calculated on the basis of the drug quantity that will produce a particular effect in 50% of the population who are between the ages of 18 and 65 and weigh about 150 lb. (70 kg.). Therefore, particularly for children and for very lean and for very obese individuals, drug dosage is frequently determined on the basis of amount of drug per kilogram of body weight or body surface area.

Sex. Differential drug effects related to the variable of sex result, in part, from size differences between men and women. Women are usually smaller than men, which will lead to high drug concentrations if dosage is prescribed indifferently. There are also demonstrable differences in relative proportions of fat and water in the bodies of men and women, and some drugs may be more soluble in one or the other. Some authorities also indicate that subjective factors regarding drug effects may vary with sexual differences, stating that women are more suggestible to drug effects than men. This, however, is a controversial hypothesis. Differential drug reactivity by sex is most pronounced during pregnancy, since drugs taken by the pregnant woman might affect the uterus and/or the fetus as a result of placental transfer. As a precaution, the use of drugs is best avoided during pregnancy unless an absolute necessity exists.

Environmental milieu. Drugs affecting mood and behavior are particularly susceptible to the influence of the patient's environment. With such drugs one has to consider effects in light of four factors: (1) the drug itself; (2) the personality of the user; (3) the environment of the user; and (4) the interaction of these three components. Sensory deprivation and sensory overload may also affect responses to drugs. Physical environment may also modify drug effects. For example, temperature affects drug activity: heat relaxes peripheral vessels and so intensifies the actions of vasodilators, while cold has the opposite effect. The relative oxygen deprivation at high altitudes may also increase sensitivity to some drugs.

Time of administration. It is well known that drugs are absorbed more rapidly if the gastrointestinal tract is free of food, while irritating drugs are more readily tolerated if there is food in the stomach.

Although admittedly highly speculative, if findings from drug research on animals are applicable to humans, the time of drug administration in relation to human biologic rhythms can significantly affect the response to various drugs. It seems quite plausible that in humans the sleep-wake rhythm, deep sleep and dreaming sleep cycle, drug-metabolizing enzyme rhythms, corticosteroid secretion rhythm, blood pressure rhythms, as well as circadian (24-hour) variation in absorption and urinary excretion contribute to the effective, ineffective, adverse, or toxic response to particular drugs. There may also be a circadian rhythm in drug receptor susceptibility. Chronopharmacology and chronotoxicology are new areas of interest, and the frequency with which drug rhythm reports are appearing in the literature is increasing. Nurses should make every effort to understand their patient's normal and abnormal rhythms and seek to determine possible relationships between the patient's reactions to drug therapy and his biologic rhythms.

Pathologic state. The presence of pathology and the severity of symptoms may call for careful consideration of the type of drug administered and for adjustment in dosage. For example, the presence of severe pain tends to increase a patient's requirement for opiates, and an extremely anxious patient can prove resistant to very large doses of tranquilizing and sedating drugs. When aspirin is administered to a patient with a fever, he will respond with a decrease in temperature, whereas a patient taking the drug for its analgesic effects will show no temperature change at all. Larger doses of insulin may be required for the diabetic patient whose condition is complicated

by fever or infection. In addition, it bears repeating that the presence of circulatory, hepatic, and/or renal dysfunctions will interfere with the physiologic processes of drug action.

Genetic factors. Genetic differences may alter greatly the response of individuals to a number of drugs. Such differences may arise from genetically conditioned deficiencies in drug metabolism or in receptor sensitivity. These pharmacogenetic abnormalities often manifest themselves as "idiosyncrasies" and may be mistakenly diagnosed as drug allergies. For example, an individual may lack pseudocholinesterase activity in his plasma. If he receives an injection of succinylcholine, which is normally hydrolyzed by plasma cholinesterase, he may remain paralyzed for a long time. The field of pharmacogenetics is of great interest since it may provide a rational explanation for many so-called drug idiosyncrasies.

Psychologic factors. The patient's symbolic investment in drugs and his faith in their effects strongly influence and usually potentiate drug effects. The placebo effect is an outstanding example of how strong motivation can influence the emergence of desired drug effects. Conversely, hostility and mistrust of medicine and health personnel can diminish drug effects. It is important for nurses to realize that their attitude and the impressions created at the time of drug administration may influence the therapeutic result.

ADVERSE RESPONSES TO DRUGS

There are many ways in which drugs may react in the body to produce unpredictable, harmful, and sometimes unexplainable responses. No drug is totally safe and absolutely free of toxic effects. Sometimes these effects are immediately apparent. At other times, they may take weeks or months to develop. Some drugs result in aberrant pharmacologic actions when administered individually; other aberrant actions are precipitated by the concurrent administration of certain chemicals. Some adverse reactions to drugs are relatively mild; others can be fatal. With the increasing numbers of drugs being utilized, the incidence of adverse reactions has increased and is presently a significant problem in medical therapeutics.

Untoward effects of drugs can be classified as iatrogenic diseases or as adverse reactions. Generally, iatrogenic diseases refer to groups of adverse effects produced unintentionally by the physician in treating the patient. Iatrogenic diseases induced by drugs manifest themselves in five major syndromes: (1) blood dyscrasias, such as agranulocytosis, thrombocytopenia, aplastic anemia, and bone marrow depression; (2) hepatic toxicity, which is common and may take the form of biliary obstruction, hepatitis-like syndromes, and hepatic necrosis; (3) renal damage, particularly glomerular damage, which is a significant toxic effect of a number of drugs, including some antibiotics; (4) teratogenic effects, or drug effects causing malformations in the fetus as a result of placental transfer of drugs taken by a pregnant woman; and (5) dermatologic effects, such as acne, psoriasis, eczema, maculopapular rashes, and, rarely, erythema multiforme.

In addition to these common and well-known drug-induced diseases, there are numerous other iatrogenic syndromes specific to certain drugs. Ulceration of the gastrointestinal tract, for example, is a common result of long-term therapy with drugs such as aspirin, steroids, and potassium chloride. The relationship being investigated between oral contraceptive agents and thromboembolic phenomena is another untoward effect that may eventually be defined as an iatrogenic disease.

Adverse drug reactions, on the other hand, refer to one way of characterizing unpredictable and sometimes unexplainable drug responses that have not been optimally, clearly, and distinctly defined. Among the most common and best defined adverse drug reactions are the following.

Drug allergy is an altered state of reaction to a drug resulting from previous sensitizing exposure and the development of an immunologic mechanism. Substances foreign to the body act as antigens to stimulate the production of antibodies or immunoglobulins. Later, when a previously sensitized individual is again exposed to the foreign substance, the antigen reacts with the antibodies in ways that are damaging to body tissues. The antigen-antibody complex is not directly responsible for the manifestations of allergy. Rather, the complex reacts with various tissues and cells of the body by processes not clearly understood and causes them to release certain substances (e.g., histamine) which then provoke the symptoms of allergy.

Allergic reactions may manifest themselves in a variety of symptoms ranging from minor skin rashes to fatal hypotension. Reactions may be localized or widespread, and the symptoms may appear immediately or within hours to days following drug administration.

Immediate reactions occur within minutes of exposure to the chemical to which the person has been previously sensitized. Immediate and severe reactions are called anaphylactic reactions and are frequently fatal if not recognized and treated quickly. Signs and symptoms are severe, occur suddenly, and produce shock. The most dramatic form of anaphylaxis is sudden, severe bronchospasm, vasospasm, severe hypotension, and rapid death. Signs are largely caused by contraction of smooth muscles and may begin with irritability, extreme weakness, nausea, and vomiting and may proceed to dyspnea, cyanosis, convulsions, and cardiac arrest. Antihistamine drugs, epinephrine, and bronchodilators are indispensable in the treatment of anaphylactic shock.

Mild allergic reactions may be characterized by the development of a rash, angioedema, rhinitis, fever, asthma, and pruritus. Some allergic reactions are delayed and may appear anywhere from 7 to 14 days after initial administration of the drug. Delayed reactions are frequently analogous to "serum sickness" and are characterized by angioedema, arthralgia, fever, lymphadenopathy, and splenomegaly. Contact dermatitis, which results from direct skin contact with the eliciting drug, is also a delayed allergic response.

An individual who has had a mild allergic response to a particular drug should avoid reexposure to that drug and, optimally, should have skin tests performed in order to more definitely diagnose his response. Reinstitution of therapy with the same drug is always dangerous to patients who manifest allergic reactions since an anaphylactoid reaction may occur.

The term *hypersensitivity* is frequently used synonymously with allergy, but it is inappropriate because it is frequently confused with other kinds of adverse drug reactions. Since there is a lack of precision to defining hypersensitivity, it may be wisest to avoid usage of the term.

Idiosyncrasy is any abnormal or peculiar response to a drug that may manifest itself by: (1) overresponse or abnormal susceptibility to a drug; (2) underresponse, demonstrating abnormal tolerance; (3) a qualitatively different effect from the one expected, such as excitation after the administration of a sedative; or (4) unpredictable and unexplainable symptoms. Idiosyncratic reactions are generally thought to result from genetic enzymatic deficiencies that lead to abnormal mechanism of metabolizing drugs. This term has been used rather vaguely to describe drug reactions that are qualitatively different from the usual effects obtained in the majority of patients and that cannot be attributed to drug allergy.

Tolerance is said to exist when there is a decreased physiologic response to the repeated administration of a drug or a chemically related substance. It is a reaction that necessitates an excessive increase in dosage to maintain a given therapeutic effect. Drugs well known for their propensity to produce tolerance are tobacco, opium alkaloids, nitrites, barbiturates, and ethyl alcohol. The actual mechanism of tolerance is unknown. Recent research indicates that prolonged administration of some drugs somehow induces the synthesis of extra drug-metabolizing enzymes in the liver, which may account for the patient's increased ability to tolerate drug doses that previously affected him. Cross tolerance between related chemicals (such as between alcohol and some anesthetics) is a well-documented phenomenon.

Cumulation occurs when the body cannot metabolize one dose of a drug before another dose is administered. In other words, when drugs are excreted more slowly than they are absorbed, each new dose adds more to the total quantity in the blood and organs than is lost in the same amount of time by excretion. Unless drug administration is adjusted, sufficiently high concentrations can be reached to produce toxic effects. Cumulative toxicity can occur rapidly, as dramatically illustrated in ethyl alcohol intoxication, or it can occur insidiously, as is the case in poisoning with heavy metals, such as lead. The latter is stored in many body tissues and deposited

in bones, therefore having prolonged effects on the body while accumulation continues.

Tachyphylaxis refers to a quickly developing tolerance to the rapid, repeated administration of a drug. It is quick in onset and the patient's initial response to the drug cannot be reproduced with even larger doses of the drug.

Drug dependence is the term preferred over the previous terminology of habituation and addiction. The World Health Organization has suggested the usage of the term *dependence* in conjunction with the drug being described (for example, barbiturate dependence or opiate dependence). Dependence can be physical or psychic. Physical dependence refers to an adaptive physiologic state to a drug that manifests itself by intense physical disturbance when the drug is withdrawn. Psychic dependence is a state of emotional reliance upon a drug in order to maintain a state of well-being. Its manifestations may range from a mild desire for a drug, to craving, and to compulsive use of the drug. Drug dependence will be explored in greater breadth and depth in Chapter 17.

Summation, additive effect, and synergism refer to different situations in which the combined effect of two or more drugs acting simultaneously is either equal to or greater than the effect of each agent given alone.

Drug antagonism occurs when the conjoint effect of two drugs is less than the sum of the drugs acting separately.

Drug interaction results from the concurrent administration of two or more drugs and may be based on several mechanisms.

Variables influencing drug interaction include the following: (1) intestinal absorption, (2) competition for plasma binding, (3) drug metabolism, (4) action at the receptor site, (5) renal excretion, and (6) alteration of electrolyte balance. The following are examples of these variables' effects: (1) Intestinal absorption: Antacids that contain calcium, magnesium, or aluminum interfere with the absorption of tetracycline. (2) Competition for plasma protein binding: Tolbutamide can be displaced from its binding on plasma proteins by bishydroxycoumarin, resulting in severe hypoglycemia. It should be recalled that many drugs are weak acids that are bound largely to plasma proteins. These weak acids may compete for binding sites on plasma proteins, thus increasing the free, active drug that may have potent effects. (3) Drug metabolism or biotransformation: The monoamine oxidase inhibitors prevent the biotransformation of tyramine, which is present in cheese and other fermented foods. As a consequence, patients taking monoamine oxidase inhibitors as antidepressants have developed severe reactions after eating cheese. (4) Action at the receptor site: There are numerous examples in therapeutics of one drug intensifying or antagonizing the action of another drug at the receptor site. For example, the antihistaminics decrease many effects of histamine, while cocaine increases the actions of epinephrine. (5) Renal excretion: Probenecid inhibits the renal clearance of penicillin. (6) Alteration of electrolyte balance: The thiazide diuretics may cause hypokalemia, which predisposes to digitalis toxicity. It should be remembered that not all drug interactions are dangerous; some are insignificant or even beneficial. Tables listing all known drug interactions are available and should be consulted by the nurse when dangerous drug interaction is suspected.

QUESTIONS

For study and review

1 Define pharmacodynamics.
2 Differentiate between structurally specific and structurally nonspecific drugs.
3 Briefly explain the receptor theory of drug action.
4 Define the terms *affinity* and *efficacy* as they relate to drug action.
5 Briefly explain the rate theory of drug action.
6 Identify and describe the four physiologic processes mediating drug action.
7 Describe how the following factors may influence drug absorption: route of drug administration, drug solubility, local conditions at the site of administration, and drug concentration.
8 Define and explain the rationale underlying the administration of drugs in "priming" and "maintenance" doses.
9 Define repository dosage forms of drugs. Identify their advantages and disadvantages
10 Explain why drug distribution in the body is unequal.
11 Explain why the term *detoxification* is not an optimally accurate conceptualization of the process of biotransformation.
12 Identify the system primarily responsible for the biotransformation of drugs.
13 Explain how drug metabolism can be depressed or stimulated.
14 Describe how the following variables influence drug action: age, body mass, sex, environmental milieu, time of drug administration, and pathologic state.
15 Define iatrogenic disease and identify the five major syndromes by which drug-induced iatrogenic disease may be manifested.
16 Define adverse drug reactions and list some of these reactions.
17 Explain how drug allergy occurs. Describe the manifestations of immediate and delayed allergic reactions.
18 Explain why drug interaction has become a vital issue in contemporary medical therapeutics.

REFERENCES

Albert, A.: Relations between molecular structure and biological activity: stages in the evolution of current concepts, Ann. Rev. Pharmacol. **11:**13, 1971.

Anders, M. W.: Enhancement and inhibition of drug metabolism, Ann. Rev. Pharmacol. **11:**37, 1971.

Aviado, D. M.: Krantz and Carr's pharmacologic principles of medical practice, ed. 8, Baltimore, 1972, The Williams & Wilkins Co.

Bush, M. T., and Sanders, E.: Metabolic fate of drugs: barbiturates and closely related drugs, Ann. Rev. Pharmacol. **7:**57, 1967.

Burgen, A. S. V.: Receptor mechanisms, Ann. Rev. Pharmacol. **10:**7, 1970.

Crossland, J.: Lewis's pharmacology, Baltimore, 1970, The Williams & Wilkins Co.

DiPalma, J. R., editor: Drill's pharmacology in medicine, ed. 3, New York, 1971, McGraw-Hill Book Co.

Goldstein, A., Aronow, L., and Kalman, S.: Principles of drug action: The basis of pharmacology, ed. 2, New York, 1974, John Wiley & Sons.

Goodman, L., and Gilman, A.: The pharmacological basis of therapeutics, New York, 1975, The Macmillan Co.

Goth, A.: Medical pharmacology, ed. 7, St. Louis, 1974, The C. V. Mosby Co.

Grollman, A., and Grollman, E.: Pharmacology and therapeutics. Philadelphia, 1970, Lea & Febiger.

LaDu, B. N., Mandel, H. G., and Way, E. L.: Fundamentals of drug metabolism and drug disposition, Baltimore, 1971, The Williams & Wilkins Co.

Levine, R. R.: Pharmacology, drug actions and reactions, Boston, 1973, Little, Brown and Co.

Meyers, F., Jawetz, E., and Goldfein, A.: Review of medical pharmacology, ed. 4, Los Altos, Calif., 1974, Lange Medical Publications.

Penn, R. G.: Pharmacology, London, 1970, Bailliere, Tindall & Cassell Ltd.

Remmer, H.: The role of the liver in drug metabolism, Am. J. Med. **49:**617, 1970.

Schreiber, E. C.: The metabolic alterations of drugs, Ann. Rev. Pharmacol. **10:**77, 1970.

Ther, L., and Winne, D.: Drug absorption, Ann. Rev. Pharmacol. **11:**57, 1971.

Vesell, E. S.: Pharmacogenetics, New Eng. J. Med. **287:**904, 1972.

CHAPTER 8

Psychologic aspects of drug therapy and self-medication

Psychologic aspects of drug therapy
Aspects of self-medication

PSYCHOLOGIC ASPECTS OF DRUG THERAPY

Every drug administered to the patient has a symbolic meaning and a potential psychologic effect in addition to its pharmacodynamic action. A drug not only alters in a useful way the function or structure of some part of the body, but it may also influence the behavior, sense of well-being, and mental state of the patient. Psychologic responses of patients to the symbol of medication may mimic pharmacologic reactions, adverse effects, or even allergic reactions to drugs. The most profound psychologic reactions may be observed in patients receiving placebos.

Medications tend to be more effective when the patient believes in his capacity to get well, when he has a strong desire to get well, and when he believes that the health personnel caring for him are sincerely interested in his health. The patient's past and present conditioning to drugs, illness, hospitals, nurses, and other health personnel as well as his health goal are determinants in his reaction to drugs. Nurses must keep in mind that one of the most important deterrents to successful drug therapy occurs when the patient and the health personnel have divergent goals. An accurate determination of the patient's goal in seeking medical advice and therapy is important to planning and implementing an effective plan of care.

A patient's reaction to the symbolic meaning and pharmacologic action of drugs is extremely complex. Only an introduction to this aspect of drug therapy can be included here. For more detailed information, the student should consult the references listed at the end of this chapter.

SYMBOLIC MEANING OF DRUGS

Medications may be a symbol of *help* to the patient. This meaning is strengthened and drug effectiveness enhanced when doctors or nurses inform a patient that a particular drug will benefit or help him. Repeated suggestions to the patient that the drug is beneficial further reinforce the therapeutic value of the drug. This is similar to the relief a mother's kiss gives to the pain of her child; the assurance it gives makes the child feel better. Investigation of the effects of drugs on the mind has resulted in the conclusion that some drugs are effective only in the presence of an appropriate mental state. The patient's faith and belief are able to confer positive benefits.

Another important symbolic meaning of a drug is related to the *power* inherent in the drug. This symbolic power is united with the patient physically and emotionally. Although the emotional unity is most often unconscious, it provides the patient with *strength* and even a temporary sense of *security*. However, it is also this symbolic power that may propel an insecure and dependent individual into a state of drug depen-

101

dence. When an individual's needs cannot be met independently, his incapacity can be overcome with the help of an external factor such as a narcotic, drug, or alcohol. One of these might be the crutch that makes the patient feel he can more successfully meet the stresses with which he is confronted.

Drugs may also be viewed as symbols of *danger.* The patient may interpret the prospect of cure as a serious threat to his emotional security if he uses illness to meet a need such as dependence. The result may be the occurrence of adverse symptoms from medications. The patient may complain of dry mouth, nausea, vomiting, palpitation, fatigue, and other vague feelings of discomfort. He may resist taking the medication, refuse to have the prescription refilled, or even throw the drug away. If he does take the medication to please his family, doctor, or nurse, or because he can no longer withstand their pleading, he may immediately feel worse.

A patient may have ambivalent feelings about medications; he may wish to regain his health and may recognize the importance of drug therapy in achieving this goal, but he may also feel that his illness is essential for the gratification of his needs. Drug therapy may then result in some of his symptoms being relieved while others are intensified.

Drug fantasies. Patients may also harbor fantasies or irrational notions about medications. A patient may think a medication is too strong and therefore refuse to take the drug, decrease the amount of drug taken at any one time, or decrease the number of times the drug is taken. This type of fantasy may be suspected when a drug known to be effective for a specific condition is ineffective in a particular patient with that condition.

If a patient believes the drug is too weak, he may take the drug too often or request the drug more often than prescribed; he may increase the amount of drug he takes or continue drug therapy for a longer period of time than prescribed. A patient with this type of fantasy is quite likely to develop symptoms of overdosage.

Some fantasies may revolve around fear. Patients tend to fear radioactive drugs such as ^{32}P

or ^{131}I and to fear dependence on drugs that have antidepressant, analgesic, or sedative effects. Although few people today believe in the claims of a cure-all remedy, there are some who believe that a certain medicament or combination of medicaments is essential to general good health and should, therefore, be taken habitually.

An honest presentation to the patient of the action of drugs and of his own responsibility in drug therapy will help alleviate the problem of drug fantasies. In addition, what the patient thinks and believes about drugs should be learned prior to instituting drug therapy; this information may be used as a basis for the teaching of positive aspects of drug therapy.

Other reactions to drugs. Not only does a patient react to the symbol of medication but also to the pharmacodynamic properties of the drug and, if they occur, to the toxic, allergenic, or other adverse effects of the drug. A patient's reaction to the side effects of a particular drug may be somewhat reduced if he has been prepared in advance of their occurrence. Medical personnel may be reluctant to warn patients of ill effects from drugs, not wanting to cause unnecessary worry and anxiety. On the whole, patients prefer knowing the potential risks of drug therapy. Failure to prepare the patient for side effects may result in anxiety, panic, or rejection of therapy when these effects occur. If a patient is harmed by a drug and he was not informed of the potential risk, litigation might ensue.

Patients who believe they are allergic to a certain drug, for real or imagined reasons, are likely to react with fear or panic when administration of that drug is contemplated. A detailed personal history and (if possible) tests for hypersensitivity should be used to corroborate or refute the patient's belief. Rejection of a patient's claim of hypersensitivity without evidence could result in dire consequences.

The route of administration of a drug and the financial cost of treatment as well as a patient's conscious and unconscious attitudes toward his drugs, doctor, nurse, illness, and so on influence the extent, duration, and intensity of the patient's response to medication. Studies indicate that when a patient is angry, resentful, or hostile, certain medications used in normal doses may not be effective.

A patient's illness may affect his emotional response to a drug. When a patient's illness is short, his recovery is complete, and medical and drug expense is not too great, he tends to have a positive reaction to drugs, hospitals, and medical and nursing personnel. Strong negative reactions toward drugs or medical personnel result when a patient has been led to believe that he will make a quick and complete recovery, and then drugs are both ineffective and expensive or symptoms of allergy, side or toxic effects, or overdosage occur. Preparing patients for limited beneficial effects of drugs, for side and toxic effects, and for drug expense tends to reduce or prevent negative reactions.

In any chronic illness a patient may suddenly rebel against ill health and may irrationally resist therapy with life-sustaining medications. When this occurs, the patient may be testing himself to see if he is really dependent on the drugs, or he may be attempting a real or symbolic act of self-destruction. Usually, the ill effects experienced from drug omission bring about reinstitution of drug therapy from which the patient does not deviate for a long time. The patient's denial of need for drug therapy is directly related to denial of illness. Rejection of medications is often associated with increase in stress. Such a patient usually needs supportive and reconstructive psychotherapy.

EFFECTS OF DRUGS ON THE MIND

Many drugs used in the treatment of nonpsychotic patients have an effect on the patient's mind. Drugs may interfere with judgment, mood, sense of values, motor ability, and coordination. Certain antihistaminics used to treat allergies may decrease the individual's alertness and cause him to be drowsy, depressed, or even accident prone. Rauwolfia compounds used to treat hypertension may cause depression. The barbiturates and tranquilizers may induce inattentiveness and confusion and reduce initiative and the ability to think creatively. Drug-induced depression calls for discontinuance of the offending drug. These patients should be watched for self-destructive tendencies, since pharmacologic

literature is abundant with examples of those with drug-induced depressions who have attempted suicide.

ASPECTS OF SELF-MEDICATION

Development of the science of public health has led to the realization that the state of a nation's health is not exclusively dependent upon the interplay between professional medical practice on the one hand and bacteria, malignancy, and other causes of disease on the other. The influence on community health of the individual's personal attempts to relieve his ailments has frequently been ignored or underestimated. Here are a few of many varied aspects that affect self-medication either positively or negatively.

In the United States nearly $2 billion is spent annually for medicines that require no prescription or physician's advice. The amount spent on drugs for self-medication has been increasing yearly in Canada, the United States, and other nations. However, in the United States, sales of nonprescription drugs have not risen as much as have sales of prescription drugs. Nonprescription drugs accounted for 80% of all pharmaceutical products sold in the United States during the 1920's; in 1967 this figure had fallen to 25%.*

Drugs sold without prescription can induce sleep or wakefulness, relieve pain or tension, or supply the body with vitamins and minerals. Remedies can be purchased for any part of the body from head to toe. Widespread use of self-medication (autotherapy) is primarily the result of advertising via mass communication media. Concern over the use of home remedies and self-medication is not new. Self-medication continues to be a controversial subject with adherents for and against it. A critical assessment of the problem should include the investigation of the realistic and practical aspects of self-medication so that the lay person's rights and obligations become apparent to the nursing student and the practicing nurse.

Autotherapy is based on the tradition of folk remedies. Among the many reasons given for the

---

*Silverman, M., and Lee, P.: Pills, profits, and politics, Berkeley, 1974, University of California Press.

continuing popularity of autotherapy are convenience, fear or embarrassment with regard to medical consultation, disappointment with professional medical methods or results, and the fact that home remedies are more economical than medical consultation.

ADVANTAGES OF SELF-MEDICATION

Historical records and present-day surveys indicate that man has a desire and a need to practice self-medication. Man insists that self-medication is an inherent right, and he has guarded this right from time immemorial. Throughout history man has searched for medicines to relieve his ailments, and he has tried almost every natural material known to him in his battle against pain, discomfort, and disease.

The public is health conscious; otherwise there would be no across-the-counter sales or use of nonprescribed drugs. Many of man's ailments are trivial and temporary, and he seeks to alleviate these discomforts in the most expedient way possible. Minor ailments do not require the time or energy of a busy physician. The success with which minor complaints are treated by members of the public attests to this fact. Indeed, if individuals sought medical advice for every minor ailment (colds, headaches, slight wounds, temporary gastrointestinal upsets, or minor burns), physicians would be unable to give attention to patients with illnesses requiring professional medical care. Although self-medication if misused or abused may harm an individual, available data indicate that there is a greater amount of harm caused by prescription drugs than by nonprescription drugs. Hazards of autotherapy can be minimized by educating the public about drugs.

DISADVANTAGES OF SELF-MEDICATION

Although man has jealously guarded his inherent right to self-medication for hundreds of years, most preparations available to him before the twentieth century were harmless vegetable concoctions. The advent of modern chemistry and pharmacology produced literally thousands of preparations for self-medication, some of which are capable of causing harm.

Today, many drugs can be bought in super-

markets, restaurants, and vending machines. The desire for self-medication can be easily gratified. Sales promotion via radio and television encourages self-medication for real or fancied ills. Since the hazards of medications are insufficiently outlined, persistent abuse of drugs may occur and toxic effects may result. Many drugs considered harmless by the general public, such as aspirin and vitamin tablets, can actually cause untoward reactions. Aspirin may depress bone marrow function, while multiple-vitamin preparations containing iron, minerals, and salts may disturb gastrointestinal function. Calcium preparations and excessive amounts of vitamin D may cause kidney damage. Persistent use of bromides may result in bromism, and habitual use of antihistaminics can cause cardiac irregularities. Habitual self-medication may also mask a serious condition, endanger the individual's life, and create a need for prolonged and expensive medical therapy. The public's lack of knowledge of drugs and illness requires restriction of availability of potentially harmful drugs.

NURSING RESPONSIBILITIES IN RELATION TO NONPRESCRIPTION DRUGS

As has been noted, self-medication is very much a part of health care. If drug abuse and misuse by laymen are to be prevented and if the potential benefits of self-medication are to be optimized, the self-medicating public must be taught to recognize the approximate boundaries of its therapeutic competence. That is, laymen must be taught the potential benefits and risks of self-medication, when to self-medicate, and when to seek professional health care.

Education of laymen regarding nonprescription drugs is the responsibility of all health professionals. Nurses in both ambulatory health care settings and in-patient settings have a unique and distinct opportunity to fulfill this responsibility. All too often, unfortunately, consumer information regarding nonprescription (or over-the-counter) drugs is derived from misleading advertising or reporting.

Prerequisite to the fulfillment of this nursing responsibility are specific knowledges and skills.

First, nurses need more information regarding the major categories of nonprescription drugs and the ingredients of those drugs. Antacids, internal and external analgesics, laxatives, sleep aids, cold medications, vitamins, and ophthalmic preparations are but a few of the categories of nonprescription drugs available. Drugs within each category may consist of many and varied ingredients, some of which may be harmful for some people. For example, aspirin is marketed under at least two dozen brand names and in combination with many other drugs such as caffeine, phenacetin, sodium bicarbonate, and aluminum hydroxide. Not only is the potential toxicity of aspirin greatly underestimated by the lay public, but combination forms of the drugs are used indiscriminately.

Second, nurses need to be skilled in interviewing techniques in order to obtain information regarding an individual's patterns of drug use. This is an especially significant skill for two reasons: (1) many laymen do not define over-the-counter preparations as medications or drugs and do not always volunteer relevant information for medical histories, and (2) symbolic investment in drug use should not be underestimated and should be assessed as part of a thorough patient-client evaluation. The nurse should understand that self-medication is complex, psychologically motivated behavior that, like all other behavior, persists when it either increases the individual's pleasure or reduces his discomfort. Practically speaking, then, interviewing regarding self-medication should explore the individual's attitude toward self-medication as well as define the types of self-medication used including herbs, roots, poultices, as well as drugstore remedies.

After nurses have fulfilled these prerequisites, consumer education (or patient teaching) may proceed. Topics appropriate for health education regarding nonprescription drugs include the following:

1 Identification of medications that can be considered permissible for home treatment (see Table 8-1)
2 Safety precautions to prevent unnecessary accidents, such as:
   a. Proper labeling of all medications (labels should be obvious and legible)
   b. Following instructions and heeding warnings on labels (e.g., Do not drive or operate machinery while taking this medication; discontinue use if rapid pulse, dizziness, or blurring of vision occurs)
   c. Checking all medications periodically for expiration date and for deterioration by heat, light, or humidity and discarding deteriorated and outdated medications
   d. Discarding unused portions of prescription drugs and never "sharing" these drugs with friends or

Table 8-1 Medications for home treatment

Medication	Use
Analgesic balm or ointment	Muscular aches
Analgesic tablets (aspirin and aspirin combinations for adults and children)	Headaches, minor aches, pains, fever
Antacids	Indigestion or upset stomach
Antidiarrheal compounds	Mild or noncomplicated diarrhea
Antiseptics	
liquid, cream, spray	Minor cuts and scrapes
mouthwash	Mild sore throat
throat lozenges	Mild sore throat
Calamine cream or lotion	Insect bites, minor itching, poison ivy
Cough syrup	Coughing caused by colds
Ipecac syrup	Accidental poisoning emergency
Laxatives, mild	Constipation
Motion or travel sickness remedies	Dizziness, nausea, vomiting from travel
Nasal decongestants	Nasal stuffiness resulting from colds or allergies
Skin creams or lotions	Chapped skin, diaper rash
Sunburn and other burn treatments	Sunburn, other minor burns
Vitamin preparations	Dietary supplement

family even if they appear to manifest similar symptoms

    e. Keeping all medications out of children's reach and never referring to medications as candy for the sake of inducement

3 Instruction that nonprescription drugs are not curative and offer only symptomatic relief, followed by instructions regarding the types of symptoms that can be treated with these drugs.

4 Counseling and instruction regarding alternative therapeutic regimens, if appropriate (e.g., the need for laxative drugs can be reduced with counseling regarding activity and food habits)

5 Instructions to seek professional health care if symptoms are chronic, persistent, unresponsive, or frequently recurring

6 Warning regarding drugs capable of producing physical and/or psychological dependence (e.g., laxatives, nonprescription analgesics, stimulants)

CONTROL OF PROPRIETARY DRUGS

An important factor in determining the limits of autotherapy is governmental control of nonprescription drugs. Control of over-the-counter drugs has increased in Canada, the United States, and most European countries in the past few decades. Home remedies have existed from time immemorial, but their legislative history is of recent vintage. Drug laws in Canada and the United States were not intended to restrict the availability of drugs for self-medication but were intended to make self-medication safer and more effective. As a result of these laws, the use of secret formulas and deceptive advertising at its worst have disappeared.

Many nonprescription drugs available to the layman have limitations of effectiveness. Thus, analgesics such as aspirin are available for the relief of minor aches and pains, but agents such as morphine that relieve visceral pain are unavailable without a prescription. A nonprescription drug, like a prescription drug, must be proved safe and effective for the conditions for which it is recommended. It is this rule that has resulted in the withdrawal of many harmful and ineffective agents from the market. Nonprescription medicines must be safe and effective within a wide range of dosage. This provides protection against misuse. Most drugs capable of causing dependence or addiction such as amphetamines and barbiturates are no longer available across the counter. Nonprescription drugs are of low toxicity and pose no threat to the average consumer when directions are followed.

According to law, all nonprescription drugs must bear these seven points on their labels:

1 Name of the product

2 Name and address of the manufacturer, packer, or distributor

3 Net contents of the package

4 Active ingredients and the quantity of certain ingredients

5 Name of any habit-forming drug contained in the prescription

6 Cautions and warnings needed for the protection of the user

7 Adequate directions for safe and effective use

Labeling and warnings that accompany nonprescription drugs help to protect the layman against misuse and potential harmful effects.

Retail sale of home remedies can also be important to proper use of autotherapy. Allowing drugs to be purchased in grocery stores or supermarkets, from mail-order houses, or vending machines promotes the use of medications without benefit of the professional advice that can be given by the pharmacist. Restricting the sale of drugs to pharmacies or stores where a registered pharmacist is employed provides an opportunity for advice on the purchase of drugs and enables the pharmacist to observe which customers repeatedly buy the same medications to treat the same ailment; he can advise these customers to see a physician.

REFERENCES

Beecher, H. K.: The powerful placebo, J.A.M.A. **159**:1602, 1955.

Dukes, M. N. G.: Patent medicines and autotherapy in society, Den Haag, Holland, 1963, Drukkerij Pasmans, v.d. Vennestraat 76.

Fischer, H. K.: Psychiatric progress and problems of drug therapy, GP **16**:92, 1957.

Fischer, H. K., and Olin, B.: The dynamics of placebo therapy, Am. J. Med. Sci. **232**:504, 1956.

Handbook of non-prescription drugs, Washington, D.C., 1973, American Pharmaceutical Association.

Jaco, E. G., editor: Patients, physicians, and illness, New York, 1970, The Free Press of Glencoe, Inc.

Kaufman, W.: Some psychological aspects of therapy with drugs, Parts I to IV, Conn. Med. **25**:300-304; 368-371; 438-441; 506-509, 1961.

Lasagna, L.: Placebos, Sci. Amer. **193**:68, 1955.

Pennes, H. H., editor: Psychopharmacology, New York, 1958, Harper & Row, Publishers.

Rome, H. P.: Doctors: drugs: patients, Med. Clin. N. Am. **34**:973, 1950.

St. Whitelock, O. V., editor: Techniques for the study of behavioral effects of drugs, Ann. N.Y. Acad. Sci. **65**:247, 1956.

Wikler, A.: The relation of psychiatry to pharmacology, Baltimore, 1957, The Williams & Wilkins Co.

Wolf, S.: Effects of suggestion and conditioning on the action of chemical agents in human subjects—the pharmacology of placebos, J. Clin. Invest. **29**:110, 1950.

CHAPTER 9

Autonomic drugs

Autonomic nervous system
The catecholamines
Indirect and direct stimulants of alpha and beta receptors
Alpha blocking agents
Beta blocking agents
Cholinergic drugs
Anticholinesterase drugs
Anticholinergic agents (belladonna group)

AUTONOMIC NERVOUS SYSTEM

Autonomic (from the Greek words *auto*, self; *nomos*, law) means a law unto itself, or self-governing. The autonomic nervous system has been known by other names. Winslow (1732) called it sympathetic because he thought it controlled the sympathies of the body; Bichat (1800) called it vegetative to designate its control over nutrition, as opposed to voluntary processes. Gaskell called it the involuntary nervous system, to contrast it with the voluntary system, which controls skeletal movement. Langley, who studied and described the structure and many of the functions and effects of the autonomic nervous system, provided much of the terminology used today to describe this system. He used the terms *sympathetic* and *parasympathetic* for the two divisions of the autonomic nervous system, and he introduced the concept of receptor.

The autonomic nervous system automatically regulates a multitude of physiologic tasks necessary for the preservation of a constant internal environment (homeostasis), emergency mecha-nisms, and repair. Digestion of a meal, heart rate, pressure of circulating blood, and many other processes are quietly supervised by a system of control whose measure of efficiency is the silence of its working.

There are a number of centers that lie in the central nervous system that are concerned with integration of all autonomic nervous system activities. There is evidence that the hypothalamus, in particular, is concerned with such integrating activities. It contains centers that function in the regulation of body temperature, water balance, carbohydrate and fat metabolism, and blood pressure. It also integrates mechanisms concerned with emotional behavior, the waking state, and sleep. The medulla oblongata integrates the control of blood pressure and respiration. In addition, the midbrain, limbic system, cerebellum, and cerebral cortex are involved in the control of and in physiologic functions regulated by the autonomic nervous system. It should be remembered that the autonomic nervous system is a part of the central nervous system, not a distinct entity.

The autonomic nervous system is composed of two systems of nerves, the parasympathetic

Table 9-1 Differentiating characteristics between the sympathetic and parasympathetic nervous systems

Characteristics	Sympathetic nervous system	Parasympathetic nervous system
Origin	Thoracolumbar	Craniosacral
Structure innervation	Cardiac muscle Smooth muscle Glands Viscera	Cardiac muscle Smooth muscle Glands Viscera
Ganglia	Near central nervous system	Near the effector (vagus, atria of heart)
Length of fibers	Preganglionics (short) Postganglionics (long)	Preganglionics (long) Postganglionics (short)
Ratio of pre- to postganglionics	High degree of divergence (1:11, 1:17)	Divergence is minimal (1:2), very discrete, fine responses
Response	Diffuse	Discrete
Ganglion transmitter	Acetylcholine (ACh)	Acetylcholine
Transmitter substance (postganglionic nerve endings)	Norepinephrine (most cases) Acetylcholine for sweat glands and blood vessels of skeletal muscles	Acetylcholine
Blocking drugs (postganglionic nerve endings)	Adrenergic blocking agents Alpha-phenoxybenzamine (Dibenzyline) Beta-propranolol (Inderal)	Cholinergic blocking agents (atropine)

and the sympathetic, whose actions are opposed in a balanced antagonism.

DIFFERENCES BETWEEN THE SYMPATHETIC AND PARASYMPATHETIC DIVISIONS

Although anatomic and physiologic differences do exist between the sympathetic and parasympathetic divisions, these differences are not always clear-cut and absolute. The anatomic concept of the autonomic, or visceral, nervous system comprises all the nerves, peripheral ganglia, and motor centers of the internal organs, or viscera (see Table 9-1).

Efferent nerves conduct messages from the central portions of the nervous system to the periphery. However, the efferent system is closely controlled by information received from the periphery via the afferent system. The efferent connections of the autonomic nervous system are built upon the principle of the two-neuron system, the two neurons being in series (see Figure 9-2).

Transmission of the impulse from one neuron to another takes place at the junction, or synapse. The peripheral synapses of the autonomic nervous system are generally to be found in the ganglia (in groups of nerve cells situated at the periphery). The neuron that conducts the impulse from the central nervous system to the peripheral ganglion is termed *preganglionic;* the neuron that transmits the impulse from the ganglion to the effector organ is termed *postgan-*

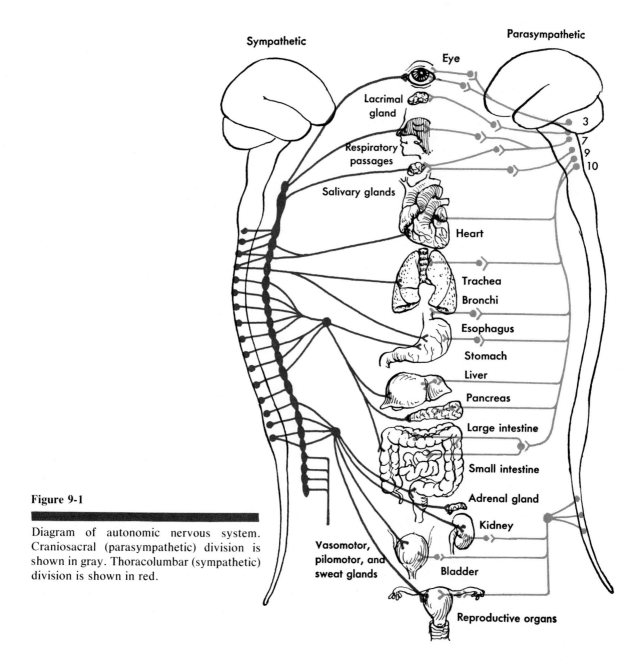

Figure 9-1

Diagram of autonomic nervous system. Craniosacral (parasympathetic) division is shown in gray. Thoracolumbar (sympathetic) division is shown in red.

glionic. A preganglionic fiber may pass through several ganglia, but it forms only a single synapse.

The effect of the sympathetic and parasympathetic systems on individual organs and functions can be seen in Table 9-2. The functions stimulated by the parasympathetic system are mainly those concerned with digestion, excretion, near vision, cardiac deceleration, and anabolism. Functions stimulated by the sympathetic system are primarily those concerned with the expenditure of energy; they are called into play

Table 9-2 Effects produced by divisions of the autonomic nervous system

Organ or function	Sympathetic effect	Parasympathetic effect
Metabolism:		
Basal metabolic rate	Increase	Decrease
Blood sugar	Increase	Decrease
Liver glycogen	Decrease	—
Body temperature	Increase	Decrease
Heart	Acceleration	Inhibition
Blood pressure (mean)	Increase	Decrease
Blood vessels:		
Skin	Constriction	—
Muscle	Dilation and constriction	—
Salivary glands	Constriction	Dilation
Lungs	Constriction and dilation	Dilation and constriction
Brain	Constriction	Dilation
Abdominal and pelvic organs	Constriction	Dilation
External genitalia	Constriction and dilation	Dilation
Smooth musculature:		
Ciliary muscle	—	Contraction
Constrictor muscle of iris	—	Contraction
Dilator muscle of iris	Contraction	—
Skin (piloerector)	Contraction	—
Bronchi	Inhibition	Constriction
Esophagus	Inhibition	Contraction
Cardia	Contraction	Relaxation
Stomach	Inhibition (or contraction)	Contraction (or inhibition)
Pylorus	Inhibition (or contraction)*	Contraction (or inhibition)
Intestine	Decrease in tone and motility	Increase in tone and motility
Sphincter ani	Contraction	—
Detrusor	Inhibition	Contraction
Vesical sphincter	Contraction	Inhibition
Uterus (human)	Mainly inhibition*	—
Glands:		
Sweat	Increase in secretion	—
Salivary	Increase in secretion†	Increase in secretion
Gastric	Decrease in secretion*	Increase in secretion
Pancreatic	Increase in secretion*	Increase in secretion
Adrenal medulla	Increase in secretion	—
Islets of Langerhans	—	Increase in secretion*

*Questionable response—uncertain about origin of response.
†Occurs at times in some glands.

Figure 9-2

Schematic representation to show the relationship between a neuron in the central nervous system, a neuron in a peripheral ganglion, and an effector organ. Note that the synapse occurs at the junction of the preganglionic and postganglionic fibers.

Nerve center   Ganglion   Effector organ

Preganglionic fiber
(with medullary sheath)

Postganglionic fiber
(without medullary sheath)

Synapse

by physical or emotional stress (pain, hemorrhage, extremes of temperature, intense emotion).

Understanding the anatomy and physiology of the autonomic nervous system facilitates understanding the pharmacology of autonomic drugs.

NERVE IMPULSE TRANSMISSION

There is now general agreement that transmission of nerve impulses at autonomic synapses and at myoneural junctions is brought about by the activity of chemical substances called mediators. These mediators are acetylcholine and the catecholamines. The classification of autonomic nerves presently in widespread use is not an anatomic one but one based on the type of chemical mediator responsible for nerve impulse transmission. Those nerve fibers that synthesize and liberate acetylcholine are known as *cholinergic* fibers; those that synthesize and secrete norepinephrine (noradrenalin) are called *adrenergic* fibers.

Drugs that bring about effects in the body similar to those produced by acetylcholine are called cholinergic drugs. An older term used to designate this group of drugs is parasympathomimetic, because they appear to mimic the action produced by stimulation of the parasympathetic nervous system. Drugs that produce effects like those produced by the adrenergic mediator are called adrenergic drugs; the older term for these drugs is sympathomimetic.

$$CH_3-\overset{\overset{\displaystyle CH_3}{|+}}{\underset{\underset{\displaystyle CH_3}{|}}{N}}-CH_2-CH_2-O-\overset{\overset{\displaystyle O}{\|}}{C}-CH_3$$

Acetylcholine

In addition to acetylcholine and norepinephrine there may be other transmitters, particularly in the central nervous system. Dopamine, gamma-aminobutyric acid, and glycine have received much interest. Nevertheless, in the peripheral portions of the autonomic nervous system, acetylcholine and norepinephrine play a predominant role which permits a rational classification of the autonomic drugs.

Epinephrine
(Adrenalin)

Norepinephrine
(Noradrenalin; levarterenol)

All preganglionic fibers of the autonomic nervous system, whether parasympathetic or sym-

Figure 9-3
Synthesis of norepinephrine and epinephrine.

pathetic, release acetylcholine at the ganglion where synapse occurs. Also, parasympathetic postganglionic fibers release acetylcholine at the effector cell. Norepinephrine is liberated from postganglionic sympathetic fibers.

THE CATECHOLAMINES

In the past great interest was evoked by confusing and conflicting reports that the effects of sympathetic nerve stimulation and the effects of epinephrine injection did not always correspond. In the mid-1940's it was shown that epinephrine had a twin, norepinephrine. With the recognition that these were separate substances that occurred naturally in the body, the confusion began to resolve. With further research one more catecholamine has been positively identified—dopamine. Dopamine is a precursor of norepinephrine and epinephrine (see Figure 9-3). However, dopamine has a transmitter role of its own in certain portions of the central nervous system. Epinephrine acts mainly as an emergency hormone, while norepinephrine is an important transmitter of nerve impulses. It is also an intermediary in epinephrine biosynthesis.

The term catecholamine originates from organic chemistry. Catechol is dihydroxybenzene, and a glance at Figure 9-2 will show that dopamine, norepinephrine, and epinephrine are all catechols as well as amines.

In 1948 Ahlquist helped to clarify the varied actions of the catecholamines by showing that in the sympathetic nervous system the adrenergic effector cells contained two distinct receptors, the alpha (α) and beta (β) receptors. Norepinephrine acts mainly on alpha receptors,

while epinephrine acts on both alpha and beta receptors. The synthetic catecholamine, isoproterenol, acts only on beta receptors. The most important alpha adrenergic activities in man are: (1) vasoconstriction of arterioles in the skin and splanchnic area, resulting in a rise in blood pressure; (2) pupil dilation; and (3) relaxation of the gut. Beta adrenergic activity includes: (1) cardiac acceleration and increased contractility; (2) vasodilation of arterioles supplying skeletal muscles; (3) bronchial relaxation; and (4) uterine relaxation. The effects of both alpha and beta stimulation will result from a summation of action where they are interrelated. That is, a change in blood pressure will depend on the degree of vasoconstriction in the skin and splanchnic area *and* the extent of vasodilation in skeletal muscles. Large arteries and veins contain both alpha and beta receptors; the heart contains only beta receptors (see Table 9-3).

While there are specific drugs that stimulate the alpha or beta receptors, there are also drugs that selectively block alpha or beta receptors. Most adrenergic blocking agents are alpha blockers; these drugs include ergot derivatives, phenoxybenzamine, and Dibenamine. In the United States in 1968 a beta receptor blocking agent, propranolol, became available for clinical use. These agents effect blockade at peripheral autonomic sites, which distinguishes them from ganglionic blocking agents that act at the ganglia.

The catecholamines norepinephrine and epinephrine are neurohormones, and they serve important functions in neural and endocrine integration. They are synthesized in the brain, in the sympathetic ganglia and nerve endings, and in the adrenal medulla. Norepinephrine and epinephrine are both produced by the adrenal me-

Table 9-3 Adrenergic receptor stimulation

Organ	Alpha receptor	Beta receptor
Heart Cardiac muscle	—	Increase contractility of atria and ventricles

Sinoatrial node
  Atrioventricular node
  Conductive tissue
		Increase heart rate
		Increase conduction velocity; shorten refractory period

Arteries	Constriction	Relaxation
Veins	Constriction	Relaxation
Bronchial smooth muscle		Relaxation

Figure 9-4

Pre- and postganglionic autonomic fibers and neurohormone transmitters.

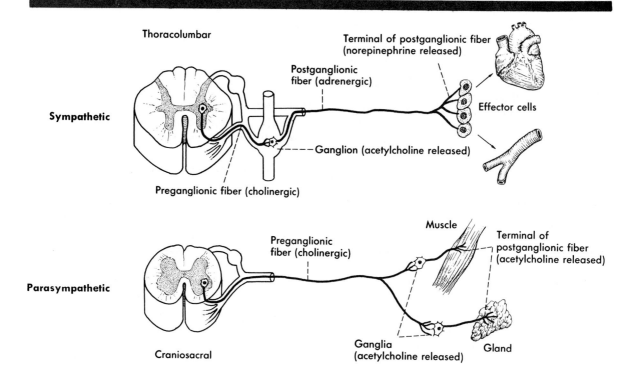

dulla and secreted into the circulation; the proportions produced vary with the nature of the physiologic stimulus. Synthesis of norepinephrine also takes place in adrenergic nerve terminals. It is achieved by the action of a series of enzymes, the most important being that of tyrosine hydroxylase. The constancy of norepinephrine in nerves is the result of a negative feedback process; norepinephrine itself inhibits tyrosine hydroxylase once the catecholamine reaches its normal level. The regulation of epinephrine synthesis is not well understood. Norepinephrine and epinephrine influence a number of physiologic target organs, which include vascular smooth muscle, the heart and liver, adipose tissue, and uterine muscle.

The catecholamines are stored in specialized subcellular particles called granules, storage granules, or granulated vesicles. These storage granules (1) take up dopamine from cytoplasm, (2) oxidize it to norepinephrine, (3) bind and store the norepinephrine to prevent its diffusion out of the cell and destruction by enzymes, and (4) release norepinephrine after appropriate physiologic stimuli. Storage of catecholamines appears to require ATP and magnesium. This uptake process serves to terminate the actions of released or administered catecholamines and to conserve norepinephrine. Metabolism of norepinephrine and epinephrine is primarily dependent on two enzymes, monoamine oxidase (MAO) and catechol-o-methyltransferase (COMT). Metabolism by MAO occurs within the neuron, while COMT catabolizes circulating catecholamines, primarily in the liver and kidney. Drugs inhibiting these enzymes may prolong the actions of catecholamines.

Norepinephrine and epinephrine are continuously present in arterial blood, although the amount varies widely during any one day. Certain physiologic stimuli such as stress and exercise significantly increase catecholamine blood levels.

Studies indicate that the major source of circulating norepinephrine comes from stimulated sympathetic nerve endings. Organs that receive a large fraction of blood and contain large numbers of sympathetic nerve endings contain the greatest amount of catecholamines. (Examples of such organs are the heart and blood vessels.) Thus the number of sympathetic nerve endings or adrenergic nerves to various organs determines the magnitude of response of these organs to increased levels or injections of catecholamines.

PHARMACOLOGIC EFFECTS OF CATECHOLAMINES

Catecholamines produce a variety of physiologic responses as evidenced by the following effects.

Cardiac effects. Epinephrine and norepinephrine produce almost the same cardiac responses when injected. These responses include the following:

Marked increase in myocardial contraction (positive inotropic effect). This increase is probably the result of an enhancement of influx of calcium into cardiac fibers. The strong myocardial contractions result in more complete emptying of the ventricles and an increase in cardiac work and oxygen consumption. The strong contractions brought about by isoproterenol and epinephrine also increase cardiac output, or minute volume. Norepinephrine, on the other hand, may not alter cardiac output and may even decrease it slightly. This effect of norepinephrine is believed to result from its potent vasoconstricting action, which increases resistance to ejection. The increased work of the heart to move the blood against increased pressure is "pressure work" rather than "volume work."

It has been shown experimentally and clinically that 0.5 mg. of epinephrine injected into arterial or venous blood and circulated by cardiac compression or massage may stimulate spontaneous and vigorous cardiac contractions. Even though the heart is in ventricular fibrillation, epinephrine increases fibrillation vigor and frequently promotes successful electric defibrillation of the patient. In these situations the drug may be repeatedly injected. Use of other drugs is also necessary, such as sodium bicarbonate to overcome acidosis. However, epinephrine cannot be used repeatedly to improve the function of a failing heart (congestive heart failure), since it increases oxygen consumption by cardiac muscle. It can also cause anginal pain in patients with angina pectoris because it increases cardiac oxygen demand. Therefore, even though it increases coronary blood flow, its use is contraindicated for patients with angina.

The production of strong contractions provided the rationale for the use of epinephrine in cardiac arrest and the injection of epinephrine directly into heart muscle.

Marked increase in cardiac rate (positive chronotropic effect). Acceleration of heart rate by the catecholamines is the result of the increased rate of membrane depolarization in the pacemaker cells in the sinus node during diastole: action potential threshold is reached sooner, pacemaker cells fire more often, and heart rate increases.

Norepinephrine with its predominantly alpha adrenergic activity may not produce as severe a tachycardia as epinephrine. The increased vasoconstriction and increased blood pressure may produce a reflex bradycardia. Dosage and patient variables affect these responses. Isoproterenol usually produces a tachycardia since its direct and reflex effects act in the same direction.

Increase in atrioventricular conduction (positive dromotropic effect). This effect accounts for the use of epinephrine in the treatment of heart block by some cardiologists.

Purkinje fiber effects. Catecholamines may produce spontaneous firing of Purkinje fibers resulting in their exhibiting pacemaker activity. This effect may produce ventricular extrasystoles and increase the susceptibility of ventricular muscle to fibrillation. These effects are more likely to occur with epinephrine than norepinephrine.

Blood pressure and blood flow effects. Vascular effects of the catecholamines depend on the dose and the vascular bed affected. Low doses of epinephrine may produce a decrease in blood pressure as a result of a decrease in total peripheral vascular resistance. In large doses epinephrine activates alpha receptors in the greater peripheral vascular system, which leads to increased resistance and an increase in blood pressure. Norepinephrine elevates blood pressure by increasing peripheral resistance and decreasing blood flow through skeletal muscles.

Norepinephrine is a vasoconstrictor and it increases total peripheral resistance. Isoproterenol is not a vasoconstrictor but a pure vasodilator; epinephrine is both a vasoconstrictor and vasodilator with vasodilation being greater in its overall net effects. For example, during great stress (fright, fight, flight phenomena) the release of epinephrine from the adrenal medulla constricts blood vessels in the skin and splanchnic areas but dilates those of muscles, thus shunting blood from noncritical to critical areas.

There is greater renal artery constriction and resistance with epinephrine than with norepinephrine. In large doses, epinephrine may actually stop blood flow through some nephrons (up to 40%) and stimulate release of ADH (antidiuretic hormone) thereby reducing urinary excretion.

Central nervous system effects. Epinephrine and isoproterenol in sufficient amounts can lead to alertness, tremulousness, respiratory stimulation, and manifest anxiety. Norepinephrine is less likely to cause anxiety and tremulousness. Beneficial cerebral effects from epinephrine and norepinephrine in cases of hypotension, are thought to be the result of increased systemic pressure with a resultant improvement in cerebral blood flow.

Smooth muscle effects. Generally, the catecholamines relax nonvascular smooth muscles. Smooth muscle of the gastrointestinal tract is relaxed, and amplitude and tone of intestinal peristalsis are reduced. This may retard propulsion of food and gastrointestinal emptying. However, this effect is rarely produced in man with therapeutic doses.

The musculature of the splenic capsule is stimulated thereby increasing contractions of that organ, which results in increasing the number of circulating red cells and blood viscosity. This effect is not of great signficance in man.

In some situations, smooth muscle of some organs react like vascular smooth muscle and contract. For example, radial and sphincter muscles of the iris contract and the smooth muscle that inserts into the lids may contract giving rise to the widened, staring eyes seen in sympathetically stimulated individuals.

In the urinary bladder, epinephrine causes tri-gone and sphincter contraction and detrusor relaxation with a delay in the desire to void.

Bronchodilator effects. Catecholamines dilate bronchial smooth muscle. Isoproterenol is a more active bronchodilator than epinephrine, which in turn is a stronger bronchodilator than norepinephrine. Epinephrine, in addition, constricts bronchial vessels and inhibits bronchial secretions, which accounts for its time-honored use in the treatment of acute bronchial asthma.

Effect on glands. Epinephrine may increase the amount of viscid saliva excreted, but as a rule sympathomimetics decrease secretion and produce a dry mouth. Catecholamines may produce local sweating on the palms of the hands and in the axillary and genital areas. The exact mechanism for these effects is not clear.

Metabolic effects. Epinephrine inhibits insulin secretion. Catecholamines have antagonistic effects on gluconeogenesis, and they decrease liver and skeletal muscle glycogen and increase lipolysis in adipose tissue. The result of these effects is a rise in blood sugar and an increase in free fatty acids. Thus in response to stress (fright, fight, flight response) there can be an abundant supply of fuel and energy.

Catecholamines also have a calorigenic effect (increased oxygen consumption) resulting from the sum of the above effects. Norepinephrine's action in relation to these effects is weaker than that of epinephrine or isoproterenol.

Other effects. Catecholamines cause a decrease in circulating eosinophils. The mechanism of this action is not known.

Drug interactions. Among the various drug interactions that can occur between the catecholamines and other drugs are the following:

1 Digitalis and the catecholamines may have an additive effect and precipitate ectopic pacemaker activity.
2 Catecholamines given to patients receiving MAO inhibitors may cause a hypertensive crisis.
3 Certain anesthetics, such as chloroform, cyclopropane, halothane, and trichloroethylene, sensitize the heart to catecholamines, and injection of these drugs during surgery is hazardous since the risk of induced arrhythmias is increased.
4 Tricyclic antidepressants, other sympathomimetic drugs, and reserpine and related drugs may potentiate the effects of the catecholamines.
5 Diuretics and antihypertensive drugs antagonize the effects of the catecholamines.
6 Epinephrine and isoproterenol should not be administered concomitantly since their combined effects may produce serious arrhythmias. Their use may be alternated if at least 4 hours have elapsed.

Epinephrine (Adrenalin)

General characteristics. Epinephrine can be prepared synthetically or obtained from the adrenal glands of domestic animals. Most of the epinephrine used in medicine at the present time is a pure synthetic preparation. Chemically, epinephrine is an amine and reacts with acids to form salts. Epinephrine hydrochloride solutions are unstable; react to light, heat, and air; turn pink and then brown when oxidized; and should be kept in the refrigerator. Discolored solutions should be discarded since there will be loss of potency.

Epinephrine acts on both alpha and beta receptors. It is a more potent alpha receptor stimulator than norepinephrine at some sites. Beta receptors are also more sensitive to epinephrine than to norepinephrine.

Action and use. The ability of epinephrine to constrict blood vessels makes it useful for topical application in stopping capillary bleeding from the nose, mouth, mucosal surfaces, and skin abrasions. It should not be used on fingers, toes, or ears since the vasoconstriction may cause tissue necrosis and sloughing. It is often added to local anesthetic solutions to delay their absorption from the site of injection by promoting local vasoconstriction, which in turn restricts the action of the anesthetic to that given area, prolongs the anesthetic action, and checks bleeding.

This same vasoconstrictor ability accounts for the use of epinephrine to relieve congestion and swelling of particular tissues—thus its use in treating allergic conditions such as urticaria and angioneurotic edema. When applied to the eye in a 2% solution, it dilates the pupil, decreases the blood flow, and reduces intraocular tension. This last effect makes it useful in treating chronic simple glaucoma.

Epinephrine may also be given by inhalation (in a 1:100 solution) to asthmatics to relieve bronchial spasm and swelling and to promote a patent airway. However, the time-honored treatment of an acute asthmatic attack is the subcutaneous injection of epinephrine, 0.2 to 0.5 ml. of a 1:1000 solution. Dosage may be repeated every 10 to 15 minutes or hourly if necessary. However, the patient may develop physiologic resistance to epinephrine. Therefore, its use should be restricted to *acute* asthmatic attacks. Asthmatics may develop an emotional dependence on epinephrine.

Epinephrine has not proved to be an effective drug in the relief of nasal congestion because of its rebound or secondary vasodilator effect, which brings about a greater swelling of the nasal mucosa than was present initially.

Epinephrine has a significant effect on beta receptors. As a consequence, it can dilate some vessels, such as those of skeletal muscle. Because of this and its potent action on cardiac beta receptors, epinephrine is not the drug of choice in most cases of shock or hypotension. On the other hand, it is the drug of choice for treating anaphylactic shock. Epinephrine may also be used to treat cardiac arrest.

Absorption and excretion. Although epinephrine is readily absorbed from mucous membranes, it is destroyed by digestive enzymes and is therefore useless if given by mouth. Rapid effects may be noted when the drug is given hypodermically or intramuscularly, and almost immediate effects occur when it is given intravenously. The drug is rapidly inactivated in the body by enzymatic alteration and is taken up by adrenergic nerves.

Preparation, dosage, and administration. The following are available preparations of epinephrine.

Epinephrine nasal solution. U.S.P. The 1:1000 aqueous solution is for topical application only. This solution is not sterile.

Epinephrine injection, U.S.P.; *adrenaline injection*, B.P. This 1:1000 solution is available in ampules and 30-ml. vials. Dosage is 0.1 to 1 ml. (25 μg. to 1 mg.) given subcutaneously or intramuscularly. This preparation is sterile and contains 1 mg. of drug in each milliliter of solution.

Subcutaneous administration is most often used. Promptness of action can be facilitated by massaging the injection site. When the intravenous route is used, the drug must be given very slowly and in a very low concentration.

Epinephrine inhalation, U.S.P. This is 1:100 (1%) epinephrine solution. It should be administered with a special nebulizer to provide a fine mist for oral inhalation. Epinephrine is well absorbed from mucous membranes. The effectiveness of this preparation for the asthmatic patient is explained on the basis of achieving a relatively high concentration of the drug in the throat and respiratory passages rather than from a systemic action. Special precautions should be observed to avoid confusing the 1:100 solution with the 1:1000 solution.

Sterile epinephrine suspension, U.S.P. (epinephrine in oil injection). Dosage for adults is 0.2 to 0.5 ml. intramuscularly. It is available in 1-ml. ampules (1:500). The duration of action is prolonged.

Epinephrine bitartrate, U.S.P. This preparation is available as a 2% ophthalmic solution.

Adrenaline injection, B.P. This is a 1:1000 solution of epinephrine tartrate for subcutaneous injection. It is a sterile solution.

Unofficial preparations of epinephrine are also available, such as epinephrine suppositories (1:1000 with cocoa butter).

Solutions of epinephrine do not keep well; deterioration is evidenced by formation of sediment and brownish discoloration.

For children the recommended subcutaneous injection dose for asthma is 0.01 ml. of 1:1000 aqueous solution per kilogram of body weight, with a maximum dose of 0.5 ml. This dosage may be repeated every 4 hours. When the intramuscular injection of epinephrine in oil (1:500) is used, the dose is 0.01 to 0.02 ml. per kilogram of body weight every 12 to 24 hours p.r.n. However, the intramuscular route is not recommended since bioavailability is not uniform and fatal cases of gas gangrene have been reported.

Because epinephrine is such a potent drug, the nurse must be particularly careful to give the correct dose. If the preparation at hand is an ampule containing 1 ml. of the drug, it does not follow that 1 ml. is the usual dose. Very often, the dose is only a few minims. The minimum fatal dose of epinephrine subcutaneously seems to be about 10 ml. of a 1:1000 solution.

Toxic effects. Toxic effects and death from epinephrine may result from overdosage caused by errors in preparation of solutions or the intravenous administration of a subcutaneous dose. Symptoms of toxicity include tachycardia, palpitations, dyspnea, pulmonary edema, severe headache, pallor, pupillary dilation, anxiety, high blood pressure, and rapid collapse. Toxic effects may be counteracted by injection of an alpha blocker and a beta blocker. Cardiac arrhythmias, which may be evoked by epinephrine, include atrial fibrillation, atrioventricular nodal rhythm, ventricular extrasystoles, ventricular tachycardia, and ventricular fibrillation.

A nurse is expected to recognize an obvious error. The strength of solution, dosage ordered, and route of administration should be carefully checked.

Contraindications. Epinephrine should not be used for patients on a regimen of digitalis, since together these drugs have a synergistic action and predispose the heart to premature beats or arrhythmias. Epinephrine should be avoided in patients with hyperthyroidism, hypertension, cerebral arteriosclerosis, and nervous instability. The drug should not be used in elderly or debilitated patients. Use of epinephrine preoperatively in patients with angle-closure glaucoma is contraindicated. Administration of epinephrine to patients with cerebral arteriosclerosis may result in cerebral hemorrhage.

Levarterenol bitartrate, U.S.P. (Levophed Bitartrate, norepinephrine); noradrenaline acid tartrate, B.P.

$$HO-\text{\raisebox{0pt}{\bigcirc}}-\overset{\overset{H}{|}}{\underset{\underset{OH}{|}}{C}}-\overset{\overset{H}{|}}{\underset{\underset{H}{|}}{C}}-\overset{\overset{H}{|}}{\underset{\underset{H}{|}}{N}} \cdot COOH-(CHOH)_2-COOH \cdot H_2O$$

Levarterenol bitartrate is a grayish white, crystalline powder, freely soluble in water. It darkens on exposure to light and air. It can be synthesized or obtained from the medullary portion of the adrenal glands of animals. It has positive inotropic and chronotropic effects on the heart and a potent constrictor action on blood vessels.

Uses. Levarterenol bitartrate is used to maintain blood pressure in acute hypotensive conditions caused by vasomotor depression, trauma, and shock. It does not take the place of intravascular fluids if the fall in blood pressure is caused by diminished blood volume.

Levarterenol may be life saving in cardiogenic shock because of its direct stimulating effect on the myocardium and its vasoconstricting action. These effects restore the cardiac output and blood pressure to a more normal level.

Preparation, dosage, and administration. Levarterenol bitartrate is available in 4-ml. ampules containing 0.2% solutions of the drug (8 mg.). Four milliliters is usually added to 1000 ml. of 5% glucose in distilled water or to 5% glucose in physiologic saline solution. Initially, it is administered slowly by intravenous infusion with a control drip bulb, 2 to 3 ml. per minute at first. The amount may be decreased to 0.5 to 1 ml. per minute, depending on the response of the patient. Vessels in the hand and ankle should not be used due to the risk of inducing gangrene. Since the drug is quickly metabolized, its pressor effects disappear within 1 to 2 minutes after the infusion is stopped. Heparin is usually added to the infusion solution to inhibit venous thrombosis. The drug is also available in 2-ml. ampules of 0.02% solution for immediate intravenous or intracardiac administration in patients with cardiac arrest. The drug is ineffective when given orally.

During administration the blood pressure of the patient must be taken frequently (every 2 to 5 minutes), since the rate of infusion is determined by changes in the patient's heart rate and blood pressure. Direct arterial measurement with an intra-arterial catheter is the preferred method of taking the blood pressure. However, the indirect measurement of blood pressure using the sphygmomanometer may be used. It should be kept in mind that blood pressure measurement obtained indirectly is significantly lower than that obtained by direct measurement; the difference may be as much as 15 mm. Hg.

Cautions. Overdosage can produce marked hypertension, severe headache, photophobia,

Table 9-4 Direct adrenergic drug effects—catecholamine type

	Epinephrine	*Norepinephrine*	*Isoproterenol*
Trade names	Adrenalin	Noradrenalin Levarterenol	Isuprel

Mode of action
  Alpha receptors
  Beta receptors
	Stimulates
	Stimulates
		Stimulates
		Stimulates the heart
			N.S.*
			Stimulates

Effects
  Cardiovascular
    Myocardium
	Increases rate and strength
	  of contractions
	Increases output
		Slows rate
		  reflexly
			Like epinephrine

Pacemaker cells	Stimulates Increases irritability May cause arrhythmias	Stimulates—like epinephrine	Like epinephrine
Coronary vessels	Dilates—increases blood flow	Dilates	Like epinephrine
Blood pressure	Increases (depending on dose)	Increases	Decreases diastolic Slightly increases systolic

Bronchi	Relaxes
	Improves airway
		Relaxes less than
		  epinephrine
			Potent bronchodilator—
			  more effective than epi-
			  nephrine

Blood vessels
    Skeletal muscle
	Dilates—increases
	  blood flow
		—	Dilates—increases
			  blood flow

Kidney	Constricts—decreases
	  blood flow
		Constricts—decreases
		  blood flow
			N.S.

Gastrointestinal tract	Relaxes smooth muscle Inhibits peristalsis	Like epinephrine	N.S.

Metabolic	Increases oxygen
	  consumption
	Mobilizes glycogen
	Causes hyperglycemia
		Increases metabolic rate
		  but less than epinephrine
			N.S.

Remarks	Tolerance does not
	  develop
		Infiltration into tissues may
		  cause necrosis and
		  sloughing	

Uses	Widely used for allergic
	  states, cardiac arrest;
	  with local anesthetics
	Given by injection or
	  inhalation
		To elevate blood pressure,
		  give by slow intravenous
		  infusion
			Heart failure
			Asthma

*N.S., Not significant.

chest pain, pallor, and vomiting. Great care must be taken that the drug does not leak into subcutaneous tissue, since its marked local vasoconstricting effect may cause the tissues to slough. If infiltration occurs, the area should be promptly infiltrated with 5 to 10 mg. of phentolamine in 10 to 15 ml. of normal saline solution.

A solution that is brown or that contains a precipitate should not be used.

Levarterenol should not be given to patients with mesenteric thrombosis, since the drug may increase ischemia and extend the area of infarction. Edema, hemorrhage, and necrosis of the intestine; hepatic and renal necrosis; focal myocarditis; subpericardial hemorrhage; and gangrene of the extremities have been reported following prolonged administration of levarterenol.

Isoproterenol

Isoproterenol has predominant beta adrenergic action. It is a synthetic catecholamine with potent cardiovascular properties. Its chemical structure resembles that of epinephrine and norepinephrine.

Its positive inotropic and chronotropic actions are greater than those of epinephrine. These effects result in increased stroke volume, cardiac output and cardiac work, and coronary flow. Therefore, it is a useful drug for patients with some types of heart disease, particularly heart block.

Uses. Isoproterenol's effects improve atrioventricular conduction and enhance the rhythmicity of the sinoatrial and ventricular pacemakers. This makes isoproterenol an important drug—and for many authorities the drug of choice—for the treatment of atrioventricular heart block and asystole. By accelerating the action of the basic pacemakers of the heart, ectopic pacemaker activity and arrhythmias are suppressed. However, its effect on cardiac automaticity can enhance ventricular irritability. Thus, some cardiologists recommend its use in atrio-

ventricular block only for patients with slow ventricular responses who do not respond to atropine. Pacemaker implantation may be preferred.

In addition, isoproterenol relaxes arterial and bronchial smooth muscles. Isoproterenol produces both pulmonary and systemic arterial dilation, which decreases vascular resistance. It can be used to reverse pulmonary hypertension caused by pressor agents, pulmonary embolism, and incompatible blood transfusion.

Isoproterenol is a more active bronchodilator than epinephrine. It shrinks swollen mucous membrane and reduces mucus secretion. This makes it a useful drug in the treatment of bronchial asthma and pulmonary emphysema and for the prevention and treatment of bronchospasm and laryngospasm during anesthesia. It is also used for the patient who is no longer benefited by the use of epinephrine and for the patient in status asthmaticus.

Isoproterenol is also used during cardiac catheterization to simulate exercise to help determine its effects on cardiovascular activity, particularly in evaluating congenital cardiac defects and acquired valvular disease. The use of isoproterenol for patients in shock is still experimental.

Preparation, dosage, and administration. The following are the preparations available of isoproterenol.

Isoproterenol hydrochloride, U.S.P. (Isuprel, Aludrine). Isoproterenol hydrochloride is available in 10- and 15-mg. sublingual tablets. However, their absorption is variable, unreliable, and at times associated with pronounced side effects such as nausea, tachycardia, and palpitations. Isoproterenol is used as a solution for inhalation in concentrations of 1:100, 1:200, and 1:400 and as a solution for injection in 1:5000 concentration. Solutions of isoproterenol turn pink on exposure to air, and patients should be told that saliva and sputum may appear pink after oral inhalation of the drug.

Isoproterenol sulfate, N.F. (Norisodrine Sulfate, Isonorin Sulfate); *isoprenaline sulfate,* B.P. This is available in the form of a powder for insufflation (10% and 25%), as a solution for inhalation (1:100), and in tablets (10 mg.) for sublingual administration.

Isoproterenol may be given intravenously. From 1 to 4 mg. per minute may be given in a continuous drip. From 5 to 40 mg. per minute have been used to arouse a pacemaker. It has been shown that isoproterenol is an effective drug in the treatment of Stokes-Adams syndrome when 1.0 mg. is administered in 200 ml. of 5% dextrose in water starting at 20 drops per minute. Thereafter, flow is regulated to maintain ventricular rate at 35 to 50 beats per minute.

Side effects and toxic effects. Untoward effects include precordial pain, heart palpitation, anginal pain, headache, nausea, tremor, and flushing of the skin. There may be a fall in arterial blood pressure. It is contraindicated for patients who have insufficient coronary blood flow and those with a history of tachycardia. Toxic effects can be counteracted by administering propranolol.

Precautions. Isoproterenol must be used cautiously in patients with valvular stenosis. Caution should also be exercised when the patient has digitalis-induced heart block.

INDIRECT AND DIRECT STIMULANTS OF ALPHA AND BETA RECEPTORS

A large number of drugs, structurally related to the catecholamines, exert effects on alpha and beta receptors by releasing catecholamines from adrenergic nerves. These are the indirectly acting sympathomimetic amines. Others act directly on the receptors, while some have both indirect and direct effects. These drugs are used widely in medicine and will be discussed below.

Ephedrine

Ephedrine is the name given to an active principle isolated from an Asiatic herb, ma huang (*Ephedra vulgaris*, var. *helvetica*), which has been used in the practice of medicine in China for more than 5000 years. In chemical composition it is an amine, closely allied to epinephrine, and it is an alkaloid. At the present time, most of the ephedrine used is produced synthetically.

Action and result. Ephedrine has both a direct and an indirect sympathomimetic action. Its indirect action is caused by its release of norepinephrine or the impairment of norepinephrine uptake by storage granules. Ephedrine is both an alpha and beta adrenergic stimulant. Like epinephrine and norepinephrine, ephedrine has positive inotropic (myocardial stimulation) and chronotropic (increased heart rate) activity, but it is a less effective vasoconstrictor. However, it does raise the blood pressure and is used for this purpose during spinal anesthesia and to treat orthostatic hypotension. It is beneficial for the treatment of hypotension caused by shock from any cause.

Ephedrine resembles epinephrine but differs from it in a number of ways. Ephedrine is more stable than epinephrine, it is well absorbed from the gastrointestinal tract, and it is effective when given orally. Its action is slower, more prolonged, but less intense than that produced by epinephrine. In addition, ephedrine stimulates the central nervous system by acting on the cerebral cortex and medulla. This accounts for its use in the treatment of narcolepsy, a state in which the patient persistently falls asleep. However, this use for ephedrine has been largely replaced by the amphetamines.

Its ability to stimulate the respiratory center in the medulla makes ephedrine a useful drug for the treatment of narcotic, barbiturate, and alcohol poisoning.

Ephedrine relaxes hypertonic muscle in the bronchioles and in the gastrointestinal tract. Emptying time of the stomach and intestine is delayed. Sphincter muscles in the urinary as well as in the gastrointestinal tracts are stimulated. The effect on metabolism is similar to that of epinephrine.

In the treatment of bronchial asthma, ephedrine is useful in preventing acute attacks. Epinephrine is preferable when attacks are acute because of its more rapid effect.

As a constituent of nasal drops, jellies, and sprays, ephedrine relieves acute congestion of hay fever, sinusitis, head colds, and vasomotor rhinitis. Shrinkage of mucous membranes begins immediately and lasts for several hours. Vasodilation does not ordinarily follow vasoconstriction, as may occur after administration of epinephrine.

Ephedrine exhibits a tendency to increase the tone of skeletal muscle. It is used in the treatment of muscle weakness associated with myasthenia gravis. It is most effective, however, when combined with prostigmine.

Ephedrine may be used in solution as a mydriatic when a cycloplegic action is not desired. It is not useful if inflammation is present. It acts as a mydriatic in the eye by acting on the radial muscles of the iris. This occurs with local application to the eye and with systemic administration of the drug.

A 3% to 4% solution is used for eyedrops, and the oral range of dosage is 20 to 50 mg. (gr. $^1/_3$ to $^3/_4$) every 3 or 4 hours. The oral dose for children is 3 mg. per kilogram of body weight daily, divided into four or six portions. Children are more resistant than adults to the stimulant effects of ephedrine.

Preparation, dosage, and administration. The following are the preparations and dosages of ephedrine.

Ephedrine sulfate capsules, U.S.P.; *ephedrine sulfate tablets.* These are available in 25 and 50 mg. for oral administration. The usual dose is 25 mg. (gr. $^3/_8$) taken three or four times daily. Effects occur 30 minutes to 1 hour after oral administration.

Ephedrine sulfate injection, U.S.P. This is available in 1-ml. ampules and 10-ml. vials containing 25 or 50 mg. (gr. $^3/_8$ to $^3/_4$) of drug per milliliter for injection. The usual dose is 25 mg. (gr. $^3/_8$).

Ephedrine hydrochloride, N.F., B.P. This is available in capsule and tablet form and the usual dose is 25 mg. (gr. $^3/_8$).

Ephedrine sulfate nasal solution, U.S.P. This is available in 1% and 3% solutions of the drug in 0.36% sodium chloride solution, to be further diluted with an equal amount of isotonic saline before use.

Ephedrine sulfate syrup, U.S.P. The usual dose is 5 ml. (20 mg. ephedrine sulfate).

Ephedrine sulfate and phenobarbital capsules, N.F. Each capsule contains 25 or 50 mg. of ephedrine sulfate and 15 or 30 mg. of phenobarbital.

(The main difference between the hydrochloride and the sulfate salts of ephedrine is that the latter are more freely soluble in water.)

Side effects and toxic effects. Older men may experience difficulty with voiding because of ephedrine's ability to relax bladder musculature. Anxiety, irritability, headache, tremor, anorexia, palpitation, and insomnia are common side effects. Nausea and vomiting may also occur. Occasionally a patient will exhibit symptoms of hypersensitivity. The same precautions are recommended for the use of ephedrine as for epinephrine. Barbiturates or some type of sedative is sometimes prescribed for the patient who is receiving the drug over a period of time. This is to counteract the central stimulating effect of ephedrine. Diminished response to the drug occurs with repeated administration. Although tolerance develops, ephedrine has not been known to cause addiction.

Phenylephrine hydrochloride, U.S.P., B.P. (Neo-Synephrine Hydrochloride)

Phenylephrine hydrochloride is a synthetic adrenergic drug chemically related to epinephrine, norepinephrine, and ephedrine.

Action and uses. Phenylephrine hydrochloride is relatively nontoxic, exhibits fewer side effects than epinephrine, and has longer lasting therapeutic effects. It has no effect on the central nervous system.

Phenylephrine hydrochloride is a powerful stimulator of alpha receptors and is therefore a potent vasoconstrictor. It elevates both the systolic and diastolic blood pressures. Its vasoconstricting action is more prolonged than that of epinephrine—it lasts 20 minutes after intravenous administration and 50 minutes after subcutaneous injection. For these reasons it is often used to treat hypotension caused by myocardial infarction, orthostatic hypotension, and hypotension resulting from loss of vasomotor tone from spinal anesthesia. It is not effective in shock caused by loss of blood volume.

Phenylephrine has very little inotropic or chronotropic effect. It does cause a reflex bradycardia as a result of its ability to elevate the blood pressure, which stimulates the baroreceptors and vagal activity. It is therefore an effective drug in converting paroxysmal tachycardia to a normal rate.

When applied topically to mucous membranes, it reduces swelling and congestion by constricting the small blood vessels.

It is useful in the treatment of sinusitis, vasomotor rhinitis, and hay fever and is used alone or with other drugs for the relief of bronchial asthma. It is sometimes combined with local anesthetics to retard their systemic absorption and to prolong their action.

Phenylephrine hydrochloride is used as a mydriatic for certain conditions in which dilation of the pupil is desired without cycloplegia (paralysis of the ciliary muscle).

Preparation, dosage, and administration. Phenylephrine hydrochloride is marketed in 10- and 25-mg. capsules for oral administration, as a solution for injection (10 mg. per milliliter in 1- and 5-ml. containers), and in a number of forms for topical application—solutions, an ophthalmic solution, a jelly, and an emulsion.

For topical application to the nasal mucous membrane, 0.25% solution is ordinarily used. As a mydriatic, 1 or 2 drops are used of the 1% solution or emulsion or the 2.5% ophthalmic solution.

The intramuscular or subcutaneous dose for adults ranges from 1 to 10 mg.; the dose for children is 0.1 mg. per kilogram of body weight. The dose for hypotensive states is 10 mg. of phenylephrine in 500 ml. of 5% dextrose by slow intravenous infusion, or 0.25 to 0.5 mg. diluted in sodium chloride injected slowly. For orthostatic hypotension the oral dose for adults is 20 mg. three times daily; for children the dose is 1 mg. per kilogram of body weight in 24 hours divided into six doses.

Side effects and precautions. Oral doses may cause mild gastrointestinal symptoms, which may be avoided by giving the drug after meals. Phenylephrine may cause tremor, insomnia, and palpitations. Intravenous doses may induce ventricular extrasystoles, paroxysmal ventricular tachycardia, a feeling of fullness in the head, and paresthesias.

Phenylephrine should be used with great caution in elderly patients or patients with hyperthyroidism, bradycardia, partial heart block, myocardial disease, or severe arteriosclerosis.

Ophthalmic solutions are contraindicated in patients with narrow-angle glaucoma.

Mephentermine sulfate, N.F., B.P. (Wyamine Sulfate)

$$CH_2-\underset{\underset{CH_3}{|}}{\overset{\overset{CH_3}{|}}{C}}-NH-CH_3 \cdot \frac{1}{2} H_2SO_4 \cdot H_2O$$

Mephentermine sulfate is a white crystalline powder that is freely soluble in water.

Action. Its effects are similar to those of ephedrine, but it brings about far less cerebral stimulation. Local application in the eye produces dilation of the pupil.

Mephentermine is an indirectly acting sympathomimetic. It releases catecholamines from storage sites in the heart and other tissues. Therefore, it tends to bring about both alpha and beta stimulating effects and inotropic and chronotropic effects on the heart.

Its vasoconstrictor effect is used to treat hypotensive states not associated with hemorrhage. In these cases the drug is given intramuscularly or intravenously. Onset of action occurs within 5 to 15 minutes and lasts 1 to 2 hours. Since it improves cardiac contraction and mobilizes blood from venous pools, thereby increasing cardiac output, it is also used in heart failure following a myocardial infarction. Mephentermine also increases cardiac conduction and shortens the refractory period of the heart. This makes it useful in treating certain cardiac arrhythmias.

Like ephedrine, mephentermine constricts the small blood vessels of the nasal mucosa and can be used topically or by inhalation to relieve nasal congestion. It does not cause rebound congestion.

It should be noted that if catecholamine

storage sites have been depleted, there may be no pressor response from mephentermine. In this case, administration of norepinephrine resupplies these depots or storage sites, which restores the action of mephentermine.

Preparation, dosage, and administration. Mephentermine sulfate is administered topically for nasal congestion and orally, intramuscularly, and intravenously for systemic effects. It is available in injection form containing 15 and 30 mg. per milliliter; as an elixir, 5 mg. per milliliter; in tablets (12.5 and 25 mg.) for oral administration; and as a solution (0.5%) for topical administration to nasal membranes (2 or 3 drops every 4 hours as needed). Dosage for systemic effect varies from 10 to 30 mg. Inhalers are also marketed that contain 250 mg. of the drug. Dose for children is 0.4 mg. per kilogram of body weight.

When given by continuous intravenous drip, 600 to 1000 mg. may be added to 1 liter of 5% glucose in water. Continuous blood pressure monitoring is required, since adverse blood pressure responses may occur.

D.E.S.I. rating for mephentermine is: *effective* for the treatment of hypotension occurring with spinal anesthesia or that which is secondary to ganglionic blockade; *probably effective* for the treatment of hypotension occurring during surgical or obstetrical procedures and shock accompanying myocardial infarction. The elixir and tablets are rated as *probably effective* for treatment of postural hypotension.

Side effects and precautions are similar to those of previously discussed sympathomimetics.

Metaraminol bitartrate, U.S.P., B.P. (Aramine Bitartrate, Pressonex Bitartrate)

$$OH \quad \overset{OH}{\underset{}{\underset{}{\text{CH}}}} \quad \overset{CH_3}{\underset{}{\text{CH}}} - NH_2$$

Metaraminol is a vasopressor agent with both direct and indirect effects on the sympathetic system. It acts indirectly by releasing norepinephrine from tissues and storage sites and directly as a neurohormone. Metaraminol also has positive inotropic effects. Since it constricts blood vessels, increases peripheral resistance, elevates both systolic and diastolic blood pressure, and improves cardiac contractility and cerebral, coronary, and renal blood flow, it is a valuable drug for the treatment of shock. It is used to overcome hypotension associated with myocardial infarction, surgical procedures, barbiturate poisoning, and trauma.

Since it exhibits beta as well as alpha adrenergic activity, it is often effective in raising blood pressure when alpha adrenergic agents are ineffective. This may be because of its ability to bring about a more effective venous flow. It does not appear to cause arrhythmias.

While the action of metaraminol is similar to that of norepinephrine, it is a less potent drug. Its onset of action is more gradual than that obtained from norepinephrine, but it is longer acting. It exerts a smoother blood pressure response than some of the other vasopressor agents, which makes it easier to determine rate of flow when given intravenously.

Preparation, dosage, and administration. Metaraminol is available in 1- and 10-ml. units containing 10 mg. per milliliter. It may be given intramuscularly in a 2- to 10-mg. dose, or by intravenous drip, 15 to 100 mg. in 500 ml. of 5% dextrose in physiologic saline. Intramuscular dose for children is 0.1 mg. per kilogram of body weight. Effects appear in 5 to 20 minutes after subcutaneous injection, 10 minutes after intramuscular injection, and within 1 or 2 minutes following intravenous administration. In emergency situations, 500 μg. to 5 mg. of metaraminol may be injected intravenously. The A.M.A. does not recommend the subcutaneous route since tissue sloughing may occur. Care should be taken to prevent tissue infiltration of intravenous infusions of metaraminol.

D.E.S.I. rating is: *effective* for hypotension occurring with spinal anesthesia, and as adjunctive treatment of hypotension resulting from hemorrhage, surgery, trauma, or drugs; *probably effective* for treatment of hypotension resulting from cardiogenic shock and septicemia.

The same precautions should be employed when giving metaraminol as when giving other powerful vasoconstrictors.

Table 9-5 Adrenergic drug effects—noncatecholamine type

	Ephedrine	Phenylephrine	Mephentermine	Metaraminol	Methoxamine
Trade names		Neo-Synephrine	Wyamine	Aramine Pressonex	Vasoxyl
Mode of action Alpha receptors Beta receptors	Stimulates Stimulates More prolonged but less intense action than epinephrine	Stimulates N.S.	Stimulates	Stimulates	Stimulates
Effects Cardiovascular Myocardium	Variable	N.S. Bradycardia may occur reflexly	Increases contractility and rate May cause bradycardia	Some increase in contractility Bradycardia may occur	— Reflex bradycardia may occur
Pacemaker cells	N.S.*	N.S.	N.S.		
Coronary vessels	Dilates—increases blood flow	Dilates—increases blood flow	Dilates—increases blood flow	—	—
Blood pressure	Increases	Increases	Increases	Increases	Increases
Bronchi	Dilates	Dilates but less than epinephrine	Dilates but less than epinephrine	N.S.	
Cerebral effects	Stimulating action	N.S.	N.S.	—	—
Blood vessels Skeletal muscle	N.S.	—†	N.S.	N.S.	—
Kidney	Constricts	Constricts	Constricts but less than ephedrine	Constricts— decreases blood flow	Decreases blood flow
Gastrointestinal tract	Decreases peristalsis	Decreases motility	Relaxes smooth muscle—inhibits	Some inhibition	Inhibits
Metabolic	Increases metabolic rate	Some increase in metabolic rate	N.S.	N.S.	N.S.
Remarks	Serious arrhythmias may occur if used with digitalis Can be given orally			Prolonged duration of action, cumulative effects may occur—give drug slowly May cause tissue sloughing—do not give subcutaneously	
Uses	Vasopressor Allergic states Nasal decongestant Enuresis Myasthenia gravis	Nasal decongestant Vasopressor Paroxysmal atrial tachycardia Mydriatic	Vasopressor Nasal decongestant	Vasopressor Nasal decongestant	Vasopressor Paroxysmal atrial tachycardia Nasal decongestant

*N.S., Not significant.
†Effect is slight, none, or unknown in man.

Methoxamine hydrochloride, U.S.P. (Vasoxyl)

$$CH_3O-\text{benzene ring}-\underset{OH}{\underset{|}{CH}}-\underset{CH_3}{\underset{|}{CH}}\cdot NH_2, \quad OCH_3$$

Methoxamine is an alpha adrenergic stimulator that appears to be devoid of beta receptor activity. Therefore, it is almost exclusively a vasoconstrictor. It is used in treating nasal congestion and hypotension. Since it has no stimulating effect on the heart, the rise in blood pressure causes a reflex bradycardia. It is this effect that makes it useful in treating paroxysmal supraventricular tachycardia.

Preparation, dosage, and administration. Methoxamine is supplied in solution form for intramuscular or intravenous injection. It is available in 1-ml. ampules containing 20 mg., in 10-ml. vials containing 10 mg. per milliliter, and in 1-ml. ampules containing 15 mg. of methoxamine and 10 mg. procaine hydrochloride. It is also available in a 0.5% nasal solution. Intramuscular dose for adults ranges from 5 to 20 mg.; for children the dose is 0.25 mg. per kilogram of body weight.

When it is given intravenously its effects occur almost immediately and last for 1 hour; intramuscularly, effects occur within 15 minutes and persist for about 90 minutes. Slow intravenous infusions of the drug may also be used—35 to 40 mg. methoxamine in 250 ml. of 5% dextrose.

Side effects. Side effects include severe headache, urinary urgency, and vomiting.

D.E.S.I. rating is: *effective* for maintaining blood pressure during anesthesia, and for terminating some episodes of paroxysmal supraventricular tachycardia; *ineffective* for treatment of shock resulting from myocardial infarction and as a vasopressor for use in poor risk candidates for emergency surgery.

Table 9-6 Principal uses of adrenergic drugs

Vasoconstrictor (pressor) action (treatment of hypotensive states)

Epinephrine	Methoxamine
Isoproterenol	Mephentermine
Levarterenol (norepinephrine)	Phenylephrine
Metaraminol	Phenylpropanolamine

Local vasoconstrictor action (hemostasis; prolong local anesthetic action)

Epinephrine	Methoxamine

Nasal decongestant action (in treatment of allergic rhinitis, common cold, hay fever)

Ephedrine	Phenylephrine
Mephentermine	Phenylpropanolamine
Methoxamine	Propylhexedrine

Bronchodilator action (in treatment of asthma)

Ephedrine	Phenylpropanolamine
Epinephrine	Protokylol
Isoproterenol	
Methoxyphenamine	

Vasodilator action (in treatment of peripheral vascular disease)

Nylidrine	

Mydriatic action (for ophthalmologic examination)

Ephedrine	Phenylephrine

ALPHA BLOCKING AGENTS

Most alpha adrenergic blocking agents are competitive blockers; that is, they compete with the catecholamines at receptor sites and inhibit adrenergic sympathetic stimulation. They are more effective against action of circulating catecholamines than against catecholamines released from storage sites. These drugs may be obtained from natural sources, such as ergot and its derivatives, or they may be synthesized.

Alpha blocking agents are used in the treatment of peripheral vascular disease; ergotamine is used to treat migraine headache. Phenotolamine is used in the diagnosis and surgical management of pheochromocytoma (tumors of the medullary portion of the adrenal gland that secrete large amounts of epinephrine and norepinephrine). Most adrenergic blocking agents are not drugs of choice in the treatment of essential hypertension, because their action is too unpredictable and side effects too troublesome.

Phenoxybenzamine hydrochloride, N.F., B.P. (Dibenzyline)

Phenoxybenzamine abolishes or decreases the receptiveness of alpha receptors to adrenergic stimuli. Its effects are predominantly those of vasodilation and inhibition of vasospasm. This drug lowers peripheral resistance and increases the size of the vascular space. For these reasons it is a useful drug in the treatment of peripheral vascular diseases, such as Raynaud's disease.

Since this agent competes with the catecholamines, it is also useful in decreasing the blood pressure of patients with pheochromocytoma. It does not block sympathetic impulses on the heart and therefore does not impair cardiac output directly. It has mild antihistaminic activity and may cause nasal drying.

Preparation, dosage, and administration. Phenoxybenzamine is available in 10-mg. capsules for oral use. The initial dose is usually 10 mg. daily. Dosage may be increased by increments of 10 mg. at 4-day intervals. Maintenance dosage is usually 20 to 60 mg. daily. Onset of action occurs in about 2 hours, and duration of action is 24 to 36 hours. Daily administration causes cumulative effects, intensifies side effects, and predisposes to toxic effects.

Side effects and toxic effects. Common side effects from phenoxybenzamine include nasal congestion, miosis, reflex tachycardia, and postural hypotension. Sedation, drowsiness, and failure to ejaculate occur occasionally.

Toxic symptoms include severe postural hypotension, vomiting, lethargy, shock, and circulatory failure.

Phentolamine hydrochloride, N.F. (Regitine Hydrochloride); phentolamine mesylate, U.S.P., B.P. (Regitine Mesylate)

Phentolamine is a direct vasodilator and an inhibitor of hypertension when there are excessive levels of epinephrine and norepinephrine. Its direct effect is more potent than its adrenergic blocking action.

Phentolamine is used in the diagnosis of pheochromocytoma. Since this tumor secretes large amounts of catecholamines, which produce elevated blood pressure, a marked fall in blood pressure following administration of phentolamine suggests the presence of pheochromocytoma. However, the test lacks precision. A false positive test may occur if the patient recently received a sedative, narcotic, or antihypertensive drug.

This drug is also used to reverse the vasoconstrictive action of an overdose or excessive response to injected norepinephrine (levarterenol). The subcutaneous injection of phentolamine following extravasation of intravenous norepinephrine will prevent tissue necrosis if prompt action is taken.

Preparation, dosage, and administration. Phentolamine hydrochloride is available in 50-mg. tablets for oral use. The usual adult dose is 50 mg. four to six times daily; for children the dose is 5 mg. per kilogram of body weight daily divided into four or six doses.

Phentolamine mesylate is administered intramuscularly or intravenously. It is prepared in 5-mg. vials to which 1 ml. of diluent is added for injection. The amount used in the test for pheochromocytoma is 5 mg. A decrease in blood pressure of more than 35 mm. Hg systolic and 25 mm. Hg diastolic implies pheochromocytoma. The preoperative dose for removal of the adrenal tumor is 2 to 5 mg. given 1 or 2 hours before surgery. For children the dose is usually 1 mg. or 0.1 mg./kg.

Side effects. Side effects include tachycardia, orthostatic hypotension, nausea and vomiting, diarrhea, weakness, dizziness, and flushing. Phentolamine should be used with caution in patients with gastritis or peptic ulcer, since it has a stimulant action on the gastrointestinal tract, and in patients with coronary artery disease.

ERGOT ALKALOIDS

Alkaloids found in extracts of a fungous disease of rye called *ergot* are derivatives of lysergic acid; some of these alkaloids cause alpha receptor blockade. The ergot alkaloids have many other effects. They are powerful constrictors of vascular or uterine smooth muscle. This action has nothing to do with the slight adrenergic effect they possess.

Ergotamine tartrate

Ergotamine has marked vasoconstrictor activity. All ergot alkaloids stimulate uterine smooth muscle; both tone and amplitude of uterine contractions are increased. However, ergotamine is no longer used as an oxytocic. It is now used chiefly to treat migraine headache and is considered almost a specific for this condition. Its efficacy in migraine is thought to result from ce-

rebral vasoconstriction, which decreases the amplitude of the pulsations of cranial arteries. The earlier the drug is taken, the smaller the dose needed and the more rapid the effect. Administration of the drug should be followed by bed rest in a quiet, darkened room for an hour or two.

This drug also has been used to relieve intense itching and hives associated with jaundice, cirrhosis of the liver, or Hodgkin's disease.

Since this drug has a cumulative action, it must be used with caution. It is capable of producing all the symptoms of ergotism: numbness and tingling of the fingers and toes, muscle pains and muscle weakness, as well as gangrene and blindness. Thus, daily use is not advised. Its use is contraindicated in patients with diabetes mellitus, hepatic and renal disease, peripheral vascular disease, and in pregnancy.

Preparation, dosage, and administration. The following are the ergotamine preparations available.

Ergotamine tartrate, U.S.P., B.P. (Gynergen). The usual oral dose is 2 mg., and the usual intramuscular or subcutaneous dose is 0.25 mg. Oral dose for children over 5 years of age is 1 mg. Ergotamine tartrate is available in tablets for oral administration (1 mg.), 2-mg. sublingual tablets, in ampules of solution for parenteral administration (0.25 mg. in 0.5 ml. and 0.5 mg. in 1 ml.), as a solution for inhalation (9 mg. per milliliter in 2.5-ml. containers; a single inhalation contains 0.36 mg.), and as suppositories for rectal administration.

Ergotamine with caffeine, N.F. (Cafergot). Each tablet contains 1 mg. ergotamine tartrate and 100 mg. caffeine. Usual dose is one to two tablets for headache. Dosage may be repeated if necessary every 30 minutes; no more than six tablets should be taken per attack. The caffeine presumably increases the effectiveness of ergotamine because of its own vasoconstrictor action.

Dihydroergotamine, N.F. (D.H.E. 45). This compound is prepared by hydrogenating ergotamine. It is available in 1-ml. ampules that contain 1 mg. of the drug. Administration is intramuscular or intravenous. Dose is 1 mg. at onset of attack; this may be repeated in 1 hour. It is said to produce fewer side effects than ergotamine tartrate. However, effects are less predictable.

Methysergide maleate, U.S.P. (Sansert)

Methysergide maleate, a drug related structurally to the ergot alkaloids, is effective for the prophylactic treatment of vascular headaches, such as migraine, cluster headaches, and others. It is of no value for treating acute attacks or in preventing tension headache. Each tablet contains 2 mg. of methysergide maleate. The drug is a serotonin antagonist.

Retroperitoneal fibrosis has been noted in a small number of patients on methysergide therapy. Its signs and symptoms usually present themselves as urinary tract obstruction. Pleuropulmonary and cardiac fibroses have also been reported. If symptoms of peripheral vascular insufficiency occur, such as cold, numb, or painful extremities and diminished pulse, the drug should be discontinued to prevent severe tissue ischemia. Because of these serious complications and numerous side effects, the approved package insert should be consulted before the drug is used. The usual dose is two to four tablets, preferably one tablet with each meal. Because of the potential dangers of prolonged therapy, treatment with methysergide should not exceed 6 months without a rest period of 3 to 4 weeks. Dosage should be gradually reduced to avoid rebound headache. In addition, patients should be instructed to report promptly any dysuria, back pain, dyspnea, or chest pain.

BETA BLOCKING AGENTS

In the United States, the only beta blocking agent presently in clinical use is propranolol (Inderal). This drug is chemically related to isoproterenol. Other drugs, Sotalol and oxprenolol

(Trasicor), are undergoing experimental clinical trials.

Beta blockers inhibit the beta receptors by competing with the catecholamines at the effector site. The exact mode of action is not known. These agents *block* beta receptors in the myocardium, bronchial, and vascular smooth muscle.

Propranolol hydrochloride, U.S.P., B.P. (Inderal)

Propranolol inhibits the inotropic and chronotropic actions caused by beta adrenergic stimulation and has a quinidine-like effect and local anesthetic effect. Propranolol inhibits pacemaker activity (normal as well as ectopic), decreases atrioventricular conduction, and prolongs cardiac diastole. It also decreases heart rate and myocardial activity, suppresses myocardial automaticity, increases systolic ejection time, and increases cardiac volume. These actions account for its clinical effectiveness in controlling various ventricular arrhythmias including digitalis-induced arrhythmia when hypokalemia is not present. It may be used in the preparation of patients for cardioversion when digitalis must be withheld prior to cardioversion.

Propranolol has been found effective in the treatment of some cases of angina, which is probably due to its ability to prevent an increase in cardiac rate during exercise. There is evidence that patients treated with propranolol can undertake a greater amount of exercise before experiencing anginal pain.

In addition, propranolol increases airway resistance, inhibits glucogenolysis in skeletal and cardiac muscles, and blocks adrenergic release of free fatty acids and insulin. It also has a hypotensive effect when taken orally for a prolonged period. Propranolol may cause EKG changes such as higher voltage T waves and an increase in the Q-T interval. Propranolol is being used experimentally in antihypertensive therapy either alone or with another hypotensive agent.

Dosage and administration. Propranolol may be administered orally or intravenously. It may be used alone or in conjunction with other antiarrhythmic agents. When given orally, it is most readily absorbed in the fasting state and therefore should be given before meals. It is effective within 30 minutes, peak action occurs in 60 to 90 minutes, and the effect lasts about 6 hours. The usual oral dose is from 30 to 120 mg. daily. The drug is available in 10- and 40-mg. tablets. Propranolol is metabolized by hepatic enzymes. Optimal dosage for children has not been determined.

When propranolol is administered intravenously, maximal effect occurs within 3 to 5 minutes; duration of effect is 2 to 4 hours. The range of dose for intravenous administration is usually 1 to 5 mg. The drug is available in 1-ml. ampules containing 1 mg. of drug per milliliter. This drug *must* be given slowly with careful monitoring of vital signs with the electrocardiogram. Administration should be discontinued when a desirable change in heart rate or rhythm is noted.

Side effects. Side effects include nausea and vomiting, lightheadedness, lethargy, mental depression, and mild paresthesia.

Toxic effects. These include hypotension, bradycardia, heart block, congestive heart failure in patients with limited cardiac reserve, and intensified hypoglycemia in diabetic patients receiving insulin or oral hypoglycemic drugs. The latter effect occurs because beta-receptor activity is necessary for a rise in blood sugar and free fatty acids. Special precautions should be taken when propranolol is used along with other adrenergic blocking agents, since the effects are additive, or when used with MAO inhibitors, since the enhanced alpha effect may lead to hypertension.

Contraindications. Propranolol is contraindicated in patients with congestive heart failure, hypotension, asthma, and atrioventricular heart block.

CHOLINERGIC DRUGS

Acetylcholine plays an important role in transmission of nerve impulses in both the sympa-

$$CH_3-\overset{\overset{\displaystyle CH_3}{|}}{\underset{\underset{\displaystyle CH_3}{|}}{N^+}}-CH_2-CH_2-O-\overset{\displaystyle O}{\underset{\displaystyle \|}{C}}-CH_3$$

Acetylcholine

$$CH_3-\overset{\overset{\displaystyle CH_3}{|}}{\underset{\underset{\displaystyle CH_3}{|}}{N^+}}-CH_2-\overset{\overset{\displaystyle }{|}}{\underset{\underset{\displaystyle CH_3}{|}}{CH}}-O-\overset{\displaystyle O}{\underset{\displaystyle \|}{C}}-NH_2$$

Bethanechol
(carbamyl-β-methylcholine)

$$CH_3-\overset{\overset{\displaystyle CH_3}{|}}{\underset{\underset{\displaystyle CH_3}{|}}{N^+}}-CH_2-\overset{\overset{\displaystyle }{|}}{\underset{\underset{\displaystyle CH_3}{|}}{CH}}-O-\overset{\displaystyle O}{\underset{\displaystyle \|}{C}}-CH_3$$

Methacholine

thetic and parasympathetic divisions of the autonomic nervous system.

Acetylcholine has two major actions on the nervous system: (1) it has stimulant effects on the ganglia, adrenal medulla, and skeletal muscle, and (2) it has stimulant effects at postganglionic nerve endings in cardiac muscle, smooth muscle, and glands. The first action resembles the effects of nicotine and therefore is referred to as the "nicotinic action" of acetylcholine. The effects of acetylcholine at the effector cell are like that of muscarine (an alkaloid obtained from the toadstool *Amanita muscaria*), and they are referred to as the "muscarinic action" of acetylcholine. These terms are used in describing acetylcholine effects because both nicotine and muscarine and their effects on nerve impulses were studied long before acetylcholine was identified or synthesized. See Table 9-7 for these actions.

Those drugs chemically related to acetylcholine that produce similar effects are cholinergic drugs. These drugs may be obtained from plant sources or synthesized. The synthetic drugs are more stable and have a more selective action on particular organs.

Cholinergic fibers are widespread; they are present in heart, spleen, uterus, vas deferens, and colon and in the vessels of the skin and muscles. It is quite likely that cholinergic fibers are present in many more tissues of the body. In

Table 9-7 Muscarinic and nicotinic actions of acetylcholine

	Muscarinic action	Nicotinic action
Cardiovascular Blood vessels Heart rate Blood pressure	Dilation Slowed Decreased	Constriction ⎫ With large doses Increased ⎬ after atropine Increased ⎭
Gastrointestinal Tone Motility Sphincters	Increased Increased Relaxed	Increased Increased —
Glandular secretions	Increased salivary, lacrimal, intestinal, and sweat secretion	Initial stimulation then inhibition of salivary and bronchial secretions
Skeletal muscle	—	Stimulated
Autonomic ganglia	—	Stimulated
Eye	Pupil constriction Decreased accommodation	—
Blocking agent	Atropine	Tubocurarine
Remarks	Effects increase as dosage increases	Increased dosage inhibits effects and causes receptor blockade

the gastrointestinal tract parasympathetic innervation predominates; it stimulates both motor and secretory action.

Acetylcholine (ACh) is synthesized in motor nerve terminals under the control of the enzyme choline-acetylase. ACh is stored in vesicles within the nerve terminals and released by (1) spontaneous rupture of small numbers of vesicles or (2) rupture of large numbers of vesicles simultaneously with nerve impulse stimulation. The former action releases amounts of ACh too small to generate a propagated muscle contraction; the latter action releases ACh in amounts sufficient to initiate muscle fiber contraction. Influx of calcium ions into the nerve apparently increases the fragility of the vesicles, promoting

their rupture. When released from nerves the ACh is hydrolyzed within milliseconds by cholinesterase located on the surface of the end plate to allow for rapid transmission of the next impulse. Hence, the effect of acetylcholine is brief. When the enzyme is made ineffective, as it is by certain drugs (anticholinesterase drugs), the effect of acetylcholine is intensified and prolonged.

Cholinergic drugs are used:

1 To stimulate the intestines and bladder postoperatively
2 To lower intraocular pressure in glaucoma
3 To promote salivation and sweating
4 To dilate peripheral blood vessels in conditions of vasospasm

5 To terminate curarization
6 To symptomatically treat myasthenia gravis

The use of cholinergic agents to treat cardiac arrhythmias has been almost abandoned, since newer and more effective antiarrhythmic agents have been developed. Therapeutic effectiveness of cholinergic drugs depends primarily upon their muscarinic action; however, some of them also possess nicotinic action. This latter action usually requires doses much larger than those used therapeutically. However, some drugs may exhibit more nicotinic than muscarinic effects.

The ideal cholinergic or anticholinesterase drug would:

1 Mimic or inhibit the effect of acetylcholine on a particular structure or organ
2 Be effective when administered orally
3 Be more stable and less easily inactivated than the drugs now available
4 Produce a therapeutic effect with minimal side effects

While these ideal drugs are not yet available, progress has been and is being made in this direction.

Cholinergic drugs used primarily to lower intraocular pressure will be discussed in Chapter 22; these include pilocarpine and carbachol.

Bethanechol chloride, N.F. (Urecholine Chloride)

Bethanechol is a cholinergic agent that has rather selective effects on the smooth muscle of the gastrointestinal and urinary tracts, where it promotes motility of the intestines and contraction of the bladder. Its action is primarily muscarinic. It does not exhibit any ganglion-stimulating effect. Bethanechol is not destroyed by cholinesterase; therefore, its action is comparatively long. It is less potent than some of the other choline derivatives but it is also less toxic. Cardiovascular effects are minimal.

Uses. This compound is useful in conditions in which stimulation of the parasympathetic nervous system is indicated. It is used to treat gastric retention after vagotomy or gastric surgery, for postoperative abdominal distention, and for nonobstructive urinary retention. It is sometimes used to prevent paralytic ileus and urinary retention in patients receiving certain drugs for hypertension (ganglion-blocking agents).

Preparation, dosage, and administration. Bethanechol chloride is available in 1-ml. ampules containing 5 mg. of the drug and also in 5-, 10-, and 25-mg. tablets. Bethanechol chloride is administered orally, sublingually, or subcutaneously. It must not be given intramuscularly or intravenously.

Oral and sublingual doses of 10 to 30 mg. three or four times daily will usually control symptoms. The effect of the drug can usually be observed in about 30 minutes. When given orally it should be administered with meals since it increases volume and acidity of gastric secretions. The usual subcutaneous dose is 2.5 to 5 mg.

When used in children and infants the dose is 0.6 mg. per kilogram of body weight divided into three oral doses. For subcutaneous use the dose is one third to one fourth the oral dose.

D.E.S.I. rating for bethanechol is: *effective* for treatment of acute postoperative and postpartum nonobstructive urinary retention and for neurogenic atony of the bladder with retention of urine; *possibly effective* for stimulating gastrointestinal motility in postoperative abdominal distention; *ineffective* (and dangerous) in the treatment of obstructive urinary retention and of the chronically distended and atrophic urinary bladder. The oral tablets have received a "probably effective" rating.

Side effects and toxic effects. Side effects include headache, flushing, abdominal cramps, sweating, asthmatic attacks, and sometimes a drop in blood pressure. Parenteral administration of atropine promptly abolishes side effects. The major advantage of bethanechol over other choline derivatives is its greater margin of safety and low incidence of severe toxic effects.

Contraindications. Bethanechol should not be used after gastrointestinal anastomosis until healing has occurred; it should not be used when peritonitis is present or when there is vesical neck obstruction. Its use is also contraindicated during pregnancy or in patients with coronary disease, hyperthyroidism, asthma, and urinary obstruction.

Methacholine chloride, N.F. (Mecholyl Chloride)

At the present time methacholine is not a popular drug. It has been used for many different conditions—to improve muscle tone of various organs, increase secretions, treat paroxysmal atrial tachycardia—and in the diagnosis of pheochromocytoma. For the latter, a positive test results when the patient responds to a subcutaneous injection of methacholine with a rise in blood pressure caused by catecholamine release from the tumor. It has primarily muscarinic action and little nicotinic action.

Pilocarpine, U.S.P.

Pilocarpine is found in the leaves of the plant *Pilocarpus jaborandi*. It is employed in ophthalmology because it constricts the pupil. The drug also causes considerable salivation and sweating when given orally or by subcutaneous injection.

ANTICHOLINESTERASE DRUGS

Some drugs act as cholinergic agents, not by directly affecting the cells innervated by postganglionic cholinergic nerves but by inactivating or inhibiting the enzyme cholinesterase that normally degrades acetylcholine. In this way the activity of acetylcholine is prolonged and its concentration at the myoneural junction increased.

DRUGS USED FOR TREATMENT OF MYASTHENIA GRAVIS

Myasthenia gravis is a rare chronic disease manifested by extreme fatigability of the skeletal muscles. Although any skeletal muscle may be involved, those concerned with movement of the eyeballs, eyelids, and face and those used in chewing, swallowing, and speech are most likely to show involvement. Ptosis of the eyelids is an almost constant symptom. Diplopia is also likely to be present. The cause of this disease is not known, although recent studies suggest that the synaptic vesicles of motor nerves have a lower than normal acetylcholine content. The disease is usually subject to remissions and exacerbations (periods of improvement followed by periods of decline). Judicious use of neostigmine or other anticholinesterase drugs may produce dramatic results, but overdosage tends to aggravate the muscular fatigue and cause side effects such as nausea and vomiting, abdominal cramps, diarrhea, and muscle twitching. It is important

Table 9-8 Prominent cholinergic agents including the anticholinesterase drugs*

Generic name	Trade name	Single adult dose	Usual route of administration
Ambenonium	Mytelase	5-25 mg.	Oral
Benzpyrinium	Stigmonene	2 mg.	Intramuscular
Bethanechol	Urecholine	10-30 mg.	Oral
			Sublingual
		2.5-5 mg.	Subcutaneous
Isoflurophate	Floropryl	1-3 gtt. 0.1% solution	Topical (eye)
Neostigmine	Prostigmin		
Bromide	Bromide	15 mg.	Oral
Methylsulfate	Methylsulfate	0.5 mg. (1-2 mg.)	Intramuscular
Physostigmine	Eserine	0.02%-1% solution	Topical (eye)
Pilocarpine		0.5%-4% solution (1 gtt.)	Topical (eye)
Pyridostigmine	Mestinon	Highly variable	Oral

*Effects to be expected are similar to those that can be expected from stimulation of the parasympathetic nervous system (see Table 9-2). Drugs are listed in alphabetical order. The majority of drugs mentioned are administered in the form of their salts.

that the patient have sufficient therapy to maintain function of the chewing and swallowing muscles to avoid malnutrition.

Neostigmine (Prostigmin)

Neostigmine is a synthetic drug available only in the form of its salts, which are freely soluble in water and stable in aqueous solutions. Neostigmine has become the standard drug for therapy of myasthenia gravis. It has both muscarinic and nicotinic actions. Neostigmine preserves endogenous ACh and has a direct cholinomimetic action. This results in increased muscle power and relief from characteristic signs and symptoms of myasthenia gravis (ptosis, dyspnea, difficulty in swallowing, and so on).

Uses. Neostigmine is used to relieve abdominal distention caused by accumulation of gas and insufficient peristaltic activity after surgical operations. It is also used for the prevention and treatment of atonic conditions of the urinary bladder. It will enable the patient to empty the bladder completely. Neostigmine is used as an antidote for excessive curarization with muscle relaxants such as tubocurarine, which act by inhibiting ACh depolarization of the skeletal neuromuscular junction.

When given for diagnosis of myasthenia gravis, improvement in muscle strength should occur in 10 minutes and last 3 to 4 hours. Atropine should be given before administration of neostigmine to control side effects.

Neostigmine is also used as a test for pregnancy. It is given intramuscularly for 3 days, and if the patient is not pregnant bleeding will occur usually within 72 hours.

Neostigmine (ophthalmic solution) is sometimes used as a miotic for patients with glaucoma.

Preparation, dosage, and administration. The following are the preparations available of neostigmine.

Neostigmine bromide, U.S.P., B.P. (Prostigmin Bromide). This drug is available in 15-mg. tablets and also in the form of a slow-release tablet for oral administration. Some patients will require only one 15-mg. tablet two or three times a day and other patients may require twenty or more tablets a day. Increased physical activity and/or emotional strain usually causes the patient to require more medication. The usual dosage is 15 mg. three times a day. This drug is also available as a 5% ophthalmic solution. The slow-release dosage form decreases the need for administration of the drug at night.

Neostigmine methylsulfate injection, U.S.P., B.P. This is available in 1-ml. ampules containing 0.25-mg. (1:4000), 0.5-mg. (1:2000), and 1-mg. (1:1000) solution. The total daily dosage must be determined in accordance with the severity of the symptoms and the response of the patient. A dose of 0.5 mg. of neostigmine intramuscularly is said to be equivalent to 15 mg. given orally. In the treatment of myasthenia gravis 1 to 2 mg. given intramuscularly every 3 hours is generally satisfactory when the patient is unable to swallow. Sometimes neostigmine bromide is given orally and neostigmine methylsulfate is given intramuscularly to reinforce the oral dosage when symptoms are severe.

Side effects and toxic effects. Side effects include nausea and vomiting, diarrhea, abdominal cramps, muscle twitching, excessive salivary secretion, urinary urgency, rapid weak pulse, and low blood pressure. In addition the patient feels faint and apprehensive. With acute toxicity pulmonary edema and respiratory failure may occur (cholinergic crisis). Excessive doses of any of the anticholinesterase compounds may cause severe weakness accompanied by parasympathetic side effects and various degrees of muscular tightness and twitching. Atropine is the physiologic antidote and should be given intravenously or subcutaneously.

Precautions. Neostigmine is contraindicated for patients with mechanical obstruction of the intestinal or urinary tract. It must be used with extreme caution and in small doses in patients with bronchial asthma.

Pyridostigmine bromide, U.S.P., B.P. (Mestinon Bromide); ambenonium chloride (Mytelase)

Pyridostigmine and ambenonium are two anticholinesterase compounds that are being used for myasthenia gravis. They differ from neostigmine mainly in their longer action and decreased severity of side effects. The longer duration of their action often makes it possible for the patient to sleep undisturbed without the administration of the drug during the night.

Both drugs are available in tablet form for oral administration. Mestinon Bromide is available in a slow-release dosage form. Dosage is determined by the severity of the disease and the response of the patient. Both drugs have been rated *effective* for treatment of myasthenia gravis.

Edrophonium chloride, U.S.P., B.P. (Tensilon Chloride)

Edrophonium is a cholinergic drug that is discussed further in Chapter 15. It is mentioned here because its action resembles that of neostigmine and because it is used in the emergency treatment of patients with myasthenia gravis and as a diagnostic agent. When it is given to a patient suspected of having myasthenia gravis, he will show prompt improvement in muscular strength should the disease be present. The duration of the action of the drug is too brief to be of value for maintenance therapy.

It is also used to differentiate a myasthenic crisis from a cholinergic crisis. An intravenous dose of the drug will produce a brief relief of symptoms if they are caused by exacerbation of the disease, but it will increase the weakness of patients suffering from medication overdose.

As a diagnostic agent, 10 mg. of the drug is administered intravenously. In myasthenia crisis, the drug is given by continuous intravenous drip. Edrophonium chloride is available in 1-ml. ampules and in 10-ml. vials that contain 10 mg. per milliliter.

NICOTINE

Nicotine is a liquid alkaloid, freely soluble in water. It turns brown on exposure to air. It is the chief alkaloid found in tobacco.

It has no therapeutic use but is of great pharmacologic interest and toxicologic importance. Its use in experiments performed on animals has helped to increase understanding of the autonomic nervous system.

Absorption. Nicotine is readily absorbed from the gastrointestinal tract, respiratory mucous membrane, and skin.

Action and result. Nicotine produces a temporary stimulation of all sympathetic and parasympathetic ganglia. This is followed by depression, which tends to last longer than the period of stimulation. It affects skeletal muscle in a way similar to the way it affects the ganglia; that is, a depressant phase follows stimulation. During the depressant phase nicotine exerts a curare-like action on skeletal muscle.

In addition, nicotine stimulates the central nervous system, especially the medullary centers (respiratory, emetic, and vasomotor). Large doses may cause tremor and convulsions. Stimulation is followed by depression. Death is caused by respiratory failure, although it may be caused more by the curariform action of nicotine on nerve endings in the diaphragm, which prevents respiratory muscles from responding, than by action on the respiratory center.

The actions and effects of nicotine on the blood-vascular system are complex. The rate of the heart is frequently slowed at first, but later it may beat faster than usual. Various disturbances in rhythm have been observed. The small blood vessels in peripheral parts of the body constrict but may later dilate, and the blood pressure will fall. The latter condition is observed in nicotine poisoning. Nicotine also has an antidiuretic action.

Repeated administration of nicotine causes tolerance to develop to some of its effects.

Toxic effects. Acute or chronic poisoning can result.

Acute poisoning. Nicotine is a rapid-acting, extremely toxic drug. Cases have been reported of gardeners who were poisoned while handling the drug as an insecticide. Death occurred in a few minutes. Black Leaf 40 is a commerical preparation that contains nicotine and is used as a spray to kill various types of insects.

Symptoms of poisoning include increased flow of saliva, nausea, vomiting, abdominal cramps, diarrhea, cold sweat, confusion, fainting, drop in blood pressure, rapid pulse, prostration, and collapse. Convulsions sometimes occur. Death results from respiratory failure.

Treatment is directed toward keeping the patient breathing. Artificial respiration with oxygen is said to be more effective than central respiratory stimulants. If life can be prolonged to give the tissues an opportunity to detoxify the drug, the patient may recover.

If the poison has been swallowed, gastric lavage with a solution of potassium permanganate (1:10,000) is recommended. Other forms of treatment will depend upon the symptoms presented.

Tobacco smoking and nicotine. The effect of tobacco in the individual who smokes is a subject about which there is considerable difference of opinion. The effects of excessive smoking seem to afford more agreement than the effects of mild or moderate use of tobacco. Excessive smoking is known to cause irritation of the respiratory tract, and it is now generally accepted that tobacco smoke exerts carcinogenic effects in the lungs of man. Chronic dyspepsia may develop in heavy smokers, and patients with gastric ulcer are usually advised to avoid overindulgence. Of considerable importance is the fact that sufficient nicotine is absorbed by smokers to exert a variety of effects on the autonomic nervous system.

In patients with peripheral vascular disease such as thromboangiitis obliterans (Buerger's disease), nicotine is generally believed to be a contributing factor in the disease and may precipitate spasms of the peripheral blood vessels and thus reduce the blood flow through the affected vessels. Vasospasm in the retinal blood vessels of the eye, associated with smoking of tobacco, is thought to be the cause of a serious disturbance of vision.

Roth found that nicotine in cigarettes must be reduced more than 60% before vascular effects of smoking fail to appear or are only slight.

Some physicians recommend that patients with hypertension and peripheral vascular disease sharply limit their smoking habits or discontinue smoking entirely. The adverse effects of cigarette smoking on the cardiovascular system are increasingly emphasized.

ANTICHOLINERGIC AGENTS (BELLADONNA GROUP)

The anticholinergic drugs that act selectively on postganglionic sites and block the muscarinic effects of acetylcholine have many important uses in medicine. These drugs are also known as antimuscarinics and their prototype is atropine, a belladonna alkaloid.

Anticholinergics relax smooth muscle, inhibit secretions of duct glands, and dilate the pupils. In toxic doses these agents will produce skeletal muscle paralysis. Anticholinergic agents may be obtained from natural sources or they may be synthesized. The synthetic drugs tend to have fewer side effects.

A number of plants belonging to the potato family (Solanaceae) contain similar alkaloids. Included are *Atropa belladonna* (deadly nightshade), *Hyoscyamus niger* (henbane),* *Datura stramonium* (Jimson weed or thorn apple),† and several species of scopola. The principal alkaloids of these plants are atropine, scopolamine (hyoscine), and hyoscyamine.

Atropa belladonna was the name conferred on one of these plants by Linnaeus in 1753. The first part of the name was selected because of the poisonous qualities of the plant and is called Atropa after Atropos, the eldest of the Greek Fates who supposedly cut the thread of life. The second part of the name, belladonna, means beautiful lady and was chosen because of the custom practiced by certain Roman women who placed belladonna preparations in their eyes to make them appear larger and more lustrous.

Atropine and scopolamine resemble each other closely, both in effects and in chemical structure, as can be seen in the accompanying formulas.

Atropine

---

*Henbane is thought to be a corruption of hennebell, which suggests a musical instrument. In medieval Latin, henbane was referred to as *Symphoniaca herba*, symphoniaca being a rod with many bells on it. (Wootton.) Henbane is the bane of domestic fowl.

†Jimson weed is a corruption of Jamestown weed, so called because it was early observed as a weed in Jamestown, Virginia. It is given its other name, thorn apple, because of its spiny capsule.

Scopolamine

Atropine

Atropine is the chief alkaloid of the plant *Atropa belladonna,* which is grown for commercial purposes in Germany, England, Austria, and North America. It is also synthesized.

Atropine is the prototype of the anticholinergic drugs. It has been in use for over half a century and continues to be a popular drug because of its therapeutic effectiveness.

Action and result. There may be a local, central, or peripheral action.

Local. There is a slight amount of absorption when atropine or belladonna is applied to the skin, especially if it is an oily or alcoholic preparation or in the form of a plaster. Belladonna ointment or suppositories were sometimes used on mucous surfaces.

When an aqueous solution of atropine is dropped into the conjunctival sac of the eye, it quickly produces dilation of the pupil, diminished secretion of tears, and impaired ability to focus objects close to the eye. If the eye is normal there is little change in intraocular tension, but it may increase in patients who have glaucoma.

Central. Atropine has prominent effects on the central nervous system and in large doses causes excitement and maniacal behavior. These behavioral effects suggest the existence of important cholinergic pathways and receptors within the central nervous system.

CEREBRUM. Small or moderate doses of atropine have little or no effect. Large or toxic doses cause the patient to become restless, wakeful, and talkative. This condition may develop into delirium and finally stupor and coma. The exalted, excited stage has sometimes been called a "belladonna jag." A rise in temperature is sometimes seen, especially in infants and young children. This is probably the result of suppression of sweating rather than action on the heat-regulating center.

Atropine has been used to diminish tremor in Parkinson's disease. It probably reduces cholinergic synaptic transmission.

MEDULLA. Therapeutic doses of atropine stimulate the respiratory center and make breathing faster and sometimes deeper. When respiration is seriously depressed, atropine is not always reliable as a stimulant; in fact, it may deepen the depression. Large doses stimulate respiration but they can also cause respiratory failure and death.

Small doses stimulate the vagus center in the medulla, causing primary slowing of the heart. The vasoconstrictor center is stimulated briefly and then depressed. Because depression follows rather soon after stimulation, atropine has been called a borderline stimulant of the central nervous system.

Peripheral. The main therapeutic uses of atropine are the result of its peripheral action rather than its central action. The more important effect is on the smooth muscle, cardiac muscle, and gland cells, which are supplied by postganglionic cholinergic nerves. Atropine is a competitive antagonist of acetylcholine; by occupying receptor sites, atropine prevents or reduces the muscarinic action of acetylcholine. To some extent, atropine brings about effects similar to those produced by stimulation of postganglionic fibers in the sympathetic nervous system. The following results of peripheral action are seen.

EYE. The pupil is dilated (mydriasis) and the muscle of accommodation is paralyzed (cycloplegia). The sphincter muscle of the iris and the ciliary muscle are both innervated by cholinergic nerve fibers and therefore are affected by atropine. Since the sphincter muscle is unable to contract normally, the radial muscle of the iris causes the pupil to dilate. Pupil dilation may reduce outflow of aqueous humor, causing a rise in intraocular pressure, a hazardous situation for patients with glaucoma. These effects in the eye are brought about by both local and systemic administration of atropine, although the usual single therapeutic dose of atropine given orally or parenterally has little effect on the eye. After the pupil is dilated photophobia occurs, and when the drug has reached its full effect the usual reflexes to light and accommodation disappear.

RESPIRATORY TRACT. Secretions of the nose,

pharynx, and bronchial tubes are decreased. The muscles of the bronchial tubes relax and the airway widens to ease breathing. Atropine and scopolamine are less effective than epinephrine as bronchodilators and are seldom used for asthma.

HEART AND BLOOD VESSELS. When the usual clinical doses are given, the cardiac rate is temporarily and slightly slowed because of the central action of the drug on the cardiac center in the medulla. Moderate-to-large doses accelerate the heart by interfering with the response of the heart muscle to vagal nerve impulses. The latter is a peripheral action. The ability of atropine to interfere with vagal stimuli explains its use in the treatment of sinus bradycardia and atrioventricular heart block. In therapeutic doses atropine has little or no effect on blood pressure, although large and sometimes ordinary doses cause vasodilation of vessels in the skin of the face and neck. This may result from a direct dilator action or from histamine release. Reddening of the face and neck is seen, especially after large or toxic doses.

GLANDS. Since the sweat glands of the skin are supplied by cholinergic nerves, atropine decreases or abolishes their activity. This causes the skin to become hot and dry. The flow of saline and mucus from glands lining the respiratory tract is reduced, and drying of the mucous membranes of the mouth, nose, pharynx, and bronchi occurs. Patients who have been given atropine, particularly for preoperative preparation, often complain of a dry mouth and thirst. Some of this discomfort may be relieved by frequent rinsing of the mouth.

Although some difference of opinion exists among authorities as to the effect of atropine on the activity of gastric glands, it appears that the amount and character of the gastric secretion are little affected by atropine when given in ordinary therapeutic doses. The secretion of acid in the stomach is presumably less under vagal control than under hormonal or chemical control. The effect of atropine on the secretion of the pancreas and intestinal glands is not therapeutically significant.

SMOOTH MUSCLE. Atropine and other belladonna alkaloids decrease tone as well as peristalsis in the stomach and small and large intestine.

Atropine does not affect the secretion of bile, but it exerts a mildly antispasmodic effect in the gallbladder and bile ducts. It exerts a relaxing effect on the ureter, especially when it has been in a state of spasm. Therapeutic doses decrease the tone of the fundus of the urinary bladder. When the detrusor muscle is hypertonic, it is relaxed by atropine.

The power of atropine to decrease the activity of uterine muscle is thought to be negligible. It is at best only mildly antispasmodic.

USES. Atropine is especially useful as a preliminary medication prior to surgical anesthesia. It decreases secretions of the mouth and respiratory passages and is effective in the prevention of laryngospasm.

Atropine and shorter-acting anticholinergics may be used as mydriatics and cycloplegics in examinations of the eye and in the treatment of certain eye conditions. Atropine is used especially for refraction of the eyes of children who need a potent drug to paralyze the muscle of accommodation. Homatropine, a shorter-acting cycloplegic and mydriatic, is usually satisfactory for adults.

Atropine is sometimes given with morphine to relieve biliary and renal colic. Atropine tends to relieve the muscular spasm induced by morphine.

Preparations of belladonna or its alkaloids are administered for their antispasmodic effects in conditions characterized by hypermotility of the stomach and bowel—pylorospasm, spastic colon, biliary and renal colic, and hypertonicity of the urinary bladder and ureters. These drugs are also found in certain cough remedies (antiasthmatic mixtures), in which case they are given to relieve mild conditions of bronchial spasm and excessive secretions. Atropine has a mild antihistaminic effect.

Symptoms in selected cases of Parkinson's disease are also relieved—the tremor, muscular rigidity, and cramps. However, other drugs are superior to atropine for this use.

Preparation, dosage, and administration. The following are the preparations available of atropine.

Atropine sulfate, U.S.P., B.P. Tablets containing 0.3, 0.4, and 0.6 mg. of drug are available. These correspond to gr. $^1/_{200}$, $^1/_{150}$, and $^1/_{100}$, respectively. The drug is also available in multiple-dose vials (gr. $^1/_{150}$ per milliliter) for injection and in the form of atropine sulfate ophthalmic ointment. Atropine sulfate is usually administered subcutaneously, orally, or topically (in the eye). The usual subcutaneous or oral dose is 0.5 mg. (gr. $^1/_{120}$), although 0.4 mg. (gr. $^1/_{150}$) is frequently ordered. The ophthalmic solution and the ointment are usually used in a 0.5% or 1% concentration.

Belladonna extract, N.F., B.P. The extract is prepared from belladonna leaf and contains alkaloids of the leaf. It is given orally, usually in doses of 15 mg. (gr. $^1/_4$).

Belladonna tincture, U.S.P., B.P. The usual dose is 0.6 ml. (10 minims), although the range of dosage may be from 0.3 to 2.4 ml. It is given orally.

Absorption, distribution, and excretion. Atropine (and also scopolamine) is readily absorbed after oral and parenteral administration. It is also absorbed from mucous membranes, as is noted when ophthalmic solutions escape through the lacrimal ducts to the mucous membrane of the nose. To a lesser extent, atropine is also absorbed from the skin. The drug is widely distributed in the fluids of the body and easily passes the placental barrier to the blood of the fetus. It is excreted chiefly by way of the kidney. Some is excreted through the bile. The remainder is apparently metabolized in the liver. Traces are found in other secretions, such as the milk.

Side effects and toxic effects. Atropine is a potent alkaloid, but it has a wide margin of safety. Poisoning occurs but is rarely fatal. The fatal dose is said to be about 100 mg. for adults and 10 mg. for children. Survival has occurred after much larger doses.

Symptoms develop rapidly after overdosage and consist of dry mouth, great thirst, and difficulty in swallowing and talking. Vision becomes blurred, pupils are dilated, and photophobia is present. A rash may develop, which is seen chiefly over the face, neck, and upper trunk. Rash is seen particularly in children, although it may occur in adults. The body temperature is elevated, and in young children and infants it may reach 107° F. and more. The skin of the face and neck is flushed; the pulse becomes rapid and may be weak. Urinary urgency and difficulty in emptying the bladder may be noted. The patient becomes restless, excited, talkative, and confused. This may progress to delirium and mania and may be mistaken for an acute psychosis. The patient may also experience giddiness, staggering, stupor, coma, and respiratory and circulatory failure.

Young children who are given atropine or scopolamine as a preanesthetic medication often have a pronounced cutaneous flush after administration of the drug. Parents may be much disturbed about this and think that the child is ill with an acute disease. This is a side effect and is not seen as often in adults as in children.

Contraindications. Atropine and related alkaloids are usually contraindicated for patients with glaucoma because of the tendency of mydriatics to increase intraocular tension.

Treatment of overdosage. If the drug has been taken by mouth, the stomach should be lavaged promptly with tannic acid solution. Administration of syrup of ipecac or activated charcoal will help to inhibit further absorption of the drug. Neostigmine or pilocarpine is sometimes ordered to be given subcutaneously in doses of 10 mg. until the mouth is moist. Physostigmine has also been recommended. Artificial respiration, oxygen, or oxygen and carbon dioxide may be indicated. Short-acting barbiturates, chloral hydrate, or paraldehyde may be given to relieve excitement. Cautious use of central nervous system stimulants is recommended should the patient become stuporous. Ice bags and alcohol sponge baths aid in reducing the fever.

Scopolamine (Hyoscine)

Action. Scopolamine resembles atropine in its peripheral effects but differs in its central action, since doses of the drug given parenterally depress the central nervous system, producing drowsiness, euphoria, relief of fear, relaxation, sleep, and amnesia. Some "over-the-counter" sleeping pills (for example, Sleep-Eze) contain small amounts of scopolamine.

Uses. Scopolamine is used as a preanesthetic medication, usually along with morphine or one of the barbiturates, to check secretions and to prevent laryngospasm, as well as for its sedative (twilight sleep) and its amnesic effects.

It is used for motion sickness because of its depressant action on vestibular function, but this use has largely been supplanted by newer drugs. It is employed as a sedative for certain maniacal and delirious patients and also for postencephalitic parkinsonism and paralysis agitans.

It is also used as a mydriatic and cycloplegic. Its effects appear more promptly and disappear more rapidly than those of atropine. Scopolamine is less likely to cause irritation in the eyes than atropine.

Preparation, dosage, and administration. The following are the available preparations of scopolamine.

Scopolamine hydrobromide, U.S.P.; *hyoscine hydrobromide*, B.P. This drug is available in 0.6-mg. (gr. $\frac{1}{200}$) tablets, which can be given orally or parenterally. Usual adult dose is 0.6 mg. orally or subcutaneously; range of dose is 0.3 to 0.8 mg. Dose for children is 0.006 mg. per kilogram of body weight orally or subcutaneously. Ophthalmic solutions are applied topically to the eye in 0.2% concentration.

Hyoscine eye ointment, B.P. The ointment contains 0.25% hyoscine hydrobromide.

Scopolamine hydrobromide injection, U.S.P.; *hyoscine injection*, B.P. The injection is available in ampules containing 0.3, 0.4, and 0.6 mg. in 1 ml. and 0.4 mg. in 0.5 ml. Dosage is 0.3 to 0.8 mg. subcutaneously.

SYNTHETIC SUBSTITUTES FOR ATROPINE (ANTISPASMODICS)

The usefulness of atropine is limited by the fact that it is a complex drug and produces effects in a number of organs or tissues simultaneously. When it is administered for its antispasmodic effects it will also produce prolonged effects in the eye, causing dilated pupils and blurred vision, as well as dry mouth and possibly rapid heart rate. When the antispasmodic effect is the one desired, other effects become side effects, which may be distinctly undesirable.

A large number of drugs have been synthesized in an effort to capture the antispasmodic effect of atropine without its other effects. Drugs of this type are frequently used to relieve hyper-

tonicity and hypersecretion in the stomach and to treat patients with gastric and duodenal ulcers.

The ideal drug for the management of peptic ulcer should block the mechanism of gastric secretion without producing blockage in the autonomic ganglia and without causing curariform effects (muscular weakness). It should be relatively nontoxic and palatable and should reduce both the volume and the acidity of the gastric secretion over long periods of time. It should be effective when given orally. It should not produce troublesome or adverse side effects. The ideal drug has not been found, which probably explains why so many different preparations are available. Seemingly no single preparation excels.

Continued synthesis of new anticholinergic drugs takes place, and if the claims for longer action and greater effectiveness are substantiated after long trial, more useful therapeutic agents may become available.

Like most of the cholinergic blocking agents, they are contraindicated for patients with glaucoma, pyloric obstruction, and prostatic hypertrophy.

Methscopolamine bromide, N.F. (Pamine Bromide)

Action. Methscopolamine bromide is an anticholinergic drug that produces antispasmodic and antisecretory effects. It can suppress both volume and acidity of gastric secretion if large enough doses are given. It slows the emptying of the stomach and reduces peristalsis in the bowel. It decreases secretion of saliva and sweat. Tolerance to the medication does not seem to develop.

Uses. Methscopolamine bromide is used as an antispasmodic in the treatment of patients with peptic ulcer and forms of gastritis associated with hypermotility and hyperacidity. It is also occasionally used to relieve excessive salivation and sweating.

Preparation, dosage, and administration. Methscopolamine bromide is available in 2.5-mg. tablets and in solution for injection (1 mg. per milliliter). The usual dosage for adults is 2.5 mg. administered before meals and at bedtime. The usual parenteral dose is 0.5 mg. intramuscularly or subcutaneously every 6 to 8 hours as needed to control symptoms. It is also available as a syrup and as an elixir containing phenobarbital.

Side effects and toxic effects. The side effects most frequently encountered include dry mouth, constipation, and blurred vision. Other effects encountered less frequently may include dizziness, palpitation, flushed dry skin, difficult urination, headache, and nausea.

Overdosage may bring about a ganglionic blocking action and a curare-like effect on skeletal muscle.

Methantheline bromide, N.F. (Banthine Bromide)

Action. Methantheline bromide has an anticholinergic action similar to that of atropine. It has a ganglionic blocking action in the autonomic nervous system, as well as a curare-like effect on skeletal muscle. It inhibits motility of the stomach and delays emptying time, inhibits motility of the small intestine and genitourinary tract, and diminishes secretions.

It is used as an antispasmodic in the treatment of patients with pylorospasm, hypermotility of the intestine, spastic colon, and spasm of the ureter and urinary bladder. Some degree of pupillary dilation accompanies the antispasmodic effect.

Preparation, dosage, and administration. Methantheline bromide is available in 50-mg. tablets for oral administration and in ampules, each containing 50 mg. The content of the ampule is dissolved in physiologic saline solution for the purpose of injection (intramuscularly or intravenously). Parenteral administration is not recommended if the patient can take the drug orally. The tablets should not be chewed because they have an unpleasant taste. Antacids with adsorbent action, such as aluminum hydroxide, should not be given with methantheline.

The usual initial dose for adults is 50 mg., although the usual effective dose is 100 mg. four times a day, before meals and at bedtime. Some patients require more, some less, than this amount. The recommended dosage is the smallest amount that will effectively relieve the symptoms. Onset of action occurs within 30 to 45 minutes and persists for 4 to 6 hours. Dose for children is 6 mg. per kilogram of body weight daily in four divided doses.

Side effects and toxic effects. Patients may experience side effects in the form of dryness of the mouth, dilated pupils, and inability to read fine print. Some may develop constipation and require a laxative. Varying degrees of urinary retention have been observed in patients with prostatic hypertrophy. A small percentage of patients complain of general malaise and weakness and do not tolerate the drug well.

Propantheline bromide, U.S.P., B.P. (Pro-Banthine Bromide)

Action. Propantheline bromide is an analogue of methantheline bromide and is said to be more effective than the latter drug to reduce the volume and acidity of gastric secretions. It is also said to produce less severe side effects. It has come to replace the older drug to a great extent.

Preparation, dosage, and administration. Propantheline is available in 7.5- and 15-mg. tablets, 30-mg. prolonged action tablets, and 30-mg. vials as a powder for intramuscular or intravenous injection. The content of the vial is dissolved in not less than 10 ml. of water for injection prior to intravenous administration. Parenteral administration is reserved for patients who cannot take the drug orally. Propantheline bromide is also available in tablets that contain phenobarbital.

The dosage of propantheline must be carefully adjusted to the needs of individual patients. The initial recommended dose is one tablet (15 mg.)

Table 9-9 Side effects characteristic of cholinergic blocking agents

Dryness of mouth	Mental confusion
Dilation of pupils (mydriasis)*	Excitement
Blurred vision	Dizziness; headache
Heart palpitation	Constipation
Flushing and dryness of skin	Urinary retention

*It must be understood that a symptom such as mydriasis is not a side effect when this is the purpose for which a drug is given.

with meals and two tablets at bedtime, with subsequent adjustment depending on the patient's reaction and tolerance to the medication. The bitter taste of methantheline bromide has been controlled by sugar-coating the Pro-Banthine tablet. Dose for children is 1.5 mg. per kilogram of body weight daily in four divided doses.

Side effects. Propantheline is thought to show less severe but not less frequent side effects than methantheline bromide.

Homatropine methylbromide, N.F. (Novatrin, Mesopin)

Action. Homatropine methylbromide is one of the older cholinergic blocking agents used in the United States. Its effects are similar to those of atropine, but it is without the latter drug's effect on the central nervous system. Its anticholinergic potency is said to be considerably less than that of atropine, but it is also less toxic. Its effect on gastric secretion and motility, and the duration of action are said to be much the same as that for atropine.

Uses. Homatropine methylbromide is used for the treatment of gastrointestinal spasm and as an adjunct in the treatment of patients with peptic ulcer.

Preparation, dosage, and administration. Homatropine methylbromide is available in 2.5-, 5-, and 10-mg. tablets and as an elixir containing 5 mg. in 5 ml. The usual oral dose is 2.5 to 5 mg. three or four times daily. Solutions are also available for injection and for oral administration. Dose for children is 3 to 6 mg. in chewable tablets four times daily. Dose for infants with colic is 1 mg. (elixir) four times daily.

Side effects. Side effects include dryness of the mouth and blurring of vision.

Table 9-10 Summary of some of the anticholinergic agents*

Generic name	Trade name	Usual single adult dose	Usual route of administration
Atropine		0.5 mg. 0.5%-1% ophthalmic solution	Oral or subcutaneous Topical
Scopolamine		0.6 mg.	Oral or subcutaneous
Hyoscine		0.2% ophthalmic solution	Topical
Synthetic mydriatics and cycloplegics Homatropine hydrobromide		1%-2% ophthalmic solution	Topical
Synthetic antispasmodics Homatropine methylbromide	Novatrin, Mesopin	5-10 mg.	Oral
Methscopolamine bromide	Pamine, Lescapine	2.5-5 mg. 0.25-1 mg.	Oral Subcutaneous or intramuscular
Methantheline bromide	Banthine	50 mg.	Oral
Propantheline	Pro-Banthine	15 mg.	Oral
Pipenzolate	Piptal	5 mg.	Oral

*Drugs listed are usually administered in the form of their salts.

Pipenzolate bromide (Piptal)

Action and result. Pipenzolate bromide is a synthetic anticholinergic drug with effects comparable to atropine. It diminishes gastric acidity and gastric motility and relieves spasms. It is used to treat peptic ulcers. The ability of pipenzolate to relax spasms of the lower gastrointestinal tract and of the sphincter of Oddi makes it useful in the treatment of ileitis, irritable colon, and biliary colic.

Side effects and toxic effects. Pipenzolate has a minimum of side effects and those are chiefly atropine-like in nature. No serious toxic reactions have been reported to date.

Preparation, dosage, and administration. Pipenzolate bromide is available in 5-mg. tablets for oral administration. The average adult dose is 5 mg. three times daily before meals and 5 to 10 mg. at bedtime. Onset of action is about 1 hour; duration of effect is 4 hours.

QUESTIONS

For study and review

1 Explain what is meant by the muscarinic action of a drug; by the nicotinic action of a drug.
2 What is the difference between cholinergic fibers and adrenergic fibers? Between cholinergic drugs and adrenergic drugs?
3 Explain why epinephrine should not be administered to patients receiving digitalis.
4 Explain the important nursing care aspects for patients receiving intravenous infusion of powerful vasoconstrictors such as levarterenol, metaraminol, or methoxamine.
5 Explain why after prolonged use of a pressor drug the drug may no longer have a vasoconstrictor effect.

Multiple choice

6 Choose the correct answer(s).
Acetylcholine:
a. promotes sympathetic stimulation by releasing norepinephrine at postganglionic fibers
b. promotes a rise in calcium concentration within nerve fibers to enhance muscle activation
c. is the transmitter substance for both the sympathetic and the parasympathetic nervous systems
d. is inactivated by cholinesterase
7 Which of the following are correct statements about anticholinergic drugs?
a. They are also known as antimuscarinics.

b. Natural sources of these drugs have fewer side effects than the synthetic drugs.
c. The most widely used anticholinergic is atropine.
d. They block the action of norepinephrine.
8 Choose the *incorrect* answer(s).
The use of epinephrine in local anesthetic solutions is for the purpose of:
a. prolonging the anesthetic action by vasoconstriction
b. delaying absorption from the site of injection
c. promoting distribution of the drug
d. inhibiting bleeding
9 Choose the correct answer(s).
Epinephrine:
a. stimulates vascular beta receptors
b. is a catecholamine secreted from the adrenal medulla
c. has a direct cardioaccelerator action
d. is therapeutically effective in the treatment of heart failure because it increases myocardial oxygen uptake
10 Which of the following are toxic effects of high doses of epinephrine?
a. reflex bradycardia   d. cardiac arrhythmias
b. anxiety   e. hypotension
c. palpitation
11 Choose the *incorrect* answer(s).
Epinephrine:
a. has both excitatory and inhibitory effects on the autonomic nervous system
b. is used in treating simple glaucoma by reducing intraocular pressure via pupil and blood vessel dilation
c. is an effective drug for relieving nasal congestion since it does not produce a rebound vasodilator or mucosal swelling effect
d. is effective in treatment of acute asthmatic attacks by its dilating effect on bronchial smooth muscle, which promotes a resistant airway
12 Which of the following effects does epinephrine have on the heart?
a. It brings about more complete emptying of the ventricles by increasing myocardial contraction.
b. It increases the heart's refractory period.
c. It inhibits stimulation of the vagus nerve causing cardiac acceleration.
d. It inhibits atrioventricular conduction.
13 In comparing the effects of ephedrine and epinephrine it will be noted that:
a. both are adrenergic drugs; ephedrine also stimulates the central nervous system
b. ephedrine is effective orally; epinephrine is not
c. the actions of ephedrine are slower and weaker but more prolonged than those of epinephrine
d. both drugs cause rebound vasodilation after their vasoconstricting effect
14 Choose the *incorrect* answer(s).
When the effects of norepinephrine and epinephrine are compared it is noted that:
a. epinephrine brings about a greater increase in oxygen consumption by the heart
b. norepinephrine is a more potent systemic vasoconstrictor

c. epinephrine is a less toxic substance than norepinephrine

d. the effects of norepinephrine are more easily reversed than those of epinephrine

15 Choose the correct answer(s).

Norepinephrine

a. has little or no effect on beta receptors of the heart

b. will cause tissue sloughing if infiltration occurs with an intravenous infusion

c. is predominantly an activator of alpha receptors of smooth muscle, which accounts for its vasoconstrictor effect

d. has a positive inotropic effect

16 Which of the following statements about the alpha and beta adrenergic receptors of the sympathetic nervous system are *incorrect?*

a. Drugs affecting the alpha receptors cause an inhibitory action.

b. Large arteries and veins contain both alpha and beta receptors.

c. The heart contains only beta receptors.

d. Norepinephrine acts mainly on alpha receptors.

17 Atropine:

a. produces dilation of the pupil and diminished secretion of tears when instilled into the eye

b. decreases gastric secretion

c. has an antispasmodic effect on the gastrointestinal tract

d. decreases muscle tremor in Parkinson's disease

18 Atropine is frequently given as a preanesthetic drug not only to inhibit oral and bronchial secretions but also to prevent:

a. cardiac arrest

b. respiratory failure

c. laryngospasm

d. hypotension

19 If the stock supply of atropine sulfate is in solution and the vial is labeled 0.4 mg. per milliliter, how many minims (approximately) would be required to give gr. $1/200$?

a. 11

b. 15

c. 20

d. $7^1/_2$

20 Anticholinesterase drugs are used therapeutically for:

a. glaucoma

b. increasing intestinal peristalsis

c. urinary retention

d. atropine poisoning

21 Anticholinergic drugs are frequently given to patients with peptic ulcer for which of the following reasons?

a. to control the gastric acidity

b. for their direct analgesic effect

c. to soothe and coat the ulcer

d. to diminish hypermotility and hypersecretion of the stomach

22 Patients with hypertension and cardiovascular disease are often encouraged to stop smoking for which of the following reasons?

a. Nicotine stimulates the central nervous system.

b. Nicotine has a tendency to cause vasospasm.

c. Tobacco smoke contains substances thought to be carcinogenic.

d. Tobacco smoke is irritating to the respiratory mucous membrane.

REFERENCES

A.M.A. drug evaluations, ed. 2, Acton, Mass., 1973, Publishing Sciences Group, Inc.

Aviado, D. M.: Krantz and Carr's pharmacologic principles of medical practice, ed. 8, Baltimore, 1972, The Williams & Wilkins Co.

Di Palma, J. R., editor: Drill's pharmacology in medicine, New York, 1971, McGraw-Hill Book Co.

Goodman, L. S., and Gilman, A., editors: The pharmacological basis of therapeutics, ed. 4, New York, 1970, The Macmillan Co.

Goth, A.: Medical pharmacology, ed. 7, St. Louis, 1974, The C. V. Mosby Co.

Grollman, A., and Grollman, E. F.: Pharmacology and therapeutics, ed. 7, Philadelphia, 1970, Lea & Febiger.

Meyers, F. H., Jawetz, E., and Goldfien, A.: Review of medical pharmacology, ed. 4, Los Altos, Calif., 1974, Lange Medical Publications.

Modell, W., editor: Drugs of choice 1976-1977, St. Louis, 1976, The C. V. Mosby Co.

Osol, A., and Pratt, R.: The United States dispensatory, ed. 27, Philadelphia, 1973, J. B. Lippincott Co.

Turner, P., and Richens, A.: Clinical pharmacology, Edinburgh, 1973, Churchill Livingstone.

Periodicals

Amsterdam, E. A., and others: Evaluation of long term use of propanolol in angina pectoris, J.A.M.A. **210:**103, 1969.

Axelrod, J.: Noradrenaline: Fate and control of its biosynthesis, Science **173:**598, 1971.

Axelsson, J.: Catecholamine functions, Ann. Rev. Pharmacol. **33:**1, 1971.

Catecholamines, Brit. Med. Bull. **29:**91, 1973.

Chandler, J. G.: The physiology and treatment of shock, R.N. **34:**42, 1971.

Dollery, C. T., and others: Clinical pharmacology of beta-receptor blocking drugs, Clin. Pharmacol. Ther. **10:**765, 1969.

Flacke, W.: Treatment of myasthenia gravis, New Eng. J. Med. **288:**27, 1973.

Fitzgerald, J. D.: Perspectives in adrenergic beta-receptor blockade, Clin. Pharmacol. Ther. **10:**292, 1969.

Geffen, L. B., and Livett, B. G.: Synaptic vesicles in sympathetic neurons, Physiol. Rev. **51:**98, 1971.

Gravenstein, J. S., and others: Atropine on the electrocardiogram, Clin. Pharmacol. Ther. **10:**660, 1969.

Greenblatt, D. J., and Shader, R. I.: Anticholinergics, New Eng. J. Med. **288:**1215, 1973.

Havard, C. W. H.: Progress in myasthenia gravis, Brit. Med. J. **3:**437, 1973.

Koelle, G. B.: Acetylcholine—current status in physiology, pharmacology and medicine, New Eng. J. Med. **286:**1086, 1972.

Pohorecky, L. A., and Wurtman, R. J.: Adrenocortical control of epinephrine synthesis, Pharmacol. Rev. **23:**1, 1971.

Roth, G.: The effects of smoking tobacco on the cardiovascular system of normal persons and patients with hypertension. Collected papers of the Mayo Clinic **45:**435, 1953.

Shore, P. A.: Transport and storage of biogenic amines, Ann. Rev. Pharmacol. **12:**209, 1972.

Sodeman, W. A., Jr., and others: Physiology and pharmacology of belladonna therapy in acid-peptic disease, Med. Clin. N. Am. **53:**1379, 1969.

Sulser, F., and Sanders-Bush, E.: Effects of drugs on amines in the CNS, Ann. Rev. Pharmacol. **11:**209, 1971.

Thadani, U., and others: Comparison of adrenergic beta-receptor antagonists in angina pectoris, Brit. Med. J. **1:**138, 1973.

Weiner, N.: Regulation of norepinephrine biosynthesis, Ann. Rev. Pharmacol. **10:**273, 1970.

CHAPTER 10

Cardiovascular drugs

Cell metabolism and the circulatory system
The heart muscle

Drugs that affect the heart

Cardiac glycosides
Antiarrhythmic drugs

Drugs that affect blood vessels

Vasodilators
Antihypertensives
Vasoconstrictors

Drugs that act on the blood and blood-forming tissue

Antianemic or hemopoietic drugs
Whole blood and its constituents
Drugs that affect blood coagulation
Antilipemic agents

The development of microelectrode techniques and recordings has resulted in new knowledge and greater understanding of cardiovascular activity. The resulting anatomic, electrophysiologic, and pharmacologic information has permitted greater precision in diagnosing and treating cardiac disease, particularly the arrhythmias. Concomitant with these advances has been the increasing use of electrocardiographic monitoring of acutely ill patients and of those with known or suspected cardiovascular disorders. In addition, the nurse's clinical role has continued to expand and now includes responsibility for the care of patients on monitoring equipment. This in turn requires the nurse to be able to recognize and understand abnormal electrocardiographic patterns and in some cases to institute therapy, including pharmacologic therapy, to prevent serious complications and unnecessary deaths. Therefore, it is necessary for nurses to understand electrophysiology of the heart and drug effects on cardiac activity if they are to keep their knowledge current and their nursing care therapeutically effective.

CELL METABOLISM AND THE CIRCULATORY SYSTEM

Vital processes in living cells involve the use of oxygen and metabolic fuels and simultaneous elimination of metabolic waste products. In unicellular organisms such as the ameba, exchange of these substances occurs primarily by the process of diffusion (the movement of particles from regions of high concentration to regions of low concentration). For example, as a single cell uses oxygen, the oxygen concentration in the protoplasm decreases, and oxygen from regions of higher concentration outside the cell diffuses into the cell. The exchange of gases and metabolic products can occur rapidly since the distance of diffusion from the surface to the center of the cell or simple organism is not great.

In complex organisms, cells are grouped together, which increases the distance of diffusion to the center of the cell mass. To maintain rapid diffusion, a circulatory system is necessary—thus, the need in man for billions of thin-walled capillaries. If capillary flow is not interrupted, diffusion distances are small and diffusion gradients are steep. When the need for oxygen and nutrients by cells is increased, faster capillary flow is required. The heart, through its pumping action, distributes blood to the capillaries by means of the numerous ramifications of the arterial system. Blood leaving the capillaries returns to the heart via numerous venous channels.

Fundamental requirements of the cardiovascular system are circulation of blood flow without interruption and regulation of blood flow in response to varying tissue demands. The heart must continuously adapt its output to balance blood flow through the billions of capillaries in the body. To meet these requirements there must be an adequate pump, effective peripheral vascular resistance, and an effective circulating blood volume.

THE HEART MUSCLE

From a physiologic standpoint the heart consists of atrial and ventricular muscle and a specialized system for the generation and conduction of electrical impulses. The heart contracts rhythmically because of the intrinsic property of the sinoatrial node for the generation of impulses. This normal pacemaker function of the sinoatrial node may be taken over, under pathologic conditions, by other portions of the conduction system.

Normally, atrial contraction is followed in about a fifth of a second by ventricular contraction. The whole contraction forms the systole, which occurs about seventy-two times each minute in the adult. Each systole is followed immediately by a period of relaxation called diastole. Heart muscle differs from skeletal muscle in that its refractory period is relatively long, which helps to preserve the cardiac rhythm.

ELECTROPHYSIOLOGY OF THE HEART

Current information on cardiac electrophysiology is organized around the action potential, automaticity or impulse generation, the velocity of conduction of impulses, and the refractory periods. Understanding these concepts is necessary before there can be understanding of drug effects.

The action potential. As shown in Figure 10-1, the resting membrane potential of the myocardium is approximately 90 millivolts. This resting potential is the consequence of the unequal distribution of ions inside and outside of the cells. Outside the cell the sodium concentration is high and the potassium level is low. Within the resting cell potassium concentration is high and the sodium level is low.

The depolarization phase of the action potential is the result of a fast inward current carried by sodium ions. Much of the current is inactivated at the peak of the action potential but some is inactivated more slowly. Shortly after the onset of the inward sodium current another inward current occurs; this is probably carried by calcium ions. The slow inactivation of the calcium current plus the residual sodium current accounts for the plateau phase of the action potential. At the peak of the action potential the interior of the cell is positive in relation to the exterior. An outward current now occurs carried by the concentrated potassium ions as they diffuse across the cell membrane into extracellular fluid, establishing the repolarization phase.

Reestablishment of the resting membrane potential and ionic differences is due to an active metabolic process that extrudes sodium and probably calcium from within the cell (via the sodium pump) and reaccumulates potassium.

Automaticity. Automaticity refers to the capacity for spontaneous, repetitive self-excitation

Figure 10-1
Potentials in single myocardial fiber.

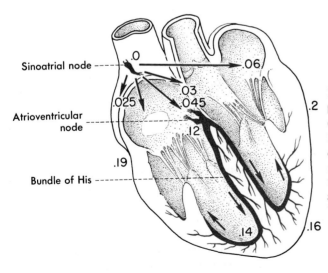

Figure 10-2

General ramification of conductive tissue in the heart and normal time sequence in seconds of depolarization (or electric conduction) from the sinoatrial node through the atria, to the atrioventricular node down the bundle of His (including right and left branches), to the terminal Purkinje fibers. Ventricular contraction then occurs.

or generation of impulses. Cells with automaticity have a resting membrane potential that undergoes spontaneous diastolic depolarization. When the threshold potential is reached the muscle undergoes a self-sustaining depolarization and contraction results.

Automatic or *pacemaker* cells are clustered in (1) the sinoatrial node and adjacent tissue, (2) the other automatic atrial cells, and (3) the His-Purkinje system (see Figure 10-2). The nonautomatic fibers of the heart include atrial and ventricular muscle fibers. The speed at which spontaneous depolarization proceeds in pacemaker cells is a primary factor in determining which cells will initiate the cardiac impulse. The fastest rate occurs in automatic cells of the sinoatrial node and adjacent tissue, and these are the primary pacemakers of the heart. Rhythms originating here are called *sinus rhythms.* The rate of depolarization is slower for the automatic cells of the His-Purkinje system. The atrioventricular node which merges with the bundle of His serves as a reserve pacemaker; it takes over when impulse generation of the sinus node is suppressed. Rhythms originating here are termed *nodal rhythms.* Any factor that significantly changes the firing rate of the automatic cells can cause arrhythmia. If the automaticity of normal pacemaker tissue is decreased, other tissue with *latent* or *potential* pacemaker ability will function as the pacemaker.

Velocity of conduction. The speed with which electrical activity is spread within the sinus node is quite slow, about 0.05 m./sec. The impulse then spreads out rapidly over the atrial musculature at a rate of about 1.0 m./sec. When the impulse reaches the atrioventricular node a delay of about 0.05 m./sec. occurs and atrial systole takes place. The impulse then spreads rapidly, 2 to 4 m./sec. along the right and left bundle branches and Purkinje fibers. Studies indicate that no more than 22 msec. may elapse during this time. This rapid activation of contractile elements evokes a synchronous contraction of the ventricles. Figure 10-2 shows the time of appearance of the impulse to various portions of the heart.

Refractory periods. Cardiac muscle is refractory to stimulation during the early phases of the action potential. *Absolute refractory period, relative refractory period,* and *functional refractory period* are commonly used terms in cardiac electrophysiology. During the absolute refractory period the heart is completely resistant to restimulation. During the relative refractory period, in the latter phases of the action potential, a strong stimulus is capable of eliciting a response. The *functional refractory period* is defined as that period during which an action potential from another part of the heart fails to reexcite an already excited area of the myocardium. This period is about 0.15 second in atrial muscle and about 0.25 second in the ventricles.

BLOOD SUPPLY

The entire blood supply to the myocardium is provided by the right and left coronary arteries, which arise from the base of the aorta (Figure 10-3). The right ventricle and atrium are supplied with blood from the right coronary artery. The left coronary artery divides into the anterior descending branch and the circumflex branch and supplies blood to the left ventricle and atrium. These main coronary vessels continue to divide, forming numerous branches. The result is a profuse network of coronary vessels. The major arterial vessels are located on the external surface of the ventricles. Arterial branches penetrate the myocardium toward the endocardial surface.

Increased oxygen delivery to the myocardium is supported almost exclusively by increased coronary blood flow. When there is increased demand for oxygen and nutrients by body tissues, the heart must increase its output. At the same time, the heart itself must be supplied with enough oxygen and nutrients to replace the energy expended. In other words, a balance must be maintained between energy expenditure and energy restoration.

During systole the myocardial contraction compresses the coronary vascular bed. This restricts coronary inflow but increases coronary outflow. Coronary inflow occurs primarily during diastole when the ventricles have relaxed and the coronary vessels are no longer compressed. Blood is driven through the coronaries by aortic pressure, perfusing the myocardium.

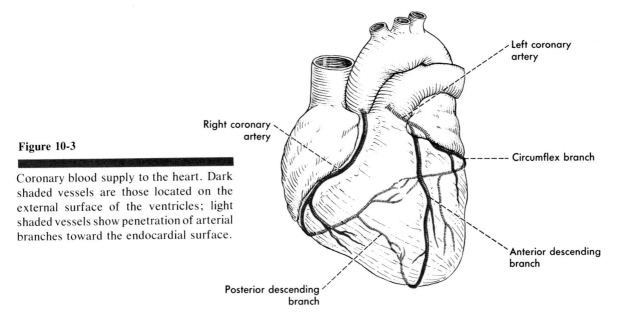

Figure 10-3

Coronary blood supply to the heart. Dark shaded vessels are those located on the external surface of the ventricles; light shaded vessels show penetration of arterial branches toward the endocardial surface.

A change in heart rate is accomplished by shortening or lengthening diastole. With tachycardia the increased amount of time required for the increased number of systolic contractions per minute reduces the time available for diastole and coronary inflow. There is also an increase in the metabolic needs of the rapidly beating heart. Coronary dilation occurs in an attempt to overcome restricted blood inflow. With bradycardia, the decreased number of systolic contractions per minute prolongs the diastolic period. There is a decrease in resistance to coronary flow and a decrease in the metabolic requirements of the myocardium.

Whenever the delivery of oxygen to the myocardium is inadequate to meet the heart's oxygen consumption needs, myocardial ischemia occurs. One of the major causes of ischemia is coronary artery disease.

NERVE SUPPLY

Normally, the heart rate is primarily controlled by the parasympathetic and sympathetic divisions of the autonomic nervous system. Cardiac parasympathetic fibers (vagal fibers) originate in the medulla and synapse with ganglionic cells located near the sinoatrial node and atrioventricular conduction tissue. The right vagus nerve has its greatest effect on the sinoatrial node, and right vagal stimulation inhibits sinoatrial nodal activity, which causes a slowing of the heart rate. The left vagus nerve primarily influences atrioventricular conduction tissue, and stimulation of this nerve produces various degrees of atrioventricular block. Parasympathetic control is usually more dominant than sympathetic control.

Sympathetic fibers originate in the upper fourth, fifth, or sixth thoracic segments of the spinal cord. Some fibers synapse with corresponding spinal sympathetic ganglia; others ascend to the cervical ganglia. Postganglionic fibers from the superior, middle, and inferior cervical ganglia travel to the heart as the superior, middle, and inferior cardiac accelerator nerves. Accelerator fibers to the heart are also supplied by the thoracic ganglia. Stimulation of sympathetic fibers to the right side of the heart (accelerator fibers) elicits greater cardiac acceleration than does stimulation of the left sympathetic fibers, while stimulation of the left sympathetic fibers (augmentor fibers) has a more profound effect on myocardial contractility than upon heart rate.

NEUROHORMONES

Neurohormonal agents are chemical substances relased from nerve endings to transmit information to adjacent cells. In man, neurohormonal transmission involves autonomic innervation (the vagus and sympathetic nerves) and two chemical agents (acetylcholine and norepinephrine). The vagus nerves are inhibitory and the sympathetic nerves are accelerator nerves. Norepinephrine is the primary catecholamine involved in the transmission of neural impulses.

Acetylcholine is released from the vagal nerve endings in the heart at the sinoatrial and atrioventricular nodes and the bundle of His. It slows the heart rate by inhibiting impulse formation and atrioventricular conduction.

Norepinephrine exists in inactive bound form in sympathetic nerve endings of the heart and with appropriate stimuli it can be released as free active norepinephrine. The catecholamines have a potent positive inotropic effect on myocardial contractility. They speed impulse formation, increase atrioventricular conduction velocity, decrease the refractory period of the atrioventricular node, and induce spontaneous depolarization in Purkinje fibers. Catecholamines increase the work load on the heart and cause a shorter systole with more complete systolic ejection of blood.

ELECTROCARDIOGRAM

Electrocardiograms are graphic representations of the sequence of cardiac excitation. Nurses caring for patients on monitor equipment should be able to detect and interpret changes in the cardiac rate or rhythm or in the conduction of the wave of electric activity or excitation. The electrocardiogram is a useful tool in determining the therapeutic effectiveness of certain drugs. Drugs used in the treatment of cardiovascular disease may alter the electric activity of the heart. The electrocardiogram may provide the earliest objective evidence of a drug's effectiveness or its toxic manifestations. A knowledgeable and observant nurse can use the information obtained from the electrocardiogram for assessing the effectiveness of drug therapy in the treatment of various cardiac arrhythmias.

Electric activity always precedes mechanical contraction. Immediately after a wave of electric activity moves through atrial muscle, the muscle contracts and blood flows from the atria into the ventricles. (See Figure 10-4 for the graphic illustration of the normal electrocardiogram.) The P wave is produced by a wave of excitation through the atria (atrial depolarization). The

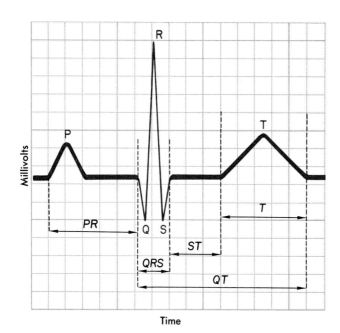

Figure 10-4

Graphic representation of the normal electrocardiogram. Vertical lines represent time, each square represents 0.04 second, and every five squares (set off by heavy black lines) represents 0.20 second. The normal P-R interval is less than 0.20 second; the average is 0.16 second. The average duration of the P wave is 0.08 second; the QRS interval is 0.08 second; the S-T segment is 0.12 second; the T wave is 0.16 second; and the Q-T interval is 1.36 seconds. Each horizontal line represents voltage; every five squares equals 0.5 millivolt.

onset of the P wave follows the firing of the sino-atrial node. After the P wave, a short pause or interval (P-R interval) occurs while the electric activity is transmitted to the atrioventricular node and conduction tissue and the ventricles. The electrocardiogram now records the QRS complex, or ventricular depolarization. This leads to contraction of the ventricles. Repolarization, or recovery, of the ventricles is indicated by the T wave. Atrial recovery or repolarization does not show on the EKG because of being hidden in the QRS complex. The EKG records receding activity as a negative potential, downward deflection; activity approaching an exploring electrode is recorded as a positive potential, an upward stroke on the graph paper or oscilloscope.

Drugs that affect the heart

Drugs may change the rate, force, and rhythm of the heart. Pharmacologic terms that have specific meaning for the actions of drugs on the cardiovascular system include the terms *inotropic, chronotropic, dromotropic,* and *pressor effects.*

Drugs with an *inotropic* (Gr. *inos,* fiber; *tropikos,* a turning or influence) effect influence myocardial contractility. If the drug has a positive inotropic effect it strengthens or increases the force of cardiac contraction. A drug with a negative inotropic effect weakens or decreases the force of muscular contraction.

Drugs with *chronotropic* (Gr. *chronos,* time) action affect the rate of the heart. If the drug increases the heart rate by increasing the rate of impulse formation in the sinoatrial node, it has a positive chronotropic effect. A negative chronotropic drug has the opposite effect and slows the heart rate by decreasing impulse formation.

When drugs have a *dromotropic* (Gr. *dromos,* a course) effect, they affect conduction through the specialized conducting tissues. A drug having a positive dromotropic action speeds conduction. A drug with negative dromotropic action delays conduction.

Drugs with *pressor* effect increase blood pressure by increasing peripheral arteriolar resistance through vasoconstriction.

CARDIAC GLYCOSIDES
DIGITALIS AND DIGITALIS-LIKE DRUGS

Drugs in the digitalis group are among the oldest and most effective therapeutic agents available to the physician for treatment of congestive heart failure. Cardiac glycosides act with specificity and rapidity and have unrivaled value in the treatment of congestive heart failure. Their use in medicine dates from the thirteenth century. However, it was not until 1785, when the English physician and botanist William Withering published his rigorous and systematic observations on the treatment of various ailments with digitalis, that cardiac glycosides became indispensable to a physician's drug armamentarium.

Chemically, all cardiac glycosides are closely related; each is composed of a sugar, a steroid, and a lactone. This is illustrated in the structural formula of digitoxin, one of the therapeutically important glycosides present in purple foxglove *(Digitalis purpurea).*

(Digitoxose)$_3$ | Sugar portion Steroid portion Lactone portion

Digitoxin

The sugar portion of the molecule will vary in different glycosides. These sugars increase the substance's water solubility and cell penetrability, alter absorption, and modify toxicity. Removal of the sugar portion from the glycoside leaves a molecule known as an aglycone or genin. An aglycone retains its digitalis-like activity but to a lessened degree. However, the lactone portion is essential to the characteristic cardiotonic properties of the molecule. The basic digitalis nucleus, the steroid portion, is similar to that of the sex hormones and corticosterones. The difference in this portion from other steroids is responsible for the inability, to date, to synthesize digitalis. The primary therapeutic use of digitalis glycosides is in treatment of congestive heart failure.

Many substances, of which digitalis is the most important, are characterized by their action on the heart. These substances belong to many different botanical families. For ages they have been used empirically in therapeutics. The action of each is fundamentally the same, so that the description for digitalis, with minor differences, will apply to all.

The most important plants that contain digitaloid substances are as follows:

Digitalis purpurea—purple foxglove
Digitalis lanata—white foxglove
Strophanthus hispidus, *S. kombé*—an African arrow poison
Scilla maritima—squill or sea onion

Digitalis

Digitalis is the dried leaves of *Digitalis purpurea*, or purple foxglove. This plant is cultivated for the drug market in England, North America, and Germany and grows wild in Europe, the United States, and Australia. Early investigators gave the plant the name *Digitalis purpurea* because the flower is purple and resembles a finger. Digitalis leaves contain a number of glycosides; the most important are digitoxin, gitoxin, and gitalin.

While all cardiac glycosides have similar pharmacologic properties, they differ in absorption and rate of elimination, time of onset of action, and duration of action. Selection of which cardiac glycoside to use is based on the needs of a particular individual and his reactions to the drug.

The primary circulatory actions of digitalis have been established only within the past few decades. However, the underlying cellular mechanisms remain uncertain.

Digitalis affects cardiac function through two important mechanisms:

1 Digitalis has positive inotropic action. It influences the mechanical performance of the heart by increasing the strength of myocardial contraction.
2 Digitalis alters the electric behavior of heart muscle through its actions on myocardial automaticity, conduction velocity, and refractory period.

Inotropic action. The inotropic action of digitalis results from direct action on the myocardium independent of extracardiac factors. Digitalis does not alter the amount of energy available for myocardial contraction; the increased contractility is associated with more efficient use of available energy. The exact mechanism by which digitalis affects the complex phenomenon of myocardial contraction remains to be established. However, present evidence suggests that digitalis increases myocardial contractility by potentiating excitation-contraction coupling. There is evidence that digitalis brings this about by:

1 Increasing the influx of calcium ions across the membrane
2 Releasing intracellular bound ionized calcium during depolarization
3 Decreasing outward movement or binding of intracellular calcium ions during and after depolarization

Electrophysiologic action. It has long been known that digitalis affects the movement of monovalent ions (Na^+, K^+) across the cell membrane. This permits digitalis to alter the electric properties of myocardium. (See Figure 10-5 for typical changes in the electrocardiographic pattern resulting from digitalization.) Membrane ATPase is concerned with active transport of sodium and potassium. Digitalis inhibits membrane ATPase, resulting in a rise in intracellular sodium and a fall in potassium. This action has been used to explain the inotropic and toxic effects of digitalis.

Automaticity of cardiac tissue is not directly affected by therapeutic concentrations of digi-

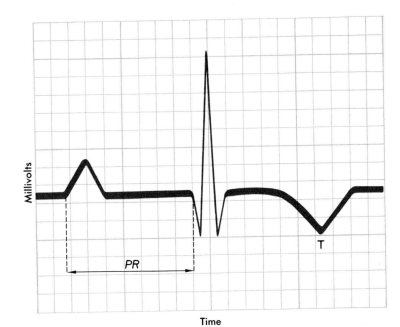

Millivolts

PR

T

Time

Figure 10-5

Representation of typical effects of digitalization on the electric activity of the heart as shown on the electrocardiogram. Note the prolonged P-R interval, the shortened Q-T interval, and the T wave inversion. (Compare with Figure 10-4.)

talis. However, toxic concentrations of digitalis can directly increase automaticity in all cardiac tissues capable of self-excitation. The result is an increased rate of both action potentials and spontaneous depolarization. This is one of the mechanisms responsible for digitalis-induced ectopic arrhythmias. Toxic doses of digitalis may significantly increase impulse formation in latent or potential pacemaker tissue.

Conduction velocity is decreased with all concentrations of digitalis. The atrioventricular conduction system is particularly affected. This slowing of conduction is partly caused by the direct action of digitalis but mostly by an increase in vagal action. This is shown on the electrocardiogram by a prolonged P-R interval.

The refractory period effects of digitalis vary in different parts of the heart. Reduction of the refractory period in the ventricles requires nearly toxic amounts of digitalis. A prolonged refractory period occurs in the atrioventricular conduction system, which is very sensitive to digitalis action. This action is partly direct and partly caused by increased vagal tone. Toxic doses of digitalis may prolong the refractory period and depress conduction in the atrioventricular conduction system to the point where a complete block occurs.

Clinical or therapeutic use of digitalis. As stated previously, the primary therapeutic use of digitalis is to treat congestive heart failure. However, digitalis is also a valuable drug in the treatment of atrial fibrillation and in the management of atrial flutter and paroxysmal tachycardia.

Congestive heart failure. Congestive heart failure is also referred to as cardiac insufficiency, heart or pump failure, and cardiac decompensation. Heart failure most often occurs as a late event of various congenital or acquired disorders of the heart or blood vessels, which place the heart under constant stress. A heart in failure is no longer capable of supplying body tissue with adequate oxygen and nutrients or of removing metabolic waste products. When pump failure occurs, there is usually failure of both sides of the heart, although failure of one side may have preceded and precipitated failure of the other side. Most of the signs and symptoms are caused by pulmonary and systemic congestion, the result of inadequate systolic outflow, and delayed venous return. The mortality for congestive heart failure is high.

The positive inotropic effect of digitalis that results in increased myocardial contractility has many important benefits for the patient with a failing heart. The increased force of systolic contraction causes the ventricles to empty more completely. This permits a slower heart rate and more complete filling, which result in the following:

1 Venous pressure falls, and the pulmonary and systemic congestion and their accompanying signs and symptoms are either diminished or completely abolished.
2 Coronary circulation is enhanced, myocardial oxygen demand is reduced, and the supply of oxygen and nutrients to the myocardium is improved.
3 Heart size is often decreased toward normal.

It has been demonstrated that some of the cardiac glycosides have a true but mild diuretic effect. However, marked diuresis in the edematous patient is primarily the result of improved heart action, improved circulation to all body tissue, and improved tissue and organ function including renal function. When digitalis is effective, the patient is noticeably improved and has an increased sense of well-being.

Atrial fibrillation. During atrial fibrillation several hundred impulses originate from the atria but only a fraction of them are transmitted through the atrioventricular node. (See Figure 10-6 for electrocardiographic pattern of atrial fibrillation.) Digitalis is ideal for slowing the ventricular rate because it increases the refractory period of the atrioventricular node and also impairs conduction. It is important to know that the purpose of using digitalis in atrial fibrillation is to slow the ventricular rate, which may prevent or eliminate cardiac failure. Digitalis does not convert the fibrillating atria into normally contracting ones.

Protective and prophylactic use. There is no general agreement concerning the value of prophylactic digitalization in the absence of congestive heart failure. Some authorities believe the cardiac glycosides may exert a protective effect on myocardial function in the absence of cardiac failure when: (1) an unusual work load is to be

Figure 10-6

Graphic representation of atrial fibrillation as seen on the electrocardiographic monitor or tracing paper. No true P waves are noted; but f (fibrillation) waves consisting of rapid, small, and irregular waves are noted. The QRS complex is normal in configuration and duration but occurs irregularly.

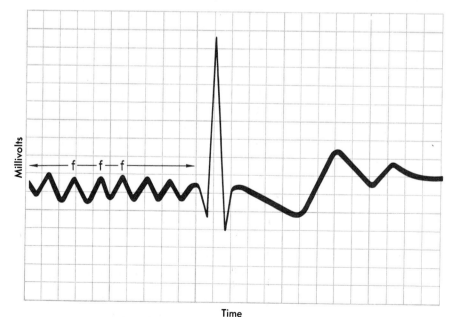

placed on the heart or (2) when a patient is to be subjected to the risk of having myocardial function depressed. Patients who may be digitalized in the absence of cardiac failure by the proponents of prophylaxis include prepartum cardiac patients and elderly or cardiac patients who are to undergo the acute stress of anesthesia and major surgery. More extensive studies are needed before the therapeutic effectiveness of prophylactic digitalization can be established.

Absorption and excretion. The absorption of various cardiac glycosides varies from a minimal amount to almost 100% after oral administration. Digitoxin is almost completely absorbed, digoxin is 80% to 90% absorbed, less than 50% of lanatoside C is absorbed, while ouabain is even less completely absorbed. Oral preparations are absorbed from the intestinal tract. Distribution is widespread throughout body tissues. The liver is the major organ for detoxifying cardiac glycosides. Since the drugs are eliminated gradually, repeated doses produce accumulation. This accounts for the persistence of digitalis' cardiac effects for several days or weeks after discontinuance of the drug.

Only a small percentage of a cardiac glycoside is excreted unchanged. Most of the drug is excreted in the urine; some is excreted in the feces. Since digitalis excretion is primarily by the kidneys, patients with renal insufficiency retain the drug longer and show greater sensitivity to the drug.

Administration. The preferred route of administration of digitalis and the cardiac glycosides for congestive heart failure is oral. Because of variation in rapidity of onset of action, duration of action, and individual response, the oral route is safest to use. It is also least expensive. Local gastric mucosal irritation is decreased by giving the drug with or just after meals.

It is not recommended that digitalis preparations be given subcutaneously because of the local irritating effect of the drugs (producing pain and abscess formation) and uncertain absorption, especially in the presence of congestive heart failure. The intravenous route is usually reserved for cases of emergency (such as patients with pulmonary edema or acute ventricular failure) or when the patient has a condition preventing the

use of oral medications (such as vomiting). Rectal administration has been used for patients who have difficulty tolerating the drug orally. However, this is an uncommon route of administration.

Standardization of digitalis preparations. Preparations of digitalis are assayed biologically. The U.S. Digitalis Reference Standard contains 1 unit of activity in 0.1 Gm. This is equal to the International Digitalis Standard. While many digitalis preparations must be assayed by the official U.S.P. method in pigeons, the pure glycosides such as digitoxin, digoxin, or deslanoside, U.S.P., are assayed colorimetrically.

Digitalization and choice of preparations. In the treatment of heart failure, the aim is to give digitalis until optimum cardiac effects are achieved and most of the signs and symptoms of heart failure have disappeared. When the patient has reached that state in which he has profited all that he can from the drug, he is said to be digitalized. The amount of drug required for digitalization may vary with each patient.

Usually digitalization is accomplished by giving the patient, over a period of hours or days, a total amount necessary to produce the desired cardiac effect—the digitalizing dose—and then keeping him on a smaller daily dose—the maintenance dose—designed to replace the daily loss of the drug from his body by destruction or excretion to maintain the desired effect. For example, a common schedule for an average adult, using whole-leaf digitalis, would include a digitalizing dose of 1 to 1.5 Gm., given in divided doses over 1 to 2 days, followed by a maintenance dose of 0.1 Gm. daily. Naturally, both the digitalizing and the maintenance doses must be adjusted to the particular patient in terms of toxic reactions and clinical signs of adequate digitalization. If digitoxin were administered orally, 1 to 1.5 mg. would constitute an average digitalizing dose of the drug and 0.1 to 0.2 mg. the maintenance dose. The rate of drug destruction following adequate digitalization is about one tenth the digitalizing dose per 24 hours. This is the rationale usually used for determining the maintenance dose. Many patients who receive digitalis must continue to take the drug the rest of their lives. In children, the dose of digitalis and the rapidity of administration depend on weight and age, body surface, severity of cardiac impairment, and response of the patient.

Differences among the preparations available occur chiefly in absorption from the gastrointestinal tract, local emetic action, and speed of excretion. The glycosides of digitalis are poorly absorbed when the whole drug is administered, which accounts for the fact that only one fifth as much of the intravenous preparation is required as the oral preparation. The digitalis glycosides are irritating to mucous membranes and subcutaneous tissues. Large oral doses of whole drug may produce nausea and vomiting shortly after administration. Smaller doses are less likely to produce emesis from local irritation. The nausea and vomiting occasioned by small doses result from a central effect on the vomiting center. All preparations capable of exerting cardiac effects are capable of emetic action, and this untoward effect cannot be avoided by changing to other members of the digitalis group or by changing the method of administration. All preparations of digitalis or digitalis-like drugs have a cumulative action, although some are more cumulative than others. Digitoxin and digitalis leaf have an especially pronounced cumulative action.

In spite of differences of opinion, the use of the whole drug in the form of digitalis tincture or powdered digitalis has to a certain extent been replaced by the use of refined preparations or by the use of the crystalline glycosides. These are frequently preferred because they are more stable and can be injected and because dosage can be determined more accurately. They are absorbed much more readily when given by mouth and cause less gastrointestinal irritation. Several glycosides are available in a high degree of purity, such as digitoxin, digoxin, and lanatoside C. These make rapid digitalization by oral administration possible with a minimum of local irritant action caused by nonabsorbable glycosides.

It should be emphasized that some of the purified digitalis glycosides are extremely potent compounds, and if looked upon as poisons they are among the most powerful poisons known. Some of the glycosides have a lethal dose for man of about 0.1 mg. per kilogram of body weight. The nurse should therefore handle these compounds with great care and respect.

Purple foxglove—preparation, dosage, and administration

Powdered digitalis, N.F.; *prepared digitalis*, B.P. This preparation is available in tablets and capsules. Range of maintenance dose is 50 to 200 mg. daily. Onset of action occurs in 2 to 6 hours; maximal effect occurs in 12 to 24 hours. Trade names include Digifortis, Digiglusin, and Digitora.

Digitalis tincture, N.F. This is the only acceptable form of liquid preparation for oral use; 1 ml. is equal to 1 U.S.P. digitalis unit. Calibrated medicine droppers or medicine glasses should be used to ensure accuracy.

Gitalin (amorphous), N.F. (Gitaligin). This is a mixture of glycosides obtained from *Digitalis purpurea*. Its action and uses are the same as those of digitalis, and the same precautions should be taken with its administration. The rate of elimination or destruction is slower than that of digoxin but faster than that of digitoxin. Gitalin is administered orally or intravenously. It is marketed in 0.5-mg. tablets. Average maintenance dose is 0.5 mg. daily; range of dose is 0.25 to 0.75 mg. daily.

Digitoxin, U.S.P., B.P. Digitoxin is the chief active glycoside of *Digitalis purpurea*. It is available in crystalline form and is readily absorbed from the intestinal tract. One milligram of digitoxin has the same effect as 1 Gm. of N.F. digitalis when given by mouth. It is available in tablet form as well as in ampules for intravenous therapy. It is extremely poisonous. Digitoxin is sold under a number of trade names: Crystodigin, Unidigin, Purodigin, and Digitaline Nativelle. *Digitoxin tablets*, U.S.P., are available in amounts of 0.1 and 0.2 mg.

Its chief disadvantage is its slow onset of action and prolonged half-life when compared to digoxin. Two to 3 weeks may elapse before digitoxin is eliminated from the body. Range of maintenance dose is 0.1 to 0.2 mg. daily. With oral administration onset of action occurs in 2 to 4 hours; maximal effect occurs within 12 to 24 hours. After intravenous injection, onset of action occurs in $\frac{1}{2}$ to 2 hours; maximal effect occurs in 8 to 9 hours. Digitoxin should be avoided for patients with severe liver disease.

White foxglove—preparation, dosage, and administration

Digilanid. This is a mixture of the crystallized cardioactive glycosides, lanatoside A, lanatoside B, and lanatoside C, obtained from the leaves of white foxglove, *Digitalis lanata.* The three components are present in this preparation in the same proportion as found in the crude drug. When these glycosides are hydrolyzed, they yield, respectively, digitoxin, gitoxin, and digoxin. The actions and uses of digilanid are similar to those of digitalis. It can be administered orally, intramuscularly, intravenously, and rectally. Dosage is 0.67 to 1.33 mg. (two to four tablets). It is usually given daily in tablet form until desired effects are obtained and then one to two tablets are given daily as maintenance dosage. Precautions to be observed are the same as those for any digitalis preparation. It is marketed in solution for injection (0.4 mg. in 2 ml.) and in tablets (0.33 mg.).

Acetyldigitoxin (Acylanid). This is a cardiac glycoside derived from lanatoside A. It resembles digitoxin in many ways but has a more rapid onset and a shorter duration of action than digitoxin. It is available in 0.1- and 0.2-mg. tablets for oral administration. Onset of action occurs in 1 to 2 hours. Maintenance dose for adults ranges from 0.1 to 0.2 mg. daily.

Lanatoside C, N.F., B.P. (Cedilanid). This glycoside of *Digitalis lanata* is thought to be more active, therapeutically, than the other two glycosides of the white foxglove. Lanatoside C is a white powder that is practically insoluble in water. Absorption after oral administration is said to be irregular. It is marketed in tablets for oral administration. Lanatoside C tablets usually contain 0.5 mg. of the drug, and 0.5 mg. (gr. $^{1}/_{120}$) is the usual dose.

Deslanoside (deacetyllanatoside C), U.S.P., B.P. (Cedilanid-D). This preparation is derived from lanatoside C and has the advantage of being more soluble and more stable than the parent substance. For practical purposes it constitutes the injectable form of lanatoside C. *Deslanoside injection,* U.S.P., is marketed in 2- and 4-ml. ampules containing 0.4 mg. and 0.8 mg. of the drug, respectively. Initial loading dose for adults is 0.8 to 1.6 mg. One half the dose may be given immediately with the remainder given in divided doses at 2-hour intervals. Maintenance dose is 0.25 to 0.5 mg. daily until a longer-acting preparation can be substituted.

Digoxin, U.S.P., B.P. (Lanoxin). This is a hydrolytic product formed from lanatoside C. It has an advantage over digitalis for the patient who must be rapidly digitalized. Some patients seem to tolerate digoxin better than digitalis. The drug may be given intravenously, in which case saturation of the tissues may be accomplished much more rapidly than with digitalis. Digoxin may also be given orally. It should be administered with caution because it is extremely poisonous. After oral administration effects appear in 1 hour, and maximal effect occurs in 6 to 7 hours. After intravenous administration effects occur in 5 to 10 minutes and reach a maximum in 1 to 2 hours. Official (U.S.P.) preparations of digoxin are available in tablets (0.125, 0.25 and 0.5 mg.) and as an injectable solution (0.1 mg. in 1 ml. and 0.5 mg. in 2 ml.). Average maintenance dose for adults is 0.25 to 0.75 mg. daily. The proprietary name Lanoxin has an advantage in that it helps to differentiate digoxin and digitoxin, which are sometimes mistaken one for the other by the student. Digoxin (Lanoxin) is widely used in pediatrics and is available as an elixir (0.05 mg. per millimeter) for oral administration to children.

Contraindications and precautions. Digitalis is contraindicated in heart block and usually when ventricular tachycardia is present. Valvular disease, diphtheria, and thyrotoxicosis are not in themselves considered indications for digitalis therapy.

Digitalis must be used with great caution in patients with acute or toxic myocarditis since the potential for glycoside-induced arrhythmias is increased in these patients. If congestive heart failure occurs in patients with acute myocarditis, digitalis may be used but in smaller than usual doses and with close observation. Ordinary doses usually do not slow the often associated tachycardia, and high doses produce arrhythmias.

Table 10-1 Dosage of digitalis and cardiac glycosides (adults)

Preparation (generic name and trade name)	Administration	Usual digitalizing quantity (given in divided doses)	Usual daily maintenance dose
Purple foxglove			
Powdered digitalis (leaf)	Oral	1.5 Gm. (1 to 2 Gm.)	0.1 Gm. (100 to 200 mg.)
Digitalis tincture	Oral	10 to 15 ml.	1 ml.
Cardiac glycosides			
Acetyldigitoxin (Acylanid)	Oral	1.8 mg. (0.6 to 2 mg.) over 24 hr.	0.15 mg. (0.1 to 0.2 mg.)
Digitoxin (Crystodigin, Digitalline Nativelle, Purodigin)	Oral	1.0 to 1.5 mg. over 24 to 48 hr.	0.1 to 0.2 mg.
	Intravenous	0.5 mg. (0.5 to 1.2 mg.)	0.1 mg. (0.1 to 0.2 mg.)
Digoxin (Lanoxin)	Oral	1.5 mg. (0.5 to 2 mg.)	0.5 mg. (0.25 to 0.75 mg.)
	Intravenous	1 mg. (0.5 to 1.5 mg.)	0.5 mg. (0.25 to 0.75 mg.)
Lanatoside C (Cedilanid)	Oral	8 mg.	1.0 mg.
Gitalin (Gitaligin)	Oral	6.5 mg. (2.5 mg. initially and then 0.75 mg. every 6 hr.)	0.5 mg.
	Intravenous	2.5 to 3.0 mg. in two injections at 24-hr. intervals	2.5 mg. two times per week
Ouabain	Intravenous only (slowly)	0.5 mg. (0.12 to 0.25 mg.)	
Deslanoside (deacetyl-lanatoside C, Cedilanid-D)	Intravenous only (slowly)	1.6 mg. (1.2 to 1.6 mg.)	0.4 mg. (0.2 to 0.6 mg.)

Side effects and toxic effects. Not all undesired effects of digitalis are toxic effects. While anorexia, nausea, and vomiting can occur with digitalis toxicity, these symptoms can also be caused by gastric irritation from oral digitalis preparations and stimulation of the vomiting center. These effects are often self-limiting and disappear as the patient adjusts to the drug.

Additional signs and symptoms of digitalis toxicity include diarrhea, headache, visual disturbances, weakness, restlessness, and nervous irritability. These are *extracardiac* manifestations of digitalis excess. These toxic effects, while troublesome to the patient, are rarely serious and are often eliminated by omission of the drug for several days. Once the toxic signs or symptoms are gone, drug therapy can again be reinstituted at a lower dosage.

Almost every type of arrhythmia can be produced by digitalis toxicity. The type of arrhythmia produced varies with the age of the patient and other factors. Premature ventricular contractions and bigeminal rhythm (two beats and a pause) are common signs of digitalis toxicity in adults, while children tend to develop ectopic nodal or atrial beats. Digitalis-induced arrhythmias are caused by depression of the sinoatrial and atrioventricular nodes. This results in various conduction disturbances (first- or second-degree block or complete heart block). Digitalis may also cause increased myocardial automaticity, producing extra systoles or tachycardias by activating latent pacemakers.

Predisposing factors to digitalis toxicity. Nurses need to be aware of the predisposing factors to digitalis toxicity. Presence of any of these factors in patients indicates need for close observation of these patients for signs and symptoms of digitalis intoxication.

POTASSIUM LOSS. Hypokalemia is a common cause of digitalis cardiotoxicity. Since potassium inhibits the excitability of the heart, a depletion of body or myocardial potassium increases cardiac excitability. Low extracellular potassium is synergistic with digitalis and enhances ectopic pacemaker activity (arrhythmias). The following are causes of potassium loss:

1 Hypokalemia occurs if large amounts of body fluids are lost as a result of vomiting, diarrhea, or diuresis from administration of diuretics. The use of various diuretic agents (mercurials, carbonic-anhydrase inhibitors, ammonium chloride, and thiazide preparations) induce potassium diuresis along with sodium and water diuresis.

2 Poor dietary intake or severe dietary restrictions decreasing electrolyte intake can cause loss of potassium.

3 Adrenal steroids cause potassium loss and sodium retention.

4 Surgical procedures associated with severe electrolyte disturbances such as abdominal-perineal resection, colostomy, ileostomy, colectomy, and ureterosigmoidostomy can cause loss of potassium.

5 Use of potassium-free intravenous fluids can cause hypokalemia.

PATHOLOGIC CONDITIONS. Kidney, liver, and severe heart disease are major factors in digitalis toxicity. From 60% to 80% of the digitalis glycosides are excreted by the kidneys. Therefore, renal disease promotes digitalis cumulation and intoxication. Since the liver is the primary organ for inactivating digitalis, any impairment of liver function decreases an individual's tolerance to digitalis. Severe cardiac disease impedes the function of all body organs and increases myocardial sensitivity to digitalis.

ADMINISTRATION OF PURIFIED GLYCOSIDES. Because purified glycosides produce fewer side effects than the whole leaf, there may be continued administration of digitalis without awareness that toxicity is occurring.

SLOWER BODY FUNCTION. Elderly persons have a slowing of body functions and often a decreased tolerance to drug therapy. Older patients often show signs of toxicity with small doses of digitalis.

INTRAVENOUS ADMINISTRATION OF DIGITALIS AND RAPID DIGITALIZATION. The risk of digitalis overdosage is increased by intravenous administration and rapid digitalization.

Treatment of digitalis intoxication. The treatment of digitalis toxicity may consist entirely of omitting administration of digitalis until toxic signs and symptoms have disappeared, or it may include the administration of other drugs such as potassium chloride or rarely EDTA. Administration of potassium chloride will tend to decrease myocardial excitability and abolish arrhythmias. Disodium ethylenediamine tetra-acetic acid (EDTA) is a calcium chelating agent. Successful treatment of digitalis toxicity has also been reported with the use of phenytoin and propranolol. There is no specific antidote for digitalis intoxication.

Ouabain, U.S.P.; G-Strophanthin

This preparation is obtained from *Strophanthus gratus*. For many years it was the standard against which all digitalis preparations were measured. It is not absorbed well from the gastrointestinal tract and hence must be given parenterally (usually intravenously). Its action is relatively rapid. Effects appear within about 30 minutes after intravenous injection, and the peak of effect is secured in about 90 minutes. Most of its effects have disappeared within 24 hours. It is one of the preparations of choice for rapid digitalization. It is relatively soluble and not likely to cause venous thrombosis when given intravenously. It is available in 1- and 2-ml. ampules containing 0.25 mg. per milliliter of solution.

NURSING MEASURES FOR CARE OF PATIENTS RECEIVING DIGITALIS PREPARATIONS

Of great importance is the careful observation by the nurse of patients receiving digitalis preparations who have one or more of the predisposing factors to digitalis intoxication. If the patient is being monitored, careful observation should be made of his electrocardiogram before and after the institution of or reduction or increase in digitalis dosage. The pulse, preferably apical pulse, should be checked prior to giving each dose to determine any marked change in rate or rhythm. It is still a safe precaution to report and record a pulse below 60 in the adult or 90 to 110 beats per minute in the child. A decision may be made to withhold the drug.

Understanding on the part of the nurse of the relationship between dosage and potency is fundamental to intelligent cooperation with the physician in the care of the patient who is receiving digitalis or related drugs. When medication is ordered in terms of a small fraction or a decimal fraction, the inference is not only that the drug is potent but also that a mistake in dosage can be especially dangerous even if the amount is small in terms of milligrams. Considerable difference exists among dosages of 1 mg., 0.1 mg., 0.15 mg., and 0.2 mg. Differences of a fraction of a milligram can make a great deal of difference when dealing with a potent preparation. The nurse must exert particular care to see that the correct dosage is given.

Figure 10-7

Counting the pulse. This is done as a precautionary measure by the nurse when administering drugs that are likely to slow the action of the heart, such as members of the digitalis group. Radial artery is shown in relation to the bones of the hand and radius and ulna.

ANTIARRHYTHMIC DRUGS

Antiarrhythmic agents are used in the prevention and treatment of disorders of cardiac rhythm. They exert their effects by reversing the electrophysiologic abnormalities that elicit the arrhythmias. Most antiarrhythmic agents are cardiac depressants and they can produce dangerous effects. It is important to keep in mind also that not all arrhythmias need to be treated.

It is believed that most arrhythmias are a consequence of (1) increased automaticity leading to activation of latent pacemakers or (2) disorders of impulse conduction. Evidence indicates that some drugs, such as the catecholamines or digitalis, increase automaticity and may produce arrhythmias. On the other hand, antiarrhythmic agents, such as quinidine, decrease automaticity, although they may depress other properties of the heart also. Procainamide, lidocaine, propranolol, and potassium salts are also employed as antiarrhythmic agents.

Quinidine

Quinidine is considered to be the prototype of antiarrhythmic drugs. Like quinine, quinidine is contained in cinchona bark and was used by Peruvian Indians for the treatment of malaria. It was introduced as an antiarrhythmic drug early in the twentieth century following a demonstration by a patient of Wenckebach's that he could control his atrial fibrillation by self-administration of quinine. It was not until 1962 that the electrophysiologic mechanisms of quinidine were identified. Of the antiarrhythmic agents now available, quinidine is the one most widely used.

Action. Quinidine depresses automaticity, has a negative inotropic effect, and influences conduction velocity. In addition, quinidine is known to have vasodepressor and vagolytic action, as well as a weak curare-like effect. Some quinidine effects may result from quinidine decreasing cell membrane permeability to the outward flow of potassium from within the cells.

Quinidine inhibits the rate of electric impulse formation from the pacemakers and thereby decreases heart rate. Abnormal or ectopic pacemaker tissue appears to be more sensitive to quinidine than normal pacemaker tissue (sinoatrial node). The blocking of abnormal electric impulses permits the sinoatrial node to reestablish control over cardiac impulse formation, which abolishes ectopic arrhythmias. Quinidine prolongs the effective refractory period which helps to protect the myocardium from rapid repeated stimuli.

Quinidine's dromotropic action is a negative one since it delays or depresses atrioventricular and intraventricular conduction velocity. This is reflected in the electrocardiogram by prolongation of the P-R interval and widened QRS complex. With increased drug effect more advanced degrees of heart block can occur.

The negative inotropic action is not a serious hazard when therapeutic doses of quinidine are used. However, marked depression of myocardial contractility may be associated with a reduction of cardiac output.

Quinidine has an effect on smooth muscle that accounts for its vasodepressor action resulting in vasodilation. The resultant decrease in peripheral vascular resistance may cause hypotension and/or decreased cardiac output. This is more likely to occur with intravenous administration of quinidine.

The vagolytic effect of quinidine inhibits vagal action on the sinoatrial and atrial ventricular nodes. This accounts for the tachycardia seen in some patients. It should be noted that hyperkalemia enhances the depressive effects of quinidine—hypokalemia counteracts the antiarrhythmic effect of quinidine.

Uses. Quinidine is effective against many arrhythmias—atrial tachycardia, atrial flutter and fibrillation, ventricular tachycardia, and premature systoles. Quinidine has proved to be a valuable drug in the treatment of recurrent paroxysmal atrial tachycardia. Electric cardioversion may be the agent of choice to convert

Figure 10-8

Tracings of action potentials recorded from a spontaneously depolarizing conducting fiber showing a comparison between the normal and the quinidine effect on the fiber.

▬ ▬(Quinidine effect)
  A Slowing of depolarization
  B Prolonged action potential (in large doses)
  C Decrease in diastolic depolarization

certain arrhythmias to a normal sinus rhythm. However, quinidine continues to have an important role in the management of chronic and paroxysmal arrhythmias.

Absorption and excretion. Quinidine is readily absorbed from the gastrointestinal tract. Therefore, effective concentrations of the drug can be achieved by the oral as well as parenteral route. It is rapidly taken up by body tissue (with the exception of brain tissue). It is excreted from the body via the urine. From 10% to 50% of a given dose is excreted within 24 hours after administration. Degradation of quinidine takes place in the liver.

Preparation, dosage, and administration. The maximal effect of an oral dose of quinidine occurs within 1 to 3 hours after administration and the effect persists for 6 to 8 hours. Quinidine sulfate is used for oral administration and the hydrochloride, lactate, gluconate, or sulfate preparations are used for intramuscular administration. Intravenous administration should only be used for emergency situations because of the potentially dangerous effects of the drug. Quinidine should not be given rectally because it has a severe irritating effect on rectal mucosa.

Quinidine sulfate, U.S.P., B.P. This drug is available in 100-, 200-, and 300-mg. capsules, and 100-, 130-, 200-, and 325-mg. tablets. Quinidine sulfate is given orally in doses of 200 to 300 mg. and repeated every 2, 4, or 6 hours. When given every 2 hours, peak blood levels are usually achieved after the fifth dose; when given orally every 4 hours peak blood levels are achieved within 48 to 72 hours; when given every 6 hours, or four times a day, peak blood levels may not be reached until the fifth day of administration. The oral maintenance dose is usually from 200 to 600 mg. daily. The dosage for children is 6 mg. per kilogram of body weight every 4 to 6 hours.

Quinidine gluconate, U.S.P. This drug is sometimes administered intramuscularly. The initial dose is from 300 to 500 mg. The drug begins to act within 15 to 30 minutes; maximum effect is reached within 1 to 3 hours. Quinidine gluconate is also given orally. In acute situations, 200 mg. of quinidine gluconate in dilute solution may be given intravenously, very slowly, with continuous monitoring of the EKG and blood pressure.

Toxic effects. Quinidine is a potentially hazardous drug. A number of sudden deaths have been reported in patients on quinidine therapy.

The toxic effects of quinidine in approximate order of frequency of occurrence include cinchonism (nausea, vomiting, diarrhea, tinnitus, vertigo, and visual disturbances), thrombocytopenic purpura, rashes and urticaria, hypotension, and ventricular fibrillation.

Some of these effects, such as thrombocytopenic purpura, are thought to be a true allergic hypersensitivity to the drug. Therefore, some clinicians give a test dose of the drug before instituting intensive therapy.

Quinidine can cause cardiac arrest since it is a depressant of myocardial excitability. In patients with conduction defects, a complete block may occur. Since quinidine depresses atrioventricular and intraventricular conduction and ventricular impulse formation, an intrinsic ventricular rhythm may fail to develop and the patient may die of cardiac arrest. Reducing or stopping the dosage of quinidine may be sufficient to overcome toxic or side effects. A true hypersensitivity to the drug necessitates absolute withdrawal of the drug.

The most effective treatment of quinidine toxicity at the present time appears to be intravenous administration of angiotensin alone or in combination with disodium calcium versenate. These drugs significantly increase peripheral vascular resistance and enhance myocardial contractility.

Contraindications. Quinidine is contraindicated in patients who are hypersensitive to the drug. Its use is also contraindicated in patients with second-degree or complete heart block, since it can further enhance conduction delay and lead to asystole.

Drug interactions. The following drug interactions may occur:

1 Action of anticoagulants may be enhanced since quinidine prolongs prothrombin time.
2 Quinidine may potentiate the hypotensive effect of antihypertensive drugs and diuretics.
3 Quinidine has a weak curare-like action and therefore it may intensify the action of neuromuscular

blocking agents (e.g., tubocurarine), and enhance the action of drugs that can depress conduction at the myoneural junction (e.g., polymyxin B, neomycin, kanamycin).

4 Quinidine may antagonize the action of neostigmine, physostigmine, and related drugs.

5 The concomitant use of quinidine with reserpine or other rauwolfia alkaloids may produce arrhythmias.

Nursing measures. Patients with liver disease, congestive heart failure, or renal insufficiency should be closely observed for toxic reactions, since interference with metabolism of quinidine or its excretion from the body can greatly increase the body's response to any given dose of the drug.

Since the drug can cause thrombocytopenic purpura, patients on quinidine therapy should be closely observed for bleeding tendencies, petechiae, or ecchymotic or purpuric areas. Patients with decreased platelets require protection from injury that could result in hemorrhage.

Early evidence of quinidine toxicity is best detected by having the patient monitored electrocardiographically and observing for changes in the patient's cardiac electric activity pattern. Abnormal prolongation of the QRS complex, evidence of second-degree or complete heart block, or appearance of premature ventricular contractions precludes continued quinidine administration.

It is recommended that the patient's blood pressure be checked before administration of quinidine. If hypotension is noted, the physician should be notified.

Procainamide hydrochloride, U.S.P., B.P. (Pronestyl Hydrochloride)

$$H_2N-\underset{}{\underset{}{\bigcirc}}-CONH-CH_2CH_2-N\underset{C_2H_5}{\overset{C_2H_5}{<}} \cdot HCl$$

Procainamide is a synthetic drug that is an effective antiarrhythmic agent with fewer toxic effects than quinidine. Procainamide is the result of investigations to produce a drug similar to the local anesthetic procaine, but with fewer central nervous system effects. It had been demonstrated that topical application of procaine to the

myocardium during thoracic surgery reduced the occurrence of premature cardiac contractions during surgery.

Action. The cardiac effects of procainamide are similar to those of quinidine. Procainamide has a negative chronotropic effect since it depresses the rate of pacemaker discharge. It has negative dromotropic action since it slows down conduction in the atria, across the atrioventricular node, through the atrioventricular conducting tissue, and within the ventricles. It has a negative inotropic action since it depresses myocardial contractility. Procainamide has the same effect on ion transfer as does quinidine. Its ability to prolong the refractory period helps to terminate circus movement.* Also, like quinidine, procainamide can cause hypotension.

Electrocardiographic changes that may be noted are prolonged P-R and QT intervals and widening of QRS complex.

Uses. Procainamide is used to treat a wide variety of ventricular and supraventricular arrhythmias. It is inferior to quinidine in the treatment of atrial fibrillation and flutter.

Absorption and excretion. When given orally procainamide is readily absorbed from the gastrointestinal tract and is rapidly excreted in the urine. Intravenously its action is almost immediate; orally, it acts within 30 to 60 minutes, with peak action occurring in 1 to 2 hours.

Preparation, dosage, and administration. The following is the available preparation of procainamide.

Procainamide hydrochloride, U.S.P., B.P. (Pronestyl Hydrochloride). This preparation is available in 250- and 500-mg. capsules and in solution for injection (100 mg. per milliliter). It is usually administered orally or intravenously, although it can be administered intramuscularly. A continuous intravenous drip of procainamide in 5% glucose in water may be used to control acute arrhythmias. Usual oral dose for adults

---

*Circus movement or rhythm refers to a widely held reentry theory that states that flutter and fibrillation occur when initial impulses meet a local block during transmission and the impulses return to the original pacemaker when the latter is no longer refractory; thus constant firing of the pacemaker occurs.

and children is 50 mg. per kilogram of body weight daily in divided doses every 3 hours.

Side effects and toxic effects. Side effects of procainamide include gastrointestinal and central nervous system disturbances and hypotension. Bone marrow depression has been reported as well as allergic reactions. Tachycardia or other arrhythmias may result from use of procainamide. More than forty cases have been reported of patients developing a systemic lupus erythematosus type syndrome while on prolonged oral maintenance doses of procainamide. If the drug is discontinued at onset of symptoms, they disappear in a few days or weeks. It is not known what the outcome would be if procainamide administration were continued.

Vasopressor drugs or molar sodium lactate may be required to overcome the hypotensive effect of procainamide. Frequent blood examinations should be done to determine the drug's effect on the leukocytes and agranulocytes.

Drug interactions. Procainamide may enhance the action of drugs with neuromuscular blocking action (curariform drugs and various antibiotics, such as neomycin). This interaction may cause respiratory depression.

Procainamide may also potentiate the hypotensive effect of antihypertensive drugs and thiazide diuretics.

Contraindications. Procainamide is usually contraindicated in patients with severe heart damage and shock, since increasing the hypotension may result in fatality. It is also contraindicated in patients with complete heart block and in patients manifesting allergic reactions. Increased widening of the QRS complex caused by procainamide contraindicates further administration of the drug.

Nursing measures. When the drug is given intravenously, electrocardiographic and blood pressure monitoring is required. Further administration of the drug should be questioned when hypotension, progressive widening of the QRS complex, or undesirable changes in the EKG pattern occur. Vasopressors, such as norepinephrine, should be readily available if hypotension occurs. Patients should be observed for and told to report symptoms of arthralgia and fever (lupus syndrome).

Lidocaine, U.S.P. (Xylocaine); lignocaine hydrochloride, B.P.

$$\text{CH}_3\text{—}\underset{\underset{\text{CH}_3}{}}{C_6H_3}\text{—}\underset{H}{N}\text{—}\underset{\underset{O}{\parallel}}{C}\text{—}CH_2\text{—}N\underset{C_2H_5}{\overset{C_2H_5}{}}$$

Lidocaine is better known and extensively used as a local and topical anesthetic agent. However, in recent years it has become one of the most frequently used drugs and in some institutions it is the drug of choice in the treatment of ventricular arrhythmias. It has gained considerable acclaim as an effective antiarrhythmic agent. Lidocaine apparently does not depress conduction in the heart, and it has less negative inotropic action than either quinidine or procainamide.

Action. The action of lidocaine is similar to that of procainamide. Lidocaine has greater antiarrhythmic potency. A dose of 100 mg. of lidocaine is pharmacologically equivalent to 400 to 500 mg. of procainamide.

Uses. Lidocaine is used to treat ventricular arrhythmias that occur during surgery or cardiac diagnostic procedures or that are caused by acute myocardial infarction or cardioversion. It may be used preoperatively in patients with a history of ventricular arrhythmia for prophylaxis. Lidocaine is effective in decreasing the frequency of premature ventricular beats.

Preparation, dosage, and administration. Lidocaine is available in a variety of preparations —solutions, jelly, ointment—and in a variety of ampule and multiple dose vial solutions. A 2% solution without epinephrine is available in 5- and 50-ml. containers for use in cardiac arrhythmias. Lidocaine is administered intravenously, 1 mg. per kilogram of body weight, and by slow intravenous injection or continuous intravenous drip. The onset of action of lidocaine occurs within 2 minutes. Duration of action of a single dose is 10 to 20 minutes; 20 minutes after discontinuing intravenous administration, none of lidocaine's effects persists. If an injection of 50 to 100 mg. does not produce a desired response, additional injections may be given every 5 minutes for a total dosage of 200 to 300 mg. For intravenous infusion, lidocaine is added to 1 liter of 5% dextrose in water and infused at a rate of 15 to 45 μg. per kilogram per minute; action occurs in 10 to 20 minutes. Therapeutic blood levels for lidocaine range from 2 to 5 μg. per milliliter. Lidocaine may be given intramuscularly into the deltoid muscle; 4 mg. per kilogram of body weight will produce a plasma level of 1 μg. per milliliter in 5 minutes, a peak level of 3 μg. per milliliter in 15 minutes, and a plasma level of 1 μg. per milliliter in 90 to 120 minutes. Intramuscular administration is controversial. Lidocaine is metabolized by the liver and rapidly excreted by the kidneys.

Side effects and toxic effects. Drowsiness is a very common side effect but this is often desirable, particularly in patients with acute myocardial infarction.

Some investigators report central nervous system disturbances (agitation, disorientation, muscle twitching, and convulsions), heart block, and hypotension, particularly with high dosage or rapid rate of administration. Blurred vision, nausea, paresthesias, tinnitus, euphoria, respiratory depression, bradycardia, and respiratory and cardiac arrest may occur. Toxic effects rapidly disappear upon discontinuance of drug administration.

Patients undergoing infusion of lidocaine should be carefully monitored for cardiac depressant effects. The blood pressure should be checked for hypotensive effect, and the patient should be carefully observed for other undesirable effects. Lidocaine must be used cautiously in patients with severe liver disease since cumulative effects can occur.

Phenytoin sodium, U.S.P., B.P. (DPH, Dilantin)

Phenytoin (formerly known in the United States as diphenylhydantoin) was introduced over 30 years ago for control of epilepsy. In 1950 phenytoin was found effective in controlling arrhythmias in experiments on dogs. During the 1960's the drug was found useful for treating arrhythmias in man.

The structure of phenytoin is related to that of the barbiturates.

Action. Phenytoin apparently decreases the excitability of myocardial tissue. The electrophysiologic mechanisms of phenytoin are similar to those for quinidine. Phenytoin prolongs the effective refractory period, reduces ventricular automaticity, and has a direct vasodilating effect.

Uses. It is used almost exclusively for patients with digitalis-induced arrhythmias. It is also used in patients unable to tolerate quinidine or procainamide.

Absorption and excretion. Phenytoin is readily absorbed from the gastrointestinal tract. Only a small amount of the drug is excreted in the urine; most is excreted from the body via the gastrointestinal tract. The liver is the major site for detoxification of phenytoin. It is available in 100-mg. capsules and as a powder for injection in vials containing 250 mg.

Preparation, dosage, and administration. When given for prevention of recurrent tachycardia or suppression of premature beats, the oral maintenance dose is usually from 200 to 400 mg. daily.

Given intravenously constant EKG monitoring is required. Clinical doses may range from 5 to 10 mg. per kilogram of body weight. The average dose is 250 mg. The drug should *not* be administered in less than 10 minutes. Slow intravenous injections of 50 to 100 mg. may be repeated every 10 to 15 minutes until a therapeutic response is obtained or maximum dose has been given.

When given intravenously, phenytoin is effective within 5 minutes. When given orally, peak action is not reached for 8 hours.

Toxic effects. The drug's ability to depress conduction may result in heart block; its ability to reduce the sinus rate and to cause vasodilation may result in bradycardia and hypotension. Rapid intravenous administration may result in cardiac or respiratory arrest. Phenytoin may cause extracardiac toxic effects including nervousness, confusion, drowsiness, ataxia, tremors, visual disturbances, cutaneous eruptions, and hyperplasia of the gums after prolonged administration.

Heart block or bradycardia caused by phenytoin may be reversed with intravenous administration of atropine.

Contraindications. Phenytoin is contraindicated in patients with bradycardia or second-degree or complete heart block.

Propranolol hydrochloride, U.S.P., B.P. (Inderal)

The beta blocker propranolol exerts an antiarrhythmic effect by two mechanisms: (1) it opposes the actions of catecholamines, and (2) it has a direct effect on the myocardium, depressing the rate of diastolic depolarization, decreasing conduction velocity, and exerting a negative inotropic effect.

It is used to control supraventricular tachycardia and arrhythmias. It may be used alone or with digitalis to slow ventricular response when atrial flutter or atrial fibrillation is present.

The major disadvantage of the beta blockers is cardiac depression, and propranolol should be used preferably when adrenergic mechanisms contribute to the arrhythmia.

Propranolol may be given orally or intravenously. The oral dose is 10 to 30 mg. three to four times a day before meals. Intravenously, 1 to 2 mg. may be given every 5 minutes without exceeding 10 mg. After oral dosage blockade occurs within 30 minutes and lasts about 3 to 8 hours. Given intravenously, onset of action occurs in 2 minutes and peak action in 3 to 5 minutes; duration of action is 2 to 4 hours.

Patients should be observed for symptoms of impending cardiac failure, hypotension, bradycardia, hypoglycemia, and other undesirable effects. The drug may cause an increase in blood urea and SGOT levels. Atropine and isoproterenol are antagonists of propranolol.

Drugs that affect blood vessels

Some drugs that affect the circulatory system have effects primarily on blood vessels. Drugs producing vasoconstriction tend to increase the blood pressure, whereas those producing vasodilation tend to lower blood pressure. Increased blood flow to the extremities—often desirable in case of arteriosclerosis or of abnormal constriction of blood vessels—may be promoted by drugs that increase the lumen of arterioles.

Drugs acting on the peripheral circulation can do so either directly or indirectly. (The mechanism by which drugs affect the alpha and beta receptors in blood vessels, thereby effecting vasodilation or vasoconstriction, is discussed in Chapter 9.) Other drugs affect vascular tone by action at still higher centers; reserpine produces vasodilation and lowers blood pressure by acting at centers in the hypothalamus and also by depleting catecholamines. Still other compounds, of which the nitrites are examples, do not appear to act on blood vessels through their nervous control but relax the muscle cells by direct action. As with many classes of other drugs, it should therefore be kept in mind that the same physiologic effect, such as vasodilation with a resultant drop in blood pressure, may result from the action of a drug at one of several different sites—brain, autonomic ganglia, or the muscle cell itself.

Drugs are also used to sclerose and obliterate the lumen of blood vessels (veins) and in this way alter the course of the circulating blood in veins that have developed varicosities.

VASODILATORS

Drugs that bring about vasodilation have a number of uses. They play a part in the treatment of coronary disease, peripheral vascular disease, and hypertension. A number of drugs act either on the smooth muscle of the blood vessels or on the vasomotor center in the medulla. Some agents exhibit other actions or combinations of actions. These are indicated under the discussion on the individual drug.

CORONARY VASODILATORS

The term *angina pectoris* refers to intermittent myocardial ischemia (temporary interference with the flow of blood, oxygen, and nutrients to heart muscle). Angina is characterized by substernal pain usually occurring with exercise or stress and relieved by rest. Angina pectoris occurs when the work load on the heart is too great and oxygen delivery is inadequate. Since coronary flow is very responsive to oxygen requirements of the heart, inadequate myocardial oxygenation implies inadequate coronary flow in relation to need. This inadequate oxygenation may be caused by coronary atherosclerosis or various disorders of the coronary vessels, such as vasomotor spasm.

Drug therapy of angina pectoris is based on the belief that relaxation of coronary smooth muscle will bring about coronary vasodilation, which in turn will improve blood flow to the myocardium. There are three therapeutic objectives for the use of antianginal drugs:

1 To decrease the duration and intensity of pain during an attack
2 To prophylactically decrease frequency of attacks and improve work capacity even though angina may occur
3 To prevent or delay the onset of myocardial infarction

While evidence exists that the first objective may be achieved, less evidence exists that the second objective can be attained, and no real proof exists that the third objective is attainable. The ideal antianginal drug would:

1 Establish a balance between coronary blood flow and the metabolic demands of the myocardium
2 Have a local rather than a systemic effect—it would act directly on coronary vessels to promote coronary vasodilation with absence of effects on other organ systems
3 Promote myocardial oxygen extraction from arterial flow
4 Have oral effectiveness with sustained action
5 Have absence of tolerance

No drug at the present time meets these criteria. Drugs presently available provide only temporary relief. Evidence is increasing that the nitrites exert their effect not so much by coronary vasodilation but by lowering blood pressure and decreasing venous return and cardiac work.

Nitrites

Certain members of the nitrite group of drugs have been used clinically for more than 100 years. Organic and inorganic nitrites and organic nitrates possess the pharmacologic effect of vasodilation. However, the exact mechanism of action of the organic nitrates remains obscure.

Since the nitrites and organic nitrates exert similar qualitative effects on the blood and circulatory system, the term *nitrite* as used in the following discussion will include both nitrates and nitrites.

Action and use. The nitrites have a direct cellular action that causes relaxation of most smooth muscles in the body including bronchial, biliary, ureteral, uterine, and gastrointestinal smooth muscle. The most important pharmacologic effects are on vascular smooth muscle. The nitrites dilate all large arteries (temporal, radial, and coronary arteries) as well as arterioles (retinal, skin, meningeal, and splanchnic), capillaries, and venules. For this reason they can be called universal vasodilators. The nitrites are used extensively for patients with angina pectoris.

Because of the vasodilating effect, there is a reduction in vascular resistance and blood pressure, resulting in decreased work load on the heart. In patients with advanced coronary arteriosclerosis there may be an absence of response to the nitrites; no change in coronary resistance is noted, since blood vessel elasticity has been severely diminished.

Sublingual preparations of the nitrites have a D.E.S.I. rating of *probably effective;* oral preparations (including sustained-release tablets) have been rated as *possibly effective.*

The rapid-acting nitrites (nitroglycerin) remain the drug of choice for treatment of angina pectoris.

Side effects. The side effects of the nitrites result from their vasodilator action. Severe headache, flushing of the skin, nausea and vomiting, hypotension, and vertigo may occur. Nitrites should be used with caution in patients with glaucoma since dilated retinal vessels may increase intraocular pressure.

Tolerance. Tolerance to the nitrites is easily developed and necessitates the employment of the smallest dose of the drug that will give satisfactory results so that dosage may be increased as tolerance develops. Tolerance begins to appear within a few days and is well established within a few weeks. On the other hand, tolerance is rather easily broken by stopping administration, and the patient is again susceptible to the effects of the drug.

Preparation, dosage, and administration. The following are available preparations of nitrates.

Nitroglycerin tablets, U.S.P.; *glyceryl trinitrate tablets,* B.P. The drug is available in 0.3-,

0.4-, and 0.6-mg. tablets for sublingual administration, and in 2.5- and 6.5-mg. timed-release capsules for oral administration. The usual sublingual dose is 0.4 mg. (gr. $^{1}/_{150}$) and may be repeated several times during the day. Oral dose is 2.5 or 6.5 mg. at 8- or 12-hour intervals. Hypodermic tablets of this preparation are used when it is desirable to give the drug subcutaneously.

$$CH_2-O-NO_2$$
$$CH-O-NO_2$$
$$CH_2-O-NO_2$$

Nitroglycerin

When taken sublingually the drug appears in the blood in about 2 minutes; peak blood level is reached in 4 minutes; the effect begins to disappear in 10 minutes and is virtually dissipated within 30 minutes. Fall in blood pressure occurs in 1 to 5 minutes after administration and maximum fall occurs in 5 to 10 minutes. There is a return to initial blood pressure readings within 15 to 40 minutes.

During an acute anginal attack, if pain is not relieved within 5 to 10 minutes, the dose may be repeated. If pain persists after two or more tablets have been taken the physician should be notified. However, some patients take as many as thirty tablets per day without harm.

For prophylactic use the patient should be instructed to insert a nitroglycerin tablet sublingually prior to undertaking any effort that may cause him to have an anginal attack.

EKG patterns are unchanged by nitroglycerin.

Nitroglycerin readily deteriorates, for it is inactivated by time, light, heat, air, and moisture. Patients should be instructed as follows:

1 A *fresh* supply of drug should be kept on hand. A fresh supply should be obtained at least every 3 months.
2 The drug should always be kept in a dark, airtight container.
3 All but a few days' supply of drug should be kept refrigerated.
4 The drug should not be kept close to the body to protect it from body heat.

Ineffectiveness of nitroglycerin may be caused by failure to adhere to these few simple rules.

Nitroglycerin ointment (Nitro-Bid). Nitroglycerin ointment contains 2% nitroglycerin in a lanolin-petrolatum base. A special dose-measuring applicator is provided for measuring the amount of and spreading the ointment on the skin; this prevents absorption through the fingers during application. A thin layer of ointment is applied over the chest, abdomen, or anterior thighs without rubbing it in. Nitroglycerin is continuously absorbed through the skin into the circulation producing prolonged vasodilation. The ointment may be applied every 3 to 4 hours and at bedtime. Dosage is usually 1 to 2 inches of ointment. The ointment is available in 60-gm. tubes which should be kept tightly closed and stored in a cool place. Discontinuation of treatment should be gradual over a period of 4 to 6 weeks to prevent sudden withdrawal reactions. If headache and postural hypotension occur, dosage should be reduced.

Mannitolhexanitrate (Nitranitol). This drug is one of the longer-acting nitrites. It is given orally, and the usual dose range is 16 to 64 mg. every 4 to 6 hours. It is available in 32-mg. tablets.

Pentaerythritol tetranitrate, N.F., B.P. (Peritrate, Pentritol, Quintrate, Vasitol, Pentafin). This preparation is available in 10- and 20-mg. tablets and in sustained-release preparations of 60 and 80 mg. The usual oral dose is 10 to 20 mg. four times a day, or one sustained-release tablet on arising and another 12 hours later. Onset of action of the tablets occurs within 30 to 60 minutes and disappears in 4 to 5 hours. Sustained-release preparations persist for about 12 hours. Tolerance rapidly develops with continuous administration.

Amyl nitrite, N.F. This preparation is available in glass ampules (pearls) that are fitted into a loosely woven material so that the pearl can be crushed and the drug inhaled. Each pearl contains about 0.3 ml. (5 minims). It has a strong unpleasant odor, and the patient should not inhale more than two or three times to prevent overdosage. The drug is effective within 30 to 60 seconds; effects last about 3 minutes. Amyl nitrite is very flammable. It is more likely to cause a throbbing headache, facial flushing, nausea, vomiting, hypotension, and reflex tachycardia than nitroglycerin.

Table 10-2 Coronary vasodilators

Generic name	Trade name or synonym	Route of administration	Dose*	Onset of action	Duration
Amyl nitrite	—	Inhalation	0.3 ml.	30 to 60 sec.	3 min.
Nitroglycerin	Glyceryl trinitrate	Sublingual	gr. $^1/_{150}$; 0.4 mg.	2 min.	15 to 30 min.
		Oral	2.5 to 6.5 mg.	30 to 60 min.	8 to 12 hr.
Pentaerythritol tetranitrate	Peritrate	Sublingual	10 mg.	10 min.	30 min.
	Pentritol	Oral	60 mg.	30 min.	12 hr.
	Pentafin	Oral	10 to 20 mg.	30 to 60 min.	4 to 5 hr.
	Vasitol	Sustained-release	80 mg.	30 to 60 min.	12 hr.
Erythrityl tetranitrate	Cardilate	Sublingual	5 to 30 mg.	5 to 10 min.	2 to 4 hr.
	Tetranitrol	Oral	5 to 30 mg.	30 min.	4 hr.
	Erythrol tetranitrate	Oral	5 to 30 mg.	30 min.	2 to 4 hr.
Isosorbide dinitrate	Isordil	Sublingual, oral	5 to 10 mg.	2 min.	$1^1/_2$ to 2 hr.
			5 to 30 mg.	15 to 30 min.	4 hr.
Trolnitrate phosphate	Metamine	Oral	2 to 10 mg.	Slow, 3 days	Up to 1 week
Dipyrimadole	Persantin	Oral	25 to 50 mg.	2 to 5 min.	20 to 30 min.

*Single dose only; dose may be repeated three or four times a day or as necessary.

Erythrityl tetranitrate. N.F. (Cardilate, Erythrol Tetranitrate, Tetranitrol). This drug is available in 5-, 10-, and 15-mg. tablets for oral or sublingual use. Initial dose is usually 5 to 10 mg. three times a day. Dosage may be increased to 30 mg. three times a day. When taken sublingually onset of action occurs within 5 to 10 minutes, orally within 30 minutes. Duration of action for either route is 2 to 4 hours. Oral route is less likely to cause headache.

Isosorbide dinitrate, U.S.P. (Isordil). This drug is available in 2.5- and 5-mg. sublingual tablets and 5- and 10-mg. tablets for oral use. Dose range is 5 to 30 mg. four times daily. Onset of action sublingually is 2 minutes; orally it is 15 to 30 minutes and lasts about 4 hours. Sustained-release tablets of 40 mg. are also available (Isordil Tembids). These provide onset of action in 30 minutes with the effect lasting for 12 hours.

Trolnitrate phosphate (Metamine, Nitretamin). This drug is marketed as 2- or 10-mg. tablets for oral use only, one to two tablets four times a day. Sublingual administration produces stomatitis. Sustained-release tablets are also available.

Ethyl alcohol

It has been common practice to permit and even recommend the use of alcoholic drinks for patients with angina. The beneficial action of alcohol probably results from its sedative action; there is no evidence that alcohol dilates the coronary arteries.

Xanthines

The xanthine derivatives (caffeine, theobromine, theophylline, and aminophylline) have been widely used for many years for treatment of angina. However, their use in angina has been steadily decreasing.

Propranolol hydrochloride (Inderal)

Propranolol, a beta adrenergic blocking drug, has produced beneficial effects in patients with angina pectoris. These effects may result from decreased sympathetic stimulation of the heart, which causes a decrease in cardiac work thereby reducing cardiac oxygen requirement. The beneficial effects reported include decreased frequency of attacks, decrease in intensity of pain, and increased tolerance to exercise.

Side effects include nausea, vomiting, light-headedness, diarrhea, constipation, rash, and mental depression. Hypotension and bradycardia may also occur. (See p.130 for other uses, contraindications, etc.) There is some evidence that propranolol can induce congestive heart failure in patients with low cardiac reserve.

Propranolol is available in 10- and 40-mg. oral tablets. Used as an antianginal agent, dose range is from 10 to 80 mg. every 6 hours.

PERIPHERAL VASODILATORS

The use of vasodilating drugs in chronic occlusive arterial disease or peripheral vascular disease has to date been very discouraging. Adrenergic blocking agents are frequently used to treat peripheral vascular diseases.

However, several drugs that are not adrenergic blocking agents have been used with some success in the treatment of these diseases.

The D.E.S.I. rating for these drugs is: *possibly effective* for treatment of peripheral vascular diseases.

Nicotinyl tartrate (Roniacol Tartrate)

Nicotinyl tartrate is the tartrate salt of nicotinyl alcohol. By its conversion to nicotinic acid in the body, nicotinyl tartrate produces direct peripheral vasodilation and increases blood flow to the extremities. Since it is oxidized slowly, it has a more prolonged effect than nicotinic acid.

Nicotinyl tartrate is used in the treatment of peripheral vascular diseases. It has been reported to be beneficial in relieving intermittent claudication of peripheral arteriosclerosis and thromboangiitis obliterans.

Side effects include flushing of face and neck, gastrointestinal disturbances, and allergic reactions.

It is available in 50-mg. tablets and 150-mg. timed-release tablets and as an elixir, 50 mg. per 5 ml. It is given in doses of 50 to 150 mg. three times a day after meals. Dose of timed-release tablets is 150 or 300 mg. morning and evening.

Cyclandelate (Cyclospasmol)

Cyclandelate has a direct relaxation effect on the smooth muscles of peripheral arterial walls. It increases peripheral circulation of the extremities and digits and elevates skin temperature of the extremities.

The drug is available in 100-mg. tablets and 200-mg. capsules for oral use. The usual dose is 100 mg. four times a day given before meals and at bedtime.

Side effects include tingling, flushing, sweating, dizziness, and headache.

Isoxsuprine hydrochloride, N.F. (Vasodilan)

Isoxsuprine hydrochloride has potent inhibitory effects on vascular and uterine smooth muscle. It is used in the treatment of peripheral vascular spasm, Raynaud's and Buerger's diseases, and arteriosclerotic vascular disease.

Side effects are relatively mild and include lightheadedness, dizziness, nausea, and vomiting. These effects usually subside with a reduction in dosage. Transient hypotension and tachycardia have also been reported.

It is available in 10-mg. tablets. Oral dosage is 10 to 20 mg. three or four times daily. Action occurs within 1 hour and persists for 3 hours after oral administration. An intramuscular preparation of 5 mg. per milliliter in 2-ml. containers is also available for acute and severe symptoms of arterial insufficiency. However, for prolonged use oral therapy is preferred.

ANTIHYPERTENSIVES

Arterial hypertension is characterized by increased peripheral vascular resistance resulting in a consistent elevation of the diastolic pressure above the accepted range of normal (above 90 mm. Hg) and pathologic changes in the retinal arterioles. Hypertension is associated with a variety of cardiac, cerebrovascular, and renal complications and decreased life expectancy. When there is no known cause for the elevated blood pressure (such as no preexisting kidney disease or atherosclerosis) the condition is termed essential or primary hypertension. For this form of hypertension, the only possible means for adequate control is drug therapy.

Evidence indicates that successful therapy in essential hypertension may result in a decrease in free norepinephrine available for vasoconstriction. Drugs may decrease free norepinephrine by:

1 Inhibiting release of norepinephrine
2 Depleting stores of norepinephrine
3 Competing with norepinephrine effector sites

The belief that norepinephrine is a contributory agent in essential hypertension is based on the following findings:

1 The hypertensive patient's blood pressure is lowered by blocking sympathetic nerve transmission surgically (via lumbar sympathectomy) or medically (via drug therapy).
2 All tissues innervated by the sympathetic nervous system contain norepinephrine.
3 Transmission of impulses from postganglionic fibers to arteriolar muscles requires the release of norepinephrine at the neuromuscular junction.
4 Maintenance of a constant level of stored norepinephrine is dependent upon its extraction from blood and its synthesis in nerve tissue.
5 Hypertensives are more reactive than normotensives to norepinephrine and other vasoactive substances.

Figure 10-9
Site and method of action of various antihypertensive drugs based on reported clinical and experimental evidence.

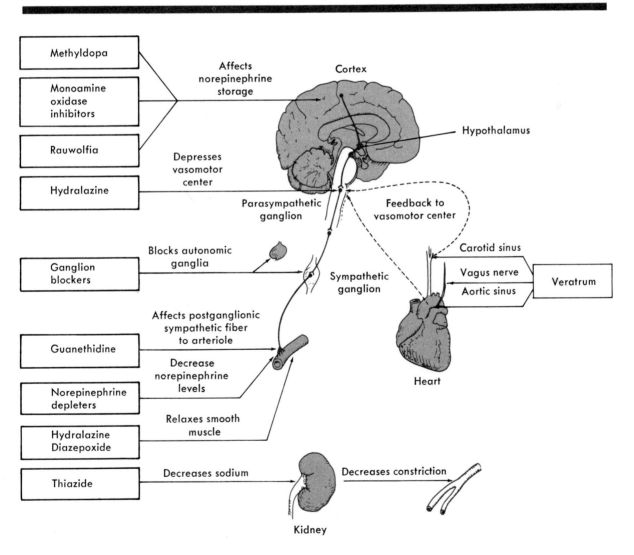

Evidence is available that a relationship exists between excess salt ingestion and human essential hypertension; susceptibility is undoubtedly on a genetic basis. However, the exact role of sodium as a causative factor in human essential hypertension is not known. It is claimed that high blood pressure is more prevalent in cultures with a high salt intake, and it has been demonstrated that children fed large amounts of salt developed hypertension. It is well known that drastic salt restriction or use of a salt-depleting diuretic like chlorothiazide reduces the blood pressure of some hypertensive individuals. A high salt intake, or retention of sodium and fluids, may cause ionic disturbances in peripheral arterioles, which may in turn increase vascular tone and vascular reactivity (particularly to adrenergic agents).

The judicious use of antihypertensive drugs can effectively control the blood pressure in a majority of hypertensive individuals with less risk of serious complications and intolerable side reactions than was true for older methods of treatment (especially sympathectomy). However, antihypertensive drug therapy remains empirical since essential hypertension is a disease of unknown etiology and the mechanism of action of many antihypertensive drugs also remains unknown.

The ideal antihypertensive drug would:

1 Maintain blood pressure within normal limits for various body positions
2 Maintain or improve blood flow, not compromise tissue perfusion or blood flow to brain
3 Reduce the work load on the heart
4 Have no undesirable effects
5 Permit long-term administration without development of tolerance

The use of sedatives, diets low in sodium chloride, and weight reduction continue to be advocated for hypertensive patients, although these measures alone are insufficient for many patients. Some patients, such as those with severe renal insufficiency or severe psychiatric disturbance, do not respond well to treatment of hypertension with drugs. On the other hand, many patients benefit from therapy and are spared damage to the heart, kidneys, and brain. The severity of hypertensive disease is often estimated in terms of the level of the diastolic blood pressure and the degree of change in the retinal vessels of the eye.

Figure 10-9 shows the action sites of various antihypertensive drugs discussed in the following sections.

ANTIHYPERTENSIVES

DRUGS ACTING ON THE SYMPATHETIC NERVOUS SYSTEM

Drugs that most effectively reduce blood pressure are those inhibiting sympathetic nervous system function. The distinction between depressants of sympathetic function and ganglionic blocking agents is that the former agents do not interfere with parasympathetic innervation. This characteristic explains why clinicians prefer depressants of sympathetic functions to ganglionic blockers for lowering blood pressure.

The action of rauwolfia compounds is typical of the pharmacologic effects of a number of depressants of sympathetic functions.

ALKALOIDS OF RAUWOLFIA

Rauwolfia serpentina is a large climbing or twining shrub that grows in India and various tropical regions of the world. The botanical name given to a whole group of these plants was *Rauwolfia*, after an early German physician and botanist, Leonard Rauwolf. The root of the shrub from which the drug is obtained resembles a snake, hence the term *serpentina*. Extracts of the root of the plant have been used for a long time (in countries where the plant is indigenous) for a variety of ills, including snake bites, hypertension, and emotional disturbances. A report of its effectiveness in treating hypertension and mental disorders first appeared in an Indian medical journal in 1931. In 1952, the alkaloid reserpine was isolated. In 1953, western investigators began using the drug and publishing their findings on the sedative and antihypertensive effects of the drug. The rauwolfia compounds are still widely used, particularly for their antihypertensive effect. Their use as sedatives for emotional disorders has declined as other more effective psychotropic drugs have become available.

Individual rauwolfia alkaloids differ in chemical structure and pharmacologic action but in general have similar actions, uses, and cautions. These agents have a cumulative action; maximum response takes several days to 2 weeks after treatment is initiated. Upon discontinuance of drug administration effects from the drug may last 4 weeks. No tolerance or dependence has been reported.

These drugs are not recommended for patients with peptic ulcer, colitis, or mental depression. Parkinsonian rigidity may occur when large doses are administered. This symptom disappears when administration of the drug is discontinued.

Reserpine, U.S.P., B.P. (Serpasil, Sandril, Serfin, Reserpoid, Rau-Sed)

Reserpine is an ester-containing alkaloid obtained from the root of a certain species of *Rauwolfia*. It is a complex heterocyclic compound that was first synthesized in 1956, although the principal source continues to be the plant. It is a whitish crystalline powder, slightly soluble in water and alcohol but very soluble in organic acids such as acetic acid. It is considered the most potent of the alkaloids of *Rauwolfia*.

Action. Reserpine greatly reduces norepinephrine levels in sympathetic postganglionic nerves (peripheral nerve endings). This action is thought not to be caused by interference with norepinephrine synthesis but by an increased release of norepinephrine resulting in storage depletion. Released norepinephrine within the nerve is inactivated by monoamine oxidase. Studies indicate that reserpine alters the ability of storage granules in nerve cells to take up and bind norepinephrine. Without adequate norepinephrine available for release, discharges of impulses from the sympathetic nervous system produce little or no effect on the effector organ (blood vessels). Since stimulation of vascular smooth muscle is inhibited, vasomotor tone is lowered, vascular relaxation occurs, and blood pressure is decreased. Reserpine is used in the treatment of moderate forms of hypertension.

Reserpine also depletes norepinephrine from various organs. Depletion of brain norepinephrine and serotonin may account for the sedative action of reserpine and also for some of its antihypertensive effect. It does not alter the brain waves (EEG); it produces calm and quietude without undue drowsiness and without mental confusion or difficulty in movement. When given it, hostile and vicious animals become gentle, calm, and manageable, without loss of alertness and muscle coordination. The animal may go to sleep if undisturbed, but it is easily aroused. The drug seems to reduce attention and responsiveness to outside stimuli, but it does not produce general centralized depression. It potentiates the central nervous system depressant actions of drugs such as barbiturates and alcohol. Depletion of cardiac norepinephrine results in bradycardia. In addition there are constriction of the pupil and increased secretion and motility of the gastrointestinal organs. These effects are believed to be the result of suppression of sympathetic centers that allow the activity of the parasympathetic centers to be more prominent and noticeable. Reserpine is not an analgesic, and it does not potentiate the effects of analgesics.

Preparation, dosage, and administration. Reserpine is available in tablets, in sustained-release spansules, as an elixir, and in liquid forms for oral use. It is available in solutions for injection and in preparations containing a thiazide diuretic, potassium chloride, and other antihypertensive agents.

Reserpine is administered orally or by intramuscular or intravenous injection. The usual dose for adults for mild hypertension is 0.1 to 0.5 mg. daily, in two or three divided doses. It is a preparation of choice for most hypertensive emergencies, in which case doses of 2.5 to 5 mg. may be given parenterally every 6 to 12 hours. Blood pressure should be determined before each injection of reserpine to avoid marked hypotension.

Side effects. Reserpine is considered to have

a low level of toxicity, but undesirable effects may occur as dosage levels rise. Nasal stuffiness, gain in weight, and diarrhea are common side effects. A Parkinsonism state may occur. Other effects include dryness of mouth, nosebleeds, insomnia, itching, and skin eruptions. The drug sometimes causes gastric irritation, and occasionally it brings about reactivation of old gastric ulcers or causes a new one to form. Postural hypotension may occur after parenteral administration.

Rauwolfia serpentina, N.F. (Raudixin, Rautina, Rautotal, Rauwoldin)

This drug is the powdered whole root of *Rauwolfia serpentina*, N.F. It is administered orally. The daily oral dose for adults is 50 to 300 mg. It is usually divided into two doses. If larger doses are required, a more potent antihypertensive drug is indicated. It is available in 50- and 100-mg. tablets. It is also available in preparations containing a thiazide diuretic and potassium chloride.

Alseroxylon (Rauwiloid, Rautensin)

This preparation is the fat-soluble alkaloidal fraction extracted from the root of *Rauwolfia serpentina*. It is administered orally. The average adult dose is 2 to 4 mg. daily. It is available in 2-mg. tablets.

Syrosingopine (Singoserp)

Syrosingopine is a derivative of reserpine. It is the least potent of the rauwolfia derivatives and has minimal central action. It is available in 1-mg. tablets. Maintenance dose is 0.5 to 3 mg. daily.

Deserpidine (Harmonyl)

Deserpidine's pharmacologic action is like that of reserpine. It is administered orally and is available in 0.1- and 0.25-mg. tablets and in combination with a thiazide diuretic. Average daily dose is 0.25 to 1.0 mg.

Rescinnamine (Moderil)

The pharmacologic actions of rescinnamine are indistinguishable from those of reserpine, with the exception that sedation and bradycardia are less common. It is available for oral adminis-tration in 0.25-, 0.5-, and 1-mg. tablets. Average initial adult dose is 0.5 mg. once or twice daily for 2 weeks. Maintenance dose is usually 0.25 to 2 mg. daily.

GUANETHIDINE AND METHYLDOPA
Guanethidine sulfate, U.S.P., B.P. (Ismelin)

$$\left[\bigcirc N-CH_2-CH_2-NH-C \begin{matrix} NH \\ \\ NH_2 \end{matrix} \right]_2 -H_2SO_4$$

Guanethidine depletes norepinephrine from the heart and other peripheral organs. It causes a release and subsequent depletion of norepi-nephrine from adrenergic nerve endings. Unlike the rauwolfia compounds it does not have addi-tional central action since it probably does not penetrate the central nervous system; and unlike the ganglionic blocking agents it does not inhibit the parasympathetic system. Therefore, it does not produce a definite sedative effect or the serious side effects of parasympathetic blockade (urinary retention, paralytic ileus).

Guanethidine's blocking actions are very se-lective. It is a potent antihypertensive agent with fewer side effects than the older ganglionic blocking agents (pentolinium tartrate and hexa-methonium chloride). Its prolonged therapeutic effect and the need for only one dose daily make it a clinically advantageous drug in the treatment of severe and malignant hypertension. The drug is only partially absorbed from the gastrointes-tinal tract and is primarily excreted by the kid-ney.

Venodilation occurs in addition to arteriolar dilation, which causes blood to pool in the splanchnic and peripheral areas. This results in some reduction in cardiac, renal, cerebral, and coronary flow. It must be kept in mind that these effects are increased in the standing position, and the drug may cause serious side effects in pa-tients with cerebrovascular, coronary, or renal disease.

Preparation, dosage, and administration. Guanethidine is available in 10- and 25-mg. tab-lets for oral administration. Initial dose is often 10 to 25 mg. daily, which is increased by 10 mg. weekly until a desirable antihypertensive re-sponse is attained. No increased dosage should be given until the patient's blood pressure has been taken in the supine and standing positions and after mild exercise. Average daily dose may range from 10 to 75 mg. Maintenance dose must always be individualized.

The onset of action of guanethidine is slow, and the antihypertensive effect may not be noted for 48 to 72 hours after treatment has been started. The action of the drug is prolonged and the hypotensive effect may persist for 7 to 10 days after drug discontinuation.

A thiazide diuretic is usually given with guanethidine to enhance the antihypertensive effect and to prevent sodium and water retention.

Side effects. The most frequently noted side effects from guanethidine are lightheadedness and weakness, especially when the patient first gets out of bed in the morning. This is caused by orthostatic hypotension, the arteriolar and venodilation permitting pooling of the blood in the lower extremities with a reduction in cerebral flow. These symptoms will disappear as the day progresses. (See section on nursing care measures and instructions for patients with orthostatic hypotension, p. 184.) Some patients receiving guanethidine show marked variation in blood pressure during the day, going from orthostatic hypotension in the morning to severe hypertension by late afternoon or evening. This effect may be alleviated by rest periods during the afternoon or early evening. The orthostatic hypotension actually reflects the therapeutic potency of the drug and is not a true side reaction. This effect may be lessened or eliminated by reduced drug dosage.

Other common side effects are diarrhea occurring after meals and at night and ejaculation failure. Impotence has been reported in a few cases. It appears that ejaculation is a sympathetic function while erection is a parasympathetic function.

Bradycardia occurs with guanethidine since the drug blocks the sympathetically innervated cardioaccelerator nerves and leaves the vagal influence unopposed. Other side effects include abdominal distress, fatigue, nausea, nasal stuffiness, and weight gain. These symptoms may be relieved by reducing drug dosage. Sodium and water retention occur if a diuretic is not also given.

Precautions. Guanethidine should be used cautiously in patients with coronary insufficiency, recent myocardial infarction, cerebrovascular disease, renal disease with nitrogen retention, or history of peptic ulcer. The increased parasympathetic tone resulting from guanethidine therapy may aggravate these conditions.

In addition, guanethidine should not be used in conjunction with monoamine oxidase inhibitors.

Methyldopa, U.S.P., B.P. (Aldomet)

$$HO \underset{HO}{\overset{}{\diagdown}} \text{—} CH_2\text{—}\underset{\underset{CH_3}{|}}{\overset{\overset{NH_2}{|}}{C}}\text{—}COOH$$

Methyldopa lowers brain and heart norepinephrine. Some investigators claim that in the body, methyldopa is converted to methyldopamine and then to methylnorepinephrine. Methylnorepinephrine may then function as a false transmitter.

Methylnorepinephrine is stored in the norepinephrine storage sites and, therefore, it is methylnorepinephrine that is released when sympathetic nerve stimulation occurs. This false neurotransmitter is a less potent pressor substance than norepinephrine, and the result is reduced sympathetic activity. The precise antihypertensive mechanism of methyldopa remains unidentified.

Methyldopa reduces blood pressure by lowering peripheral vascular resistance. Since it also reduces renal vascular resistance it is often used in patients with renal hypertension and in hypertensive patients with impaired renal function. The drug has little or no effect on cardiac output. Lowered blood pressure occurs in both the lying and standing positions. Although the standing response is greater, the difference between the standing and lying blood pressures is not as great as that obtained with guanethidine or ganglionic blocking agents.

Sedation does occur with methyldopa since it readily penetrates brain tissue and lowers norepinephrine levels. Methyldopa is absorbed from the gastrointestinal tract and excreted by the kidney.

Preparation, dosage, and administration. Methyldopa is available in 250-mg. tablets for oral use. The usual starting dose is 500 mg. daily with increments of 250 mg. weekly or biweekly until an optimum blood pressure response is obtained. Daily dosage may range from 500 to 3000 mg. (0.5 to 3.0 Gm.). Effect occurs within 4 to 6 hours; duration of action is 8 to 12 hours. Upon discontinuance of the drug, pretreatment blood pressure levels return within 24 to 48 hours.

Methyldopa is also available in 5-ml. ampules containing 50 mg. per milliliter for intravenous use in hypertensive crises. From 250 to 500 mg. of the drug is given at 6-hour intervals. Blood pressure begins to fall about 2 hours after injection. The drug may also be given by intravenous infusion in 100 to 200 ml. of 5% dextrose in water over a period of 30 to 60 minutes. Frequent blood pressure monitoring is highly recommended. In addition to a diuretic, hydralazine may be added as a third agent to achieve the desired antihypertensive effect.

Side effects. Side effects from the use of methyldopa are sedation, depression, dry mouth, nasal congestion, fever, altered liver function tests (although no liver toxicity has been reported), and decreased white and platelet cell counts. Sodium and water retention occur if a diuretic is not given along with methyldopa. Liver function tests and blood cell determinations should be done at regular intervals. Numerous other side effects may occur, and their elimination may be brought about by a reduction of dosage.

Precautions. Methyldopa is contraindicated in patients with liver disease, eclampsia, or a history of mental depression.

ANTIHYPERTENSIVES

DRUGS ACTING ON VASCULAR SMOOTH MUSCLE

Several drugs used in the treatment of hypertension exert their effect directly on the vascular smooth muscle causing vasodilation. Hydralazine, diazoxide, and some new experimental drugs belong to this class. When the blood pressure is lowered by drugs that act on the vascular smooth muscle, this effect is generally accompanied by reflex cardiac stimulation. In some current investigations some of these direct vasodilators are combined with propranolol in order to prevent the reflex cardiac stimulation that is mediated by sympathetic nerves that release norepinephrine which in turn acts on beta receptors in the heart.

Hydralazine hydrochloride, U.S.P. (Apresoline Hydrochloride)

Hydralazine hydrochloride is an effective antihypertensive agent, particularly when used in combination with other drugs for treating the patient with moderately severe hypertension. Hydralazine is thought to produce its effects by direct action on blood vessels. These actions reduce vascular resistance by producing arteriolar vasodilation. In combination with a rauwolfia preparation or a thiazide, it often lowers diastolic blood pressure in both the recumbent and upright positions, and toxic effects from hydralazine are decreased.

Preparation, dosage, and administration. Hydralazine hydrochloride is usually administered orally, although it may be given intravenously or intramuscularly when the patient is unable to take the drug orally. It is available in 10-, 25-, 50-, and 100-mg. tablets and as a sterile solution for injection of 20 mg. per milliliter. As with other antihypertensive drugs, medication is started with small doses and the dosage increased gradually until desired effects are obtained or symptoms of toxicity appear. The initial oral dose for patients with moderate to severe hypertension is 10 mg. given after meals and at bedtime. Patients may receive larger doses, depending on the severity of the hypertension and their response to the drug. Maximal daily dose is 200 mg. which is usually given in four divided doses. Repeated blood pressure readings must be taken not only to determine the effect of the drug but also to avoid serious side effects.

Side effects and toxic effects. Side effects associated with hydralazine hydrochloride vary all the way from merely unpleasant effects to those that are serious and require cessation of administration. Headache, heart palpitation, anxiety, mild depression, dry mouth, unpleasant taste in the mouth, and nausea and vomiting are symptoms that are unpleasant but may not necessitate discontinuance of administration. More serious symptoms include symptoms of coronary insufficiency, edema, chills, fever, and severe depression. Toxic symptoms that may result from prolonged administration of hydralazine hydrochloride in large doses resemble those of early rheumatoid arthritis or acute systemic lupus erythematosus.

Antihistaminic drugs, salicylates, or barbiturates are useful to control headache, palpitation, anxiety, and nausea and vomiting. The more severe symptoms require cessation of therapy with this drug. Fortunately, most symptoms subside when the drug is withdrawn. However, the lupoid state may persist for an indefinite period.

Diazoxide (Hyperstat I.V.)

Diazoxide is a chlorothiazide derivative but it has no diuretic activity. It does have marked antihypertensive action due to a direct vasodilator action on peripheral arterioles. Its basic mechanism of action remains uncertain. Diazoxide has been used to effectively treat patients with severe or malignant hypertension refractory to other antihypertensive agents. Some clinicians consider it the drug of choice for treatment of hypertensive crisis. Advantages of diazoxide include: (1) it has rapid onset of action, with maximal blood pressure fall usually occurring within 5 minutes after intravenous injection, (2) it does not require continuous infusion, (3) it does not cause extreme hypotension, (4) it does not cause sedation, and (5) drug resistance apparently does not occur.

Preparation, dosage, and administration. Diazoxide is available in solution for intravenous injection containing 15 mg. per milliliter in 20-ml. containers. The usual adult dose is 300 mg. (20 ml. of injectable solution) given intravenously within 30 seconds or less to the recumbent patient. Rapid injection ensures maximal response. Blood pressure should be monitored at 1-minute intervals for the first 5 minutes, then at 5-minute intervals until blood pressure is stabilized, then at hourly intervals. In ambulatory patients, blood pressure should be measured with the patient standing before monitoring is completed. The injection may be repeated in $^1/_2$ to 24 hours if necessary. Oral hypotensive therapy should be started as soon as the blood pressure is stabilized. Dosage for children or adults is 5 mg. per kilogram of body weight.

Side effects. Numerous side effects can occur with diazoxide, the more common ones being nausea, vomiting, abdominal discomfort, tachycardia, and a sensation of warmth or burning along the injected vein. Phlebitis and cellulitis may result from extravasation.

Other adverse effects include sodium and water retention and hyperglycemia. Use of a diuretic will help prevent fluid overload and decrease the risk of precipitating congestive heart failure. The hyperglycemia effect is usually mild and subsides without treatment, but oral hypoglycemic agents or insulin may be indicated. Orthostatic hypotension may occur, especially if diuretics are given; it is recommended that these patients remain recumbent for 8 to 10 hours.

Precautions. Blood glucose levels should be monitored in patients with diabetes or a family history of diabetes and in patients requiring multiple injections of the drug. Diazoxide should be used with caution in patients with cerebrovascular or coronary artery disease and those with impaired cardiac reserve. Safe use in pregnancy has not been established; adverse effects on the fetus have been reported. Mothers receiving the drug should not breast feed their infants.

Drug interactions. Diazoxide may increase the action of other hypotensive agents. It displaces warfarin from its protein binding sites, and its use in patients receiving coumarin anticoagulants may potentiate hypoprothrombinemia, necessitating reduction in anticoagulant dosage.

Sodium nitroprusside (Nipride)

Sodium nitroprusside is a potent direct-acting vasodilator used for treatment of hypertensive crisis when other drugs have been ineffective. It acts rapidly, within 2 minutes, but continuous infusion is necessary to maintain the hypotensive effect. Other antihypertensives should be started as soon as the blood pressure is under control. Solutions are reddish-brown in color; deterioration by light is evidenced by a change in color to blue. Solutions that change color should be discarded. Adverse reactions include restlessness, agitation, muscle twitching, and rash. Bone marrow depression has been reported.

Sodium nitroprusside must be prepared by the hospital pharmacy using 50 mg. of drug per liter of 5% dextrose injection. A fresh solution must be prepared every 4 hours; the solution should be protected from light by covering the bottle with aluminum foil or opaque material. The solution is administered at a rate of 10 to 30 drops per minute; the patient, his blood pressure, and the flow rate must be monitored frequently.

ANTIHYPERTENSIVES

DRUGS ACTING ON REFLEXES
VERATRUM PREPARATIONS

Veratrum viride and *Veratrum album* (green and white hellebore) are two species of plants that contain alkaloids with the capacity to slow the heart and lower blood pressure.

The hypotensive effect of veratrum alkaloids results from their rather unique ability to reflexly depress the vasomotor center and sympathetic activity by stimulating receptors in the carotid sinus and aortic arch. The veratrum compounds also stimulate the vagus, which slows the heart and dilates peripheral blood vessels with a fall in blood pressure.

The veratrum alkaloids all have a central emetic effect and the resulting nausea and vomiting is a serious disadvantage. In addition, the range between toxic and therapeutic dose is narrow. These disadvantages have limited their usefulness.

Veratrum preparations such as alkavervir (Veriloid), protoveratrine (Protalba, Beralba), or cryptenamine (Unitensin) have been used effectively for hypertensive emergencies.

They reduce blood pressure almost immediately upon intravenous use. Constant expert supervision and blood pressure monitoring are required to regulate the dose according to blood pressure response and to avoid serious side effects such as respiratory depression and collapse.

Side effects. Side effects of the veratrum preparations include epigastric distress, increased flow of saliva, nausea, vomiting, hiccoughing, and slow pulse. These effects may be stopped with atropine. Overdosage causes bradycardia, hypotension, respiratory depression, and collapse. Ephedrine is useful in overcoming the hypotension.

Contraindications. Veratrum products are contraindicated in patients with high intracranial pressure (which is not secondary to hypertension), digitalis intoxication, uremia, or cerebrovascular disease.

ANTIHYPERTENSIVES

GANGLIONIC BLOCKING AGENTS

Among the earliest effective agents for treatment of hypertension (and still the most potent of the antihypertensive drugs) are the ganglionic blocking agents. These drugs block transmission of both sympathetic and parasympathetic nerve impulses at the ganglia. The parent compound of this group of drugs is a quaternary ammonium compound, tetraethylammonium chloride. It is not well suited for the treatment of hypertension because of its short duration of action, its ineffectiveness when given orally, and its distressing side effects.

In 1950 the methonium derivatives were introduced and hexamethonium chloride became the drug of choice in managing severe and malignant hypertension. Despite the difficulties in managing patients receiving hexamethonium because of its erratic absorption and action and severe side effects, its use demonstrated that severe hypertension could be controlled with an improvement in morbidity and mortality. Since 1961, however, the ganglionic blocking agents have been seldom used. Newer antihypertensive drugs that have more selective action and less severe side effects are preferred.

Ganglionic blocking agents block the action of acetylcholine (ACh) upon the ganglion cells by competing with acetylcholine at the synapse of autonomic ganglia. This results in reduced transmission of impulses from preganglionic to postganglionic fibers in both sympathetic and parasympathetic nerves. Blocking transmission of impulses through the sympathetic ganglia abolishes vasoconstrictor tone; the blood vessels dilate and arterial pressure falls. This is the desired clinical effect. The greatest antihypertensive effect occurs when the patient stands, since compensatory vasoconstrictor reflexes regulating blood pressure with position change are suppressed. The result is that blood pools in the leg veins, venous return to the heart is decreased, and cardiac output falls. If blood supply to the brain is inadequate, fainting occurs. These are of course undesired effects but a natural result of the drugs' pharmacologic action. Sympathetic block also causes loss of body heat and lowered body temperature as a result of vasodilation in the skin. Sweating is also inhibited.

Major disadvantages in the use of ganglion blockers result from parasympathetic blockade. This causes dry mouth, reduced gastric secretion, paralytic ileus, constipation, urinary retention, blurred vision, and loss of visual accommodation.

Impotence may also occur, owing to the combined sympathetic and parasympathetic block. Erection is prevented by the latter, while the former prevents ejaculation.

These drugs do not penetrate the blood-brain barrier and therefore do not exert central nervous system actions.

Ganglion blockers still have a place in modern medicine in the treatment of hypertensive emergencies when it is necessary to lower the blood pressure rapidly, in management of the patient resistant to other antihypertensive therapy, and in combination with other less potent drugs. Withdrawal of these drugs must be gradual to avoid a rebound in pressure and the possibility of a vascular accident. Tolerance may develop with prolonged administration of any of the ganglionic blocking agents.

Hexamethonium chloride (Methium Chloride); hexamethonium tartrate

Hexamethonium is rarely used today except in emergencies. Many of its previous dosage forms are no longer available. It is not given orally since it is poorly and irregularly absorbed from the gastrointestinal tract. When it is given parenterally its effects are achieved rather promptly and last 4 to 6 hours.

Pentolinium tartrate, N.F., B.P. (Ansolysen Tartrate)

Pentolinium is administered orally, subcutaneously, and intramuscularly. It is available in 20-, 40-, 100-, and 200-mg. tablets and as a sterile solution, 100 mg. in 10 ml. The total daily oral

Figure 10-10

Determining the blood pressure prior to the administration of antihypertensive drugs such as hexamethonium chloride or pentolinium tartrate (Ansolysen) in order that adjustments in dosage may be made according to the patient's response to the drug. Dosage may need to be increased, decreased, or omitted. The blood pressure may need to be taken with the patient in standing, sitting, and lying positions.

dosage may vary from 60 to 600 mg. The initial oral dose is usually 20 mg. The initial dose is made as small as possible and increased gradually while the patient is under careful medical supervision. The initial parenteral dose recommended is 2.5 to 3.5 mg.

Pentolinium is about five times more potent than hexamethonium and has a longer duration of action (8 to 12 hours).

Chlorisondamine chloride (Ecolid Chloride)

Chlorisondamine is more potent than hexamethonium or pentolinium but less potent than mecamylamine. It is available in 25-mg. tablets for oral administration. The initial dose is 12.5 mg.; daily increments are determined by the patient's response. The average daily dose is 50 to 100 mg. twice daily. Duration of action is 8 to 12 hours.

Mecamylamine hydrochloride, N.F. (Inversine Hydrochloride)

Mecamylamine is marketed in 2.5- and 10-mg. tablets for oral administration. The dosage recommended is that which will reduce the blood pressure and maintain it without the appearance of severe side effects. Treatment is usually started with a dosage of 2.5 mg. twice daily and is gradually increased. The average total daily maintenance dose is about 25 mg. (divided into three portions). Dosage must be determined in relation to blood pressure readings.

Mecamylamine is well absorbed from the intestinal tract. It lowers the blood pressure of both normal persons and hypertensive patients. Its duration of action is 6 to 12 hours. Mecamylamine is absorbed by the central nervous system; confusion, tremors, and psychologic difficulties have been observed in some patients being treated with the drug.

Trimethaphan camsylate, U.S.P. (Arfonad Camsylate)

Trimethaphan camsylate is a rapid-acting ganglionic blocking agent that lowers blood pressure in both normotensive and hypertensive persons. The duration of its action is brief, which makes it unsuited to the treatment of hypertension.

This drug is used for the production of controlled hypotension during certain types of surgical procedures in which the production of some degree of hemostasis in capillary beds, arterioles, and venules helps to prevent excessive bleeding and increases visualization and exposure of the surgical field. It is used especially in neurosurgery and peripheral vascular surgery.

Preparation, dosage, and administration. Trimethaphan camsylate is administered by continuous intravenous infusion as a 0.1% solution in 5% dextrose in water or in isotonic salt solution. It is available in 10-ml. ampules containing 500 mg. Blood pressure returns to normal levels about 5 minutes after administration is stopped.

The use of this drug is recommended for administration only by experienced anesthetists. Respiratory depression is a complication, particularly when a muscle relaxant has been used. Tachycardia is a potential complication.

ANTIHYPERTENSIVES

AMINE OXIDASE INHIBITORS

The monoamine oxidase inhibitors have the paradoxical ability to lower blood pressure. Monoamine oxidase is an enzyme active in the metabolic breakdown of catecholamines. The precise mechanism by which these drugs reduce blood pressure remains undetermined.

Pargyline hydrochloride, N.F. (Eutonyl)

$$\text{C}_6\text{H}_5-\text{CH}_2-\underset{\underset{\text{CH}_3}{|}}{\text{N}}-\text{CH}_2-\text{C}\equiv\text{CH} \cdot \text{HCl}$$

Pargyline is used for moderate to severe hypertension. It is a potent amine oxidase inhibitor that, like guanethidine and ganglionic blocking agents, exerts a predominant orthostatic antihypertensive effect. Onset of action is slow, about 3 to 4 days. It takes 7 days for the cumulative effect to be sufficient to bring about a decrease in blood pressure. Maximum response to the drug may take as long as 3 weeks.

Upon discontinuance of the drug, blood pressure returns to pretreatment levels in 10 to 14 days.

Preparation, dosage, and administration. The drug is available in 10-, 25-, and 50-mg. tablets. The usual initial dose is 10 to 25 mg. daily. Because of the cumulative effect, drug dosage should be increased slowly by increments of 10 mg. at weekly or biweekly intervals until the desired blood pressure response is obtained. The usual maintenance dose is 25 to 75 mg. per day. Pargyline is not recommended for children under 12 years of age.

Pargyline is usually used along with an oral diuretic since this reduces the amount of pargyline required, reduces side effects, and promotes more effective lowering of blood pressure in the supine position.

Side effects. The most common side effects are dry mouth, insomnia, daytime drowsiness, nervousness, weight gain, and impotence or inability to ejaculate. Reducing drug dosage may eliminate these side effects. For some patients a different antihypertensive drug may be needed. Nightmares and psychotic reactions may occur.

Pargyline has been known to exert a euphoric action in some patients; this is particularly helpful for the depressed hypertensive patient.

Cautions. Since pargyline is an amine oxidase inhibitor, the patient must be cautioned against ingesting foods or liquids that contain large amounts of tyramine. Since monoamine oxidase inhibitors increase the concentration of norepinephrine and tyramine is a precursor of norepinephrine, a "flooding" of the body with norepinephrine may result. Severe vasoconstriction can occur with marked blood pressure elevation. Several deaths reported in the literature have been attributed to this effect. Foods known to contain high tyramine content are cheese products, particularly cheddar cheese; excluded are cream and cottage cheese. The more aged and the less acid the cheese, the greater its tyramine content. Some alcoholic beverages, beer and wine (especially chianti), and some meats, fruits, and vegetables have sufficient concentrations of tyramine and tyrosine to cause the patient on monoamine oxidase inhibitors to have extreme headaches, serious blood pressure elevation, and tachycardia. Since these reactions can occur with use of pargyline and amphetamines, amphetamines and antidepressants should not be taken concomitantly. Fortunately these reactions disappear in 1 to 2 hours in most cases, but these reactions may be serious and caution must be exercised.

Since pargyline may potentiate action of drugs affecting the central nervous system, it should not be given with imipramine, amitriptyline, ganglionic blocking agents, or sympathomimetic amines. If barbiturates are used, they must be given in reduced dosage.

ANTIHYPERTENSIVES

THE THIAZIDES
Chlorothiazide, U.S.P., B.P. (Diuril); hydrochlorothiazide, U.S.P., B.P. (HydroDiuril, Esidrix, Oretic)

The effectiveness of chlorothiazide and certain related compounds, when given alone or in conjunction with other antihypertensive agents in the treatment of hypertension, has now been established.

Action. Although introduced and primarily useful as a diuretic agent, chlorothiazide has been found to have significant blood pressure lowering action in hypertensive subjects, perhaps because of its effect in reducing the amount of water, sodium, and chloride in the body and possibly because of certain inherent properties of the drug. It also augments the effects of other drugs used in treatment of hypertension.

Uses. Chlorothiazide is used either alone, in cases of mild hypertension, or in combination with other antihypertensive drugs. This permits lower drug dosage, reduction of unpleasant side effects, and enhanced hypotensive effects.

Preparation, dosage, and administration. Chlorothiazide is available in tablets of 250 and 500 mg. for oral administration. When given alone, doses of 500 mg. may be prescribed to be given from one to three times daily. When combined with other antihypertensive drugs, the dosage is lower, usually 250 mg. twice daily.

Hydrochlorothiazide is available in tablets of 25 and 50 mg. for oral administration. There are also tablets containing hydrochlorothiazide and potassium. Some pharmaceutical companies market a combination of this drug and another antihypertensive in the same tablet. The usual antihypertensive dose is 25 to 50 mg. one or two times a day, but doses as high as 200 mg. a day may be used.

Side effects. Unlike many antihypertensive drugs, chlorothiazide produces few unpleasant side effects. Patients occasionally experience weakness, fatigue, nausea, abdominal pain, distention, and diarrhea. A fairly high percentage of patients has been known to show some disturbance of blood electrolytes. The blood uric acid level may be elevated and the level of serum potassium lowered. Chlorothiazide is administered cautiously to patients with renal insufficiency. Some physicians recommend that the patient on prolonged therapy with this drug be given supplemental amounts of potassium chloride. Skin rash has been observed occasionally. Leukopenia, thrombocytopenia, and agranulocytosis have occurred but are rare.

Other thiazide compounds. A number of preparations chemically related to chlorothiazide have been marketed, such as polythiazide, N.F. (Renese), and bendroflumethiazide, N.F. (Naturetin). These drugs have helped to eliminate need for parenteral injection of mercurial diuretics and have permitted liberalization of sodium chloride intake. (See Table 11-2 for comparison of the various thiazides and Chapter 11 for more detailed information on the thiazides.)

NURSING MEASURES FOR CARE OF PATIENTS ON ANTIHYPERTENSIVE THERAPY

Instructions to patients to avoid or decrease orthostatic hypotensive effect. The nurse should give the patient on antihypertensive therapy the following instructions:

1 The patient should rise slowly from a lying to a sitting position and from a sitting to a standing position. This allows for physiologic adjustment of the vascular system. It also allows vasoconstriction of lower extremity vessels to occur, which prevents pooling of blood and syncope.
2 The patient should never stand perfectly still in one place for any length of time, especially within 2 hours after taking the drug. Standing still causes

relaxation of leg vessels with pooling of blood and may result in syncope or weakness. This is particularly true in the early morning since this is the time when postural hypotension is often most severe. The patient should avoid standing still in church, waiting in line, standing on buses and subway trains, and in telephone booths. He should use caution while shaving or showering.
3 If weakness and dizziness occur they can be relieved by muscular activity or recumbency.
  a. If standing or sitting, the patient should flex his calf muscles, wiggle his toes, rise up on his toes, and allow his feet to return to flat position. This results in alternate vasoconstriction and vasodilation and prevents blood from pooling in lower extremities.
  b. If possible, the patient should lie flat with his legs slightly higher than his head to promote cerebral flow and decrease pooling of blood in legs.
4 The patient should be instructed to be careful within 2 hours after taking drugs. He should avoid driving a car if blurred vision or hypotension occurs. He should be cautious when working with or around heavy and dangerous machinery.
5 The patient should not take hot baths or steambaths since this promotes peripheral vasodilation and may cause a hypotensive reaction.

Other instructions to patient

1 The patient should take precautions in the heat or when in the sun, or at the beach, since heat increases peripheral blood flow through vascular relaxation from heat dissipation, and since some antihypertensive drugs cause decreased sweating, hypotension, heat stroke, and other serious side effects from vasodilation can occur.
2 If impotency occurs he should consult his doctor. Omission of an occasional dose or a decrease in dosage may overcome this effect.
3 The patient should *not suddenly omit drug therapy.* If the drug is suddenly discontinued blood pressure tends to rise higher because of increased sensitivity to pressor substances. Gradual withdrawal of the drug is therefore necessary.
4 The patient should carry an identification card with the name of the drug, dosage, and the times the drug is taken.
5 If chest pain occurs after taking the drug, the patient should discontinue taking the drug and consult his doctor. This is especially important in patients with history of angina pectoris.
6 Alcohol in moderation is acceptable.
7 If headache occurs at night or early in the morning,

the patient should sleep with his head elevated or in a sitting position.

8 When the patient is on a monoamine oxidase inhibitor he should be cautioned to avoid foods or beverages high in tyramine or tyrosine (see p. 183). In addition, he should not take any medicine not prescribed for him by his physician, since drug incompatibilities may occur.

9 Another important aspect is moderation with salt intake or the ingestion of foods high in sodium content. Such foods include bacon, ham, sausage, tuna, crabmeat, various cheeses, and crackers.

Nursing care of patients with orthostatic hypotension. An Ace bandage or an elastic stocking can be used to overcome vascular relaxation in lower extremities. It should be applied with the legs slightly elevated or horizontal. Bandages or stockings should be snug but not excessively constricting. The bandages need be applied only when the patient is up and about; they should be removed when he returns to bed. A snug girdle may help overcome orthostatic hypotension.

The patient's blood pressure should be checked in lying, sitting, and standing positions. The readings should be charted and reported. Dosage is often regulated according to blood pressure obtained in standing or upright position. With some drugs blood pressure is lowest in standing position and highest in lying position. Blood pressure in the sitting position may be lower than that obtained in the lying position but higher than that recorded for the standing position. The patient should be upright for at least 3 minutes before reading is taken. Patients on bedrest should be in a semireclining position with the head of the bed elevated.

Nursing care of patients with side effects. Visual disturbances may occur with the use of some drugs such as ganglion blockers. There may be interference with pupillary response and sensitivity to light because of poor accommodation. The patient may need to wear sunglasses and avoid bright lights.

Constipation is a common effect with some antihypertensive drugs such as ganglion blockers. Daily elimination is very important when antihypertensive drugs are given orally or if the drug is primarily eliminated via the intestinal tract. Constipation may cause either irregular or constant absorption of the drug, and cumulative effects may occur. Adequate diet, liquids, and exercise are important to avoid this effect. Cathartics (such as 30 to 45 ml. daily of milk of magnesia) or enemas may be necessary during early stages of treatment. The antihypertensive agent may need to be changed if regular and unassisted elimination cannot be established.

Other side effects include diarrhea, urinary retention, and dry mouth and nasal mucosa. Diarrhea is likely to occur with guanethidine therapy. This may require changing the drug or use of antidiarrheic agents. Urinary retention is likely to occur in the older male with prostatic hypertrophy. These patients should be placed on recorded intake and output. Dry mouth is likely to occur with any drug that inhibits sympathetic activity, since the salivary glands are innervated by the sympathetic nerves. Dry mouth interferes with carbohydrate digestion. In addition, the patient is more prone to oral infections. Good oral hygiene is essential for these patients. Dry nasal mucosa is not a serious side effect, but it is an annoying one. Nonirritating lubricants, such as lanolin or glycerine, may be used to relieve this effect.

Teaching the patient to take his own blood pressure. Some authorities believe that the patient should be taught to take, record, and graph his own blood pressure at home. This often lessens nonadherence to the therapeutic program and serious side effects from overdosage.

VASOCONSTRICTORS

Vasoconstrictor drugs usually exert their effects by bringing about contraction of the muscle fibers in the walls of the blood vessels or by stimulation of the vasomotor center in the medulla. They may be used to stop superficial hemorrhage, relieve nasal congestion, raise and sustain the blood pressure, and sometimes increase the force of the heart action.

Angiotensin amide (Hypertensin)

Since 1898 it has been known that a relationship exists between the kidneys and elevated blood pressure. Research revealed that a substance released from the kidneys was converted in the bloodstream to a vasoconstrictor. In 1940 reports appeared in the United States and Argentina describing this vasopressor substance. In the United States it was named angiotonin and in South America, hypertensin. In 1957 this agent was synthesized and renamed angiotensin.

It has been shown experimentally that ischemic kidneys release an enzyme-like substance known as renin, which acts on a globulin in plasma in the blood to form angiotensin I, which is vasoinactive. Angiotensin I is then converted by a plasma enzyme to angiotensin II which is the most powerful vasoconstrictor known.

Angiotensin II is destroyed by an enzyme called hypertensinase (an antipressor substance) produced by both the normal kidney and gut and found in red blood cells and pancreas and in small amounts in the liver.

The renin-angiotensin system appears to be a homeostatic mechanism for regulating blood pressure. A drop in blood pressure results in release of renin and the eventual formation of angiotensin II. Angiotensin amide is the synthetic preparation of angiotensin II with identical pharmacologic properties.

Angiotensin amide acts directly on the smooth muscle of arterioles, causing vasoconstriction. It has no effect on venules. Its ability to elevate blood pressure is probably the result of (1) its arteriolar vasoconstricting effect, and (2) its ability to stimulate aldosterone release, which causes renal tubular absorption of sodium and an increase in body sodium and water, with a resultant rise in blood volume.

Angiotensin has no direct stimulating effect on the heart, and a rise in blood pressure may cause a reflex bradycardia and decreased cardiac output.

Angiotensin amide is a controversial substance. It is used by some clinicians to treat hypotension, particularly refractory hypotension when the other vasopressor agents have been ineffective.

Angiotensin acts immediately; *continuous monitoring of the blood pressure is required.*

Drugs that act on the blood and blood-forming tissue

The following information includes only those drugs used to treat certain anemias, to replace blood volume, or to influence blood clotting.

ANTIANEMIC OR HEMOPOIETIC DRUGS

The formation of both red cells and hemoglobin is a complex process, and deficiency in any one of a number of constituents may result in failure to produce the needed number of red cells or an adequate amount of hemoglobin. The hemoglobin molecule is composed of globin (a protein) and hematin (an iron-containing pigment). A related protein (myoglobin) is found in the muscle cells of mammals.

Some of the factors that promote formation of red blood cells are:

1 A diet adequate in essentials for production of mature red blood cells; namely, iron, vitamin C, vitamin B complex, the antianemic factor (vitamin B$_{12}$), and animal protein
2 Normal gastrointestinal tract activity to assure adequate digestion and absorption of needed essentials
3 A liver able to store iron as well as the antianemic factor. It has been observed that chronic disease of the liver leads to anemia. Much of the iron needed for synthesis of hemoglobin is salvaged from erythrocytes. The antianemic factor is vital for the maturation and formation of normal red blood cells.
4 Normal activity of blood-forming tissues, particularly the red bone marrow of the adult

Although an adequate diet is the preferable way to acquire the essential constituents for blood formation, various disease conditions require treatment that brings about more rapid results than can be obtained from diet alone.

Antianemic drug therapy is aimed at eliminating the cause of the anemia or at symptomatic relief. Vitamin or hormonal deficiency may lead to anemia; specific examples are deficiency of ascorbic acid or of thyroid or adrenocortical hormones. Replacement of any of these missing substances can be considered specific therapy for the corresponding anemia. The major antianemic substances under this heading are iron, vitamin B_{12}, and folic acid.

Iron

Iron is a metallic element that is rather widely distributed in the body. It is found not only in hemoglobin but also in the cytochrome pigments of cells and as a reserve supply in the blood-forming organs. Iron is essential to the normal transport of oxygen and to normal tissue respiration.

Iron deficiency results in a form of anemia in which the red blood cells are hypochromic and microcytic—the red blood cells contain less hemoglobin (and therefore have a low color index) and are smaller than normal. Iron-deficiency anemia is associated with symptoms of low vitality, pallor of the skin and mucous membrane, fatigue, and poor appetite.

Absorption, metabolism, and excretion of iron compounds. Absorption of iron is influenced by a number of factors: (1) the presence of acid in the gastric content (the acid is thought to favor dissociation of iron compounds and the reduction of ferric to ferrous iron, although some doubt has been expressed about this); (2) the presence of reducing substances in the alimentary canal, such as ascorbic acid, which helps to keep iron in a soluble form; and (3) the dietary intake of iron.

Iron is absorbed primarily from the upper part of the duodenum where the acidity prevents formation of insoluble iron compounds. Iron is stored in the form of ferritin or hemosiderin in bone marrow, liver, spleen, and other reticuloendothelial tissue. Both forms can be mobilized and used for hemoglobin synthesis. Iron transport is carried on by transferrin, a specific iron-binding protein in plasma. The transfer of iron to maturing erythrocytes occurs by release of iron from transferrin to specific receptor sites on the membranes of immature red blood cells.

Most iron used for new erythrocyte formation comes from disintegrated red blood cells, whose life span is about 120 days. Approximately 25

mg. of iron daily comes from this source. At best the amount of iron actually absorbed from the gastrointestinal tract is small, about 1 to 2 mg. daily. This is usually adequate since the body is extremely protective of its iron supply.

Iron is not readily eliminated from the body; that which is eliminated was probably not absorbed. It is primarily excreted via the intestinal tract. Only minute traces of iron are excreted via the urinary tract.

Uses. Iron therapy is indicated by hypochromic (iron-deficiency) anemia that occurs following hemorrhage or in persons with an inadequate supply of iron. The major and only significant way of losing iron from the body to such an extent that anemia develops is by blood loss resulting from a sudden acute large hemorrhage or a slow insidious loss from menorrhagia, hemorrhoids, or a silent ulcer or tumor of the gastrointestinal tract.

Iron is used prophylactically in pregnancy, for premature infants, and for those whose diet contains an inadequate amount of iron (such as a diet for peptic ulcer).

Iron requirements in man. Since much of the iron salvaged from worn-out red cells is reused in the body, only a small amount (1 to 2 mg.) needs to be absorbed from the diet to maintain a positive iron balance. During periods of rapid growth and development the body's need for iron is correspondingly increased. Pregnancy, early childhood, early adolescence (especially in girls), and menopause constitute periods when the iron content should probably be increased either by increased dietary intake or medicinal iron or both. Women up through the age of menopause require two to four times as much iron as the adult male because of pregnancy and loss of menstrual blood. The body requirements are ordinarily met by a diet adequate in red meats, green vegetables, eggs, whole wheat, and other foods rich in iron.

Action and result. The local action of iron salts constitutes a side action.

Local. When inorganic iron compounds are administered orally, iron acts as an irritant and astringent. It reacts with tissue proteins and forms an insoluble iron compound. Irritation and astringent effects along the gastrointestinal tract may cause nausea and vomiting, constipation or diarrhea, and abdominal distress. Solutions of ferric iron are sometimes used for their strong astringent properties. They are applied externally as styptics. Ferric solutions are also occasionally used as gargles for their astringent effects. Organic forms do not cause the same irritation because of the fact that they dissociate with difficulty.

Systemic. The action for which iron is most often administered is its hematopoietic one. If iron reserves of the body are depleted, they are restored when ample amounts are administered. It is believed that the action of iron in conditions of deficiency is largely to supply that which is needed for the hemoglobin molecule. The exact mechanism by which iron is utilized by the bone marrow is unknown. Iron is of value only in hypochromic anemias or those in which the color index is low. Iron therapy in this condition can be expected to result in increased vigor on the part of the patient, increased resistance to fatigue, improved condition of the skin and nails, improved appetite, and general feeling of well-being. In other words, it brings about a tonic effect. When administered to individuals with normal blood values it does not bring about an increase in the hemoglobin but only increases the reserve supply of iron in the body.

Maximum response may be expected in the case of hypochromic anemias between the second and the fourth week. Favorable response may, however, be inhibited by vitamin deficiency, infection, achlorhydria, hepatic disorder, or disorders of absorption in the intestine. If the iron deficiency is a severe one, other forms of therapy may be needed to supplement the iron therapy. Blood transfusion will restore the blood more rapidly than anything else that can be done. The physician is likely to maintain that the major medical indication, apart from replacing iron, however, is to find the source of blood loss. To treat iron-deficiency anemia without investigating the possible cause has been vigorously criticized by leading hematologists.

Chlorosis, an iron-deficiency condition in its classic form, has largely disappeared, but a similar although mild grade of anemia in girls of adolescent years (ages 14 to 20) is still a common finding. It responds well to iron therapy.

Preparation, dosage, and administration. It is widely accepted that ferrous salts are better absorbed than ferric salts, and that oral administration is preferable to parenteral. Large doses of iron are usually given, since only 15% of an oral dose is absorbed. Administration after meals tends to reduce gastrointestinal irritation. The concomitant administration of orange juice or ascorbic acid is sometimes used since either acts as a reducing agent to aid absorption.

Oral iron preparations. Ferrous sulfate, U.S.P., B.P., is the most widely used form of iron and is very economical. It is always given orally as a tablet, extended-release capsule, or elixir. The tablets are often enteric coated, since ferrous sulfate rapidly oxidizes in air to form ferric sulfate. The average dose of ferrous sulfate for adults is 300 mg. daily. Dosage range for infants and children is usually 300 to 600 mg. daily. Dosage must be individually determined according to the severity of anemia.

Ferrous gluconate, N.F., B.P. (Fergon). This preparation of iron is available in tablet, capsule, and liquid forms. Dosage is usually the same as that for ferrous sulfate. It is said to have less tendency to cause gastric distress and is better tolerated by some patients than is ferrous sulfate.

Ferrous fumarate, U.S.P., B.P. (Ircon). It is claimed that this oral preparation of iron is better tolerated than either the sulfate or gluconate preparations. It is available as tablets, chewable tablets, and sustained-release forms. Usual adult dose is 200 mg. three or four times daily.

Ferrocholinate (Chel-Iron, Ferrolip). This preparation is a chelated (bound) form of iron, which is believed to be less toxic and better tolerated than some of the older preparations such as ferrous sulfate and ferrous gluconate. At the same time it is said to be clinically effective in the treatment of iron-deficiency anemia. It is administered orally and can be given between meals. It is available in tablets, as a syrup, and as a solution. The proposed dose is 330 mg. three times daily for adults and children.

Side effects and toxic effects. Long-continued administration of iron may cause headache, loss of appetite, gastric pain, nausea, vomiting, and constipation or diarrhea. Patients should be forewarned of the possibility of experiencing abdominal cramps and diarrhea when taking certain preparations of iron. If only the latter symptoms develop, the drug can be stopped for a day or two and then resumed. Patients should also be told that oral preparations will usually cause the stool to be dark red or black. If many untoward symptoms develop, it may be necessary to take a longer rest period before resuming administration. Tolerance to iron is apparently not developed.

Serious acute poisoning can result from ingestion of large doses of iron compounds. Most cases of severe poisoning have occurred in young children who have swallowed many tablets of ferrous sulfate. Some deaths have been reported. Preparations of iron should be kept out of the reach of children. The signs and symptoms of poisoning are those of gastrointestinal irritation, destruction of tissue, and shock.

Precautions. To avoid injury or staining of the teeth, solutions should be well diluted with water or fruit juice and taken through a glass tube or straw.

Iron stains on linen and clothing may be removed with oxalic acid.

Parenteral iron preparations. The preferable route of administration of iron is usually the oral one. However, the following conditions are indications for parenteral administration: (1) for patients with hypochromic anemia who do not tolerate oral iron preparations, (2) for those who do not absorb iron well from the gastrointestinal tract or have gastrointestinal complications such as ulceration or severe diarrhea, (3) for those who for one reason or another cannot be relied upon to take the iron orally, such as the aged or the mentally disturbed, and (4) for those in whom a maximal rate of hemoglobin regeneration is needed, such as patients with severe iron deficiency (patients prior to surgery for which there is immediate need or for patients in the last trimester of pregnancy).

Iron-dextran injection, U.S.P., B.P. (Imferon). This is a colloidal suspension of ferric hydroxide in complex with partially hydrolyzed low molecular weight dextran. The preparation is stable, has a pH of 6, and contains 50 mg. of elemental iron per milliliter. It is available in 2- and 5-ml. ampules and 10-ml. vials. D.E.S.I. rating is *effective* for treatment of iron-deficiency

anemia. Total dosage is calculated by determining the approximate extent of the hemoglobin deficit and adjusting the daily dose accordingly. The initial intramuscular dose is usually 50 mg. on the first day, and amounts up to 250 mg. may be given every day or every other day thereafter until the amount needed has been given. Dosage for children is 25 to 100 mg. daily. The intramuscular preparation is given by deep injection into the gluteal muscle. The subcutaneous tissue should be pushed aside before insertion of the needle to prevent leakage along the tract of the needle. Initial intravenous dose is 15 to 30 mg.; this is increased by 10 mg. daily until hemoglobin returns to normal. Maximum dose is 100 mg. It should be given slowly, 1 ml. in 2 minutes, and the patient should rest 15 to 30 minutes after each dose.

Dextriferron injection (Astrafer). This preparation is an iron-carbohydrate complex that is administered intravenously. It is recommended that the initial dose not exceed 1.5 ml. of a 2% solution (30 mg. of iron).

Iron sorbitex, N.F. (Jectofer); *iron sorbitol,* B.P. This is an intramuscular preparation of iron in combination with sorbitol and citric acid. It is available in 2-ml. ampules that contain 50 mg. of iron per milliliter. Iron sorbitex is rapidly absorbed (50% to 70% within 3 hours and up to 95% within 24 hours after injection). It is primarily excreted in the urine, and the urine of patients receiving this drug may turn dark. Dosage must be determined individually for each patient.

Side effects. Side effects from parenteral administration of iron include headache, nausea, vomiting, muscle ache, fever, and mild urticaria. Severe anaphylactic reactions can also occur.

Pain is sometimes experienced at the site of intramuscular injection, and there may be permanent brownish discoloration of the skin at the injection site. Injection of an iron preparation outside a vein may cause a severe local reaction. When iron is administered orally there is a limit to which it will be absorbed, but when it is injected into the bloodstream an overdose may be serious, partly because there is no satisfactory way for the body to excrete the amount taken in, over and above what the body can use or can store as a normal reserve. It is deposited in organs such as the liver or pancreas, causing hemochromatosis.

Iron antidote

Deferoxamine (Desferrioxamine B, Desferal). Deferoxamine is a polyhydroxamic acid found in combination with iron in certain microorganisms. Deferoxamine is an iron-chelating agent; that is, it has great affinity for iron, removes iron from its tissue storage form (ferritin), binds the iron, and blocks its absorption.

Deferoxamine is used to treat iron overloading that may result from ingestion of large quantities of iron over a long period of time or from a metabolic abnormality that permits absorption of large amounts of iron from the diet, thereby increasing iron storage. This condition is termed hemosiderosis if no tissue damage occurs and hematochromatosis if tissue damage results. Deferoxamine is also used to treat iron poisoning.

Deferoxamine may be given orally, intramuscularly, or intravenously and by direct instillation into the stomach via gastric tube. Rapid urinary excretion of iron occurs after parenteral administration.

Vitamin B$_{12}$ (cyanocobalamin)

One of the major developments in nutrition in the past 50 years began with the recognition by Minot and Murphy in 1926 that a substance in liver could cure the hitherto fatal disease pernicious anemia. Their discovery led to the eventual isolation by other scientists of the pure compound, at first called "antianemic factor" in 1948, and in 1956 the elucidation of the structure of this molecule—vitamin B$_{12}$. Vitamin B$_{12}$ is an extremely complex and large organic molecule containing the metal cobalt. It has a structure similar to heme, the iron-bearing porphyrin in the hemoglobin molecule.

Today it is believed that persons with pernicious anemia (now a misnomer since the disease can be arrested) lack the ability to absorb vitamin B$_{12}$ from dietary sources, at least at the normal rate. They must therefore be supplied with enormous doses of the vitamin by mouth (so that a sufficient amount can be absorbed) or else be given rather small doses parenterally (since by this route all is made available to the tissues).

The exact role of the vitamin in body chemistry is not well understood, but it is clearly required for some chemical step in the formation and normal development of the mature red cell.

Vitamin B$_{12}$ is believed to act as a coenzyme in certain biologic reactions necessary for the normal synthesis of methionine, deoxynucleic acids, and other essential constituents of all cells.

The exact nature of the disease process in pernicious anemia that prevents the absorption of vitamin B$_{12}$ is not well understood. There is good evidence, however, that these patients fail to manufacture in their gastric mucous membrane a specific substance required for the normal absorption of vitamin B$_{12}$. The absorption factor has been called the intrinsic factor to distinguish it from vitamin B$_{12}$, which, before its chemical nature was understood, used to be somewhat mysteriously identified as "extrinsic factor."

There is no lack of vitamin B$_{12}$ in a normal diet. Even without a dietary supply, evidence shows that there is sufficient formation of the vitamin by bacteria normally present in the intestine of man and other mammals. The patient with pernicious anemia therefore, in a sense, starves in the midst of plenty since he lacks the substance necessary for absorption of vitamin B$_{12}$.

For this reason, it is also possible to supply the vitamin indirectly by giving the patient a preparation of dried gastric mucosa containing the intrinsic factor and thereby enabling him to absorb his own vitamin B$_{12}$ from the diet. The surest way of remedying a deficiency, however, is to give the vitamin directly by injection, and this is the most common way of treating pernicious anemia.

When the body is deficient in vitamin B$_{12}$ over a period of time, a series of characteristic symptoms and pathologic changes develop. The onset is gradual, and the early symptoms are usually fatigue, sore tongue, and achlorhydria. The patient develops a peculiar yellowish pallor and complains of increasing weakness, breathlessness, itching, dyspepsia, and diarrhea. Degenerative changes in the nervous system also occur, giving rise to incoordination of movement, loss of vibratory sense (as a result of changes in the dorsal columns of the spinal cord), peripheral neuritis, optic atrophy, and, sometimes, psychosis. Death may result from the changes associated with pernicious anemia unless the changes are arrested, which is accomplished effectively with the administration of vitamin B_{12}.

Uses. Pernicious anemia is one of the macrocytic hyperchromic anemias for which the administration of vitamin B_{12} is effective either as the pure vitamin or in a preparation of liver. It constitutes a form of replacement therapy, and administration must be continued indefinitely. It corrects the abnormalities of the red blood cells, relieves the sore mouth and tongue, restores normal function of the peripheral nerves, and arrests the progression of changes in the central nervous system. In some cases the changes in the nervous system are reversed if the irreversible stage of degeneration has not been reached. Vitamin B_{12} is also used in certain nutritional macrocytic anemias and for tropical and nontropical sprue. Beneficial effects have been reported in a number of neurologic disorders, such as trifacial neuralgia. These effects have been secured only after very large doses.

Preparation, dosage, and administration. Cyanocobalamin is a red crystalline substance that contains cobalt; it is obtained from cultures of *Streptomyces griseus* as a by-product in the manufacture of antibiotics. Because there is a group of closely related B_{12} factors, the activity of any preparation coming from natural sources may result from several members of this group. Prior to the availability of pure vitamin B_{12}, liver was administered extensively since it contains B_{12}, but it is now considered scientifically obsolete since liver preparations have no advantage over the pure vitamin but have several distinct disadvantages—liver is more expensive, may be painful to receive, and is allergenic in some persons.

Cyanocobalamin (vitamin B_{12}), U.S.P., B.P. This is available in a variety of preparations for oral administration and in powder or solution for injection. Parenteral dosage for adults is 100 to 1000 μg. daily for 1 week followed by the same dose one to three times weekly until remission occurs. Remission maintenance dose is 100 to 1000 μg. every 4 weeks. For patients with neurological damage, 1000 μg. may be given one or more times weekly for several months, then once or twice weekly for a year. If neurological dam-

age is not reversed by this time it is probably irreversible. Dosage for children is 1000 to 5000 μg. given in doses of 100 μg. over a period of 2 or more weeks, then 30 to 50 μg. every 4 weeks. Oral therapy is less satisfactory than parenteral treatment. Oral dosage for adults is 1000 μg. daily until remission occurs, then 1000 μg. as often as necessary to maintain remission.

Vitamin B_{12} with intrinsic factor concentrate. This is a mixture of vitamin B_{12} with preparations of gastric mucosa obtained from the stomachs of domestic animals used for food. It is available in capsule and tablet form. It may be desirable for an occasional patient for whom parenteral therapy is difficult or undesirable. However, the administration of vitamin B_{12} by injection is considered more dependable. It is no longer an official preparation.

Side effects and toxic effects. No undesirable side effects or toxic effects have been reported following administration of vitamin B_{12}, even after large parenteral doses.

Use of hydrochloric acid. Since nearly all patients with pernicious anemia have a lack of hydrochloric acid in the stomach, full doses of the official dilute hydrochloric acid may be prescribed for the patient, to be given with meals not only to aid digestion but also to act as a gastric antiseptic. The usual dose is $1/2$ to 1 fluidram, which is well diluted with water (one-third to one-half glass).

Folic acid

The chemical name for folic acid is pteroylglutamic acid. It is a member of the vitamin B complex and can be prepared synthetically. It is found only in small amounts in the free state in a number of foods.

Folic acid is an important growth factor for a large number of cells. It participates in the synthesis of amino acids and deoxyribonucleic acid (DNA). DNA deficiency interferes with cell mitosis, and this may result in the development of large cells (megaloblasts) that are characteristic of megaloblastic anemias.

Folic acid has been used as a supplement to liver therapy in the treatment of pernicious anemia. It produces a response in blood similar to that produced by liver extract. The hemoglobin and red cells increase to normal, and bone marrow returns to its normal state. The appetite improves, and the patient feels better in general. In most patients the blood response is apparently maintained indefinitely with folic acid. It does not, however, prevent the development or the progression of neurologic changes that are often a part of the disease, and it may in fact make them worse. Because of this, it cannot be recognized as adequate therapy for pernicious anemia and cannot replace vitamin B_{12}. Its use is therefore dangerous when used alone for this condition, and the presence of folic acid in many multivitamin preparations adds to the hazard of this type of irrational therapy when it is used in the treatment of an undiagnosed anemia.

Uses. Although folic acid should not be employed in the treatment of pernicious anemia except possibly as a supplement to adequate therapy with vitamin B_{12}, it is used for the treatment of selected cases of macrocytic anemias and of nutritional and metabolic disorders associated with such anemia. It frequently is useful in the treatment of an anemia of pregnancy. It is sometimes used in the treatment of anemia associated with tropical sprue and celiac disease, although there is some question as to whether it constitutes complete therapy.

Preparation, dosage, and administration

Folic acid, U.S.P., B.P. (Folvite). This preparation is marketed in 0.25- and 1-mg. tablets and as an elixir, 1 mg. per milliliter, for oral administration, and as a solution for injection, 15 mg. per milliliter. The usual oral and parenteral dose for adults and children is 0.25 to 1 mg. daily. Folic acid injection, U.S.P., is the same as sodium folate. It is the preparation preferred for parenteral therapy.

WHOLE BLOOD AND ITS CONSTITUENTS

Transfusions of whole blood are of value not only to replace red cells but also to restore blood volume and blood pressure. The latter value is seen particularly in the treatment of shock.

Blood transfusion plays an important although passive role in the treatment of anemic conditions. Transfusions do not apparently stimulate the bone marrow to greater activity but in times of crises they may save the patient's life when the patient cannot wait for iron or liver to become effective.

For blood transfusions to be used satisfactorily, it is important that the blood be readily available and of the suitable type. It is also essential that a careful technique be developed and strictly adhered to in order to help prevent reactions. The blood should be administered slowly, particularly if the patient's anemia is severe. Sometimes one transfusion of whole blood will suffice, but under other conditions a series of small transfusions may accomplish better results.

TREATMENT OF HYPOVOLEMIC SHOCK

Adequate blood volume is absolutely essential to maintain viability of cells, normal tissue function, and life itself. Extensive trauma and hemorrhage that seriously lower blood volume usually require blood replacement. Whenever 30% of the blood volume is lost, prompt treatment is essential. Fresh whole blood replaces not only blood volume but vital clotting factors (platelets) and essential cellular elements (red and white blood cells). Stored blood rapidly loses its platelets and clotting factors. In cases of severe and continued blood loss, blood may need to be administered under pressure and even through more than one infusion route. Need for blood volume replacement may be determined not only by estimating blood loss when hemorrhage is visible and blood loss is measurable, but also by severity of shock, serial measurement of arterial blood pressure and blood volume, central venous pressure, hematocrit, pulse, and hourly urine output. Blood pressure alone, without the use of other physiologic parameters, is a very unreliable criterion for the presence or severity of shock. Prompt control of bleeding as well as blood replacement is essential.

It is important, of course, that blood used for replacement match the patient's specific type of blood. While blood may not always be the fluid of choice for volume replacement, it is usually the most dependable. If the loss of blood volume is the result of hemorrhage, whole blood replacement is the therapy of choice, along with control of hemorrhage. Whole blood contains all the necessary fluid-holding constituents and does not pass out of the vascular system as rapidly as most parenteral fluids. The use of plasma expanders and noncolloid fluids, such as isotonic saline, offers only temporary support. Blood should not be used for transfusion if more than 21 days have passed since it was obtained from the donor. With massive transfusions, hypocalcemia may occur from the citrate used to prevent the blood from clotting. Citrate binds and inactivates calcium. Calcium gluconate is given to replace the calcium content.

If lost blood volume is replaced promptly with adequate amounts of blood, there is no problem. However, if treatment is delayed, more and more blood is required to maintain blood pressure and other vital signs. Actually more blood will be required than has been lost from hemorrhage. The reason for this is that some of the blood remaining in the circulatory system becomes trapped in the capillaries and small blood vessels, particularly in the liver and splanchnic area. The trapped cells may form microclots or small thrombi. Trapping is probably caused by increased resistance to blood flow from compensatory vasoconstriction. In addition, with decreased velocity of flow, there is increased viscosity. As blood viscosity increases, the plasma cannot keep red cells in suspension, and they settle out of the plasma causing sludging or aggregation of cells in the microcirculation. As blood flow slows and red blood cells bump into one another in the small vessels, a sticky substance forms on the outside of the red blood cell, and this further promotes sludging or red cell aggregation.

The use of high molecular weight dextran (see p. 194) may further increase viscosity as well as red blood cell aggregation. Clinical studies have shown that low viscosity dextran infusions help to mobilize noncirculating red cells, thus its use along with whole blood for treatment of shock caused by hemorrhage.

Avoidance of sludging. The following are methods used to avoid aggregation of red blood cells:

1 Adequate mechanical respiratory movements should be maintained by encouraging the patient to breathe deeply and regularly or by using mechanical assistance. These respiratory movements help to bring blood into the thorax and assist blood flow. (From 30% to 50% of the patients who die following shock show signs of pulmonary insufficiency and pulmonary emboli.)
2 Muscle movement is promoted by having the patient contract and relax the muscles in his extremities, shoulders, and buttocks. Circulation can be assisted by massaging and moving the patient's muscles and by position movement of the patient (if this is not contraindicated by his condition).

Use of vasoconstrictors and vasodilators in shock therapy. The use of vasoconstrictors (such as norepinephrine) is considered by researchers to be *contraindicated* in hypovolemic shock. These drugs will further reduce capillary blood flow and hasten cell death.

In some cases where significant vasoconstriction is present, vasodilators such as phenoxybenzamine or phentolamine have been used to reduce peripheral resistance to blood flow and to increase capillary perfusion. The use of vasodilators plus volume replacement has resulted in a decrease in mortality from hypovolemic shock.

Since hypovolemic shock can be more successfully treated than other forms of shock, its prompt recognition and safe management are of great importance.

HUMAN RED BLOOD CELLS, U.S.P.

Human red blood cells are citrated whole blood from which plasma has been removed. Its use is indicated when blood cell replacement is necessary but an increase of plasma volume is unnecessary or undesirable. It is used for treating certain cases of anemia. Expiration date should be noted.

BLOOD PLASMA

Blood plasma is the fluid part of the blood that may be procured by separating the blood cells from the whole citrated blood. Plasma may be given irrespective of the donor's group. Many authorities believe that blood plasma, since it contains fibrinogen, albumin, gamma globulins, hemagglutinins, prothrombin, sugar, and salts, is an ideal transfusion medium to restore effective blood volume in the treatment of peripheral circulatory failure associated with severe burns, traumatic shock, or hemorrhage. It is also used to maintain colloid osmotic pressure and to supplement blood proteins. Blood plasma can be used as it is for transfusions or it can be concentrated, dehydrated, and stored for long periods of time without deterioration. The addition of sterile distilled water is all that is needed to make it ready for immediate use. Plasma in the dried form is particularly stable and useful when transportation, storage, and contamination are problems that must be considered.

Normal human plasma. Normal human plasma is obtained by pooling equal parts of citrated whole blood from eight or more adult human beings who qualify as donors by virtue of their having passed physical examinations and various clinical tests. Procedures are carried out under definite aseptic conditions, and the cell-free plasma is obtained by centrifugation or by sedimentation. It is dispensed in liquid, dried, or frozen form. The usual amount given whole or restored is 500 ml. It is administered to combat surgical and traumatic shock, in the treatment of burned persons when much plasma has been lost, and in cases in which whole blood is not immediately available for the treatment of hemorrhage.

A serious problem with the use of pooled human plasma is the transmission of viral hepatitis. Since plasma from one infected donor may appear in many bottles of plasma, the incidence of transmitting viral hepatitis is far greater than when whole blood is used.

BLOOD PROTEINS

Blood plasma can be further broken down to many useful parts. Albumin is just as effective as plasma in shock treatment, and effective treatment requires less of the albumin than of the plasma.

Thrombin and fibrinogen also can be separated from plasma and then purified and concentrated into fine white powders. When put into solution they coagulate to form fibrin. The solution is sometimes applied locally to stimulate blood clotting and to provide a sort of glue in skin grafting.

Human fibrinogen, U.S.P.: *dried human fibrinogen,* B.P., is available as a powder for injection with a suitable amount of diluent.

Normal human serum albumin, U.S.P., is a brownish, viscous, clear, relatively odorless liquid obtained from the blood of healthy human donors. It is made free of the hazard of the virus of serum hepatitis by heating at 60° C. for 10 hours. It is available in a solution (25 Gm. in 100 ml.) or as a dried preparation. The normal unit is composed of 25 Gm. of human albumin to which sterile water or physiologic saline solution can be added before use. This is then equivalent to about 500 ml. of whole human plasma, in terms of protein osmotic pressure. It is used in the treatment of shock and in situations in which it is important to raise the serum protein of the blood. It is administered intravenously.

Human antihemophilic human factor, U.S.P., B.P. (dried form), is normal human plasma that has been processed promptly to preserve the antihemophilic globulin component. Hemophilia is the result of a congenital deficiency in a particular globulin, and this reduces the ability of the blood to clot. Antihemophilic human plasma is administered to bring about temporary relief of the dysfunction of the clotting mechanism in the patient with hemophilia. It is dispensed in the frozen or the dried form.

PLASMA SUBSTITUTES
Dextran (Expandex, Gentran); dextran 70 injection, B.P.

Dextran is a glucose polymer made by the action of special bacteria *(Leuconostoc mesenteroides)* on sucrose. The resulting polysaccharide does not easily pass through capillary walls. The molecules are like those of serum albumin and have a molecular weight of about 75,000.

Uses. Dextran is used to expand plasma volume and maintain blood pressure in emergency conditions resulting from shock and hemorrhage. It is not a substitute for whole blood or its derivatives when the latter are needed for the treatment of anemia secondary to hemorrhage or when it is essential to restore blood proteins after traumatic injuries, burns, and so forth. It has no oxygen-carrying property. The effect of an injection of 500 to 1000 ml. of dextran (6%) usually persists for a period of 24 hours. From 30% to 50% is excreted in the urine and the remainder is metabolized in the body.

Preparation, dosage, and administration. Dextran is administered intravenously in isotonic solution of sodium chloride. The usual dose is 500 ml. of 6% solution infused at the rate of 20 to 40 ml. per minute. Repeated infusions can be given when necessary, if blood or its derivatives are not at hand or if their use is not indicated. Solutions of dextran do not require refrigeration and are easily stored. The 6% solution of dextran is osmotically equivalent to serum albumin.

Although high molecular weight dextran is effective in replacing lost blood volume, it has been shown clinically and experimentally that this form of dextran has an adverse effect on flow in minute vessels and capillaries because it increases blood viscosity. Another disadvantage of this form of dextran is that it interferes with normal clotting by coating platelets.

Side effects and toxic effects. Untoward effects are rare with the exception of an antigen-antibody type of reaction in certain persons. It has been established that bleeding time of recipients may be increased. This seems to be a temporary effect. Patients with cardiovascular disease who receive dextran infusions should be watched for congestive heart failure and pulmonary edema. Temporary depression of renal tubule functioning has been reported.

Dextran 40, B.P.
(LMD, Rheomacrodex)

Low molecular weight dextran with a molecular weight of 40,000 is a less effective expander of plasma volume than high molecular dextran. However, it has been used effectively to restore flow in the microcirculation and to improve tissue perfusion by reducing blood viscosity and sludging and preventing intravascular coagulation.

Dextran 40 is also used as a priming agent for pump oxygenators or bypass machines used for open-heart surgery.

Action. Dextran 40 may reduce blood viscosity by drawing fluid from the tissues into the vascular system, and therefore patients should be watched for signs of dehydration (warm dry skin and mouth, thirst, rise in body temperature). Pre-

vention of intravascular clotting is theorized by some researchers to result from the ability of dextran 40 to maintain the electronegativity of red blood cells, which causes the cells to repel one another. In addition, red blood cell rigidity may be decreased, which promotes flow of red cells through the small blood vessels.

Absorption and excretion. Dextran 40 is rather rapidly excreted by the kidneys in patients with normal renal function. The viscosity and specific gravity of the urine may be increased during the administration of dextran 40 and throughout the duration of its effects, particularly in patients with decreased urine flow. A low specific gravity of urine with dextran 40 may indicate inability of the kidneys to remove dextran and is an indication for discontinuance of therapy. This drug should not be used in patients with renal disease. Its use is not contraindicated in patients with reduced urine output caused by shock. However, its use should be discontinued if no improvement in urine flow occurs. Unexcreted dextran is slowly degraded to glucose, which is then metabolized to respiratory carbon dioxide and water.

Preparation, dosage, and administration. Dextran 40 is available for intravenous injection as a 10% solution in 500- and 1000-ml. bottles in combination with dextrose 5% or sodium chloride 0.9%. When used in shock therapy total dosage in the first 24 hours should not exceed 2 Gm. per kilogram of body weight (10 ml. of a 10% solution equals 1 Gm. of dextran). Thereafter, total dosage should not exceed 1 Gm. per kilogram of body weight per 24 hours. It is not recommended that therapy be continued for longer than 5 days.

Side effects and toxic effects. Adverse effects to dextran 40 include urticarial reactions, nausea, vomiting, wheezing, a tight feeling in the chest, and hypotension. However, these are not common reactions, but are anaphylactoid.

DRUGS THAT AFFECT BLOOD COAGULATION

Drugs affecting the clotting of blood are used both to hasten clotting (hemostatics) and to retard clotting (anticoagulants). In some instances normal components necessary for blood clotting must be supplied.

DRUGS THAT AFFECT BLOOD COAGULATION

HEMOSTATICS

Absorbable gelatin sponge, U.S.P., B.P. (Gelfoam)

Absorbable gelatin sponge is a specially prepared form of gelatin having a porous nature. It is used to control capillary bleeding and may be left in place in a surgical wound. It is completely absorbed in 4 to 6 weeks. It should be well moistened with isotonic saline solution or thrombin solution before it is applied to a bleeding surface. Its presence does not induce excessive scar formation.

The hemostatic action is the result of its action as a tampon and liberation of thromboplastin from damaged platelets traumatized by contact with the sponge.

Human fibrin foam

This is a sterile dry preparation of human fibrin that, when applied to a bleeding surface, acts as a mechanical coagulant. In combination with thrombin it gives a chemical as well as a mechanical matrix for coagulation. It is used in surgery of organs such as the brain, liver, or kidneys where ordinary methods for the control of bleeding are ineffective or inadvisable.

It is absorbed within a short period of time and need not be removed after bleeding has stopped.

Oxidized cellulose, U.S.P., B.P. (Oxycel, Hemo-Pak)

This is a specially treated form of surgical gauze or cotton that exerts a hemostatic effect but is absorbable when buried in the tissues. The hemostatic action is caused by the formation of an artificial clot by cellulosic acid. Absorption of oxidized cellulose occurs between the second and the seventh day following implantation, although absorption of large amounts of blood-soaked material may take 6 weeks or longer. Oxidized cellulose is of value in the control of bleeding in surgery of such organs as the liver, pan-

creas, spleen, kidney, thyroid, and prostate. Its hemostatic action is not increased by the addition of other hemostatic agents. It should not be used as a surface dressing except for the control of bleeding, because cellulosic acid inhibits the growth of epithelial tissue. Since it interferes with bone regeneration it should not be implanted in fractures.

Thrombin, U.S.P.; dried human thrombin, B.P.

This is a preparation of thrombin isolated from bovine plasma. It is intended as a hemostatic agent for *topical application* to control capillary bleeding. It may be applied as a dry powder or dissolved in sterile isotonic saline solution. It is not injected.

Vitamin K

Vitamin K was discovered by Dam of Copenhagen in 1935 as a result of a study of newly hatched chicks that had a fatal hemorrhagic disease. This condition, he found, could be prevented and cured by the administration of a substance found in hog liver and in alfalfa. It was later discovered that the delayed clotting time of the blood was caused by deficiency of prothrombin content. Vitamin K occurs naturally in two forms known as K_1 and K_2. Both have a naphthoquinone nucleus and exhibit similar physiologic properties.

Vitamin K–like compounds

In natural vitamin K (K_1 or K_2), R is a long alkyl chain of twenty or thirty carbons. In synthetic vitamin K (Menadione), R is only hydrogen. These compounds are called naphthoquinones from the parent nucleus. The synthetic analogues greatly resemble the natural vitamin. Certain of the analogues are water soluble, whereas the natural vitamin is fat soluble. The fat-soluble vitamin requires the presence of bile in the intestine to ensure adequate absorption after oral administration. This is not essential for the water-soluble preparations.

Vitamin K is widely found in foods; deficiency is rarely caused by lack of it in the diet. It is also synthesized by intestinal bacteria.

Action and result. Vitamin K is essential to the synthesis of prothrombin by the liver. The exact mechanism of its action is not known, although it is thought to contribute to the activation of an enzyme necessary to the formation of prothrombin.

Prothrombin deficiency may occur because of inadequate absorption of vitamin K from the intestine (usually because of biliary disease in which bile fails to enter the intestine) or because of destruction of intestinal organisms, which may occur with antibiotic therapy. It is also encountered in the newborn, in which case it is probably caused by the fact that the intestinal organisms have not yet become established. It may result from therapy with certain anticoagulants.

Uses. Vitamin K is useful only in conditions in which the prolonged bleeding time is the result of low concentration of prothrombin in the blood, which is not in turn the result of damaged liver cells. Vitamin K is routinely administered to newborns to help prevent hemorrhage. Although prothrombin may be normal at birth, it declines until about the sixth day, when the liver is able to form prothrombin. Vitamin K may be given to the mother prior to delivery.

It is also indicated in the preoperative preparation of patients with deficient prothrombin, particularly those with obstructive jaundice. In addition, it is given as an antidote for overdosage of systemic anticoagulants such as bishydroxycoumarin, as well as for hemorrhagic disorders and hypoprothrombinemia secondary to large doses, or overdosages, of drugs such as salicylates, quinine, sulfonamides, arsenicals, and barbiturates. Hemorrhagic conditions not caused by deficiency of prothrombin are not successfully treated with vitamin K.

The natural concentrates have, to a great extent, been replaced by the synthetic preparations. It is important that the prothrombin activity of the blood be measured frequently when the patient is receiving a preparation of vitamin K. Parenteral preparations should be administered if for some reason the intestinal absorption is impaired.

Preparation, dosage, and administration. The following are the preparations of vitamin K available.

Menadione, N.F. This drug is a synthetic substitute for natural vitamin K. The presence of bile is essential for adequate absorption after oral administration. Menadione tablets, N.F., and menadione injection, N.F., are official preparations. The usual dose is 1 to 2 mg. daily.

Menadione sodium bisulfite, N.F. (Hykinone). This form is similar to menadione but it is water soluble, and oral doses need not be accompanied by bile salts. It is available in tablet form for oral administration as well as in solution for subcutaneous, intramuscular, and intravenous injection. Menadione sodium bisulfite injection, N.F., and menaphthone sodium bisulfite injection, B.P., are official preparations for injection. Average daily dose is 0.5 to 2 mg. daily. Dosage is determined in relation to the prothrombin level of the blood.

Various other commercial water-soluble vitamin K analogues are also available. Synkamin is marketed in 1-ml. ampules containing 1 mg. of the drug and in capsules containing 4 mg. of the drug.

Menadiol sodium diphosphate, N.F. (Synkayvite). This is a derivative of menadione and has the same action and uses as other analogues of vitamin K. It is water soluble and is adequately absorbed after oral administration without bile salts. It is administered orally, subcutaneously, intramuscularly, and intravenously. The dosage is approximately three times that of menadione. It is available in 5-mg. tablets for oral administration and in solution for injection. The usual dose is 4 to 75 mg.

Phytonadione, U.S.P. (vitamin K_1, Mephyton, Konakion); *phytomenadione*, B.P. This preparation acts more promptly and over a longer period of time than the vitamin K analogues. It is a fat-soluble vitamin, and the presence of bile salts in the intestine is essential to adequate absorption. It will stop bleeding 3 to 4 hours after intravenous administration and produces a normal prothrombin level in 12 to 14 hours. It is useful to reverse the effects of anticoagulant therapy that have produced a serious deficiency of prothrombin in the blood. Phytonadione is available in 5-mg. oral tablets and as an emulsion for intravenous injection. The emulsion is diluted with isotonic salt solution or sterile water before it is injected. The dosage varies greatly; 2 to 20 mg. may be given daily, although much larger doses have been given in emergency situations. However, small doses of vitamin K_1 orally administered will effectively correct the reduced prothrombin activity induced by certain anticoagulants (coumarin drugs). Effects are said to be less predictable when severe liver damage is present. The dosage must be determined according to the level of prothrombin activity, the length of time during which the patient has received anticoagulant therapy, and the hazard of restoring the risk of thrombosis. Large doses of vitamin K_1 are said to make subsequent regulation of anticoagulant therapy with coumarin drugs more difficult.

Phytonadione solution (Aqua Mephyton, Konakion). This preparation is a water-soluble form of vitamin K_1 that may be given subcutaneously or intramuscularly.

DRUGS THAT AFFECT BLOOD COAGULATION

ANTICOAGULANTS

Diseases associated with abnormal clotting within vessels take a great toll of lives. It is estimated that over a million persons suffer from thrombosis or embolism in the United States each year. Diseases caused by intravascular clotting include some of the major causes of death from cardiovascular sources—coronary occlusion and cerebrovascular accidents. Drugs that inhibit clotting are therefore important.

Anticoagulation therapy is directed toward preventing intravascular thrombosis by decreasing blood coagulability. This therapy has no direct effect on a blood clot that has already formed or on ischemic tissue injured by an inadequate blood supply because of the clot.

Anticoagulants are indicated in:

1 Occlusive vascular disease, such as thromboangiitis obliterans
2 Sudden arterial occlusion
3 Venous thrombosis
4 Pulmonary embolism
5 Cerebrovascular thrombosis
6 Coronary artery occlusion or myocardial infarction

Anticoagulants are used prophylactically in:

1 Major surgery where there is previous history of thrombosis or when prolonged immobilization will be necessary
2 Pelvic surgery in the male or female, since pelvic surgery is notorious for its high incidence of postoperative thrombophlebitis
3 Patients on bedrest for more than 2 or 3 days, since this predisposes them to vascular stasis
4 Rheumatic heart disease

Anticoagulants are also used to prevent clotting of blood to be used for transfusion, laboratory, or experimental work. The mechanism of blood coagulation is very complex. During the past two decades many new coagulation factors

Table 10-3 Blood coagulation factors

Name	Factor
Fibrinogen	I
Prothrombin	II
Tissue thromboplastin	III
Calcium	IV
Proaccelerin (labile factor, accelerator globulin)	V
(Accelerin)*	VI
Proconvertin (stable factor, serum prothrombin conversion accelerator, SPCA)	VII
Antihemophilic factor	VIII
Plasma thromboplastin component, Christmas factor	IX
Stuart-Prower factor	X
Plasma thromboplastin antecedent (PTA)	XI
Hageman factor	XII
Fibrin stabilizing factor	XIII

*Existence of factor VI is disputed. It was previously called accelerin, but it is no longer believed to be involved in hemostasis. There is no name or function now assigned to "factor VI."

have been discovered and new terminology has come into existence. Three stages of blood coagulation are recognized:

Stage I—formation of thromboplastin

Stage II—conversion of prothrombin to thrombin

Stage III—conversion of fibrinogen to fibrin

It is stage I that is most complex, and at least eight of the twelve blood coagulation factors (IV, V, VIII, IX, X, XI, XII, and phospholipid) are essential for formation of intravascular thromboplastin (see Table 10-3). Formation of extravascular or tissue thromboplastin requires only factors IV and VII. Tissue or extrinsic thromboplastin is released from injured tissue; intravascular or intrinsic thromboplastin is released from platelets. Factor XIII aids in maintenance of an insoluble fibrin clot.

The following is a summary of the last stages of the coagulatory process:

$$\text{Prothrombin} \xrightarrow{\text{Thromboplastin + Calcium}} \text{Thrombin}$$

$$\text{Fibrinogen} \xrightarrow{\text{Thrombin}} \text{Fibrin}$$

Local trauma, vascular stasis, and systemic alterations in coagulability of blood are still considered the principal etiologic factors in the initiation of thrombosis.

Arterial thrombosis is most frequently associated with atherosclerotic plaques, high blood pressure, and turbulent blood flow that damages the inner lining of the blood vessel and causes platelets to stick and aggregate and release thromboplastin. Arterial thrombi are platelet or white thrombi.

Venous thrombosis occurs most often in areas where blood flow is reduced or static. This appears to initiate clotting and produce a red thrombus. Current anticoagulants are more effective in preventing venous than arterial thrombosis. To prevent arterial thrombosis will require a drug that will control platelet aggregation, and such a drug is not yet available.

Anticoagulant therapy is primarily prophylactic. These agents act (1) by preventing fibrin deposits, (2) by preventing extension of a thrombus, and (3) by preventing thromboembolic complications. Anticoagulation therapy is still empirical and is based largely on clinical experience. Long-term anticoagulant therapy remains controversial. Nevertheless there is evidence that anticoagulant therapy reduces the incidence of thrombosis and therefore prolongs life.

Bleeding tendencies constitute the most important side effect of the anticoagulants. Hematuria, epistaxis, ecchymosis, and bleeding gums may occur as well as other signs of bleeding.

Contraindications to the use of anticoagulants include blood dyscrasias, liver or kidney disease, peptic ulcer, chronic ulcerative colitis, and active bleeding. Patients undergoing spinal cord or brain surgery should not use anticoagulants since even minor bleeding may cause serious consequences. Certain drugs such as salicylates, cincophen, phenylbutazone, and reserpine increase the risk of bleeding and should not be given with anticoagulants. Use of barbiturates and oral anticoagulants is also somewhat hazardous; discontinuance of the barbiturate with continued administration of the anticoagulant may result in active bleeding. In the presence of barbiturates, higher doses of the anticoagulants are required for optimum effect. Unless the anticoagulant dosage is reduced when barbiturates are discontinued, excessive loading of the anticoagulant may occur, resulting in toxic or bleeding effects.

Sodium citrate

Sodium citrate is used as an anticoagulant in blood that is to be used for a transfusion or that is to be stored for a time. Anticoagulant sodium citrate solution, N.F., is an approximately 4% sterile solution of sodium citrate in water. It is used as an anticoagulant for blood plasma and for blood for fractionation. Anticoagulant citrate dextrose solution, U.S.P., is used as an anticoagulant for storage of whole blood. Sodium citrate acts by binding plasma calcium and preventing the formation of thrombin.

Heparin sodium injection, U.S.P.; heparin injection, B.P.

Heparin is a mucopolysaccharide that is strongly acidic because of the presence of sulfate groups in the molecule. Heparin, as the name implies, was first found in the liver and subsequently in the lungs and intestinal mucosa. It is present in the mast cells of these tissues; it has also been found in the tunica intima of blood vessels.

Action and uses. Heparin prevents coagulation by (1) interfering with the formation of thrombin from prothrombin, (2) preventing thrombin from acting as a catalyst in converting fibrinogen into fibrin, and (3) preventing agglutination and disintegration of platelets and release of their thromboplastin. Therefore heparin increases the clotting time of blood. The effects of heparin are thought to be caused by its strong electronegative charge by which it blocks enzymatic reactions. The action of heparin can be inhibited or reversed by protamine sulfate, which has a strong positive charge. Heparin is also known to be antilipemic; that is, it reduces blood lipids or fats. It has been shown to dissolve clots in the sludge stage.

Heparin is the drug of choice for sudden arterial occlusion since its action is immediate and readily reversible if surgery becomes necessary for clot removal. In thrombophlebitis there is evidence that heparin is superior to the coumarin drugs in preventing pulmonary complications. It is also preferred for treating thrombophlebitis occurring during pregnancy since it does not cross the placental barrier. Heparin is not excreted in the mother's milk. Since coumarin drugs can go through these channels they can cause fetal complications and hemorrhage in the newborn.

Heparin is usually used when rapid anticoagulant action is desired. It is used prior to the use of oral anticoagulants (coumarin derivatives). Heparin approaches the ideal anticoagulant—it is rapidly absorbed, readily excreted, and almost nontoxic. Its main disadvantages are its short action, high cost, need for parenteral injection, and local reactions at injection sites. Hypersensitivity to heparin is rare but allergic reactions have been reported. Alopecia may occur, but it is reversible after withdrawal of the drug. Osteoporosis has been reported in patients on large doses of heparin for long periods of time (6 months or more).

Preparation, dosage, and administration. Heparin is inactive orally and must be administered parenterally. It is obtained commercially from domestic animals slaughtered for food. It may be given by a single injection or continuous intravenous drip. The response to heparin occurs almost immediately and lasts for a relatively short time (3 to 4 hours) unless the dose is repeated. When administration is discontinued, the clotting time returns to normal rather quickly, and there is danger of massive clot formation should the drug be discontinued too soon. Dosage needs to be determined for each individual patient and maintained at a level that keeps the clotting time well above normal (15 to 20 minutes). The potency of heparin sodium is expressed in units. When it is given intravenously at spaced intervals, 50 mg. (5000 units) may be given at a time. For continuous drip, 100 to 200 mg. (10,000 to 20,000 units) are added to 1000 ml. of 5% sterile glucose solution or to isotonic saline solution and the flow started at about 20 to 25 drops per minute.

Subcutaneous injections of 10,000 to 12,000 units every 8 hours or 14,000 to 20,000 units every 12 hours are also acceptable. Different injection sites should be used to avoid producing a massive hematoma.

Intramuscular injection of heparin in a slowly absorbed medium repository form has been recommended, and this does reduce the frequency of the injections to one every 48 hours. Dosage for the repository form is 20,000 to 40,000 units. There are accompanying disadvantages, however. The injections may be painful and the absorption may not be even, so that sometimes there is inadequate heparinization and at other times an excessive effect may be obtained. Nurses need to check the injection site carefully because of the possibility that a local hematoma will develop, which may result in tissue slough.

Heparin antagonist—protamine sulfate injection, U.S.P., B.P.

Protamine sulfate is a protein-like substance derived from the sperm and mature testes of the salmon and other fish. Protamine by itself is an anticoagulant and will cause prolongation of clotting time; it is an antithromboplastin but is not as active as heparin. When protamine is given in the presence of heparin, they are attracted to each other instead of to the blood elements, and each neutralizes the anticoagulant activity of the other. Because it is a basic protein (many free amino groups), it is able to combine with the sulfuric acids of heparin and inactivate them.

Uses. Protamine is used as a heparin antagonist to combat the bleeding tendency from an overdosage of heparin.

When given intravenously to treat the bleeding tendency resulting from an overdose of heparin, protamine acts almost instantaneously, and its effects persist for about 2 hours. Its availability is therefore essential for safe management of a patient having anticoagulant therapy with heparin. It has been used experimentally to treat certain bleeding states believed to be characterized by increased amounts of heparin or heparin-like substances in the circulation.

Preparation, dosage, and administration. Protamine sulfate is administered intravenously and, occasionally, intramuscularly. In the treatment of overdosage of heparin, the extent of the overdosage can be determined from the amount of heparin given over the previous 3 or 4 hours; the amount of protamine needed is approximately equal to the amount of heparin over-

dosage. The commercial preparation of protamine sulfate consists of a solution containing 10 mg. in 1 ml.

COUMARIN DERIVATIVES

When cattle are allowed to eat improperly cured sweet clover, they may develop a hemorrhagic disorder believed to be caused by a deficiency of prothrombin. In 1941 Link and his associates at the University of Wisconsin were able to show that the substance responsible for the prothrombin deficiency was a coumarin derivative. These workers later synthesized dicumarol and since that time other coumarin derivatives have been synthesized. These compounds differ mainly in their speed and duration of action. (See Table 10-4, below, for comparison of various anticoagulants.)

Action and result. Although the coumarin drugs are referred to as anticoagulants, they do not appreciably affect coagulation time or bleeding time when they are administered in therapeutic amounts. Dosage is computed on the basis

Table 10-4 Comparison of various hypoprothrombinogenic agents

Generic name	Trade name	Peak effect	Recovery	Average initial dose	Average maintenance dose	Route of administration
Acenocoumarol	Sintrom	24 to 48 hr.	48 hr.	16 to 28 mg.	2 to 10 mg.	Oral
Anisindione	Miradon	36 to 72 hr.	24 to 72 hr.	300 mg.	50 to 100 mg.	Oral
Dicumarol	—	24 to 72 hr.	7 to 9 days	200 to 300 mg.	25 to 100 mg.	Oral
Diphenadione	Dipaxin	48 hr.	20 days	20 to 30 mg.	2.5 to 5 mg.	Oral
Ethyl biscoumacetate	Tromexan	18 to 24 hr.	48 hr.	1.5 to 1.8 Gm.	0.6 to 0.9 Gm.	Oral
Phenindione	Danilone Hedulin Eridone	18 to 24 hr.	24 to 48 hr.	200 to 300 mg.	50 to 100 mg.	Oral
Phenprocoumon	Liquamar	36 to 48 hr.	7 to 14 days	20 to 30 mg.	0.75 to 6 mg.	Oral
Warfarin sodium	Coumadin Sodium Panwarfarin	12 to 18 hr.	5 to 7 days	10 to 50 mg.	2.5 to 10 mg.	Oral Intramuscular Intravenous

of the plasma prothrombin time. Decreased prothrombin activity seems to act as a deterrent to intravascular clotting. Adequate and safe therapy therefore depends in part on accurate determinations of the patient's plasma prothrombin time.

Coumarin derivatives are prothrombin depressants, and they depress hepatic synthesis of factors II, VII, IX, and X. These agents probably compete with vitamin K, which functions enzymatically in the clotting process.

Vitamin K and a coumarin compound like dicumarol show similarity of structure, as indicated in the accompanying formulas. This has led to the supposition that the coumarin compounds act as competitors to prevent the utilization of vitamin K by the liver. Thus, the antagonist to the anticoagulant effect of coumarin agents is vitamin K.

Dicumarol

Menadione (vitamin K)

Uses. Coumarin derivatives are the drugs of choice for long-term anticoagulant therapy to protect against sudden acute arterial occlusion or thromboembolic phenomena from any predisposing factor that may cause loss of limb or life. They are the drugs of choice for recurrent phlebitis, chronic occlusive arterial disease, and myocardial infarction.

Major advantages of these drugs are: (1) they are effective with oral administration, (2) they are inexpensive, and (3) they need be given only once a day when the maintenance dose has been established.

However, coumarin drugs depress factors other than prothrombin, and this may account for unexplained bleeding at "safe" levels of prothrombin. Since it is impractical to measure each factor separately, and since it is not known which factor when excessively depressed results in bleeding, Quick's prothrombin test remains the standard test in most clinical laboratories. Prothrombin time is usually maintained at a "safe" level of 35 to 60 seconds, or 15% to 30% of normal.

Dicumarol, U.S.P.

Official preparations of dicumarol are available in 25-, 50-, and 100-mg. tablets and also in capsules. It is administered orally. The usual initial dose is 200 to 300 mg. daily. Subsequent dosage for a day or two depends on the prothrombin time of the patient and may vary from 50 to 200 mg. Some authorities attempt to keep prothrombin activity between 10% and 30% of normal and others between 15% and 25% of normal. In most patients, 25 to 50 mg. daily are required as maintenance doses. Dosage is determined not only by the prothrombin time but also by the direction in which it is changing. Dicumarol requires 24 to 72 hours for its action to develop, and its action persists 24 to 72 hours after its administration is discontinued.

Ethyl biscoumacetate, N.F. (Tromexan)

This synthetic derivative of dicumarol produces a similar anticoagulant action. It is available in 150- and 300-mg. tablets for oral administration. Its action and uses are similar to those of dicumarol, but it is more rapidly absorbed, acts over a shorter period of time, is detoxified and excreted faster, and has less cumulative effect than dicumarol. Average initial dose for a 24-hour period is 1.5 Gm. given at one time or in divided dosage. Subsequent doses of 600 to 900 mg. per day are usual, but maintenance dosage is regulated by determinations of prothrombin activity. This compound is more expensive than dicumarol.

Warfarin sodium, U.S.P.
(Coumadin Sodium, Panwarfin)

Warfarin sodium is available in 5-, 10-, and 25-mg. tablets for oral administration and as a powder from which a solution is made for injection (intravenous and intramuscular). Its action is more rapid than that of dicumarol and is more prolonged. The initial oral and intravenous dose is 25 to 50 mg., then 5 to 10 mg. daily, depending on prothrombin activity.

Acenocoumarol (Sintrom)

Acenocoumarol is a synthetic coumarin type of anticoagulant. Its action is faster than that of dicumarol but less rapid than that of ethyl biscoumacetate. It is available in 4-mg. tablets for oral administration. The initial dose is 16 to 28 mg. on the first day of therapy followed by 8 to 16 mg. on the second day. The average maintenance dose is 2 to 10 mg. daily, depending on the response of the patient as measured by frequent determinations of the prothrombin time.

PHENINDIONE DERIVATIVES
Phenindione, B.P. (Danilone, Hedulin, Eridone)

Phenindione is a synthetic anticoagulant similar in action to dicumarol but unrelated chemically. It acts more promptly than dicumarol and in smaller doses. Therapeutic levels are obtained within 18 to 24 hours usually, and prothrombin time usually returns to normal 24 to 48 hours after administration of the drug has been discontinued.

This drug may produce an orange or reddish discoloration of the urine that patients may mistake for hematuria. Phenindione is administered orally in initial doses of 200 to 300 mg.; one half is given in the morning and one half at bedtime. Continued dosage is adjusted as determinations of prothrombin activity indicate.

Periodic examinations of the blood, liver, and kidneys have been recommended because this drug has been known to cause agranulocytosis and hepatic and renal damage.

Diphenadione, N.F. (Dipaxin)

Diphenadione is closely related to phenindione and is one of the most potent and long-acting depressants of prothrombin activity. It is therefore effective in smaller doses than most oral anticoagulants. The initial dose is 20 to 30 mg. orally, followed by 10 to 15 mg. on the second day. Subsequent dosage is determined in accordance with the prothrombin time. The precautions to be observed for these drugs are much the same as those for the coumarin derivatives.

EFFECTIVE ANTICOAGULANT THERAPY

Both heparin and coumarin derivatives are important anticoagulants. They can be used to complement each other. In some instances the administration of both heparin and one of the synthetic anticoagulants such as dicumarol is started simultaneously. The heparin is discontinued as soon as the prothrombin activity has been sufficiently reduced and the coumarin compound is producing a full therapeutic effect. Heparin is needed when rapid anticoagulant effect is required or when adequate facilities for determining the prothrombin time are not available (this prevents the use of one of the synthetic anticoagulants).

In certain conditions when a rapid but not immediate anticoagulant effect is desired, dicumarol and ethyl biscoumacetate are given together on the first day of therapy and only the former drug is given on successive days.

NURSING MEASURE FOR PATIENTS ON ANTICOAGULANT DRUG THERAPY

The following are aspects of care for patients taking anticoagulant drugs.

1 Patients should be observed for bleeding
   a. Nosebleeds or bleeding gums

b. Petechiae, purpura, or ecchymotic areas
c. Blood in urine or stools
2 Patients on anticoagulant therapy should be instructed to carry an identification card that lists the patient's and physician's names and phone numbers and the name and dosage of drug.
3 Dietary factors, especially the ingestion of fat, are associated with increased tendency to thrombosis. It may be of benefit to advise the patient of a diet with moderate to low fat content. The relationship between high fat content and thrombosis has not been proved, however.
4 Patients should be advised to protect themselves from injury.
5 When heparin is used, blood should be drawn for clotting time when heparin activity is least, just before another injection of heparin is to be given.
6 Vitamin K should be readily accessible if bleeding occurs. Outpatients should carry vitamin K with them, and 5 to 20 mg. should be taken at once if bleeding occurs. Statistics show that bleeding occurs in approximately 10% of all patients on long-term anticoagulant therapy. However, fatalities are rare.
7 Patients on long-term therapy must be instructed to take their medication *as prescribed* and to report without fail for their blood tests. Cooperation of the patient is important for safe and effective anticoagulation therapy. Some physicians do not advocate long-term anticoagulant therapy for unreliable patients—those patients who do not eat properly, go on alcoholic binges, do not take their medicine as directed, and do not report for the test of their prothrombin activity (prothrombin time) as they have been directed to do.

ANTILIPEMIC AGENTS

From both clinical and experimental studies there is evidence that an important relationship exists between atherosclerosis and high levels of circulating blood lipids or fats (glycerides, phospholipids, and cholesterol). Atherosclerosis is a causative factor in coronary artery disease and myocardial infarction, in cerebral arterial disease that results in senility or cerebral vascular accidents, in peripheral arterial occlusive disease (which may cause gangrene and loss of limb), and in renal arterial insufficiency. It is also a factor in hypertension. Therefore there is intensive research to develop antilipemic drugs. If serum lipid levels could be controlled within normal limits, the development and progression of atherosclerosis might be inhibited or prevented.

That a positive relationship exists between high serum lipid levels and atherosclerosis is controversial; some individuals with high serum lipid levels have no objective evidence of atherosclerosis, while others with marked atherosclerotic signs and symptoms have normal serum lipid levels. However, more persons with high blood lipid levels have atherosclerosis than those with so-called normal blood lipid levels. Consequently, some researchers and clinicians believe that if lipid levels can be controlled, so can the atherosclerotic process. At the present time the available antilipemic drugs are also controversial, and their place in drug therapy requires more long-term critical studies. None of the antilipemic drugs is thought to have any effect on reversing the atherosclerotic process once it has begun. Means of preventing atherosclerosis remain obscure. Multicausative factors are undoubtedly involved and include dietary saturated fats, faulty fat metabolism, genetic influence, and other factors as yet unknown.

Clofibrate, U.S.P., B.P. (Atromid)

Clofibrate is a preparation of p-chlorophenoxyisobutyric acid. It is particularly effective in lowering serum triglycerides, serum cholesterol, and phospholipids. The exact mode of action of clofibrate is unknown, but the drug appears to block the synthesis of blood lipids. It is administered orally in doses of 500 mg. three or four times daily. Several weeks or even 2 or more months of therapy are required before the serum lipid level is reduced to the desirable level. Clofibrate has also been shown to enhance the action of anticoagulants. Side effects reported include nausea, abdominal discomfort, urticaria, abnormal liver function tests, and alopecia. Further clinical trials are necessary before the role of clofibrate in the control of atherosclerosis can be determined.

Cholestyramine resin, U.S.P. (Cuemid, Questran)

Cholestyramine is a chloride salt of a quaternary ammonium anion exchange resin. In the intestinal lumen it exchanges chloride ions for bile acids. Since the resin and the bile acids bound to the resin are nonabsorbable, there is increased fecal excretion of bile acids. To compensate for this loss of bile acids, the body increases the rate of oxidation of cholesterol to convert the sterol to bile acids. This in turn lowers serum cholesterol levels.

Cholestyramine was originally introduced for the treatment of pruritus associated with biliary stasis. It is now used clinically in the treatment of some types of hyperlipidemia.

Preparation, dosage, and administration. Cholestyramine is available as a powder for oral administration. The powder should be mixed with fruit juice, soup, milk, water, or pureed fruit prior to administration and given with the patient's meal. Adult dosage is 3.33 to 4 Gm. given three or four times daily. It should not be given simultaneously with other drugs, particularly acid drugs such as aspirin, because of its ability to bind acids. A period of 1 to 4 hours should intervene between the administration of cholestyramine and other oral medications.

Side effects. Side effects from cholestyramine include nausea, vomiting, constipation, diarrhea, and skin reactions. Bleeding tendencies have been noted during prolonged treatment with cholestyramine. This effect is thought to be caused by hypoprothrombinemia associated with vitamin K deficiency. It is recommended that fat-soluble vitamins be given intramuscularly to patients receiving cholestyramine.

Niacin, N.F.; nicotinic acid, B.P.

Nicotinic acid decreases serum lipids. Its exact mode of action is unknown. Niacin is the generic name now used for nicotinic acid.

Reductions in serum lipids have been sustained for 2 to 5 years with nicotinic acid therapy. However, with discontinuance of therapy, serum lipid levels return to pretreatment levels within 2 to 6 weeks. Resistance to nicotinic acid therapy occurs in about 25% of patients.

Preparation, dosage, and administration. Nicotinic acid is available in tablets of varying strengths for oral administration. The usual adult dose is 1 to 2 Gm. three times daily with meals.

Side effects. Numerous and often disagreeable side effects may occur from nicotinic acid. Common side effects include severe gastrointestinal upset, flushing, pruritis, nervousness, and urticaria. The drug should be used cautiously in patients with allergies and peptic ulcers since nicotinic acid causes a release of histamine and stimulates hydrochloric acid secretion. Giving the drug with meals or with antacids may reduce the incidence and severity of side effects. Prolonged treatment with niacin has resulted in hepatic disease.

Dextrothyroxine sodium, N.F. (Choloxin, D-thyroxine Sodium)

It has long been known that a definite relationship exists between thyroid function and serum cholesterol levels. Hypothyroidism is associated with high serum cholesterol levels, and administration of thyroid hormones lowers serum cholesterol. Dextrothyroxine apparently increases the rate of oxidation of cholesterol, increases biliary excretion of cholesterol, and promotes intestinal excretion of cholesterol and other lipids.

Preparation, dosage, and administration. Dextrothyroxine sodium is available in 2- and 4-mg. tablets for oral administration. The initial dose is usually 1 to 2 mg. daily, with increments of 1 to 2 mg. every 4 weeks until the desired response is obtained. Maintenance dosage usually ranges from 4 to 8 mg. daily for adults.

Side effects. Numerous side effects from dextrothyroxine have been reported. The most frequent side effects are caused by the metabolic effects of the drug and include insomnia, palpitation, tremor, loss of weight, diuresis, and menstrual irregularities. Other less common side effects include headache, dizziness, tinnitus, malaise, muscle pain, and other subjective complaints.

Precautions. Since dextrothyroxine may potentiate anticoagulant therapy, dosage of anticoagulant drugs should be decreased, prothrombin times should be determined weekly, and patients should be observed for bleeding tendencies.

Dextrothyroxine also tends to elevate blood sugar levels in diabetic persons, which necessitates increased dosage of insulin or hypoglycemic agents.

Because dextrothyroxine increases the metabolic rate, it must be used cautiously for patients with angina pectoris; the drug may precipitate attacks. An increase in incidence or severity of anginal attacks indicates need to discontinue the use of dextrothyroxine.

This drug is contraindicated for patients with advanced liver or kidney disease, hypertension, or organic heart disease and in pregnant women and nursing mothers.

QUESTIONS

For study and review

1 What do you think you need to understand about digitalis and its preparations in order to give intelligent nursing care to the patient getting the drug?

2 What special precautions would you observe and what observations would you be expected to make when caring for a patient getting digitalis for congestive heart failure?

3 What should a patient who is to be on long-term anticoagulant therapy with dicumarol have in the way of instruction before treatment is begun?

4 Explain how quinidine can cause cardiac arrest.

5 For what condition are anticoagulants used prophylactically?

6 Why are the coumarin or phenindione drugs the drugs of choice for long-term anticoagulant therapy?

7 What electrocardiographic changes would contraindicate further administration of quinidine? of procainamide? of Dilantin?

8 What instructions would you provide a patient on nitrate therapy?

9 Explain how the monoamine oxidase inhibitors effect a lowering of the blood pressure.

10 What instructions should be given to the patient who experiences orthostatic hypotension from antihypertensive therapy?

11 Under what circumstances would vasoconstrictors be used to treat hypotension accompanying shock? When would vasodilators be used?

12 Why are different drugs used in treatment of hypochromic anemia and pernicious anemia?

13 What is thought to be the role of vitamin B_{12} in the treatment of anemia? When is its use indicated rather than a preparation of iron? of folic acid?

14 Why would you encourage a patient to continue taking vitamin B_{12} when he says that he feels perfectly well and

sees no reason for spending his money this way, in spite of the fact that the doctor says he should continue taking it?

15 What is the rationale for the use of antilipemic agents? What precautions must be taken when certain antilipemic agents are used?

Multiple choice

16 Of the following, choose the *incorrect* answer:
   a. Digitalis toxicity may be caused by the drug's ability to lower potassium levels.
   b. A decrease in body sodium is responsible for digitalis toxicity.
   c. Nausea and vomiting from digitalis may result from digitalis' stimulating effect on the vomiting center in the medulla.
   d. All cardiac glycosides have the same type of effects on the heart.

17 Which of the following are the most common effects seen on the EKG tracing or monitor with therapeutic doses of digitalis?
   a. S-T segment depression
   b. P-R interval lengthening
   c. peaked P wave
   d. T wave inversion

18 Select the desired effects of digitalis on the heart.
   a. decreased vagal stimulation
   b. increased amount of energy available for myocardial contraction
   c. prolonged refractory period of the heart
   d. increased impulse formation in potential pacemakers

19 Digitalis intoxication is most likely to occur:
   a. with intravenous rather than oral administration of digitalis
   b. in patients with severely impaired heart function
   c. with rapid digitalization
   d. when diuretic agents are not used

20 The action of digitalis is enhanced by:
   a. potassium   c. sodium
   b. chloride   d. calcium

21 Longest duration of drug action occurs with:
   a. lanoxin   c. gitalin
   b. digitoxin   d. lanatoside C

22 Which one of the following does not occur in digitalis intoxication?
   a. heart block
   b. bradycardia
   c. decreased urinary output
   d. visual disturbances

23 Desirable effects of digitalis in treatment of heart failure include:
   a. increased venous pressure
   b. decreased heart size
   c. slowed conduction
   d. increased urinary output

24 Digitalization of the patient refers to:
   a. the development of early symptoms of digitalis poisoning

b. a state in which the patient is free of symptoms of heart failure

c. a state in which the failing heart is receiving maximum benefits from the digitalis preparation

d. a condition in which the heart has been slowed to normal

25 Symptoms that may indicate cumulative effects of digitoxin are:

a. marked increase in urine output

b. pulse rate below 60

c. nausea and vomiting

d. diarrhea

26 Which of the following statements about quinidine are *incorrect?*

a. Quinidine often causes ventricular arrhythmias because of its ability to depress conduction and the sinoatrial node.

b. Quinidine depresses the excitability of the heart.

c. Quinidine increases the refractory period of the heart.

d. Administration of potassium counteracts the antiarrhythmic effect of quinidine.

27 Desirable effects from quinidine include:

a. increased heart rate

b. delayed conduction of impulses

c. blocking impulses from latent pacemaker tissue

d. increasing depolarization time

28 Which of the following do not occur with the use of quinidine?

a. thrombocytopenic purpura

b. heart block

c. premature ventricular contractions

d. a lupus erythematoid reaction

29 Procainamide has which of the following actions?

a. slows conduction

b. depresses cardiac excitability

c. depresses myocardial contractility

d. has a hypertensive effect

30 Nitrites have which of the following desirable actions?

a. dilation of retinal vessels and increase of intraocular pressure

b. reduction in blood pressure from the vasodilating effect

c. decreased coronary vascular resistance

d. overcoming of decreased vascular elasticity

31 Which of the following statements about nitrites is *incorrect?*

a. Nitroglycerine is ineffective when taken orally.

b. Amyl nitrite is the most rapidly acting of the nitrites.

c. Nitroglycerine increases blood flow through the skin capillaries.

32 Which of the following statements are true?

a. Hydralazine used in combination with other antihypertensive drugs helps reduce the high incidence of toxic effects from hydralazine.

b. Hydralazine interferes with the vasoconstricting effects of norepinephrine.

c. Peripheral resistance refers to resistance of blood flow through the systemic circulation.

d. Hydralazine has a marked effect on the parasympathetic nervous system.

33 Antihypertensive drugs that lower blood pressure by depleting the body of stored norepinephrine include:

a. reserpine　　　　　c. guanethidine

b. veratrum preparations　　d. methyldopa

34 Choose the *incorrect* answer.

Veratrum preparations:

a. may cause bradycardia as a result of their vagal-stimulating ability

b. have a central emetic effect that causes nausea and vomiting

c. have a wide margin of safety

d. reduce blood pressure by reflex inhibition of vasomotor activity

35 Select the correct statement:

a. Suppressing the sympathetic nervous system also decreases the activity of the parasympathetic nervous system.

b. Dosage for antihypertensive drugs is based on the blood pressure obtained in the sitting rather than standing or lying positions.

c. Ganglionic blocking agents are the most potent antihypertensive drugs.

d. Withdrawal of antihypertensive drugs is not likely to cause a pressure rebound.

36 Repeated prothrombin time determinations are required with administration of:

a. dicumarol　　　　c. vitamin K

b. heparin　　　　　d. protamine

37 Which of the following is used to counteract the effects of dicumarol?

a. thrombin　　　　c. vitamin K

b. whole blood　　　d. protamine sulfate

38 Heparin therapy is regulated by determining the patient's:

a. prothrombin time　　c. platelet count

b. clotting time　　　d. bleeding time

39 Which of the following statements are *not* true?

a. Heparin inhibits the conversion of prothrombin to thrombin.

b. Normal blood clotting requires calcium for conversion of prothrombin to thrombin.

c. Heparin prevents agglutination of platelets.

d. Heparin is not effective in preventing clot extension.

40 The use of heparin is based on:

a. its inability to cross the placental blood barrier

b. its low toxicity

c. the ease with which vitamin K reverses its anticoagulant effects

d. the need for rapid anticoagulant action

41 Which of the following laboratory findings would indicate a favorable response of a patient to treatment with vitamin B_{12}?

a. increased hemoglobin

b. increased reticulocyte count

c. increased color index

d. increased white blood cell count

42 Which of the following preparations may produce a favorable hematopoietic response in a patient with pernicious anemia but will not arrest degenerative changes in nervous system?

    a. vitamin B_{12} **c.** liver extract
    b. folic acid   **d.** defatted hog stomach

43 Iron is best absorbed from the duodenum for which of the following reasons?
    a. The duodenum has a better absorbing surface than the rest of the bowel.
    b. The duodenal secretions are alkaline in reaction.
    c. Iron is best absorbed from an acid medium.
    d. The jejunum and ileum excrete the salts of heavy metals rather than absorb them.

44 If a patient has developed a thrombosis, which of the following drugs would you expect the physician to order first?
    a. menadione sodium bisulfite
    b. dicumarol
    c. heparin
    d. ethyl biscoumacetate (Tromexan)

REFERENCES

General

A.M.A. drug evaluations, ed. 2, Acton, Mass., 1973, Publishing Sciences Group, Inc.

Aviado, D. M.: Krantz and Carr's pharmacologic principles of medical practice, ed. 8, Baltimore, 1972, The Williams & Wilkins Co.

Bartels, C. C.: Occlusive arterial emergencies, Med. Clin. N. Am. **53:**335, 1969.

Bellet, S.: Clinical disorders of the heartbeat, ed. 3, Philadelphia, 1971, Lea & Febiger.

Brogan, E., and others: Glucagon therapy in heart failure, Lancet **1:**482, 1969.

Di Palma, J. R., editor: Drill's pharmacology in medicine, New York, 1971, McGraw-Hill Book Co.

Goodman, L. S., and Gilman, A., editors: The pharmacological basis of therapeutics, ed. 5, New York, 1975, The Macmillan Co.

Goth, A.: Medical pharmacology, ed. 7, St. Louis, 1974, The C. V. Mosby Co.

Grollman, A., and Grollman, E. F.: Pharmacology and therapeutics, ed. 7, Philadelphia, 1970, Lea & Febiger.

Hudak, W. J., and others: Cardiovascular pharmacology of perhexiline, J. Pharmacol. Exp. Ther. **173:**371, 1970.

Meyers, F. H., Jawetz, E., and Goldfien, A.: Review of medical pharmacology, ed. 4, Los Altos, Calif., 1974, Lange Medical Publications.

Modell, W., editor: Drugs of choice 1976-1977, St. Louis, 1976, The C. V. Mosby Co.

Osol, A., and Pratt, R.: The United States dispensatory, ed. 27, Philadelphia, 1973, J. B. Lippincott Co.

Prasod, K., and Callaghan, J. C.: Electrophysiologic basis of use of a polarizing solution in the treatment of myocardial infarction, Clin. Pharmacol. Ther. **12:**666, 1971.

Rodman, M. J.: Drugs used in managing cardiac emergencies, R. N. **36:**55, 1973.

Rodman, T., and others: The physiologic and pharmacologic basis of coronary care nursing, St. Louis, 1971, The C. V. Mosby Co.

Spann, J. F., Jr., et al.: Recent advances in the understanding of congestive heart failure, Mod. Con. Cardiovasc. Dis. **39:**73, 79, 1970.

Spencer, R.: Problems of drug therapy in congestive heart failure, R.N. **35:**46, 1972; Nurs. Outlook **18:**30, 1972.

Turner, P., and Richens, A.: Clinical pharmacology, Edinburgh, 1973, Churchill Livingstone.

Cardiac glycosides

Doherty, J. E.: Digitalis glycosides. Pharmacokinetics and their clinical implications, Ann. Int. Med. **79:**229, 1973.

Gould, L., and others: Clinical studies on proscillaridin, a new squill glycoside, J. Clin. Pharmacol. **11:**135, 1971.

Langer, G. A.: The mechanism of action of digitalis, Hosp. Pract. p. 49, Aug. 1970.

Ogilvie, R. I., and Ruedy, J.: An educational program in digitalis therapy, J.A.M.A. **222:**50, 1971.

Smith, T. W., and Haber, E.: Digitalis. Parts I to IV. New Eng. J. Med. **289:**945; **289:**1010; **289:**1063; **289:**1125, 1973.

Antiarrhythmic drugs

Bacaner, M.: Experimental and clinical effects of bretylium tosylate on ventricular fibrillation, arrhythmias, and heart block, Geriatrics **26:**132, 1971.

Bassett, A. L., and Hoffman, B. F.: Antiarrhythmic drugs: Electrophysiological actions, Ann. Rev. Physiol. **11:**143, 1971.

Bigger, J. T., and Mandel, W. J.: Effect of lidocaine on the electrophysiological properties of ventricular muscle and Purkinje fibers, J. Clin. Invest. **49:**63, 1970.

Bigger, J. T.: Antiarrhythmic drugs in ischemic heart disease, Hosp. Pract. p. 69, Nov. 1972.

Bloomfield, S. S., and others: Quinidine for prophylaxis of arrhythmias in acute myocardial infarction, New Eng. J. Med. **285:**979, 1971.

Davis, C. W., and Halliday, R. P.: Cardiac drugs. In Burger, A., editor: Medicinal chemistry, Part II, New York, 1970, Wiley Interscience, pp. 1065-1091.

Escher, D. J. W., and Furman, S.: Emergency treatment of cardiac arrhythmias, J.A.M.A. **214:**2028, 1970.

Fors, W. J., Vanderark, C. R., and Raynolds, E. W.: Evaluation of propanolol and quinidine in the treatment of quinidine-resistant arrhythmias, Am. J. Cardiol. **27:**190, 1971.

Fowler, N. O.: Modern treatment of cardiac arrhythmias: A perspective, Mod. Treat. **7:**13, 1970.

Gettes, L. S.: The electrophysiologic effects of antiarrhythmic drugs, Am. J. Cardiol. **28:**526, 1971.

Hayes, A. H.: The actions and clinical use of the newer antiarrhythmic drugs, Rat. Drug Ther. **6:**1, July, 1972.

Lemberg, L., and others: The treatment of arrhythmias following acute myocardial infarction, Med. Clin. N. Am. **55:**273, 1971.

Levey, G. S.: Catecholamine sensitivity, thyroid hormone and the heart, Am. J. Med. **50:**413, 1971.

Levitt, B., and others: The nervous system as a site of action for digitalis and antiarrhythmic drugs, Mt. Sinai J. Med. **37:**227, 1970.

Nevins, M. A.: Drug-pacemaker interactions, J. Thorac. Cardiovasc. Surg. **61:**610, 1971.

Rosen, M. R., and Gelband, H.: Antiarrhythmic drugs, Am. Heart J. **81:**428, 1971.

Selzer, A., and Cohn, K. E.: Treatment of ventricular extrasystoles and tachyarrhythmias in acute myocardial infarction, Ann. Rev. Physiol. **21:**47, 1970.

Wasserman, A. J., and Proctor, J. D.: Pharmacology of antiarrhythmias: Quinidine, beta blockers, diphenylhydantoin, bretylium, Med. Coll. Va. Quart. **9:**53, 1973.

Vasodilators

Aronow, W. S.: Drug therapy: Management of stable angina, New Eng. J. Med. **289:**516, 1973.

Aviado, D. M.: Sympathomimetic drugs, Springfield, Ill., 1970, Charles C Thomas, Publisher.

Bogaert, M. G., and others: Metabolism of nitroglycerin in man: Influence of phenobarbital, Arch. Int. Pharmacodyn. Ther. **192:**198, 1971.

Charlier, R.: Antianginal drugs, New York, 1971, Springer-Verlag.

Epstein, S. E., and others: Angina pectoris: Pathophysiology, evaluation and treatment, Ann. Intern. Med. **75:**263, 1971.

Haas, H.: Studies with coronary-active drugs, Brux. Med. **50:**665, 1970.

Haddy, F. J.: Pathophysiology and therapy of the shock of myocardial infarction, Ann. Intern. Med. **73:**809, 1970.

Haddy, F. J.: Physiology and pharmacology of the coronary circulation and myocardium, particularly in relation to coronary artery disease, Am. J. Med. **47:**274, 1969.

Hilger, H. H.: The influence of coronary vasodilators on coronary blood flow in man, Brux. Med. **50:**557, 1970.

Kadatz, R.: The pharmacology of coronarotropic drugs using dipyridamole as an example, Brux. Med. **50:**609, 1970.

Launchbury, A. P.: Some recently introduced drugs, Progr. Med. Chem. **7:**1, 1970.

Mason, D. T., and Amsterdam, E. A.: Action of the nitrates on the peripheral circulation and myocardial oxygen consumption: Significance in the relief of angina pectoris, Chest **59:**296, 1971.

Melville, K. I.: The pharmacological basis of antianginal drugs, Pharmacol. Phys. **4:**1, Mar. 1970.

Muller, O.: The effect of nitroglycerine and amyl nitrite on central haemodynamics in patients with coronary heart disease, Adv. Cardiol. **4:**267, 1970.

Oglesby, P.: Angina pectoris, Rat. Drug Ther. **6:**1, Dec. 1972.

Parmley, W. W., and Sonnenblick, E. H.: Glucagon: A new agent in cardiac therapy, Am. J. Cardiol. **27:**298, 1971.

Sandler, G.: Investigation of verapamil in the treatment of angina pectoris, Brux. Med. **50:**669, 1970.

Antihypertensives

Aagaard, G. M.: Treatment of hypertension, Am. J. Nurs. **73:**620, 1973.

Bourne, H. R., and Melmon, K. L.: Guides to the pharmacologic management of hypertension, Rat. Drug Ther. **5:**4, 1971.

Davis, J. O.: What signals the kidney to release renin? Circ. Res. **28:**301, 1971.

Foley, M. L.: Variations in blood pressure in the lateral recumbent position, Nurs. Res. **20:**64, 1971.

Fries, E. D.: Hypertensive crisis, J.A.M.A. **208:**338, 1969.

Fries, E. D.: Medical treatment of chronic hypertension, Mod. Conc. Cardiovasc. Dis. **40:**17, 1971.

Gilmore, H. R.: The treatment of chronic hypertension, Med. Clin. N. Am. **55:**317, 1971.

Hamilton, M.: Management of hypertension, Nurs. Mirror **132:**33, 1971.

Laverty, R.: The mechanism of action of some antihypertensive drugs, Br. Med. Bull. **29:**152, 1973.

Ledingham, J. M.: Mechanisms in renal hypertension, Proc. Roy. Soc. Med. **64:**409, 1971.

Li, D. M. P., and Bentley, G. A.: The effects of various antihypertensive drugs on the reflex responses to vasoactive substances, Eur. J. Pharmacol. **12:**24, 1970.

Rodman, M. J.: Drugs used in treating hypertension, R. N. **36:**41, 1973.

Rodman, M. J.: Managing high blood pressure, R. N. **32:**73, 1969.

Romero, J. C., and Hoobler, S. W.: The renin-angiotensin system in clinical medicine, Am. Heart J. **80:**701, 1970.

Thorn, G. W.: Approach to the patient with hypertension, Perspect. Biol. Med. **14:**578, 1971.

Vaamonde, C. A., and others: Hypertensive emergencies, Med. Clin. N. Am. **55:**325, 1971.

Antianemic or hemopoietic drugs

Castle, W. B.: Current concepts of pernicious anemia, Am. J. Med. **48:**541, 1970.

Corcino, J. J., and others: Absorption and malabsorption of vitamin B_{12}, Am. J. Med. **48:**562, 1970.

Crieghton, R. R.: Ferritin: Structure, synthesis and function, New Eng. J. Med. **284:**1413, 1971.

Erslev, A. J.: The search for erythropoietin, New Eng. J. Med. **284:**849, 1971.

Fisher, J. W.: Erythropoietin: Pharmacology, biogenesis and control of production, Pharmacol. Rev. **24:**459, 1972.

Giorgio, A. J.: Current concepts of iron metabolism and the iron deficiency anemias, Med. Clin. N. Am. **54:**1399, 1970.

Kahn, S. B.: Recent advances in the nutritional anemias, Med. Clin. N. Am. **54:**631, 1970.

Neuvonen, P. J., and others: Interference of iron with the absorption of tetracyclines in man, Br. Med. J. **4:**509, 532, 1970.

Rodman, M. J.: Drugs for treating nutritional anemias, R. N. **35:**61, 1972.

Rothman, D.: Folic acid in pregnancy, Am. J. Obstet. Gynecol. **108:**149, 1970.

Waxman, S., and others: Drugs, toxins and dietary amino acids affecting vitamin B_{12} or folic acid absorption or utilization, Am. J. Med. **48:**599, 1970.

Whole blood and its constituents (treatment of shock)

Alexander, S., and Fonad, G. A.: Treatment of cardiogenic shock, Med. Clin. N. Am. **53**:309, 1969.

Chandler, J. G.: The physiology and treatment of shock, R. N. **34**:42, 1971.

Christy, J. H.: Treatment of gram-negative shock, Am. J. Med. **50**:77, 1971.

Dietzman, R. H., and others: Drugs in the treatment of shock, Pharmacol. Phys. **4**:1, 1970.

Greenbaun, R.: The blood and transfusion fluids in shock, Int. Anesthesiol. Clin. **7**:775, 1969.

Haljamoe, H.: "Hidden" cellular electrolyte responses to hemorrhagic shock and their significance, Rev. Surg. **27**:315, 1970.

Lambert, K., and others: Pathophysiology and management of bacteremic shock, A.O.R.N.J. **10**:67, 1969.

Lefer, A. M., and Verrier, R. L.: Role of corticosteroids in the treatment of circulatory collapse states, Clin. Pharmacol. Ther. **11**:630, 1970.

Morris, D. G.: The patient in cardiogenic shock, Cardiovasc. Nurs. **5**:15, 1969.

O'Donohue, W. J., Jr.: Current concepts in the pharmacologic approach to shock, So. Med. J. **62**:1402, 1969.

Payne, J. P.: The management of shock in primitive conditions, Int. Anesthesiol. Clin. **7**:949, 1969.

Shoemaker, W. C., and others: The dilemma of vasopressors and vasodilators in the therapy of shock, Surg. Gynec. Obstet. **132**:51, 1971.

Drugs that affect blood coagulation

Anticoagulants in acute myocardial infarction: Results of a cooperative clinical trial, J.A.M.A. **225**:724, 1973.

Borden, C. W.: The current status of therapy with anticoagulants, Med. Clin. N. Am. **56**:235, 1972.

Conn, W. W., and Willis, P. W.: Some aspects of the pharmacology of oral anticoagulants, Clin. Pharmacol. Ther. **11**:312, 1970.

Deykin, D.: The use of heparin: Current concepts, New Eng. J. Med. **280**:937, 1969.

Deykin, D.: Warfarin therapy, New Eng. J. Med. **283**:691, 801, 1970.

Di Palma, J. R.: Precautions with anticoagulants, R. N. **34**:57, 1971.

Diveld, S., and Joullie, M. M.: Coagulants and anticoagulants. In Burger, A., editor: Medicinal chemistry, New York, 1970, Wiley Interscience, pp. 1092-1122.

Ebert, R. V., and others: Long-term anticoagulant therapy after myocardial infarction, J.A.M.A. **207**:2263, 1969.

Eipe, J.: Drugs affecting therapy with anticoagulants, Med. Clin. N. Am. **56**:255, 1972.

Griner, P. F., and Rickles, F. R.: Chloral hydrate and warfarin therapy, Ann. Intern. Med. **75**:142, 1971.

Koch-Weser, J., and Sellers, E. M.: Drug interactions with coumarin anticoagulants. Parts I and II, New Eng. J. Med. **285**:487; **285**:547, 1971.

Koprowicz, D. C.: Drug interactions with coumarin derivatives, Am. J. Nurs. **73**:1042, 1973.

Macon, W. L., and others: Significant complications of anticoagulant therapy, Surgery **68**:571, 1970.

Mitchell, J. R. A.: The search for an anti-thrombotic agent, Adv. Cardiol. **4**:233, 1970.

Ogston, D., and Douglas, A. S.: Anticoagulant and thrombolytic drugs, Drugs **1**:228, 1971.

O'Reilly, R. A., and others: Determinants of the response to oral anticoagulant drugs in man, Pharmacol. Rev. **22**:35, 1970.

Stormorlsen, H., and Owren, P. A.: Physiopathology of hemostasis, Semin. Hematol. **8**:3, 1971.

Tributt, D. A., and others: Comparison by controlled clinical trial of streptokinase and heparin in treatment of life-threatening pulmonary embolism, Br. Med. J. **1**:343, 1974.

Wright, I.: Anticoagulant therapy, Drug Ther., Jan. 1971.

Antilipemics

Bach, F. L.: Antilipemic agents. In Burger, A., editor: Medicinal chemistry, New York, 1970, Wiley Interscience, pp. 1123-1171.

Bagdale, J. D., and Bierman, E. L.: Diagnosis and dietary treatment of blood lipid disorders, Med. Clin. N. Am. **54**:1383, 1970.

Bricker, L. A.: A clinical approach to the hyperlipidemias, Med. Clin. N. Am. **55**:403, 1971.

Ho, K-I, and Taylor, C. B.: Control mechanisms of cholesterol biosynthesis, Arch. Pathol. **90**:83, 1970.

Lees, R. S., and Wilson, D. E.: The treatment of hyperlipidemia, New Eng. J. Med. **284**:186, 1971.

Rodman, M. J.: Drugs that reduce blood cholesterol, R. N. **32**:77, 1969.

Weiss, P.: The treatment of hyperlipidemia, Rat. Drug Ther. **6**:1, Sept. 1972.

CHAPTER 11

Central nervous system drugs

The central nervous system

Depressants

Analgesics
Hypnotics and sedatives
Alcohols
Anticonvulsant drugs

Stimulants

THE CENTRAL NERVOUS SYSTEM

Drugs act to increase or decrease the activity of nerve centers and conducting pathways. Stimulants and depressants of the brain, the spinal cord, or specific centers of each have been developed, and their effects, on the whole, are highly predictable.

Physiologically man is constituted of numerous cells that have been organized into tissues, the tissues into organs, and the organs into systems; and all of these taken as a whole provide man with his structure and vital functions. All of man's functions, from the most basic (respiration and elimination) to the most complex and highly developed (abstract reasoning and creative thought), require coordination if he is to function as a whole. The main coordinator of man's body functions is his nervous system.

The central nervous system is composed of the brain, spinal cord, and numerous nerve cells called neurons. It is often referred to as the somatic or cerebrospinal nervous system. Striated muscle (skeletal or voluntary muscle) control and the unique functions of the brain (reasoning and memory) are primary concerns of the central nervous system.

The central nervous system of man functions much like a computer. Information from the external world (such as that related to sight, sound, touch, smell, and taste) and from the internal world (such as that related to oxygen or carbon dioxide blood levels, muscle tension, and body temperature) is sent to the appropriate part of the central nervous system. The information is integrated and instructions relayed to appropriate cells or tissues to produce the necessary actions and environmental adjustments. Information concerning these actions and adjustments is again fed back into the central nervous system. The constant feeding of information into the central nervous system permits continuous adjustment to be made in the instructions sent to various tissues to ensure effective control of body functions.

THE CENTRAL NERVOUS SYSTEM AND DRUG ACTION

The *cerebral cortex* constitutes the outer layer of gray matter covering each of the two hemispheres of the brain and the four lobes into which each hemisphere is divided. These lobes

211

are named for the bones of the skull under which they lie—frontal, parietal, occipital, and temporal. The frontal lobe contains the motor and speech areas. The sensory cortex is located in the parietal lobe, the visual cortex in the occipital lobe, and the auditory cortex in the temporal lobe. Association areas lie near these areas and act in conjunction with them. In addition, large parts of the cortex are concerned with higher mental activity—reasoning, creative thought, judgment, memory—those attributes that are unique to man and separate him from other animals.

Drugs that depress cortical activity may decrease acuity of sensation and perception, inhibit motor activity, decrease alertness and concentration, and even promote drowsiness and sleep. Drugs that stimulate the cortical areas may cause more vivid impulses to be received and greater awareness of the surrounding environment. In addition increased muscle activity and restlessness may occur. The specific response brought forth by a drug depends to a large extent on the personality of the individual, his emotional and physiologic state, the specific attributes of the drug, and a host of other factors.

The *thalamus* is composed of sensory nuclei and serves as a relay center for impulses to and from the cerebral cortex. It also serves as a center of unlocalized sensations. It enables the individual to have impressions of agreeableness or disagreeableness about a sensation. Drugs that depress cells in the various portions of the thalamus may interrupt the free flow of impulses to the cerebral cortex. This is one way pain is relieved.

The *hypothalamus* lies below the thalamus and contains centers that regulate body temperature, carbohydrate and fat metabolism, water balance, and autonomic function. There is evidence that there is also a center for sleep and wakefulness here. Some of the sleep-producing drugs are thought to depress centers in the hypothalamus. The thalamus and hypothalamus constitute important regions of the brain known as the diencephalon.

The *medulla oblongata* contains the so-called vital centers, the respiratory, vasomotor, and cardiac centers. If the respiratory center is stimulated, it will discharge an increased number of nerve impulses over nerve pathways to the muscles of respiration. If it is depressed, it will discharge fewer impulses, and respiration will be correspondingly affected. Other centers in the medulla that respond to certain drugs are the cough center and the vomiting center. The medulla, pons, and midbrain constitute the brainstem and contain many important correlation centers (gray matter) as well as ascending and descending pathways (white matter).

The *reticular formation* is a part of the central nervous system that has been studied increasingly in recent years. Its importance is only beginning to be appreciated. It is made up of cells and fine bundles of nerve fibers that extend in many directions. The formation extends from the upper part of the spinal cord forward through the brainstem to the diencephalon. It exhibits both inhibitory as well as excitatory functions in relation to other parts of the nervous system. It receives afferent impulses from all parts of the body and relays impulses to the cortex to promote wakefulness and alertness, which affects many cerebral functions, such as consciousness and learning. It also inhibits or excites activity in motor neurons, promoting both reflex and voluntary movements. Its overall function is thought to be that of an integrating system that influences activities of other parts of the nervous system. Depression of the reticular formation produces sedation and loss of consciousness. Many drugs are believed to exert an effect on the reticular formation. It is particularly sensitive to certain depressant drugs, such as barbiturates and anesthetics.

The *cerebellum* contains centers for muscle coordination, equilibrium, and muscle tone. It receives afferent impulses from the vestibular nuclei as well as the cerebrum and plays an important role in the maintenance of posture. Drugs that disturb the cerebellum or vestibular branch of the eighth cranial nerve cause loss of equilibrium and dizziness.

The *spinal cord*, a center for reflex activity, also functions in the transmission of impulses to and from the higher centers in the brain and may be affected by the action of drugs. Large doses of spinal stimulants may cause convulsions; smaller doses may increase reflex excitability.

When a drug is described as having a central action, it means that it has an action on the brain or the spinal cord.

SYNAPTIC TRANSMISSION IN THE CENTRAL NERVOUS SYSTEM

There is evidence that transmission of impulses at synapses in the central nervous system is humoral. For example, it is known that some parts of the central nervous system contain acetylcholine (ACh) and acetylcholinesterase. Since acetylcholine is a known chemical transmitter of nerve impulses, it can be assumed that its presence in the central nervous system is for the purpose of transmission of nerve impulses. Not all parts of the central nervous system contain acetylcholine. Those areas that contain high concentrations are the motor cortex, thalamus, hypothalamus, geniculate bodies, and anterior spinal roots; very low concentrations are found in the cerebellum, optic nerves, and dorsal roots of the spine. Atropine blocks the action of acetylcholine and is used in treating some of the symptoms of Parkinson's disease, which is characterized by rigidity, tremors, and disturbance of voluntary and involuntary movements.

The extent and strength of muscle contractions depend on the number of motor neurons involved and the frequency with which they discharge impulses. Inhibition of motor neuron activity may be presynaptic or postsynaptic.

Studies indicate that presynaptic inhibition occurs in the brain and is widespread at the spinal level affecting transmission in afferent fibers from skin and muscle. The function of presynaptic inhibition is probably to suppress weak inputs that would otherwise cause unnecessary responses. This modulation of nerve impulses results in less transmitter substance being liberated. The net effect is a limiting or "inhibiting" of impulses to postsynaptic nerve fibers. Inhibition is important for orderly function. The convulsant drug picrotoxin is known to reduce presynaptic inhibition. Strychnine reduces postsynaptic inhibition.

Postsynaptic inhibition may be the result of changes in the membrane permeability of the postsynaptic cells caused by release of chemical transmitters from presynaptic nerve endings.

Lower motor neurons release acetylcholine at the neuromuscular junction, causing contraction in striated (voluntary) muscle. The concentration of acetylcholine must be high since a large number of muscle fibers must respond synchronously for striated muscle contraction to occur, and also because acetylcholine is very rapidly destroyed by the enzyme cholinesterase. In all likelihood this constitutes a protective mechanism for the body and prevents man from being a constantly quivering organism.

Renshaw cells are special interneurons. Nerve fibers that innervate skeletal muscle give off side branches that synapse with the Renshaw cells. These cells in turn synapse with the large anterior horn cells in the spinal cord. They are inhibitory cells and cause muscle contraction to be less vigorous and to terminate sooner than would otherwise be possible. When a motor neuron is stimulated, the Renshaw cell is also excited, thereby dampening any excessive activity in the motor neurons. The inhibitory mediator released by the Renshaw cell may be glycine.

Upper motor neurons are scattered throughout the cerebral cortex; a number of them are located in the motor cortex. About three fourths of the nerve fibers from these motor neurons cross to the opposite side at the level of the medulla, descend to the spinal cord, and synapse with interneurons, which in turn synapse with the lower motor neurons. Almost all motor neurons of one side are controlled by the motor cortex of the other side. Therefore, injury to the motor cortex of the right side causes paralysis on the left side of the body (hemiplegia). Systems other than the upper and lower motor neuron systems are concerned with voluntary movement, but lower motor neurons form the common final pathway for stimuli for voluntary movement.

Catecholamines (dopamine, norepinephrine, and epinephrine) and serotonin are synthesized, stored, and metabolized in the brain. These substances do not easily penetrate the blood-brain barrier, but their precursors do. The effect of injected catecholamines on the central nervous system is slight in comparison to the effect on the autonomic nervous system. However, an increase in catecholamines and serotonin causes cerebral stimulation. Drugs, such as reserpine, that release catecholamines and reduce amine concentration in the brain have a depressing or sedative action. Methyldopa lowers the serotonin and norepinephrine levels and this, too, has a cerebral depressing effect.

Special staining techniques indicate that there are adrenergic and serotoninergic tracts within the central nervous system. Dopamine, a catecholamine, is especially concentrated in the basal ganglia. The low level of dopamine at this site in individuals suffering from Parkinson's disease led to the new therapeutic approach of utilizing its precursor L-dopa with good results in many cases.

The blood-brain barrier prevents drug penetration to the brain and spinal cord. This has impeded both physiologic and pharmacologic research on the central nervous system. Therefore, less is known about the central nervous system than about the autonomic nervous system.

Depressants

Mild drug-induced depression of the central nervous system is frequently characterized by lack of interest in surroundings, inability to focus attention on a subject, and lack of inclination to move or talk. The pulse and respiration may become slower than usual, and as the depression deepens, acuity of all sensations such as touch, vision, hearing, heat, cold, and pain diminish progressively. Psychic and motor activities decrease; reflexes become sluggish and finally are abolished. If the depression is not checked, it progresses to unconsciousness, stupor, coma, respiratory failure, and death. Some depressant drugs, such as the general anesthetics, act upon the entire central nervous system; others, such as the anticonvulsant drugs, are more selective in their action. The depressants include the following: (1) analgesics, drugs that relieve pain; (2) hypnotics and sedatives, which produce sleep

and rest; and (3) general anesthetics, which produce loss of sensation and unconsciousness.

ANALGESICS

Analgesics are drugs that relieve pain without producing loss of consciousness and reflex activity. Physical pain is a part of a larger experience called "pain experience," which includes, in addition to the sensation of pain, all the associated emotional sensations for a particular person under particular circumstances. This accounts for the wide variation in individual response to the sensation of pain. It is known that stimuli causing pain must be more intense than those evoking other sensations. There is a strong link between pain and tissue damage.

Pain perception and response are influenced by such psychologic factors as past experience, attention, and emotion. In addition, the intensity, duration, and location of harmful stimuli also influence pain perception and response. Pain that increases rapidly in intensity (such as that accompanying acute myocardial infarction or extensive partial thickness burns) does not usually permit the individual to achieve any control over pain. Pain that is less severe with a slow rise in intensity permits the individual to exert some control over it. The latter may be achieved by the person thinking about something else or engaging in activity that diverts his attention.

There appears to be a relatively constant pain threshold for each individual. Although the pain threshold varies from individual to individual, tolerance to pain appears to be far more variable than pain threshold. For example, certain stimuli, such as heat applied to the skin at an intensity of 45° to 48° C., will initiate the sensation of pain in almost all individuals. Pain threshold is the minimum intensity of a harmful stimulus that produces the sensation of pain, while tolerance to pain refers to the point beyond which the pain can no longer be endured. There is evidence that some sensitization or adaptation to pain occurs, that is, there is a diminution of response with constant stimulation.

Action. Analgesics act in several ways: (1) by elevating the pain threshold; (2) by altering the

Morphine

Codeine
(methylmorphine)

Papaverine

attitude or mood of the patient from one of concern to one of detachment, promoting a sense of well-being or mild euphoria; and (3) by producing sedative and soporific effects.

Opium and its derivatives, related synthetic compounds, and the analgesic antipyretics, such as aspirin and phenacetin, belong to the analgesic group of drugs.

The search for an ideal analgesic continues, but it is difficult to find one that does all desired of it. It should (1) be potent, so that it will afford maximum relief of pain; (2) not cause dependence; (3) exhibit a minimum of side effects, such as constipation, respiratory depression, nausea, and vomiting; (4) not cause tolerance to develop; (5) act promptly and over a long period of time with a minimum amount of sedation, so that the patient is able to remain awake and be responsive; and (6) be relatively inexpensive. Needless to say, no present-day analgesic has all of these qualifications, and so the search continues.

NONSYNTHETIC NARCOTIC ANALGESICS—OPIATES

Opium is one of the oldest analgesics about which there is any record. Opium is described in Chinese literature written long before the time of Christ. The name comes from the Greek *opos*, meaning "juice of plants."

Opium is the hardened dried juice of the unripe seed capsules of *Papaver somniferum*, a species of poppy grown largely in China, India, Iran, Turkey, and Asia Minor. The poppy plant is indigenous to Asia Minor, and from there knowledge of opium spread to Greece and Arabia, where physicians became well versed in its use. Arabian traders were responsible for its introduction into the Orient, where it was known

as "smoking dirt." The Chinese used it chiefly to control some of the symptoms of dysentery until its cultivation was exploited for commercial reasons by European powers, and the opium habit spread through many parts of the Orient.

Paracelsus is credited with compounding the preparation "laudanum." Paregoric was first used as an elixir for asthma and was prepared by a chemistry professor at Leyden. Thomas Dover, an English physician, used the powder as a sweating agent for gout in 1732.

Opium in the crude form was used until well into the nineteenth century, before the chief alkaloid, morphine, was isolated. The discovery of other alkaloids soon followed, and their use came to be preferred to that of the crude preparations.

Composition. The active principles of opium are alkaloids, of which there are some twenty in number, although only three are used widely in the practice of medicine—morphine, codeine, and papaverine.

The alkaloids of opium belong to two distinct classes. Morphine and codeine belong to the phenanthrene group, and papaverine is known as a benzylisoquinoline derivative. This helps to explain why papaverine has a much different effect in the body from other alkaloids. Papaverine has little effect on the nervous system but produces relaxation of certain smooth muscles in the body. (See Table 11-1.) Morphine and codeine act mainly on the central nervous system, where they produce a combination of depressing and stimulating effects. Both promote contraction of smooth muscle, especially muscle in organs of the gastrointestinal tract.

The alkaloids form 25% of the active constituents of opium; the rest are such substances as gums, oils, resins, and proteins.

Table 11-1 Selected effects of opiates

	Morphine	Codeine	Dilaudid	Papaverine
Potency of analgesic action	Potent	One-sixth to one-tenth that of morphine	Ten times more potent than morphine	None
Effects Respiration	Markedly depressed Carbon dioxide retention	Depression one-fourth that of morphine	Like morphine	None or slight bronchial relaxation
Gastrointestinal	Decreased activity, spasm, and constipation	Like morphine but less prominent	Like morphine but less constipating	Relaxes
Biliary	Increased intrabiliary pressure Possibility of spasm	Less intense spasms than from morphine	Like codeine	Relaxes
Genitourinary Ureters	Possibility of spasms Increased tone, decreased motility	Increased tone, decreased motility	Like morphine	Relaxes
Bladder	Increased sphincter tone Retention of urine	Increased tone, decreased motility	Like morphine	Relaxes
Uterus	Tone increased Contractions decreased	Not significant	Like morphine	None
Eyes	Pupil constriction	Less than morphine	Like morphine	None
Cerebral	Stimulation of vomiting center—nausea and vomiting Depressed cough center Cortical sedation Rise in pain threshold Euphoria	Less than morphine Large doses required to produce euphoria	Less than morphine	None

Action and result of opium and morphine. The effects of opium result chiefly from the morphine that it contains; therefore, the two preparations will be considered together.

Cerebrum. Morphine exerts a narcotic* action

---

*The word *narcotic* can be confusing because it is used in at least three different ways: (1) a central nervous system depressant, (2) a dependence-producing drug, and (3) a drug that may be neither of these but that may come under the restrictions of the federal narcotic law (Controlled Substances Act). In this chapter the term *narcotic* will be used to mean a depressant of the central nervous system with dependence-producing properties.

which results in analgesia and sleep. Morphine elevates the mood, causing euphoria in many patients, relieves fear and apprehension, and produces feelings of peace and tranquility. Its pronounced dependence liability is explained by its ability to cause a relatively intense euphoric state. Prolonged concentration becomes difficult, and the patient becomes apathetic, with a slowing of both mental and physical activities. The exact mode of action is still not known. The most outstanding effect of morphine is relief of pain. This is highly specific because pain may be effectively relieved without affecting other sensations appreciably. Continuous dull pain is more effectively relieved than sharp intermittent pain. It is especially effective for visceral pain, although when used in large enough doses it will abolish almost all forms of pain.

Morphine continues to be the most valuable analgesic in medicine, and ordinarily a nurse does not need to fear morphine dependence in a patient who is receiving the drug over a short period for severe pain.

In small doses morphine seems to have little or no effect on the motor areas of the brain. The diminished restlessness is probably caused by the drowsiness and sleep that is produced.

Brainstem and hypothalamus. Morphine has a highly selective action on the respiratory center. Doses that have little or no effect on other parts of the brain will depress respiration, causing a decrease in rate and minute volume, retention of carbon dioxide, and decreased sensitivity to carbon dioxide's stimulating effects. Toxic doses cause slow shallow respiration. Death from poisoning is caused by respiratory failure. Therapeutic doses of morphine and related alkaloids have little or no effect on the medullary centers concerned with blood pressure, heart rate, or rhythm.

Morphine acts as a miotic—it constricts the pupil of the eye. The exact mechanism or site of action is not clear, although there seems to be agreement that the action is central with an effect on the oculomotor nerve, since instillation of morphine in the eye does not cause miosis. Tolerance to this effect of morphine does not develop. In poisoning, pupils become pinpoint in size. It is believed that this is caused at least partly by increased sensitivity of the pupil to light, although pupil constriction occurs even in darkness.

After administration of morphine the cough center is depressed and coughing is relieved. Morphine and related compounds will abolish the cough reflex, but codeine is the drug of choice for this effect since it is less likely to cause respiratory depression and dependence.

The heat-regulating center is slightly depressed after therapeutic doses of morphine. Reduction of body temperature may be caused in part by this effect, but it is also caused by increased perspiration, decreased physical activity, and increased loss of heat because of peripheral vasodilation.

Nausea and vomiting may occur after administration of morphine and related alkaloids. This is thought to be caused by stimulation of a chemoreceptor emetic trigger zone in the medulla. Patients who remain in a recumbent position have nausea and vomiting less often than patients who are ambulatory.

Spinal cord. There is evidence that in laboratory animals morphine may stimulate the spinal cord to the extent that convulsive seizures result. In man the action of morphine on the spinal cord is complex. There is some spinal stimulation, but the depressant action of morphine on higher centers prevents a convulsive reaction at the cord level. Morphine may also exert an indirect suppression of spinal reflexes.

Cardiovascular system. Toxic amounts of morphine or related alkaloids are required to produce significant changes in heart rate and blood pressure. With large doses of morphine, the T wave of the electrocardiogram may be depressed or inverted, which may interfere with electrocardiographic interpretations of patients with suspected myocardial infarctions. This is important to remember since these patients often receive large doses of morphine to reduce chest pain, anxiety, and restlessness.

Changes that occur after therapeutic doses are believed to be the result of decreased physical activity and sleep. Toxic amounts will stimulate the vagal center and depress the vasomotor center, causing a lowering of blood pressure and a slowing of the heart rate. Diminished oxygen to the brain greatly contributes to the hypotension that develops in morphine intoxication. Therapeutic doses of morphine will produce relaxation of small blood vessels in the face, neck, and upper chest, making the patient feel flushed and warm. Sweating is common. Itching of the nose is frequently observed and is thought to be caused by histamine release. It indicates an allergic reaction and need for a different drug.

Gastrointestinal tract (smooth muscle and glands). Many of the effects of morphine on the gastrointestinal tract are probably the result of morphine's preventing the release of mediators from nerves innervating the smooth muscle of the gastrointestinal tract.

In general, glandular activity throughout the length of the alimentary tract is diminished. Gastric, biliary, and pancreatic secretions are decreased, and the digestion of food in the small intestine is hindered. The tone of smooth muscle in the sphincters is increased, and this delays the emptying of the stomach and small intestine. Although the nonpropulsive type of rhythmic contractions in the intestine are increased, propulsive peristalsis is decreased and a type of spasm has frequently been observed. The tendency to increased tone extends also to the biliary ducts and the sphincter of Oddi. The defecation reflex is depressed as a result of diminished sensitivity of the bowel and rectum and increased tone and spasticity of the muscle of the large bowel.

Many of the actions mentioned explain why patients receiving opiates, and especially morphine, are prone to develop gas pains, constipation, and sometimes abdominal distention. The stomach empties more slowly, peristalsis fails to keep the intestinal contents moving, water continues to be absorbed from the intestinal content, and the feces gradually become hardened. When the rectum does fill, there is little or no inclination to empty it. Decreased peristaltic activity may give rise to local accumulation of gas, which causes a painful stretching of the intestine. These effects are observed particularly in the postoperative patient who has had not only several doses of morphine but also an anesthetic and one or more doses of a sedative.

The effect of morphine on the smooth muscle of the gastrointestinal organs also explains why morphine does not always alleviate the pain and distress in these organs when, for some reason, the muscle already has become hypertonic. The presence of a stone in the common bile duct may cause the muscle of the duct to contract painfully, and this may be intensified rather than relieved by the effect of morphine, unless the dose of morphine is large enough to make the analgesic effect more pronounced than the effect on the smooth muscle.

These effects also help to explain the kind of diet that should be given to a patient who has had morphine. It is obvious that the patient is not likely to have either the inclination or ability to enjoy or digest a full meal. Tolerance to the effects of morphine on the gastrointestinal muscle develop slowly if at all.

The papaverine group of alkaloids differs in their effect on the muscle of the gastrointestinal tract in that they produce relaxation.

Genitourinary tract. The tone of the muscle in the ureters and the detrusor muscle of the urinary bladder is said to be affected much the same as the tone of the muscle in the gastrointestinal organs. Increased tone in the sphincter muscle of the bladder may contribute to difficulty in urination. In addition there is decreased perception of the stimulus to void. This sometimes explains a patient's inability to void and the need for catheterization. Morphine also releases the antidiuretic hormone and therefore has an antidiuretic effect. This is an important factor to keep in mind when checking the patient's urinary output.

Other smooth muscle. Morphine promotes contraction of the bronchial musculature, but this effect is significant only in persons subject to allergic reactions and asthma. Allergic reactions to morphine and related alkaloids are said to be rather common. Morphine may release histamine.

Although there seems to be no direct action of morphine on uterine muscle, normal labor may be delayed because of central depression, and the respiration of both the mother and the child will be depressed.

Therapeutic uses and the natural alkaloids. Morphine is used primarily as an analgesic for control of severe pain. It should not be used if other analgesics will suffice, but when pain is severe, the narcotic analgesics have no rival. When morphine is given to a patient who is already in severe pain, the chief effect seems to be that the patient's emotional reaction to the pain is altered. He is no longer afraid of the pain or thrown into a panic because of it. If the nurse asks such a patient about his condition half an hour or so after he has been given a hypodermic of morphine, he is likely to say: "I still have pain, but I can stand it."

If morphine is given before the patient begins to experience pain, its effect seems to be somewhat different; a better blocking of the pain impulses occurs and the patient may experience no pain. This explains why, on the first or possibly the second postoperative day, a patient should not be allowed to wait until he is in full pain if the greatest analgesic effect of morphine is to be achieved.

In surgical conditions in which the alleviation of severe pain may make diagnosis more difficult and lead to undue delay in operating, morphine should not be used or it should be employed only in very small doses and with great caution. It should not be used in chronic conditions in which there is pain, since prolonged administration is almost certain to result in dependence. Exceptions to this rule are to be found in cases of inoperable cancer in which the patient cannot recover and may be spared much unnecessary suffering by its use. The administration of a drug such as chlorpromazine or promethazine can be used to potentiate the action of morphine and reduce the amount of morphine needed. Morphine is not recommended for the relief of pain in persons of neurotic or hysteric temperaments unless its use is absolutely necessary.

Ordinarily, morphine or related alkaloids are not given to produce sleep unless sleeplessness is caused by pain or dyspnea. There are conditions in which the relief of restlessness and apprehension is essential, such as the patient suffering from a myocardial infarction.

Morphine is used to check peristalsis in conditions such as hemorrhage and severe diarrhea and after surgery on the stomach and bowel. Preparations of opium are prescribed more often than morphine to check diarrhea because of opium's slow absorption and effect on smooth muscle.

Morphine is frequently used as premedication prior to the administration of a general anesthetic to relieve apprehension and facilitate induction.

Codeine is the opiate of choice in relieving a cough because it effectively depresses the cough center and is less likely to produce dependence than morphine.

Tolerance. Different individuals require varying periods of time before the repeated administration of opium derivatives fails to have the effect that it originally produced. This condition is known as tolerance. A patient who suffers considerable pain may be relieved at first by 15 mg. (gr. $^1/_4$) of morphine, but if the painful condition persists, the time will come when he requires an ever-increasing dose to experience the same relief. The person who has developed tolerance may eventually take doses that would have caused death if given as an initial dose. Tolerance does not develop uniformly—tolerance is developed to the hypnotic, analgesic, and respiratory depressant effects of opiates but not to their effects on the pupil of the eye and on the gastrointestinal muscle. Tolerance develops faster when the dosage is administered regularly and is large and may occur after 2 weeks of repeated administration. The exact mechanism of action whereby tolerance develops is not known.

Side effects. Side effects may include one or more of the following.

Nausea and vomiting may be caused by pronounced stimulating effects on the vomiting center. These effects may be counteracted by some phenothiazine derivatives, but these drugs should not be given in the presence of hypotension, since they will augment it.

Constipation may outlast the analgesic effect. Cathartics and enemas are frequently required. *Urinary retention* may require catheterization.

Postural hypotension with dizziness and faintness may occur. These patients should be instructed to arise or change positions slowly to allow compensatory mechanisms to become effective. These symptoms may not occur if the patient remains recumbent.

Depression of respiration and coughing tends to result in retained secretions and predisposition to atelectasis. Coughing and deep breathing should be encouraged in these patients. Mechanical assistance with intermittent positive pressure breathing (IPPB) may be necessary to promote adequate respiratory excursions.

Behavioral changes, such as increased restlessness and excitement, tremors, delirium, and insomnia, may occur. These usually require use of a different analgesic.

Allergic reactions, which include urticaria, skin rash, itching (itching of the nose is a common occurrence), or activation of other allergic phenomena such as asthma, may occur in the allergic individual. In these cases the drug should be discontinued and another analgesic substituted.

Contraindications. Because of its depressant effect on respiration, its tendency to increase intracranial pressure, and its tendency to make the patient less responsive, morphine is contraindicated or used cautiously for patients with head injuries and for patients who have had a craniotomy performed. Other persons for whom it may not be indicated are those with bronchial asthma, hypertrophy of the prostate gland, or stricture of the urethra (because of the effect on smooth muscle). Morphine is also contraindicated in acute alcoholism and in convulsive disorders, and it must be used with caution for patients with inadequate oxygen–carbon dioxide exchange.

Acute poisoning. Poisoning with opium or morphine occurs from overdoses taken as a medicine or with suicidal intent. As a rule, the toxic dose of morphine for the adult who is not in pain is about 60 mg. (gr. 1), and the lethal dose is approximately 250 mg. (gr. 4). Death may come within the hour after ingestion of a fatal dose, or the patient may linger for 6 to 12 hours. The longer the patient lives, the better his chances for recovery since the drug is being destroyed and excreted and restorative measures can be instituted. The nurse is often in a position to detect the early symptoms of poisoning.

Symptoms begin with depression, which progresses into a deep sleep from which the patient at first is easily aroused; then it becomes increasingly difficult to arouse him (stupor); and finally he cannot be aroused at all (coma). A significant early symptom of overdosage is slow respirations (10 to 12 per minute). In advanced poisoning the respirations may be 2 to 4 per minute, and Cheyne-Stokes breathing may be observed. Death usually results from asphyxia brought on by a developing respiratory failure; hence, this condition becomes a focal point toward which therapy must be directed. The pupils of the eyes are at first constricted, later they become pinpoint sized, and as the asphyxia deepens, the pupils dilate. The patient, as a rule, perspires freely and increasingly as poisoning advances. In early stages the skin is warm as well as moist, and the color is fairly normal, but later the body temperature falls and the skin feels cold and clammy and appears cyanotic or gray. The heart action is not much affected at first, but later the pulse becomes weak and irregular. The blood pressure is usually maintained near normal until the lack of oxygen becomes pronounced and shock develops.

Figure 11-1

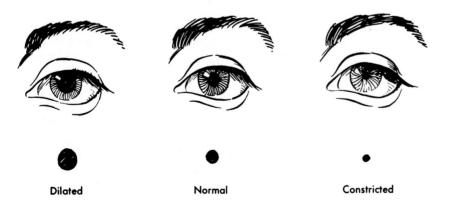

Salts of morphine produce constriction of the pupil. Pinpoint pupils occur only in advanced states of poisoning.

Dilated   **Normal**   **Constricted**

The symptoms of poisoning that the nurse should regard as particularly significant are slow respirations (fewer than 12 per minute), deep sleep, and constricted pupils. Further doses of morphine should be withheld when these symptoms appear and the patient carefully watched to prevent development of more serious symptoms. If a toxic dose has already been taken, however, prompt treatment is necessary to save the patient's life. Attention must be focused on respiration. The older respiratory stimulants have been replaced by the morphine antagonists, which give very good results. (See the discussions on nalorphine hydrochloride, levallorphan tartrate, and naloxone later in this chapter.) Artificial respiration should be given without delay if breathing has become dangerously slow.

Treatment is directed toward elimination of the poison from the body. If the drug has been taken orally, the stomach should be emptied. Repeated lavage, however, is not recommended. Tannic acid or dilute potassium permanganate solution (1:2000) may be used to wash out the stomach, since these agents attack alkaloids chemically and thereby inactivate them. Strong black coffee, as hot as may be given with safety, may be administered by tube, by mouth, and also by rectum. Additional measures consist largely of keeping the patient awake, as warm and dry as possible, and by changing the patient's position frequently to prevent development of hypostatic pneumonia. Prolonged stupor also requires that attention be given to food intake, fluids, and bladder distention. Measures that uselessly exhaust the patient should be avoided.

Opium

The following are the preparations of whole opium drugs.

Opium tincture, B.P. (Laudanum). The usual dose is 0.6 ml. (10 minims) and the range of dosage 0.25 to 2 ml. It is used to check intestinal peristalsis. It contains approximately 10 mg. of morphine per milliliter.

Paregoric, U.S.P.; *camphorated opium tincture*, B.P. The usual dose is 5 ml. and range of dosage 5 to 10 ml. This is a 1:250 solution of opium together with benzoic acid, camphor, oil of anise, glycerin, and diluted alcohol. Paregoric is given to check intestinal peristalsis to relieve diarrhea. It contains approximately 0.4 mg. of morphine per milliliter. It has a very bitter taste. It must be stored in light-resistant, air-tight containers away from heat.

The foregoing preparations of whole opium must be given by mouth and are not suited to parenteral injection. This is partly because the two tinctures contain alcohol and because preparations of whole opium contain resins and other substances that are not readily soluble in water and tissue fluids.

Opium and belladonna suppositories. These are no longer official preparations, but they continue to be prescribed for the analgesic action of opium and the antispasmodic effect of belladonna. Some physicians prescribe them for relief of painful hemorrhoids and for patients who have had a transurethral resection. The usual dose is one suppository inserted rectally every 3 to 4 hours. Each suppository contains 65 mg. (gr. 1) of opium and 8 mg. (gr. $\frac{1}{8}$) of belladonna in a suitable base.

Morphine

Morphine sulfate, U.S.P., B.P. Morphine sulfate is available as tablets, capsules, and a solution for injection in vials or ampules. The injection form may also contain atropine or scopolamine. The usual dose is 10 mg. (gr. $\frac{1}{6}$); the range of dosage is 5 to 15 mg. (gr. $\frac{1}{12}$ to $\frac{1}{4}$).

Morphine hydrochloride, B.P. The usual dose is 15 mg. (gr. $\frac{1}{4}$); the range of dosage is 8 to 20 mg. (gr. $\frac{1}{8}$ to $\frac{1}{3}$). However, investigators are of the opinion that 10 mg. (gr. $\frac{1}{6}$) per 70 kg. of body weight comes closer to being an optimal dose for both morphine sulfate and morphine hydrochloride. Larger doses may be needed sometimes, but they are associated with a higher incidence of untoward effects. The action and uses of these two salts are the same.

Morphine is readily absorbed after subcutaneous or intramuscular injection; more than half the drug is absorbed within 30 minutes after injection. Onset of action occurs within 5 to 10 minutes, a euphoric action (pleasant drowsiness, freedom from anxiety and fear) occurs within 30 minutes, and peak action (rise in pain threshold) or maximum analgesic action occurs in 60 to 90 minutes. Actual increase in the pain threshold may last only a few hours, but the decreased emotional reaction to pain may permit the patient to endure the pain for 4 to 6 hours or more. This, of course, depends upon the patient's reaction to the drug, dosage given, and severity of pain. About 90% of the drug is excreted in the urine within 24 hours. The drug is inactivated by the liver.

Morphine may be given orally, and onset of action then occurs in 10 to 15 minutes. However, since absorption from the gastrointestinal tract is highly variable, this route is less dependable for therapeutic effectiveness and is seldom used.

Morphine may be given intravenously; peak action occurs in 5 minutes. The drug must be administered slowly to avoid severe reactions in patients with hypersensitivity to morphine.

Dosage for children is 0.1 to 0.2 mg. per kilogram of body weight given subcutaneously.

Morphine injection, U.S.P., B.P. This is a sterile solution of a suitable salt of morphine in water for injection.

Codeine

Codeine phosphate injection, U.S.P., B.P.; *codeine phosphate tablets,* U.S.P., B.P. The usual dose is 30 mg. (gr. $1/_2$); the range of dosage, 15 to 60 mg. (gr. $1/_4$ to 1). After subcutaneous injection peak effect is reached in 30 to 60 minutes; duration of effect is 3 to 4 hours. Codeine is a natural alkaloid of opium, but it is made from morphine. Codeine sulfate, N.F., is like the phosphate, except that it is less soluble in water. Codeine is about one sixth as analgesic as morphine. It is also less constipating (although it does cause constipation) and less depressing to respiration. Codeine is less habit-forming than morphine, although drug dependence does occur. It is a preparation of choice in cough mixtures for the treatment of a dry, unproductive cough. Doses beyond 60 mg. are thought to be inadvisable because if effect is not secured with 60 mg. it will not be accomplished with a higher dosage. Large doses of codeine tend to stimulate

the brainstem. Codeine has a greater tendency to excite nerve centers than morphine.

Dosage for children for pain is 3 mg. per kilogram of body weight for a 24-hour period in divided doses; for cough the dose is one third to one half that for pain.

Codeine is available in a variety of forms as tablets or capsules, in solution for injection in vials and ampules, and in elixir and syrup form for coughs. Codeine is also prepared in combination with other drugs such as aspirin.

Terpin hydrate and codeine elixir, N.F. Usual dose is 5 ml., which contains 10 mg. of codeine (gr. $1/_6$). This is used to relieve coughing.

Dihydrocodeinone bitartrate (Dicodid, Hycodan, Tussionex). This is similar in action to codeine sulfate (or phosphate) but more active and more likely to cause drug dependence. It is used to relieve cough. The dose is 5 to 15 mg. (gr. $1/_{12}$ to $1/_4$). It is marketed in oral tablets and as a syrup.

Pantopon

Pantopon is an artificial mixture composed of the purified alkaloids of opium in the same proportion as they are found in opium but in about five times the concentration. It is free from gums, resins, and the like. Some think it is more valuable than opium itself; however, this is questionable. Pantopon has an advantage in that it can be injected and opium cannot. It is used for the same reasons as morphine. Patients who are hypersensitive to morphine can sometimes tolerate pantopon satisfactorily. The dosage is twice that of morphine. It may be administered orally or subcutaneously. The usual therapeutic dose is 20 mg. (gr. $1/_3$).

Hydromorphone hydrochloride, N.F. (Dilaudid)

This is prepared from morphine. The usual dose of hydromorphone is 2 mg., which is about five times as analgesic as morphine. It may be given orally, subcutaneously, or by suppository. The last preparation allows for slower absorption and more prolonged effect, which is an advantage because the duration of analgesic effect is shorter than that of morphine. Its analgesic effect is accompanied by minimal hypnotic effect, which is desirable when the drug is given to patients in whom it is important to relieve pain without producing a stupefying effect. It depresses respiration, but side actions such as euphoria, nausea, vomiting, and constipation seem to be less marked than with morphine. Both drug dependence and tolerance can occur. Federal narcotics regulations apply to this drug.

SYNTHETIC NARCOTIC ANALGESICS

Mention has been made that morphine falls short of being an ideal analgesic, not because it is not sufficiently potent but because it depresses respiration, produces constipation, and may produce drug dependence. Consequently, there has been an almost continuous search for an analgesic with fewer of the disadvantages of morphine. Some of the newer agents have been found to exhibit some advantages over morphine. For a comparison of dosage and action time of various nonsynthetic and synthetic narcotic analgesics administered subcutaneously or intramuscularly, see Table 11-2.

Meperidine hydrochloride, U.S.P. (Demerol Hydrochloride); pethidine hydrochloride, B.P.

Meperidine hydrochloride is a synthetic substitute for morphine discovered by two German scientists who were searching for a substitute for atropine. It is a stable, white crystalline powder soluble in alcohol and very soluble in water.

Action and result. Meperidine depresses the central nervous system, probably at both the cortical and subcortical levels. The exact mechanism of action is unknown. Its most outstanding effect is to produce analgesia. It is especially effective for visceral pain, although it also relieves pain in structures of the body wall. Its analgesic potency is said to be slightly greater

Table 11-2 Comparision of narcotic analgesics for subcutaneous or intramuscular administration

Generic name	Trade name	Average adult dose	Usual range of single dose	Onset of action	Peak action	Duration of action
Nonsynthetic narcotic analgesics						
Morphine	—	10 mg. (gr. $1/6$)	5 to 15 mg. (gr. $1/12$ to $1/4$)	5 to 10 min.	1 hr.	4 to 6 hr.
Codeine	—	30 mg. (gr. $1/2$)	15 to 60 mg. (gr. $1/4$ to 1)	5 to 10 min.	30 to 60 min.	3 to 4 hr.
Hydromorphone	Dilaudid	2 mg.	1 to 4 mg.	5 to 10 min.	1 hr.	3 to 4 hr.
Pantopium	Pantopon	20 mg. (gr. $1/3$)	5 to 20 mg. (gr. $1/12$ to $1/3$)	5 to 10 min.	1 hr.	3 to 4 hr.
Synthetic narcotic analgesics						
Meperidine	Demerol Pethidine	50 to 100 mg.	50 to 150 mg.	15 min.	1 hr.	2 to 4 hr.
Anileridine	Leritine	25 to 50 mg.	25 to 100 mg.	15 min.	1 hr.	2 to 4 hr.
Methadone	Adanon Amidone Dolophine	7.5 mg.	2.5 to 10 mg.	10 min.	1 to 2 hr.	4 to 6 hr.
Phenazocine	Prinadol	2 mg.	1 to 3 mg.	5 to 20 min.	1 hr.	2 to 6 hr.
Alphaprodine	Nisentil	40 to 60 mg.	40 to 60 mg.	5 min.	30 min.	2 hr.
Levorphanol	Levo-Dromoran	2 to 3 mg.	1 to 3 mg.	15 min.	1 to $1 1/2$ hr.	4 to 8 hr.

than codeine and lasts 2 to 4 hours, depending on the dosage. The onset of action occurs in 15 minutes, and peak action occurs in 1 hour. It is about one tenth as analgesic as morphine; hence, severe pain is not well controlled by meperidine. Euphoria is produced in some patients and lasts for an hour or so. Compared to morphine it is less likely to cause sleep and sedation unless large doses are given. There is little depression of the respiratory center with the usual therapeutic doses; however, toxic doses can produce marked depression. Compared to morphine, it is less likely to cause nausea and vomiting and it does not produce pupillary constriction or depress the cough center.

Meperidine in therapeutic doses has little or no effect on the cardiovascular system, particularly if the patient is in a recumbent position. When given to patients who are up and about or when given by rapid intravenous injection, postural hypotension and fainting may result. Like morphine it is prone to cause an elevation of intracranial pressure and must be used cautiously in patients with head injuries or conditions in which there is an elevation of cerebrospinal pressure.

Meperidine was formerly thought to be a useful agent to relieve the spasm of smooth muscle, but it has been found that it resembles morphine in some of its effects on smooth muscle; it has been found to promote spasm of muscle in the biliary tract. It exerts a rather weak antispasmodic effect on the bronchial musculature and can more safely be used than morphine for the asthmatic patient who has need for an analgesic. The tendency to produce spasm in the smooth muscle of the gastrointestinal tract is said to be somewhere between that of morphine and codeine. It is rather mildly spasmogenic and does not produce constipation; therefore, it is of no value in the therapy of severe diarrhea. It has more effect on the small intestine than on the colon. The emptying of the stomach is somewhat retarded.

Uses. Meperidine is used primarily as a substitute for morphine to produce analgesia. When so used it has the advantage of producing much less sedation and constipation. However, it does not take the place of morphine for the relief of severe pain. It is quick acting and short acting. It is suited to the management of intermittent pain such as renal colic.

Meperidine is widely used as a preanesthetic agent.

In obstetrics it is frequently combined with scopolamine, promethazine, or one of the short-acting barbiturates to produce obstetric amnesia.

Preparation, dosage, and administration. Meperidine hydrochloride is available for oral use in 50- and 100-mg. tablets and in ampules, vials, and disposable injection units for parenteral administration. The single oral or parenteral dose usually varies from 50 to 100 mg. For severe pain doses up to 150 mg. may be given. The usual dosage for children is 6 mg. per kilogram of body weight for 24 hours, given in divided doses. It is also available as a syrup. Although meperidine can be given orally, it is more effective when given intramuscularly. Occasionally it is given rectally, and it is rarely administered intravenously. It may be given orally for relief of chronic pain. It is irritating to subcutaneous tissue.

Side effects and toxic effects. Side effects include dizziness, nausea and vomiting, dry mouth, sweating, headache, fainting, and drop in blood pressure. Toxic effects include dilated pupils, mental confusion, tremor, incoordination, convulsions, and respiratory depression. Death may result. Toxic effects are said to produce more physical impairment than that caused by other narcotic drugs.

Meperidine has a distinct capacity to produce drug dependence. Some physicians are of the opinion that dependence develops more rapidly than with morphine. Withdrawal symptoms develop more rapidly but are thought to be less severe. At one time tolerance was thought to develop more slowly than with morphine, but if pain is to be controlled, the drug must be given more often because of the short duration of action, and therefore tolerance develops more quickly. It is subject to provisions of the Controlled Substances Act.

Treatment of acute intoxication depends upon severity of symptoms. If respiratory depression becomes severe it can be antagonized by the administration of nalorphine.

Contraindications. Meperidine is contraindicated in severe dysfunction of the liver (since the drug is inactivated in the liver), in certain conditions involving the gallbladder and the bile ducts (since meperidine causes contraction of these structures), and in cases in which there is increased intracranial pressure. Severe toxic reactions have occurred following use of meperidine in patients receiving MAO inhibitors; hypotension, cyanosis, and respiratory depression occur.

Anileridine hydrochloride, N.F. (Leritine)

Anileridine is a ~~synthetic analgesic~~ closely ~~related to meperidine~~. It is available as a dihydrochloride for oral use and as a phosphate for parenteral administration.

Action and result. The action of anileridine is like that of meperidine. Its analgesic activity is three to six times greater than that of meperidine but less than that of morphine. Duration of action is slightly less than that of meperidine and considerably less than that of morphine.

Uses. Anileridine is used to relieve moderate to severe pain in many medical, surgical, obstetric, and dental situations.

Preparation, dosage, and administration. Anileridine hydrochloride is available in 25-mg. tablets for oral use. Anileridine phosphate is available as a solution in which 25 mg. is contained in each milliliter for parenteral administration. The usual adult dose is 25 to 50 mg. subcutaneously or intramuscularly every 4 to 6 hours. Peak action occurs in 1 hour and duration of action is up to 4 hours.

Side effects and toxic effects. Side effects are similar to those of meperidine. Nervousness and restlessness caused by cerebral excitement have been reported. Toxic effects include respiratory and circulatory depression. Its dependence po-

tential is equivalent to that of morphine. Anileridine is antagonized by nalorphine.

Methadone hydrochloride, U.S.P., B.P. (Dolophine)

Methadone was synthesized during World War II by German chemists. It occurs as a white crystalline substance that has a bitter taste; it is soluble in both alcohol and water.

Action and result. Methadone resembles morphine in a number of respects. It also depresses the central nervous system and acts as a potent analgesic, although it has a weaker sedative effect than morphine. Only in minimal doses does it cause less respiratory depression than morphine. Euphoria is less intense than that produced by morphine. The effects of methadone on smooth muscle are somewhat more variable than morphine, but, on the whole, the results are similar. Given parenterally it produces analgesia in 10 to 15 minutes; duration of action is 4 to 6 hours. Given orally analgesia occurs in 20 to 30 minutes.

Uses. Methadone is used primarily as an analgesic. The duration of its effect is about the same as for morphine. It is somewhat more satisfactory for the relief of chronic pain than morphine, but it is not as useful as a preanesthetic medication.

It is given to relieve cough because of its depressant effect on the cough center (antitussive effect).

Methadone can prevent or relieve acute withdrawal symptoms of morphine-like drugs and therefore it is used in the treatment of patients dependent on heroin or other morphine-like drugs. Methadone also produces withdrawal symptoms but dependence develops more slowly and the withdrawal symptoms are less severe than those associated with morphine or heroin.

Preparation, dosage, and administration. Methadone hydrochloride is available in 2.5-, 7.5-, and 10-mg. tablets and in solutions dispensed in ampules or multiple-dose vials containing 10 mg. per milliliter. It is also available as an elixir (1 mg. per milliliter) and as a syrup (0.34 mg. per milliliter). The usual oral or parenteral dose is 7.5 mg. every 4 hours as necessary; the range of dosage is 2.5 to 10 mg. To relieve cough 1.5 to 2 mg. is given. Methadone is sometimes administered orally but more often parenterally. It is more effective than morphine when given orally. Subcutaneous injections sometimes cause local irritation, in which case intramuscular injection is preferred. If it is given intravenously the patient should be in recumbent position.

Side effects and toxic effects. Methadone exhibits some of the same disadvantages as morphine. It causes nausea and vomiting, itching of the skin, constipation, light headedness, and respiratory depression. Death results from respiratory failure.

Both tolerance and dependence occur following repeated doses of methadone. The same precautions need to be observed in the administration of methadone as for morphine. Nalorphine acts as an antagonist to methadone as it does for morphine and meperidine. The use and administration of methadone is subject to restrictions of the Controlled Substances Act.

Phenazocine hydrobromide, B.P. (Prinadol)

Phenazocine is a potent synthetic narcotic analgesic similar to morphine, although it is effective in smaller doses and is said to be more rapid in producing analgesia. Its analgesic potency is three to four times that of morphine. Given intramuscularly it acts within 5 to 20 minutes; duration of action varies from 1 to 6 hours. It seems to produce less sedation than morphine, but its capacity to produce respiratory depression and dependence is very similar to the older drug. It is said to have no effect on uterine contractions.

It is employed as a preanesthetic narcotic and used in obstetrics and in the control of severe pain. It is reported to be useful as an analgesic for patients who are to have angiograms under local anesthesia.

Preparation, dosage, and administration. Phenazocine hydrobromide is available in 10-ml. vials and 1-ml. ampules (2 mg. per milliliter) for intramuscular and intravenous administration. The usual intramuscular dose is 1 to 3 mg. every 4 to 6 hours. It is incompatible with a number of drugs; therefore, it should not be administered in the same syringe with another medication.

Side effects and toxic effects. Side effects other than those mentioned previously include nausea and vomiting, headache, hypotension, and mild constipation. Severe respiratory depression is relieved by administration of levallorphan or nalorphine.

Alphaprodine hydrochloride, N.F. (Nisentil)

Alphaprodine hydrochloride is a white crystalline powder with a bitter taste and a fishy odor. It is a synthetic narcotic analgesic that is chemically related to meperidine.

Action and result. Its analgesic potency is said to be between that of meperidine and morphine. It resembles morphine in that it produces euphoria, mild sedation, slight dizziness, itching, and sweating. It is less likely to cause depression of respiration, nausea, and vomiting than morphine. Its analgesic and general depressant actions are less intense than those of morphine, but it acts more quickly and over a shorter time (about 2 hours). It passes the placental barrier easily, especially if given in conjunction with a barbiturate, and can depress respiration in the fetus unless it is given long enough before the time of delivery. Its effect on smooth muscle is similar to that of morphine. It has little or no cumulative action.

Uses. Alphaprodine is said to be suited for use as an analgesic for obstetric patients and patients undergoing urologic examination. It is also useful as a preanesthetic narcotic prior to minor surgery involving the musculoskeletal system and the eyes, nose, or throat.

Preparation, dosage, and administration. Alphaprodine hydrochloride is available in 1-ml. ampules containing 40 or 60 mg. and 10-ml. vials of solution containing 60 mg. per milliliter. The usual dose is 40 to 60 mg., depending on the size of the patient. The dose may be repeated at 2-hour intervals. Alphaprodine hydrochloride is

Table 11-3 Selected effects of some synthetic narcotic analgesics

	Meperidine (Demerol)	Methadone	Levorphanol (Levo-Dromoran)
Analgesic potency	Between that of codeine (60 mg.) and morphine (15 mg.)	Like morphine	Five times that of morphine Hypnotic effect similar to morphine
Action Onset	15 min.	20 to 30 min.	60 to 90 min. (intra- muscular)
Duration	2 to 4 hr. (intramuscular)	4 to 6 hr.	4 to 8 hr.
Effects Respiratory	Mild depression Bronchodilation Sometimes bronchospasm	Depression—similar to morphine Bronchial constriction	Depression—like morphine Apnea caused by overdose
Gastrointestinal	Decreased motility Spasm No constipation effect	Increased tone Decreased motility Spasms—like morphine	Decreased motility Spasms Moderate constipation
Genitourinary Ureters	Decreased motility and tone	Spasms—like morphine	—
Bladder	Increased tone Retention uncommon	—	—
Kidney	Not significant Some decrease in urinary output	Antidiuretic action Reduced urinary output	Reduced urinary output
Uterus	Decreased tone and contractions	No relief of pain of labor or uterine contractions	Reduced motility
Eyes	No pupil change with therapeutic dose Blurred vision	Miosis with large dose	Miosis
Salivary glands	Moderate decrease in secretions Dryness of mouth	Stimulation Slight increase in secretions	—
Cerebral	Euphoria Mild depression Drowsiness Dizziness Giddiness	Not significant with therapeutic dose Cortical depression with large doses	—

usually administered subcutaneously. When very rapid and brief analgesia is desired, it is given intravenously; action occurs in 1 to 2 minutes and persists for 30 to 60 minutes.

Side effects and toxic effects. The undesirable effects are similar to those of morphine. Death can result from respiratory failure. Nalorphine is an effective antidote. Drug dependence may develop, although this is considered unlikely under conditions in which this drug is used.

Levorphanol tartrate, N.F., B.P. (Levo-Dromoran Tartrate)

Levorphanol tartrate is a white, odorless crystalline powder. It has a bitter taste and is slightly soluble in water. It is a synthetic analgesic pharmacologically and chemically related to morphine.

Action and result. Its analgesic potency is comparable to that of morphine but in smaller dosage. The analgesic effect is said to last somewhat longer than in the case of morphine (4 to 8 hours). Maximum analgesic effects are obtained in 60 to 90 minutes after subcutaneous injection. In man, 2 to 3 mg. of levorphanol tartrate is said to relieve pain as effectively as 10 to 15 mg. of morphine. It has less effect than morphine on the smooth muscle of the gastrointestinal tract. Tolerance develops slowly. (See Table 11-3.)

Uses. This drug is useful to relieve severe visceral pain, such as that associated with terminal carcinoma, renal and biliary colic, myocardial infarction, and gangrene. It is also used as a preanesthetic narcotic as well as for the relief of postoperative pain. It can be used for practically all the same conditions for which morphine is employed.

Preparation, dosage, and administration. Levorphanol tartrate is available in solution, dispensed in 1-ml. ampules and 10-ml. vials of solution containing 2 mg. per milliliter. It is also available in scored 2-mg. tablets for oral administration. Recommended average dose for adults is 2 to 3 mg. The initial dose should be as small as possible to delay the development of tolerance. This drug is usually given subcutaneously, but, unlike morphine, it is almost as effective after oral administration as when given subcuta-

Table 11-4 Comparison of analgesic dose of certain narcotic compounds

Generic name	Trade name	Equivalent analgesic dose (mg.)
Morphine		10
Codeine		60
Dihydromorphinone	Dilaudid	2
Meperidine	Demerol	100
Methadone	Dolophine (and others)	10
Alphaprodine	Nisentil	40
Levorphanol	Levo-Dromoran	2
Phenazocine	Prinadol	2

neously. This constitutes a possible advantage over morphine.

Side effects and toxic effects. The side effects are the same as those for morphine except for a lower incidence of constipation. As is true of most narcotics, dizziness and vomiting are observed more in ambulatory patients than in those who must remain in bed. The drug is capable of causing drug dependence and must be used with the same precautions that are observed in the use of other such drugs. It is subject to the restrictions of the Controlled Substances Act.

Oxycodone hydrochloride (Eucodal, Percodan)

Oxycodone is a derivative of morphine and related to codeine. It is five to six times more potent than codeine and also has a greater dependence potential than codeine, but it is less potent with less dependence potential than morphine. It is used as an analgesic for the treatment of moderate pain and as a cough suppressant. Oxycodone has therapeutic side and toxic effects similar to the other narcotic analgesics. The usual oral dose is 3 to 20 mg. The same precautions should be used when administering oxycodone as when giving other narcotics. Onset of action occurs in 10 to 15 minutes and peak action in 30 to 60 minutes, with duration of action lasting 3 to 6 hours after oral administration.

Oxymorphone hydrochloride, N.F. (Numorphan)

Oxymorphone is a semisynthetic narcotic with a pharmacologic action resembling that of morphine. It is a potent drug useful for treating severe pain. The dose of oxymorphone is about one tenth that of morphine. Oxymorphone is said to cause fewer untoward effects (constipation, nausea, and vomiting) than morphine. Precautions are necessary to prevent respiratory depression and other toxic effects. It may be administered orally in 5- or 10-mg. doses or parenterally in 0.75- to 1.5-mg. doses. Rectal suppositories are also available containing 2 and 5 mg. of the drug. When given subcutaneously the drug acts in 5 to 10 minutes, peak action occurs in 10 to 20 minutes, and duration of action is 3 to 6 hours. Its margin of safety, dependence-producing potential, and duration of analgesic action are comparable to that of morphine.

SYNTHETIC NONNARCOTIC ANALGESICS
Pentazocine, N.F. (Talwin)

Pentazocine is a potent nonnarcotic analgesic for parenteral use. It is a synthetic compound that may be used in place of morphine and other narcotic analgesics. It is not classified as a narcotic. With repeated and frequent use some tolerance develops. Drug dependence potential appears to be less than that of codeine. Precautions are the same as for other potent analgesics.

Uses. Pentazocine has been used for the relief of pain in connection with surgical procedures, during labor, in urologic procedures, and in many medical disorders.

Preparation, dosage, and administration. Pentazocine is supplied in ampules of 1 ml. containing 30 mg. of the base. It is also available in disposable syringes and multiple-dose vials and in 50-mg. tablets for oral use. Pentazocine

should not be mixed in a syringe with soluble barbiturates because precipitation will occur.

Usual oral dose is 50 mg. every 3 to 4 hours, but due to relatively poor absorption, the dose may need to be 100 mg. Usual parenteral dose is 30 mg. every 3 to 4 hours as necessary. Daily dose should not exceed 600 mg. Following subcutaneous or intramuscular administration, pentazocine acts in 10 to 30 minutes with a duration of effect of 2 to 3 hours. For patients in labor a single intramuscular 30-mg. dose has been found useful. An intravenous 20-mg. dose may give adequate pain relief to some patients in labor when contractions become regular. This dose may be given two or three times at 2- to 3-hour intervals, as needed. Because of limited clinical experience, the use of pentazocine in children is not recommended.

Side effects and toxic effects. Nausea, vertigo, dizziness, lightheadedness, vomiting, and euphoria may occur following the use of pentazocine. Respiratory depression was reported in about 1% of the patients. The usual narcotic antagonists are not effective in the treatment of respiratory depression produced by pentazocine but naloxone is effective.

Propoxyphene hydrochloride, U.S.P. (Darvon); dextroproxyphene hydrochloride, B.P.; propoxyphene napsylate (Darvon-N)

Propoxyphene hydrochloride is a synthetic analgesic compound with about half the potency of codeine. Like codeine, it does not depress respiration when given in ordinary therapeutic amounts, but unlike codeine, it produces little or no relief of cough. It relieves mild to moderate pain better than severe pain. Onset of action and duration of effects are similar to codeine. It does not act as an antipyretic. Next to aspirin it is the largest selling analgesic.

Uses. It is used alone or along with certain other analgesics, such as aspirin, for the relief of pain associated with chronic or recurring diseases like rheumatoid arthritis and migraine headache.

Preparation and dosage. Propoxyphene hydrochloride is available in 32- and 65-mg. capsules. The usual dose for adults is 65 mg. four times a day with or without other medication for the relief of pain. Dose for propoxyphene napsylate is 100 mg. three or four times daily.

Darvon compound contains the following: propoxyphene hydrochloride, 32 mg. (65 mg. in Darvon Compound-65); phenacetin, 162 mg.; aspirin, 227 mg.; and caffeine, 32.4 mg. Dosage is one to two capsules three or four times a day. Darvon and Darvon Compound are given orally. Propoxyphene hydrochloride is not suited to parenteral administration because of a local irritating action.

Side effects and toxic effects. Therapeutic doses do not produce euphoria, tolerance, or physical dependence. Abuse with morphine-like dependence has been reported, however. Sudden cessation of administration has not been known to produce withdrawal symptoms. It appears to have a low level of toxicity. Side effects of nausea, vomiting, and constipation are considered minimal. Large doses may cause drowsiness and dizziness. Patients are occasionally hypersensitive to this drug. There are no known contraindications except hypersensitivity. It is not subject to the restrictions of the Controlled Substances Act.

Overdosage may cause confusion, respiratory depression, coma, pupil constriction, and muscle fasciculations. Convulsions are prominent in most cases of propoxyphene poisoning, and arrhythmias and pulmonary edema have been reported. Apnea, cardiac arrest, and death have occurred. The narcotic antagonists may be used to overcome respiratory depression. Analeptics or other central nervous system stimulants should not be used because of their potential for precipitating fatal convulsions.

The 32-mg. dose of propoxyphene hydrochloride has been given a D.E.S.I. rating of *ineffective.* The 65-mg. dose and the mixture with 325 mg. of aspirin have been rated as *effective.* Some clinicians believe propoxyphene to be inferior to aspirin.

Ethoheptazine citrate (Zactane)

Ethoheptazine is a synthetic nonnarcotic analgesic structurally similar to meperidine. It is without antipyretic and sedative effects and seemingly has no effect on cough and respiration. It is said to be more effective than aspirin when given alone. It is used for its analgesic effects for mild to moderate pain rather than for severe pain. Its greatest use seems to be for the control of pain associated with musculoskeletal disorders, for postpartum and postoperative patients, and for patients in the early stages of neoplastic disease. It is not particularly effective for headaches. It has been combined with aspirin to enhance its effectiveness. This combination is marketed under the name of Zactirin.

Preparation, dosage, and administration. Ethoheptazine citrate is marketed in 75-mg. tablets for oral administration. The dosage may be from 75 to 150 mg. three or four times daily. Its D.E.S.I. rating is *possibly effective;* unless new evidence of its efficacy is produced it must be withdrawn.

Ethoheptazine citrate with aspirin contains 75 mg. of ethoheptazine citrate and 325 mg. (gr. 5) of aspirin in each tablet. Dosage is one to two tablets three or four times a day.

Side effects and toxic effects. Side effects are not often seen. Epigastric distress, dizziness, and pruritus are effects that are observed occasionally. It does not cause dependence.

NARCOTIC ANTAGONISTS

The antinarcotic drugs comprise nalorphine, levallorphan, and the newer naloxone. Nalorphine and levallorphan are weak narcotics that compete with the stronger narcotics for central nervous system receptor sites and thus act as antagonists. Naloxone has no depressant action of its own but acts as a pure antagonist. All of these drugs antagonize the actions of the opiate-like drugs, but naloxone is unique in being effective against pentazocine also.

Nalorphine hydrochloride, N.F. (Nalline Hydrochloride); nalorphine hydrobromide, B.P.

Nalorphine, a synthetic congener of morphine, acts as an antagonist of morphine, meperidine, and methadone in the event of narcotic poisoning. There is evidence that it also reverses the respiratory depression caused by overdoses of hydromorphone, levorphanol, and alphaprodine. It does not reverse the respiratory depression caused by barbiturates or some general anesthetics.

Uses. Nalorphine is of value in the treatment of acute poisoning from morphine and related analgesics, but its use should not exclude the use of other supportive measures for the patient. In narcotic-depressed patients it increases respiratory rate and volume in 1 or 2 minutes, helps to restore decreased blood pressure, abolishes pupil constriction, and counteracts gastrointestinal spasm. Sedative effects are less markedly affected. Nalorphine is not recommended for the treatment of drug abuse. It can be used to prevent respiratory depression in the newborn when given to mothers shortly before delivery, provided they have been given morphine or one of the related analgesics.

Large doses of nalorphine hydrochloride cause drowsiness, lethargy, sweating, and dysphoria (misery). In morphine abusers it produces rapid onset of withdrawal symptoms and can therefore be used in diagnosing cases of dependence. Doses beyond 40 mg. are not recommended.

Preparation, dosage, and administration. Nalorphine hydrochloride is a white powder, and nalorphine injection, N.F., B.P., is a solution suited for parenteral administration. It is available in 1- and 2-ml. ampules and in 10-ml. vials. The concentration of the solutions varies from 0.2 to 5 mg. per milliliter. It can be given subcutaneously, intramuscularly, or intravenously.

The usual adult dose is 5 to 10 mg., which can be repeated if the respirations are not adequate. Since it is a derivative of morphine, it had been subject to the restrictions of the federal narcotics law, but it has now been reclassified and is no longer under such restrictions.

Levallorphan tartrate, U.S.P., B.P. (Lorfan)

Levallorphan is a narcotic antagonist chemically related to levorphanol. It relieves the respiratory depression caused by the action of narcotics but not the depression that may result from the action of anesthetics, barbiturates, or pathologic conditions. It is said to abolish the respiratory depression without affecting the state of analgesia. When given alone, however, it acts as a respiratory depressant and produces slight analgesia.

Uses. The action and uses of levallorphan are much the same as those of nalorphine. When given after or together with narcotics it relieves or prevents respiratory depression. It is fully as effective as nalorphine to antagonize the respiratory depression of morphine, and some physicians consider it more effective. It is less expensive than nalorphine.

Preparation, dosage, and administration. Levallorphan tartrate is available for adults as a solution in which 1 mg. is contained in each milliliter; for children, it is available in concentration of 0.05 mg. per milliliter. Total dosage varies with the patient and the degree of depression. One or more doses of 0.4 to 0.6 mg. may be given as necessary. In acute poisoning with morphine, 1 mg. may be the initial dose. Levallorphan is administered intravenously, as a rule, although it may be given subcutaneously and intramuscularly.

Naloxone hydrochloride, U.S.P. (Narcan)

Naloxone hydrochloride is an important new narcotic antagonist. Naloxone reverses the respiratory depressant action of narcotics such as morphine, meperidine, and methadone. An important feature of the pharmacology of naloxone is its lack of respiratory depressant action and its failure to cause sedation or analgesia. It is essentially a pure narcotic antagonist. It also antagonizes the actions of pentazocine. Similarly to the other narcotic antagonists, naloxone precipitates an abstinence syndrome when administered to addicts who are taking a narcotic.

Naloxone hydrochloride is available in ampules and vials containing 0.4 mg. per milliliter. The drug is administered intravenously, intramuscularly, or subcutaneously. Usual adult dose is 0.4 mg., which may be repeated at intervals of 2 to 3 minutes.

NONNARCOTIC ANALGESICS THAT ARE ALSO ANTIPYRETICS

Antipyretics were more in demand when effort was made to cure fevers by antipyresis. Today many physicians look upon fever as a reaction of the body that helps the individual combat infection, and therefore reduction of the fever is not always desirable. Antipyretic drugs are still used for the relief of high fever, especially in children. Aspirin is probably used more than any other single agent for this purpose.

During the latter part of the nineteenth century, when chemists were trying to find a cheaper source of quinine than the natural source, they discovered a number of compounds that differed in some respects from quinine but resembled it in their ability to reduce fever and relieve pain. Several of these compounds have survived chiefly because of their analgesic properties.

Salicylates

The natural source of salicylic acid is willow bark, although it is now made synthetically from phenol. The cheaper synthetic product is identical with, and therefore as effective as, the natural product. Salicylic acid itself is irritating and can be used only externally, necessitating the synthesis of derivatives for systemic uses. All of these compounds will be referred to as "salicylates" and will be discussed as a group. Usefulness of the various members of the group depends upon their solubility, their salicylic acid content, and their tendency to cause local irritation.

Salicylic acid   Aspirin

Sodium salicylate   Methyl salicylate

Aspirin is by far the most widely used of all the salicylates. In 1971, Americans spent $104.6 million for aspirin, $387 million for combinations of aspirin with other pain relievers, and $63.1 million for products to relieve arthritic and rheumatic pains.

Salicylates are rapidly absorbed from the stomach and upper small intestine, and are rapidly excreted by the kidney. Rapid excretion explains the need for large and frequent dosage. Alkalinizing the urine increases the rate of excretion of free salicylate.

Systemic action. These drugs are used systemically for their analgesic, antipyretic, and anti-inflammatory actions.

Analgesic. The major use of salicylates (aspirin and sodium salicylate) is for the relief of pain (analgesia). When compared on the basis of weight, the former compound is said to be the more potent analgesic. These preparations are especially effective for headache, neuralgia, dysmenorrhea, myalgia, fibrositis, neuritis, rheumatoid arthritis, and rheumatic fever. Aspirin is probably more widely used than any other single therapeutic agent. The estimated amount used yearly in the United States is approximately 10,500 tons.

Analgesic doses of the salicylates do not produce dulling of consciousness, mental sluggishness, or disturbances of memory. Unlike the opiates, analgesia produced by the salicylates is not accompanied by euphoria or sedation. They do not cause drug dependence.

There is evidence that salicylates have a selective peripheral action that protects pain receptors against bradykinin, which may be a mediator of the inflammatory process. Salicylates are therefore effective in treating peripheral pain (musculoskeletal pain or muscle and joint pain) and in relieving headache. Salicylates are not effective in relieving visceral pain or severe traumatic pain. Their analgesic potency is less than that of codeine.

The preparations are helpful in the symptomatic treatment of gout. They are less valuable for this purpose than certain other agents, but they are also less toxic. They decrease the renal threshold of uric acid and promote its excretion.

Antipyretic. Little or no effect is observed in persons with a normal body temperature, but in the febrile patient, a marked fall in temperature may be brought about. The salicylates seem to reduce fever by increasing the elimination of heat. It is believed that they act upon the heat-regulating center in the hypothalamus. As a result of this action, peripheral blood vessels dilate, and heat is lost from the body by radiation and by evaporation of increased perspiration. There is evidently no effect on heat production.

However, care must be exercised to avoid giving any of these preparations if the patient is benefiting from the fever or if the cause of illness would be obscured by reduction of temperature.

Unpleasant symptoms associated with a cold or attack of influenza may be relieved by one or more of the salicylates since they relieve muscular aching, headache, and fever, but their use should be accompanied by rest in bed. They exert no effect on the progress of the infection. In other words, it is impossible to "break up" a cold with aspirin as is commonly believed.

Anti-inflammatory action and the prostaglandins. Prostaglandins are synthesized and released by nearly all cells and tissues. Their production is not limited to specialized cells. Unlike the hormones, they are ubiquitous. They are not stored in the body, but are synthesized and released under certain conditions such as cell damage. Precursors of the prostaglandins are the long-chain fatty acids. To date, five groups of prostaglandins have been isolated and are referred to by the letters E, F, A, B, and C. The E and F groups are usually referred to as primary prostaglandins (PGE, PGF). They were originally isolated from seminal vesicle extracts.

During the past few years, intensive research on the prostaglandins has resulted in the following findings:

1 Prostaglandin E compounds:
   a. increase vascular permeability
   b. induce vasodilation
   c. may cause pain
   d. release lysosomal enzymes
   e. prevent the release of histamine from sensitized leukocytes
   f. are released during antigen-antibody reactions
2 Nonsteroid anti-inflammatory drugs (aspirin, indomethacin) inhibit prostaglandin synthesis.

It is hypothesized that inhibition of prostaglandin synthesis by aspirin and other nonsteroid anti-inflammatory drugs may account for some of their ability to decrease inflammation. It is not known if the prostaglandins are the primary mediators of inflammation. Interestingly, the anti-inflammatory steroids (dexamethasone, hydrocortisone, and others) inhibit prostaglandin synthesis only slightly.

Experiments indicate that aspirin inhibits formation of excess prostaglandins in the brain. Since aspirin relieves headache, this suggests that aspirin has a central action. It has also been shown that the E compounds elevate body temperature, and it is a well-known fact that in ordinary doses aspirin can reduce fever.

There is some speculation that preoperative treatment with aspirin-like drugs may inhibit some of the effects of surgical trauma. Much more research is needed, however, before the primary role of the prostaglandins and the basic mechanisms of action of the anti-inflammatory, analgesic, and antipyretic drugs are elucidated.

Respiratory. Therapeutic doses of aspirin and sodium salicylate do not affect respiration. Large or toxic doses at first stimulate the respiratory center, producing increased depth and rate of respiration and can cause *respiratory alkalosis*. Later, toxic doses can cause respiratory acidosis and respiratory depression.

Cardiovascular. In patients receiving large doses of salicylates, the plasma volume of the blood increases as much as 20%, hematocrit falls, and cardiac output and work are increased. If the patient has cardiac insufficiency, these effects may lead to cardiac failure and pulmonary edema.

Gastrointestinal. Salicylates in large doses are prone to produce gastrointestinal irritation (gastric distress, nausea, and vomiting). This effect is attributed to both a local and a central action—the gastric mucosa may be affected and also the vomiting center in the brain. The administration of sodium bicarbonate with the oral doses of salicylates helps to prevent irritation, but it also promotes excretion via the kidney. This is not an advantage when the maintenance of a definite blood level is desirable. It is claimed that gastric irritation is decreased appreciably when aspirin is buffered with aluminum glycinate and magnesium carbonate and that it is also absorbed more rapidly. A subsequent study fails to support this latter claim, however. Unlike sodium bicarbonate, these substances do not increase the sodium intake, which is an advantage in certain instances.

Gastric ulceration can occur and occult blood has been found in the stools of patients on salicylate therapy. Extent of blood loss is dose related. Gastric irritation may be reduced by taking the drug with milk, food, or large amounts of water.

Metabolic effects. Salicylates lower blood sugar levels in diabetics, and the drugs have been shown to deplete liver glycogen. However, normal doses of salicylates can be used by diabetics without their interfering with the action of antidiabetic drugs or insulin. With very large doses of aspirin, adjustment in the dose of antidiabetic drugs and insulin may be necessary. Salicylates interfere with protein binding of thyroxine and can alter certain thyroid function tests (PBI).

Platelet aggregation and prothrombin synthesis. Aspirin inhibits platelet aggregation, weakly inhibits prothrombin synthesis, and prolongs bleeding time. For these reasons it is being investigated for the prevention of thrombosis. Aspirin displaces coumarin anticoagulants from protein-binding sites, which leads to higher concentrations of active anticoagulant drug, which in turn

can result in active bleeding. Patients on both drugs should have frequent prothrombin and bleeding time determinations to ascertain if anticoagulant dose needs to be reduced.

Local action. Salicylic acid is irritating to both skin and mucous membrane. It softens epidermis without producing inflammation. Salicylic acid is a constituent of some corn and callus removers, and it is used to remove warts and upper layers of the skin in the treatment of certain skin diseases. It is also used for the treatment of fungal infections. Whitfield's ointment contains benzoic acid and salicylic acid; it loosens the outer horny layers of the skin and is known as a *keratolytic.*

The salts of salicylic acid have no effect on skin, but after their oral ingestion the salicylic acid that is released is likely to cause gastric irritation, nausea, and vomiting. Methyl salicylate produces irritation of both skin and mucous membranes and at one time was used for its counterirritant effects. It was rubbed on sore and painful joints and muscles to produce some degree of redness and improved circulation. It now is rarely prescribed for this purpose. In solution the salicylates are weakly bacteriostatic and are capable of inhibiting certain fermentative and putrefactive processes. Sodium salicylate is sometimes used as a sclerosing agent in the treatment of varicose veins.

Side effects and toxic effects. The safety range of the salicylates is wide, and most cases of poisoning are mild. However, the indiscriminate use of these drugs by lay persons for every kind of ache or pain has resulted in numerous instances of toxic reactions. Also, aspirin poisoning is common in children. Mild poisoning is called salicylism and consists of ringing in the ears, dizziness, disturbances of hearing and vision, sweating, nausea, vomiting, and diarrhea. The so-called salicylic jag results from stimulation of the central nervous system and may progress to a state of delirium. Skin eruption and other allergic manifestations as well as deaths from salicylate poisoning have been reported. Intensive therapy with salicylates and massive doses can produce a decreased prothrombin level in the blood and hemorrhagic manifestations. This appears to accompany a deficiency or diminished intake of vitamin K. There is little likelihood of hemorrhage if the dosage is kept at 1 Gm. or less a day. Other dangerous symptoms of salicylate poisoning include depression, coma, irregular pulse, first a rise and then a fall in blood pressure, and deep, labored respirations that become slower and slower until respiratory failure results. Hyperthermia may occur since salicylate can have a thermogenic effect. Hyperthermia should be treated vigorously with tepid or alcohol sponges, ice packs, or hypothermal blanket. Poisoning and untoward reactions to the salicylates are frequently a matter of personal idiosyncrasy.

There is no specific antidote for salicylate poisoning; hence, treatment is largely symptomatic. All that is usually necessary in mild cases of poisoning is to stop administration of the drug and give plenty of fluids. If massive doses have been taken, it may be necessary and desirable to empty the stomach, preferably with gastric lavage, and then instill a saline evacuant. If the symptoms are those of depression, stimulants may be ordered; if the symptoms are those of overstimulation, mild sedatives may be prescribed. The artificial kidney may be useful in eliminating some of the salicylate from the body.

Overdosage in children. Although aspirin and aspirin compounds are among the safest analgesics known, the ease with which they can be purchased has contributed to carelessness in their use. The so-called baby aspirin, which is available in 1-gr. flavored tablets or dulcets, has been responsible for a high incidence of poisoning in young children. Children eat it thinking it is candy. This has produced severe and sometimes fatal poisoning. The younger the child, the more dangerous overdosage is likely to be. Methyl salicylate should not be left where children can obtain it. Doses as small as 6 ml. has caused death in children. The fact that it is used as a flavoring agent suggests to the child that it is good to eat.

All salicylates should be kept out of the hands of children and in child-resistant containers. Mothers should be helped to understand that indiscriminate administration of these drugs to children, and particularly to young children, can be dangerous.

Preparation, dosage, and administration. The following are the preparations and dosages of salicylates.

Aspirin, U.S.P., B.P. This is a white, crystalline, odorless powder. It has a bitter taste and is poorly soluble in water. In the presence of moisture it hydrolyzes slowly to acetic acid and salicylic acid. It is available in capsule and tablet form. Enteric-coated tablets are available for patients with gastric or duodenal ulcers who would not tolerate the plain tablets well. The usual dose is 600 mg. (gr. 10) every 3 to 4 hours as necessary. It is available in 150-, 300-, and 600-mg. tablets (gr. $2\frac{1}{2}$, 5, and 10) for adults and 65-mg. (gr. 1) tablets for children. The latter are coated with a sweet-tasting material that may lead the child to think of aspirin as candy. Aspirin Suppositories, U.S.P., are also available.

Sodium salicylate, N.F., B.P. This preparation is a white or pinkish powder with a sweetish saline taste. The usual dose is 600 mg. (gr. 10) every 2 to 4 hours as needed. It is relatively soluble in water and is absorbed more rapidly than aspirin. It is available in 300- and 600-mg. tablets (gr. 5 and 10) plain or enteric coated. It is also available in ampules of sterile solution for injection.

Both aspirin and sodium salicylate may be given in large doses to patients with acute rheumatic conditions (as much as 1 Gm. every hour until untoward symptoms appear, such as ringing in the ears). The route of administration is usually oral, and both preparations should be accompanied by ample amounts of water. Sodium salicylate is occasionally given intravenously when high concentrations in the blood are desired and it is difficult to attain them with oral administration.

Salicylamide (Salamide). Salicylamide, the amide of salicylic acid, shares the actions and uses of aspirin. It has no advantage over aspirin with the exception that it can be used effectively for patients who are allergic to aspirin. Administration and dosage are essentially the same as for aspirin.

Salicylic acid, U.S.P., B.P. This form is too irritating for oral administration, but it is a component of many ointments and preparations for external use.

Methyl salicylate, U.S.P., B.P. (Wintergreen Oil). This preparation is too irritating to be used internally except in low concentrations as a flavoring agent.

Drugs that may be combined with salicylates. Codeine and aspirin are frequently given together, and aspirin is also combined with other analgesics and sedatives. Such combinations are believed to bring more effective relief of pain than any one of the drugs given alone. Carefully controlled studies may in time cause a reversal of this opinion.

APC Capsules contain aspirin, phenacetin, and caffeine (see under Phenacetin). The aspirin and phenacetin have added analgesic action. Caffeine reduces cerebral blood flow and may counteract cerebral vascular dilation and excessive pulsation, which are implicated in headache pain. The clinical superiority of APC Capsules over aspirin alone has not been demonstrated.

Para-aminobenzoic acid (PABA), when administered with sodium salicylate, was found to raise the level of salicylate in the blood plasma. It acts by inhibiting the metabolism of the salicylates as well as their excretion from the kidney. Para-aminobenzoic acid can be given orally for this purpose.

Phenacetin; acetaminophen

$$H_5C_2-O-\langle\text{ring}\rangle-\overset{H}{N}-\overset{O}{\overset{\|}{C}}-CH_3$$

Phenacetin

$$HO-\langle\text{ring}\rangle-\overset{H}{N}-\overset{O}{\overset{\|}{C}}-CH_3$$

Acetaminophen

These drugs are often referred to as coal-tar analgesics and antipyretics. They are phenol derivatives. Acetaminophen is a metabolic product of phenacetin.

Action and result. The two chief effects of these drugs are to produce analgesia and to reduce fever. Their effects are the same as those described for aspirin but they do not have the anti-inflammatory or antirheumatic effects of aspirin. They do not cause gastric irritation or uricosuria nor do they affect carbohydrate metabolism or respiration.

Uses. These drugs have been used as analgesics especially for the relief of headache, and have been the active ingredient of many headache remedies. They also have been used to relieve muscular aches and pains of various kinds.

Preparation, dosage, and administration

Phenacetin (Acetophenetidin), B.P. Phenacetin is available in 300-mg. tablets. The usual dose is 600 mg. for adults every 3 to 4 hours. Daily dose should not exceed 2.4 Gm.

Acetaminophen, U.S.P. (Apamide, Tylenol); *paracetamol,* B.P. These are available in drops, tablets, and syrup. The usual dose for adults is 300 to 600 mg. The dose for children age 6 to 12 years is 150 to 300 mg.; for children age 1 to 6 years, 60 to 120 mg. The dose for infants under 1 year is 60 mg. The B.P. preparation is available in 0.5-Gm. tablets.

Aspirin, phenacetin, and caffeine capsules. Each capsule contains 200 to 250 mg. aspirin, 120 to 150 mg. phenacetin, and 15 to 30 mg. caffeine. These same drugs are found in combination and marketed as Empirin Compound, Aspirin Compound, APC Capsules, and a number of others. These three drugs are also combined with codeine or with one of the barbiturates. These preparations are preferably given orally.

Side effects and toxic effects. Side effects are negligible, but the toxic effects are serious and have caused a number of deaths. Poisoning may occur from a single dose or overdose, but it is usually the result of the prolonged use of some proprietary headache remedy. Symptoms include profuse sweating, nausea and vomiting, skin eruption, weakness, cyanosis caused by the formation of methemoglobin, slow weak pulse, and slow respirations. Most severe cases of poisoning show subnormal temperature, leukopenia, and collapse. Large doses of phenacetin administered over a long period may cause renal papillary necrosis.

Phenacetin may cause hemolytic anemia after prolonged use. Phenacetin produces allergic reactions. Considerable individual susceptibility to these drugs seems to exist; some persons are unharmed by them, whereas others develop severe‘ reactions.

These drugs can damage the blood, bone marrow, kidneys, (analgesic nephrotoxicity) and liver if the patient is adversely susceptible to the drug. This constitutes a strong point against prolonged self-medication. Recently dementia has been reported after prolonged use of phenacetin.

In cases of mild poisoning it is usually sufficient simply to discontinue the drug and wait for its elimination from the body. In more severe cases gastric lavage may be indicated if the drug has been recently ingested. Blood transfusions and shock therapy may be necessary. Oxygen is sometimes indicated if the patient is cyanotic.

OTHER ANTI-INFLAMMATORY DRUGS
Phenylbutazone, U.S.P., B.P. (Butazolidin)

Phenylbutazone is a white or light yellow powder with a slightly bitter taste and a slight aromatic odor. It is a synthetic preparation that is chemically related to aminopyrine and antipyrine and exhibits similar analgesic and antipyretic actions. It is absorbed rapidly and completely from the digestive tract and more slowly from intramuscular sites of injection. It is likely to cause some irritation regardless of the channel of administration. Renal excretion of sodium and chloride is reduced, causing retention of fluid. In patients with gout the drug brings about a reduction of uric acid in the blood.

Uses. Phenylbutazone is regarded as a potent analgesic to relieve the pain of rheumatoid arthritis and associated conditions (bursitis, peritendinitis, painful shoulder). It is said to suppress inflammation, to relieve stiffness and swelling, and to shorten the period of disability. However, because of the high incidence of toxic effects, its use is recommended only for those patients who do not respond to less toxic drugs.

It is used particularly to relieve symptoms of gout when the patient has an acute episode of this disease and does not respond well to conservative measures.

Preparation, dosage, and administration. Phenylbutazone is available in 100-mg. enteric-coated tablets. The initial daily dose for adults is 300 to 600 mg., given in divided portions. The minimal effective dose is then determined and may be as low as 100 to 200 mg. It should not be used longer than 10 days. To avoid gastric irritation it should be given at mealtime, just after a meal or with a glass of milk. Nonsodium antacids also help to minimize irritation without increasing the ingestion of sodium. A diet restricted in sodium chloride is recommended while the patient is receiving this drug.

Side effects and toxic effects. The administration of phenylbutazone is accompanied by a rather high incidence of side effects (approximately 40% of the patients). Side effects include edema, nausea, gastric distress, stomatitis, rash, and dizziness. Toxic effects include hepatitis, hypertension, temporary psychosis, leukopenia, thrombocytopenia, and agranulocytosis. Chronic ingestion of the drug may be associated with acute leukemia and renal and liver necrosis. Some patients experience a reactivation of peptic ulcers with bleeding, and others complain of nervousness, confusion, visual disturbances, and fever and may develop cardiac arrhythmias.

Contraindications. Phenylbutazone is contraindicated for patients with edema, cardiac insufficiency, a history of peptic ulcer or blood dyscrasia, or hepatic or renal dysfunction. Patients receiving this drug should be under close medical supervision, and periodic examination of their blood is recommended to detect early indications of toxic effects even if the drug has only been given for 10 days.

Drug interactions. Phenylbutazone causes the following drug interactions:

1 Potentiates the action of warfarin; initially potentiates but later inhibits action of coumarin-type anticoagulants
2 Potentiates hypoglycemic action of sulfonylurea compounds and insulin; potentiates the action of penicillin and sulfonamides

3 With barbiturates the activity of both drugs is inhibited

4 Inhibits action of steroids, sex hormones, aminopyrine, antipyrine, and dipyrone

Oxyphenbutazone, N.F., B.P. (Tandearil)

Oxyphenbutazone is a metabolic product of phenylbutazone. Its uses and toxic effects are similar to those of the parent drug. It is available in tablets containing 100 mg. The average daily dose for adults is 300 to 400 mg. given in three to four equal portions. The administration of the drug after meals is preferable to minimize gastric irritation. Like phenylbutazone, oxyphenbutazone can cause liver damage and depression of the bone marrow. Its use should also be restricted.

Indomethacin, N.F., B.P. (Indocin)

$$H_3C{-}O \cdots \quad CH_2{-}COOH \quad CH_3 \quad N \quad C{=}O \quad Cl$$

Indomethacin is an antirheumatic drug chemically unrelated to the previously discussed analgesic agents or the corticosteroids. It has potent anti-inflammatory, analgesic, and antipyretic activity, but it may cause some serious adverse effects. It should not be used as an antipyretic or analgesic.

Uses. The drug has been found effective in the treatment of rheumatoid arthritis, degenerative joint disease of the hip, and gout, particularly when salicylates are ineffective or not tolerated.

Preparation, dosage, and administration. Indomethacin is supplied in capsules of 25 and 50 mg. each. The average dose for adults is 25 to 50 mg. two or three times daily by mouth.

Side effects and toxic effects. Indomethacin is a potent drug that can cause serious side effects and toxic effects. It may cause peptic ulceration and gastric irritation and is contraindicated in patients who have peptic ulcer, gastritis, or ulcerative colitis. The safety of the drug in pregnant women and the pediatric age group has not been established. Adverse effects also include headache, dizziness, nausea, vomiting, anorexia, skin rashes, and bone marrow depression.

DRUGS USED IN THE TREATMENT OF GOUT

Gout is a metabolic disease of unknown origin. Heredity is thought to have a bearing on the incidence of the disease since it occurs more often in relatives of persons with gout than in the general population. It is seen mostly in males. It is characterized by defective purine metabolism and manifests itself by attacks of acute pain, swelling, and tenderness of joints such as those of the great toe, ankle, instep, knee, and elbow. The amount of uric acid in the blood becomes elevated, and tophi, which are deposits of uric acid or urates, form in the cartilage of various parts of the body. These deposits tend to increase in size. They are seen most often along the edge of the ear. Chronic arthritis, nephritis, and premature sclerosis of blood vessels may develop if gout is uncontrolled.

Drugs given to relieve gout are those given to relieve pain and increase elimination of uric acid. The latter are called *uricosuric agents*. Salicylates, probenecid, and colchicine are drugs of choice at the present time. Colchicine, however, is not uricosuric. Other drugs that are used are phenylbutazone and indomethacin. They are effective in relieving attacks of acute gouty arthritis and may be used when the administration of colchicine is not feasible.

The salicylates increase urinary output of uric acid and, in milder cases of gout, may afford considerable relief. The dosage must be large to accomplish this effect. The recommended dose is 5 or 6 Gm. a day in divided portions for 3 to 5 consecutive days of the week with omission of the drug for the remainder of the week. Dosage must be determined according to the needs of the patient. The effect and dosage of aspirin and sodium salicylate in the treatment of gout are the same. The former preparation is preferable for patients who must have a diet restricted in sodium. The salicylates should not be administered with probenecid, since each is said to counteract the uricosuric effect of the other.

Since uric acid is not very soluble in acid urine but is readily soluble in alkaline urine, the use of an alkalinizing agent is indicated in conjunction with uricosuric agents. The maintenance of an alkaline medium in the kidney prevents the deposit of uric acid and the formation of renal stones and gravel. The amount needed differs with individual patients.

Colchicine, U.S.P., B.P.

$$CH_3O$$

$$CH_2 — CH_2$$

$$C$$

$$CHNHCOCH_3$$

$$CH_3O$$

$$CH_3O$$

$$C$$

$$C$$

$$C$$

$$CH$$

$$HC$$

$$C=O$$

$$HC == COCH_3$$

Colchicine is an alkaloid obtained from the seeds and corm (bulbous root) of the *Colchicum autumnale* (meadow saffron), which belongs to the lily family of plants. Extracts of this plant have been used for hundreds of years in the treatment of gout.

Action and result. Locally, colchicine is an irritant. The mechanism of its systemic action remains unknown. It does not affect the amount of uric acid in the blood or in the urine (thus it is not uricosuric) and it has no effect on the size of tophi. It does not effectively relieve pain other than that of acute gouty arthritis. It is an interesting drug not only because of its potent analgesic effect in gout but also because of its ability to arrest mitotic division of cells when they are in metaphase. During this phase it prevents the development of the spindle. This occurs in both normal and cancer cells. It has been suggested that colchicine may relieve gout by arresting the formation of lactic acids. Inflammation of synovial tissues is associated with lactic acid production, and this favors a local decrease in pH, which promotes uric acid deposition. Colchicine decreases lactic acid production and the inflammatory response. These effects are apparently caused by colchicine-inhibiting leukocyte mobility and phagocytoses.

Uses. Colchicine is used to prevent or relieve acute attacks of gout. The response is often dramatic, and pain may be relieved within a few hours, the fever and swelling often diminishing after the relief of pain. It frequently must be used in doses large enough to cause some gastrointestinal irritation. Tolerance does not seem to develop. It is sometimes given every night or every other night to prevent the development of an acute attack.

Preparation, dosage, and administration. Colchicine is available in 0.5- and 0.6-mg. tablets and in ampules containing 1 mg. in 2 ml. of solution for intravenous infection. The initial dose of 1 mg. is usually followed by 0.5 mg. every hour or every 2 hours until the pain is relieved or the patient begins to have diarrhea, nausea and vomiting, or abdominal pain. Camphorated opium tincture or bismuth subcarbonate may be required to control the diarrhea. Colchicine is usually administered orally. Inflammatory symptoms usually subside in 12 hours and are completely gone in 48 to 72 hours. The drug should not be administered for the next 3 days to avoid toxic effects from accumulation. Occasionally, it is given by intravenous injection when rapid relief is important or when oral administration is not feasible. It is very irritating if injected outside a vein and therefore cannot be given subcutaneously or intramuscularly.

To be effective, colchicine must be given promptly at the first indication of an oncoming attack, and dosage must be adequate. Once the dose that will cause diarrhea has been determined, it is often possible to reduce subsequent doses to prevent diarrhea and still achieve satisfactory relief of pain. Caution should be used when this drug is given to elderly or feeble persons and those with cardiac, renal, or gastrointestinal disease.

Side effects and toxic effects. Prolonged use can cause agranulocytosis, peripheral neuritis, and aplastic anemia. In acute poisoning the patient complains of abdominal pain, nausea, vomiting, and diarrhea, which may become bloody as poisoning advances. Excessive loss of fluid and electrolytes and the dilation of capillaries result in shock. Scanty urine and blood in the urine indicate damage to the kidney. The pulse becomes rapid and weak, and the patient becomes exhausted.

The main measures used in the treatment of poisoning depend upon the patient and the symptoms that are presented. Treatment is directed toward removal of the poison if possible (gastric lavage) and the prevention of shock. Atropine and morphine will relieve abdominal pain. Artificial respiration and the administration of oxygen are indicated should there be symptoms of respiratory involvement.

Probenecid, U.S.P., B.P. (Benemid)

$$CH_3CH_2CH_2 \diagdown NSO_2 \diagdown \bigcirc \diagdown COOH$$
$$CH_3CH_2CH_2 \diagup$$

Probenecid is a white crystalline powder that is soluble in alcohol but relatively insoluble in water. Chemically, it is related to the sulfonamides and was first introduced as an agent to inhibit the excretion of penicillin by the kidney.

Action and result. It has been found to inhibit renal excretion of a number of other substances including para-aminosalicylic acid (which is used in the treatment of tuberculosis) and uric acid. It inhibits the reabsorption of urate in the kidney tubules, and this results in reduction of uric acid in the blood. This uricosuric action helps to prevent or retard formation of tophi and joint changes in chronic gouty arthritis. Probenecid is not an analgesic.

Uses. Probenecid is especially useful for the treatment of chronic gout and gouty arthritis. It is not effective in acute attacks of gout. Precipitation of urates in the kidney can be prevented by keeping the urine alkaline. It is also used in penicillin therapy when it is desirable to maintain high levels of the antibiotic in the blood plasma.

Preparation, dosage, and administration. Probenecid is available in 500-mg. tablets. The usual dose is 250 mg. twice daily for 1 week; then 500 mg. twice daily. This may be increased to 500 mg. four times daily.

From 3 to 7.5 Gm. of sodium bicarbonate is administered orally to maintain alkalinity of the urine. In gout, probenecid should not be given with salicylates because their effects are said to be antagonistic. A high fluid intake to produce copious volumes of urine is recommended to minimize formation of uric acid stones and occurrence of renal colic and hematuria.

Side effects and toxic effects. Probenecid is well tolerated by most patients. A few persons may experience nausea, constipation, or skin rash. Blood dyscrasias, liver necrosis, and serious hypersensitive reactions have been reported, but these are rare. Precautions should be taken against formation of renal calculi.

Sulfinpyrazone, U.S.P., B.P. (Anturane)

Sulfinpyrazone, a drug related to phenylbutazone, is useful in the prevention of attacks of gout because of its potent uricosuric action. The drug is available in 100-mg. tablets and 200-mg. capsules. The drug is administered in doses of 200 to 400 mg. daily in two divided doses, preferably with meals. Uricosuric effects may last for 10 hours after oral administration. The dose may be gradually increased. If acute attacks occur, it may be necessary to add colchicine, phenylbutazone, or other medications. Its interactions with other drugs are similar to those of phenylbutazone.

Side effects. Sulfinpyrazone may provoke renal colic because of the precipitation of uric acid. It may increase incidence of acute attacks of gout in the early weeks of treatment. The drug may activate peptic ulcers and may cause some blood dyscrasias.

Allopurinol, U.S.P., B.P. (Zyloprim)

Allopurinol represents an entirely different approach to the treatment of gout. It blocks the terminal steps in uric acid formation by inhibiting xanthine oxidase.

Uses. Allopurinol is intended for the treatment of either primary or secondary gout.

Preparation, dosage, and administration. Allopurinol is supplied in 100-mg. scored tablets. The dosage varies with the severity of the disease, but the average dose for adults is 200 to 300 mg. per day divided into two or three doses. Larger doses have been used for severe cases of gout. Fluid intake should be sufficient to maintain urinary output of 2 liters.

Side effects and toxic effects. Allopurinol should not be used in pregnant women and in children except in those children whose hyperuricemia is caused by a malignant disease. Allopurinol should not be used in nursing mothers. Nausea, vomiting, diarrhea, headache, drowsiness, and a metallic taste may occur. Toxic effects include liver damage, skin rash, fever, and leukopenia. If skin rash appears the drug should be stopped. Allopurinol is not an innocuous drug, and strict attention should be given to the approved package insert before it is used.

HYPNOTICS AND SEDATIVES

A hypnotic is a drug that produces sleep, and as a group these drugs have been widely used both for hospitalized patients and by the public at large. Sedatives are drugs that soothe and relieve anxiety.

Hospitalized patients often find it difficult to obtain rest and sleep for a variety of reasons. The surroundings are unfamiliar; they may be subjected to sensory overload or sensory deprivation, and their anxiety level is usually increased. In addition, pain or discomfort may prevent them from sleeping. Equally important as a deterrent to sleep are minor discomforts, such as cold feet, an aching back, a wrinkled bed, lack of sufficient ventilation, too few or too many blankets, a full bladder, or a distended rectum. Occasionally, a patient cannot sleep because he is hungry. It would be a poor nurse who would rely entirely on the effects of a hypnotic or sedative to remedy such discomforts.

The only difference between a hypnotic and a sedative action is one of degree. When a drug is given at the hour of retirement and in full dosage, producing sleep soon after administration, it is known as a hypnotic. When it is given in reduced dosage several times during the day and perhaps again at bedtime, it is called a sedative. Sedation is a calming, quieting effect, and the patient who is calm and relaxed during the day usually sleeps better at night. The terms *soporific* and *somnifacient* are synonymous with *hypnotic*. Many of the drugs known as tranquilizers are used for some of the same effects as the sedatives. Hypnotics act much like general anesthetics if large enough doses are given. They characteristically spare the medullary centers until large doses have been given.

SLEEP AND VARIOUS ASPECTS OF NURSING CARE

Sleep can be defined as a recurrent, normal condition of inertia and unresponsiveness during which an individual's overt and covert responses to stimuli are markedly reduced.

During sleep a person is no longer in sensory contact with the immediate environment, and stimuli that have bombarded the senses of sight, hearing, touch, smell, and taste during waking hours will no longer attract attention or exert a controlling influence over the individual's voluntary and involuntary movements or functions. It certainly is not difficult to understand that everyone needs to escape from constant stimuli.

Present-day knowledge about sleep has been obtained from research on normal subjects using the electroencephalogram (EEG) and electro-oculogram (EOG). The electroencephalogram provides graphic illustrations of brain waves, and this permits comparisons to be made between brain wave patterns of sleep and wakefulness. Brain waves are, of course, an indication of the electric activity occurring in the brain. The electric activity is greater during wakefulness than during sleep; during sleep the greatest electric activity occurs during dreaming sleep, with the least activity occurring in deep sleep. The electro-oculogram provides graphic illustrations of eye movements. Electrodes placed near the outer canthus of each eye monitor the amount, rate, and size of eye movements. These are also recorded as wave patterns. Rapid eye movements during sleep are associated with dreaming sleep.

Sleep research has shown that sleep is not one level of unconsciousness; it actually consists of four main sleep stages that occur in regular cyclic patterns characterized by variations in depth of sleep and variations in brain waves and eye movements (see Figure 11-2).

Onset of sleep is a drowsy period, and brain wave activity is similar to that seen in normal

Figure 11-2

Cyclic variation of a night of sleep.

awake individuals, that is, the brain waves are relatively fast and frequent. As sleep gradually deepens to Stage II sleep, a change in brain waves is seen, with the waves becoming slower in frequency. Stages III and IV are deep sleep stages—the brain waves are slow and have great height and depth. In other words, large brain wave deflections are seen.

From the standpoint of dreaming, sleep consists of two main functional states. One is called "slow wave," nondreaming, or non–rapid eye movement (NREM) sleep. The other is referred to as "paradoxical," dreaming, or rapid eye movement (REM) sleep. It should be kept in mind that REM sleep is not synonymous with light sleep, since it takes a bigger stimulus to arouse an animal or person from REM sleep than from synchronous slow wave sleep.

Sleep research indicates that there is both a psychologic and physiologic need for the body to maintain an equilibrium between the various stages of sleep. Physiologic functions of the body tend to be depressed during nondreaming sleep. For example it is known that:

1 There is a fall in blood pressure (10 to 30 mm. Hg)
2 Pulse rate is slowed
3 Metabolic rate is decreased
4 Activity of the gastrointestinal tract is slowed
5 Urine formation slows
6 Oxygen consumption and carbon dioxide production are lowered
7 Body temperature decreases slightly
8 Respirations are slower and more shallow
9 Body movement is minimal

Dreaming sleep tends to increase most of these parameters, and body movements are more noticeable—turning, jerking, arm and leg movements, talking, crying, or laughing—and of

course, eye movements can be seen under the closed lids. The dynamic physiologic equilibrium of the body continues to be maintained even during sleep. Depression of physiologic functions occurs during deep sleep and an increase in functions occurs during dreaming. Repeated studies have shown that when individuals are deprived of deep sleep, they become physically uncomfortable, tend to withdraw from society and their friends, are less aggressive and outgoing, and manifest concern over vague physical complaints and changes in bodily feelings. The overall impression made by persons deprived of deep sleep is that of a depressive and hypochondriac reaction.

However, dreaming sleep is also important. From studies during which individuals were deprived of dreaming sleep (every time the subjects attempted to dream, as evidenced by rapid eye movements, they were awakened and not permitted to dream) the following results were observed. The individuals during their waking hours became less well integrated and less effective. They showed signs of confusion, suspicion, and withdrawal. They appeared anxious, insecure, and irritable, they had greater difficulty concentrating, they had a marked increase in appetite with a definite weight gain, and they were introspective and unable to derive support from other people.

It is the belief of many psychologists and psychiatrists that wish fulfillment finds expression in dreams, and potentially harmful thoughts, feelings, and impulses are released through the dream so as not to interfere in the functioning of the personality during waking hours.

It is also known that in dream deprivation studies, the longer dream deprivation continues, the greater the increase in attempts to dream, until the individual begins to dream almost upon falling asleep. When subjects are finally permitted to dream, a marked increase of dreaming is noted for the entire night, and as much as 75% of the night may be spent in dreaming. This amount diminishes for each succeeding recovery night until the individual has once again established his normal sleep pattern.

Research has shown that deep sleep takes priority over dreaming sleep when there has been prolonged sleep deprivation. In other words, deep sleep needs will be met first, after which dreaming sleep needs will be met. The body attempts to reestablish the normal equilibrium between the sleep stages.

Each individual establishes his own normal sleep pattern, which will vary somewhat from night to night and which is influenced by the individual's emotional and physical state. For most individuals, any alteration in sleeping habits will cause problems in falling asleep, staying asleep, or both. Since drugs affect an individual's physical or emotional state, they also influence his sleep pattern.

Sleep research has also provided important knowledge about drugs and their effects on sleep and dreaming. Drugs commonly used in the hospital and in the home to promote rest and muscle relaxation and to ensure a good night's sleep actually alter the occurrence and length of sleep stages. The stage particularly affected is Stage I in which rapid eye movement occurs.

The drugs known to definitely affect the sleep pattern of man are:

1 Sleeping medications—hypnotics or sedatives (such as glutethimide or pentobarbital)
2 Tranquilizers (such as chlorpromazine)
3 Amphetamines
4 Ethyl alcohol (such as that contained in whiskey or cocktails)

In no study reported in the literature up to the present time has any sleep medication failed to alter the individual's pattern of sleep, and these patterns continue to be disrupted long after the sleeping medication has been discontinued. Sleep research studies also show that it may take as long as 3 to 5 weeks after sleeping medications have been discontinued before the individual's sleep pattern returns to its predrug or normal pattern.

Since both the amphetamines and barbiturates reduce dreaming time, when both these drugs are administered to the same individual the effect on dreaming is an additive one; that is, dreaming sleep is more greatly reduced than when either drug is used alone. Some drugs, such as reserpine, increase dreaming time, which may account for the bizarre dreams reported by patients receiving this drug. Other drugs, such as tranylcypromine parnate (an antidepressant), when withdrawn have been known to cause nightmares, suggesting they may markedly decrease dreaming sleep, which is made up upon withdrawal of the drug. It is theorized by some researchers that the chronic alcoholic has hallucinations upon withdrawal because whiskey reduces total dreaming sleep and he is making up for lost dream time.

Side effects from alteration in sleep pattern include irritability, tremors, tenseness, agitation, confusion, decreased attentiveness, sluggishness or lethargy, and many other symptoms. A newer hypnotic, Dalmane, does not decrease dream time. However, it does decrease Stage IV sleep (deep sleep). The significance of this is yet to be determined.

It is therefore important for nurses to remember:

1 Sleeping medications (hypnotics or sedatives) cause dreaming sleep to be less than normal.
2 When sleeping medications or hypnotics are discontinued, a rebound occurs, and dreaming sleep increases markedly until the loss has been overcome.
3 Sleeping medications cause a prolonged alteration in the individual's normal sleep pattern, which may still be present 3 to 5 weeks after the sleeping medication has been discontinued.
4 Altering the sleep pattern affects the individual physically and emotionally.

Since nurses are in a strategic position to influence the sleep their patients receive, it cannot be stressed enough that nurses must exercise caution when making decisions about giving or repeating an h.s. or p.r.n. order for a sleeping medication, hypnotic, or sedative. Nurses who immediately resort to administering a sleeping medication when a patient complains of being unable to sleep may be doing the patient more harm than good. It is important for nurses to keep informed about the drugs they administer, since there continues to be new knowledge about drugs, and this includes the so-called old drugs.

Nurses must also teach patients and their families ways to promote good sleep without resorting to drugs—including over-the-counter drugs.

Nurses should find out from their patients

what their sleep habits are and what they do to ensure good sleep at home. For example:

1 What do they do about environmental control, which includes ventilation, lighting, and noise?
2 What do they do about physical care? Do they shower before retiring or go for a walk?
3 What do they do about food? Do they ingest a snack before retiring?
4 What do they do about quiet recreation before sleep such as reading?

The patient's sleep history and drug history can be valuable aids to help plan the nursing care for the patient that will best promote good sleep.

Another very important factor is that every effort should be made not to disrupt the patient while he is sleeping, if at all possible. Numerous interruptions for various aspects of care can do nothing but alter the patient's sleep pattern.

CHARACTERISTICS OF A SATISFACTORY HYPNOTIC

Since rest and sleep are so important to relieve the effects of fatigue, stress, and strain in everyday life, it is equally if not more important that the sick person have adequate help in securing the benefits of sleep and relaxation. A hypnotic should produce sleep that is refreshing and as much like natural sleep as possible. In addition, the hypnotic should act within a reasonable length of time after administration and allow the patient to awaken somewhere near his usual time of awakening with no hangover effects. The hypnotic should not be dependence producing and should not produce adverse effects on body organs. Some investigators would add as a desirable characteristic a lack of influence on rapid eye-movement (REM) sleep, but this may be premature.

BARBITURATES

The barbiturates were among the first drugs to be synthesized. The first one was introduced into medicine by Emil Fischer and Joseph von Mehring in 1903 under the name of Veronal. Phenobarbital, known also as Luminal, is the second oldest of the barbiturates. Since the time of their introduction, hundreds of similar compounds have been synthesized, but only a limited number have proved clinically useful. New compounds have resulted from slight changes in the basic barbiturate molecule, and these changes have resulted in compounds that vary from the earlier compounds mostly in speed and duration of action. The formulas on the following page show the relationship of certain present-day compounds with the basic structure of barbituric acid and barbital. Various members of this family of drugs are made by substituting other substances for hydrogen atoms at position 5.

Some of the barbiturates have stood the test of time very well. Large amounts of these drugs are prescribed and used, as is evident from the fact that thousands of pounds are produced annually. Nevertheless, flurazepam is rapidly increasing in popularity and replacing the barbiturates in the treatment of sleep problems.

The barbiturates are all colorless, white crystalline powders that have a more or less bitter taste. They are sparingly soluble in water but freely soluble in alcohol. The sodium salts of these compounds are freely soluble in water.

Action and result. Important actions of the barbiturates are those of sedation and hypnotic effect. Barbiturates have been shown to depress the neurons and synapses of the ascending reticular formation of the brainstem, and this effect may be responsible for the reduction in electric activity of the cortex. Since the ascending reticular formation receives stimuli from all parts of the body and relays impulses to the cortex (thus promoting wakefulness and alertness), depression of the ascending reticular formation decreases cortical stimuli, reducing the need for wakefulness and alertness.

There is evidence that the barbiturates act at all levels of the central nervous system. The extent of effect varies from mild sedation to deep anesthesia, depending upon the drug selected, method of administration, dosage, and the reaction of the individual's nervous system. The barbiturates are not usually regarded as analgesics and cannot be depended upon to produce restful sleep when insomnia is caused by pain. However, when combined with an analgesic the sedative action seems to reinforce the action of the analgesic and to alter the patient's emotional reaction to pain. Therapeutic doses of the longer-acting barbiturates may result in depression and lowered vitality on the following day ("hangover effect").

All of the barbiturates used clinically depress the motor cortex of the brain in large doses, but phenobarbital, mephobarbital, and metharbital exert a selective action on the motor cortex, even in small doses. This explains their use as anticonvulsants.

Ordinary therapeutic doses have little or no effect on medullary centers, but large doses, especially when administered intravenously, depress the respiratory and vasomotor centers. Death from overdosage is caused, as a rule, by respiratory failure accompanied by hypotension.

Smooth muscles of blood vessels and of the gastrointestinal organs are depressed after large amounts of barbiturates, but clinical doses do not usually produce untoward effects. Motility of the gastrointestinal organs may be reduced and emptying of the stomach delayed slightly, but there is apparently little interference with the ability to respond to normal stimuli. Uterine muscle is affected little by hypnotic doses of barbiturates, and the force of uterine contractions at the time of childbirth is not diminished unless anesthesia has been produced by one of these drugs.

Uses. The barbiturates have many uses and are very popular drugs.

Hypnotics. For best effects the barbiturates should be administered at such times as will coincide with the usual hour of retirement. Long-, short-, or intermediate-acting barbiturates are chosen to meet the needs of individual patients.

Sedatives. The barbiturates have, for purposes of sedation, a wide range of therapeutic

Barbituric acid (contains no carboxyl group but is capable of forming a salt)

Secobarbital (Seconal)

Barbital (diethyl barbituric acid)

Pentobarbital (Nembutal)

Amobarbital (Amytal)

Phenobarbital (Luminal)

uses. Although the tranquilizing drugs have come into a position of great prominence, the barbiturates are still used to calm and sedate the nervous patient and for patients who have physical illness in which there is usually an emotional factor, as in the case of hypertension, chronic ulcerative colitis, and gastric ulcer.

Anticonvulsants. Barbiturates are used to prevent or control convulsive seizures associated with tetanus, strychnine poisoning, cerebral pathology, and epilepsy. Phenobarbital has been especially valuable in the prevention and control of grand mal epilepsy. It may be prescribed alone or in conjunction with other anticonvulsant drugs. Mephobarbital and metharbital are also effective in the symptomatic treatment of certain types of epilepsy.

Anesthetics. For selected forms of surgical procedures, and especially for surgery of short duration, the rapid-acting barbiturates are employed. Thiopental sodium is the preparation most widely used in the United States. These barbiturates are further discussed under "Intravenous anesthetics" (see p. 346).

Preanesthetic medications. The short-acting barbiturates, such as pentobarbital sodium, are selected for this effect. They are often ordered to be given the night before surgery to enable the patient to sleep and may also be ordered to be given the morning of the operation. They are frequently supplemented by other medications just before the patient is taken to the operating room.

Obstetric sedation and amnesia. For obstetric sedation and amnesia the barbiturates are used either alone or in combination with other drugs, such as scopolamine or meperidine. However, drugs that cause respiratory depression of the mother are likely to cause respiratory depression in the infant as well.

Psychiatry. Barbiturates are sometimes used in psychiatry to temporarily release a patient from strong inhibitions and enable him to cooperate more effectively with his therapist. Amobarbital, pentobarbital, and thiopental are the barbiturates likely to be chosen for this purpose.

Absorption and excretion. Barbiturates are readily absorbed after both oral and parenteral administration. The more soluble sodium salts are more rapidly absorbed than the free acids. Most of the barbiturates, with the exception of barbital, undergo change in the liver before they are excreted by the kidney. Some are excreted partly in an altered form and partly unchanged, and others are excreted in a completely altered form. The longer-acting barbiturates are said to be metabolized or chemically altered more slowly than the rapidly acting members. The more slowly a barbituate is altered or excreted, the more prolonged is its action. If excretion is slow and administration prolonged, cumulative effects will result.

Classification. The barbiturates are classified according to the duration of their action as long-, intermediate-, short-, and ultrashort-acting. This means that the short-acting drugs produce an effect in a relatively short time (10 to 15 minutes) and also act over a relatively short period (3 hours or less). Short-acting barbiturates are used in the treatment of insomnia, for preanesthetic sedation, and in combination with other drugs for psychosomatic disorders. Long-acting barbiturates require 30 to 60 minutes to become effective and act over a period of 6 hours or more. Long-acting barbiturates are used for treating epilepsy and other chronic neurologic disorders and for sedation in patients with high anxiety. Ultrashort-acting barbiturates are used as intravenous anesthetics. Thiopental sodium, which belongs to the ultrashort-acting group of barbiturates, acts rapidly and can produce a state of anesthesia in a few seconds. See Table 11-5 for dosage, methods of administration, and length of action.

Administration. The oral channel of administration is preferred and should be used whenever possible. Certain preparations may be given subcutaneously, intramuscularly, intravenously, or rectally, depending on the purpose to be achieved and the general condition of the patient. The intravenous route is the most dangerous and used only for production of anesthesia or in emergencies. Parenteral administration is also used when a patient is too ill to take the drug orally or has nausea and vomiting or when it is important to have a rapid depressant action.

Contraindications. Barbiturates should be avoided for patients who manifest hypersensi-

Table 11-5 Dosage, administration, and length of action of barbiturates

Preparation	Usual adult dose	Usual method of administration	Length of action
*Barbital (Veronal); barbitone sodium, B.P.	300 mg. (gr. 5)	Oral	Long
*Phenobarbital, U.S.P. (Luminal); pheno-barbitone, B.P.	30 to 100 mg. (gr. $1/2$ to $1^1/_2$)	Oral	Long
Mephobarbital, N.F. (Mebaral)	400 to 600 mg. (gr. 6 to 10)	Oral	Long
Metharbital, N.F. (Gemonil)	100 mg. (gr. $1^1/_2$)	Oral	Long
*Amobarbital, U.S.P. (Amytal)	100 mg. (gr. $1^1/_2$)	Oral	Intermediate
Aprobarbital (Alurate)	60 to 120 mg. (gr. 1 to 2)	Oral	Intermediate
Probarbital sodium (Ipral Sodium)	120 to 250 mg. (gr. 2 to 4)	Oral	Intermediate
Butethal (Neonal)	100 mg. (gr. $1^1/_2$)	Oral	Intermediate
Butabarbital sodium, N.F. (Butisol Sodium)	8 to 60 mg. (gr. $1/8$ to 1)	Oral	Intermediate
Pentobarbital sodium, U.S.P. (Nembutal Sodium); pentobarbitone sodium, B.P.	100 mg. (gr. $1^1/_2$)	Oral, rectal	Short
Secobarbital sodium, U.S.P. (Seconal); quinalbarbitone sodium, B.P.	100 to 200 mg. (gr. $1^1/_2$ to 3)	Oral, rectal	Short
Calcium cyclobarbital (Phanodorn); cyclobarbitone, B.P.	200 mg. (gr. 3)	Oral	Short
Butallylonal (Pernoston)	200 mg. (gr. 3)	Oral	Short
Sodium hexobarbital (Evipal Sodium)	2 to 4 ml. 10%	Intravenous	Ultrashort
Thiopental sodium, U.S.P. (Pentothal Sodium); thiopentone sodium, B.P.	2 to 3 ml. 2.5% in 10 to 15 sec.; repeated in 30 sec. as required	Intravenous	Ultrashort

*Sodium salts are available.

tivity toward them or who have been previously dependent on them. If a patient tells the nurse that he is hypersensitive to this group of drugs, the statement should be recorded and the information made known to the physician. Seriously impaired hepatic or renal function may also constitute a contraindication for the use of these drugs, although only the physician can decide whether the degree of damage warrants the use of a different type of drug.

Side effects and toxic effects. Unusual effects or reactions may be exhibited as one or more of the following: (1) marked symptoms of hangover—listlessness, prolonged depression, nausea, and emotional disturbances; (2) skin rash, urticaria, swelling of the face, and asthmatic attack; and (3) bad dreams, restlessness, and delirium.

This last category of symptoms may be experienced especially by elderly or debilitated patients. Night nurses find that they need to watch older patients carefully when they have been given a hypnotic dose of a barbiturate. Such patients tend to go to the bathroom more frequently than younger adults and under the influence of a barbiturate may become confused and have difficulty orienting themselves. Barbital, amobarbital, and pentobarbital are said to exert this effect more often than phenobarbital.

Restlessness is also produced when barbiturates are administered to patients in severe pain. The drug, in this instance, does not relieve pain but depresses the higher centers that normally serve as control centers. Mental confusion and delirium may result. An analgesic is usually prescribed to be given with a barbiturate if the patient has pain.

Acute poisoning. Because barbiturates are widely known and obtained with comparative ease, they have been one of the agents of choice for suicide. Poisoning also occurs accidentally and can occur when these drugs are given intravenously by persons insufficiently experienced in giving anesthetics. The fatal dose varies, but when fifteen to twenty times the usual therapeutic dose is absorbed, severe poisoning and possibly death will result. The lethal dose is said to be 1 to 1.5 Gm. or more. When seen in the earlier stages of poisoning, the patient is usually in a deep sleep or stupor. Occasionally, confusion and excitement precede heavy sleep. When poisoning is fully advanced, the patient is comatose and many of his reflexes are sluggish or absent. Respiration is either slow or rapid and shallow. Lack of oxygen affects the cardiovascular system and results in shock. The blood pressure drops; the pupils may become pinpoint in size; and the pulse is rapid and weak. Death is usually the result of respiratory failure, especially if a rapidly acting barbiturate has been taken. If death is delayed, it is more likely to be caused by hypostatic pneumonia or pulmonary edema.

TREATMENT. The treatment for acute poisoning will vary with the condition and needs of the patient. Sometimes little more than general supportive measures are required (keeping the patient warm and turned periodically, providing for adequate fluids and nutrition, and so on). If the patient is deeply comatose and unresponsive and having serious difficulty with respiration, great effort may be required to save his life.

If the drug has been swallowed and there is reason to think that part or most of it remains in the stomach, prompt gastric lavage may be done. A saline cathartic is sometimes instilled, after lavage, to hasten elimination of the drug. The danger of aspiration of gastric content at the time of lavage is always a calculated risk. The nurse should have some of the gastric washings saved in the event that a toxicologic examination becomes necessary. At all times the maintenance of an open airway is of primary importance. In severe depression the physician may plan to use an endotracheal tube or a respirator and administer oxygen or oxygen and carbon dioxide. The nurse will be expected to keep a careful check and to monitor the respirations, pulse, blood pressure, and degree of responsiveness.

Use of analeptic drugs (central nervous system stimulants that antagonize the action of depressants is looked upon with disfavor at the present time because many of these drugs are themselves capable of producing toxic symptoms. Supportive therapy, a patent airway, and mechanical ventilation are more effective in overcoming respiratory depression. Levarterenol, amphetamines, and phenylephrine may be used to combat circulatory collapse. Hemodialysis is an effective procedure for removing the drug from the patient's system; this procedure may be resorted to only if renal failure occurs. Shock from barbiturates causes a decrease in intravascular volume, and reversal of this phenomenon requires intravenous infusion of volume expanders such as dextran or concentrated albumin.

Chronic poisoning. Drug dependence to the barbiturates can develop. Tolerance is said to develop slowly and to a lesser degree than it does to morphine and related drugs. Occasional doses of barbiturates in quantities of 0.1 Gm. (gr. $1\frac{1}{2}$) do not cause drug dependence. In fact, it takes an appreciably larger daily dose, of 0.4 to 0.8 Gm. or more, over a period of time to establish drug dependence.

In recent years the abuse of barbiturates has become a problem of increasing concern. The seriousness of the situation is reflected in the large number of state laws passed to regulate the sale of barbiturates and in the continued effort for federal control.

Symptoms of chronic intoxication include slowness of thought, mental depression, incoherent speech, failing memory, skin rash, weight loss, gastrointestinal upsets, and anemia. There is frequently an ataxic gait; coarse tremor of the lips, fingers, and tongue; increased emotional instability; and mental confusion. The clinical manifestations are similar to those of chronic alcoholism. Because of the poor motor coordination, patients may fall and be injured. They are likely to fall asleep while smoking and set the bed or room furnishings on fire. They are unable to work, and they constitute a real hazard if they attempt to drive power machinery. Their judgment may be so impaired that they take additional doses of drug when they are already seriously intoxicated; this may account for some cases of reported suicide with barbiturates. Long-continued use of the short-acting barbiturates in large doses results in withdrawal symptoms characterized by great weakness, tremor, anxiety, nausea and vomiting, and a series of grand mal convulsions or psychosis or both. Withdrawal symptoms are precipitated when the drug dosage is appreciably reduced or stopped altogether.

Many opium users are also barbiturate users. They resort to barbiturates when they have difficulty getting their supply of opiates. The barbiturates most commonly selected seem to be pentobarbital, secobarbital, and amobarbital or the sodium salts of these compounds. Some authorities feel that the dependence resulting from the overuse of the barbiturates is, in some respects, more dangerous and undesirable than the dependence resulting from the misuse of opiates.

TREATMENT. The best treatment results are obtained in an institution with well-prepared personnel, and even then there is a rather high percentage of discouraging results. Abrupt withdrawal of the drug is quite dangerous since convulsive phenomena may occur.

Advantages and disadvantages encountered in the use of barbiturates. Barbiturates lend themselves to a variety of uses. They are anticonvulsants, anesthetics, hypnotics, and sedatives, although no one of them excels in all of these actions. They are easily administered in tablets or capsules, and may be given rectally or parenterally. They have a reasonably wide margin of safety.

The main disadvantages are that in large doses they all depress the respiratory center and they are often used for suicide. In addition, they have a high dependence potential. These are drugs that should never be left at the bedside for the patient to take at will. Patients have been known to hoard barbiturates until they had enough to commit suicide.

In the past these drugs had wide use and were easily obtained, which resulted in indiscriminate use and use for suicidal purposes. State laws restrict the sale of hypnotic drugs and prohibit the sale or possession of barbiturates except under proper licensure. Barbiturates may not be purchased or dispensed without a physician's prescription, and the prescription may not be refilled without the physician's personal sanction.

Choice of barbiturate. In choosing barbiturate preparations, consideration is given primarily to the duration of effect produced by the drug and to individual needs of patients. Phenobarbital is an outstanding member of the group of barbiturates because of its anticonvulsant action. Secobarbital and pentobarbital are good examples of short-acting barbiturates, and the ultrashort-acting ones are described under anesthetics.

Barbiturates may be combined in the same capsule so that a long-acting and a short-acting or moderately long-acting preparation can be used to advantage for the patient who has difficulty both in getting to sleep and remaining asleep for the desired number of hours. Tuinal is an official combination of secobarbital sodium and amobarbital sodium, U.S.P. It is available in capsules containing gr. $3/_4$ (0.05 Gm.) of each barbiturate (total 0.1 Gm., gr. $1^1/_2$) or gr. $1^1/_2$ of each (total 0.2 Gm., gr. 3).

Phenobarbital (Luminal)

Phenobarbital not only requires a relatively long time to take effect but also exerts an effect over a long period (6 or more hours) and is used when prolonged sedation is required. It is used as a hypnotic as well as a sedative for a variety of nervous conditions, such as chorea, gastrointestinal neuroses, and preoperative and postoperative states of tension. It is also used as a sedative for patients with hypertension and coronary artery disease. Because its action is rather slow, it is not the best drug for certain kinds of insomnia or for use as a preanesthetic medication. Adult hypnotic dose is 100 mg. (about gr. $1/_2$);

sedative dose is 30 mg. (gr. $\frac{1}{2}$). Sedative dose for children is 1 to 6 mg. per kilogram of body weight daily divided into three doses.

Phenobarbital has a selective depressant action on the motor cortex of the brain when given in sedative doses to epileptic patients. However, when effective anticonvulsant doses are given, some degree of central depression also results. (The patient feels tired, relaxed, and perhaps dull and sleepy.) In this respect phenobarbital is inferior to the anticonvulsant drug phenytoin (Dilantin). On the other hand, phenobarbital is regarded as one of the least, if not the least, toxic of the antiepileptic drugs. The dosage range for adults is 50 to 200 mg. for convulsive disorders; for children the range is 3 to 5 mg. per kilogram of body weight. This may be given in one dose at bedtime or it may be given in divided doses throughout the day. Should it be necessary to discontinue the drug for an epileptic patient, it should be done gradually and never stopped suddenly or severe epileptic seizures may be precipitated. Phenobarbital is often given to patients after surgical operation on the brain to minimize the irritating effect of the procedure. Patients may continue to take the drug for a year or more under medical supervision.

The action and uses of phenobarbital sodium are the same as those of phenobarbital except that it can be injected when phenobarbital either cannot be given by mouth or the desired effects are not being secured following oral administration.

CAUTION: Errors sometimes occur if the nurse forgets, or does not understand, that phenobarbital (Luminal) and phenobarbital sodium (Sodium Luminal) are not one and the same drug. The latter, the sodium salt, can be given parenterally but the former cannot.

Preparation, dosage, and administration. The following preparations are available.

Phenobarbital tablets, U.S.P.; *phenobarbitone tablets*, B.P. Tablets containing 15, 30, 60, or 100 mg. are available for oral administration.

Phenobarbital elixir, U.S.P. The elixir is for oral use only. Each 5 ml. contains 7.5 or 20 mg. of drug.

Phenobarbital sodium, U.S.P.; *phenobarbitone sodium*, B.P. The usual dose is 100 mg. (gr. $1\frac{1}{2}$). This is a powder dispensed in ampules for parenteral or oral administration.

Phenobarbital sodium injection, U.S.P. The usual parenteral dose is 100 mg. (gr. $1\frac{1}{2}$). A sterile solution of phenobarbital sodium in a suitable solvent (50 mg. in 1 ml., 125 mg. in 1 or 5 ml., and 300 mg. in 2 or 5 ml.) for intramuscular or subcutaneous injection. Aqueous solutions of phenobarbital sodium decompose upon standing.

Phenobarbital sodium tablets, U.S.P.; *pheno-*

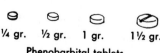

Phenobarbital sodium ampules
Injection

¼ gr.   ½ gr.   1 gr.   1½ gr.
Phenobarbital tablets
Oral only

Figure 11-3

These illustrations emphasize the point that phenobarbital and sodium phenobarbital are not the same drug. Sodium phenobarbital is suitable for parenteral administration, whereas plain phenobarbital is not.

barbitone sodium tablets, B.P. Tablets containing 30, 60, or 100 mg. are available. The usual dose is 30 mg. (gr. $\frac{1}{2}$) orally.

Phenobarbital is also available in 50-, 65-, and 100-mg. sustained-release dosage forms.

Secobarbital sodium, U.S.P. (Seconal); quinalbarbitone sodium, B.P.

Secobarbital sodium is a short-acting barbiturate, more active than barbital, and given in correspondingly smaller doses. Small doses produce a sedative effect and larger doses, a hypnotic effect.

Preparation, dosage, and administration. Dosage of secobarbital sodium is 100 mg. (gr. $1\frac{1}{2}$) at bedtime for adults. As a preanesthetic agent, 100 to 200 mg. are given 30 minutes to 1 hour before the patient goes to the operating room. Sedative dose for children is 6 mg. per kilogram of body weight daily divided into three doses; anticonvulsant dose is 3 to 5 mg. per kilogram given intramuscularly or intravenously. It is available in 30-, 50-, and 100-mg. capsules and in 30-, 65-, 130-, and 200-mg. rectal suppositories.

Pentobarbital sodium (Nembutal Sodium)

Pentobarbital sodium, the most widely used short-acting barbiturate, acts over a rather brief period of time (3 to 6 hours), which is sometimes an advantage, particularly if large doses have been given. It is used as a hypnotic and as a sedative prior to anesthesia.

Pentobarbital and pentobarbital calcium are similar in action and use to pentobarbital sodium. Pentobarbital calcium has no advantage except that it is better suited for making compressed tablets than sodium pentobarbital.

Preparation, dosage, and administration

Pentobarbital sodium elixir, U.S.P. (Nembutal Sodium Elixir). The elixir contains 20 mg. in 5 ml. It is used for sedation of children or elderly patients.

Pentobarbital sodium, U.S.P. (Nembutal Sodium); *pentobarbitone sodium*, B.P. The usual hypnotic adult dose is 100 mg. (gr. $1\frac{1}{2}$). Range of sedative dose for adults is 15 to 50 mg., which may be given 3 or 4 times daily. Sedative dose for children is 6 mg. per kilogram of body weight divided into three doses. Anticonvulsant dose is 3 to 5 mg. per kilogram of body weight. The preparation is available in capsules, ampules containing the drug in powder form or in solution for injection, suppositories for rectal administration, and sustained-release dosage forms for slow, continuous absorption. Pentobarbital sodium injection, U.S.P., may be given intravenously if prompt action is essential to control convulsive seizures associated with some types of drug poisoning, rabies, tetanus, chorea, and eclampsia. Aqueous solutions of pentobarbital are not stable and decompose on standing or after boiling.

NONBARBITURATE SEDATIVES AND HYPNOTICS

Although several nonbarbiturate sedatives and hypnotics are available, it should be emphasized that all are habit forming, may cause physical dependence, and are subject to abuse.

Ethchlorvynol, N.F., B.P. (Placidyl)

$$CH\equiv C - \overset{\displaystyle OH}{\underset{\displaystyle CH_2CH_3}{C}} - CH = CHCl$$

Ethchlorvynol is a colorless-to-yellow liquid with a pungent odor. It is a mild hypnotic somewhat less predictable than the barbiturates. It acts within 15 to 30 minutes after administration, and the duration of its effects is about 5 hours.

Uses. Ethchlorvynol is said to be useful in the treatment of insomnia if pain and anxiety are not complicating factors. It is also useful for patients who are unable to take barbiturates. It may be used as a daytime sedative. In addition it has anticonvulsant and muscle-relaxing actions.

Preparation, dosage, and administration. Ethchlorvynol is available in 100-, 200-, and 500-mg. capsules. The usual adult hypnotic dose is 500 mg.; sedative doses are correspondingly smaller. It is administered orally. Dosage for elderly and debilitated patients should be reduced to the smallest effective amount.

Side effects. This drug seems to have a wide margin of safety. Side effects include headache, fatigue, ataxia, dizziness, mental confusion, nightmares, and nausea and vomiting. Hypotension, mild hangover, and mild excitation have been reported.

Ethinamate, N.F. (Valmid)

Ethinamate exerts a mild sedative effect upon the central nervous system. The duration of its effect is shorter than that produced by the barbiturates. It is effective within 15 to 25 minutes, and the duration of its effect is about 4 hours. It has not been known to cause habituation or addiction, and tolerance does not seem to develop. It is readily absorbed from the gastrointestinal tract and rapidly destroyed or excreted from the body.

Uses. It is used chiefly as a rapid-acting hypnotic for the treatment of simple insomnia. It can be used for patients with impaired function of the liver and kidney. It is not a hypnotic of choice for patients requiring heavy or continuous sedation.

Preparation, dosage, and administration. Ethinamate is available in 500-mg. tablets. The minimal effective hypnotic dose for adults is 500 mg. Larger and repeated doses may be required to produce a full night's sleep. It is administered orally.

Side effects. Excitement in children, mild gastrointestinal symptoms, and skin rash have occurred with use of ethinamate. Use in children is not recommended. Patients who receive the drug over long periods of time should be under careful observation.

Glutethimide, N.F., B.P. (Doriden)

Glutethimide is a hypnotic and sedative that depresses the central nervous system and produces effects similar to those produced by the short-acting barbiturates. The main advantage claimed for it is that it can be used for patients who do not tolerate the barbiturates. It is effective in 15 to 30 minutes and its effects last 4 to 8 hours. Hangover effects do not seem to be noticeable unless the drug is administered late at night or unless the dose is repeated in the course of the night. It is not considered an addicting agent in the same sense as morphine, but dependence has occurred. Its abuse has led to many cases of chronic and acute intoxication with a number of fatalities.

Uses. At present, the greatest use for glutethimide seems to be for relief of simple or nervous insomnia, provided it is uncomplicated by pain or severe agitation. It can be used both as a preoperative and as a daytime sedative.

Preparation, dosage, and administration. Glutethimide is marketed in 125-, 250-, and 500-mg. tablets. The usual hypnotic dose for adults is 500 mg. given orally at bedtime. For daytime sedation, 125 to 250 mg. may be given orally three times daily after meals. For preoperative sedation 500 mg. the night before surgery and 500 to 1000 mg. 1 hour before anesthesia may be given.

Side effects. The principal side effects seem to be nausea and, occasionally, skin rash. Toxic effects and treatment are much the same as those for poisoning with the barbiturates. Treatment of poisoning may be quite difficult.

Methyprylon, N.F., B.P. (Noludar)

Methyprylon depresses the central nervous system in a manner similar to the barbiturates except that it has less tendency to depress the respiratory center. The onset of action is about 30 minutes and duration of action is about 7 hours. Its capacity to cause dependence is thought to be less than that of the barbiturates, although further study may prove otherwise.

Uses. Methyprylon is used in the treatment of simple and nervous insomnia.

Preparation, dosage, and administration. Methyprylon is marketed in 50- and 200-mg. tablets and as an elixir containing 10 mg. per milliliter. Doses of 50 to 100 mg. three or four times daily are prescribed to produce sedation, and 200 to 400 mg. is the usual adult hypnotic dose given at bedtime.

Side effects. The incidence of side effects is thought to be low, although the following have been observed: nausea, vomiting, constipation, diarrhea, headache, itching, and skin rash. No serious toxic effects on the kidney, liver, or bone marrow have been reported.

Flurazepam, N.F. (Dalmane)

Flurazepam is related to the benzodiazepine compounds, which are widely used as minor tranquilizers. Numerous side effects have been reported. In elderly persons dizziness, staggering, ataxia, and falling have occurred. Flurazepam has become a very popular drug. It is claimed that flurazepam is useful in the therapy of all sleep disorders in that it does not suppress dream or REM sleep. However, it does decrease deep sleep. It reduces sleep induction time and increases sleep duration time. Hypnotic effects occur in 20 to 45 minutes and last 7 to 8 hours. It is available in 15- and 30-mg. capsules. Usual adult dose is 30 mg. at bedtime; for elderly patients initial dose is 15 mg.

OLDER HYPNOTICS

There are a number of hypnotics that were almost abandoned when the barbiturates became popular. They seem to be gradually regaining some of their lost popularity. They include chloral hydrate and paraldehyde as well as a number of others.

Chloral hydrate, U.S.P., B.P. (Noctec)

$$Cl_3-CHOH$$
$$|$$
$$OH$$

Chloral hydrate was first synthesized in 1862. It is the oldest of the hypnotics and is still used. It is a chlorinated derivative of acetaldehyde, or it may be described as a hydrate of trichloracetaldehyde. It is a crystalline substance that has a bitter taste and a penetrating odor. It is readily soluble in water, alcohols, and oils such as olive oil.

Action and result. Locally, chloral hydrate is an irritant. Systemically, it depresses the central nervous system and decreases awareness of external stimuli. It acts promptly (10 to 15 minutes) and produces sleep that lasts 4 to 8 hours or more. The sleep greatly resembles natural sleep; the patient can be awakened without difficulty. It produces little or no analgesic effect, and it is neither an anesthetic nor an anticonvulsant.

In therapeutic doses there is little or no effect on the heart and respiratory center. The pulse and blood pressure are not lowered more than

can be observed in ordinary sleep. In large doses chloral hydrate depresses the respiratory and vasomotor centers, resulting in slowed respiration and dilation of cutaneous blood vessels. Effect on the heart is said to be similar to that of chloroform. Overdoses will cause cardiac depression, especially in patients with heart disease.

Uses. Chloral hydrate is used as a sedative. It produces sedation similar to paraldehyde and the barbiturates. It is sometimes used to relieve symptoms during the withdrawal phase of drug dependence (alcoholism, opiate, or barbiturate).

Chloral hydrate is used as a hypnotic when insomnia is not the result of pain. It is one of the cheapest hypnotics. Its chief disadvantage is that it can produce gastric irritation. It also has an unpleasant taste, but this problem is remedied by administering the drug in capsule form.

Preparation, dosage, and administration. The usual adult hypnotic dose of chloral hydrate is 500 mg. Larger doses may also be prescribed (250 mg. to 2 Gm.). Adult sedative dose is 250 to 500 mg. three times daily after meals. Hypnotic dose for children is 50 mg. per kilogram of body weight; sedative dose is 25 mg. per kilogram divided into three or four doses. It is marketed in soft gelatin capsules containing 250 and 500 mg. and in suppository form. It can be prepared as an aqueous solution or a syrup.

If the liquid solution is administered it should be well diluted with water or given in a syrup or milk to disguise the taste. It is sometimes given to children in the form of a retention enema (dissolved in oil). It is too irritating to be given parenterally. It should not be given with alcohol to avoid the additive effects of two depressant drugs. Such a combination is sometimes referred to as a "Mickey Finn" or knockout drops.

Side effects and toxic effects. Symptoms of both acute and chronic toxicity are sometimes observed. The local effects of the drug may cause nausea and vomiting when it is taken orally.

Although chloral hydrate has a wide safety range, acute poisoning can occur. Symptoms are similar to those of any central depressant and include deep sleep, stupor, coma, lowered blood pressure, slow weak pulse, slow respiration, and cyanosis. Death is usually caused by respiratory depression or it may result from sudden heart failure in patients who have cardiac damage. If the patient survives, there is a possibility that damage may have been done to the liver and kidneys.

Treatment is essentially the same as that for acute poisoning with barbiturates.

Chloral hydrate habitues develop some tolerance to the drug, but habit formation is not common. It sometimes results in chronic poisoning, manifested by degenerative changes in the liver and kidneys, nervous disturbances, weakness, skin manifestations, and gastrointestinal disturbances. Treatment is gradual withdrawal of the drug and rehabilitative measures similar to those used in the treatment of the alcoholic.

Contraindications. Chloral hydrate is contraindicated for patients with serious heart disease or impaired function of the liver and kidney and sometimes for patients with gastric or duodenal ulcer.

Petrichloral (Periclor)

Petrichloral is a derivative of chloral that exhibits a hypnotic and sedative action similar to chloral hydrate. It is better tolerated than the latter drug because it has no odor or aftertaste, and it does not produce gastric irritation. It has a wide margin of safety.

Preparation, dosage, and administration. Petrichloral is available in 300-mg. gelatin capsules. The usual hypnotic dose is 600 mg., and the sedative dose for daytime effect is 300 mg. every 6 hours.

Chloral betaine, N.F. (Beta-Chlor) tablets

This is a formulation providing chloral betaine in tablet form. Each tablet contains 870 mg. of chloral betaine, equivalent to 500 mg. of chloral hydrate. It is administered by mouth in a dose of one to two tablets as a hypnotic 15 to 30 minutes before bedtime. The effects, uses, toxic actions, and contraindications are the same as for chloral hydrate.

Paraldehyde, U.S.P., B.P.

Paraldehyde has been used as a hypnotic since 1882, when it was introduced into medicine. It is a colorless, transparent liquid with a strong odor and a disagreeable taste. It is only slightly soluble in water but freely soluble in oils and in alcohol.

Action and result. Paraldehyde depresses the central nervous system, producing drowsiness and sleep in 10 to 15 minutes after a hypnotic dose. The sleep closely resembles a natural sleep and lasts for 4 to 8 hours. Therapeutic doses do not depress the medullary centers and do not affect the heart and respiration. It is less potent than chloral hydrate but also less toxic. It is not an analgesic, but it may compel sleep in spite of pain.

Paraldehyde is rapidly absorbed from the mucosa of the gastrointestinal tract and also from intramuscular sites of injection, although it may cause some irritation when given parenterally. The fate of paraldehyde in the body is not known, but a large part of it is thought to be destroyed in the liver. It is therefore contraindicated for patients who have serious impairment of liver function. It is not contraindicated for patients with renal disease. A part of the drug is excreted by the lungs, where it tends to increase bronchial secretions, and for this reason it is avoided for patients with bronchitis or pneumonia.

Uses. Paraldehyde is employed for its hypnotic and sedative effects in treatment of conditions in which there is a threat of convulsive seizures or nervous hyperexcitability. It is used therefore in delirium tremens, tetanus, strychnine poisoning, and mania. It is sometimes used as a basal anesthetic, particularly for children; when so used it is given rectally.

Preparation, dosage, and administration. Paraldehyde is available as a plain liquid for oral administration or as a sterile solution dispensed in ampules (2 and 10 ml.) for parenteral use. The usual adult oral dose is 8 ml. (2 fluidrams) but may be increased to 10 or 15 ml. in some instances. When paraldehyde is given orally it should be disguised in a suitable medium such as a flavored syrup, fruit juice, wine, or milk, and it should be very cold to minimize the odor and taste. It can also be given as a retention enema (mixed with a thin oil). When given intramuscularly a pure sterile preparation should be used. The usual intramuscular dose is 5 ml. It is rarely given intravenously. Paraldehyde must be stored in tight, light-resistant containers in a cold place. Paraldehyde from a container opened longer than 24 hours must be discarded since it can be completely converted to acetic acid, and fatality may occur if the converted drug is administered.

Side effects and toxic effects. The chief disadvantages of paraldehyde are its obnoxious odor, disagreeable taste, and irritating effect on the throat and stomach if the drug is not well diluted in a suitable medium. Because of the odor it is not suitable for patients who are up and about, for they will reek with the odor of the drug. Fortunately, if the patient is capable of noticing the odor, his sense of smell becomes dulled after a time. Paraldehyde is not as safe a drug as was once thought; it is now known that the margin between an anesthetic and a lethal dose is very narrow. Symptoms of overdosage resemble those of alcohol overdosage in that mild poisoning can usually be "slept off." The incidence of acute toxicity is low, although deaths from paraldehyde depression have been reported. The symptoms of poisoning and treatment are essentially the same as those for chloral hydrate. In spite of the taste and odor, some patients do become dependent on paraldehyde.

Bromides

The term *bromides* frequently refers to sodium bromide, although a number of bromide salts have been popular. They have been used for their sedative, hypnotic, and anticonvulsant effects, but their range of usefulness has been narrowed because of the appearance of better drugs. They are slow-acting depressants of the

nervous system. Bromide intoxication, however, is still encountered. A number of headache remedies contain bromides and are easily procured as over-the-counter drugs.

ALCOHOLS

Although there are many alcohols that vary physically from liquids to solids, the alcohol usually meant, unless otherwise specified, is ethyl alcohol. Methyl alcohol, propyl alcohol, butyl alcohol, and amyl alcohol are examples of other alcohols. Chemically speaking, they are hydroxy derivatives of aliphatic hydrocarbons.

Ethyl alcohol

$$H-\underset{\underset{H}{|}}{\overset{\overset{H}{|}}{C}}-\underset{\underset{H}{|}}{\overset{\overset{H}{|}}{C}}-OH$$

Ethyl alcohol has been known in an impure form since earliest times, and it is the only alcohol used extensively in medicine. It was formerly thought to be a remedy for almost any disease or disorder. It is a colorless liquid and lighter than water with which it mixes readily. It lowers surface tension and acts as a good solvent for a number of substances. In concentrations above 40% it is flammable. Ethyl alcohol, also referred to as grain alcohol, is the product of the fermentation of a sugar by yeast. If the carbohydrate used for fermentation to alcohol is a starch, the starch must first be broken down to a sugar before the molecules can be fermented.

Action and result. Ethyl alcohol may have either a local or systemic action.

Local. Ethyl alcohol denatures proteins by precipitation and dehydration. This is said to be the basis for its germicidal, irritant, and astringent effects. It irritates denuded skin, mucous membranes, and subcutaneous tissue. Considerable pain may be experienced from a subcutaneous injection of alcohol, and slough of the tissue may result. When it is injected into or near a nerve it may produce degeneration of the nerve and anesthesia. Alcohol evaporates readily from the skin, produces a cooling effect, and reduces the temperature of the skin. When rubbed on the surface of the body it acts as a mild counter-irritant. It dries and hardens the epithelial layer of the skin and helps to prevent bed sores when used externally. However, its use on skin that is already dry and irritated is usually contraindicated. Solutions of ethyl alcohol that measure 70% by weight seem to exert the best bactericidal effects. High concentrations have a marked dehydrating effect but do not necessarily kill bacteria. Ethyl alcohol in proper concentration is considered an effective germicide for a number of uses, but it does not kill spores.

Systemic. According to modern scientific authorities alcohol is not considered a stimulant (popular ideas to the contrary). It is thought to interfere with the transmission of nerve impulses at synaptic connections, but how this is accomplished is not known. It exerts a progressive and continuous depression on the central nervous system (cerebrum, cerebellum, cord, and medulla). Its action is comparable to that of the general anesthetics. The excitement stage, however, is longer, and when the anesthetic stage is reached, definite toxic symptoms are present. Also, when alcohol is taken socially, attempts are usually made to stay in an early stage rather than to pass rapidly to unconsciousness. The margin between the anesthetic and fatal dose is a narrow one. What sometimes appears to be stimulation results from the depression of the higher faculties of the brain and represents the loss of learned inhibitions acquired by socialization. The results of the action of alcohol vary with the individual, one's tolerance, the presence or absence of extraneous stimuli, and the rate of ingestion. Small or moderate quantities produce a feeling of well-being, talkativeness, greater vivacity, and increased confidence in one's mental and physical power. The personality becomes expansive, and there is a general loss of inhibitions. The finer powers of discrimination, concentration, insight, judgment, and memory are gradually dulled and lost. Large quantities of the drug may cause excitement, impulsive speech and behavior, laughter, hilarity, and in some cases, pugnaciousness. Others may become melancholy or unduly sentimental. The individual usually becomes ataxic, mutters incoherently, has disturbance of the special senses,

is often nauseated, may vomit, and eventually lapses into stupor or coma.

The respiratory center is not depressed except by large doses.

CARDIOVASCULAR. Alcohol depresses the vasomotor center in the medulla and in this way brings about dilation of the peripheral blood vessels, especially those of the skin. This causes a feeling of warmth. Because of the dilation of the capillaries, heat is lost from the surface of the body and more must be brought from the interior. This accounts for the fact that an intoxicated person may freeze to death more quickly than a normal person. Alcohol also depresses the heat-regulating mechanism in a manner similar to the antipyretics, and before the advent of the modern antipyretics it was used to reduce fever.

Small doses (10 to 25 ml.) in man produce an insignificant increase in the pulse rate, caused mainly by the excitement and the reflex effect on the gastrointestinal tract. Larger doses produce the same effect but may be followed by lowered blood pressure caused by the effect on the vasoconstrictor center. Only high concentrations of alcohol depress the heart.

GASTROINTESTINAL. The effect of alcohol upon the function of the digestive organs depends upon the presence or absence of gastrointestinal disease, the degree of alcoholic tolerance, and the concentration of the beverage used as well as the type and amount of food present. Small doses in the patient who likes alcohol will stimulate the secretion of gastric juice rich in acid. Salivary secretion is also reflexly stimulated. Large and concentrated doses of alcohol tend to inhibit secretion and enzyme activity in the stomach, although the effect in the intestine seems to be negligible. However, when large quantities of alcohol are taken over a period of time, gastritis, nutritional deficiencies, and other untoward results have been observed.

Absorption and excretion. Since alcohol does not require digestion in the stomach or intestine it is readily absorbed from both organs. Ninety percent or more of the alcohol that is absorbed is metabolized, chiefly in the liver. It is oxidized first to acetaldehyde and eventually to carbon dioxide and water. It is oxidized at the rate of about 10 grams per hour, which amounts to

Table 11-6 Relation between clinical indications of alcoholic intoxication and concentration of alcohol of the blood and urine

Stage	Blood alcohol (%)	Urine alcohol (%)	Clinical observations
Subclinical	0 to 0.11	0 to 0.15	Normal by ordinary observations, slight changes detectable by special tests
Emotional instability	0.09 to 0.21	0.13 to 0.29	Decreased inhibitions; emotional instability; slight muscular incoordination; slowing of responses to stimuli
Confusion	0.18 to 0.33	0.26 to 0.45	Disturbance of sensation; decreased pain sense; staggering gait; slurred speech
Stupor	0.27 to 0.43	0.36 to 0.58	Marked decrease in response to stimuli; muscular incoordination approaching paralysis
Coma	0.36 to 0.56	0.48 to 0.72	Complete unconsciousness; depressed reflexes; subnormal temperature; anesthesia; impairment of circulation; possible death
Death (uncomplicated)	Over 0.44	Over 0.60	

about 70 calories. Alcohol does not form glycogen and hence it cannot be stored, so that it is a food only in the sense that it contributes calories. It supplies no minerals or vitamins.

Alcohol that escapes oxidation is excreted by way of the lungs and kidneys, and some is found in a number of excretions such as sweat.

Alcohol produces an increased flow of urine because of increased fluid intake, which ordinarily accompanies the drinking of alcoholic beverages. It has been suggested that alcohol may also act as a diuretic through central nervous system depression and inhibition of ADH (antidiuretic hormone) release. If the patient has preexisting renal disease, there may be further damage to the kidney. Large and concentrated doses of alcohol are thought to injure the renal epithelium.

Since alcohol, after absorption, is distributed in the tissues of the body in approximately the same ratio as their water content, a rough estimate of the quantity taken may be obtained from an analysis of the blood and urine (Table 11-6). The National Safety Council regards concentration of alcohol in the blood up to 0.05% as evidence of unquestioned sobriety. Concentrations between 0.051% and 0.149% are regarded as grounds for suspicion and for use of performance tests, and anything more than 0.15% is evidence of unquestionable intoxication. The states differ as to what is accepted as a legal limit.

Effects of alcohol that may not be discernible to the casual observer become apparent when the individual who has had a number of doses of alcohol attempts to operate a piece of power machinery such as an automobile. Visual acuity (especially peripheral vision) is diminished, reaction time is slowed, judgment and self-control are impaired, and the individual tends to be complacent and pleased with himself. Many drivers will take chances when under the influence of alcohol that they would never take ordinarily. This leads to disaster, as statistics reveal.

Uses. Ethyl alcohol is used topically as an astringent and antiseptic. It is rubbed on the backs and buttocks of patients to prevent decubiti. It is used to cleanse the skin, and it is poured on dressings over wounds. It is a popular disinfectant for the skin.

It is an excellent solvent and preservative for many medicines and medicinal mixtures (spirits, elixirs, fluidextracts).

Alcohol sponges are given to lower the temperature of the patient with a high fever since it increases heat dissipation. Caution must be exercised when alcohol sponges are given, particularly to children, since alcohol intoxication can occur.

At times alcohol is injected into a nerve to destroy sensory nerve fibers and relieve pain associated with a severe and protracted neuralgia, such as trifacial neuralgia (tic douloureux) or inoperable cancer. An injection of 80% ethyl alcohol is used. Effects may persist for 1 to 3 years or until regeneration of the peripheral nerve fibers takes place.

Alcohol is used to produce vasodilation in peripheral vascular disease. Concentrated solutions often produce greater peripheral vasodilation than any other drug. The pain associated with Buerger's disease may be relieved with the use of ethyl alcohol administered orally. It may be prescribed to decrease the frequency of anginal attacks but effects are said to be unreliable. Benefits to the cardiac patient, if they occur, are believed to result from the rest and relaxation that the alcohol produces.

Alcohol is also used as an appetizer for patients with poor appetite during periods of convalescence and debility. From 5% to 10% solutions of alcohol have also been given in intravenous fluids (5% dextrose and isotonic saline solution) to supplement the caloric intake.

The use of some form of alcohol has long been advocated to thwart the development of a head cold, perhaps because it makes the patient more comfortable, drowsy, and sleepy, thereby promoting sleep and rest. Increased circulation of blood through the skin will relieve feelings of chilliness. It seems to have no effect on the course of the cold itself.

It may be used as a hypnotic for older persons who do not tolerate other hypnotics. It is used as a home remedy or for a hospitalized patient who requests it. It is occasionally given in intravenous fluids for its sedative effects—to reduce the amount of opiate or barbiturate needed to keep a patient comfortable.

Preparations and dosage. The following are various preparations of ethyl alcohol. Dosage varies with the purpose for which the alcohol is administered. When whiskey is prescribed as a vasodilator, 30 ml. may be ordered to be given two or three times a day. When an alcoholic beverage is given for its effects as an appetizer, it should be given before meals. From 30 to 60 ml. are usually given.

Alcohol (ethyl alcohol, ethanol), U.S.P., B.P. Alcohol contains not less than 92.3% by weight corresponding to approximately 94.9% by volume of C_2H_5OH.

Diluted alcohol, U.S.P. The diluted form contains not less than 41% and not more than 42% by weight of ethyl alcohol. The B.P. lists a number of dilute alcohols.

Whiskey (spiritus frumenti). Whiskey is an alcoholic liquid that is obtained by the distillation of the fermented mash of wholly or partly malted cereal grain and contains approximately 50% by volume of ethyl alcohol. It usually is stored in charred wood containers for a period of not less than 2 years.

Brandy (spiritus vini vitis). Brandy is an alcoholic liquid obtained by the distillation of the fermented juice of sound, ripe grapes. It contains approximately 50% by volume of ethyl alcohol. It is stored in wood containers, frequently as long as 2 years.

Other spirits are solutions of volatile substances in alcohol. In most cases the dissolved substance has a more important action than the alcohol, which is used merely as a solvent.

Wines. Wines are fermented liquors made from grapes or other fruit juices. Besides alcohol, wines may contain various acids, such as tartaric, tannic, or malic.

Dry wines are those that contain no added sugar. They contain about 10% alcohol.

Sweet wines are those to which sugar has been added. They contain about 15% alcohol.

Sparkling wines contain carbon dioxide, which makes them effervescent. Examples are champagne and sparkling burgundy.

Acute alcoholism. In states of acute intoxication the patient is stuporous or comatose, the skin is cold and clammy, respirations are noisy and slow, and pupils are dilated or normal. The breath is usually heavy with alcoholic fumes. Death may result if the coma is prolonged or if injury, hypostatic pneumonia, or infection complicates the picture.

Ordinary intoxication treats itself with time and sleep. In severe intoxication the stomach should be emptied. Emetics in cases of deep narcosis are inactive and worse than useless because they add to the depression. The stomach, therefore, should be emptied with a stomach tube. Difference of opinion exists as to the use of analeptic drugs, but if the depression is deep and the patient cannot be aroused, drugs such as amphetamine phosphate, pentylenetetrazol, methylphenidate hydrochloride, and others have been recommended. In case of threatened respiratory failure, artificial respiration and the inhalation of oxygen and carbon dioxide may be beneficial. The patient's position should be changed frequently to combat development of hypostatic pneumonia. As the patient emerges from a comatose state he may become acutely active and require the administration of a sedative. (Chlorpromazine should *not* be given; it potentiates the effects of alcohol.) Recovery is comparable to recovery from an anesthetic.

The headache, nervousness, and gastric irritability that frequently follow acute alcoholism are best relieved by antacids and demulcents, such as sodium bicarbonate and bismuth subcarbonate. The combined use of glucose and insulin therapy has been advocated by some because it promotes slightly the detoxication of alcohol. The administration of isotonic saline solution intravenously will help the dehydrated patient by reestablishing the electrolyte pattern of the blood.

Chronic alcoholism. The more common manifestations of chronic alcoholism are redness of the face, nose, and conjunctivae caused by the injection of the blood vessels, gastroenteritis, cirrhotic changes in the liver, nephritis, arteriosclerosis and chronic myocardial changes, amblyopia caused by orbital optic neuritis, dulling of the mental faculties, tremors caused by degeneration, and muscular weakness. Not infrequently, the prolonged use of alcohol leads to mental change, which may manifest itself in the gradual weakening of the mental powers, with hallucinations and delusions or other forms of psychosis. To be successfully treated the chronic alcoholic must want to be treated and must want to get well. Early establishment of rapport between the patient and the physician as well as with the nurse is very important. Treatment must include rehabilitation and help in making better adjustments to the patient's living conditions. The best results are probably obtained in a hospital.

Careful attention should be given to the patient's physical needs, such as diet, fluid balance, and general hygiene, since optimal physical fitness makes the patient feel better and increases his ability to deal with the problems that have contributed to his illness or have caused it to continue. Particular attention is given to supplying adequate amounts of vitamin B complex and ascorbic acid.

Sedatives and tranquilizing agents make the patient more comfortable, help him to sleep better, and relieve anxiety. The patient is also likely to eat better.

There is need for adequate medical supervision at all times as well as for good nursing care if good results are to be attained. Although relapses are frequent, fewer alcoholics relapse after treatment than those who are treated for morphine dependence.

In the treatment of chronic alcoholism, two additional aspects of treatment are deserving of mention because of the success that has been attained. The first is the psychologic approach to the problem or problems of the chronic alcoholic as made by Alcoholics Anonymous. This is an organization composed entirely of rehabilitated alcoholics who are, therefore, in a unique position to understand the problems of other alcoholics. The organization has its headquarters in New York and has many local groups in cities and towns throughout the United States. Frequent meetings, mutual assistance and understanding, and a definite program of constructive rehabilitation have resulted in the fact that approximately 50% of those who enter the organization with a sincere desire to stop drinking do so. Another 25% are reclaimed after one or more failures, and most of the remaining 25% are for one reason or another never successfully reclaimed. Another technique has involved the administration of a drug (disulfiram; Antabuse) that the subject knows will produce unpleasant symptoms if he then takes alcohol.

Delirium tremens is a form of psychosis that sometimes develops in the chronic alcoholic. It usually occurs after prolonged excessive drinking followed by abstinence and can be viewed as a type of withdrawal syndrome comparable to that seen after withdrawal of barbiturates in persons addicted to them. In the alcoholic who has been drinking for some time it may be precipitated by exposure, surgical operation, or serious illness, especially pneumonia. There may be warning symptoms such as restlessness, insomnia, anorexia, anxiety, fear, and tremor. Chronic alcoholics refer to the first stage of delirium tremens as the "shakes." During the attack the patient continues to have tremor, insomnia, delirium, and terrifying hallucinations of such things as snakes and small animals creeping over him. The patient may have a temperature of 102° to 103° F. Death may result from collapse, traumatism, or infection.

Many methods of treatment have been tried. Sedatives such as paraldehyde, amobarbital sodium, mephobarbital, and some of the tranquilizing agents are tried when the patient is maniacal. Symptomatic treatment of the patient includes attention to fluids, nutrition, and vitamins. Some physicians have found ACTH and cortisone beneficial in promoting recovery.

Contraindications. Ethyl alcohol is contraindicated for certain persons and should be avoided by others. This includes the following:

1 Patients who have ulceration of the gastrointestinal tract, especially patients with hyperacidity and gastric or duodenal ulcers
2 Patients with acute infections of the genitourinary organs
3 Pregnant women
4 Epileptic persons
5 Patients with liver or kidney disease
6 Persons with personality problems, maladjusted persons, or those who have at one time been alcohol or drug dependent

Alcohol and life span. The effect of alcohol on resistance to infection and on the life span has been a subject of controversy for many years. It is believed that evidence is lacking to prove that moderate amounts of alcohol have much effect one way or the other. Statistics show, however, that chronic alcoholics and heavy drinkers have a shorter life span than those who abstain from alcohol. Some of the ill effects that have been attributed to alcohol have been found to be caused by general impairment of health, which in turn is caused by malnutrition and poor hygiene. Apparently, it often is not so much the direct effect of alcohol that injures the person as the inability of the alcoholic to take care of himself and others.

Methyl alcohol (wood alcohol)

Methyl alcohol is prepared on a large scale by the destructive distillation of wood. It has also been prepared synthetically. It is important in medicine chiefly because of the cases of poisoning that have resulted from its ingestion. The main effects are on the central nervous system. However, intoxication does not occur as readily as with ethyl alcohol unless large amounts are consumed. Methyl alcohol is oxidized in the tissues to formic acid, which is poorly metabolized. This is the basis for the development of a severe acidosis. Symptoms of poisoning include nausea and vomiting, abdominal pain, headache, dyspnea, blurred vision, and cold clammy skin. Symptoms may progress to delirium, convulsions, coma, and death. In nonfatal cases the patient may become blind or suffer from impaired vision. Treatment is directed toward the relief of acidosis since this seems to be related to the severity of the visual symptoms. Large amounts of sodium bicarbonate may be needed to treat acidosis successfully. Obviously, methyl alcohol is much more toxic than ethyl alcohol. One dose of 60 ml. has been known to cause permanent blindness. Fluids containing methyl alcohol usually bear a "Poison" label.

Isopropyl alcohol, N.F., B.P.

Isopropyl alcohol is a clear, colorless, liquid with a characteristic odor and a bitter taste. It is miscible with water, chloroform, and ether but insoluble in salt solutions. It is a good solvent for creosote and compares favorably with ethyl alcohol in its antiseptic action. It has been recommended for disinfection of the skin and for rubbing compounds and lotions to be used on the skin. Its bactericidal effects are said to increase as its concentration approaches 100%. It differs in this respect from ethyl alcohol.

It is occasionally misused as a beverage. It can cause severe poisoning and death. The first symptoms are similar to intoxication from ethyl alcohol, but the symptoms progress to coma from which the patient may not recover.

Butyl and amyl alcohols

Butyl and amyl alcohols are said to be several times as toxic as ethyl alcohol.

DRUGS USED IN TREATMENT OF CHRONIC ALCOHOLISM
Disulfiram (Antabuse)

$$H_5C_2 \diagdown \quad S \quad S \quad \diagup C_2H_5$$
$$\underset{H_5C_2}{\diagup} N - \overset{\parallel}{C} - S - S - \overset{\parallel}{C} - N \underset{C_2H_5}{\diagdown}$$

Disulfiram is used to sensitize an individual to alcohol by bringing about an unpleasant alcohol-disulfiram reaction. This reaction begins with flushing in the face, which develops into intense vasodilation of the face and neck and upper part of the body. Hyperventilation and increased pulse rate may occur. Nausea may occur in 30 to 60 minutes along with facial pallor, hypotension, and copious vomiting. There is usually an intense feeling of discomfort, pulsating headache, palpitations, dyspnea, and a constrictive feeling in the neck. The reaction lasts 30 minutes to several hours followed by drowsiness and sleep. This experience is so unpleasant that alcohol tends to repel the individual who does not wish to reexperience the discomforting symptoms.

In the body alcohol is oxidized to acetaldehyde. Disulfiram inhibits the enzyme aldehyde dehydrogenase, which converts acetaldehyde to acetate. This permits acetaldehyde to accumulate and cause toxic effects. Disulfiram has few effects unless the person ingests alcohol. A 50% success rate in the treatment of alcoholism has been reported by some study groups.

Administration. Patients must be carefully selected, and given a thorough explanation of the treatment and unpleasantness they will experience, and must give full consent for treatment. All signs of alcohol intoxication must be absent, and the patient should not have ingested alcohol for at least 12 hours prior to initiation of therapy. A daily dose of 500 mg. of disulfiram is given in the morning for a period of 1 to 2 weeks. The physician may then administer a dose of alcohol to produce the typical symptoms that will repel the individual from ingesting alcohol. The alcohol test may not be given at all, and it is usually omitted for patients over age 50. A maintenance dose of 250 mg. (range of dosage is 125 to 500 mg.) may then be given for months or years depending upon the individual. The act of taking the daily dose of disulfiram serves as a daily re-dedication to avoid use of alcohol. Effects persist for 2 weeks after discontinuance of therapy, and patients should be warned not to ingest alcohol during this time. Psychotherapy aimed at mental and social rehabilitation should accompany disulfiram therapy.

Side effects. During early weeks of therapy, drowsiness, impotence, headache, peripheral neuritis, and a metallic taste may occur. About 20% of patients experience fatigability. High doses may cause a confusional state and convulsions. Deaths have occurred following the "test drink." The abstinence from alcohol may cause anxiety, hostility, and even experimentation with other drugs.

Contraindications. Disulfiram is contraindicated if there is serious cardiovascular disease, epilepsy, cirrhosis of the liver, nephritis, or pregnancy.

Calcium carbimide (Temposil, Abstem)

This drug has actions similar to those of disulfiram. Its effects develop more rapidly and are dissipated in 12 to 24 hours; it produces fewer side effects than disulfiram. Usual dosage is 50 to 100 mg. daily.

ANTICONVULSANT DRUGS

Epilepsy is regarded as a symptom of disease or disorder of the brain rather than a disease in itself. It is associated with marked changes in the electric activity of the cerebral cortex, and these alterations are often detected in the electroencephalogram. Therefore, the EEG is often a valuable aid to the physician in making a diagnosis. Sometimes the convulsive seizure is associated with a brain tumor, growth of scar tissue, or the presence of a toxin or a poison, but at other times no specific cause can be found. Epileptic seizures vary and are often grouped according to grand mal seizures, petit mal seizures, jacksonian epilepsy, and psychomotor attacks. There are about 1 million epileptic persons in the United States.

Grand mal epilepsy is the type most frequently seen. Such attacks are characterized by sudden loss of consciousness. The patient falls forcefully and experiences a series of tonic and clonic muscular contractions. The eyes roll upward, the arms are flexed, and the legs are extended. The force of the muscular contractions causes air to be forced out of the lungs, which accounts for the cry which the patient may make as he falls. Respiration is suspended temporarily, the skin becomes cyanotic, perspiration and saliva flow, and the patient may froth at the mouth and bite his tongue if it gets caught between his teeth. When the seizure subsides the patient regains partial consciousness and may complain of aching. He then tends to fall into a deep sleep.

Petit mal seizures are most often seen in childhood and consist of temporary lapses of consciousness that last for a few seconds. Patients appear to be staring into space and may exhibit a few rhythmic movements of the eyes or head. They do not convulse. They may experience many attacks in a single day. Sometimes an attack of petit mal is followed by one of grand mal.

Jacksonian epilepsy is described by some authorities as a type of focal seizure; it is associated with irritation of a specific part of the brain. A single part, such as a finger or an extremity, may jerk and such movements may end spontaneously or spread over the whole musculature. Consciousness may not be lost unless the seizure develops into a generalized convulsion.

Psychomotor attacks are characterized by brief alterations in consciousness, unusual stereotyped movements (such as chewing or swallowing movements) repeated over and over, temperamental changes, confusion, and feelings of unreality. It is often associated with grand mal seizures and is likely to be resistant to therapy with drugs.

Some patients have more than one type of seizure or have mixed seizures. This is significant because different types of seizures respond rather specifically to certain anticonvulsant drugs. The aim of therapy is to find the drug or drugs that will effectively control the seizures and will at the same time cause a minimum of undesirable side effects.

Mechanism of action of the anticonvulsant drugs. The effectiveness of anticonvulsant drugs is often measured by the amount of increased voltage necessary to provoke an electroconvulsion in an animal who has previously received the anticonvulsant to be tested or by the degree of their antagonism to chemical substances capable of producing convulsions. Pentylenetetrazol is a drug against which anticonvulsants are measured for effectiveness.

The mode and site of action of these drugs are still regarded as uncertain. The convulsive seizure may be effectively suppressed, but the abnormal brain waves may or may not be altered. All clinically useful drugs for epilepsy inhibit the seizure.

Although there is no ideal anticonvulsant drug, if one could be synthesized to order, a number of characteristics would be considered highly desirable:

1 The drug should be highly effective but exhibit a low incidence of toxicity.
2 It should be effective against more than one type of seizure and for mixed seizures.
3 It should be long acting and nonsedative so that the patient is not incapacitated with sleep or excessive drowsiness.
4 It should be well tolerated by the patient and inexpensive, since the patient may have to take it for years or for the rest of his life.
5 Tolerance to the therapeutic effects of the drug should not develop.

The present-day drugs that are considered especially satisfactory and safe are phenobarbital, phenytoin sodium, and trimethadione. The bromides are among the oldest anticonvulsants known, but because they tend to cause states of chronic toxicity, they seldom are used. The barbiturates have been discussed but their use as anticonvulsants will be emphasized again. They are an important group of drugs for this purpose, especially the longer-acting members. Phenobarbital is effective against all types of epileptic seizures except certain petit mal types. It is considered one of the safest of the anticonvulsants. Its chief disadvantage is that it must often be given in doses that produce apathy and sleepiness. Amphetamines or methylphenidate may be ordered to counteract the drowsiness. Mephobarbital and metharbital are similar to phenobarbital, especially when given in comparable doses.

Phenytoin sodium, U.S.P., B.P. (Dilantin)

$$C_6H_5 - \underset{\underset{O=C-N}{|}}{\overset{\overset{C_6H_5}{|}}{C}} - NH \diagdown \underset{}{C-O-Na}$$

Phenytoin is a synthetic agent chemically related to the barbiturates. It is an odorless white or cream-colored powder with a bitter taste.

Action and result. Phenytoin exerts a selective action on the cerebral cortex of the brain without appreciably affecting the sensory areas. It is an anticonvulsant but not a hypnotic. It is somewhat more effective in controlling grand mal seizures than phenobarbital, although patients vary in their response to these drugs. It is strongly alkaline in solution and may produce gastric irritation.

Uses. In the treatment of epilepsy it is more effective for grand mal than petit mal seizures. It may increase the attacks of petit mal. Psychomotor seizures are sometimes controlled. It does not cure the mental deterioration sometimes found in the epileptic. On the other hand, it does not cause mental deterioration. It is frequently prescribed in combination with phenobarbital. It may be prescribed for patients following surgical operations upon the brain to prevent convulsive seizures.

Preparation, dosage, and administration. Phenytoin is marketed in 30- and 100-mg. capsules (delayed action), in 50-mg. scored tablets, and in an oral suspension (100 mg. per 4 ml.). It is also available for parenteral administration in "Steri-Vials," each containing 100 to 250 mg. of the drug. When used alone, the beginning daily dose for adults is 100 mg. orally with one-half glass of water three times a day. The dosage may be gradually increased until optimum effects are obtained. Most adults seem to tolerate 300 to 400 mg. daily without toxic effects. Dosage for children is 3 to 8 mg. per kilogram of body weight. Increase in dosage is made slowly and with careful observation of the patient. When the drug is combined with one or more other anticonvulsants, the dosage of individual drugs is often reduced. The transition from phenobarbital and other hypnotics to phenytoin is made gradually, with some overlapping of drugs to prevent the precipitation of convulsive seizures.

There are a number of preparations available that are mixtures of barbiturates and one of the hydantoins. Phelantin contains diphenylhydantoin, phenobarbital, and methamphetamine hydrochloride. Hydantal contains methylphenyl-ethyl hydantoin and phenobarbital. Mebroin contains phenytoin and methobarbital. These preparations have the advantages of convenience (two or more drugs in one tablet) and slightly lower cost, but there is the disadvantage of always having a fixed amount of each drug. It is advantageous for the physician to be able to make adjustments of dosage when several drugs are taken together.

Side effects and toxic effects. The incidence of toxic reactions with phenytoin is greater than with phenobarbital. The less serious side effects include apathy, nervousness, dizziness, ataxia, blurred vision, hyperplasia of the gums (excessive formation of gum tissues), and hirsutism (excessive growth of hair, especially on the face). Other reactions that sometimes occur are tremor, excitement, hallucinations, psychosis, nausea, and vomiting. If the patient is particularly sensitive to the drug he may develop skin rash, exfoliative dermatitis, fever, and difficult breathing. Hepatitis, blood dyscrasias, periarteritis nodosa, and lupus erythematosus from phenytoin have been reported.

Drug interactions. Phenytoin and its derivative participate in many drug interactions:

1 Drugs that can potentiate the action of phenytoin include: aspirin, phenylbutazone, chloramphenicol, cycloserine, isoniazid, estrogens, griseofulvin, chlordiazepoxide, sulfonamides, and anticoagulants.
2 Drugs that inhibit the action of phenytoin include: alcohol, antihistamines, barbiturates, glutethimide, sedatives, and hypnotics. The effects of other central nervous system depressants may be additive.
3 Phenytoin potentiates the action of the following drugs: antihypertensives, folic acid antagonists,

methotrexate, propranolol, quinidine, and tubocurarine.

4 Phenytoin inhibits the action of corticosteroids and digitalis.

Mephenytoin, N.F. (Mesantoin); methoin, B.P.

$$C_6H_5$$
$$C_2H_5-C-NH$$
$$C=O$$
$$O=C-N-CH_3$$

Mephenytoin is an anticonvulsant drug similar in chemical structure and activity to phenytoin. It is less potent as an anticonvulsant than the latter preparation. It produces more sedation than phenytoin but less than phenobarbital. Tolerance develops with this drug.

Uses. Mephenytoin seems to be more effective for grand mal and psychomotor seizures than for petit mal seizures since it may provoke attacks of petit mal. Certain patients who do not respond favorably to phenytoin or to phenobarbital may benefit from this drug.

D.E.S.I. rating is *effective* for grand mal and focal, jacksonian, and psychomotor seizures refractory to other drugs.

Preparation, dosage, and administration. Mephenytoin is available in 100-mg. tablets for oral administration. The average daily dose for adults is 200 to 600 mg.; for children, 100 to 400 mg. As for all anticonvulsants, the optimum daily dosage must be calculated to meet the needs of each patient.

Side effects and toxic effects. Side effects during initial therapy include nausea, vomiting, nervousness, sleeplessness, and dizziness. This is a drug that can produce serious toxic effects and therefore caution in its use is recommended. In cases of hypersensitivity to the drug, destruction of blood cells can occur, which may vary from leukopenia to agranulocytosis and aplastic anemia. Some patients become jaundiced, indicating damage to the liver. Other symptoms of toxicity include fever and dermatitis.

Ethotoin, B.P. (Peganone)

$$H$$
$$C_6H_5-C-N-H$$
$$C=O$$
$$O=C-N-C_2H_5$$

Ethotoin belongs to the hydantoin group of anticonvulsants.

Uses. It is said to be less effective than phenytoin, but it is also less toxic. It is effective in grand mal epilepsy but does not always bring about complete relief of seizures. To be satisfactory it may need to be used with other anticonvulsants.

D.E.S.I. rating is *effective* for the control of grand mal and psychomotor seizures.

Preparation, dosage, and administration. The average daily adult dose of ethotoin is 2 to 3 Gm. given orally after meals in four to six divided portions. Dosage for children is 500 mg. to 1 Gm. daily in divided doses. It is available in 250- and 500-mg. tablets.

Trimethadione, U.S.P. (Tridione); troxidone, B.P.

$$CH_3$$
$$CH_3-C-O$$
$$C=O$$
$$O=C-N-CH_3$$

Trimethadione belongs to a group of compounds known as the oxazolidine diones.

Action. Its primary action is on the central nervous system, although it is not restricted to the motor cortex. It exerts an analgesic effect in some instances as well as an anticonvulsant action. It is said to surpass all other anticonvulsants in raising the threshold to pentylenetetrazol-induced seizures. The precise mechanism of action, however, is unknown.

Uses. Trimethadione is used chiefly in the treatment of petit mal epilepsy. It appears to be more effective for petit mal in children than in adults. It is not effective for grand mal seizures. It is frequently given with phenytoin or phenobarbital if the patient has attacks of both petit mal and grand mal. It rarely seems to be adequate to control psychomotor seizures. Because of its toxicity the A.M.A. recommends its use be reserved for refractory cases. D.E.S.I. rating is *effective* for control of petit mal seizures.

Preparation, dosage, and administration. Trimethadione is available in 150-mg. tablets, 300-mg. capsules, and solution (37.5 mg. per milliliter) for oral administration. The dose for children is 300 to 900 mg. daily and for adults, 900 to 1200 mg. daily, in divided portions. Dosage may need to be increased.

Side effects and toxic effects. Symptoms of toxicity appear infrequently, but they may be serious and fatal. Nausea and vomiting, skin eruption, blurring of vision, and sensitivity to light are considered indications for reduction of dosage or temporary withdrawal of the drug. Careful medical supervision of the patient receiving the medication is essential. Rare instances of aplastic anemia explain why it is thought advisable for the patient to have periodic examinations of the blood to detect early signs of toxic effects.

The drug is not recommended for patients with hepatic or renal disease, with disease of the optic nerve, allergic reactions to drugs, or blood dyscrasias. Its use in pregnant women may cause malformation of the fetus.

Paramethadione, U.S.P., B.P. (Paradione)

Action and uses. The action and uses of paramethadione are similar to those of trimethadione. It belongs to the same chemical group, and no significant pharmacologic difference between them is known. Some patients not benefited by trimethadione are benefited by paramethadione and vice versa. D.E.S.I. rating is *effective* for petit mal.

Preparation, dosage, and administration. The initial dose of paramethadione for adults is 900 mg. given orally in divided doses. Thereaf-

ter, dosage is adjusted to the minimum effective dose. Initial dosage for children varies from 300 to 600 mg., depending on size.

Side effects. Side effects are similar to those of trimethadione, except the incidence of skin rash and photophobia is said to be less with paramethadione. Neutropenia has been reported.

Phenacemide, N.F. (Phenurone)

Phenacemide bears a close chemical relationship to the hydantoin compounds, as can be seen in the accompanying formulas.

Phenacemide

Phenytoin

Uses and toxic effects. Phenacemide is a synthetic anticonvulsant that has the advantage of being effective in the treatment of grand mal, petit mal, psychomotor epilepsy, and mixed seizures. It is often effective when other anticonvulsants are not, but it is one of the more toxic agents and may cause personality changes, liver damage, and depression of bone marrow. Deaths have been reported. Some physicians regard it as being too toxic for routine use.

Preparation, dosage, and administration. Phenacemide is available in 300- and 500-mg. tablets for oral administration. It may be prescribed alone or with other anticonvulsants. The dosage recommended is as small as will permit control of seizures.

Ethosuximide, U.S.P., B.P. (Zarontin)

Ethosuximide is the drug of choice for treating petit mal. It is as a rule ineffective for psychomotor or grand mal epilepsy. A single dose produces peak blood levels in 2 to 4 hours which last for 24 hours. Large daily doses produce a peak on the fourth day, which is maintained until the drug is discontinued. It is eliminated from the blood 2 days after the drug is stopped.

Side effects. Side effects to ethosuximide include nausea, vomiting, drowsiness, vertigo, headache, diarrhea, and weight loss. Blood dyscrasias and neurologic and psychologic reactions have occurred rarely. Mental and physical abilities may be impaired, and patients should be cautioned about performing potentially hazardous tasks.

Preparation and dosage. Ethosuximide is available in 250-mg. capsules. Dosage for adults and children over 6 years of age is 500 mg. initially. The dose thereafter is individualized by increments of 250 mg. every 4 to 7 days until seizures are controlled with minimal untoward effects. For children under 6 initial dose is 250 mg. daily with gradual increase in dosage as above.

Other anticonvulsants

There are a number of other anticonvulsants that are in current use. These include phensuximide (Milontin) and methsuximide (Celontin), which are effective for petit mal seizures. Primidone (Mysoline) is chemically similar to phenobarbital. It is about as effective as phenobarbital for the management of grand mal seizures and is quite effective in psychomotor epilepsy. Acetazolamide, U.S.P. (Diamox), is sometimes used as a supplement to routine medication with anticonvulsants. It is primarily a diuretic and a carbonic anhydrase inhibitor. In addition to these antiepileptic drugs diazepam administered intravenously is the current initial therapy of choice in status epilepticus.

Role of the nurse

The nurse sometimes plays an important role in helping the patient with epilepsy to learn how to live with his handicap. The patient often needs encouragement and help to enable him to understand why strict adherence to the routine the physician has worked out for him is so important. The patient may never be cured, but with care he may experience minimal symptoms and be able to lead a full and useful life. The patient or a family member should be instructed to keep a record of the frequency, duration, and symptoms of attacks and to report signs and symptoms of undesirable drug effects. Urinalyses and blood counts should be performed every 1 to 3 months.

Stimulants

Drugs included under the heading of stimulants will be limited, for the most part, to those whose major effect is on the central nervous system. There are drugs, such as atropine, cocaine, and ephedrine, that are central nervous system stimulants but, medically, they have more important actions on other systems of the body.

The central nervous system stimulants may produce dramatic effects, but their therapeutic usefulness is limited because of the multiplicity of their actions and side effects. Also, repeated administration and large doses are prone to precipitate convulsive seizures, coma, and exhaustion. The number of drugs that stimulate the central nervous system is large, but the number actually employed for this purpose is limited. Those having particular therapeutic value are the respiratory stimulants and the analeptics. Although analeptics restore consciousness and mental alertness, they are little used now because of the danger of precipitating convulsions.

Stimulants are classified on the basis of where in the nervous system they exert their major effects—on the cerebrum, on the medulla and brainstem, or on the spinal cord. Amphetamine is mainly a stimulant of the cerebral cortex; nikethamide acts mainly on the centers in the medulla and the brainstem; and strychnine is a spinal stimulant. These drugs may also affect other parts of the nervous system. The drugs that act primarily on the medullary centers are said to be the best analeptics.

XANTHINES

Caffeine, theobromine, and theophylline are known as methylated xanthines. Their actions are similar, although their effect on specific structures varies in intensity.

Caffeine is a trimethylxanthine (three methyl

groups) and theobromine and theophylline are dimethylxanthines (two methyl groups). Caffeine, theophylline, and theobromine are alkaloids that all act on the central nervous system, the kidney, the heart, the skeletal muscle, and the smooth muscle, but the degree of their action on these structures varies considerably. Of the three xanthines, caffeine is the most effective stimulant of the central nervous system, theophylline is less effective, and theobromine has little effect. On the kidney, theophylline ranks first in effectiveness, theobromine second, and caffeine third. Aminophylline (a theophylline compound) is the xanthine preparation of choice to produce relaxation of the bronchial tubes.

Xanthine   Theobromine

Caffeine   Theophylline

Caffeine

Caffeine is a white crystalline powder commercially obtained from tea leaves. It is the active alkaloid occurring in a number of plants used as beverages—coffee, the seed of *Coffea arabica;* tea, the leaves of *Thea sinensis;* the kola nut of Central America; and guarana, derived from the seeds of a Brazilian plant and from yerba maté or Paraguay tea. Tea contains from 1% to 5% caffeine*; coffee, from 1% to 2%. Tea contains 10% to 24% tannin. Coffee contains a variable amount of caffetannic acid (average, about 12%), which is not very astringent.

*Although tea contains more total methylated xanthines than coffee, less tea is usually used in preparing the beverage (at least in the United States), and it therefore usually contains less caffeine.

Action and result

Cortical and medullary. Caffeine stimulates the central nervous system, especially the cerebral cortex. Its action is a descending one; small doses (100 to 150 mg.) stimulate the cerebrum, and larger doses stimulate the medullary centers and the spinal cord. Doses large enough to stimulate the spinal cord are never ordered. As a result of the cortical stimulation the individual is more alert, thinks faster, has a better memory, forms judgments more quickly, learns faster (temporarily), and has a decreased reaction time. Drowsiness and fatigue disappear. The sense of touch may be more discriminating and the sense of pain more keen. Stimulation is not necessarily followed by depression, except as it brings about exhaustion of natural reserves.

Caffeine, when taken orally in ordinary therapeutic doses, has little or no effect on medullary centers. Large doses given parenterally will stimulate the respiratory center, especially if it is moderately depressed. There is some stimulation of the vagus and vasoconstrictor centers of the medulla, although this is partially masked by the peripheral action on the heart and blood vessels.

Decreased susceptibility to fatigue has also been observed, but whether the action is a direct one on the striated muscle cells or whether the effect is produced by masking the sense of fatigue through cerebral stimulation is not fully understood.

Large doses of caffeine stimulate the entire central nervous system, including the spinal cord. There is first an increased reflex excitability that may, with increasing dosage, result in muscle twitching, especially in the limbs and face.

Cardiovascular. Caffeine stimulates the myocardium, bringing about both an increased cardiac rate and an increased cardiac output. This effect is antagonistic to that produced on the vagus center; consequently, a slight slowing of the heart may be observed in some individuals and an increased rate in others. The latter effect usually predominates after large doses. Overstimulation may cause tachycardia and cardiac irregularities.

A slight and somewhat transitory elevation of blood pressure is sometimes noted. Some investigators are of the opinion that caffeine constricts the intracranial blood vessels and brings about some lowering of intracranial pressure.

Renal. Like the other xanthines, caffeine increases the flow of urine, but its action is relatively weak. The mode of action seems to be that of depressing the tubule cells and preventing reabsorption of fluid although increase in glomerular filtration may be more important therapeutically.

Metabolic. The metabolic rate is slightly increased by caffeine. An appreciable tolerance to certain effects of caffeine is readily established, although apparently not to the cerebral effects. Caffeine is also used to relieve fatigue, depression, and headache.

Gastric. Caffeine stimulates the output of pepsin as well as hydrochloric acid in the gastric juice. Thus coffee is usually omitted from the diet of patients with gastric or duodenal ulcer.

Uses. Caffeine is used as a mild cerebral stimulant. It is used also occasionally as a respiratory stimulant, provided the depression of the medullary center is not severe. In cases of severe respiratory depression there are better respiratory stimulants. Caffeine is no longer used for the relief of narcotic depression unless more effective drugs are not available.

Caffeine is used with one or more analgesic drugs or with ergotamine tartrate for the relief of headache. Its effect in such cases is thought to be caused by its effect on cerebral blood vessels.

Preparation, dosage, and administration. The following are the preparations and dosages of caffeine.

Caffeine, U.S.P., B.P. The usual dose is 200 mg. (gr. 3).

Caffeine and sodium benzoate injection, U.S.P. It is available in 2-ml. ampules and 10-ml. vials, 250 mg. per milliliter. The usual dose is 0.5 Gm. (500 mg.) to 1 Gm.

Citrated caffeine. This is available in 60- and 120-mg. tablets. The average dose is 60 to 120 mg. orally.

Ergotamine tartrate with caffeine, N.F. (Cafergot). Each tablet contains 1 mg. of ergotamine tartrate and 100 mg. of caffeine. The drug is given orally for migraine headache (one to two tablets).

Caffeine is usually prescribed as citrated caffeine or caffeine and sodium benzoate because they are more soluble than caffeine itself. Caffeine and sodium benzoate is usually given intramuscularly, whereas the citrated form is given orally. Caffeine may also be given in the form of a liquid, either orally or by rectum. The caffeine content of an average cup of coffee as made in the United States is between 100 and 150 mg. Twelve ounces of a cola drink contains 35 to 55 mg. of caffeine, while a cup of cocoa may contain as much as 50 mg. of caffeine. Caffeine sometimes exhibits a local irritant action on the gastric mucosa, resulting in nausea and vomiting or gastric distress. Sick persons often do not tolerate coffee well as a beverage especially if they are slightly nauseated. Weak tea is often better tolerated.

Side effects and toxic effects. Fatal poisoning by caffeine is rare, partly because it is readily excreted. The fatal dose is presumably about 10 Gm. Toxic doses produce excessive irritability, restlessness, insomnia, nervousness, profuse flow of urine, nausea, vomiting, headache, and heart palpitation, particularly in susceptible individuals. The more chronic symptoms of poisoning include insomnia, anxiety, and functional cardiac symptoms. The signs of chronic caffeine poisoning are more commonly seen among workers such as night nurses, who use coffee to keep awake and continue to work when physically tired. The symptoms of nervousness disappear when the overuse of coffee is remedied. Stopping the intake of caffeine and providing rest and quiet are sufficient treatment measures. In certain individuals a short-acting sedative may be indicated. The use of coffee to combat fatigue is like a whip to a tired horse, and it would be better to get needed rest than to continue using coffee to keep going.

The question is sometimes raised as to whether or not caffeine causes physical and psychic dependence. Many persons note that if they do not have their usual cup or two of coffee in the morning, they feel irritable and nervous and develop a headache. This probably indicates psychic dependence.

AMPHETAMINES

Amphetamines are synthetic sympathomimetic amines. Amphetamines are weak inhibitors of monoamine oxidase (MAO). However, their central nervous system stimulation is not thought to be a result of monoamine oxidase inhibition. They release catecholamines which exert a stimulating effect on the cerebral cortex and probably on the reticular activating system. This effect produces feelings of wakefulness, alertness, and euphoria or elation.

Amphetamines can produce emotional dependence but physical dependence does not occur. Prolonged use of amphetamines leads to tolerance. Amphetamines may be used to treat nonpsychotic, mild depressive states, but they are of little or no value in psychotic depressive states. They have been largely replaced by the tricyclic antidepressants. They are widely, but questionably, used for their ability to depress appetite and reduce obesity.

Amphetamine

Amphetamine is prepared synthetically from ephedrine. The accompanying formulas indicate points of similarity and difference.

Ephedrine   Amphetamine

Action and result. Amphetamine stimulates the central nervous system, particularly the cerebral cortex. The effects depend upon the personality and mental state of the individual and the amount of drug administered. The results of action seen after oral administration usually include an elevation of mood that may become a true euphoric exhilaration, decreased feeling of fatigue, increased willingness to work, increased confidence, alertness, power of concentration, and sometimes talkativeness. Continued use may cause irritability, sleeplessness, dizziness, and anorexia. Large doses tend to be followed by fatigue and mental depression. Amphetamine may fortify a person for prolonged physical and mental exertion, but the end result in terms of fatigue is correspondingly greater and requires a longer period for rest than usual. When the respiratory center is depressed, amphetamine exerts a stimulating effect upon it; this may be significant in treatment of poisoning from depressant drugs.

Uses. Currently, amphetamine has three principal uses: to treat narcolepsy, hyperkinetic behavior disorders, and obesity. Its D.E.S.I. rating is *effective* for the treatment of these three conditions. Amphetamine is effective in controlling the symptoms of narcolepsy (e.g., overpowering desire to sleep) but it is not curative. These patients do not appear to develop tolerance to amphetamine.

Hyperkinetic behavior, a manifestation of minimal brain dysfunction in children, is thought to be the result of faulty norepinephrine metabolism. Amphetamines may improve the behavior and performance of these children. A government appointed panel of experts has concluded that amphetamines are safe and proper treatment for hyperkinesis and that no dangers (e.g., dependence, toxicity) exist with proper treatment.

As an anorexigenic, amphetamine is less effective than dextroamphetamine, and the latter drug is usually preferred for this effect. Tolerance to the anorectic effect does occur, and the drug should not be used for periods longer than 6 to 10 weeks. Some clinicians advocate 2-week periods of amphetamine therapy alternating with 2-week periods without therapy rather than continuous treatment. The basic mechanism for depressing the appetite is not known.

Drug interactions. Amphetamine or its derivatives used during or within 14 days after administration of an MAO inhibitor may result in hypertensive crisis. Tricyclic antidepressants can potentiate the effects of amphetamine. Amphetamine blocks the uptake of guanethidine at nerve endings and loss of control of blood pressure may occur. The hypotensive action of methyldopa and of reserpine is also inhibited by amphetamines.

Preparation, dosage, and administration. The drug is available with the hydrochloride, sulfate, or phosphate salt and in combination with analgesics or barbiturates to depress excessive irritability and tension.

Amphetamine sulfate, B.P. (Benzedrine). This drug is marketed in tablets of 5 and 10 mg., in solution for injection (20 mg. per milliliter), and in 15-mg. sustained-release capsules. It is marketed under the trade name of Benzedrine. Amphetamine sulfate is usually administered orally and given in divided doses—the total daily dose is divided into several smaller doses and distributed through the day. To prevent interference with sleep the final dose of the day should not be given after 4:00 P.M. When injected, it is given intramuscularly or by slow intravenous drip.

Amphetamine phosphate (Raphetamine Phosphate). This form is available in 2- and 5-mg. tablets for oral administration and in solution for injection (100 mg. per 10 ml.). Small initial doses, 5 mg. or less, are recommended, to be followed with gradually increased amounts if necessary. Amphetamine phosphate has the same effects and uses as amphetamine sulfate, but its physical property of increased solubility in water makes it better suited for parenteral administration.

Side effects and contraindications. There is danger in the promiscuous use of amphetamine to overcome sleepiness and lack of alertness, because the natural warning signs associated with fatigue may be eliminated. Furthermore, amphetamine has high drug abuse potential. It is to be avoided by persons with hypertension and cardiovascular disease and by persons who are unduly restless, anxious, agitated, and excited. Side effects include dryness of the mouth, headache, insomnia, irritability, a sense of intoxication, anxiety, and even paranoia.

Elevated blood pressure, tachycardia, and gastrointestinal disorders may occur. Abrupt withdrawal after prolonged use may cause depression and lethargy. Some clinicians advocate gradual withdrawal of the drug to avoid these effects. Despite the numerous side effects caused by these drugs, there is a wide margin of safety between therapeutic and toxic doses.

Dextroamphetamine sulfate, U.S.P. (Dexedrine); dexamphetamine, B.P.

Action and uses. Dextroamphetamine sulfate, for the most part, has the same action and uses as amphetamine sulfate, although it exhibits a greater stimulating effect on the central nervous system. It is considered to be less toxic than amphetamine sulfate because of its diminished sympathomimetic activity. It seldom causes rapid pulse, changes in blood pressure, or tremor. However, the same dangers attend its indiscriminate use as is true of other amphetamines.

Preparation, dosage, and administration. Dextroamphetamine sulfate is available in 5- and 10-mg. tablets, as an elixir (5 mg. per 5 ml.), and in sustained-release capsules (Spansules) containing 5, 10, or 15 mg. of drug. It is also marketed in combination with analgesics, such as aspirin or phenacetin, or with one of the barbiturates, such as amobarbital. The latter combination is sometimes used when elevation of blood pressure and insomnia constitute problems. The usual dose of dextroamphetamine is 2.5 to 15 mg. daily given orally.

It may be taken three times a day 30 minutes to 1 hour before meals. The last dose should be taken at least 6 hours before retiring to avoid insomnia. Sustained-release forms are taken once daily in the morning.

In the treatment of barbiturate intoxication, 10 to 20 mg. of dextroamphetamine is administered intramuscularly or intravenously. This dosage may be repeated at 30-minute intervals until the desired response has been obtained. It is available for injection as dextroamphetamine sulfate in 10- and 30-ml. vials containing 20 mg. of dextroamphetamine per milliliter.

Methamphetamine hydrochloride (Desoxyephedrine Hydrochloride); methylamphetamine hydrochloride, B.P.

Methamphetamine hydrochloride greatly resembles amphetamine sulfate; the two drugs differ in their action only in degree. The central stimulant action of this drug is slightly greater, and the cardiovascular action is slightly less than that of amphetamine. Like amphetamine, it is used in the treatment of narcolepsy, as part of the treatment of alcoholism or barbiturate poisoning, and for treatment of hyperkinesis. Because it allays hunger and depresses motility in the gastrointestinal tract, it has been used in the treatment of obesity.

It is contraindicated for patients with hypertension, cardiovascular disease, hyperthyroidism, anxiety states, or undue restlessness. Severe toxic psychoses have occurred in individuals who abuse methamphetamine, commonly referred to as "speed" (see Chapter 13).

Preparation, dosage, and administration. Methamphetamine hydrochloride is marketed in 5- and 10-mg. capsules, 2.5-, 5-, 7.5-, and 10-mg. tablets, as an elixir (0.667 and 1 mg. per milliliter), and in solution for injection (20 mg. per milliliter). Methamphetamine is given parenterally as well as orally. The beginning oral dose is 2.5 mg. daily; this is increased to 2.5 to 5 mg. two or three times a day until the desired response is obtained. In case of emergency, 10 to 15 mg. may be given slowly by intravenous injection. In emergency, the usual dose is 15 to 30 mg. when the drug is given intramuscularly.

Phenmetrazine hydrochloride, N.F., B.P. (Preludin)

Phenmetrazine hydrochloride resembles amphetamine pharmacologically, especially in its ability to depress appetite. It should be used along with calorie restriction and moderate exercise when taken as an appetite depressant. It is a mild stimulant of the central nervous system, and it rarely causes changes in pulse rate and blood pressure. It is administered orally in 25-mg. doses two or three times a day, an hour before meals, or in an oral extended-release form containing 50 or 75 mg. of the drug, which is taken once daily.

Other central nervous system stimulants used primarily as appetite suppressants are diethylpropion hydrochloride (Tenuate, Tepanil), phendimetrazine tartrate (Plegine), phentermine (Ionamin, Wilpo), and chlorphentermine (Pre-Sate).

Methylphenidate hydrochloride, U.S.P. (Ritalin)

Methylphenidate is a central nervous system stimulant that is less potent than amphetamine but more potent than caffeine. It does not appreciably affect blood pressure, heart rate, circulation time, or respiration. Although it is widely used in the treatment of mild depression, it has received a D.E.S.I. rating of *possibly effective*

in the treatment of apathetic senile behavior and mild depression; and *ineffective* in increasing response to psychotherapy and in treating psychiatric conditions associated with depression.

Its most important use is in the treatment of hyperkinetic children and those with certain behavioral and learning problems. It has been found to significantly improve task performance in children in both groups probably because it improves mood, causes euphoria, and increases motor and mental activity, cognitive ability, and motor functions. D.E.S.I. rating is *effective* for treating hyperkinetic behavior disorders, and for treating narcolepsy. It is rated as *probably effective* for treating drug-induced lethargy caused by tranquilizers, barbiturates, antihistamines, and anticonvulsants.

Preparation, dosage, and administration. Methylphenidate is available as tablets containing 5, 10, or 20 mg., and in 10-ml. vials containing 100 mg. of drug for parenteral administration. Usual dose for adults is 10 to 60 mg. two or three times daily given 30 to 45 minutes before meals. If the patient is unable to sleep at night, the last dose should be taken before 6 P.M.

For hyperkinetic children, dose is 5 mg. before breakfast and lunch; dosage may be increased gradually by 5 to 10 mg. weekly. Dosage above 60 mg. is not recommended.

Parenteral administration (subcutaneously, intramuscularly, intravenously) is used primarily to overcome drug-induced lethargy and sedation. Usual dosage range is 10 to 50 mg. given one or more times as required.

Side effects. Nervousness and insomnia are common reactions, which can usually be controlled by reducing dosage or omitting the afternoon or evening dose. Numerous other side effects can occur and include anorexia, nausea, dizziness, palpitations, headache, and skin rash. Hypertension, hypotension, and arrhythmias have occurred. Prolonged therapy has caused abdominal pain and weight loss, particularly in children.

Precautions. Methylphenidate must be used with caution in patients with epilepsy since the drug can lower the convulsive threshold. It should also be used cautiously in patients with hypertension. Long-term therapy should be accompanied by repeated medical examination and complete blood and platelet counts. Its use in pregnant or lactating women is not recommended.

Tolerance and psychic dependence has occurred with long-term use, and abnormal behavior and psychotic episodes have been observed. When the drug is withdrawn careful supervision is required since severe depression may result.

Methylphenidate must be used cautiously in emotionally unstable persons and in those with a history of drug dependence or alcoholism. It has been used as a substitute for amphetamines by drug abusers.

Overdosage. Signs and symptoms of acute intoxication are primarily the result of overstimulation of the central nervous system and sympathetic nervous system and include vomiting, agitation, tremors, muscle twitching, convulsions, euphoria, confusion, hallucinations, delirium, sweating, tachycardia, arrhythmias, hypertension, mydriasis, hyperpyrexia, and dryness of mucous membranes.

Treatment consists of supportive measures, evacuation of gastric contents if possible, a short-acting barbiturate, cooling procedures for high body temperature, and adequate maintenance of circulation and respiration. The effectiveness of dialysis for methylphenidate overdosage has not been established.

Drug interactions. Methylphenidate can potentiate the action of many drugs including angiotensin, anticholinergics, anticonvulsants, anticoagulants, MAO drugs, pressor drugs, phenylbutazone, and tricyclic antidepressants. It decreases the hypotensive effect of guanethidine. Dosage of these drugs should be readjusted when given with methylphenidate.

QUESTIONS

For study and review

1 Differentiate between the "short-acting," "ultrashort-acting," and "long-acting" barbiturates. Give five examples of each.
2 How should narcotics be stored in hospital clinical units?
3 Explain what is meant by the term *narcotic.*
4 Define alcoholism. What, if any, are the therapeutic uses of alcohol?
5 Explain the following statement: "Drugs that decrease

or release catecholamine concentration in the brain have a depressing or sedative action."
6 What rationale is used by some clinicians for not using analeptics for treatment of barbiturate poisoning?
7 Explain how a drug may be used as a sedative, a hypnotic, or an anesthetic.
8 What are the signs of salicylate poisoning?
9 Discuss the pros and cons of administration of sleeping medications.

Multiple choice questions

10 Which of the following statements about central nervous system stimulants are *not* correct?
   a. Since caffeine stimulates the output of pepsin and hydrochloric acid, coffee is often restricted for patients with peptic ulcers.
   b. Theophylline has a greater stimulant effect on the central nervous system than caffeine.
   c. Caffeine's ability to increase mental alertness is a result of cerebral cortical stimulation.
   d. Caffeine is a drug of choice for respiratory depression.
11 A cup of coffee before writing an examination may be considered a good use of caffeine because:
   a. caffeine depresses the higher centers and thus relieves worry and tension
   b. caffeine stimulates the cerebral cortex
   c. caffeine stimulates the myocardium and thus improves circulation
   d. caffeine stimulates fatigued muscle
12 Choose the *incorrect* answer.
   The amphetamines:
   a. are contraindicated in patients with cardiovascular disease or hypertension
   b. may be used to overcome respiratory depression from depressant drugs
   c. are anorexigenic agents
   d. are not known to cause depression upon withdrawal
13 The nausea and vomiting that may accompany the administration of morphine are caused by:
   a. stimulation of cerebral cortex
   b. irritation of gastrointestinal tract
   c. stimulation of chemoreceptor emetic trigger zone in the medulla
   d. stimulation of stomach contractions
14 Choose the *incorrect* answer.
   Morphine poisoning is indicated by the following signs:
   a. hypotension
   b. abnormally slow respiratory rate
   c. tachycardia
   d. pinpoint pupils
15 Important factors for the nurse to know about morphine include:
   a. Morphine has an antidiuretic effect.
   b. Morphine may cause intestinal spasms or "gas pains."
   c. Constipation is likely to be a postoperative complication when morphine is given pre- and postoperatively.
   d. Morphine is the most valuable analgesic available.
16 The greatest use of morphine lies in its ability to act as a(n):

a. antispasmodic   c. cough remedy
b. analgesic   d. antidiarrheic

17 The habit-forming quality of opium is explained by its effect on:
   a. higher centers of the cerebral cortex
   b. respiratory center
   c. vasomotor center
   d. smooth muscle of the bowel

18 Select the correct statements about meperidine.
   a. With therapeutic doses, meperidine depresses respirations to the same degree as morphine.
   b. Severe pain is not well controlled with meperidine.
   c. Syncope may occur when meperidine is given to an ambulatory patient.
   d. Meperidine is an effective antispasmodic.

19 Which of the following statements about salicylates are true?
   a. Aspirin can cause erosion of the gastric mucosa resulting in gastric bleeding because of its poor solubility in gastric juice.
   b. Salicylates are better tolerated when given with an alkaline substance such as sodium bicarbonate because salicylate excretion is increased.
   c. Since salicylates lower the prothrombin level, patients receiving both salicylates and anticoagulants should be on reduced anticoagulant therapy.
   d. For more rapid absorption, buffered salicylates should be administered.

20 Select the correct statements.
   a. Salicylate poisoning is more likely to occur from accidental ingestion than from administration of salicylates for therapeutic effect.
   b. Therapeutic doses of aspirin will not lower the temperature of nonfebrile individuals.
   c. Salicylates do not cause euphoria, sedation, or addiction.
   d. Salicylates will effectively relieve visceral as well as peripheral pain.

21 Choose the *incorrect* answer.
Barbiturates:
   a. have a depressant effect on the entire central nervous system
   b. primarily depress the motor areas of the cerebral cortex
   c. are not effective analgesic agents when used alone
   d. do not enhance the analgesic action of salicylates

22 Phenobarbital is one of the best of the barbiturates to prevent convulsive seizures because it:
   a. depresses the motor centers in the brainstem
   b. depresses the entire cerebral cortex
   c. exerts a highly selective depressant action on the motor cortex
   d. acts as an anticonvulsant in ordinary doses

23 Indicate which of the following channels of administration you would expect to use to give phenobarbital sodium.
   a. oral   c. sublingual
   b. rectal   d. intramuscular

24 Indicate which of the following statements are correct.
   a. The effects of alcohol can be reduced by caffeine.
   b. Nutritional complications are commonly found in the alcoholic.

   c. Episodic use of alcohol is not characteristic of the chronic alcoholic.
   d. An alcoholic has psychologic dependence on alcohol but not physical dependence.

25 Which of the following statements about alcohol are *incorrect?*
   a. When applied locally alcohol may denature proteins.
   b. A 70% by weight solution of ethyl alcohol is bactericidal.
   c. Alcohol is a stimulant.
   d. Toxic amounts of alcohol will impair respiration.
   e. Alcohol injected into a nerve only temporarily destroys the sensory nerve endings.

26 The method by which alcohol exerts a vasodilator effect is by:
   a. depression of muscle in the blood vessels
   b. depression of vasomotor center
   c. general cerebral depression
   d. depression of motor cortex

27 Which of the following statements about anticonvulsant therapy are *incorrect?*
   a. Sudden withdrawal of antiepileptic drugs may precipitate epileptic seizures.
   b. Preferred antiepileptics decrease muscle tone without loss of voluntary control.
   c. Phenacemide is the least toxic of the clinically available antiepileptics.
   d. Phenytoin suppresses grand mal seizures.

REFERENCES

General

A.M.A. Drug Evaluations, ed. 2, Acton, Mass., 1973, Publishing Sciences Group, Inc.

Aviado, D. M.: Krantz and Carr's pharmacologic principles of medical practice, ed. 8, Baltimore, 1972, The Williams & Wilkins Co.

Cuthbert, M. F., editor: The prostaglandins, Philadelphia, 1973, J. B. Lippincott Co.

Goodman, L. S., and Gilman, A., editors: The pharmacological basis of therapeutics, ed. 4, New York, 1970, The Macmillan Co.

Goth, A.: Medical pharmacology, ed. 7, St. Louis, 1974, The C. V. Mosby Co.

Meyers, F. H., Jarvetz, E., and Goldfien, A.: Review of medical pharmacology, ed. 4, Los Altos, Calif., 1974, Lange Medical Publications.

Osol, A., and Pratt, R.: The United States dispensatory, ed. 27, Philadelphia, 1973, J. B. Lippincott Co.

Narcotic analgesics

Jick, H., Slone, D., Shapiro, S., Lewis, G. P., and Siskind, V.: A new method for assessing the clinical effects of oral analgesic drugs, Clin. Pharmacol. Ther. **12:**456, 1971.

Lewis, J. W., Bentley, K. W., and Cowan, A.: Narcotic analgesics and antagonists, Ann. Rev. Pharmacol. **11:**241, 1971.

Miller, R. R., Feingold, A., and Paxinos, J.: Propoxyphene hydrochloride: A critical review, J.A.M.A. **213**:996, 1970.

Moertel, C. G., Ahmann, D. L., Taylor, W. F., and Schwartau, N.: A comparative evaluation of marketed analgesic drugs, New Eng. J. Med. **286**:813, 1972.

Pert, C. B., and Snyder, S. H.: Opiate receptors: Demonstration in nervous tissue, Science **179**:1011, 1973.

Potter, D. R., and Payne, J. P.: Newer analgesics: with special reference to pentazocine, Br. J. Anaesth. **42**:186, 1970.

Rodman, M. J.: Drugs for pain problems, R. N. **34**:59, 1971.

Sturner, W. Q., and Garriott, J. C.: Deaths involving propoxyphene: A study of 41 cases over a two-year period, J.A.M.A. **223**:1125, 1973.

Sunshine, A., Laska, E., Slaftas, J., and Fleischman, E.: A comparative analgesia study of propoxyphene hydrochloride, propoxyphene napsylate, and placebo, Toxicol. Appl. Pharmacol. **19**:512, 1971.

Vandam, L. D.: The potent analgesics, New Eng. J. Med. **286**:249, 1972.

Young, D. J.: Propoxyphene suicides, Arch. Intern. Med. **129**:62, 1972.

Nonnarcotic analgesics

Atkins, E., and Bodel, P.: Fever, New Eng. J. Med. **286**:29, 1972.

Barr, W. H., and Penna, R. P.: Internal analgesics. In Griffenhagen, G. B., and Hawkins, L. L., editors: Handbook of nonprescription drugs, American Pharmaceutical Association, 1971.

Davison, C.: Salicylate metabolism in man, Ann. N.Y. Acad. Sci. **179**:249, 1971.

Hunter, J.: Study of antipyretic therapy in current use, Arch. Dis. Child. **48**:313, 1973.

Kingsley, D. P. E., and others: Analgesic nephropathy, Br. Med. J. **4**:656, 1972.

Krane, S. M.: Action of salicylates, New Eng. J. Med. **286**:317, 1972.

Langman, M. J.: Epidemiological evidence for the association of aspirin and acute gastrointestinal bleeding, Gut **11**:627, 1970.

Smith, J. B., and Willis, A. L.: Aspirin selectively inhibits prostaglandin production in human platelets, Nature (New Biol.) **231**:235, 1971.

Vandam, L. D.: Analgesic drugs—the mild analgesics, New Eng. J. Med. **286**:20, 1972.

Vane, J. R.: Inhibition of prostaglandin synthesis as a mechanism of action of aspirin-like drugs, Nature **231**:232, 1971.

Narcotic antagonists

Evans, L. E. J., and others: Treatment of drug overdosage with nalokane, a specific narcotic antagonist, Lancet **1**:452, 1973.

Maugh, T. H.: Narcotic antagonists: The search accelerates, Science **177**:249, 1972.

Hypnotics and sedatives

Baekeland, F., and Hartmann, E.: Sleep requirements and the characteristics of some sleepers, Int. Psych. Clin. **7**:33, 1970.

Bellville, J. W., Forrest, W. H., Shroff, P., and Brown, B. W.: The hypnotic effects of codeine and secobarbital and their interaction in man, Clin. Pharmacol. Ther. **12**:607, 1971.

Devenyi, P., and Wilson, M.: Barbiturate abuse and addiction and their relationship to alcohol and alcoholism, Canad. Med. Ass. J. **104**:215, 1971.

Johns, M. W.: Methods for assessing human sleep, Arch. Int. Med. **127**:484, 1971.

Kales, A., and Kales, J. D.: Evaluation, diagnosis and treatment of clinical conditions related to sleep, J.A.M.A. **213**:2229, 1970.

Kales, A., editor: Sleep: Physiology and pathology, Philadelphia, 1970, J. B. Lippincott Co.

Mautner, H. G., and Clemson, H. C.: Hypnotics and sedatives. In Burger, A., editor: Medicinal chemistry, New York, 1970, Wiley-Interscience, Inc.

Alcohols

Brunt, P. W.: Progress report: Alcohol and the liver, Gut **12**:222, 1971.

Cahn, S.: The treatment of alcoholics: An evaluative study, New York, 1970, Oxford University Press.

Israel, Y.: Cellular effects of alcohol, Quart. J. Stud. Alcohol. **31**(2):293, 1970.

Mendelson, J. H.: Biologic concomitants of alcoholism, New Eng. J. Med. **283**:24, 71, 1970.

Rubin, E., and Lieber, C. S.: Alcoholism, alcohol and drugs, Science **172**:1097, 1971.

Anticonvulsant drugs

Ausman, J. J.: New developments in anticonvulsant therapy, Postgrad. Med. **48**:122, 1970.

Geller, M., and Christoff, N.: Diazepam in the treatment of childhood epilepsy, J.A.M.A. **215**:2087, 1971.

Griggs, W. L.: Epilepsy: Practical medical treatment, Mod. Treatm. **8**:258, 1971.

Kutt, H., and Louis, S.: Untoward effects of anticonvulsants, New Eng. J. Med. **286**:1316, 1972.

Rodman, M. J.: Drugs for treating epilepsy, R. N. **35**:63, 1972.

Stimulants

Griffith, J. D., Cavanaugh, J., Held, J., and Oates, J. A.: Dextroamphetamine: evaluation of psychomimetic properties in man, Arch. Gen. Psychiat. **26**:97, 1972.

Safer, D., Allen, R., and Barr, E.: Depression of growth in hyperactive children on stimulant drugs, New Eng. J. Med. **287**:217, 1972.

Sroufe, L. A., and Stewart, M. A.: Treating problem children with stimulant drugs, New Eng. J. Med. **289**:407, 1973.

CHAPTER 12

Psychotropic drugs

Role of drug therapy in psychiatry
Anatomy and physiology of emotions
Central nervous system

Psychotropic drugs

Major tranquilizers—antipsychotic agents
Minor tranquilizers—antianxiety agents
Antidepressants

ROLE OF DRUG THERAPY IN PSYCHIATRY

Drugs play an important role in contemporary approaches to psychiatric care. The development of the tranquilizing drugs opened many avenues of treatment that were not available before. Although emphasis in therapy is placed on milieu factors by many workers in the field, drug therapy is a valuable adjunct to providing comprehensive psychiatric care. The effect of drug therapy in psychiatric illness can be neither ignored nor overestimated. Because the use of the psychotropic drugs is not presently thought of as a "cure," consideration is given to the patient's total life situation as an important determinant of his health status. The use of drugs alleviates symptoms and allows the patient an opportunity to participate more easily in other forms of treatment. Drugs temporarily modify behavior while other therapies, such as psychotherapy, can shape behavior and produce a permanent change. Some drugs disrupt patterns of behavior or modify the electric patterns or fields within the brain that produce changes. However, any enduring effects on behavior are more likely to result from the individual's concurrent inter-

action with the environment. Since incoming information must be translated into biochemical changes before it can affect the nervous system function, environmental transactions, like drugs, may affect similar pathways before influencing behavior. Their effects can be additive, potentiating, or antagonistic, depending on their nature and direction. The milieu may potentiate the effectiveness of the drug or detract from it.

Drugs affect behavior indirectly as the chemical composition of a drug interacts with other chemicals, enzymes, or enzyme substrates. The alteration of the biochemical cell environment produces a change in cellular, tissue, and organ function. A modification of the behavior state of the patient results and determines the nature of his interaction with the environment. Drugs affect various levels of integration, from simple to complex—from cellular activity to psychosocial interaction.

ANATOMY AND PHYSIOLOGY OF EMOTIONS

In order to understand the action of drugs in alleviating the symptomatology of mental illness, the nurse must have knowledge of the function-   **275** ing of the nervous system. The trend in nursing toward a holistic view of man and his phenomenologic experience no longer allows the practitioner to separate out the functions of the mind from the body. Neurophysiologists have traditionally identified each part of the nervous system by a specific function or made tentative architectonic maps of the cerebral cortex, allocating specific functions to various areas of the brain. Recent research has indicated a change in this perspective. The brain is considered to be a single organ composed of various structures that produce a final unified effect when they react on each other in a normal fashion. The interrelationship of various structures is extremely intricate, and it is difficult to allocate special functions to each structure. Papez in 1937 was one of the first to suggest the function of a reverberating circuit in the brain as an explanation of emotional experience. Research has revealed methods for measuring certain types of brain activity, and such information has made it possible to speculate in some detail on the physiologic substrates of emotional activity. For purposes of clarity in discussing the neuroanatomic and neurophysiologic bases of emotions, the various aspects of the nervous system will be discussed under the following headings:

1. Central nervous system
2. Autonomic regulation
3. Biochemical mechanisms

CENTRAL NERVOUS SYSTEM

The central nervous system functions in the coordination and direction of activities in the tissues and organs of the body. The various parts and levels of the central nervous system form a closely related and integrated series of mechanisms and systems through which the human being achieves adjustment and adaptation to his environment. The central nervous system is responsible for consciousness, behavior, memory, recognition, learning, and the more highly developed attributes of human beings such as imagination, abstract reasoning, and creative thought. In addition, it serves to coordinate such vital regulatory functions as blood pressure,

heart rate, respiration, salivary and gastric secretions, muscular activity, and body temperature. Discussion will be limited to consideration of the functions of the central nervous system that are believed to affect the emotions and behavior.

The cerebrum, the largest part of the brain, is divided into two hemispheres. The outer surface of the cerebral hemispheres is composed of gray matter known as the cerebral cortex. It is thought to be the site of consciousness and is divided into sensory, motor, and association areas. These areas receive sensations from organs of special sense (sight, hearing, smell, and taste) as well as from the skin, muscles, joints, and tendons (touch, pain, and temperature). Large parts of the cortex now appear to function as a whole in providing the anatomic basis for such mental attributes as recognition, memory, intelligence, imagination, and creative thought.

Beneath the cortex are tracts of fibers comprising the white matter, which connect the lower centers of the brain, spinal cord, and associated areas of the cortex with each other. The basal ganglia (corpus striatum, claustrum, and amygdaloid nucleus) are located near the lateral ventricle of the cerebrum. The hippocampus, a mass of gray matter lying close to the lateral ventricle, is connected by a tract of fibers (the fornix) to the mamillary bodies in the hypothalamus. The hippocampus, the fornix, the amygdaloid nucleus, the hippocampal gyrus, and the uncus are collectively referred to as the limbic system. This system is believed to be concerned with the conscious experience of emotion.

The midbrain, pons, and medulla form the part of the brain below the cerebrum. The midbrain contains the nuclei of cranial nerves III and IV. The pons is mainly a pathway for ascending and descending tracts of the fibers. The medulla oblongata is continuous with the spinal cord. It contains vital groups of synapses that are concerned with the reflex control of blood pressure (vasomotor center), heart rate and force (cardiac center), respiration (respiratory center), vomiting (vomiting center), and temperature. The reticular formation consists of a complex network of cell bodies and interlacing fibers in the medulla, pons, midbrain, and diencephalon.

Figure 12-1

Reticular activating system.

Reticular activating
system and tracts

Main motor tract
(pyramidal)

Main sensory tracts
(spinothalamic and thalamocortical)

Figure 12-2

Papez circuit.

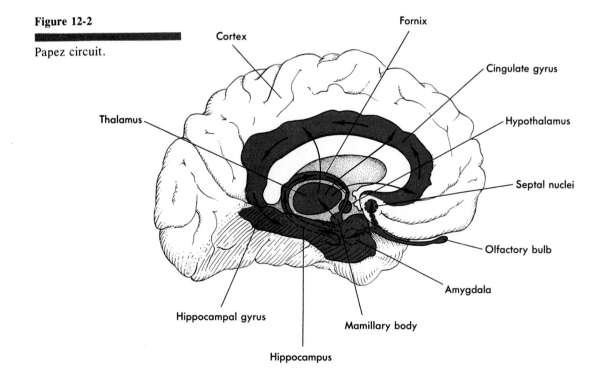

Cortex

Fornix

Cingulate gyrus

Thalamus

Hypothalamus

Septal nuclei

Olfactory bulb

Amygdala

Hippocampal gyrus

Mamillary body

Hippocampus

The reticular activating system is thought to function in alerting the cortex to sensory stimuli and in originating the emotional reactions associated with somatic sensory experiences (pain, touch, hearing, sight). Experimental stimulation of this system produces alertness in behavior, whereas decrease in its activity leads to relaxation and drowsiness. The reticular activating system has its upper end in the posterior hypothalamus and lower thalamus.

The cerebellum lies on the dorsal side of the pons and is attached to the brainstem. It functions as part of the feedback mechanisms concerned with subconscious control of equilibrium, posture, and movement.

The thalamus and hypothalamus are located in the region of the brain that is called the diencephalon (the between brain). Most sensations are relayed through the thalamus to the cerebral cortex. The conscious appreciation of pain is said to be located in the thalamus. In recent years there has been a gradual increase of knowledge relative to the functions of the hypothalamus. In spite of extensive research and experimentation there still seems to be some question of its specific mode of function. It has been conjectured that the hypothalamus contains integrative mechanisms that, in addition to their effect on behavior patterns, also aid in regulating the basic life functions of man (control of water excretion, appetite, sleep-wake mechanisms, temperature, and blood pressure). The hypothalamus seems to function through its relationships with other parts of the nervous system and endocrine system. It is part of a system of complex circuits within the brain so strategically placed that its derangement may have profound effects. These interrelationships between cerebral cortex, thalamus, hypothalamus, and various other circuits in the brain produce patterns of behavior that are modifiable by situations and autonomic adjustments to adapt the individual to changes in both external and internal environments.

Papez proposed that "the hypothalamus, the anterior thalamic nuclei, the gyrus cingulum, the hippocampus, and their interconnections constitute a harmonious mechanism which may elaborate the functions of central emotion as well as participate in emotional expression."* The Papez circuit functions in the following sequence:

On stimulation of the hippocampus this structure relays impulses via the fornix to the mammillary bodies of the hypothalamus. From that area they continue to the anterior thalamic nuclei and to the cingulate gyrus of the cerebral cortex. The functional circuit is completed by fibers leaving the cingulate gyrus by way of the cingulum and returning to the hippocampus via the hippocampal gyrus.*

This proposed circuit provides an understanding of the anatomic basis for the expression of emotion and behavior. The intricate balance of positive and negative controls leads to a better conceptualization of the function of the central nervous system in the regulation of emotions and behavioral patterns in human beings. There is increasing evidence that these areas of the central nervous system have some control over behavior and emotions; however, at best, these data have been superficial, inconclusive, and theoretical.

AUTONOMIC REGULATIONS

The functions of the sympathetic and parasympathetic visceral nervous system are discussed in Chapter 9. The importance of the reactions of these systems in the production of behavior is paramount in gaining an understanding of drug action and/or the behavioral manifestations of side effects from the use of drugs. Since the central nervous system functions in the regulation of integrated behavior, considerable effort has been extended toward locating and defining the integrative centers. Scientific evidence is accumulating for grouping the functions of the subcortical systems into two separate and antagonistic divisions. Two such systems have been identified in the hypothalamus and have been labeled the "ergotropic division" and the "trophotropic system." Much of the work in defining and locating these divisions is based on the behavioral and physiologic responses elicited by their stimulation.

BIOCHEMICAL MECHANISMS

The functions of the central nervous system are dependent upon the actions of certain neuro-

---

*Marks, J.: Scientific basis of drug therapy, New York, 1965, Pergamon Press, Inc., p. 5.

hormonal agents located in the brain and peripheral tissues. These neurohormones are stored in inactive forms, and at the right moment nerve impulses release their free forms, which then stimulate transmission of appropriate reactions.

There is evidence that acetylcholine is released from central neural tissue, such as the surface of the cerebral cortex, into the cerebrospinal fluid during activity. The rate of release is proportional to the level of activity. Thus it is known that some central synapses are cholinergic. However, others are not.

Norepinephrine has also been found to be present in the central nervous system. Tyrosine and dopamine are normal constituents of the brain and known precursors of norepinephrine synthesis. High concentrations of norepinephrine are located in the hypothalamus, medulla, limbic system, and cranial nerve nuclei. Low concentrations of norepinephrine are found in the striatum and caudate nucleus where dopamine, the immediate precursor of norepinephrine, is found in high concentration. It is believed that both norepinephrine and dopamine function as transmitters. They have widespread inhibitory and excitatory effects on a wide variety of centrally mediated functions such as sleep and arousal, affect, and memory. Thus, some central synapses are adrenergic.

Serotonin is another transmitter substance found in the central nervous system. Areas rich in serotonin include the hypothalamus, pineal gland, midbrain, and spinal cord. Serotonin is synthesized in the brain and stored in the subcellular particles. Alteration of the level of serotonin in the nervous system is associated with changes in behavior. Many drugs mimic or block the action of serotonin on peripheral tissues and produce changes in mood and behavior, which suggests that they interfere with the action of serotonin and norepinephrine in the brain.

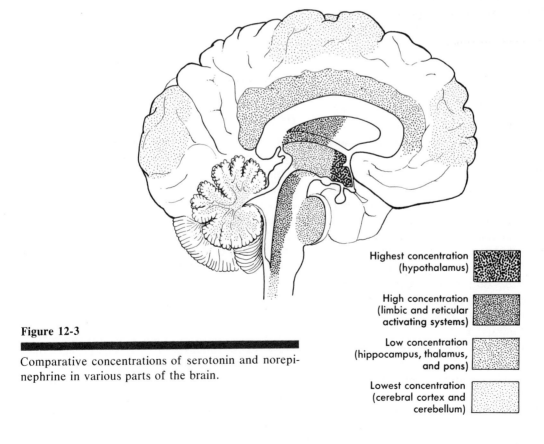

Highest concentration
(hypothalamus)

High concentration
(limbic and reticular
activating systems)

Low concentration
(hippocampus, thalamus,
and pons)

Lowest concentration
(cerebral cortex and
cerebellum)

Figure 12-3

Comparative concentrations of serotonin and norepinephrine in various parts of the brain.

Other proposed central neurotransmitters include histamine, amino acids (e.g., glutamate, GABA), substance P (a polypeptide composed of thirteen different amino acids), and the prostaglandins.

Psychotropic drugs

The two major drug groups that comprise the classification of psychotropic drugs are the *tranquilizers* and the *antidepressants.* The term *tranquilizer* reflects the action of this group of drugs in effecting a change toward tranquility in the affective and behavioral state of the individual. Tranquilizers have a direct effect on the levels of anxiety that create a pathologic adjustment to intrapersonal and interpersonal experiences. Anxiety is reduced without subsequent impairment of consciousness, and hyperactivity is controlled. The delusions, hallucinations, and confusion associated with psychopathology are decreased to a tolerable level. The tranquilizers are commonly classified as *major* and *minor* tranquilizers. The major tranquilizers are sometimes referred to as "neuroleptics" or "ataractics" (from the Greek word *ataraktos* meaning "undisturbed" or "peace of mind"). The major tranquilizers or "antipsychotic" agents are those substances that affect psychotic symptoms and autonomic regulations. Minor tranquilizers, or "antineurotic" agents, are those substances that are characterized by their action in the relief of mild or moderate anxiety and that are not usually known to be effective as antipsychotic agents. The main therapeutic action of the minor tranquilizers seems to be in treatment of anxiety that accompanies neurotic symptomatology. The minor tranquilizers do not evoke extrapyramidal symptoms such as tremor, rigidity, or dystonic reactions; they produce few autonomic symptoms and tend to raise the convulsive threshold.

The antidepressant drug group has led to an effective psychopharmacologic treatment of depression states. The antidepressants, also called "psychostimulants" or "psychic energizers" because of their stimulating and energy-producing action, have replaced some of the older drugs (amphetamine, caffeine) in the treatment of depressive states. The older drugs were found to cause rise in blood pressure, increase in heart rate, and loss of appetite. Drugs such as the amphetamines are high-risk drugs for causing psychic dependency, which reduces their effectiveness for long-term treatment.

Another group of drugs, the psychotomimetics, are included in the psychotropic drug classification. This group of drugs will not be given consideration in this discussion of the psychotropic drugs since their mechanism of action is unknown and their usefulness in the treatment of mental illness is still in the experimental stages. The action of these drugs has been known to mimic or produce psychotic states and therefore they are sometimes called *hallucinogenic drugs.* The most publicized and best known of these drugs is lysergic acid diethylamide (LSD). These drugs cause initial autonomic disturbances (tachycardia, dilation of the pupil, tightness in the chest and abdomen, and nausea) followed by vivid visual hallucinations, severe anxiety, and delusions. Use of these drugs should be restricted to controlled experimental research because of the grave danger of irreversible sequelae.

SELECTION AND USE OF PSYCHOTROPIC DRUGS

In the past physicians selected psychotropic agents on the basis of diagnostic category—schizophrenia, manic-depressive syndrome, or psychoneurosis. More recent proposals have indicated a radical change in the physician's approach to selecting drugs for the mentally ill person. The pharmacologic treatment of psychiatric disorders would appear to be similar to that of somatic disorders—modification of the most disabling components of the patient's behavior so that the patient may more effectively cope with his environment and take advantage of the therapeutic milieu available. It would seem more rational to deemphasize the diagnostic classifications of psychiatric disorders as a basis for drug selectivity and to consider instead the most disabling behavioral manifestations that can be observed. This implies a thorough assessment of the patient prior to the administration of drugs. This assessment should include the specific disabling features of the patient's behavior, a decision as to the goals of therapy, the dynamics involved, and the specific directional changes sought. Other factors helpful in making an accurate assessment of the patient's need for drug therapy are:

1 The degree of agitation or behavioral arousal
2 The degree of over- or underactivity
3 Patterns of affective response to stress (avoidance or escape, aggression, fear, inhibited withdrawal)
4 The degree of social withdrawal
5 The nature and dynamics of depressive elements present
6 Sleep problems
7 Need for environmental control
8 Medical complaints
9 Possible drug dependence
10 Past drug history—effectiveness of response to drugs

When the physician establishes the need for drug therapy, it must then be decided what agent or combination of agents is best suited for the behavioral and medical needs of the patient. Since there are many drugs available, it is judicious for the physician to become familiar with a few drugs rather than make a haphazard selection of several agents. This requires an intimate knowledge of the behavioral actions, the pharmacologic effects, and the potential adverse reactions of the agents used, as well as an awareness of the many individual and environment-related factors present. Upon selection of the agent or agents to be used, the dosage is then increased until the desired and expected effects are produced. Continuous reevaluation based on observation of the effects of the drug selected is needed. Increase or reduction of dosage may be indicated in order to gain the desired effects. The nurse plays an important role in the evaluation and reassessment of a patient's response to drug therapy. It is important to be aware of the criteria the physician uses in selecting psychotropic drugs and the expected effects so that the patient's progress may be observed and reported. Knowledge of the action of drugs also assists the nurse in understanding the interpersonal responses that take place in the therapeutic nurse-patient relationship.

MAJOR TRANQUILIZERS— ANTIPSYCHOTIC AGENTS
RAUWOLFIA ALKALOIDS

The first of the drugs to play an important part in the pharmacologic treatment of mental illness were the rauwolfia alkaloids. These drugs came into prominence around 1953, although they have been used in India for many years for the treatment of mental disorders. The most widely used of these compounds is reserpine. The principal use of the rauwolfia alkaloid compounds today is in the treatment of hypertension. Their use in this respect is described in Chapter 10. The rauwolfia alkaloids are still considered as antipsychotic agents; however, they are not widely used because of the toxic side effects present with large single doses. It is necessary to administer these compounds in small daily dosages that prolong the effects of their action and delay their therapeutic effectiveness. As a tranquilizer, reserpine produces many of the same effects as the phenothiazine drug groups; however, its use is now restricted to those patients who do not respond to phenothiazine treatment. Since the phenothiazine drugs achieve the same tranquilizing effects, the rauwolfia compounds have been replaced by these drugs.

PHENOTHIAZINE DERIVATIVES

Discovery of the phenothiazine derivatives arose out of research in the area of the antihistamines. Chlorpromazine hydrochloride was introduced in 1951 and has found wide acceptance in the treatment of mental illness. Additional investigation of the action of chlorpromazine in producing undesirable side effects led to the development of numerous derivatives, which comprise the largest group of psychotropic agents.

About two thirds of all antipsychotic drugs are phenothiazine derivatives. They are commonly divided chemically into the following four subgroups: (1) the dimethylamine compounds (chlorpromazine, promazine, and triflupromazine); (2) the piperidyl compounds (thioridazine, mesoridazine, piperacetazine, and mepazine); (3) the piperazine compounds (acetophenazine, fluphenazine, perphenazine, prochlorperazine, thiopropazate, trifluoperazine, carphenazine, and butaperazine); and (4) thioxanthene derivatives (thiothixene and chlorprothixene). The chemical structure of these compounds and specific information regarding their action, effects, and adverse reactions will be presented separately following the general discussion of commonalities that have been identified. The type of action is essentially similar with all phenothiazine derivatives; individual compounds vary chiefly in their potency and in the nature and severity of their side effects.

Site and mechanism of action of phenothiazine derivatives. It has been suggested that the cause of schizophrenia may be related to an excess of dopamine in the central nervous system. The antipsychotics increase the rate of dopamine turnover (synthesis and destruction) and may block dopamine-mediated transmission. These actions could also account for the extrapyramidal side effects (parkinsonism-like effects) of the antipsychotics.

Since the behavioral effects of chlorpromazine are reversed by cholinesterase inhibitors (e.g., physostigmine), some antipsychotic drugs may have a central cholinolytic effect. In addition, chlorpromazine and related antipsychotic drugs have adrenergic blocking effects. Thus some antipsychotic drugs may centrally affect catecholamine action or uptake. Laboratory electrographic studies show the limbic system to be electrically sensitive to the antipsychotics; seizures caused by very large doses of these drugs begin here and spread to cortical structures. It would appear that antipsychotics have a stimulating neurophysiologic action even though the behavioral manifestation of the tranquilizers is reduction in activity.

Antipsychotics depress lower levels of the central nervous system. Depression of the vomiting center accounts for the antiemetic effect of these drugs. Alteration of the temperature regulating center results in a minor fall in body temperature except in the extremities where vasodilation occurs. Shivering is also suppressed. Thus chlorpromazine and related drugs can be used

when it is desirable to induce hypothermia. The phenothiazines are thought to act centrally as antinorepinephrine drugs, blocking the adrenergic synapses.

The administration of phenothiazines to the human being leads to a widespread reduction of sympathetic tone in the body. There is vasodilation and hypotension with compensatory tachycardia, relaxation of smooth muscle, alteration of pupillary size, and decreased salivary and gastric secretions. Because the phenothiazines act to suppress central sympathetic activity without significantly depressing the reticular activating system, their use is favored in the control of psychomotor agitation, since this effect is produced without significant loss of cortical functioning or consciousness. The hallucinations and delusions associated with psychosis are mitigated or eliminated by the action of the phenothiazines.

Pharmacologic characteristics and uses. The most important pharmacologic characteristics of these substances are: (1) antipsychotic activity (an ability to calm aggressive, overactive, disturbed patients); (2) failure of large doses to produce deep coma and anesthesia (patients show both behavioral and electroencephalographic arousal when stimulated); (3) production of reversible and irreversible effects on the extrapyramidal system, leading to the development of related signs and symptoms; and (4) lack of any notable tendency to cause psychogenic or physical dependence.

Behavioral effects. The phenothiazine derivatives are used to reduce psychotic symptoms and therefore are useful in the treatment of acute and chronic psychoses. Control of deeply disturbed patients is achieved without causing depression of vital centers. Psychotic conditions marked by excessive psychomotor activity, panic, fear, and hostility respond well to the administration of the phenothiazines. Relief of emotional tension, excitement, and agitation lessens the patient's response to hallucinations and delusions. Destructive and combative behaviors are notably reduced. On the other hand, some of the piperazine compounds are useful in stimulating the withdrawn apathetic patient so that he becomes more alert, sociable, and communicative. The phenothiazines may make some depressive reactions worse and do not seem to be of value in treating hysteria or obsessive-compulsive reactions. However, phenothiazines seem to be helpful in allaying the agitation and anxiety that occur prior to electroconvulsive treatments.

Small doses of the antipsychotic agents are sometimes used to control the anxiety, tension, and emotional disturbance in the psychoneurotic patient. Anxiety that often accompanies diseases with psychogenic components is easily controlled with small doses of the phenothiazine derivatives. However, the risk involved from the side effects does not seem to warrant their use in these instances. The minor tranquilizers appear to be more useful in these conditions.

Some of the phenothiazine derivatives have been used in nonpsychiatric settings because of their secondary actions (antiemesis; potentiation of hypnotic, analgesic, and anesthetic agents).

Adverse behavioral effects. Antipsychotics can cause unpleasant effects. For the most part, antipsychotic therapy is not a subjectively pleasant experience. The feelings of lassitude and fatigability limit the patient's ability to engage in many otherwise normal and nonexhausting activities. The depressing effects may decrease the patient's willingness to take medication. Depression may also account for the greater incidence of suicide in psychotics on drug therapy than in those receiving only institutional care.

Some patients experience feelings of excitement and restlessness. These reactions are more likely to occur early in treatment and after administration of piperazine derivatives.

All antipsychotics affect sleep. Chlorpromazine may inhibit or enhance REM sleep, depending on dosage. Lithium is a REM suppressant, and REM rebound may occur after withdrawal.

Side effects. The phenothiazine derivatives produce a wide variety of untoward effects. Individuals vary in their ability to tolerate these compounds, and difficulty with side effects may determine the effectiveness of the compound. The pattern of adverse reactions is one of the important factors that the physician considers in choosing among the compounds. Some of these side effects result from the secondary action of the drugs on the central and autonomic nervous systems, while others are idiosyncratic or allergic in nature.

Quinidine-like effect. Antipsychotics have effects on the heart similar to those of quinidine. EKG findings show T wave changes and prolonged P-R interval and QRS complex, reflecting slowed conduction. Ventricular ectopic pacemaker activity may occur, which can lead to ventricular fibrillation and death. Thioridazine (Mellaril) is particularly hazardous in this regard.

Autonomic effects. The autonomic effects are as follows.

Parasympatholytic effects—Tranquilizers have atropine-like properties that can be very prominent with large doses. Manifestations of this effect include dry mouth, failure of accommodation for near vision, constipation, and urinary retention.

Beta-adrenergic effects—Phenothiazines and related drugs intensify beta-adrenergic effects of sympathetic nerve stimulation. This action accounts for the vasodilating and postural hypotensive effects.

Convulsant effect—Extremely high doses of tranquilizers may cause convulsions, although this is rare clinically. Epileptics are more susceptible to this effect.

Patients should be cautioned against driving an automobile, operating dangerous machinery, or performing tasks that require absolute precision, motor coordination, and mental alertness.

Decreased libido may be a troublesome side effect for patients on a maintenance dosage of these drugs. Careful explanation of the cause of this side effect may alleviate the patient's anxiety. Some patients refuse medications before home visits for this reason.

Liver. Cholestatic hepatitis with obstructive jaundice is the most frequent form of liver disorder observed. It usually develops within the first 5 weeks of treatment. If bilirubinuria and icterus are detected in liver function tests, the drug should be withdrawn immediately. Since the subsequent changes in the liver persist for a much longer time, it is not advisable to change treatment to another phenothiazine compound. Fatality is rare, and recovery from phenothiazine jaundice usually occurs within a few weeks. It is undesirable to use these drugs in patients who have known liver disease. Such patients are probably no more susceptible to such reactions than other patients, but the consequences might be more serious should they occur.

Hematologic complications. Leukopenia, granulocytopenia, agranulocytosis, purpura, and pancytopenia are hematologic complications that occur. The incidence of their occurrence is low; however, the mortality rate is high. Physicians and nurses should be alert to the appearance of such signs as sore throat, fever, or weakness in patients taking these drugs. With the appearance of these symptoms the drug is usually discontinued and a white blood cell and differential count are made to determine the cause of the disturbance. Some physicians order routine monthly or bimonthly laboratory tests to avoid such complications. However, most physicians believe that this precaution is of little value, since blood dyscrasias occur so rapidly that it is impractical to do blood counts frequently enough to protect the patient.

Postural hypotension. Postural hypotension is usually mild and occurs with initial dosage of the phenothiazines. Compensatory adjustment usually takes place in a few days. It can be especially serious, though, with patients in whom a sudden drop in blood pressure would be undesirable (elderly patients with evidence of arteriosclerosis or patients with cardiovascular disease). If this side effect is causing an unusual amount of difficulty or serious hazards, the following remedial measures may be instituted: (1) a change of medication to one of the phenothiazine derivatives that is not known to produce this side effect with such frequency, (2) reduction of dosage, or (3) discontinuation of medication for a 24-hour period with a gradual buildup of dosage as tolerated. The patient who complains of dizziness, lightheadedness, or palpitation may be experiencing orthostatic (postural) hypotension. This can easily be confirmed by comparing the patient's blood pressure in the prone and standing positions. The nurse may instruct the patient to rise slowly from the recumbent position and to sit on the edge of the bed for a few minutes before attempting to stand. Support and reassurance may be necessary to allay the patient's anxiety. Explanation of this phenomenon may also aid in the patient's understanding of this experience and reduce his anxiety. Patients should be encouraged to remain in a recumbent position for 1 hour after initial doses, parenterally administered doses, or large oral doses of the phenothiazines.

Dermatoses. Dermatoses are usually mild and can be controlled by discontinuing the drug. It is often possible to resume treatment later with another compound, or even the same one, without recurrence of the allergic skin reaction. If photosensitivity develops, the patient should stay out of the sunlight or wear protective clothing to prevent solar erythema. Nurses should instruct patients regarding this side effect and/or assist them in providing the necessary protective measures to avoid exposure. A dark purplish-brown skin pigmentation, induced by light, has been reported in hospitalized psychiatric patients who were given large dosages of phenothiazines for 3 to 10 years.

Endocrine imbalance. Endocrine imbalance is caused by depression of hypothalamic functions. These symptoms have been reported infrequently and include delayed ovulation and menstruation, amenorrhea with false positive results from pregnancy tests, lactogenic response in female patients, and weight gain. These symptoms may cause unwarranted anxiety and compound the patient's problems. After ordinary steps are initiated to determine other possible causative factors for these symptoms without positive results, the patient should be reassured that the medication she is receiving is the causative factor. Depending on the patient's current symptomatology, reinforcement of these facts may be necessary.

In pregnancy the risk of administration of these drugs should be weighed against the expected therapeutic outcome.

Extrapyramidal symptoms. Extrapyramidal symptoms may appear after the administration of a single dose of phenothiazines or after prolonged usage. Extrapyramidal symptoms are considered to be a rather normal consequence of drug action. These reactions are of four general types: pseudoparkinsonism, akinesia, akathisia, and dyskinesia. Pseudoparkinsonism resembles true parkinsonism and manifests

Figure 12-4

Persistent dyskinesia (abnormal movements of extremities). Complication of long-term therapy with tranquilizers.

A

B

C

Figure 12-5

Persistent dyskinesia. **A,** In-and-out movements of the tongue. **B,** Sucking and smacking of the lips. **C,** Lateral jaw movements.

symptoms such as tremor, mask-like facial expression, rigidity, drooling, loss of associated movements of the arms, and some restlessness. Akinesia is usually less distressing to the patient and becomes evident to medical personnel when the patient complains of fatigue and weakness of the arms and legs. Akathisia (motor restlessness) becomes apparent when the patient is observed to be extremely restless, continually moving his hands, mouth, and body. Dyskinesia is a less common disturbance that takes many forms such as torsion spasm, opisthotonos, oculogyric crises, drooping of the head, protrusion of tongue, and other facial disturbances (Figure 12-5). Patients complain of stiff neck and inability to swallow and usually become very frightened with the onset of these symptoms. The dramatic suddenness of onset is often frightening to nursing personnel as well. Recognition of the cause of this symptomatology is helpful in allaying the anxiety of both nurse and patient. Immediate action should be instituted to reverse this extrapyramidal reaction. The administration of an antiparkinsonian agent orally (when possible) or parenterally will produce a reversal of symptoms in as dramatic a fashion as the onset of the symptoms. The nurse should stay with the patient and reassure him that the symptoms will subside, which also gives the nurse an opportunity to observe the patient closely. Pseudoparkinsonism, akathisia, and akinesia may have a more gradual onset than dyskinesia; however, they may be just as troublesome to patients. Generally these extrapyramidal symptoms are easily controlled by lowering the dosage or discontinuing the medication, using a compound that has a low incidence of these reactions (see Table 12-1), or controlling these reactions with use of antiparkinsonian drugs. Occasionally, the symptoms persist. Antiparkinsonian agents most commonly used are benztropine mesylate, biperiden, and procyclidine.

Precautions. There are several precautions that should be observed in the use of phenothiazine compounds.

Autonomic blockade may occur as one of the most serious effects resulting from the adrenergic blocking action of the phenothiazines. If circulatory collapse occurs, a vasopressor agent

Table 12-1 Frequency of incidence of extrapyramidal symptoms from antipsychotic agents

	Generic name	*Trade name*
Highest incidence	Fluphenazine	Permitil; Prolixin
	Trifluoperazine	Stelazine
	Perphenazine	Trilafon
	Prochlorperazine	Compazine
	Thiopropazate	Dartal
	Acetophenazine	Tindal
	Triflupromazine	Vesprin
	Chlorpromazine	Thorazine
	Carphenazine	Proketazine
	Butaperazine	Repoise
	Piperacetazine	Quide
	Thiothixene	Navane
Lowest incidence	Mepazine	Pacatal
	Thioridazine	Mellaril
	Mesoridazine	Serentil

such as levarterenol or angiotensin amide should be given. *Epinephrine* should *never* be used since its administration to a patient with partial adrenergic blockade may result in further fall of blood pressure.

Potentiation of other drugs is a common effect produced by the phenothiazine derivatives. They should be used cautiously in patients who are under the influence of alcohol, barbiturates, or morphine-like analgesics. Dosage of anesthetics should be reduced. These drugs should also be used with care in patients who are taking antihypertensive drugs. They should be used cautiously in patients receiving atropine or related drugs due to the additive anticholinergic effects.

Antiemetic effects of these agents may complicate the diagnosis of nausea and vomiting related to organic disorders.

Other adverse reactions that have been observed are melanosis of internal organs such as the heart, liver, and kidneys after the administration of chlorpromazine in large doses. Electrocardiographic alterations resembling those caused by quinidine or by hypokalemia and pigmentary retinopathy have been noted, especially when large doses of thioridazine have been administered. These drugs should be administered

Table 12-2 Major tranquilizers (phenothiazine derivatives and thioxanthines)

Generic name	Trade name	Side effects*	Dosage range† per 24 hour period (mg.)
Dimethylamine subgroup			
Chlorpromazine hydrochloride	Thorazine	1-9, 11, 12-15, 23	30 to 1200
Triflupromazine	Vesprin	1-12	60 to 150
Piperidyl subgroup			
Thioridazine	Mellaril	1-3, 6, 7, 12, 13, 17-19	30 to 800
Mepazine	Pacatal	1-11, 13, 14	50 to 400
Mesoridazine	Serentil	1-7, 13, 19, 21	100 to 400
Piperacetazine	Quide	1, 6, 7, 10, 11, 19, 20, 23, 29	20 to 160
Piperazine subgroup			
Acetophenazine	Tindal	1, 6	40 to 80
Butaperazine	Repoise	6, 7, 11	15 to 100
Carphenazine maleate	Proketazine	1, 6, 8, 9	75 to 400
Fluphenazine	Permitil; Prolixin	1-9, 11, 12, 15, 18	1 to 20
Perphenazine	Trilafon	1-9, 11, 12	6 to 64
Prochlorperazine	Compazine	1-7, 9, 11, 12, 15, 20	15 to 150
Thiopropazate	Dartal	1, 3-7, 11, 12, 14, 15	15 to 100
Thiothixene	Navane	1, 3, 5-7, 10, 12-14, 18, 23	6 to 60
Trifluoperazine	Stelazine	1, 2, 4-9, 11, 12, 15, 18	2 to 20

_—40 mg._

Key to table
1. Sedation or sleep
2. Ataxia
3. Dry mouth
4. Constipation
5. Dermatitis
6. Extrapyramidal symptoms
7. Hypotension
8. Blood dyscrasia (usually agranulocytosis)
9. Jaundice
10. Convulsions
11. Antiemetic
12. Blurred vision

13. Hypothermia
14. Tachycardia
15. Nasal congestion
16. Menstrual irregularities
17. Nausea and vomiting
18. Edema
19. Impotence
20. Increased appetite
21. Bradycardia
22. Increased gastric secretions
23. Photosensitivity

*Side effects here are not intended to be a complete account of possible adverse reactions.
†Since drug dosage varies with the patient's response and the severity of the disease, consult drug digest for dosage schedules.

cautiously to patients with suspected heart disease. Because of the pronounced anticholinergic action of these agents, they should not be administered to patients with a history of glaucoma or prostatic hypertrophy. During the summer months, instances of hyperthermia and heat prostration have been reported. The phenothiazines should be used cautiously and in small doses in patients with a history of convulsive disorders because of their action in reducing the convulsive threshold. These drugs are contraindicated in comatose patients because of their central nervous system depressive effect.

Cardiac findings in sudden death after prolonged use of the phenothiazines have been inconclusive. Patients have been known to die suddenly and unexpectedly. Postmortem examinations of these patients have revealed the presence of a brown granular pigment in the heart and other viscera. It has been hypothesized that death is caused by ventricular arrhythmia or asphyxia during a convulsive seizure.

DIMETHYLAMINE SUBGROUP
Chlorpromazine hydrochloride, U.S.P., B.P. (Thorazine Hydrochloride)

The structural formulas of phenothiazine and chlorpromazine are represented as follows.

Phenothiazine

Chlorpromazine

Chlorpromazine was introduced for clinical trial in 1951. It is a grayish white, crystalline powder that is soluble in water. It is chemically related to the antihistaminic promethazine (Phenergan) but in comparison chlorpromazine has little antihistaminic activity. It was introduced in Europe under the name of Largactil.

Preparation, dosage, and administration. Chlorpromazine hydrochloride is marketed in sustained-release capsules (30, 75, 150, 200, and 300 mg.); in solution, in ampules, and in multiple-dose vials (25 mg. per milliliter); in syrup (2 mg. per milliliter); in tablets (10, 25, 50, 100, and 200 mg.); and as a concentrate (30 mg. per milliliter). Chlorpromazine is available also in suppository form (25 and 100 mg.).

The smallest effective dose is the one recommended. Oral adult dosage varies from 10 mg. to 1 Gm. or more per day. Total daily amounts are usually given in three evenly spaced doses. For children the oral dose is 2 mg. per kilogram of body weight daily in divided doses. Intramuscular dose is 0.5 mg. per kilogram every 6 to 8 hours.

Chlorpromazine hydrochloride is administered orally, intramuscularly, and intravenously. It is usually given orally unless for some reason the patient is unable to take the dose by mouth. Often patients will conceal tablets in the back of their mouth or around the teeth and lip area. The concentrate may be used effectively in this case. The taste of chlorpromazine hydrochloride concentrate can become more palatable when given in fruit juice; however, the patient should be told there is medication in the juice. If chlorpromazine concentrate is used for long periods of time, close attention must be given to proper oral hygiene. The concentrate is a highly irritating substance on contact with skin and eyes. Care should be taken to wash areas of the body that come into contact with this substance immediately. Nurses have been known to contract very uncomfortable dermatologic conditions as a result of their contact with this substance. Chlorpromazine hydrochloride is considered too irritating to be given subcutaneously. When given intramuscularly it should be injected deeply and slowly in divided doses of not more than 1 ml. per injection site. Massage of the site of injection helps to reduce local irritation. Some patients have been known to develop abscesses at the injection site, which are thought to result from large doses of this substance in one area. Use of the intramuscular route of administration of chlorpromazine is usually indicated when the patient refuses the tablet or concentrate form or when the most immediate effect of the drug is desired. If the patient is severely agitated, combative, or struggling, care should be taken to follow safe administration technique. This technique usually requires enough well-trained personnel to adequately restrain the patient while the medication is being given.

Chlorpromazine has a D.E.S.I. rating of *effective* for use in psychotic conditions associated with moderate to severe anxiety, tension, and agitation; for preoperative use to relieve restlessness and apprehension; as an adjunct in the treatment of tetanus; and for control of nausea and vomiting. It is rated *probably effective* for use in other types of agitation and tension (e.g., alcohol withdrawal) and hyperactivity and aggressiveness in disturbed children. It is rated as *ineffective* in treatment of severe personality disorders or of somatic conditions associated with emotional stress, such as neurodermatitis, arthritis, severe asthma, and degenerative states.

Triflupromazine hydrochloride, N.F. (Vesprin)

Action and uses. This compound is at least twice as active as chlorpromazine but otherwise is similar to chlorpromazine in its spectrum. It has been found to be useful in the management of pernicious vomiting of pregnancy, postoperative emesis, and the nausea and vomiting following encephalograms or ventriculograms.

Triflupromazine has a D.E.S.I. rating of *effective* for control of serious agitation and of severe nausea and vomiting. It is rated as *probably effective* as a preoperative medication and as an adjunct for withdrawal from habitual use of alcohol or barbiturates. It is rated *ineffective* in the treatment of mental disorders characterized by delirium.

Preparation, dosage, and administration. Triflupromazine hydrochloride can be administered orally in tablets of 10, 25, and 50 mg., in a suspension of 50 mg. per 5 ml., and intramuscularly in solutions of 10 and 20 mg. per milliliter. Oral therapy should be substituted for parenteral administration as soon as possible. The usual dose for hospitalized psychotic adults is 100 to 150 mg. daily. Dosage for children is 30 to 150 mg. daily in divided doses. The initial daily dosage for elderly patients with psychoses is 10 mg. three times a day. For prevention and treatment of nausea and vomiting in adults, the oral dose is 20 to 30 mg. daily.

PIPERIDYL SUBGROUP
Mepazine hydrochloride and mepazine acetate (Pacatal)

Mepazine base

Action and uses. Mepazine is a phenothiazine compound that has not appeared to be too effective in treating psychotic disorders. It has been noted to have a slight euphorigenic effect. Its administration is associated with rather severe atropine-like effects, and bladder dysfunction commonly occurs. Because of these side effects

and its apparent inability to control psychotic symptoms, its use has been limited.

Preparation, dosage, and administration. Mepazine hydrochloride is administered orally. The initial dose for psychiatric patients varies from 25 to 100 mg. per day, depending upon the nature and severity of the symptoms. Antiemetic doses range from 50 to 100 mg. daily. The drug is marketed in 25-, 50-, and 100-mg. tablets.

Mepazine acetate is like mepazine hydrochloride except that it is suited for parenteral administration (intramuscular or intravenous). Dosage varies from 50 to 200 mg.

Thioridazine hydrochloride, U.S.P., B.P. (Mellaril)

This phenothiazine derivative is chemically similar to mepazine. It is not a highly potent tranquilizer. It does not exert an antiemetic effect, and it seems to have no effect on temperature regulation. It has a broad spectrum of useful antipsychotic activity and is considered by many to be a good all-round tranquilizer. It is believed to have the advantage of producing minimal extrapyramidal effects. However, patients taking large doses have been known to develop pigmentary retinopathy. Sudden death has been reported in some patients after prolonged usage of this drug.

Preparation, dosage, and administration. Thioridazine hydrochloride is available in 10-, 25-, 50-, 100-, 150-, and 200-mg. tablets and as a concentrate (30 mg. per milliliter) for oral administration. Adult dosage varies from 20 to 800 mg. daily. Dosage for children 2 years of age or over is 1 mg. per kilogram of body weight in three or four divided doses. Dosage for this preparation as well as for other tranquilizers is adjusted to meet the needs of the individual.

Side effects and toxic effects. Drowsiness is a frequent side effect, especially after large doses. Many other side effects associated with therapy with the phenothiazine compounds have been seen after the administration of this drug, but on the whole, toxic effects are said to occur less often than after the administration of chlorpromazine. Visual impairment and blindness have occurred. Therefore, patients should be closely observed for signs of diminished visual acuity, impaired night vision, and brown discoloration of objects. (For other side effects see discussion of phenothiazine derivatives, p. 283.)

Mesoridazine besylate, N.F. (Serentil)

Mesoridazine is a metabolite of thioridazine. It was introduced in 1970 and is used for treating acute and chronic schizophrenia, the manic phase of manic-depressive psychosis, and involutional, senile, organic, or toxic psychosis with the exception of delirium tremens. Its actions, side effects, precautions, and drug interactions are the same as for thioridazine and the antipsychotic phenothiazines (see chlorpromazine).

Preparation and dosage. It is available in oral tablets of 10, 25, 50, and 100 mg., and as a solution for injection containing 25 mg. per milliliter. Oral dosage for adults and for children over 12 years is 100 to 400 mg. daily in divided doses. For elderly patients dosage is one fourth to one half the usual dose. Intramuscular dosage is 25 to 200 mg. daily in divided doses.

Piperacetazine, N.F. (Quide)

Piperacetazine is an antipsychotic drug of the piperidyl group of the phenothiazines. It is closely related to acetophenazine. It is used for the control of hyperactivity, agitation, and anxiety states associated with acute and chronic schizophrenic reactions in adult patients under adequate medical supervision. It is more effective in acute than chronic schizophrenia. Piperacetazine causes a higher incidence of extrapyramidal effects than other piperidine compounds and resembles the piperazine drugs in this respect. Side effects and precautions are the same as for the phenothiazines and chlorpromazine.

Contraindications. Piperacetazine is contraindicated for pregnant women or those who may become pregnant, for patients who are comatose or markedly depressed, and for patients with blood dyscrasias or liver disease.

Preparation and dosage. Piperacetazine is available in 10- and 25-mg. tablets. Dosage for adults and children over 12 years of age is 20 to 40 mg. daily in divided doses initially. Maintenance dose is up to 160 mg. daily in divided doses. Elderly patients should receive one fourth to one half the usual dose.

PIPERAZINE SUBGROUP
Acetophenazine maleate, N.F. (Tindal)

Action and uses. Acetophenazine maleate is a member of the piperazine group of phenothiazine derivatives and may be effective in the management of patients with chronic brain syndrome. Large doses have been effective in the treatment of psychotic patients. It has limited usefulness in the treatment of patients whose anxiety is associated with psychosomatic conditions (peptic ulcer, hypertension). It is much less potent than other derivatives. It is more sedative and produces fewer extrapyramidal phenomena. It is rated (D.E.S.I.) *effective* for control of agitation and anxiety of schizophrenia; and *ineffective* for treatment of insomnia, anorexia, and hypertension.

Preparation, dosage, and administration. Acetophenazine maleate is available for administration in tablets of 20 mg. only. It is not available for parenteral administration. The usual oral dosage is 40 to 80 mg. a day. In patients who have insomnia, the last tablet should be taken 1 hour before retiring. Dosage for children is 0.8 to 1.6 mg. per kilogram of body weight divided into three doses.

Fluphenazine hydrochloride, U.S.P., B.P. (Permitil, Prolixin)

In terms of potency fluphenazine hydrochloride is one of the most active compounds and is considered more than twenty times as potent as chlorpromazine. It offers the advantage of sustained and prolonged action as an antipsychotic agent. D.E.S.I. rating is the same as for acetophenazine. It is the prototype of the piperazine compounds.

Preparation, dosage, and administration. Fluphenazine hydrochloride can be administered either orally or intramuscularly. An initial daily dose of 2.5 to 10 mg. is suggested for adults with psychotic conditions. The dosage may be gradually increased to 20 mg. a day; however, the usual maintenance dose is 1.5 to 5 mg. Elderly patients may require much less than the average amounts. Children should rarely receive more than 2 mg. per day. Oral preparations include a concentrate of 5 mg. per milliliter (Permitil); an elixir of 2.5 mg. per 5 ml. (Prolixin); 0.25-, 1-, 2.5-, 5-, and 10-mg. tablets (Permitil or Prolixin); and repeat-action tablets of 1 mg. (Permitil Chronotab). The intramuscular preparation is in a solution of 2.5 mg. per milliliter in 10-ml. containers. Parenteral injection has an average duration of action of 2 weeks.

Fluphenazine enanthate, U.S.P. (Prolixin Enanthate)

Fluphenazine enanthate is an esterified derivative of fluphenazine hydrochloride. It maintains all the properties and actions of the pheno-

thiazines; however, it has gained increasing popularity because of its prolonged action. One injection of 25 mg. per milliliter solution maintains its action and effects for 1 to 3 weeks. This effect seems to facilitate its use with outpatients or individuals who might not otherwise be disposed to taking medication on a daily basis. Because of its potency and the high incidence of extrapyramidal symptoms, some physicians feel concomitant treatment with antiparkinsonian agents is necessary. The risk of irreversible extrapyramidal symptoms seems to be the greatest in elderly female patients with organic brain disease or damage who have received fairly high dosages of phenothiazines for prolonged periods.

Oral and parenteral dosage for adults is 2.5 to 10 mg. daily in divided doses at 6 to 8 hour intervals. In hospitalized patients 20 mg. may be given. Dose for children is 0.25 to 3.0 mg. in divided doses.

Perphenazine, N.F., B.P. (Trilafon)

Perphenazine is similar to chlorpromazine in action and clinical uses. Milligram for milligram it is said to be six times more potent than chlorpromazine. It has an antiemetic effect. D.E.S.I. rating is *effective* for antipsychotic and antiemetic use; *ineffective* for treating behavioral disorders in children or for treating chronic alcoholism.

Preparation, dosage, and administration. Administration of perphenazine may be oral, rectal, intramuscular, and, occasionally, intravenous. The oral dosage for psychotic adults varies from 16 to 64 mg. daily given in two to four divided doses. It is marketed in solution for injection, 5 mg. per milliliter in 1- and 10-ml. containers; as a syrup of 2 mg. per 5 ml.; as a liquid concentrate, 16 mg. per 5 ml.; and in tablets of 2, 4, 8, and 16 mg. Rectal suppositories are available in 2, 4, and 8 mg. Perphenazine should not be administered intravenously except during surgery to counteract retching, hiccoughs, and vomiting; this route is not recommended for psychiatric conditions.

Prochlorperazine, U.S.P., B.P. (Compazine)

Prochlorperazine is approximately four times as potent as chlorpromazine. It has a rapid and stimulating effect, which makes it useful in the treatment of psychomotor retardation, apathy, and withdrawal. It shares all the additional effects of the phenothiazines in antipsychotic activity. In small doses it has been effective in controlling nausea and vomiting associated with some somatic conditions. D.E.S.I. rating is the same as for perphenazine.

Preparation, dosage, and administration

Prochlorperazine suppositories, U.S.P. (Compazine). Prochlorperazine is administered rectally. The suggested dose for adults is one 25-mg. suppository twice daily. Suppositories are available in 2.5, 5, and 25 mg.

Prochlorperazine edisylate, U.S.P. (Compazine Edisylate). Administration may be oral in doses similar to those given for the maleate salt. Intramuscular injection is given of 10 to 20 mg., repeated at intervals of 1 to 6 hours, for control of psychotic symptoms. Intramuscular dose for adults with nonpsychiatric conditions is 5 to 10 mg., repeated once if necessary. It is available in solution for injection, 5 mg. per milliliter in 2- and 10-ml. containers; the solution concentrate contains 10 mg. per milliliter and the syrup contains 5 mg. per 5 ml.

Prochlorperazine maleate, U.S.P., B.P. (Compazine Maleate). This preparation is administered orally to psychotic adults. It is given initially in divided doses that range from 30 to 40 mg. daily. Dosage is gradually increased to 75 to 150 mg. a day. Tablets come in 5-, 10-, and 25-mg. strengths and sustained-release capsules of 10, 15, 30, and 75 mg.

Thiopropazate hydrochloride (Dartal)

Thiopropazate hydrochloride shares its therapeutic effectiveness with prochlorperazine. It is useful in the management of psychotic symptoms marked by agitation and aggression.

Preparation, dosage, and administration. Thiopropazate hydrochloride is administered only through the oral route. The usual dose for adults with psychotic conditions is 10 mg. three times a day. The dosage may be increased to 100 mg. as a maximal dose to produce the desired effects. Increments or decreases in dosage are recommended at 3- or 4-day intervals at 10 mg. per day. Tablets of 5- and 10-mg. strengths are available.

Trifluoperazine hydrochloride, N.F., B.P. (Stelazine)

Trifluoperazine is fast acting and approximately ten times as active as chlorpromazine. It has been successful in stimulating patients with symptoms of psychomotor retardation, apathy, and withdrawal. Its use in psychoneurotic and psychosomatic conditions has not been established. It has been proved to be an effective antipsychotic agent. D.E.S.I. rating is: *effective for psychotic conditions*; *probably effective* for involutional melancholia; *ineffective* for chronic brain syndrome or mental deficiency.

Preparation, dosage, and administration. Trifluoperazine hydrochloride is available in concentrate solution of 10 mg. per milliliter and in 1-, 2-, 5-, and 10-mg. tablets for oral administration. A solution is also available for intramuscular injection, 2 mg. per milliliter in 10-ml. containers.

Dosage varies considerably, depending upon the severity of symptoms to be controlled. For mild anxiety reactions, oral dosage may range from 1 to 4 mg. daily. The dosage for patients with major psychosis may start at 2 to 5 mg. daily, but the optimum dosage may become 15 to 20 mg. daily. Some patients require as much as 40 mg. daily. For children 6 to 12 years of age the dosage is 1 mg. once or twice daily, which may be increased up to 15 mg. daily.

Carphenazine maleate, N.F. (Proketazine)

Carphenazine has a spectrum of activity similar to that of other piperazine phenothiazines. Uses, side effects, precautions, and drug interactions are like those of other phenothiazines. It is available in 12.5-, 25-, and 50-mg. tablets and as an oral liquid concentrate containing 50 mg. per milliliter. Initial oral dose for adults is 75 to 50 mg. daily in divided doses. Dosage may be increased by 25 to 50 mg. daily every 7 to 14 days. Maximal dosage is 400 mg. daily. For elderly patients dose is one fourth to one half the usual dose.

Butaperazine maleate (Repoise)

Butaperazine is an antipsychotic drug of the piperazine subgroup useful for treatment of acute and chronic schizophrenia. Clinical evidence that it is more effective than chlorpromazine for chronic schizophrenia is inconclusive. It has antiemetic, spasmolytic, antihistaminic, and weak hypotensive activity. Side effects, precautions, and contraindications are the same as for phenothiazines and chlorpromazine.

Preparation and dosage. Butaperazine is available in 5-, 10-, and 25-mg. tablets. Initial dose for adults and for children over 12 years of age is 15 to 30 mg. daily in three divided doses; this may be increased gradually to 100 mg. daily. Reduced dosage is advised for elderly and debilitated patients.

THIOXANTHENE DERIVATIVES
Thiothixene, N.F. (Navane)

Thiothixene, a thioxanthene derivative, resembles the piperazine phenothiazines in its tranquilizing and antiemetic actions and to a lesser degree the spasmolytic and hypotensive effects. Its indications for use, side effects, precautions, and drug interactions are the same as those for the phenothiazines. Extrapyramidal symptoms and insomnia occur frequently with this drug. It is available in 1-, 2-, 5-, and 10-mg. capsules; as a liquid concentrate, 5 mg. per milliliter, and as a solution for injection containing 2 mg. per milliliter in 2-ml. ampules.

Oral dosage for adults and for children over 12 years of age is 6 to 15 mg. daily in divided doses initially, which may be gradually increased to a maximum dosage of 60 mg. daily. Intramuscular dosage is 8 to 16 mg. daily in divided doses, which may be increased to a maximum dosage of 30 mg. daily.

Chlorprothixene, N.F. (Taractan)

Action and uses. Although chlorprothixene is not a phenothiazine, its action and effects are very similar to the phenothiazine compounds. It is used in similar conditions, and adverse reactions associated with phenothiazine therapy should be borne in mind when this agent is used. This compound is thought to be less likely to produce troublesome side effects such as extrapyramidal symptoms, agranulocytosis, and cholestatic hepatitis. However, a few incidences of these effects have been reported. This agent has also been reported to be useful as an antiemetic.

Preparation, dosage, and administration. Chlorprothixene is administered orally and intramuscularly. Oral dosages range from 30 to 600 mg. per day. The drug is administered orally in tablets of 10, 25, 50, and 100 mg. Dosage for children over 6 years of age is 30 to 100 mg.

daily in divided doses. Intramuscular dosage for the acutely agitated patient with a psychotic condition is 75 to 200 mg. per day; for treatment of nausea and vomiting 12.5 to 25 mg. seems to be adequate. Preparations for injection come in a solution of 12.5 mg. per milliliter in 2-ml. containers.

BUTYROPHENONE DERIVATIVE
Haloperidol, U.S.P., B.P. (Haldol)

$$Cl-\langle\bigcirc\rangle-\underset{\underset{OH}{|}}{C}\langle\bigcirc\rangle N-CH_2-CH_2-CH_2-CO-\langle\bigcirc\rangle-F$$

Action and uses. Haloperidol was introduced in the United States as an antipsychotic agent in 1967. Research conducted in Europe in the area of anesthesia brought this compound into view as a possible antipsychotic agent. Subsequent use indicated its effectiveness in the control of hyperactivity associated with the manic phase. Extrapyramidal symptoms occur frequently and, as the manic phase becomes controlled, severe depressive elements may be seen in some patients, precipitating a suicide risk. Adverse reactions discussed earlier in regard to the phenothiazines also apply to this compound.

Preparation, dosage, and administration. Haloperidol is administered orally in tablets of 0.5, 1, and 2 mg. and as haloperidol concentrate of 2 mg. per milliliter. A solution for injection contains 5 mg. per milliliter in 1-ml. ampules. Initial dosages should be gradually increased in increments of 0.5 to 1 mg. every 3 days until the desired effects are attained. Daily doses greater than 15 mg. are not recommended. Maintenance dose is usually 2 to 8 mg. daily. Dosage is the same for adults and children over 12 years of age.

PSYCHOTHERAPEUTIC DRUG FOR MANIC PSYCHOSIS
Lithium carbonate, B.P. (Lithane, Eskalith, Lithonate)

Lithium was introduced in 1970 to terminate manic and hypomanic episodes in patients with manic-depressive psychosis, evidenced by motor hyperactivity, reduced need for sleep, flight of ideas, grandiosity, elation, poor judgment, ag-

gressiveness, and hostility. Difference of opinion exists concerning lithium as a drug of choice for treating the mania of manic-depressive illness. Some clinicians consider phenothiazines (e.g., chlorpromazine) to be superior to lithium, particularly for highly active patients. Some prefer to initiate therapy with the phenothiazines for their more rapid action and then use lithium alone or with a phenothiazine. Others prefer treatment solely with lithium. More controlled studies are needed to determine the merits of single-drug treatment, sequential therapy, and combination therapy.

Lithium has been found to calm the patient and control acute symptoms. Seven to 10 days are required for the drug to take effect after initiation of therapy. Results are inconclusive concerning the ability of lithium to prevent or decrease the frequency of manic episodes.

Since a small range exists between therapeutic and toxic doses, lithium serum levels should be monitored weekly or twice weekly initially and monthly during maintenance therapy. Blood samples should be drawn 8 to 12 hours after the last dose. Serum lithium levels should be maintained at 1 to 1.5 mEq. per liter for acute symptoms and 0.6 to 1.2 mEq. per liter after the acute attack subsides. If serum levels of lithium exceed 1.5 mEq. per liter, the drug should be discontinued for 24 hours and then resumed at a lower dosage.

Preparation, dosage, and administration. Lithium is available in 300-mg. capsules and tablets. Dose is individualized according to serum levels and clinical response. If satisfactory effects are not obtained in 14 days, the drug should be discontinued. Recommended dosage is 600 mg. three times a day for acute episodes and 300 mg. three times a day for maintenance therapy. However, larger or smaller doses may be required.

Side effects. Severity of side effects parallels the rise in lithium serum levels. During initial phase of treatment fine hand tremor, polyuria, and mild thirst may occur and persist during therapy. Nausea and general discomfort may also occur.

Early signs of lithium intoxication include diarrhea, vomiting, drowsiness, muscle weakness, and ataxia. As toxicity increases blurred vision, slurred speech, tinnitus, nystagmus, weight loss, muscle hyperirritability, abdominal pain, and dizziness may occur.

With moderate to severe toxicity the following effects occur in addition to those previously listed: hyperactive reflexes, choreoathetoid movements, hyperextension of limbs, grunts, gasps, epileptiform convulsions, toxic psychosis, syncope, EEG changes, circulatory failure, stupor, and coma. Many other adverse effects may also occur. No specific antidote for lithium poisoning is known.

Precautions. The patient and members of his family should be warned to discontinue therapy if signs of toxicity occur and to notify the physician immediately.

Since lithium may impair mental and physical ability, the patient should be cautioned about driving a car or operating hazardous equipment. Because toxicity of lithium is increased when sodium intake is restricted, the patient should maintain a normal diet and normal salt and water intake. If excessive diarrhea, vomiting, or sweating occurs, lithium should be discontinued and supplemental salt and fluid administered.

Thyroid involvement has been reported, and patients who develop a diffuse nontoxic goiter may need to be treated with small doses of thyroid. Use of lithium is not recommended for pregnant women since the fetus may be affected; two women on lithium delivered infants with congenital malformations. Its use for children under 12 years is not recommended because of inadequate experience with the drug in that age group.

Contraindications. Lithium is contraindicated in patients with cardiovascular or renal disease, in those with brain damage, and in pregnancy.

Drug interactions. Diuretics should not be used with lithium since the fluid and sodium loss potentiates the effects of lithium.

MINOR TRANQUILIZERS— ANTIANXIETY AGENTS

Minor tranquilizers, also known as antianxiety drugs, have been recommended for the treatment of symptoms associated with psychoneurotic and psychosomatic conditions. The advantage of their use in these conditions is their effect in allaying moderate anxiety states and the muscle tension associated with psychomotor agitation. Psychoneurotic conditions with severe disabling symptoms are treated more effectively with the stronger phenothiazine derivatives. In milder forms of psychoneuroses, the minor tranquilizers act as a valuable adjunct to psychotherapy by diminishing anxiety and tension associated with the treatment process. The antianxiety agents are not recommended for the long-term treatment of psychotic conditions; however, large doses have been effective in controlling the psychomotor hyperexcitability of acute psychotic episodes. Chlordiazepoxide has been especially effective in treating hyperactive alcoholic patients with withdrawal reactions or delirium tremens. Most of the compounds in this group can be given alone or in conjunction with antispasmodics, analgesics, vasodilators, adrenal corticosteroids, and estrogens. They have been effective in relieving the symptoms of certain gastrointestinal, musculoskeletal, and cardiovascular disorders as well as menopausal discomforts. They differ in their sedative effects from barbiturates in that they do not produce a significant loss of mental acuity.

Chemical structure, site, and mechanism of action. The antianxiety agents share similar central depressant action, but their secondary central and peripheral effects vary. Chemically they can be divided according to the following subgroups: (1) diphenylmethanes, (2) benzodiazepines, and (3) propanedol. One action of these drugs that accounts for their antianxiety response is their depressive effect on the polysynaptic reflexes of the spinal cord. This effect suggests that their main mode of action is that of reducing skeletal muscle tension, which indirectly reduces the number of afferent proprioceptive impulses aggravating existing anxiety.

These drugs are thought to exert very little effect, if any, on the neocortex and neurotransmitter centers. However, their antianxiety action seems to parallel their depressant action on the limbic structures (septum, amygdala, and hippocampus). Since it has been postulated that the

Table 12-3 Comparison of effect of major and minor tranquilizers

Major tranquilizers	Minor tranquilizers
Antipsychotic effect	Antianxiety effect
Depress activity of lower brain centers (e.g., vomiting center); antiemetic effect	Do not depress lower brain centers; significant antiemetic effect
Extrapyramidal effects (e.g., tremors and spasticity)	No extrapyramidal effects; tend to produce general muscular relaxation
Autonomic effects	No autonomic effects
Monophasic effect	Biphasic effect: small doses tend to produce a euphoric state; large doses tend to produce a sedative effect
Low abuse potential	High abuse potential
No tolerance	Tolerance may develop
No withdrawal syndrome	Withdrawal symptoms can occur
Suppress active avoidance behavior but not escape response	Suppress both avoidance behavior and escape response
No anticonvulsive activity	Anticonvulsive activity
No reduction of conflict	Reduction of conflict
Depress general motor activity	Little effect on motor activity

Table 12-4 Minor tranquilizers (antianxiety agents)

Generic name	Trade name	Side effects*	Average daily dosage range (mg.)
Diphenylmethane group			
Hydroxyzine hydrochloride	Atarax	2-5, 8, 13, 14, 17, 18	50 to 400
Hydroxyzine pamoate	Vistaril	2-5, 8, 13, 14, 17, 18	50 to 400
Benactyzine	Suavitil	1-7, 8, 16, 22, 26, 27	3 to 10
Benzodiazepine group			
Chlordiazepoxide	Librium, Libritabs	1-3, 6, 7, 9-11, 14, 16, 20, 22, 23, 25	15 to 300
Diazepam	Valium	1-3, 5, 7, 9-11, 16, 23, 27	4 to 10
Oxazepam	Serax	2, 3, 8-10, 16, 21	30 to 200
Clorazepate	Tranxene	1-7, 16, 21-23	7.5 to 60
Propanediol group			
Meprobamate	Equanil, Miltown	1-4, 7, 8, 10, 11, 13, 15, 16, 18, 19, 22-24	200 to 1200

Key to table
1. Anxiety or agitation
2. Sedation and sleep
3. Ataxia
4. Dry mouth
5. Blurred vision
6. Constipation
7. Dermatitis
8. Hypotension
9. Blood dyscrasias
10. Jaundice
11. Convulsive seizures
12. Hypothermia
13. Antiemetic
14. Increased appetite
15. Edema
16. Nausea and/or vomiting
17. Bradycardia
18. Increased gastric motility or diarrhea
19. Activation of peptic ulcer
20. Decreased libido
21. Depressive symptoms
22. Mental confusion
23. Dependence
24. Hyperthermia
25. Menstrual irregularities
26. Mydriasis
27. Hallucinations

*Side effects here are not intended to be a complete account of possible adverse reactions.

amygdala and the hippocampus influence behavior, the action of these drugs may inhibit their stimulation and thus inhibit the subsequent behavioral responses that they regulate. A similar reduction of sensitivity brought about by their depressant effect reduces reactions to stressful influences and stimuli. They have the ability to produce mild sedation without adversely affecting the level of consciousness or the quality of psychomotor performance.

Side effects and precautions. The minor tranquilizers are relatively safe when used in small dosages. They have fewer disabling side effects than the phenothiazine derivatives; however, numerous reports of untoward effects have appeared. Drowsiness, ataxia, dizziness, and headache occur occasionally after initial doses. Patients should be cautioned against driving an automobile, operating dangerous machinery, or performing tasks that require absolute precision, motor coordination, and mental alertness. Drowsiness, ataxia, and confusion are more commonly seen in the elderly. These reactions can be avoided by gradually increasing the dosage until the desired effects are produced. Some patients have been known to exhibit mild forms of inappropriate behavior that were not related to their current condition after initial doses. Other signs of drug hypersensitivity have been noted such as rash, fever, chills, nausea, vomiting, and dry mouth. Blood dyscrasias and jaundice have been reported occasionally. Some of these drugs are habit-forming, and withdrawal of the drug may cause mild to severe withdrawal reactions including delirium and convulsions. Caution should be taken to avoid dependence on these drugs. Physicians should maintain close supervision of individuals who are taking these drugs for prolonged periods, especially individuals who have a history of alcoholism, drug addiction, or severe dependency problems. Overdosage with massive amounts of these drugs produces coma, shock, and death. Patients with a history of blood dyscrasias, impaired renal function, hepatic disease, or allergies should be evaluated carefully before the administration of these drugs is initiated, even though there have been relatively few reports of adverse effects in these conditions. Use of any drug in pregnancy or lactation requires that the potential benefit of the drug be weighed against its possible hazards to mother and child.

Phenothiazine compounds and antidepressant drugs that potentiate the action of other drugs should not be used concomitantly with the antianxiety agents.

Paradoxic reactions of rage, excitement, stimulation, hostility, confusion, and depersonalization have occurred when these agents have been administered to severely disturbed or psychotic patients.

DIPHENYLMETHANES
Hydroxyzine hydrochloride, N.F. (Atarax); hydroxyzine pamoate, N.F. (Vistaril)

Hydroxyzine is an antianxiety agent that also has antiemetic and antihistaminic actions. It has been useful in the management of acute and chronic urticaria and other manifestations of allergic dermatoses. It has also been used to treat the nausea and vomiting associated with pregnancy and motion sickness. It produces sedation preoperatively and postoperatively; however, it usually potentiates the action of opiates and barbiturates used during these periods, which necessitates reduction of their dosage. Incidence of side effects is low; any drowsiness that develops tends to be transient and does not induce sleep unless large doses are given.

Preparation, dosage, and administration. Both drugs may be administered orally, intravenously, and intramuscularly. The usual dosage for adults is 25 to 100 mg. given three or four times daily. Parenteral administration should be reserved for emergency situations only and oral dosages should be substituted as soon as possible. Dosage for sedation of children is 1 mg. per kilogram of body weight.

Hydroxyzine hydrochloride comes in 10-, 25-, 50-, and 100-mg. tablets and in syrup, 10 mg. per 5 ml. It is also prepared in solution for injection, 25 and 50 mg. per milliliter.

Hydroxyzine pamoate is available in capsules

of 25, 50, and 100 mg.; as a suspension of 25 mg. per 5 ml.; and in solutions for injection of 25 and 50 mg. per milliliter.

Benactyzine hydrochloride (Suavitil)

Benactyzine hydrochloride has been used in the treatment of mild psychoneurotic conditions. This drug has no apparent sedative or hypnotic action and tends to cause blocking of thought processes (apathy, indifference, and retarded mental activity). These actions differentiate it from other antianxiety agents.

Action and uses. This agent is an autonomic suppressant and is capable of blocking certain conditioned reflexes. Its use in the treatment of psychoneurotic conditions has not been widely accepted. Some patients experience a sense of unreality and an inability to concentrate, while others who manifest a frankly hostile attitude have been known to deteriorate considerably after the administration of this drug.

Precautions. This drug is contraindicated before electroshock therapy and in patients with glaucoma or benign prostatic hypertrophy.

Preparation, dosage, and administration. The oral route is used in the administration of this drug. Tablets of 1 mg. are available. The suggested initial dose is 1 mg. given three times daily for 2 or 3 days, with a gradual increment to 3 mg. three times a day until the desired effect is attained. Dosages over 10 mg. per day are undesirable. Therapeutic response may be delayed for several weeks.

BENZODIAZEPINES

Benzodiazepines are among the most widely used drugs in clinical medicine. More than 77 million prescriptions for these antianxiety drugs were filled in the United States in 1972; two-thirds of these prescriptions were for diazepam. A drug surveillance program in Boston in 1973 revealed that in two teaching hospitals 30% of all medical inpatients were given diazepam and 32% received flurazepam. The popularity of these drugs probably results from the fact that their antianxiety effects occur at nontoxic doses. Drowsiness and undesirable central nervous system depression occur less frequently with benzodiazepine agents than with comparable doses of meprobamate or barbiturates.

Effects. The site of antianxiety activity appears to be the limbic system. Electrical discharges and transmission in the limbic system are inhibited by low doses of benzodiazepines that do not depress the rest of the brain. Benzodiazepines have a disinhibiting effect; major tranquilizers do not produce disinhibition at any dosage level. Benzodiazepines can precipitate hostility, rage, and physical violence. This paradoxical reaction may represent a disinhibition or release of "anxiety bound" hostility.

Other effects of benzodiazepines include the following.

Muscle relaxation. The exact mechanism for this is unknown. The benzodiazepines probably have more than one site of muscle relaxant activity.

Anticonvulsant effect. Benzodiazepines prevent or arrest generalized seizure activity caused by electric shock, systemic administration of analeptics, or local anesthetics. How the action occurs has not been established.

Circulation and respiration. Benzodiazepines even in large doses produce only minor circulatory and respiratory depression. Rapid intravenous injection of diazepam can cause transient bradycardia, hypotension, and apnea. Recent studies indicate that diazepam can dilate coronary blood vessels and enhance coronary blood flow. This is a local rather than central effect and has been reported only after diazepam was injected intravenously. Oral doses of benzodiazepines provide symptomatic relief for some patients with angina pectoris, but it is believed that this results from their central antianxiety effects rather than from a direct influence on coronary blood flow.

Clinical uses. Chlordiazepoxide and diazepam are long-acting compounds with pharmacologically active metabolites. More than two daily doses are seldom necessary. Clorazepate's metabolite, nordiazepam, also has a long duration of action. Many patients need only a single dose at bedtime for promotion of sleep at night and reduced anxiety during the day. If necessary, a second smaller dose can be added during the day. This schedule is particularly useful for patients with sleep disturbances associated with anxiety.

Nurses need to know that even with single daily doses, the drugs or their metabolites can accumulate in the body after several days of therapy; therapeutic effects may not appear for 5 to 10 days after initiation of therapy, and clinical effects may persist for several days after termination of therapy. Oxazepam is more rapidly converted to inactive metabolites and therefore is short acting and nonaccumulating. Most patients need three or four daily doses of oxazepam.

Antianxiety drugs are most effective during short-term use, such as for periodic anxiety, but are ineffective or unnecessary when given continuously for months.

Emotional disorders. Benzodiazepines are used for patients with neurotic anxiety. They are also beneficial for patients with neurotic or reactive depression. They are not of value for treatment of schizophrenia; they have no specific effect in disordered thought of psychotic patients, and some schizophrenics appear to deteriorate from chronic treatment with chlordiazepoxide or diazepam.

Neuromuscular disease. Benzodiazepines produce partial relief of spasticity in patients with cerebral palsy, multiple sclerosis, parkinsonism, amyotrophic lateral sclerosis, cerebrovascular accident, or traumatic spinal cord lesions. Effective muscle relaxant doses are relatively high for these conditions, and many patients experience drowsiness or sedation.

Diazepam is used extensively for acute, reversible musculoskeletal disorders, such as back strain and "slipped disc." It does not supplant the need for analgesics, local heat, and rest, but it is superior to other muscle relaxant drugs such as methocarbamol and carisoprodol. It has also been used in treatment of tetanus.

Seizures. When intractable, repetitive seizures occur (status epilepticus) intravenous diazepam appears to be the drug of choice. It is effective for grand mal, petit mal, psychomotor, and myoclonic seizures. Oral diazepam is of no value in the treatment of grand mal epilepsy. Clonazepam is being tested for its usefulness in preventing petit mal seizures.

Alcohol withdrawal. Chlordiazepoxide is very popular for treatment of the alcohol withdrawal syndrome. Benzodiazepines do not share potential hazards of the phenothiazines to produce seizures and hypotension or of the barbiturates to cause respiratory depression; nor do they have the noxious odor and serious injection site complications associated with paraldehyde. Benzodiazepines are not effective in preventing chronic alcoholics from returning to alcoholism.

Sleep disorders. Benzodiazepines seem to interfere less with rapid eye movement (REM), or dreaming, sleep than barbiturates and certain other hypnotics. REM rebound does not occur when the benzodiazepines are discontinued. Addiction to benzodiazepines is rare, and the danger of serious poisoning after intentional overdosage is minimal.

Benzodiazepines inhibit slow-wave, or deep, sleep and are being tested for their effectiveness to control somnambulism (sleep-walking), enuresis, and night terrors which occur during slow-wave sleep.

Flurazepam (Dalmane) is a benzodiazepine marketed specifically for use as a hypnotic.

Cardioversion. Diazepam can be given intravenously for cardioversion. If countershock is performed within 5 minutes of the injection, patients are in a state of light sleep and will not remember the shock. Adverse cardiovascular and respiratory effects are less frequent with diazepam than with thiopental or methohexital. However, full recovery is delayed because of diazepam's long duration of action.

Labor and delivery. Diazepam and chlordiazepoxide given parenterally are suitable adjuncts to local and systemic analgesics used during labor and delivery. They enhance analgesia, reduce opiate requirements, enhance amnesia, and with adequate precautions have no serious adverse effects on the infant. However, diazepam readily crosses the placenta and reaches higher concentrations in fetal circulation that in maternal blood. High doses of diazepam may produce lethargy, hypothermia, and respiratory depression in the newborn.

Preoperative medication. Benzodiazepines can be effectively used as preoperative sedatives. The drugs are more effective after intramuscular injection than after oral administration. They are less toxic than the opiates.

Induction. Diazepam is commonly used as an induction agent just before administration of general anesthesia. It produces more amnesia and has fewer adverse effects than the barbiturates. However, recovery from general anesthesia is more delayed with diazepam than with barbiturates.

Adverse effects. Like all drugs, the benzodiazepines are not without their adverse effects and hazards.

Neurologic. The central nervous system depressant effects include fatigue, drowsiness, somnolence, muscle weakness, nystagmus, ataxia, and dysarthria. The effects are dose dependent and subside when dosage is decreased or discontinued. These effects are more likely to occur in elderly patients and less likely to occur in heavy cigarette smokers. Impairment of motor and cognitive performance may also occur. Patients should be cautioned about automobile driving and working with hazardous equipment.

Psychiatric. Benzodiazepines can cause sleep disturbances and nightmares. There are two reports in the literature of self-destructive ideation leading to successful suicide by patients on diazepam therapy.

Benzodiazepines may produce paradoxical excitement, hostility, rage, and violent, destructive behavior. The frequency of these reactions is not established.

Injection site complications. Intravenous injection of diazepam causes local pain and irritation in many patients, which may lead to phlebitis. Intramuscular administration of diazepam is also painful.

Abuse, dependence, and overdosage. Any drug can be abused and this is true for the benzodiazepines. Physiologic and psychologic dependence may occur if large doses are taken over a long period of time. Their abuse and dependence potentials are less than those of other sedatives such as the barbiturates. Serious effects from overdosage or fatal poisoning are rare.

Other effects. It has not been substantiated whether the benzodiazepines are toxic to the liver, cause hematologic toxicity, or are teratogenic.

These drugs do not alter microsomal enzyme function and can be given without danger of interaction with oral anticoagulants and other drugs metabolized by liver microsomal enzymes.

Chlordiazepoxide hydrochloride, N.F., B.P. (Librium, Libritabs)

Action and uses. The actions and uses are similar to all antianxiety agents. Chlordiazepoxide has been effective in controlling the acute withdrawal symptoms of chronic alcoholic conditions (delirium tremens and agitation). However, since alcoholics in general are addiction-prone, caution should be exerted in its use for these patients over prolonged periods. It is known to have a muscle relaxant effect and has been beneficial in treating musculoskeletal conditions in which anxiety and tension intensify the symptoms. Its direct action in these instances is unknown and may well be the result of its sedative effect. It has found a wide range of uses as an antianxiety agent in nonpsychiatric settings, mainly for the control of mild to moderate anxiety associated with psychosomatic conditions. This drug should be limited to small dosages in elderly patients.

Chlordiazepoxide is slightly more effective than meprobamate, but in comparison to diazepam it is less potent as an antianxiety agent, has less anticonvulsant action, and produces less drowsiness.

Preparation, dosage, and administration. This drug can be administered orally, intramuscularly, or intravenously. It is prepared as capsules and tablets of 5, 10, and 25 mg.; and as a powder for injection of 100 mg. per ampule. The average daily dosage should not exceed 300 mg. The usual daily adult dosage for relief of mild to moderate anxiety is 15 to 40 mg. and 10 to 20 mg. for elderly or debilitated patients. For children over 6 years of age, dosage is 0.5 mg. per kilogram of body weight daily in divided doses. It is well absorbed after oral administration, and peak blood concentration is reached in about 4 hours. Absorption by the intramuscular route is slow and erratic. For rapid and reliable sedative effects the oral or intravenous route should be used. Repeated dosages of chlordiazepoxide can produce cumulative effects due to accumulation in the body of the drug and its two active metabolites. Half-life of the drug is from 20 to 24 hours. In the patient with alcoholic agitation or delirium tremens, intramuscular or intravenous injections initially may be as high as 50 to 100 mg.

Adverse reactions. Paradoxic reactions of rage, excitement, stimulation, hostility, confusion, and depersonalization have resulted from the administration of this drug to severely disturbed psychotic patients.

Drowsiness, ataxia, and lethargy occur frequently. Rash, nausea, headache, increased or decreased libido, an increase in vivid dreams, agranulocytosis, and jaundice occur less frequently.

Diazepam, U.S.P., B.P. (Valium)

Diazepam is effective in the treatment of anxiety and tension related to organic or functional conditions. Diazepam is slightly more effective than meprobamate and five times more potent than chlordiazepoxide. Long-term use may result in psychic and physical dependence. Sudden

cessation of the drug can result in withdrawal symptoms. It has been found to be useful in treating mild to moderate depression occurring alone or with anxiety and tension. Because of its muscle relaxant properties, it is a useful adjunct in the treatment of muscle spasms (conditions such as cerebral palsy and athetosis). It is becoming the drug of choice in the treatment of status epilepticus.

Preparation, dosage, and administration. This drug is available in tablets of 2, 5, and 10 mg. and in 2- and 10-ml. containers, 5 mg. per milliliter, for injection. Daily doses for adults range from 4 to 40 mg. When given intramuscularly, diazepam is absorbed slowly, erratically, and probably incompletely. Given orally, diazepam is rapidly and completely absorbed; peak blood concentrations are reached in 2 hours. Thus this drug should be given either orally or intravenously.

After a single oral or intravenous dose, clinical effects may seem to "wear off" rapidly, due to rapid and extensive tissue distribution. Diazepam is metabolized slowly and has a half-life between 20 and 40 hours in most patients, but it may be as long as 50 hours in some individuals. Repeated dosage leads to cumulative effects. Steady-state concentrations are usually obtained after 5 to 10 days of therapy. Diazepam or its metabolite can still be detected in the blood a week or more after termination of therapy. Diazepam should not be mixed or diluted with other solutions or drugs, or added to intravenous fluids.

Oxazepam, N.F. (Serax)

Oxazepam is closely related in its effects to chlordiazepoxide. It has been effective in the treatment of patients with anxiety, tension, and irritability associated with psychoneurotic conditions. It is said to be particularly valuable in the management of anxiety in elderly patients; however, scientific data have not validated this belief as yet. Oxazepam is less effective than either chlordiazepoxide or diazepam; it also has a lower incidence of adverse reactions. Its half-life in normal subjects ranges between 3 and 21 hours. Oxazepam is relatively rapidly metabolized to a psychopharmacologically inactive substance and, therefore, cumulative effects are less important during prolonged therapy than is true for chlordiazepoxide or diazepam.

Preparation, dosage, and administration. This drug is administered orally in capsules of 10, 15, and 30 mg. or 15-mg. tablets. Daily doses range from 30 to 120 mg. for adults. Parenteral preparations are not available.

Clorazepate dipotassium (Tranxene)

Clorazepate, the newest benzodiazepine antianxiety drug, was marketed in 1972. Its actions and uses are similar to those of the other benzodiazepine derivatives. Controlled studies indicate that it is an effective antianxiety drug. It is rapidly hydrolyzed in the body to nordiazepam, which is very slowly biotransformed and thus long lasting; cumulative effects occur with clorazepate. Peak plasma levels of nordiazepam occur within 1 hour after oral administration; the half-life of nordiazepam is about 24 hours. Clorazepate and diazepam appear to be equally effective. Most common side effects are drowsiness and ataxia. Adverse effects are the same as for other benzodiazepine compounds.

Preparation and dosage. Clorazepate is available in 3.75-, 7.5-, and 15-mg. capsules. Oral dose for adults is 15 to 60 mg. daily in divided doses; for elderly patients dose is 7.5 to 15 mg. daily; for children over 6 years of age dose is 7.5 to 60 mg. daily in divided doses.

PROPANEDIOL COMPOUNDS
Meprobamate, U.S.P., B.P. (Equanil, Miltown)

$$H_2N-\overset{\overset{\displaystyle O}{\|}}{C}-O-CH_2-\overset{\overset{\displaystyle C_3H_7}{|}}{\underset{\underset{\displaystyle CH_3}{|}}{C}}-CH_2O-\overset{\overset{\displaystyle O}{\|}}{C}-NH_2$$

Meprobamate is a synthetic drug that is chemically related to mephenesin, a skeletal muscle relaxant. As can be observed from the formula, the chemical structure differs markedly from that of reserpine or the phenothiazine derivatives. Meprobamate is a straight-chain aliphatic compound. It is a crystalline white powder with a bitter taste.

Action and result. The effects of meprobamate depend on the dosage employed. When used in large doses, as in animal experiments, the drug is not only an antianxiety agent but also a muscle relaxant and anticonvulsant. It acts as an interneuronal blocking agent and causes relaxation of skeletal muscle. It is also referred to as a centrally acting muscle relaxant. It is believed by some investigators, however, that meprobamate as employed in ordinary doses acts mainly as a sedative. Some even believe that its action under these circumstances does not differ significantly from that of phenobarbital.

Uses. Meprobamate has been effective in bringing about relief of anxiety and tension, abnormal fears, psychosomatic disorders, behavior disorders, and insomnia. It is not a potent hypnotic, but the relief of tension that it produces is conducive to sleep. Improvement after administration of this drug is usually characterized by decreased irritability, improved sense of well-being, and greater relaxation. It may also be used to treat musculoskeletal disorders and petit mal epilepsy.

Preparation, dosage, and administration. Meprobamate is marketed in sustained-release capsules of 200 mg., in an oral suspension of 40 mg. per milliliter, and in tablets of 200 and 400 mg. The usual adult dose is 400 mg. three or four times daily. Initial dose for children over 6 years of age is 100 to 200 mg., two or three times daily. Older children may tolerate doses as high as 2.4 Gm. Meprobamate is also available as a solution, 80 mg. in 5-ml. vials for intramuscular injection.

Side effects and toxic effects. Although meprobamate is not considered a toxic drug, it has been known to cause a number of side effects and untoward reactions. The more common reactions are drowsiness and allergic manifestations, such as skin rash, itching, and urticaria. The allergic reaction is sometimes sufficiently severe to require the administration of a corticosteroid and cessation of administration, but the symptoms usually respond well to administration of one of the antihistaminic drugs. Evidence exists that both psychic dependence and physical dependence can develop. Some patients seem to develop tolerance as well. Withdrawal symptoms, including convulsions, have been observed. Such symptoms are seen only after prolonged administration and abrupt discontinuance of administration.

Gradual withdrawal of meprobamate therapy is essential in the event that physical or psychic dependence develops.

ANTIDEPRESSANTS

Interest in psychotherapeutic agents useful for alleviating depressions has brought about a significant change in the treatment of these conditions. Depressive states appear to be unique to the human being and have been classified by psychiatrists as endogenous psychotic depressions and reactive depressions. Endogenous psychotic depressions are characterized by the absence of external causes for depression (death of a loved one, loss of employment, or debilitating illness), and the apparent grief and depression are of psychopathologic origin. Reactive depressions usually are abnormal depressive responses to environmental factors and are associated with emotional tension and instability. Psychomotor hyperexcitability (agitation) often occurs. Other behavioral manifestations characterizing depression are the expression of feelings of worthlessness, inadequacy, hopelessness, ambivalence, dependence, guilt, and suicidal tendencies. Delusions are common, the content of which express self-accusatory and guilt feelings. Initiative is lost and the patient is apathetic. The eyes are often directed downward, the corners of the mouth sag, lower eyelids droop, and the skin on the forehead may be furrowed. Depression is usually accompanied by poor appetite, loss of weight, sleep disturbances, coated tongue, foul breath, and constipation. About 30 years ago depressed patients were treated with analeptic drugs, such as pentylene tetrazole, to induce convulsions, which seemed to improve their condition. Later insulin was used to produce convulsions resulting from hypoglycemia.

Electroconvulsive therapy (ECT) was developed and found to be much safer than the aforementioned treatments. Electroconvulsive therapy is still used today, specifically for the depressed patient with manifestations of agitation.

Short-acting neuromuscular blocking agents and barbiturates are used prior to these treatments to prevent damage to the patient's limbs during the convulsions. These convulsions are induced by passing an AC current, for a fraction of a second, through electrodes fixed to the scalp. It is thought that the cycle of events leading to the depressive symptoms is broken by the electric change that allows neuronal activity to return to normal. Electroconvulsive therapy has also been known to increase the free amines in the brain. The psychoactive drugs used in the treatment of depression have not replaced electroconvulsive treatment; however, they have occasionally been a valuable adjunct to this form of treatment. Other measures such as psychotherapy, reduction of environmental stresses, and milieu therapy should also accompany electroconvulsive therapy. The psychoactive drugs commonly used in the treatment of depression are the tricyclic compounds and the monoamine oxidase inhibitors. All of these drugs appear to be most therapeutic in the treatment of endogenous depression. The monoamine oxidase inhibitors have produced favorable results in both endogenous and reactive depressions. Favorable responses to these drugs include elevation of mood, increased physical activity and mental alertness, and improved appetite and sleep patterns, accompanied by a reduction of premorbid preoccupation and delusions.

The tricyclic compounds, the monoamine oxidase inhibitors, and the amphetamines provide relief for some of the symptomatology related to depression. However, they do not treat the underlying causes of depression. They may relieve the depressive effects of temporary situational stress, but caution should be exerted to avoid using these drugs without a thorough evaluation of causative factors. The amphetamines act to stimulate the nervous system directly with little or no monoamine oxidase inhibition. Their action is brief (3 to 4 hours) and is frequently followed by a letdown. Hypertensive effect and reduced appetite are additional effects. Dependency can result from prolonged use of amphetamines. The difficulties involved with the use of these drugs should be weighed against the expected therapeutic results.

Since the amphetamines are not widely used for the treatment of depression, further discussion of antidepressant drugs will be confined to the tricyclic compounds and monoamine oxidase inhibitors.

MONOAMINE OXIDASE INHIBITORS (PSYCHIC ENERGIZERS)

Site and mechanism of action. One of the most significant discoveries in psychopharmacology was the accidental discovery of isoniazid, an antitubercular drug that produced euphoria, appetite stimulation, nervousness, insomnia, and orthostatic hypotension. It was abandoned in the treatment of tuberculosis because of these side effects. In the mid-1950's it became known for its monoamine oxidase inhibitory function. At about the same time the function of serotonin was defined in its relationship to central neuronal activity.

Monoamine oxidase is an enzyme found in the brain, blood platelets, liver, spleen, and kidneys and is responsible for destroying body chemicals such as the neurohormones epinephrine, norepinephrine, and serotonin. Monoamine oxidase inhibitors produce their central stimulation indirectly by inhibiting the monoamine oxidase enzyme. By decreasing or modifying the rate of destruction of the neurohormones, these inhibitors increase their longevity. Monoamine oxidase inhibitors act to increase psychomotor activity, increase appetite, and potentiate other drugs. They also act to prevent the release of norepinephrine from storage sites in the adrenergic neurons.

Side effects and precautions. The occurrence of a wide variety of side effects after the administration of the monoamine oxidase inhibitors has been cause for concern among most authorities. These side effects have often resulted in fatalities and/or severe medical conditions (see Table 12-5). The existence of hypertension is a contraindication for the use of monoamine oxidase inhibitors.

The suicidal tendencies present in the pa-

Table 12-5 Frequent side effects from monoamine oxidase inhibitors*

Postural hypertension	Nausea	Tachycardia
Dizziness	Vomiting	Edema
Restlessness	Diarrhea	Palpitation
Insomnia	Abdominal pain	Impotence
Weakness	Constipation	Headaches
Drowsiness	Anorexia	not from
Anxiety	Dryness of mouth	rise in
Agitation	Blurred vision	blood
Manic episodes	Chills	pressure)

*These side effects can usually be relieved with reduction of dosage. Most of the side effects reported are related to failure to recognize the cumulative action of these drugs with subsequent incorrect dosage. It is important to reduce dosage as soon as improvement of symptoms is observed to avoid precipitating side effects caused by the cumulative action of the drug.

tient's condition may compound his nursing care problem because of the delayed effect of these drugs in relieving suicidal tendencies. This effect presents an additional risk to the patient during initial phases of drug therapy. The nurse should be alert to the possibility of any impulsive ingestion of these substances.

Since the risk of suicide is frequently higher near the end of the depressive cycle, attention should be given to the possibility of suicidal attempts during this period. Overt patient behavior may indicate a remission of depressive symptomatology; however, this may be caused by drug action and not by alleviation of pathologic processes. Antidepressants should generally be continued for several months after the remission of symptoms and should never be discontinued abruptly, since a relapse may occur. Most authorities feel that these drugs should only be used in a psychiatric hospital setting for patients who are severely depressed and have serious suicidal tendencies.

Paradoxic hypertension. Paradoxic hypertension has been reported during the use of the monoamine oxidase inhibitors. Hypertensive crises have occurred after the ingestion of certain foods or beverages that are rich in amines (such as tyramine) or in amino acids (such as tyrosine) that may be decarboxylated in the body to form pressor amines normally inactivated by monoamine oxidase (see Chapter 9). Foods and beverages known to contain these amines are cheese (especially strong or aged varieties), bananas, avocados, beer, and Chianti wine. Drugs containing pressor agents (certain cold remedies, hay fever preparations, or anorexiants) should be avoided. The physician may instruct the patient initially in these precautions; however, nurses must provide the continued reassurance, support, and reinforcement of these restrictions.

During hospitalization, the depressed patient's anorexia may prompt well-meaning family members or friends to bring supplementary foods to the patient or a little wine to stimulate his appetite. Careful nursing observation during visiting hours and instruction of the family regarding these restrictions can avoid serious consequences. Communication with the hospital dietitian may also prevent these foods from appearing on the patient's hospital menu. As the patient's depression lifts or if electroconvulsive therapy is used concomitantly with drug therapy, reinstruction of the patient may be necessary. These foods and beverages should not be ingested for at least 2 to 3 weeks after discontinuance of drug therapy.

Intracranial bleeding associated with paradoxic hypertension and severe occipital headache that may radiate frontally has been known to occur. Symptoms that accompany this condition are stiffness or soreness of the neck, nausea, vomiting, sweating (with fever or with cold clammy skin), dilated pupils, photophobia, constricting chest pain, tachycardia, and bradycardia or other arrhythmias. Discontinuation of the drug immediately is recommended when any of these signs and symptoms occur. Fever is managed by external cooling and either phentolamine mesylate (5 mg. intravenously) or pentolinium tartrate (3 mg. intravenously) is used to control severe hypertensive reactions.

Hepatic toxicity. Jaundice and leukopenia are known side effects of the monoamine oxidase inhibitor compounds. It is recommended that patients receiving these drugs have periodic blood cell counts and tests of hepatic function.

Contraindications. The monoamine oxidase inhibitor compounds should be used with caution in patients who have a history of impaired kidney

Table 12-6 Contraindicated conditions for administration of monoamine oxidase inhibitors

Cardiovascular disease
Cardiac decompensation
Congestive heart failure
Cerebrovascular disorders
Pheochromocytoma
Hepatic disease
Blood dyscrasias—anemia, hepatitis
Pregnancy
Angina pectoris*
Epilepsy
Kidney dysfunction
Depressions accompanying:
  Chronic brain syndromes
  Schizophrenia
  Alcoholism
  Drug addiction
Conditions manifesting:
  Overactivity
  Overstimulation
  Agitation

*May suppress the warning signal of pain. Should be used with caution.

function or epilepsy. Overactive, overstimulated, or agitated patients usually do not respond well to these drugs. These drugs are also contraindicated in many other conditions (see Table 12-6).

Drug interactions. The effects of alcohol, barbiturates, and morphine-like analgesics are potentiated by the monoamine oxidase inhibitors thiazide and phenothiazine. Compounds that lower blood pressure should be administered carefully in conjunction with monoamine oxidase inhibitors. Reduction of dosage of both agents may be necessary.

The monoamine oxidase inhibitors should not be given with amitriptyline, desipramine, imipramine, or nortriptyline. These combinations may produce severe atropine-like reactions, tremors, hyperpyrexia, generalized clonic convulsions, delirium, and even death. Other monoamine oxidase inhibitors should not be administered concomitantly or soon after the administration of another agent in this group. Such combinations also produce hypertensive crises or convulsive seizures. A 2- to 3-week interval should follow the discontinuance of any of these drugs before another is started (Table 12-7).

Table 12-7 Drug incompatibility with administration of monoamine oxidase inhibitors

Monoamine oxidase inhibitors		
Generic name	Trade name	Incompatible drugs
Isocarboxazid	Marplan	Combination of any mono-amine oxidase inhibitor
		Other antidepressants
Nialamide	Niamid	Amphetamines
		Alcohol
		Barbiturates
		Morphine-like analgesics
		Cocaine, procaine, ether
Phenelzine	Nardil	Phenothiazine compounds
		Methyldopa, dopamine
		Tryptophan
		Antihypertensives
		Antiparkinsonian drugs
		Insulin
Tranylcypromine	Parnate	Thiazide diuretics
		Sympathomimetic amines— phenylephrine

Tranylcypromine sulfate, N.F., B.P. (Parnate)

Tranylcypromine sulfate should be reserved for use in patients with severe depressive conditions who have not responded to electroconvulsive treatment or in whom such therapy is contraindicated, and for patients who do not respond to other antidepressant therapy.

Preparation, dosage, and administration. Tranylcypromine sulfate is administered orally in 10-mg. tablets. Initial dosage per day is 20 mg. with gradual increments not to exceed 30 mg. It is recommended that the lowest effective dosage be used.

Nialamide, B.P. (Niamid)

Nialamide is an effective antidepressant used primarily in the management of endogenous depressions. It is also known to be effective in some reactive depressions.

Preparation, dosage, and administration. The only route of administration of nialamide is oral. It is marketed in tablets of 25 and 100 mg. strength. The usual dosage is 75 to 100 mg. a day in single or divided dosage with maintenance dosages as low as 12.5 mg. every other day.

Isocarboxazid, N.F., B.P. (Marplan)

Isocarboxazid is administered to patients with symptoms of depression and withdrawal, and seems to be an effective antidepressant in selected psychiatric conditions. It is useful in treating the depressed phases of anxiety or the depression of manic-depressive syndromes, as well as certain involutional, obsessive, and disassociative reactions. It does not appear to be as effective as electroconvulsive therapy in the treatment of severe psychiatric disorders. Its effects are cumulative and require 3 to 4 weeks of therapy before improvement is noted.

Preparation, dosage, and administration. Isocarboxazid is administered orally in 10-mg. tablets. The proposed initial dosage is 30 mg. daily given in single or divided doses. The average daily dosage should not exceed 30 mg., and the suggested maintenance dose is 10 to 20 mg. a day or less.

Phenelzine sulfate, N.F., B.P. (Nardil)

Phenelzine sulfate is useful in the treatment of both endogenous and reactive depressions. There is a latent period before onset of action, and the maximal effect occurs within 1 or 2 weeks.

Preparation, dosage, and administration. Phenelzine sulfate is administered orally in 15-mg. tablets. The initial daily dosage is 15 mg. three times a day. The average daily dosage should not exceed 75 mg. and maintenance dosages as low as 15 mg. every other day have been reported.

TRICYCLIC ANTIDEPRESSANTS

Tricyclic antidepressants bear close structural resemblance to the phenothiazine compounds. They produce potent antidepressant and mild tranquilizing effects. Investigations were conducted to develop an antidepressant drug that did not affect monoamine oxidase and therefore produced fewer side effects than the monoamine oxidase inhibitors. The tricyclic antidepressants have advantages that prompt many physicians to favor these drugs over monoamine oxidase inhibitors. There is very little risk of excessive stimulation (hypertensive crises and so on). There have been no reports of irreversible retinal or liver damage, and there is a higher incidence of successful therapy.

Site and mechanism of action. This group of antidepressant drugs does not inhibit monoamine oxidase or change the concentration of serotonin or other amines in the brain. Their mechanism of action is not known. However, it is hypothesized that the action of the drugs may be to affect brain amine levels by interfering with their re-uptake into nerves; thus they potentiate the action of catecholamines. The drugs have atropine-like, antihistamine, antiepinephrine, and antiserotonin actions. Autonomic side effects associated with these actions occur but are not serious and usually subside as treatment continues. They have only a slight depressant effect on the central nervous system. They antagonize the antihypertensive action of guanethidine.

Side effects. This group of drugs has been known to produce a wide variety of side effects. The most common side effects (Table 12-8) can be controlled by reduction of dosage. Skin rash has occurred and usually requires discontinuance of medication for relief.

Cardiovascular effects. Hypotension, hypertension, palpitations, tachycardia, arrhythmias, and heart block have been reported.

Central nervous system and neuromuscular effects. Confusion (particularly in the elderly), disorientation, hallucinations, delusions, anxiety, restlessness, insomnia, nightmares, exac-

Table 12-8 Common reversible side effects from tricyclic antidepressants*

Muscular hypertension	Dizziness
Drowsiness	Excitement
Dry mouth	Headache
Tremor	Numbness and tingling
Fatigue	of extremities
Weakness	Epigastric distress
Blurring of vision	Nausea, vomiting
Constipation	Insomnia
Urinary retention	Headache
Tachycardia	Flushing
Orthostatic hypotension	Impotence
Anorexia	Mild extrapyramidal
Generalized convulsions	stimulation
Excessive perspiration	

*These reactions can be relieved or controlled by reducing drug dosage.

erbation of psychosis, parkinsonian syndrome, numbness, tingling, paresthesias, ataxia, convulsions, tinnitus, and alterations in EEG patterns may occur.

Allergic reactions. Skin rash, urticaria, petechiae, photosensitivity, edema (generalized or of the face and tongue), and drug fever have been known to occur.

Anticholinergic effects. These may include dry mouth, blurred vision, disturbance of accommodation, constipation, paralytic ileus, urinary retention, and delayed micturition.

Hematologic effects. Blood dyscrasias may occur. If the patient develops fever and sore throat during therapy, leukocyte and differential counts should be performed.

Gastrointestinal effects. These include nausea and vomiting, anorexia, stomatitis, epigastric distress, and diarrhea.

Endocrine effects. These effects include testicular swelling, gynecomastia, and impotence in the male; breast enlargement and galactorrhea in the female; increased or decreased libido; and hyper- or hypoglycemia.

Other effects. Weight gain or loss, weakness, dizziness, fatigue, drowsiness, jaundice, altered liver function, headache, and alopecia may occur.

Precautions. Other agents may potentiate the action of these drugs (Table 12-9), and their use

Table 12-9 Drug incompatibility with administration of tricyclic antidepressants

Tricyclic compounds		
Generic name	*Trade name*	*Incompatible drugs*
Imipramine	Tofranil	Monoamine oxidase inhibitors
		Alcohol
		Barbiturates
Desipramine	Norpramin	Control nervous system
		depressants
		Thiazide diuretics
Nortriptyline	Aventyl	Vasodilators
		Anticholinergic agents
Amitriptyline	Elavil	Thyroid
Protriptyline	Vivactil	Guanethidine
Doxepin	Sinequan	
	Adapin	

Table 12-10 Conditions that contraindicate administration of tricyclic antidepressants

Glaucoma	Angina pectoris
Kidney disease	Congestive heart failure
Pyloric stenosis	Paroxysmal tachycardia
Epilepsy	Benign prostatic hypertrophy
Overactivity, overstimula-	Before surgery
tion, or agitation	

in selected conditions is contraindicated (Table 12-10).

The risk of suicide is the same with anticholinergic drugs as it is with monoamine oxidase inhibitors. The precautions regarding continued administration and abrupt discontinuance of the drug are also the same as for monoamine oxidase inhibitors.

The tricyclic antidepressants should not be administered concomitantly with the monoamine oxidase inhibitors. They should not be given less than 2 or 3 weeks after the discontinuance of the monoamine oxidase inhibitors. They should not be used concurrently with guanethidine.

These drugs should not be given in the late afternoon or evening because their stimulating effect can cause insomnia.

Imipramine hydrochloride, U.S.P., B.P. (Tofranil, Presamine)

Imipramine hydrochloride is an effective antidepressant drug that has found wide acceptance in the treatment of endogenous and reactive depressions. Initial improvement in depressive symptomatology may be noted within the first few days; however, maximal benefit is usually achieved in 1 to 2 weeks.

D.E.S.I. rating is *effective* for relief of symptoms of depression, particularly endogenous depression; *possibly effective* for depressions due to organic lesions and other psychotic states; and *ineffective* for enuresis.

Preparation, dosage, and administration. Imipramine hydrochloride is administered orally in tablets of 10, 25, and 50 mg. and intramuscularly in solution for injection of 12.5 mg. per milliliter. Initial dosage for hospitalized patients is 100 to 150 mg. daily in divided dosages. Gradual increment of dosage is suggested until the desired effects are observed; however, these dosages should not exceed 300 mg. per day. Outpatients may receive 75 mg. initial daily dosages in divided amounts and with gradual increments not exceeding 200 mg. per day. Reduction of dosage to a maintenance level of 50 to 150 mg. per day may be indicated as soon as desirable effects are noted. High dosages are not recommended for the elderly or adolescent patient.

Amitriptyline hydrochloride, U.S.P., B.P. (Elavil Hydrochloride)

Amitriptyline hydrochloride produces antidepressant and mild tranquilizing effects. Its uses and actions are as effective as imipramine in the treatment of endogenous depression. Reports indicate that this drug is effective in neurotic patients with excessive ruminative tendencies related to their depression; however, it has not been successful with other neurotic depressive conditions.

D.E.S.I. rating is *effective* for relief of symptoms of depression, especially those of endogenous depression; *possibly effective* for relief of anxiety; and *ineffective* for relief of headache.

Preparation, dosage, and administration. Amitriptyline hydrochloride is marketed for oral administration in 10-, 25- and 50-mg. tablets and for intramuscular uses in solution for injection, 10 mg. per milliliter. The usual initial dosage is 75 mg. a day in divided doses with gradual increments to 150 mg. per day. Additional doses may be added to the bedtime dosage in 25-mg. increments if this is necessary. Elderly and adolescent patients may find 10 mg. three times a day with 20 mg. at bedtime a satisfactory regimen.

Desipramine hydrochloride, N.F., B.P. (Norpramin, Pertofrane)

$$CH_2CH_2CH_2NHCH_3$$

Desipramine hydrochloride is thought to be as useful as imipramine in the treatment of endogenous and reactive depressions. Desipramine hydrochloride has been identified as the primary active metabolite of imipramine, and it is believed that the antidepressive action of imipramine is due to desipramine. The effectiveness of this drug may be reduced after a few weeks in some patients.

Preparation, dosage, and administration. Desipramine hydrochloride is only administered orally in 25- to 50-mg. capsules (Pertofrane) and in 25- to 50-mg. tablets (Norpramin). The average initial dosage per day is 75 to 150 mg. given in divided doses. When the desired results are achieved the average daily maintenance dose is 50 to 100 mg. in divided doses. Daily doses should not exceed 200 mg.

Nortriptyline hydrochloride, N.F., B.P. (Aventyl Hydrochloride)

$$CHCH_2CH_2NHCH_3$$

Nortriptyline hydrochloride is as effective as amitriptyline in the treatment of endogenous and reactive depressions and produces similar results. Patients who respond to this drug ordinarily indicate a change in behavior within the first week of therapy. The effectiveness of nortriptyline as an adjunct to electroconvulsive treatment is unpredictable. It is used as an antidepressant and has some tranquilizing action.

Preparation, dosage, and administration. Nortriptyline hydrochloride is administered orally in 10- and 25-mg. capsules and as a liquid of 10 mg. per 5 ml. The average initial daily dosage is 20 to 40 mg. given in divided dosages. This dosage may be continued for 5 to 7 days or until the desired results are attained. Reduction of dosage may then be necessary for maintenance therapy. Usual maintenance doses are from 30 to 75 mg. per day. Daily dosages should not exceed 100 mg. per day as adverse side effects may occur. For elderly patients 30 to 50 mg. per day may be sufficient.

Protriptyline hydrochloride, N.F., B.P. (Vivactil)

$$CH_2CH_2CH_2NHCH_3$$

Protriptyline is a tricyclic antidepressant related structurally to amitriptyline and nortriptyline. Like these other drugs its mechanism of action is unknown. It is useful for the treatment of endogenous and exogenous depression. Its psychomotor activating action makes it particularly suitable for treating withdrawn, apathetic, and lethargic patients. Depressed patients with agitation, tension, and anxiety may become more disturbed when treated with protriptyline. Side effects and precautions are the same as for other tricyclics.

Protriptyline is well absorbed from the gastrointestinal tract. Plasma levels of the drug appear in 2 hours; peak levels occur in 8 to 12 hours and then gradually decline. Rate of excrétion is slow; about 50% of the drug is excreted in 16 days.

Preparation and dosage. Protriptyline is available in 5- and 10-mg. tablets. Oral dosage for adults is 15 to 60 mg. daily in three or four divided doses; for adolescents and elderly patients dosage is 15 mg. daily in three divided doses. Any increase in dose should be made in the morning dose. The cardiovascular system of elderly patients should be monitored.

Doxepin hydrochloride (Sinequan, Adapin)

Doxepin is a tricyclic drug with pharmacologic action similar to that of amitriptyline. It has anticholinergic, antihistaminic, and antiserotonin effects. It is not recommended by the A.M.A. as the primary drug for treating anxiety and tension. Doxepin is reported to be as effective, and in some cases more effective, than amitriptyline in relieving symptoms of depression in psychoneurotic patients.

Preparation and dosage. Doxepin is available in 10-, 25-, and 50-mg. capsules. Oral dose for adults is 75 mg. daily in three divided doses initially, with an increase or decrease in dose depending upon the response of the patient. For severely depressed patients 150 to 300 mg. daily may be required.

QUESTIONS

For study and review

1 Traditionally neurophysiologists have identified each part of the nervous system by allocating specific functions to certain areas of the brain. Recent research has indicated the following change in this perspective:
  a. The brain functions as a result of the independent action of specific areas contributing to total body functioning.
  b. The brain is now considered to be an intricate system of specific structures to which unique functions can easily be allocated.
  c. The brain acts as a unit.
  d. The interrelationship of various structures of the brain are extremely intricate; however, recent research has identified specific functions for each structure.

2 The highest mental activities—recognition, memory, intelligence, imagination, and creative thought—are attributed to:
  a. the cerebral cortex only
  b. interaction of the thalamus, epithalamus, and hypothalamus
  c. interaction among the cerebral cortex, thalamus, epithalamus, and hypothalamus
  d. interreaction of the cerebral cortex and hypothalamus

3 The reticular activating system appears to function by:
  a. alerting the cerebral cortex to emotion
  b. alerting the cerebral cortex to emotional stimuli from the environment
  c. alerting the hypothalamus and cerebral cortex to somatic sensory experience
  d. alerting the cerebral cortex to sensory experience and originating emotional reactions associated with somatic sensory experience

4 The term *psychotropic drugs* encompasses which of the following drug groups?
  a. major and minor tranquilizers, antidepressants
  b. major tranquilizers and antidepressants
  c. major tranquilizers and rauwolfia drugs
  d. antidepressants, amphetamines, and minor tranquilizers

5 Nurses should be aware of the physician's criteria for selection of psychotropic drugs:
  a. so they can look up the side effects of the drugs
  b. so they can evaluate the patient's response to drug therapy in light of the physician's goals for selecting the drug
  c. so they can interpret these criteria to the patient
  d. so they can observe and report any side effects that may occur

6 Rauwolfia alkaloids are considered antipsychotic agents but are not widely used as tranquilizers because:
  a. large single doses cause severe side effects
  b. large single doses are expensive
  c. their therapeutic action is delayed for several weeks
  d. prolonged administration causes hypertension

7 Most of the antipsychotic drugs are phenothiazine derivatives. Commonalities can be identified because:
  a. the type of action is essentially similar with all phenothiazine derivatives
  b. individual compounds vary chiefly in their potency
  c. individual compounds vary slightly in the nature and severity of their side effects
  d. individual compounds vary only in number and kind of adverse reactions reported

8 The phenothiazines are thought to have which of the following modes of action on the central nervous system?

a. blocking of adrenergic synapses of the ergotrophic system
b. depression of the reticular activating system
c. stimulation of central sympathetic activity
d. acetylcholine blockage

9 The most important pharmacologic characteristics of the phenothiazines are:
a. antipsychotic activity
b. failure of large doses to produce coma or anesthesia
c. extrapyramidal symptoms
d. causes physical and psychogenic dependence with large doses

10 The phenothiazine derivatives are used to reduce psychotic symptoms and, therefore, are useful in the treatment of acute and chronic psychoses. The nurse may notice which of the following behavior changes after the administration of the phenothiazine drugs?
a. drooling, ataxia, akinesia
b. weight gain, dry mouth, blurred vision
c. increased motor activity, less frequent hallucinatory experiences
d. reduction of agitation, destructive or combative behavior, delusions

11 Measures known to be effective in the management of the most common side effects resulting from phenothiazine administration are:
a. reduction of dosage or discontinuance of drug
b. administration of antiparkinsonian drugs
c. intravenous administration of levarterenol (Levophed)
d. administration of milk of magnesia, Cepacol mouthwash, and reduction diet

12 A common side effect known to occur with the administration of large dosages of phenothiazine derivatives is photosensitivity. The nurse's responsibility in avoiding unnecessary complications is:
a. instructing the family and patient in the appropriate preventive measures
b. reporting the occurrence of dark purplish brown skin pigmentations to the doctor
c. providing protective clothing and/or keeping the patient out of the sun
d. restricting or limiting the patient's outdoor activities during times of the day when solar exposure would be maximal

13 Extrapyramidal symptoms may appear after the administration of phenothiazine drugs. The most severe and distressing extrapyramidal symptom experienced by the patient is:
a. ataxia   c. akinesia
b. dyskinesia   d. akathisia

14 Antiparkinsonian agents most commonly used are:
a. Cogentin, Kemadrin, Artane, and Akineton
b. Benadryl
c. Coramine, Dexedrine, Ritalin
d. Lorfan, Nalline, Megimide

15 Phenothiazine drugs are known to potentiate the action of other drugs. Phenothiazine drugs should be given cautiously to persons who are known to have ingested which of the following substances?

a. alcoholic beverages
b. barbiturates
c. morphine-like analgesics
d. monoamine oxidase inhibiting drugs

16 Which of the following precautions should be observed when administering chlorpromazine hydrochloride intramuscularly?
a. Slowly rotate the vial from left to right in order to diffuse the white crystalline powder before drawing the medication up for injection.
b. Avoid getting solution for injection into contact with skin or eyes.
c. Inject the medication slowly, taking care to administer only 1 ml. per injection site.
d. Massage the injection site to avoid local irritation.

17 Indicate the generic name for each of the following antipsychotic agents and number according to approximate incidence of extrapyramidal symptoms:

Tindal _____ _____
Stelazine _____ _____
Compazine _____ _____
Thorazine _____ _____
Mellaril _____ _____
Prolixin _____ _____
Vesprin _____ _____

18 Minor tranquilizers are thought to be effective for which of the following conditions?
a. some gastrointestinal, musculoskeletal, and cardiovascular conditions
b. acute psychotic episodes marked by agitation
c. psychosomatic or psychoneurotic conditions
d. withdrawal reactions or delirium tremens

19 Minor tranquilizers differ from barbiturates in their sedative effects because:
a. minor tranquilizers have longer duration of action
b. minor tranquilizers have fewer side effects
c. minor tranquilizers have little effect on levels of awareness
d. minor tranquilizers tend to cause disorganization of thought processes in high dosages

20 The mechanism of action that best explains the effect minor tranquilizers have in controlling the anxiety related to psychoneurotic conditions is:
a. their central depressant action on the neocortex
b. their stimulation of the different proprioceptive impulses
c. their depressive effects on the polysynaptic reflexes of the spinal cord
d. their stimulation of adrenergic binding sites

21 Patients taking any of the minor tranquilizers are cautioned against activities such as driving an automobile, operating dangerous machinery, or performing tasks requiring precision because of the common occurrence of which of the following side effects?
a. drowsiness, ataxia, dizziness, headache
b. rash, fever, dry mouth, chills
c. nausea, vomiting, confusion
d. jaundice, increased white blood counts, diarrhea

22 Occasionally patients taking chlordiazepoxide hydro-

chloride (Librium) experience a paradoxic reaction, which means:

a. anxiety increases instead of decreasing

b. rage, hostility, confusion, and depersonalization result

c. shock and respiratory embarrassment occurs

d. nothing happens at all

23 Physicians may hesitate to prescribe meprobamate as an antianxiety agent because:

a. it is too expensive for use in a long-term treatment program

b. it is habit-forming

c. it precipitates exaggerated behavior patterns

d. its usefulness is restricted to middle-aged persons with psychoneurotic behavior patterns

24 Antidepressant drug therapy is used in the treatment of endogenous or reactive depressions. Its effectiveness is thought to be most helpful in:

a. relief of the symptomatology of depression

b. treating depressive effects resulting from temporary situational stress

c. treating the underlying causes of reactive depression

d. relief of the underlying causes of endogenous depressions

25 Monoamine oxidase is an enzyme found in the brain, blood platelets, liver, spleen, and kidneys and is responsible for:

a. stimulation of ganglion cells releasing epinephrine from the adrenal medulla

b. destroying body chemicals such as the neurohormones epinephrine and norepinephrine

c. increasing the sympathetic tone within the hypothalamus

d. restoring the balance of serotonin, epinephrine, and norepinephrine in cortex

26 Monoamine oxidase inhibiting drugs act:

a. to decrease high concentrations of serotonin in the brain

b. to stimulate sympathetic tone in the hypothalamus

27 Check the following side effects most commonly seen with the administration of monoamine oxidase inhibitors.

a. chest pain

b. severe occipital headache

c. dizziness

d. drowsiness

e. seizures

f. postural hypotension

g. drowsiness

h. dilated pupils

i. vomiting

j. diarrhea

k. agitation

l. dry mouth

28 Which of the following drugs should not be given in conjunction with monoamine oxidase inhibitors?

a. Tofranil

b. Norpramin

c. chloral hydrate

d. Enovid

e. Elavil

f. Darvon compound

g. Aventyl

h. elixir terpin hydrate

29 Tricyclic antidepressant drugs are more widely used than monoamine oxidase inhibitors in the treatment of depression for the following reasons:

a. There is very little risk of hypertension crises.

b. There is a higher incidence of successful therapy.

c. They have fewer side effects than monoamine oxidase inhibitors.

d. They are less expensive.

30 Monoamine oxidase inhibitors and tricyclic antidepressants should only be administered in the hospital setting because:

a. the hospital diet controls the incidence of ingestion of contraband food or beverages

b. their side effects are serious

c. patients taking these medications should not be operating dangerous machinery

d. the risk of suicide is high

REFERENCES

Books

A.M.A. drug evaluations, ed. 2, Acton, Mass., 1973, Publishing Sciences Group, Inc.

Aviado, D. M.: Drantz and Carr's pharmacologic principles of medical practice, ed. 8, Baltimore, 1972, The Williams & Wilkins Co.

Childress, S. J.: Antianxiety agents. In Burger, A., editor: Medicinal chemistry, Part II, New York, 1970, Wiley Interscience, pp. 1498-1510.

Di Palma, J. R., editor: Drill's pharmacology in medicine, New York, 1971, McGraw-Hill Book Co.

Goodman, L. S., and Gilman, A., editors: The pharmacological basis of therapeutics, ed. 5, New York, 1975, The Macmillan Co.

Goth, A.: Medical pharmacology, ed. 7, St. Louis, 1974, The C. V. Mosby Co.

Grollman, A., and Grollman, E. F.: Pharmacology and therapeutics, ed. 7, Philadelphia, 1970, Lea & Febiger.

Kaiser, C., and Zirkle, C. I.: Antidepressant drugs. In Burger,

A., editor: Medicinal chemistry, Part 1, New York, 1970, Wiley Interscience, pp. 1470-1497.

Meyers, F. H., Jawetz, E., and Goldfien, A.: Review of medical pharmacology, ed. 4, Los Altos, Calif., 1974, Lange Medical Publications.

Modell, W., editor: Drugs of choice 1976-1977, St. Louis, 1976, The C. V. Mosby Co.

Osol, A., and Pratt, R.: The United States Dispensatory, ed. 27, Philadelphia, 1973, J. B. Lippincott Co.

Turner, P., and Richens, A.: Clinical pharmacology, Edinburgh, 1973, Churchill Livingstone.

Periodicals

Almy, G. L., and Taylor, M. A.: Lithium retention in mania, Arch. Gen. Psychiat. **29:**232, 1973.

Crane, G. E.: Cardiac toxicity and psychotropic drugs, Dis. Nerv. Syst. **31:**534, 1970.

Davis, J. M., and Fann, W. E.: Lithium, Ann. Rev. Pharmacol. **11:**285, 1971.

Goldfield, M., and Weinstein, M. R.: Lithium in pregnancy: A review with recommendations, Am. J. Psych. **127:**888, 1971.

Hollister, L. E.: Clinical use of psychotherapeutic drugs: Current status, Clin. Pharmacol. Therap. **10:**170, 1969.

Hollister, L. E.: Mental disorders in antianxiety and antidepressant drugs, New Eng. J. Med. **286:**1195, 1972.

Kellner, R.: Drugs, diagnoses, and outcomes of drug trials with neurotic patients, J. Nerv. Ment. Dis. **151:**85, 1970.

King, L. J.: Chemotherapy of mental depression, Ann. Rev. Med. **21:**367, 1970.

Mathysse, S.: Antipsychotic drug actions, Fed. Proc. **32:**200, 1973.

Prien, R. F., and others: Comparison of lithium carbonate and chlorpromazine in treatment of mania, Arch. Gen. Psychiat. **26:**146, 1972.

Rodman, M. J.: Drugs for managing mood disorders, R. N. **33:**64, 1970.

Schow, M., et al.: Lithium and pregnancy, Br. Med. J. **2:**135, 1973.

Schyll, W. K., and Sapira, J. D.: Critique of studies of lithium salts in the treatment of mania, Am. J. Psych. **127:**218, 1970.

Singer, I., and Rothenberg, D.: Mechanisms of lithium action, New Eng. J. Med. **289:**254, 1973.

Usdin, E.: Absorption, distribution and metabolic fate of psychotropic drugs, Psychopharmacol. Bull. **6:**4, 1970.

Drug abuse

Although most drugs are prescribed and administered with a high degree of discrimination, all drugs potentially can be misused or abused. The prescription of drugs without adequate exploration of the patient's presenting complaint, for example, is representative of drug misuse by a physician. Prolonged and unsupervised administration of drugs for symptomatic relief is another such example. In general, drug misuse refers to nonspecific or indiscriminate use of drugs. Drug abuse, on the other hand, refers to self-medication or self-administration of a drug in chronically excessive quantities, resulting in psychic and/or physical dependence, functional impairment, and deviation from approved social norms.

Drug abuse is neither a new nor a recent phenomenon. Rather, it has been known throughout history as one expression of man's search for relief of his physical and psychosocial problems. Indeed, one study suggests that epidemics of drug abuse have occurred throughout man's history.

Contemporary drug abuse has attained prominence as an issue with moral, legal, social, in-trapsychic, and medical aspects and as an issue that is difficult to examine objectively. In order to fulfill their professional responsibility to society in relation to this pressing social issue, nurses need current knowledge about drugs most frequently abused, reasons for drug abuse, crisis intervention in relation to drug abuse, and knowledge of regional treatment facilities to which they can refer patients either for emergency care or for long-term treatment.

It is beyond the scope of this chapter to explore all aspects of drug abuse in depth. Instead, this chapter will focus upon the abuse of consciousness-altering drugs. However, the nurse is urged to explore other aspects of the complex phenomenon of drug abuse independently in order to achieve a more holistic frame of reference.

DRUG DEPENDENCE

In the past, drug abuse was defined in terms of *habituation* and *addiction*. These terms, however, have been used in so many ways that no longer is there any consensus regarding their definitions. Moreover, the terms *habituation* and *addiction* are nonspecific in that they do not describe the nature of the problem. Characteristics of drug abuse will vary according to the particular agent abused, and different drugs will have entirely different patterns of dependence and different characteristics of withdrawal. In an attempt to reduce the conceptual ambiguity of "habituation" and "addiction," the World Health Organization in 1964 suggested that the use of these terms be replaced by the concepts of *physical* and *psychic dependence*. Its statement regarding this issue reads as follows:

> Drug dependence is a state of psychic or physical dependence or both on a drug arising in a person following administration of that drug on a periodic or continuous basis. The characteristics of such a state will vary with the agent involved and these characteristics must always be made clear by designating the particular type of drug dependence in each specific case—e.g., drug dependence of the barbiturate type, of the morphine type. . .

Physical dependence on a drug refers to an adaptive physiologic state that occurs after prolonged administration of that drug which manifests itself by intense physical disturbances (withdrawal symptoms) when the drug's administration is discontinued. That is, physical dependence on a drug can be demonstrated only by production of a withdrawal syndrome. This syndrome can be relieved by readministering the drug or by administering a pharmacologically related drug. (Drugs are cross-dependent when they are mutually capable of relieving withdrawal symptoms that result from the withdrawal of either drug.) Closely related to physical dependence is the production of drug tolerance with a tendency to increase the drug dose.

Psychic dependence, by contrast, is a state of emotional reliance upon a drug in order to maintain a drug-induced state that, to the involved individual, is preferable to a drug-free state of being. The manifestations of psychic dependence can range from a mild desire for a drug to "craving" to compulsive use. Either type of dependence can exist independently of the other or both can exist simultaneously. Both types of dependence potentially can lead to a compulsive pattern of drug use that, Goodman and Gilman state,* is characterized by a narrow, almost exclusive, and highly invested involvement in procuring and using the drug.

ETIOLOGIC FACTORS IN DRUG ABUSE

A characteristic common to most drugs that cause dependence is that they are initially taken because the individual believes that a desirable pharmacologic effect will result. In order to cause dependence, then, a drug must produce favorable, pleasant, unusual, or desirable effects. The person who is dependent on a drug has found something that will give him relief from his problems, and the drug is generally used as an adjustive mechanism. Since very few drugs without central nervous system effects are abused, one of the predominant factors contributing to drug abuse appears to be intrapsychic and motivated by a desire to alter one's state of mind. This desire may derive from a number of conditions. Pleasure-seeking behavior often seems to be an etiologic factor in drug abuse and, among other goals, may represent escape from inner tensions, a search for euphoria, an attempt to explore unknown aspects of cognitive function, or an attempt to discover one's self. More specifically, some psychologic hypotheses have been advanced in relation to persons prone to use drugs as escape mechanisms. Descriptions of potentially drug-dependent personalities have included characteristics of strong psychologic dependence, low threshold of frustration, fear of failure, and feelings of inadequacy. Other authorities dispute the "addiction-prone" personality hypothesis, maintaining that everyone has the potential to become dependent on something.

Other factors related to the development of drug abuse may derive from social conditions. In today's society, anxiety, tension, insomnia, and other manifestations of stress are common. Many people seek relief by self-medication with

---

*Goodman, L. S., and Gilman, A.: The pharmacological basis of therapeutics, ed. 4, New York, 1970, The Macmillan Company.

either over-the-counter agents or prescription drugs. According to Fort,* dependence upon chemically active substances to treat some problems of living has spread to almost all areas of life. Indeed, Fort cites, our society has in many ways accepted the slogan of "better living through chemistry." Drugs are available for almost every purpose—to help us to relax, to help us to awake, to promote concentration, and to prevent conception, for example—and their use is generally socially acceptable.

Other authorities have cited social factors such as peer-group pressure, the permissiveness of the present generation, and the rapid cultural-technologic changes occurring in our society as other factors influencing drug abuse. Drug abuse may also symbolize alienation from society and rejection of society's mores.

TYPES OF DRUGS ABUSED

All drugs have some abuse potential, and some sources indicate that drug abuse may be more related to the personality of the user than to the drug itself. Perhaps among the most frequently abused chemically active substances are the xanthines and theobromines, which are contained in beverages such as coffee, tea, chocolate, and colas. Although these substances are rarely perceived as drugs by the lay public, they do produce mild stimulant and euphoriant effects and their use may lead to psychic dependence. Nicotine and ethyl alcohol are also frequently abused, with consequent physical and psychic dependence. Atropine, epinephrine, steroids, belladonna alkaloids, and cardiac glycosides are examples of other drugs that may induce altered states of perception, thought, and feeling as a result of their prolonged and concentrated therapeutic use and also may be abused.

However, as previously indicated, few drugs without central nervous system effects are abused. Therefore, the four major categories of commonly abused drugs are narcotics, general central nervous system depressants, central ner-

vous system stimulants, and other mind-altering drugs that have been variably classified as hallucinogenic, psychotomimetic, and psychedelic. When used for prolonged periods of time, depressant drugs like the opiates, barbiturates, and alcohol generally produce both physical and psychic dependence. Stimulant drugs like the amphetamines and cocaine appear to produce psychic but not physical dependence. The other mind-altering drugs have variable and, at this time, questionable dependence-producing qualities, but it seems generally agreed that they all produce psychic dependence.

Before proceeding, it is necessary to differentiate among the terms *hallucinogenic, psychotomimetic,* and *psychedelic.* Although all three terms have been utilized interchangeably, they have some distinct differences. *Hallucinogenic* refers to the tendency of a drug to produce auditory and/or visual hallucinations. Hallucinogenic effects, however, are neither a uniform nor a primary property of all consciousness-altering drugs, and the term should be used with discrimination. The term *psychotomimetic* refers to the ability of a drug to chemically induce a psychotic state that mimics a "natural" psychosis. Again, this term must be used with discrimination when referring to mind-altering drugs, since not all induce psychosis. The term *psychedelic* was originally intended to be a nonjudgmental adjective referring to the "mind-manifesting" properties of a drug, that is, to a drug's ability to effect states of consciousness an individual would not usually experience. It has, however, become more ambiguous in definition and has acquired some valuational connotations. It may be used to refer to self-administered mind-altering drugs for their subjective effects of inducing states of altered perception, thought, and feeling. Because of such imprecision of terms, the broad term *mind-altering* will be used throughout this chapter.

Drug abuse may take several forms. It may be experimental abuse, in which the individual uses drugs in an exploratory way after which he may accept or reject continuing use of the drugs. Drug abuse may occur only in social contexts; drugs that are frequently abused only in social situations include alcohol, marihuana, nicotine,

*Fort, J.: The pleasure seekers, Indianapolis, 1969, The Bobbs-Merrill Company.

and caffeine. Episodic drug abuse refers to the periodic abuse of excessive amounts of a drug, as frequently occurs with ethyl alcohol. Compulsive drug abuse is characterized by irrational, compulsive abuse of a drug. Ritualistic drug abuse, on the other hand, may be related to religious or philosophical rites.

PHARMACOLOGIC BASIS OF PHYSICAL DRUG DEPENDENCE

Several hypotheses attempt to explain the pharmacologic basis of the physiologic adaptation that occurs in tolerance and physical drug dependence.

According to Martin's pharmacologic redundancy theory,* there are two or more pathways mediating the physiologic functions influenced by the opiates. Martin assumes that morphine sulfate interrupts one of the redundant pathways but does not interrupt the other. This results in hypertrophy of the uninterrupted pathway (pathway A), which then assumes the functions mediated by the interrupted pathway (pathway B). Therefore, tolerance to morphine is the result of hypertrophy of pathway A. When the drug is withdrawn, pathway B resumes its normal level of excitability but, because pathway A is still overfunctioning, the total system then functions at a level that is higher than the predrug state of function. This exaggerated function, Martin states, is the hyperexcitability that is characteristic of the abstinence syndrome.

Collier,* on the other hand, hypothesizes that tissue may contain two types of receptors for particular drugs. One of these types, the "pharmacologic receptors," produces a pharmacologic response when contact is made with the drug. The other receptors are "silent receptors" that elicit no response. The development of drug tolerance results from a change in the number and production of these receptor types, the pharmacologic receptors decreasing in number and the silent receptors increasing in number.

From a third frame of reference, Crossland* states that physical adaptation to depressant drugs simply involves an increase in the amount of excitatory transmitter that is adequate to overcome the drug-depressed condition of the nerve cells. When the drug is withdrawn, hyperexcitability (abstinence symptoms) occurs if the nerve cells return to normal condition more rapidly than the transmitter supply.

Although these and other theories of physical drug dependence are in hypothetical stages and are still being researched, they generally seem to agree that, in a state of dependence, a condition of latent hyperexcitability develops in the cells of the central nervous system following frequent and prolonged administration of depressant drugs.

ALTERED STATES OF CONSCIOUSNESS PRODUCED BY DRUGS

The effects of various mind-altering drugs are unpredictable and highly variable. The same drug in the same dose may produce quite disparate effects in two different individuals. The primary factors influencing the effects of any drug are generally defined as: (1) the pharmacologic properties of the drug itself; (2) the personality of the user; (3) the environment of the user; and (4) the interaction of these three components. The effects of mind-altering drugs, specifically, are also thought to be related to the purity of the drug used (drugs transferred illegally are frequently adulterated, or "cut," with other substances), the underlying psychopathology in the user, and the age of the user. Many drug users, for example, are adolescents who are dealing with the intrapsychic problems accompanying this stage of maturation. The tenuous emotional equilibrium of this stage may particularly predispose to negative reactions to mind-altering drugs. The effects of mind-altering drugs also appear to be particularly subject to the

*In Phillipson, R. V., editor: Modern trends in drug dependence and alcoholism, London, 1970, Butterworth & Co. (Publishers) Ltd.

*Crossland, J.: Lewis's pharmacology, ed. 4, Baltimore, 1970, The Williams & Wilkins Co.

user's mood, expectations, and social environment. Most adverse reactions to marihuana, for example, are said to occur in novice users, since they may enter the experience with a mental set of fear.

Adequate preparation for the drug experience, therefore, is a significant factor influencing the nature of that experience. In addition, the presence or lack of a supportive environment (particularly the presence and guidance of a trusted and knowledgeable person) and the presence or lack of an opportunity to understand and to reintegrate the experience following recovery from the drug are variables that may influence a drug experience either positively or negatively.

In describing the phenomenon of the "psychedelic" experience, Houston* identifies some general effects that are commonly observed and experienced after the administration of mind-altering drugs. Among the most common and repeated effects she identifies the following: changes in auditory, visual, olfactory, tactile, gustatory, and kinesthetic perception; changes in body image; changes in experiencing time and space; changes in rate and content of thought; abrupt and frequent changes in mood and affect; heightened suggestibility; possible occurrence of depersonalization and ego dissolution; possible activation of repressed materials; awareness of internal organs and body processes; multiple and fragmentized consciousness; concern with philosophic, cosmologic, and religious questions; perception of a world released from its normal ordering; a sense of capacity to communicate better through nonverbal means; and feelings of empathy.

Houston states that these are not the only effects of psychedelic drugs but that this description should serve to convey some idea of their mind-altering effects. She goes on to categorize the effects of these drugs into four major levels of consciousness as follows:

1 Sensory level. The drug user may experience a great variety of sensory awareness, including heightened awareness of visual phenomena, such as colors,

---

*Houston, J.: Phenomenology of the psychedelic experience. In Hicks, R. E., and Fink, P. J.: Psychedelic drugs, Hahnemann symposium, New York, 1969, Grune and Stratton, Inc., pp. 1-7.

lines, textures, and spatial relationships. This sensory awareness may also be focused upon internal processes of the body. It may be a pleasant heightened awareness or a frightening one. Often, Houston states, it is the only alteration in consciousness the drug user experiences.

2 Recollective-analytic level. In this level of altered consciousness, the drug user is described as experiencing psychologic involution and introspection and engaging in self-analysis of personal problems, values, and potentialities. Emergence of unconscious material may occur and the drug user may experience regression. In an unsupportive context or in a context of latent psychosis, this experience may result in an acute panic psychosis. With an appropriate, predetermined mental set and knowledgeable guidance, Houston states, the experience may be therapeutic.

3 Symbolic level. At this level of consciousness, the drug user is described as experiencing rich symbolism in which his life expands beyond the particular-personal orientation to a personal-universal orientation, and the individual may see his life in terms of a guiding pattern or goal.

4 Integral level. The experience of this level of consciousness is described as extremely rare and is characterized as being similar to religious and mystic experiences in which profound and fundamental value and behavior changes occur or in which "self-actualization" occurs.

Houston's categorization provides a conceptual tool for comprehending experiences with mind-altering drugs, although it is by no means the only frame of reference to apply to the drug experience. Again, it must be emphasized that (1) expanding and continuing research is necessary to validate information regarding drug abuse and (2) at this time the illicit drug experience appears to have as much (if not more) potential for being frightening and negative as it has for being pleasant and constructive.

CENTRAL NERVOUS SYSTEM DEPRESSANTS
CANNABIS DRUGS

The cannabis drugs are derived from the leaves, stem, fruiting tops, and resin of the female hemp plant *Cannabis sativa*. The potency of the active ingredient, tetrahydrocannabinol

(Δ^9-THC), is greatest in the resin of the plant and seems to vary according to the climatic conditions under which the plant is grown. In the United States, the plant generally grows wild rather than being cultivated and thus is generally low in potency.

Tetrahydrocannabinol (Δ^9-THC)

Preparations. Marihuana and hashish are the most common forms of cannabis drugs used in the United States. Hashish refers to the powdered form of the plant's resin, which is five to eight times as potent as marihuana. Other forms of cannabis drugs used in different parts of the world include "bhang," "ganja," and "charas," which are commonly used in India and which correspond, respectively, to American marihuana, hashish, and unadulterated resin. In Morocco, "kif" is used, while in South America, a cannabis drug often used is called "dagga."

Mode of administration. Cannabis drugs may be absorbed when administered by oral, subcutaneous, or pulmonary routes but are most potent when inhaled. Either the pure resin or the dried leaves of the cannabis plant may be smoked in pipes or cigarettes. Because the smoke is acrid and irritating, some users prefer to smoke marihuana through a water pipe. The smoke is deeply inhaled and retained in the lungs as long as possible in order to achieve maximum saturation of the absorbing surface. Powdered hashish and marihuana may also be mixed with foods, a mode of administration that delays the drug's absorption. The effects of smoking are rapid and generally last 2 to 3 hours, while the effects of the orally ingested drug may not begin for several hours.

Mechanism of action. All of the cannabis drugs seem to act as central nervous system depressants, their "high" resulting from depression of higher brain centers and consequent re-

lease of lower centers from inhibitory influence. While there is some controversy regarding their classification, the cannabis drugs are not narcotics and are more frequently classified as sedative-hypnotic-anesthetics or psychedelic drugs. Like the sedative-hypnotics, they appear to depress the ascending reticular activating system and, as their dosage increases, their effects will proceed from relief of anxiety, disinhibition, and excitement to anesthesia. If dosage is high enough, respiratory and vasomotor depression and collapse may occur.

Little is known about the metabolism of the active principle found in cannabis extracts. Research has yielded some marihuana homologs and analogs (such as synhexyl), which should permit standardization of dosage and yield more information regarding structure-activity relationships of the cannabis drugs.

Effects. The drugs have mind-altering properties and induce an anxiety-free state of relaxation characterized by a feeling of extreme well-being. Perceptions of time and space are distorted; ideas flow freely and disconnectedly; there may be interruptions in thought that are blanks or gaps similar to "epileptic absence"; and there may be states of inwardness and/or occasional excitement in the form of hilarity. Hallucinations can occur with high doses of the drug but are generally reported to be pleasant. There is little controlled research with these drugs, but some experiments suggest that impaired decision-making and psychometric performance are related to the use of these drugs. The drug experience is highly subjective and the presence of an altered state of consciousness may not be perceived by the novice until he is sensitized to it by his colleagues.

The incidence of adverse reactions to marihuana appears to be low. Minor side effects include immediate tachycardia and delayed bradycardia, delayed hypotension, conjunctival vascular congestion, dryness of the mouth and throat, hyperphagia, delayed gastrointestinal disturbances, and possible vasovagal syncope. More serious side effects that may occur are psychologic and include fear, panic, feelings of paranoia, disorientation, memory loss, confusional states, and a variety of perceptual alterations. Moreover, marihuana has been known to precipitate acute psychotic reactions in poorly organized personalities. The incidence of adverse effects appears to be highest in novice users of the drug. However, these adverse effects generally appear to be short-lived and self-limiting.

Apparently psychic dependence and tolerance to marihuana develop but not physiologic dependence. Experimentally, however, marihuana withdrawal has been demonstrated. Subjects who had been given large daily doses of synhexyl for 1 month, for example, demonstrated hyperexcitability when the drug was abruptly withdrawn; this excitability was relieved by readministration of the drug.

The effects of prolonged abuse of marihuana have not yet been scientifically proved. However, there seems to be some indication that amotivational states, apathy, memory problems, and some loss of mental acuity may occur. Physiologically, the possibility of chronic, long-term use of marihuana cigarettes leading to chronic bronchitis and emphysema cannot be discounted.

There has also been some question regarding the use of marihuana leading to the use of opiates, a progression termed the "stepping-stone" theory. This theory, however, appears somewhat controversial and some authorities state that any progression in drug use stems from personality and environmental factors rather than from the pharmacologic properties of marihuana. The multiple drug use theory lends support to this hypothesis, stating that a person predisposed to abuse one drug is also likely to abuse other, and perhaps stronger, drugs.

Withdrawal symptoms. Physiologic withdrawal symptoms after discontinuation of marihuana use have been produced experimentally. Whether or not marihuana produces physical dependence outside of experimental situations is still being explored. Some restlessness, anxiety, irritability, and insomnia may be associated with withdrawal of the drug, but these symptoms are generally mild and of short duration.

OPIATES

The opium derivatives comprise the most abused narcotics, although some other narcotics are also abused. The pharmacologic types of drugs that cause opiate-like dependence include the morphine group (heroin, Dilaudid, codeine), the morphinon group (racemorphan, levorphanol), the meperidine group (Demerol, Nisentil), and the methadone group. Of the opiates, heroin, codeine, and morphine are most often abused, heroin (diacetylmorphine) being the most potent of the three.

Mode of administration. The opium derivatives generally appear as a white powder and can be administered through the percutaneous route (absorption through the mucous membranes) by sniffing, in the form of subcutaneous injections (known in street language as "skin popping"), or directly intravenously ("mainlining"). The rate of absorption is correspondingly increased, with "mainlining" producing almost immediate drug effects.

Mechanism of action and effects. The opium derivatives, being narcotics, act as central nervous system depressants, probably acting on the sensory cortex, psychic or higher centers, and thalami. Because these drugs elevate mood, relieve fear and anxiety, and produce feelings of peace and tranquility, they are particularly likely to lead to physical and psychic dependence. Rapid intravenous injection of these drugs produces warm, flushing sensations described as being similar to sexual orgasm. This is followed by a soothing state that seems to be best characterized as a state of complete drive satiation. The individual "high" on opiates feels no need to satisfy drives for basic biologic needs and is often described as being "on the nod"—drowsy, content, and euphoric. The drugs do not produce hallucinogenic or psychotomimetic effects.

Physical dependence upon heroin is evident in the withdrawal syndrome that develops if the drug is withheld and in the marked tolerance that develops with continued use of the drug. Also, because persons dependent upon heroin so frequently feel satiated, physical, emotional, and social deterioration often occurs. The individuals may feel little need for food and may become grossly malnourished and weak. Preoccupation with obtaining the drug makes participation in the usual social and vocational aspects of life difficult, if not impossible. While the drug craving grows, tolerance to the drug is also marked and, eventually, the motivation for using the drug becomes oriented more to the avoidance of withdrawal symptoms and less to the achievement of euphoria.

Withdrawal symptoms. Symptoms of withdrawal from heroin are autonomic in origin and appear within 8 hours after the last dose in individuals who are physically dependent. They may originally be manifest as restlessness, chills and hot flashes, pilomotor erection on the skin (which gave rise to the term *cold turkey*), nasal secretions, drowsiness, lacrimation, sneezing, yawning, cramping of the abdomen, the back, and the lower extremities (the latter probably resulted in the phrase "kick the habit"), vomiting and diarrhea, perspiration, muscular twitching, and a craving for the drug. Such symptoms are usually followed by a restless sleep known as "yen" from which the patient may awaken irritable, weak, and depressed.

Occasionally, withdrawal symptoms are severe enough to result in cardiovascular collapse. If withdrawal is untreated, it may continue for up to 7 to 10 days, after which the physical dependence of the body upon the presence of opiates is eventually lost. Psychic dependence continues for a longer period; some authorities claim it continues forever.

Treatment of opiate dependence

Withdrawal programs. Generally, opiate withdrawal is a difficult task, and repeated relapses to drug abuse can be expected. Abrupt and complete withdrawal ("cold turkey") can be accomplished but is generally avoided as a dangerous and inhumane approach. Therapeutic withdrawal from an opiate may be somewhat more comfortably achieved by successively tapering the drug's dosage over a period of several days.

The choice of withdrawal program is partly influenced by the following factors: the patient's physical condition; the duration of drug dependence; the type of drug being taken and its daily dose; motivation for drug abuse; motivation for withdrawal; and whether the patient is also dependent on other drugs. In some instances, depending on these factors, opiate withdrawal may need to be accomplished within a hospital and with close medical supervision.

In identifying criteria for evaluating opiate withdrawal, the Council on Mental Health emphasizes that recovery from dependence of the morphine type is not to be equated with cure. Regardless of repeated relapses to drug abuse, therapeutic programs should continue. Progress in withdrawal may be indicated by progressively longer periods of abstinence from opiates without resort to the use of other psychoactive drugs and by the patient's growing confidence in his ability to function effectively without drugs.

METHADONE MAINTENANCE. A currently preferred method of withdrawal is immediate withdrawal with concurrent substitution of methadone hydrochloride, a program pioneered by Drs. Vincent Dole and Marie Nyswander. Methadone hydrochloride is a synthetic opiate analgesic that, by virtue of cross-tolerance, permits effective substitution of methadone dependence for heroin dependence. Its effectiveness against heroin dependence results from its ability to block the euphoriant effects of heroin and the craving for the drug without producing heroin's deleterious physical and mental effects. As long as methadone is administered, the individual will not experience the "kick" from a dose of heroin. When properly administered, methadone allows the individual to function adequately and without intellectual or emotional impairment. Methadone is taken orally, generally in daily doses of 100 to 180 mg. in a "carrier" of cherry syrup, orange juice, or the like. In its eighteenth report, the W.H.O. Expert Committee on Drug Dependence defined methadone maintenance as follows: "Methadone maintenance is the continuing daily oral administration of methadone under adequate medical supervision, the dose being adjusted to (a) prevent the occurrence of abstinence phenomena (b) suppress partially or completely any continuous preoccupation with the taking of drugs of the morphine-type and (c) establish a sufficient degree of tolerance and cross tolerance to blunt or suppress the acute effects of such agents."* Because the injection procedure of administering heroin ("fixing") itself may be one factor in producing dependence, the oral administration of methadone discourages dependence upon injections. Methadone is also available in pill form, known as dolophine.

---

*Council on Mental Health: Narcotics and medical practice, J.A.M.A. **218**(4):578-583, 1971.

Methadone dependence does occur, but it is less serious than heroin dependence and withdrawal symptoms are less severe. Methadone withdrawal programs generally include supplemental rehabilitation techniques such as vocational and social rehabilitation. After the individual has functioned free of heroin for a sufficient period of time, secured steady employment, and readjusted his life style, he theoretically can be withdrawn from methadone maintenance. Some treatment centers report having accomplished withdrawal from methadone through the use of chlorpromazine, while others maintain that methadone may need to be taken indefinitely. Whether the latter can be avoided is still being researched.

OPIATE ANTAGONISTS. Some drugs, such as nalorphine (Nalline), levallorphan (Lorfan), cyclazocine, and naloxone are opiate antagonists and block or diminish the effects of concurrently administered opiates, thereby facilitating withdrawal. These drugs are also useful in counteracting the respiratory depression found in narcotic overdose.

THERAPEUTIC COMMUNITY PROGRAMS. Therapeutic community programs include programs such as group psychotherapy, self-help approaches such as Synanon, and halfway houses. Because persons withdrawing from drugs frequently cannot make the transition easily, groups of persons who have decided to abstain from drug use can meet or live together in an attempt to support and guide one another through this transition. Ultimately, an individual should emerge from such a program with sufficient personal growth and appropriate support systems so that he will be able to manage his life satisfactorily without resorting to drug abuse.

NARCOTIC MAINTENANCE. In a number of countries, notably Great Britain, physicians have been permitted to prescribe opiates to persons who have a history of intractable dependence, thereby maintaining them and preventing withdrawal symptoms. Prescriptions are presently issued only through designated hospitals and only through the National Health Service. When such a system is implemented appropriately, it appears that the drug user can feel normal, function normally, and will seldom seek supplemental or illicit sources of drugs. There are, however, several reasons why such programs sometimes do not operate effectively and may be abused. Allowing the patient to determine his own dose of the drug and supplying the drug in such form and quantity that it can be easily resold or misused are examples of the ways in which such systems can be abused.

ETHYL ALCOHOL

Ethyl alcohol is one of the most abused drugs in the world and, contrary to popular opinion, is not a stimulant. Rather, it is a primary and continuous depressant of the central nervous system.

Mode of administration and pharmacodynamics. Ethyl alcohol is ingested orally and is well absorbed from the stomach and intestines. Distribution to all tissues including the brain is rapid. The drug is metabolized in the liver to acetaldehyde at the rate of 10 to 20 ml. per hour. Ninety percent is metabolized; 5% is excreted through the lungs and 5% through the kidneys.

Mechanism of action. Ethyl alcohol acts by depressing the reticular activating system, which is thought to be largely responsible for integration of central nervous system activity.

Effects. The drug can foster a pseudostimulant effect that is a consequence of hyperactivity of various parts of the brain that have been suddenly released from the inhibitory control of the cortex. Some of the first mental processes affected are those that depend on this control. Further effects of alcohol on the central nervous system are proportionately related to blood concentrations of alcohol. Memory, concentration, and finer discrimination abilities are successively lost with higher drug concentrations. Emotional lability may result with sensory-motor disturbances following. Incoordination may be accompanied by slurred speech and followed by stupor as the drug continues to cause irregular descending depression of the central nervous system. Large doses of alcohol will produce anesthesia, which may be followed by medullary paralysis. Alcohol has also been implicated as a causative factor in cardiac arrhythmias and cardiomyopathies. These conditions may result from individual sensitization.

Physiologically, ethyl alcohol causes diuresis because of depressed secretion of antidiuretic hormone and vasodilation as a result of depression of the vasomotor center.

Repeated and prolonged use of large doses of ethyl alcohol results in the development of marked tolerance and physical and psychic dependence. Malnutrition may result, because while alcohol contains calories, it contains no vitamins. Cirrhosis of the liver, gastritis, peripheral polyneuropathy, portal hypertension, and lowered resistance to disease are also common adverse effects of dependence of the ethyl alcohol type.

Another significant and potentially adverse effect of alcohol lies in the fact that it potentiates the actions of many drugs and may, therefore, be instrumental in many drug fatalities.

Withdrawal symptoms. The intensity of the ethyl alcohol withdrawal syndrome depends upon the duration of dependence on the drug and the degree of intoxication. Generally, within a few hours after the last dose of alcohol, the physically dependent person begins to experience weakness, tremulousness, anxiety, gastrointestinal disturbances, and hyperreflexia. Within 24 hours, acute alcoholic hallucinosis results, followed by disorientation, confusion, and delusional thinking. Convulsive seizures may occur and death from cardiovascular collapse may occur at the height of the withdrawal syndrome. If the person lives, recovery from the syndrome is complete by the fifth or seventh day of abstinence.

Treatment of the abrupt withdrawal syndrome may include the administration of longer-acting depressant drugs, such as pentobarbitone or paraldehyde, if the patient is seen in early stages of delirium tremens, when withdrawal is severe. Once the withdrawal symptoms are controlled, the drug dosage can be safely and progressively reduced at a rate that prevents the development of further symptoms.

Long-term treatment of alcohol dependence includes methods similar to treatment of dependence of the opiate type, such as halfway houses and therapeutic organizations like Alcoholics Anonymous.

Aversion therapy is also utilized in treatment of alcohol dependence and involves the administration of drugs to prevent complete metabolism of alcohol, thereby causing unpleasant physical symptoms. Drugs such as emetine, apomorphine, and disulfiram are used as adjuncts in the treatment of chronic alcoholism. If ethyl alcohol is administered after treatment with any of these drugs, the "aldehyde syndrome" is produced, with resulting bodily vasodilation, hypotension, pulsating headache, nausea, vomiting, diaphoresis, thirst, chest pain, vertigo, weakness, and blurred vision. If the patient wishes to avoid the experience of this syndrome, he must not ingest alcohol.

Barbiturates

Although it is not generally known by the lay public, the barbiturates and some nonbarbiturate sedative-hypnotics can cause physical as well as psychic dependence. It appears that short-acting barbiturates, in addition to drugs like glutethimide (Doriden), chloral hydrate, paraldehyde, and methyprylon (Noludar), are most likely to produce physical dependence, possibly because they produce sudden and forceful desired effects.

Because these drugs have been more extensively described in previous chapters, mechanisms of action and effects will not be explored. Rather, the focus of this section will relate to acute intoxication and withdrawal syndromes resulting from dependence on these drugs.

Both the acute and chronic effects of barbiturate intoxication resemble those of alcoholic intoxication. Manifestations may include emotional lability, muscular incoordination, difficulty in cognitive processes, and sedation. Toxic doses lead to stupor and respiratory depression. The reasons for barbiturate abuse are similar to those of ethyl alcohol abuse—both drugs produce disinhibition and mild euphoria.

The withdrawal syndrome accompanying cessation of barbiturate and previously identified nonbarbiturate hypnotic administration has been termed one of the most dangerous in the field of drug abuse. It may begin with weakness, tremulousness, restlessness, anxiety, insomnia, gastrointestinal disturbances, and orthostatic hypotension. Within the first 24 hours, the patient may be too weak to get out of bed. Symptoms may progress to confusion, delirium, and hallucinations. In addition, major convulsive seizures are more common in barbiturate withdrawal than in alcohol withdrawal. Agitation and hyperthermia may lead to exhaustion, cardiovascular collapse, and death. If the withdrawal syndrome is untreated, it generally ends by the eighth day of drug abstinence and its end is generally preceded by prolonged sleep. It is recommended that patients experiencing barbiturate withdrawal be hospitalized because, even when the syndrome appears mild, it may herald impending convulsions and cardiovascular collapse.

Treatment of barbiturate withdrawal generally consists of substitution of the drug with a longer-acting barbiturate such as pentobarbitone, the dosage of which is then slowly tapered over a period of several weeks until it is completely withdrawn.

Minor tranquilizers

The fact that the use of tranquilizers can lead to psychic dependence is well known. Less well known is the fact that the use of these drugs can also produce physical dependence similar to dependence of the barbiturate type.

Phenothiazine type tranquilizers, while not known to produce physical dependence, will result in anxiety, insomnia, and gastrointestinal disturbances if abruptly withdrawn. Drugs such as meprobamate, diazepam (Valium), and chlordiazepoxide (Librium), however, will frequently manifest withdrawal syndromes marked by the occurrence of major convulsions.

CENTRAL NERVOUS SYSTEM STIMULANTS
AMPHETAMINES

It is of interest to note that persons who are amphetamine abusers often begin the cycle of abuse inadvertently. Amphetamine dependence often begins as infrequent use of the drug to stay awake (such as by college students studying for exams, night shift workers, or overambitious achievement-oriented persons) or use of the drug for appetite control purposes. Although the use of the drug often begins for legitimate purposes and with legitimate prescription, its exhilarating effects may become so attractive as to lead to high rates of dependence.

Mechanism of action. The amphetamines are synthetic sympathomimetic amines that are chemically and pharmacologically related to epinephrine and norepinephrine. The exact mechanism by which amphetamines act is unknown, but they result in central nervous system stimulation, probably by stimulating the reticular activating system.

Preparations. Chemically, there are three types of amphetamines: salts of racemic amphetamines, dextroamphetamines, and methamphetamines, all of which vary in degree of potency and peripheral effects. Dextroamphetamine is said to have fewest peripheral effects, such as hypertension and tachycardia.

Other agents that have been called "psychotomimetic amphetamines" include dimethyltryptamine (DMT), dimethoxymethyl amphetamine (DOM), and diethyltryptamine (DET). These drugs seem to span the line between the amphetamines and lysergic acid diethylamide in producing their effects. DMT and DET produce short (1 to 2 hours) psychotomimetic reactions that are characterized by more pronounced autonomic nervous system effects than those produced by LSD. DOM (also called STP for Dr. Timothy Leary's slogan "serenity, tranquility, and peace" and for the brand name of a motor oil additive that promises added power) appears to produce longer psychotomimetic reactions (16 to 72 hours) with much more intense physiologic effects than the other two drugs.

Effects. The amphetamines are most commonly abused because they produce an elevation of mood, a reduction of fatigue, a sense of increased alertness, and "invigorating aggressiveness.'' It must be noted that amphetamines do not create extra physical or mental energy—rather, they promote expenditure of present resources, sometimes to the hazardous point of fatigue that is often unrecognized. Intravenous injection results in marked euphoria, an orgasmic feeling known as the ''flash'' or ''rush,'' a sense of great physical strength and capacity, and a sense of ''crystal-clear'' thinking. The user feels little or no need for rest, sleep, or food and may continually engage in vigorous activity that he may perceive as exhilarating and creative. To an objective observer, inefficient, stereotyped, and repetitious behavior is common during an amphetamine ''high,'' and the drug user may engage in perseverating behavior such as repeatedly reconstructing mechanical devices. Depending on the dosage of the drug taken (as much as 1.5 Gm. is known to have been injected in one dose by long-term users), the individual may experience a ''run'' of variable length, perhaps for several days. Some amphetamine users will force themselves to lie down and to close their eyes for a few hours during such a ''run'' and will also ''force-feed'' themselves in an attempt to prolong the ''run.'' Termination of the drug's use may result from a variety of factors, such as exhaustion, fright, or inability to obtain more of the drug. Withdrawal of the drug is followed by long periods of sleep. Upon awaking, the individual often feels hungry, extremely lethargic, and profoundly depressed, a phenomenon known as ''crashing.'' This phenomenon may be very severe, and the risk of suicide must be considered.

The stimulant properties of the amphetamines can cause dramatic cardiorespiratory effects, such as tachycardia, dyspnea, and chest pain. Users of amphetamines may panic because of association of these signs and symptoms with those of a myocardial infarction. To deal with these disturbing symptoms, amphetamine users often utilize depressants or ''downers.'' Some drugs, such as Dexamyl (dextroamphetamine sulfate and amobarbital) combine a central nervous system stimulant with a central nervous system depressant in an attempt to minimize the overstimulation produced by the amphetamine ingredient.

Amphetamines are also said to be psychotomimetic drugs. Although there is some conflicting evidence regarding the etiology of amphetamine psychosis, it is claimed that heavy users may develop psychosis characterized by delusions of persecution, paranoia, and fully formed visual and auditory hallucinations. Some authorities suggest that these phenomena may be related to the insomnia produced by prolonged amphetamine abuse because sleep deprivation, in and of itself, leads to psychologic disturbance such as deterioration in performance, misperceptions, and hallucinations.

In addition, marked tolerance to amphetamines occurs.

Withdrawal symptoms. Although amphetamines do not appear to lead to physical dependence, as identified by the criterion of a characteristic and reproducible withdrawal syndrome, some authorities maintain that the signs and symptoms characteristic of ''crashing'' may constitute just such a syndrome.

COCAINE

A potent central nervous system stimulant, cocaine is therapeutically used largely as a local anesthetic, since it is likely to cause toxic side effects when administered by other routes. When it is used for its stimulant effects, it produces euphoria and increased expenditure of energy similar to that produced by the amphetamines and may lead to a similar psychotic state with strong elements of paranoia.

Cocaine may be administered by sniffing the white, fluffy crystalline powder (that resembles snow, hence the name) or by direct intravenous injection. Sometimes it is mixed with heroin for heightened effects, this combination being known as a ''speedball.''

Adverse effects. Chronic use of cocaine results in nausea, weight loss, insomnia, gastrointestinal disturbances, and hyperexcitability of the nervous system with twitching or spasm of muscles, or convulsions. Prolonged sniffing of cocaine may result in perforation of the nasal septum, which results from ischemic necrosis produced by cocaine's vasoconstrictor properties.

Physical dependence does not seem to be characteristic of cocaine abuse, but strong psychologic dependence is evident.

HALLUCINOGENIC AGENTS

Classification of the most common hallucinogenic agents included: (1) those drugs containing the indole nucleus, such as lysergic acid diethylamide and its variants, dimethyltryptamine (DMT) and its analogs, and psilocybin and (2) those drugs containing the phenyl ring, such as mescaline, STP, and the anticholinergic hallucinogens.

Lysergic acid diethylamide

Lysergic acid diethylamide is a colorless, odorless, and tasteless substance that is a synthetic derivative of lysergic acid, a compound that naturally occurs in ergot and some varieties of morning glory seeds.

Therapeutic uses. A number of potentially therapeutic uses of LSD have been proposed, all of which merit more investigation. These include the drug's use in the treatment of chronic alcoholism and in the reduction of intractable pain as found in malignant disease and in phantom limb sensations. For a time, some psychiatrists also used the drug to induce psychosis, thereby helping the patient to revive repressed memories, the influence of which could then be dealt with by the patient and his therapist. The psychotomimetic effects of the drug have also generated the theory that some chemical imbalance may be involved in the etiology of schizophrenia. However, such preliminary data regarding the therapeutic uses of LSD merit much more research.

Mode of administration. LSD is usually distributed as a soluble powder and can be ingested in capsule, liquid, or tablet form. A frequent, but now obsolete, mode of ingestion was from an aqueous solution on sugar, although the drug can be licked off any object impregnated with it, such as a cookie, a stamp, or blotting paper. The drug may also be administered subcutaneously, intramuscularly, or intravenously. It is readily absorbed from the intestinal tract and mucous membranes as well as from body fluids.

Dosage. Pharmacologically, on a weight-for-weight basis, LSD is more active than almost any other drug and can be detected in the body at concentrations of 1 part per billion. The human body reacts to relatively minute doses of the drug, and 100 to 250 μg. administered orally can produce a potent experience up to 12 hours long in the majority of subjects.

Mechanism of action. LSD acts pharmacologically as a sympathomimetic agent. These effects, however, are secondary to the profound psychologic changes that it also produces. The drug is believed to be a serotonin antagonist and inactivates monoamine oxidase and acetylcholinesterase. Cross-tolerance to mescaline and psilocybin has been demonstrated. The exact biochemical mechanism of action, however, is not currently known.

Effects. The effects of LSD usually begin within 20 to 50 minutes after administration and, like effects of other mind-altering drugs, cannot be reliably predicted. Autonomic nervous system changes are relatively mild and may include tachycardia, hypertension, nausea, vertigo, and perspiration. Effects vary widely among individuals and are in part related to the dosage, the mental set of the individual, and the environment of the individual. The drug experience may also vary for the same individual from time to time; he may have a pleasant experience or a "good trip" one time, the next may be an unpleasant or "bad trip."

The initial reaction to the drug may be one of vague anxiety and sometimes nausea. Later, there are general changes of perception involving sound, sight, touch, body image, and time. The brightness of colors may be intensified, for example, and there is generally heightened awareness of the environment, creating a flood of sensations and impressions. There may be synesthesia, that is, the translation of one type of sensory experience into another sensory modality, such as "hearing a color." Every perception assumes an increased sense of significance and meaning. Changes in cognitive functioning and value judgment formation may occur (good and bad may become equal). There may be blurring of boundaries between the self and the environment, and an ineffable state of transcendence may be achieved.

However, unpleasant experiences with LSD are also rather frequent. Clinically, evidence of impaired judgment in the toxic state is frequent and examples of such behavior are well known, as demonstrated, for example, by LSD users attempting to stop traffic with their bodies. Some authorities state that if the previously described altered state of consciousness develops in the context of fear and disorganization, psychosis may occur. Moreover, one of the chief dangers of the drug is that it will precipitate a latent psychosis into activity. With the release of repressed material with which the individual cannot cope, an acute panic psychosis may result. Feelings of acute panic and paranoia during a toxic LSD psychosis can result in homicidal thoughts and actions. Toxic delirium, with altering and alternating levels of consciousness, follows toxic psychosis, and the experience generally resolves in a stage of exhaustion in which the user feels empty, unable to coordinate his thoughts, and depressed. During this time, suicide is a decided risk.

The chemical effects of LSD might be antidoted by administration of a tranquilizer, a barbiturate, or nicotinic acid. It is specifically recommended that the administration of chlorpromazine be avoided in LSD toxicity because it may accentuate anticholinergic-like drug effects and may, in high doses, lead to severe hypotension or confusion, further compounding the situation. However, the administration of medication is recommended only as an adjunct to psychotherapy of a crisis intervention nature. The latter is directed primarily to the restoration of a positive mental set under the guidance of a stable and consistent human point of reference whom the patient trusts. A "talk-down" approach in a quiet environment is often utilized and consists of directing the patient's attention away from perceptions producing panic, reassuring him that the experience will dissipate, and reassuring him that he has not permanently harmed himself. Hospital practices of administering massive doses of tranquilizers, applying restraints, and isolating such patients are to be avoided. The patient's dramatically heightened awareness of his environment and distorted perceptions may render these measures traumatic rather than therapeutic.

Markedly unfavorable reactions induced by LSD include prolonged, delayed, and recurrent reactions. The last have been described as "flashback phenomena," referring to the repetition of a previous LSD-induced experience that is unrelated to renewed administration of the drug. Moreover, a "bad trip" on LSD is likely to be a paranoid experience, and tendencies to violence can be characteristic of LSD intoxication. Research reports of chromosomal damage related to LSD ingestion are increasing, although there appears to be some variation in susceptibility to chromosomal breaks that is of unknown etiology. The drug does not seem to cause physical dependence, but tolerance to the drug occurs rapidly and psychic dependence is frequent.

Pregnant women should be especially cautioned against taking LSD. Because lysergic acid is the base of all ergot alkaloids, it has uterine stimulant properties that can adversely affect a pregnancy.

Withdrawal symptoms. Insofar as is known, LSD does not produce physical dependence, and there are no withdrawal symptoms following discontinuation of long-term use.

Mescaline

Mescaline is the chief alkaloid extracted from the peyote cactus, and it produces hallucinogenic effects similar to those produced by LSD. Like the amphetamines, mescaline belongs to the amine group and its chemical

Table 13-1 Signs and symptoms of acute drug intoxication

Drug abused	Signs and symptoms
Cannabis drugs	Tachycardia and postural hypotension; conjunctival vascular congestion; clear sensorium; distortions of perception; dryness of mouth and throat; possible panic
Opiates	Depressed blood pressure and respirations; fixed, pinpoint pupils; depressed sensorium; coma; pulmonary edema
Barbiturates and other general central nervous system depressants	Depressed blood pressure and respirations; ataxia; slurred speech, confusion; depressed tendon reflexes; coma; shock
Amphetamines	Elevated blood pressure; tachycardia; other cardia arrhythmias; hyperactive tendon reflexes; pupils dilated and reactive to light; hyperpyrexia; perspiration; shallow respirations; circulatory collapse; clear or confused sensorium; possible hallucinations; paranoid feelings
Hallucinogenic agents	Elevated blood pressure; hyperactive tendon reflexes; piloerection; perspiration; pupils dilated and reactive to light; anxiety; distortion of body image and perception; delusions; hallucinations

structure distantly resembles that of norepinephrine. It is usually ingested in the form of a soluble crystalline powder that is either dissolved or capsulated. The usual dose of mescaline is about 500 mg.

The effects of mescaline appear within 2 or 3 hours and may last 4 to 12 hours or longer. They are characterized by prodromal abdominal pain, nausea, vomiting, and diarrhea, which are followed by vivid and colorful visual hallucinations.

Psilocybin

Psilocybin is a drug derived from Mexican mushrooms *(Psilocybe mexicana)* that produce hallucinogenic effects similar to those produced by mescaline but of shorter duration.

PATHOPHYSIOLOGIC COMPLICATIONS RESULTING FROM DRUG ABUSE

Physical and psychic dependence on drugs is frequently associated with debilitated physical states caused by the user's extensive involvement in procuring and using the drug. Malnutrition, dehydration, and avitaminosis are often evident. Respiratory complications such as pneumonia, pulmonary emboli, and abscesses are frequently associated with neglect, debilitation, and the respiratory depression produced by central nervous system depressants. The intravenous administration of illicit drugs often leads to a high incidence of sepsis and hepatitis as a result of the use of contaminated equipment. In addition, cellulitis, sclerosis of the veins, phlebitis, and skin abscesses may occur. Last but not least, death from accidental overdose is not uncommon. Overdosage is a particularly significant potential danger because illegal drugs are notoriously unreliable in regard to the potency of their active ingredient. The drugs are frequently well adulterated, or "cut," by the time they reach the user. If an individual who has unknowingly been using "cut" drugs receives pure or stronger drugs, he runs the risk of toxicity and even death. Overdosage may also occur when an individual who has been withdrawn from drugs for some time (thereby having lost his accumulated tolerance) injects his previous usual dose, which now is in excess of his tolerance level.

Parenthetically, it must be said that the dose unreliability of most mind-altering drugs also affects research findings. Because dosage is difficult to control and because most drug abuse research is ex post facto, research results frequently may be skewed.

As a consequence of all of these factors, the life expectancy of persons who are physically dependent upon drugs is generally lower than that of nondependent individuals.

LEGAL ASPECTS OF DRUG ABUSE

In May, 1971, the Controlled Substances Act became effective, replacing the former Narcotics Acts and Drug Abuse Control Amendments. In July, 1973, the Drug Enforcement Agency (DEA) became the sole law enforcement agency for combating drug abuse. The DEA is charged with the responsibility of controlling narcotics and dangerous drug abuse through enforcement and prevention by working cooperatively with other federal agencies and with state and local governments. The DEA also registers physicians and those who are authorized to administer, dispense, and prescribe controlled substances.

The possession and distribution of hallucinogenics, opium poppy and straw, coca leaves, and certain opiates and opium derivatives are, of course, illegal. Since 1937, it has been illegal in the United States to possess or sell marihuana. Nevertheless, controversy exists about the classification of marihuana as a narcotic in the same category as the opiates and cocaine. Although the sale and traffic of marihuana are felonies, some states have passed statutes making the possession and use of marihuana a misdemeanor.

NURSING INTERVENTIONS RELATED TO DRUG ABUSE

The nurse may be called upon to function in any aspect of health care related to drug abuse: in prevention, in case-finding, in treatment of acute intoxication, and in long-term rehabilitation. To function with optimal effectiveness, the nurse not only needs current knowledge of drugs most frequently abused but must also add other aspects of nursing process, such as patient teaching, crisis intervention, administration of acute emergency care, and support of therapeutic and rehabilitative regimens. Because drug abuse is such a complex, multifaceted behavioral phenomenon, the nurse must relate to and treat the whole patient. Therefore, the nurse must take into account the patient's reality and his environment, and must evolve an understanding of what mind-altering drugs realistically can and cannot do.

In their preventive role, nurses may function either inside or outside the hospital environment. Within the hospital, they will be required to make decisions regarding a patient's need for a narcotic or any other drug that may produce dependence. Many nurses are reluctant to administer narcotics to a patient in pain, for example, for fear of producing dependence. The tendency to avoid the use of narcotics should not be carried to such extremes, but it behooves nurses to exercise their repertoire of skills in a therapeutic attempt before administering a narcotic. A large component of pain is one's subjective response to pain. Many patients experiencing pain are also anxious and/or depressed. It has been found that if these conditions are relieved, the physical pain will also be alleviated. When medication is indicated, if a nonnarcotic analgesic will relieve the pain, it should be administered in place of a narcotic analgesic. Or, when narcotic analgesics are indicated, return to drugs that do not produce dependence should be accomplished as soon as possible. It must be emphasized that, when other nursing interventions fail, prescribed drugs should never be withheld from patients who are experiencing physical or psychologic pain.

Preventive nursing roles both inside and outside the hospital environment also include education regarding drugs of all types, but particularly regarding drugs prone to producing dependence. The promotion of the use of functional coping mechanisms rather than the use of drugs is another crucial aspect of the nurse's preventive role in drug abuse. Persons who abuse drugs because of psychologic problems frequently have lost sight of their strength to deal with their problems in other ways. In such situations, the nurse can apply knowledge of crisis intervention and of supportive psychotherapy.

As a health professional the nurse also has a responsibility in identifying persons who are dependent on drugs in order to refer them to appropriate resources. The diagnosis of drug dependence usually is not difficult, and often the individual will admit to his need for drugs. Observation for physical signs of drug abuse will frequently yield substantial evidence. Needle marks and scars of abscesses along intravenous routes and pupillary dilation are some overt signs that are often indicative of chronic drug abuse. Signs of acute intoxication differ according to the drug abused and may manifest themselves variably, as indicated in Table 13-1. Striking changes in personality, interest patterns, and social relationships may also be indicative of drug abuse. A medical history of hepatitis, abscesses, or bacterial endocarditis may further substantiate an assumption, and diagnostic tests are available to detect the presence of some drugs in the bloodstream and in urine. Conclusive evidence of chronic drug dependence is the appearance of a withdrawal syndrome.

The nurse's role in acute drug intoxication, or in treatment of overdoses, can be twofold: support of medical therapy and/or interviewing the patient or his companions in an attempt to discover the specific agent that precipitated intoxication. With drugs increasingly being mixed, it is often difficult to identify the drug used and to provide an antidote. In such cases, persistent, patient, nonjudgmental, and painstaking probing of the patient's history may be necessary.

The nurse may also be called upon to care for a patient undergoing withdrawal, a most difficult physiologic phenomenon that requires astute observation of the patient's physical condition as well as a firm but supportive and reassuring interpersonal approach.

When withdrawal of the drug is completed, however, the role of the nurse does not terminate. Indeed, physiologic withdrawal may be defined as the starting point for meeting the problem of the patient's drug dependence. Continuing help and contact are necessary and must be maintained for a long period of time. If such help is not available, relapse to the abuse of drugs is almost inevitable.

QUESTIONS

For study and review

1 Differentiate between drug misuse and drug abuse.
2 Define physical and psychic drug dependence.
3 Identify the four major categories of drugs that are commonly abused.
4 Identify four factors that are significant in influencing the nature of an individual's experience after administration of a mind-altering drug.
5 Describe some factors that are believed to be causative in the development of drug abuse.
6 Differentiate among the following terms: hallucinogenic, psychotomimetic, and psychedelic.
7 Compare and contrast the primary forms of the cannabis drugs utilized in the United States.
8 Identify the active ingredient of the cannabis drugs.
9 Describe the effects and adverse effects produced by the cannabis drugs.
10 Describe the pharmacologic effects of the opium derivatives. Explain why these drugs can lead to dependence.
11 If heroin is withheld from an individual dependent upon the drug, what physiologic effects might the nurse expect the patient to experience?
12 Explain the rationale for the use of methadone hydrochloride, itself a dependency-producing drug, for accomplishing heroin withdrawal.
13 List three narcotic antagonists that may be used in the treatment of dependence of the opiate type.
14 Identify the effects for which the amphetamines are most frequently abused, and describe the experience of an amphetamine "high."
15 Identify the three most commonly used amphetamines.
16 Explain why high doses of amphetamines may be dangerous to persons with cardiac problems.
17 Explain why individuals who abuse amphetamines often use depressants in conjunction with these drugs.
18 Describe the psychologic effects produced by LSD.
19 Identify the currently known major adverse effects of LSD.
20 Explain why pregnant women should be especially cautioned against taking LSD.
21 Identify some therapeutic goals for which the use of LSD has been proposed.

22 Describe how LSD intoxication or a "bad trip" might be antidoted.

23 List the most common pathophysiologic complications that result from physical drug dependence and explain why they occur.

24 Explain the significance of dosage control in relation to frequently abused drugs.

REFERENCES

Abel, E. L.: Drugs and behavior, New York, 1974, John Wiley & Sons.

Baden, M. M.: Angiitis in drug abusers, New Eng. J. Med. **284:**111, 1971.

Beaconsfield, P., and others: Marihuana smoking: cardiovascular effects in man and possible mechanisms, New Eng. J. Med. **287:**209, 1972.

Council on Mental Health: Narcotics and medical practice, J.A.M.A. **218**(4):578-583, 1971.

Dimijian, G. C., and Radelat, F. A.: Evaluation and treatment of the suspected drug user in the emergency room, Arch. Intern. Med. **125:**162, 1970.

Dole, V. P.: Methadone maintenance treatment for 25,000 heroin addicts, J.A.M.A. **215:**1131, 1971.

Fort, J.: The pleasure seekers, New York, 1969, The Bobbs-Merrill Company.

Griffith, J. D., and others: Dextroemphatamine: evaluation of psychomimetic properties in man, Arch. Gen. Psychiat. **26:**97, 1972.

Hicks, R. E., and Fink, P. J.: Psychedelic drugs, a Hahnemann symposium, New York, 1969, Grune and Stratton, Inc.

Hollister, L. E.: Marijuana in man: three years later, Science **172**(3978):21-28, 1971.

Jacobsen, C. B., and Berlin, C. M.: Possible reproductive detriment in LSD users, J.A.M.A. **222:**1367, 1972.

Journal of Psychedelic Drugs

Kaufman, R., and Levy, S. B.: Overdose treatment. J.A.M.A. **227:**411, 1974.

Maugh, T. H.: Narcotic antagonists: The search accelerates, Science **177:**249, 1972.

Methadone maintenance, Med. Letter Drugs Therap. **16**(26):Dec. 20, 1974.

Morgan, A. J., and Moreno, J.: Attitudes toward addiction, Amer. J. Nurs. **73:**497, 1973.

Nelson, K.: The nurse in a methadone maintenance program, Amer. J. Nurs. **73:**870, 1973.

Pascarelli, E. F.: Methaqualone abuse, the quiet epidemic, J.A.M.A. **224:**1512, 1973.

Phillipson, R. V., editor: Modern trends in drug dependence and alcoholism, London, 1970, Butterworth & Co. (Publishers) Ltd.

Ray, O. S.: Drugs, society, and human behavior, St. Louis, 1972, The C. V. Mosby Co.

Russo, J. R.: Amphetamine abuse, Springfield, Ill., 1968, Charles C Thomas, Publisher.

Seixas, F. A., Cadoret, R., and Eggleston, S., editors: The person with alcoholism, Ann. New York Acad. Sci. **233:**Apr. 15, 1974.

Singer, A. J., editor: Marijuana: chemistry, pharmacology, and patterns of social use, Ann. New York Acad. Sci. **191:**Dec. 31, 1971.

Smith, D. E., editor: The new social drug: cultural, medical and legal perspectives on marijuana, Englewood Cliffs, N. J., 1970, Prentice-Hall, Inc.

Ungerleider, J. T.: The problems and prospects of LSD, Springfield, Ill., 1968, Charles C Thomas, Publisher.

Wilder Smith, A. E.: The drug users: The psychopharmacology of turning on, Wheaton, Ill., 1969, Harold Shaw Publishers.

Wittenborn, J. R., and others: Drugs and youth: proceedings of the Rutgers symposium on drug abuse, Springfield, Ill., 1969, Charles C Thomas, Publisher.

CHAPTER 14

Anesthetic agents

General anesthetics
Local anesthetics

Anesthetic drugs are central nervous system depressants that possess two characteristics: (1) they have an affinity for nervous tissue; and (2) their action is reversible, with cells returning to normal upon elimination of the drug from the cells. There are two major classifications for these drugs. *Local anesthetic agents* block nerve conduction when applied locally to any type of nerve tissue in any part of the nervous system and thereby abolish sensation in that region; they do not produce unconsciousness. *General anesthetic agents* are capable of producing *narcosis,* that is, stupor or loss of consciousness, and thereby general loss of sensation. Loss of consciousness is preceded by analgesia and accompanied by muscular relaxation.

GENERAL ANESTHETICS
DISCOVERY

It is more than 100 years since the first volatile anesthetics were used to produce relief of pain and unconsciousness during a surgical operation. Prior to that, agents to relieve pain were limited to alcoholic beverages and opium. The psychic as well as physical trauma associated with surgery without a good anesthetic definitely limited what the surgeon could do for a patient. Surgical skill was equated with speed. An English physician, Sir Clifford Allbutt, is quoted as follows: "When I was a boy, surgeons operating upon the quick were pitted one against the other like runners on time. He was the best surgeon both for the patient and the onlooker, who broke the three minute record in an amputation or a lithotomy."*

Nitrous oxide was discovered in 1772 by Joseph Priestley, who did not realize that the gas had anesthetic properties. Sir Humphrey Davy in 1799 suggested that because of its pain-relieving property, it might be tried in connection with surgery, but his suggestion passed unheeded for many years. Three hundred years elapsed from the time of the discovery of ether until it began to be used for the relief of pain during surgery. Dr. Crawford Long of Georgia in 1842 had a patient inhale ether while he removed a tumor from the neck. Dr. Long failed to publish a report of this administration and therefore failed to receive full credit for being the first to discover the value of ether as an anesthetic agent.

Horace Wells, a dentist, observed some of the properties of nitrous oxide and began to use it in connection with his dental practice. In 1845 he attempted to demonstrate its capacity to relieve pain during a surgical operation. The demonstration failed and his efforts were ridiculed, with the result that this useful agent received little attention for some time thereafter. It was not recognized in that day how difficult it is to produce a good level of anesthesia with nitrous oxide alone for the period of time required for a surgical operation.

In 1846 William Morton, another dentist, who later studied medicine, successfully anesthetized

*Beckman, H.: Pharmacology; the nature, action, and use of drugs, Philadelphia, 1961, W. B. Saunders Co., p. 272.

332

a patient with ether at the Massachusetts General Hospital in Boston. The success of this undertaking launched a new era in surgery.

Chloroform was discovered in 1831, and in 1847 James Simpson of England demonstrated its usefulness. Queen Victoria knighted him for his contribution to the relief of pain.

More than 80 years elapsed before any other general anesthetic gained a permanent place in anesthesia. Since 1935 many new anesthetic agents have been introduced.

ACTION OF GENERAL ANESTHETICS

General anesthetics affect all excitable tissues of the body. They vary widely in chemical structure, and there is also great variation in the concentrations required of different anesthetics to produce a given state of anesthesia. There are a number of interesting theories to explain the mechanism whereby anesthetics act.

Theories of action. Although many theories of narcosis have been proposed, none satisfactorily explains the basic mechanisms of action. Indeed, it is possible that different anesthetics have different modes of action and that no one theory will suffice.

The Overton-Meyer theory stresses the relationship between the lipid solubility of an anesthetic agent and its potency; the greater the solubility in fat, the greater the narcotic power. Since the nervous system has a high lipid content, this theory explains why anesthetics are preferentially taken up by the brain. However, not all lipid-soluble substances possess anesthetic activity, and some narcotics are not fat soluble.

In 1939 Ferguson proposed that anesthetic potency is related not to action on receptors but to thermodynamic activity, which depends on the drug concentration necessary to give a biologic effect and on the drug's solubility. When the drug reaches a certain saturation at the cellular level, it interferes with or impedes some metabolic function.

In 1961 Miller and Pauling put forth the theory that anesthetic action is essentially a physical event whereby an anesthetic reacts with the water in brain tissue to form microcrystals of ice, which then form an *ice cover* at nerve cell membranes. This blocks the passage of ions across the membranes, reducing their excitability and interfering with synaptic transmission. This event results in narcosis. It is also hypothesized that an ice cover is always present, even in the absence of an anesthetic, and that the ice cover increases as the body temperature falls. This theory provides an explanation for anesthesia caused solely by hypothermia and the need for less anesthetic drug with hypothermia.

Biochemical theories of anesthesia have also been proposed. These theories claim that there is interference with various biochemical processes such as oxidation, phosphate uptake, and synthesis of adenosine triphosphate (ATP) and acetylcholine (ACh), causing impaired synaptic transmission in the brain. Although there is some experimental support for these theories, there is also evidence against them.

Recent investigations show that some anesthetics inhibit sodium-stimulated ATPase activity in the brain, which could disturb the processes maintaining ion transport across nerve cell membranes, presumably at synapse sites. Theories that propose that anesthesia results from interference with energy utilization rather than energy expenditure tend to be more acceptable to physiologists.

When anesthesia is first induced, the concentration gradient from alveolar air to blood is steep and therefore absorption of the gas into the blood is rapid. With time, the concentration of gas in alveolar air, blood, and tissues approaches equilibrium and absorption of the gas slows. When the anesthetic is stopped, the reverse process occurs. Elimination is very rapid at first and then slower. Equilibrium of anesthetics in the fat depots of the body is more slowly reached than in other tissues and is more slowly eliminated. This effect is probably caused by the relatively small blood supply to fat depots. Alveolar walls are highly permeable to anesthetics, and free diffusion occurs between the alveolae and capillary membranes. A great deal of investigational work is being done, but regardless of the ultimate explanation, anesthesia is produced by progressively increasing the amount of the anesthetic agent, first in the blood and subsequently in the nervous system.

Unlike many other drugs, the anesthetics that

can be given by inhalation are absorbed, transported, and excreted by the body without undergoing significant chemical change. There is evidence, however, for some hepatic metabolism of many anesthetics, which is quantitatively minor. For the most part, they are exhaled and excreted by way of the lungs, except for small amounts lost by way of the kidneys and skin. They are therefore relatively safe agents, since their anesthetic effect can be rapidly reversed by elimination from the lungs, provided respiration is maintained satisfactorily. This possibility of rapid removal by breathing permits the safe use of drugs that show surprisingly small difference between an anesthetic dose and a fatal dose.

The pattern of depression is similar for all anesthetics—*irregular descending depression.* The medullary centers are depressed last. It is fortunate that the medulla is spared temporarily, since it contains the vital centers concerned with heart action, blood pressure, and respiration.

Balanced anesthesia. Balanced anesthesia should provide not only sleep but also analgesia, elimination of certain reflexes, and good muscular relaxation. The following is an example of how it can be achieved:

1 Premedication with a barbiturate, a narcotic analgesic (meperidine), and a parasympathetic inhibitor (atropine)
2 Induction using an intravenous or short-acting anesthetic (thiopental)
3 Maintenance of anesthesia using an anesthetic gas (nitrous oxide), possibly in conjunction with an intravenous barbiturate
4 Maintenance of muscle relaxation using a curare type drug or neuromuscular blocking agent (succinylcholine)

The advantages of this procedure are:

1 Rapid induction
2 Reduction in amount of drug required to maintain a desired state of anesthesia
3 Minimal adverse effects
4 Minimal disturbance of physiologic functions and of organs of detoxification and excretion
5 No need for deep state of anesthesia for optimal muscle relaxation

Factors influencing drug choice are the patient's physical condition and previous drug therapy, the operative procedure to be performed, and the estimated length of the operation.

PREANESTHETIC MEDICATIONS

Satisfactory anesthesia is partly dependent on the preparation of the patient. Preanesthetic medications are administered for: (1) sedative and amnesic effects (barbiturates and narcotic analgesics); (2) inhibition of salivary and mucous secretions (atropine and scopolamine); and (3) inhibition of anticipated undesirable side effects such as vagal stimulation (abolished by atropine) and spasms (relieved by succinylcholine).

Barbiturates may be administered the night before the operation to ensure a sound and restful sleep. Narcotics, barbiturates, or tranquilizers administered prior to the patient being taken to the operating room promote serenity, amnesia, and smooth induction. It is important that the nurse administer the medications at the time they are ordered to be given, since a narcotic given too close to the time of administration of the general anesthetic may achieve its full effect during anesthesia and cause severe respiratory depression.

Patients have been known to faint after receiving phenergan along with morphine or meperidine. Ambulatory patients receiving these drugs should be carefully watched.

PREPARATION OF THE PATIENT

Preparation of the patient for general anesthesia is very important. Vital signs should be carefully checked before the patient is taken to the operating room, and any alteration from normal should be recorded and immediately reported. The mental state of the patient should be noted and any undue anxiety or expressions of fear of death should be reported immediately. Severe anxiety or fear, unless allayed, affects both the autonomic and central nervous systems and may cause reactions that are deleterious physiologically and psychologically. These patients may resist relaxation and fight the anesthetic. A greater amount of anesthetic is therefore required, and toxic levels of drugs may be administered inadvertently. Preparation for surgical procedures should be carefully explained to patients. It may be helpful to highlight the safety factors incorpo-

Table 14-1 Preanesthetic agents

Drug classification	Agent most frequently used		Desired effect
	Generic name	Trade name	
Narcotic analgesics	Morphine Meperidine	Demerol	Sedation to decrease tension, anxiety, and provide analgesia
Barbiturates	Pentobarbital Secobarbital	Nembutal Seconal	Decreased apprehension Sedation Rapid induction
Phenothiazines	Promethazine Triflupromazine	Phenergan Vesprin	Sedation Antihistaminic Antiemetic Decreased motor activity
Anticholinergics	Atropine Scopolamine	– –	Inhibition of secretions, vomiting, and laryngospasms Sedation (with scopolamine)
Skeletal muscle relaxants	Succinylcholine d-Tubocurarine	Anectine	Promotion of muscular relaxation
Intravenous barbiturate	Thiopental	Pentothal	Rapid induction

rated in today's modern operative procedures.

Food is usually withheld after the evening meal, and standard procedure is to give the patient nothing to eat or drink after midnight. This procedure helps prevent aspiration if nausea and vomiting occur.

Patients may complain of dry mouth caused by the use of atropine or scopolamine to minimize secretions of saliva and mucus. Frequent rinsing of the mouth may be helpful. The necessity for coughing, deep breathing, and frequent turning during the postoperative period should be taught to the patient preoperatively. This preoperative teaching promotes patient cooperation postoperatively when he is asked to perform procedures that often induce pain.

REQUIREMENTS OF AN IDEAL GENERAL ANESTHETIC

The following are the requirements of an ideal general anesthetic:

1 It is highly desirable that the anesthetic agent have a sufficiently wide safety range; considerable difference should exist between the therapeutic and the toxic dose.
2 It should produce anesthesia rapidly and not be unpleasant to take.
3 Recovery should be rapid and free from discomfort.
4 It should be readily excreted from the body without damage to body tissues.
5 It should produce maximum muscular relaxation and should not increase capillary bleeding.
6 It should be of such potency that the levels of anesthesia are easily controlled and that oxygen may be administered freely with it.
7 It should be a stable substance and not explosive.
8 It should be a nonirritant and free from side effects.
9 It should not depress the cardiovascular system.
10 It should be compatible with catecholamines.

There is no known anesthetic that fulfills all of the foregoing requirements, but these criteria may be used to evaluate the properties of the various anesthetic agents.

STAGES OF GENERAL ANESTHESIA

Anesthetists have learned to observe a patient's reactions while under anesthesia and have come to know when conditions are satisfactory for surgical procedure and when a reaction constitutes a danger signal.

The stages of anesthesia vary with the choice of anesthetic, speed of induction, and skill of the anesthetist. Present-day practice of inducing anesthesia with an intravenously administered anesthetic prior to inhalation anesthesia promotes rapid transition from consciousness to surgical anesthesia, and the early stages of anesthesia are not seen. However, if the drug is given slowly enough, usually all stages can be ob-

Table 14-2 Stages and planes of ether anesthesia and selected central nervous system effects

| Central nervous system effects | Stage 1 | Stage 2 | Stage 3 planes | | | | Stage 4 |
			1	2	3	4	
Consciousness	Maintained Analgesia Euphoria Some distortion of perceptions Variable amnesia	Lost	Absent	Absent	Absent	Absent	Absent
Respiration	No alteration or increased rate with some irregularity	Rapid, irregular	Regular	Regular but expirations longer than inspirations	Diaphragmatic	Thoracic ceases Diaphragmatic depressed	No respiratory movement Respiratory paralysis
Skeletal muscles	Normal tone	Tone increased	Small muscles relaxed	Large muscles relaxed	Complete relaxation	Complete relaxation	Diaphragm paralyzed
Eye Pupils Movements Tear secretion	Reaction to light Unchanged	Dilated Increased	Constriction Increased	Mid-dilation None Decreased	None Decreased	Dilated None Absent	Dilated None
Reflexes Lid Corneal Pharyngeal "or gag" Laryngeal Cough	Present Present	Present Present	Absent Present Absent	Absent Absent Absent	Absent Absent Absent in large bronchi	Absent Absent Absent in small bronchi	Absent Absent
Heart rate		Increased	Decreased				
Blood pressure	Unchanged	Increased	Normal	Normal	Decreased	Decreased	Decreased
Venous pressure	Unchanged	Increased	Unchanged				Increased

served. They are most easily seen when ether is used as the only anesthetic. All stages may not be seen with all anesthetics. (See Table 14-2.)

Stage 1: analgesia. This stage begins with onset of anesthetic administration and lasts until loss of consciousness. Smell and pain are abolished before consciousness is lost. Vivid dreams and auditory or visual hallucinations may be experienced. Speech becomes difficult and indistinct. Numbness spreads gradually over the body. The body feels stiff and unmanageable. When ether is used alone its irritating effects may cause choking, coughing, a feeling of asphyxia, and increased secretions.

Stage 2: excitement. This stage varies greatly with individuals but begins with loss of consciousness. Reflexes are still present and may be exaggerated, particularly with sensory stimulation such as noise. The patient may struggle, shout, laugh, swear, or sing. There is an increase in autonomic activity, muscle tone, eye movement, and rapid and irregular breathing. Irregular respiration may be the cause of uneven absorption of anesthetic; a period of apnea followed by a few deep breaths may produce a toxic concentration of anesthetic in the blood. Most anesthetic deaths have occurred in this stage.

The variability in this stage results from: (1) amount and type of premedication; (2) the anesthetic agent used; and (3) the degree of external sensory stimuli. Since the advent of balanced anesthesia, excitement during induction is rare. However, this stage is important for classifying and analyzing drug effects in investigational studies.

Stages 1 and 2 constitute the *stage of induction.*

Stage 3: surgical anesthesia. The third stage is divided into four planes of increasing depth of anesthesia. Whether a patient is in one or the other of these four planes is determined by the character of the respirations, eyeball movement, pupil size, and degree to which reflexes are present or absent. Most operations are done in plane 2 or in the upper part of plane 3. (See Table 14-2.) As the patient moves into plane 1 the respiratory irregularities of the second stage have usually disappeared and respiration becomes full and regular. As anesthesia deepens, respiration

becomes more shallow and also more rapid. Paralysis of the intercostal muscles is followed by increased abdominal breathing; finally, only the diaphragm is active. The eyeballs, which exhibit a rolling type of movement at first, gradually move less and then cease to move at all. Normally, if the pupils were reflexly dilated in the second stage, they now constrict to about the size they are in natural sleep. The reaction to light becomes sluggish. The pupils dilate as plane 4 is approached.

The face is calm and expressionless and may be flushed or even cyanotic. The musculature becomes increasingly relaxed as reflexes are progressively abolished. Most abdominal operations cannot be performed until the abdominal reflexes are absent and the abdominal wall is soft. The body temperature is lowered as the anesthetic state continues. The pulse remains full and strong. Blood pressure may be slightly elevated, but in plane 4 the blood pressure drops and the pulse becomes weak. The skin, which was warm, now becomes cold, wet, and pale.

With an anesthetic such as ether the third stage (upper planes) may be maintained for hours with little change by the repeated administration of small amounts of the drug.

Stage 4: medullary paralysis (toxic stage). The fourth stage is characterized by respiratory arrest and vasomotor collapse. Respiration ceases before the heart action, so that artificial respiration may lighten the anesthetic state (if a gaseous agent has been used) and save the patient's life.

ADMINISTRATION OF ANESTHETICS BY INHALATION

Open-drop method. Liquid anesthetics, such as ether, are frequently given by dropping the anesthetic on gauze placed on a wire mask that fits over the patient's nose and mouth. The anesthetic vaporizes, mixes with air, and is inhaled. There is free access to air. No attempt is made to confine the vapor, and there is no rebreathing of the anesthetic mixture. Its major advantage is its simplicity; it can be used when no other equipment is available. This method is used only for operations of short duration or for obstetric delivery. Major disadvantages include inability to control rate of vaporization resulting in uneven anesthesia; waste of drug; fire and explosion hazard if drug is flammable; and irritation to mucous membranes or skin, causing increased secretions and burns. Another form of the open method is seen when a gaseous agent such as nitrous oxide merely flows over the patient's face.

Semiclosed method. This refers to the use of some means to decrease the escape of the anesthetic vapor. A mixture containing gases or vapors mixed with air or oxygen is inhaled from a closed mask that communicates with a reservoir or breathing bag. Recirculation of expired gases is prevented by valves. Exhalations pass through a valve on the top of the mask. There is greater retention of carbon dioxide than with the open method, but a higher concentration of anesthetic vapor is provided. This method sacrifices simplicity, and the exhaled gases may be a fire hazard.

Closed method. This method can be used for both gases and volatile liquids. An anesthetic machine is used and an apparatus fits over the nose and face of the patient, or an endotracheal tube connects the respiratory tract of the patient with the anesthetic machine, thus forming a closed system. Provision is made for removal of carbon dioxide, absorption of moisture, and regulation of the intake of the anesthetic agent or agents, as well as oxygen. Regulation of respiration by the anesthetist is made possible by the periodic and rhythmic compression of the breathing bag. The closed method affords better control of the anesthetic state, as well as greater economy of the anesthetic, since rebreathing of the mixture occurs. Minimal waste of drug makes it more economical and the fire hazard is decreased.

INHALATION AND INTRAVENOUS ANESTHETICS

Inhalation or *volatile anesthetics* are gases or liquids that can be administered by inhalation when mixed with oxygen and can effect a concentration in the blood and brain to depress the central nervous system and cause anesthesia or narcosis. (See Table 14-3.) They have the following characteristics:

1 They are complete anesthetics and thus can abolish superficial and deep reflexes.
2 They provide for controllable anesthesia since depth of anesthesia is easily varied by changing the inhaled concentration.
3 Allergic reactions to these agents are uncommon.
4 Rapid recovery can occur as soon as administration ceases since the anesthetic is excreted in expired air.

Intravenous or *nonvolatile anesthetics* (also called basal anesthetics) include organic solids or liquids that are water soluble and lend themselves to intravenous or intramuscular injection or rectal instillation. Although they can produce loss of consciousness, cortical activity is not completely interrupted, a number of reflexes remain active, and patients respond to painful stimuli. These are not controllable anesthetics. Nonvolatile anesthetics are suitable only for basal narcosis.

INHALATION GENERAL ANESTHETICS
Ether, U.S.P., B.P. (diethyl ether)

Ether is a clear, colorless liquid with a pungent odor and a bitter, burning taste. It is formed by the action of sulfuric acid on ethyl alcohol. It is highly volatile and very flammable. Mixtures of ether and air or ether and oxygen are explosive. It is decomposed by light, air, and moisture and should therefore be kept in sealed metal containers. Ether is a good solvent for fats, oils, resins, and adhesive plaster.

Action and result. Ether may have either a local or systemic action.

Local. When applied to the skin and allowed to evaporate, ether has a cooling effect. If it is not allowed to evaporate, it reddens the skin and acts as a rubefacient. Ether irritates mucous membranes and causes increased secretion of mucus, saliva, and tears. When moderately dilute, it acts as a carminative in the digestive tract. Nausea and vomiting may result from gastric irritation or from central stimulation of the vomiting center.

Systemic. The systemic action of ether has been described in the presentation of the stages

Table 14-3 Properties of major inhalation anesthetics

Properties	Ether (diethyl)	Chloroform	Halothane
Inflammable and explosive	Yes	No	No
Induction	Slow—unpleasant	Rapid—pleasant	More rapid than ether—pleasant
Recovery	Slow	Rapid	More rapid than ether
Mucous membrane irritant	Yes—coughing, laryngeal spasms, profuse mucous secretions	Less than ether	Nonirritant
Sympathetic stimulant	Yes	No	No
Increased capillary bleeding	Yes	No	No
Cardiovascular effects: Sensitization of myocardium to epinephrine Heart rate Blood pressure	No Decreased in plane 3 Decreased in plane 3	Yes—may cause arrhythmia Decreased Decreased	Yes Bradycardia Hypotension
Skeletal muscle relaxation	Excellent	Good	Not adequate when used alone
Postoperative effects	Nausea, vomiting	Nausea, vomiting, possibly permanent liver and kidney damage	Rare (a few cases of severe liver damage have been reported)
Use	Major and prolonged operations Obstetric labor	Not common	Widely used, often used with nitrous oxide

of anesthesia. Ether has an action similar to that of curare at the myoneural junctions (see p. 366). It is said to be the only anesthetic to possess this action. When ether and a member of the curariform drugs are used together, the dose of the latter must be reduced. The induction period is comparatively slow, and the period of recovery is longer than for a number of other general anesthetics. Nausea and vomiting are common in the recovery phase.

For a time, ether makes the heart beat faster and stronger. In the deeper planes of surgical anesthesia the myocardium is directly depressed. Ether produces peripheral vasodilation. As a result there may be oozing of blood from the cut edges of skin during and after surgery. Blood pressure is lowered as anesthesia deepens. The skin feels warm, and the face is frequently flushed. Sudden, marked pupil dilation is regarded as a danger signal, since it may mean the beginning of respiratory failure. Of course, the size of the pupil may be modified by the action of the preanesthetic drugs such as morphine and atropine.

Some effect on the kidney is indicated by the presence of albumin in the urine and scanty urine formation for several hours after anesthesia. Postoperative urinary retention may result from poor tone in the bladder. There is no evidence that ether causes any damage to the liver.

Contractions of the uterus are not much affected by moderate degrees of anesthesia, but they are slowed and decreased by deep anesthesia. Ether is not an entirely satisfactory anesthetic to relieve the pain of childbirth, because its analgesic effect cannot be obtained fast enough. There are better analgesics for this.

In the early stages of anesthesia there may be sufficient stimulation of smooth muscle of the gastrointestinal tract to cause nausea and vomiting. During moderate or deep surgical anesthesia ether produces diminished peristalsis and tone of smooth muscle of the gastrointestinal organs. This effect is sometimes responsible for the development of distention. Early ambulation helps prevent intestinal accumulation of gas.

Recovery from ether anesthesia proceeds in reverse order; the patient goes from the stage of surgical anesthesia through the stage of excitement and on through the stage of analgesia before becoming fully conscious. The nurse must make sure that the patient's face is turned to the side to prevent aspiration of mucus or vomitus. No patient should ever be left alone until he is fully conscious.

The sense of hearing returns comparatively early. This is a fact worth noting by attendants, who might discuss the patient's medical status, assuming that he is still unconscious. Postanesthetic doses of morphine or similar narcotics should be withheld until the gagging, swallowing, and coughing reflexes have fully returned. Return of function of these reflexes coincides with the return of consciousness.

Uses. Ether is now infrequently used as a general anesthetic. A combination of nitrous oxide gas, oxygen, and ether (G-O-E) is used for surgical anesthesia. Nitrous oxide is used for induction to avoid the unpleasant suffocating effects of ether and the excitement of the second stage. Ether can be used to check convulsive seizures associated with tetanus and strychnine poisoning. It is used as a fat solvent to cleanse the skin prior to surgical procedures.

Preparation, dosage, and administration. The dose of ether depends upon the patient, the length of operation, and the depth of anesthesia to be maintained. Only unopened sealed containers of ether should be used for anesthesia.

Ether is administered in any of the ways mentioned under administration of anesthetics in this chapter. It is often given by the open-drop method, although the closed system is also employed, especially if ether is combined with other agents.

Side effects and toxic effects. Acute toxicity caused by overdosage may occur during administration. If induction occurs too rapidly there may be a temporary respiratory arrest. Removal of the mask or facepiece is usually all that needs to be done. Respiration is usually resumed at the normal rate. Prolonged administration of ether may result in respiratory depression and respiratory failure. The pulse becomes feeble and irregular, and the blood pressure drops. The skin becomes cold, clammy, and gray. The pupils dilate widely and do not react to light. Other dangers associated with ether anesthesia are those that arise from aspiration of mucus or vomitus or from some other form of airway obstruction.

Treatment of overdosage is prevented by keeping the patient in the lighter planes of surgical anesthesia. Oxygen and artificial respiration will hasten elimination of the ether and lighten the anesthesia.

Advantages. Ether is considered to be a relatively safe anesthetic. There is a wide margin of safety between the anesthetic and toxic dose. It brings about excellent muscular relaxation. It is said that if anesthetists could have but one anesthetic agent they would probably choose ether.

Disadvantages. Ether is flammable and potentially explosive. It is irritating to mucous membranes and unpleasant to inhale. The recovery period from ether anesthesia may be unpleasant because of nausea and vomiting.

Contraindications. Although ether has long been thought to be contraindicated in pulmonary disease, this opinion has, to some extent, been reversed. Ether depresses activity of the vagus nerve, which is desirable in thoracic surgery. When ether is administered in a closed system with adequate amounts of oxygen and continual removal of carbon dioxide and when steps are taken to prevent accumulation of secretions in the bronchial tubes and trachea, this anesthetic seems to serve satisfactorily for thoracic surgery even when pulmonary disease is present. Its use is not recommended for patients in acidosis or for those who have advanced renal disease. Unless special precautions are taken it should not be administered when an open flame or cautery must be used.

Drug interactions. Certain antibiotics such as neomycin and polymyxin B have neuromuscular blocking action. Ether may intensify this block in patients taking these antibiotics preoperatively. This potentiation may cause respiratory arrest. Patients receiving adrenergic blocking drugs such as phenoxybenzamine or propranolol preoperatively may not be able to maintain optimal level of blood pressure or cardiac output during anesthesia.

Chloroform, N.F., B.P.

$$H-\underset{\underset{Cl}{|}}{\overset{\overset{Cl}{|}}{C}}-Cl$$

Chloroform is a heavy, clear, colorless liquid. It has a characteristic odor and a sweet taste. It is prepared by the action of chlorine on alcohol or by the direct chlorination of methane. It should be protected from bright light when stored. It is not flammable, and when mixed with oxygen it does not form an explosive mixture. It is incompatible with catecholamines.

Action and result. Chloroform, like ether, progressively depresses the central nervous system. Depth of anesthesia is difficult to judge since the classic signs of depth do not apply to chloroform. Chloroform is more pleasant to inhale than ether. It provides a faster induction and is not as irritating to mucous membranes, since a lower concentration can be used. It provides excellent muscular relaxation. It is excreted mainly from the lungs much the same as ether.

Uses. Chloroform is little used in the United States. It is used more often in tropical countries as an emergency anesthetic and for surgical or obstetric patients, where it is difficult to give ether by the open-drop method because of its high volatility. In the United States it has been replaced by safer anesthetics.

Preparation and dosage. Chloroform is marketed in brown bottles to retard decomposition.

The solution is sweet-smelling and colorless and contains 99% to 99.5% chloroform. The remainder consists of alcohol. Dosage is determined on an individual basis.

Side effects and toxic effects. Chloroform is said to have caused five times as many deaths as ether. It may disturb the rhythm of the heart and cause it to slow or to stop beating. This effect is thought to be preventable by the proper use of atropine. Chloroform has also been blamed for damage of the liver and the kidney. Some authorities are of the opinion that the dangers of chloroform have been exaggerated and believe that, because of its advantages, its status should be reevaluated. They maintain that with present-day facilities for supplying adequate oxygen and removing carbon dioxide, chloroform is not necessarily more toxic than a number of other anesthetics.

Halothane, U.S.P., B.P. (Fluothane)

$$F-\underset{\underset{F}{|}}{\overset{\overset{F}{|}}{C}}-\underset{\underset{Br}{|}}{\overset{\overset{Cl}{|}}{C}}-H$$

Halothane is a volatile, nonflammable, nonirritating general anesthetic whose potency is said to be about twice that of chloroform and four times that of ether. Induction with this agent is made rapidly and smoothly, and during recovery the return of consciousness is also rapid. Pharyngeal and laryngeal reflexes are easily suppressed; therefore, there is little likelihood of complications such as laryngospasm, coughing, or bronchospasm. Since the agent is nonirritating, and because it depresses salivary and mucous secretions, there is little or no increase in bronchial and salivary secretions. Muscular relaxation is moderately satisfactory; muscle relaxants are sometimes needed to promote adequate relaxation. There is a low incidence of postoperative nausea and vomiting.

Preparation, dosage, and administration. Halothane is administered by closed inhalation. The drug is usually vaporized with oxygen or an oxygen–nitrous oxide mixture; 1% to 2% halothane concentration will maintain surgical anesthesia.

Side effects and toxic effects. Some degree of hypotension has been noted with most patients. Severe hypotension may result from a suddenly increased concentration of the anesthetic or when deep planes of anesthesia are attempted. Alterations in the cardiac rate and rhythm are frequently produced by halothane, the most common of which is a slow pulse. This can usually be prevented by the administration of atropine or a related type of drug. Halothane sensitizes the cardiac muscle to epinephrine and levarterenol; therefore, the administration of these drugs during anesthesia with halothane is avoided. Anesthetists are using ephedrine, phenylephrine, or methoxamine to combat hypotension.

Respiration is frequently depressed, and the depression progresses with increasing depth of anesthesia. Uterine contractions during labor cease. Halothane apparently does not harm the kidneys. However, patients who develop jaundice after exposure to halothane should not be reexposed to this drug. Severe, even fatal, liver damage has occurred in a few individuals following halothane anesthesia. It is difficult to avoid the impression of a causal role of the anesthetic in some of these cases. Halothane is such a potent anesthetic that the margin of safety between the toxic dose and the therapeutic dose is not great.

Uses. Halothane is widely used. It can be used alone or with nitrous oxide and muscle relaxants for a wide variety of operations.

Advantages. Halothane is nonexplosive, does not burn, provides rapid induction and rapid recovery, is nonirritating, has a relatively pleasant odor, and depresses salivary and bronchial secretions. It is potent and can be given with adequate amounts of oxygen. Patients may need respiratory assistance, but completely controlled respiration is easily achieved.

Disadvantages. Halothane is a strong respiratory and circulatory depressant. It causes vasodilation, hypotension, and tachypnea (rapid, shallow respirations) in the upper planes of anesthesia. In addition, the drug is expensive. It is destructive to steel, rubber, and plastic materials if the liquid drug is permitted to come in contact with them.

Contraindications. Halothane is contraindicated in most obstetric deliveries, and in patients with known hepatic or biliary disease.

Nitrous oxide, U.S.P., B.P. (Nitrogen Monoxide)

Nitrous oxide, one of the oldest and safest anesthetics, is a colorless gas somewhat heavier than air, with a slight odor and a sweetish taste. It long has been known as "laughing gas." It is unique among volatile anesthetics in that it is an inorganic compound (contains no carbon atoms) and is made from ammonium nitrate. It is nonflammable and nonexplosive, but at sufficiently high temperatures it will dissociate, release oxygen, and support combustion.

Action and result. The central nervous system is the only part of the body that seems to react to nitrous oxide. When the gas is mixed with air and inhaled it produces an effect similar to that of a mild intoxicant. The patient feels merry, laughs, and talks, but he does not go to sleep.

When the pure gas is inhaled, the patient first feels warm, numb, dizzy, and confused. Vivid dreams and hallucinations may be experienced. After a few deep inspirations the patient becomes pale and soon loses consciousness. If administration is continued the patient becomes cyanosed and death results from asphyxia. The upper planes of surgical anesthesia are reached in 1 or 2 minutes, but by this time the patient is already becoming seriously depleted of oxygen. Respirations are deep and rapid, later becoming irregular and shallow. If administration is stopped before cyanosis is marked, consciousness is regained rapidly. Because many untoward effects are associated with anoxia, administration of undiluted nitrous oxide is not recommended. Anesthesia can be safely prolonged when a mixture of 35% oxygen and 65% nitrous oxide is used, but this combination is insufficiently potent to produce satisfactory surgical anesthesia without premedication for many operations. Higher concentrations may be used during induction or for brief intermittent use during labor. Nitrous oxide has no untoward effects on circulation, respiration, and the liver or kidneys unless oxygen deficiency is allowed to develop and persist. Nitrous oxide does not irritate the respiratory mucous membrane. Muscular relaxation is not as complete as it is with ether or cyclopropane, and a neuromuscular blocking agent must be used for procedures requiring muscular relaxation. It does produce excellent analgesia.

Uses. If nitrous oxide were more potent it would probably be regarded as an ideal anesthetic. Due to its excellent analgesia it can be given with oxygen to produce analgesia in dental procedures, surgical procedures that are brief and do not require muscular relaxation, and obstetrics. It is also used as an agent for induction prior to the use of other anesthetics. Its greatest use is as a component of balanced anesthesia for prolonged or complicated surgery.

Preparation and administration. Nitrous oxide is available in the compressed state in steel cylinders for closed system administration. It is also available for self-administration during childbirth. The brief use of 100% nitrous oxide during contractions and 100% oxygen between contractions can produce analgesia without decreasing uterine contractions or maternal oxygen saturation.

Side effects and toxic effects. Nitrous oxide itself is a very innocuous substance and has remarkably low side and toxic effects. It can cause bone marrow depression with prolonged administration. If anoxia occurs it is probably the result of poor technique and not the gas itself. The disadvantage of nitrous oxide is its low anesthetic potency, although this can be remedied by proper use of supplemental agents.

Ethylene

$$H_2C=CH_2$$

Ethylene is a colorless, highly volatile gas with a slightly sweet taste and an unpleasant but not intolerable odor. When mixed with a certain amount of oxygen it is highly explosive and flammable. However, it is believed to be no more explosive than ether-oxygen or ether-oxygen–nitrous oxide mixtures when comparable precautions are taken. Ethylene was first used for clinical surgery in 1923.

Action and result. Induction is smooth and rapid. Ethylene is less powerful as an anesthetic than either ether or cyclopropane but slightly more potent than nitrous oxide. It is difficult to reach more than plane 1 or possibly plane 2 of surgical anesthesia with ethylene.

Ethylene does not irritate the respiratory mucosa, and it does not increase salivary secretion. The patient awakens readily when administration of ethylene is stopped. Respiratory depression and vasomotor depression are uncommon, and postoperative complications are rare.

Uses. Because of its explosiveness, the availability of more potent anesthetics, and its slight increase in potency over nitrous oxide, the use of ethylene has been almost abandoned.

Preparation and administration. Ethylene is available in steel tanks in which the gas is kept under pressure. It is administered with oxygen in a closed system technique with a gas machine. It is important for the patient to receive a preliminary medication so that adequate amounts of oxygen may be given during anesthesia to prevent hypoxia.

Disadvantages. The chief disadvantage associated with the use of ethylene is the hazard of fire and explosion. As is true of certain other anesthetics, the time of greatest danger is at the end of the operation, when the mask is lifted from the patient's face. For this reason no one should touch the anesthetist or the anesthetic machine other than those constantly working with the patient or with the machine. A small spark of static electricity may set off an explosion. This precaution applies to all explosive mixtures.

Cyclopropane, U.S.P., B.P.

$$H_2-C \overset{\displaystyle CH_2}{\textstyle\diagup \ \ \diagdown} C-H_2$$

Cyclopropane is a colorless gas, heavier than air, flammable, and explosive in most anesthetic concentrations when mixed with air or oxygen. It has a mildly pungent but not unpleasant odor. It is stable and is stored in metal cylinders where, under pressure, it liquefies easily.

Action and result. Cyclopropane is a potent anesthetic. Adequate amounts of oxygen can be given with it, to the extent of 20% or more, and it will still produce satisfactory anesthesia. A wide margin of safety exists between the anesthetic and the toxic dose. Induction is pleasant and rapid. It does not irritate the respiratory

Table 14-4 Properties of gaseous anesthetics

Properties	Cyclopropane	Nitrous oxide
Inflammable and explosive	Yes	No—but supports combustion
Induction	Rapid	Rapid
Recovery	Rapid	Rapid
Results in increased capillary bleeding	Yes	No
Sensitization of myocardium to epinephrine	Yes—may cause arrhythmia	No
Skeletal muscle relaxation	Adequate at deep levels of anesthesia	Poor when used alone
Postoperative effects	Nausea and vomiting Excitement and laryngospasm may occur	Anoxia if oxygen supply inadequate (should be prevented)
Use	Widely used	To induce anesthesia For brief anesthesia (dental extraction) Principal agent in balanced anesthesia

mucous membrane. There is little change in respiration until deep depression is produced. Laryngospasm occasionally develops; therefore, atropine or scopolamine is likely to be prescribed as a preliminary medication. Cyclopropane produces a fair amount of muscle relaxation, although the supplemental effect of a muscle relaxant may be required. Uterine and intestinal muscles are not affected unless the patient is in the lower planes of surgical anesthesia.

Uses. Cyclopropane has been used successfully as a general anesthetic for a wide variety of operations. It has been approved as an anesthetic for chest surgery in which quiet respirations and absence of bronchial irritation are important. It is also used in obstetrics, since it can be administered in amounts that do not affect uterine activity or the respirations of the child. Its explosiveness has limited its use in favor of newer, nonflammable agents. However, it is still often selected for patients in shock or impending shock.

Preparation and administration. Stored in steel cylinders, cyclopropane is administered by inhalation preferably with the use of the closed system because it is both expensive and explosive.

Side effects and toxic effects. As anesthesia with cyclopropane deepens, disturbance of cardiac rhythm may occur. Sudden death has been known to result. This effect seems to be related to the development of hypoxia and the retention of carbon dioxide. It can be prevented by maintaining adequate ventilation. The incidence of nausea, vomiting, and postoperative distention is said to be less than after ether anesthesia but more than that seen after anesthesia with nitrous oxide or ethylene.

**Vinyl ether, N.F., B.P.
(Divinyl Ether, Vinethene)**

$$H-C=C-O-C=C-H$$
$$\quad\ |\ \ |\qquad\ |\ \ |$$
$$\quad\ H\ H\qquad H\ H$$

Vinyl ether is a clear, colorless fluid that greatly resembles ether. It is more volatile but about as flammable and explosive as diethyl ether. Partial decomposition may occur when it is exposed to light and air.

Action and result. Vinyl ether rapidly depresses the central nervous system, which means that the toxic stage is also reached rapidly. To prevent overdosage the patient must be watched with more than usual care. Induction is rapid and smooth, and surgical anesthesia is produced two or three times more quickly than with ordinary ether. Continuous administration is necessary to maintain anesthesia; otherwise, the patient promptly recovers consciousness. The effects on respiration and circulation are similar to those produced by diethyl ether. It produces satisfactory muscular relaxation with minimal respiratory irritation.

Uses. Vinyl ether is used especially for minor operations or surgical procedures of short duration. It is sometimes used as an induction agent prior to the administration of another anesthetic. It is a useful anesthetic in dentistry, for postpartum repair work, and in surgery of the ear, eye, nose, and throat.

Preparation and administration. Vinyl ether is available in 10-, 25-, 50-, and 75-ml. bottles with droppers. It can be administered by the open-drop, semiclosed, and closed methods.

Side effects and toxic effects. This drug has a narrow safety range and can cause liver and kidney damage. It may cause increased flow of saliva, even after the administration of atropine. It is contraindicated in the aged and for patients with hepatic or renal insufficiency. It may cause convulsions and should not be used in patients with a convulsive disorder. It is particularly important to prevent hypoxia during its administration, since lack of oxygen is believed to be the cause of the hepatic damage. Repeated administration of vinyl ether after short intervals or prolonged administration at any time is not recommended. Nausea and vomiting seldom occur.

Methoxyflurane, N.F., B.P. (Penthrane)

$$H-\overset{\displaystyle Cl}{\underset{\displaystyle Cl}{C}}-\overset{\displaystyle F}{\underset{\displaystyle F}{C}}-O-CH_3$$

Methoxyflurane is an inhalation anesthetic suitable for both induction and maintenance of anesthesia. It is not flammable or explosive in any concentration mixed with air or oxygen at operating room temperatures. It is a colorless liquid with a boiling point of 104.65° C. and it has a fruity odor. It is stable in light and in the presence of oxygen, moisture, and carbon dioxide absorbers. Methoxyflurane can be administered by any of the usual techniques—closed, semiclosed, and open-drop. Induction is slow and recovery prolonged. It produces as good muscle relaxation as does diethyl ether. When muscle relaxants are used with it, they should be administered in less than the usual dose. Since it is a halogenated compound, there is the possibility it may cause acute or delayed liver and kidney damage; its administration in the presence of liver disease is contraindicated.

Fluroxene, N.F. (Fluoromar)

Fluroxene is a derivative of vinyl ether with an odor similar to vinyl ether. Fluroxene is a volatile liquid. It is explosive and flammable but its flammability is thirty times less than that of ethyl ether. It provides a more rapid and pleasant induction than ethyl ether. Potency and depressant effects are less than those of halothane. It can be used alone or with nitrous oxide; it is used primarily for minor surgery not requiring profound muscle relaxation. This is not a widely used anesthetic.

Trichloroethylene, N.F., B.P. (Trilene)

This is a nonflammable, nonirritating, volatile liquid with an odor similar to chloroform. It is a potent analgesic and used primarily for this purpose in obstetrics and minor surgical procedures and as an analgesic for ambulatory patients (such as for relief of trigeminal neuralgia). It can be self-administered. It is not suitable for major surgery since it is cardiotoxic and causes arrhythmias and is a poor muscle relaxant.

Ethyl chloride, N.F., B.P.

$$C_2H_5Cl$$

Ethyl chloride is a colorless, highly volatile liquid with an agreeable odor and a sweetish, burning taste. It is flammable and explosive and should be kept from any contact with fire.

Ethyl chloride is a powerful, rapid-acting general anesthetic. It closely resembles chloroform in its effects, but it acts more rapidly. It does not provide complete muscular relaxation. Because of the ease with which the anesthesia progresses beyond the surgical stage and because of the danger of cardiac arrest associated with its administration, it is rarely used except for short and minor procedures.

Ethyl chloride also acts as a local anesthetic. After it is sprayed on the area to be anesthetized, it evaporates so rapidly that it freezes the underlying tissues and produces insensibility to pain. It thus permits incision and drainage of boils, carbuncles, and the like. The edema and erythema that result from the thawing of the tissues can be rather painful.

Enflurane (Ethrane)

Enflurane is a relatively new, nonflammable, and very stable anesthetic that has gained widespread popularity. Clinical anesthesia with enflurane resembles that of halothane and methoxyflurane but muscular relaxation is more pronounced and tachypnea is uncommon. Enflurane is thus superior to halothane for abdominal surgery. Only a small amount of the drug is metabolized, and renal and hepatic toxicity have not been reported. Enflurane sensitizes the myocardium to catecholamines. Some degree of arterial hypotension commonly occurs.

INTRAVENOUS ANESTHETICS

Intravenous anesthesia means the induction of unconsciousness by a nonvolatile anesthetic or hypnotic before the production of surgical anesthesia. Intravenous anesthetics are valuable to allay emotional distress, since many patients dread having a tight mask placed over the face while they are fully conscious. These anesthetics reduce the amount of general anesthetic required. The principal drug used for this purpose is thiopental sodium.

The intravenous anesthetics most commonly used are the ultrashort-acting barbiturates. These drugs are rapidly taken up by brain tissue because of their high oil-water solubility. For example, equilibrium between brain and blood occurs

within 1 minute after injection of thiopental. Shortness of action results from the drug being quickly redistributed into the fat depots of the body. Amount of body fat affects drug action. The greater the amount of body fat, the briefer the effect of a single intravenous dose. However, with prolonged administration or large doses, there is prolonged drug action resulting in delayed recovery; this is caused by saturation of fat depots and the slow rate of drug release (10% to 15% per hour).

Advantages for using intravenous anesthetics include the rapidity with which unconsciousness is induced, amnesic effects, prompt recovery with minimal doses, and simplicity of administration. They are nonirritating to mucous membranes and use is not accompanied by the hazard of fire or explosion.

Disadvantages of using this type of anesthetic include tissue sloughing and necrosis if drug infiltrates into tissue; thrombosis if arterial injection occurs; and hypotension, laryngospasm, and respiratory failure from overdosage or prolonged administration.

Thiopental sodium, U.S.P. (Pentothal Sodium); thiopentone, B.P.

Barbiturates are used both as general anesthetics and as basal anesthetics. Thiopental sodium is an ultrashort-acting barbiturate and seems to be the most popular. Its use has steadily increased since it was first introduced by Dr. John S. Lundy in 1934.

Action and result. Thiopental sodium produces loss of consciousness in seconds. Induction is smooth, easy, and pleasant for the patient. Recovery is uneventful and rapid, and complications are rare. Opinion has been expressed that the experienced, skillful anesthetist finds the control of anesthesia with this agent as easy or easier than with many of the anesthetics given by inhalation. Abdominal relaxation is likely to be inadequate even with deep anesthesia, and if used as a general anesthetic it is frequently supplemented with one of the curariform drugs. Due attention must be given to the possible dangers of hypoxia, obstruction of air passages, and respiratory depression.

Uses. Thiopental sodium is used as a basal anesthetic to carry the patient through the period of induction prior to the use of an anesthetic given by inhalation or injection. It is also used in combination with a number of other drugs for many kinds of minor and major surgery. It may be given by intermittent intravenous injection along with a muscle relaxant and nitrous oxide and oxygen.

Preparation, dosage, and administration. Thiopental sodium is marketed in glass ampules containing 0.5, 1, 5, or 10 Gm. of the powder with anhydrous sodium carbonate, which acts as a buffer and makes the resulting solution less irritating to tissues. Thiopental sodium is unstable when in solution and must be freshly made. The usual adult dose is 2 to 4 ml. of a 2.5% solution; it is given intravenously in about 10 to 15 seconds and is repeated in 30 to 60 seconds as required until the desired effect is obtained. A 40% solution is sometimes given rectally as a basal anesthetic for children (30 mg. per kilogram of body weight). Induction dosage of a 2% solution for children is as follows: 1.5 ml. for children weighing 15 kg.; 3 ml. for children weighing 30 kg.; 4 ml. for children weighing 40 kg.; and 5 ml. for children weighing 50 kg.

Side effects and toxic effects. The rapid onset of action of this barbiturate is both a desirable effect and a potential danger. Medullary paralysis may develop rapidly when an overdose is given. The drug also has a tendency to produce laryngospasm. This can be prevented or handled successfully with the use of atropine or succinylcholine or by the use of endotracheal intubation. Although some difference of opinion seems to exist as to how thiopental is metabolized, there seems to be agreement that it is detoxified chiefly in the liver and the metabolic products are excreted by the kidney. This accounts for the prolonged emergence phase associated with this drug. Its use is not recommended for patients with severe heart disease, hepatic disease, anemia, or respiratory difficulties. Its use is absolutely contraindicated in patients hyper-

sensitive to barbiturates and those with porphyria.

Propanidid, B.P.

Propanidid has been recently introduced by clinical investigation as an intravenous anesthetic. It is a phenoxy-acetic acid derivative. Propanidid is a water-insoluble, yellow oil available in a 0.5% solution. It has a rapid action. Onset of action usually occurs in 20 to 25 seconds. Following a single injection, consciousness is regained in about 4 minutes.

Sodium thiamylal; sodium methohexital

Sodium thiamylal (Surital Sodium) and sodium methohexital (Brevital Sodium) are ultrashort-acting barbiturates with properties similar to those of thiopental.

ADJUNCTS TO ANESTHESIA AND DISSOCIATIVE ANESTHESIA

In recent years various drugs have gained popularity as preanesthetic agents. These include droperidol (Inapsine), fentanyl (Sublimaze), and the combination of droperidol and fentanyl (Innovar). The latter combination is used to produce *neuroleptic anesthesia,* which is characterized by (1) quiescence, (2) disinterest and detachment from the environment without loss of consciousness or ability to communicate, and (3) decreased skeletal muscle activity. Droperidol may be used alone to treat nausea and vomiting.

Ketamine, a new intravenous anesthetic, has been introduced as a "dissociative anesthetic"; it has both analgesic and amnesic properties.

Droperidol, N.F. (Inapsine)

Droperidol is related to haloperidol, which is pharmacologically similar to the phenothiazine psychotherapeutic drugs. Droperidol was first synthesized in Belgium after a long period of research for a potent, short-acting, well-tolerated neuroleptic drug for use in anesthesiology.

A parenteral injection of droperidol produces tranquility and detachment without loss of consciousness, although the patient may experience considerable drowsiness. Voluntary movements are markedly decreased. As a preoperative medication, droperidol significantly decreases the incidence of postoperative nausea and vomiting in patients given strong opiate analgesics. It may cause a moderate degree of tachycardia; in large doses it may cause hypotension because of a vasodilating effect. When administered alone it has *no* analgesic effect.

After intravenous or intramuscular administration, onset of action occurs in 3 to 10 minutes and lasts 6 to 8 hours. Most of the drug is metabolized in the liver and excreted via the urinary and intestinal tracts.

Uses. Droperidol is used preoperatively, and during induction and maintenance of anesthesia as an adjunct to general or regional anesthesia.

Dosage. Adult preoperative dose, intravenous or intramuscular, is 2.5 to 10 mg. given 30 to 60 minutes before induction of anesthesia. To reduce incidence of postoperative nausea and vomiting, 1.25 to 2.5 mg. may be given.

Side effects. Common side effects of droperidol are extrapyramidal symptoms (tremors, flexed arms, extended neck, upward rotation of eyes, etc.) and hypotension. Mild to moderate hypotension and tachycardia may occur immediately after administration; severe hypotension may occur postoperatively. Patients have also experienced hallucinations and nightmares when given droperidol postoperatively. Other reported side effects include dizziness, chills, facial sweating, and restlessness.

Cautions. Droperidol should be used with extreme caution in elderly or debilitated patients and in those with cardiovascular disorders.

Drug interactions. Droperidol can potentiate the action of narcotics, barbiturates, anesthetics, tranquilizers, alcohol, and other central nervous system depressants. When droperidol is used with other depressants, dosage of each drug should be reduced.

Fentanyl citrate, U.S.P. (Sublimaze)

Fentanyl is a strong narcotic analgesic that has morphine-like action. It has a faster onset but shorter duration of action than morphine. After intramuscular injection, onset of action occurs in 5 to 15 minutes; duration of action is 1 to 2 hours. After intravenous injection, peak action occurs in 3 to 5 minutes; duration of action is 30 to 60 minutes. Most of the drug is metabolized in the liver.

Because of its short duration of action, fentanyl is not recommended for the same uses as morphine. It is used preoperatively for minor and major surgery, urologic procedures, and gastroscopy.

Dosage. Preoperative dose is 0.05 to 0.1 mg. given intramuscularly; the same dose can be given postoperatively every 2 to 3 hours.

Side effects. A variety of side effects can be produced by fentanyl including euphoria, miosis, nausea, vomiting, pruritus, constipation, hypotension, and respiratory depression. Rapid intravenous injection or large doses may cause muscle rigidity and apnea. Succinylcholine may be used to counteract these effects. Levallorphan or nalorphine can be used to counteract respiratory depression; it must be remembered, however, that these drugs will also overcome the analgesic effect of fentanyl.

Precautions. The patient must be closely observed for signs of respiratory depression and muscle rigidity. Drugs for counteracting adverse effects should be immediately available as well as equipment to support respiration.

Drug interactions. Central nervous system depressants (sedatives, hypnotics, tranquilizers, alcohol) potentiate the respiratory and sedative effects of fentanyl. If any of these drugs are used with fentanyl, dosage of each drug should be markedly reduced one fourth to one third.

Droperidol and fentanyl (Innovar)

The preparation of droperidol and fentanyl, Innovar, consists of 1 part fentanyl to 50 parts droperidol: 0.05 mg. of fentanyl to 2.5 mg. droperidol per milliliter. It is available in 2- and 5-ml. ampules.

Innovar is used to produce neuroleptic anesthesia. Droperidol is a neuroleptic drug with prolonged action; fentanyl is a narcotic analgesic with a very short duration of action. This combination produces quiescence, reduced response to painful stimuli, and decreased motor activity. This state permits the patient to undergo short procedures requiring a conscious and cooperative patient, such as bronchoscopy and cystoscopy, without pain. Innovar is also used as a premedication for anesthesia and as an adjunct for induction and maintenance of anesthesia.

Dosage. Recommended dosage for preoperative medication is 0.5 to 2.0 ml. given intramuscularly 45 to 60 minutes preoperatively depending upon the patient's weight, age, and physical status. The first two or three doses postoperatively may be one half the preoperative dose.

Side effects. The fentanyl component of Innovar may cause severe respiratory depression, and extrapyramidal symptoms (tremor, akathisia, etc.) may be caused by the droperidol component. Apnea, laryngospasm, bronchospasm, bradycardia, and hallucinations may also occur.

Cautions. Innovar should be used cautiously in children; in patients with impaired liver, kidney, or pulmonary function; and in those who are poor surgical risks. It probably should not be used for patients with parkinsonism.

Innovar should not be administered with other psychosedatives, hypnotics, or strong analgesics because of possible additive or potentiating effects increasing the risk of hypotension and respiratory depression.

The fixed-dose combination of droperidol and fentanyl is controversial and disapproved of by some authorities. Repeated injections of Innovar after induction can result in droperidol overdosage.

Ketamine hydrochloride, N.F. (Ketalar, Ketaject)

Ketamine is a rapid-acting nonbarbiturate intravenous anesthetic. It is a derivative of the psychotomimetic drug phencyclidine (Sernylan). Ketamine acts on the mid brain within the reticular formation; it produces analgesia and amnesia but not muscular relaxation. Ketamine has been called a "dissociative anesthetic"; that is, it produces a cataleptic state in which the patient appears to be awake but detached from his surroundings and unresponsive to pain. The patient's eyelids usually do not close, nystagmus is common, and there may be slight involuntary and purposeless movements. After recovery, the patient does not recall the experience. Since ketamine causes hypertonus, muscle tone in the oropharynx is maintained and airway obstruction caused by relaxation of soft tissues seldom occurs; mechanical stimulation may cause laryngospasm. Respiration is usually not depressed.

Ketamine is a potent cerebral vasodilator; it increases both cerebral blood flow and cerebrospinal fluid pressure.

Uses. Ketamine has its greatest usefulness for diagnostic studies in children and for repeated anesthesia in burned children. It is best suited for short diagnostic or surgical procedures. Ketamine is also recommended for induction of anesthesia when a barbiturate is contraindicated. Its adverse effects limit its usefulness in adults.

Preparation and dosage. Ketamine is prepared in concentrations of 10, 50, and 100 mg. per milliliter. It is usually given intravenously in doses ranging from 1 mg. to 4.5 mg. per kilogram of body weight for induction of anesthesia. Onset of action is rapid, occurring in less than 1 minute; duration of action is 5 to 10 minutes. When given intramuscularly the usual dose is 6.5 to 13 mg. per kilogram of body weight. Onset of action is about 5 minutes; duration of action from 12 to 25 minutes.

Side effects and precautions. Ketamine can cause numerous side effects and therefore a number of precautions are necessary with this drug.

Psychologic effects. Emergence from ketamine anesthesia may be accompanied by unpleasant dreams, hallucinations, and emergence delirium. Patients may show irrational behavior, excitement, confusion, or euphoria. These reactions occur more frequently in adults than in children or the elderly. These effects are less likely to occur with intramuscular administration of the drug. These psychic reactions usually last only a few hours; however, recurrences may occur up to 24 hours postoperatively. If nurses and recovery room personnel protect the patient from visual, tactile, and auditory stimuli during recovery, the incidence of psychic effects may be reduced. Ketamine should not be given to neurotic or psychotic patients.

Cardiovascular. Ketamine has pressor effects, which may result from liberation of catecholamines. It increases heart rate and cardiac output and elevates systolic and diastolic blood pressures. This necessitates caution when ketamine is given to elderly patients with arteriosclerosis; and it is contraindicated in patients with severe hypertension. Bradycardia and

Table 14-5 Drug-induced reactions to anesthetics

Type of drug	Example of drug		Reaction	Prevention
	Generic name	Trade name		
Antihypertensives	Bretylium Reserpine Guanethidine	Darenthin Ismelin	Circulatory depression Reduced cardiac output Hypotension Bradycardia	Use of vasopressors during anesthesia
Antidepressants	Pargyline Tranylcypromine Phenelzine	Eutonyl Parnate Nardil	Hypertension Potentiation of action of narcotics, hypnotics	Avoid use of narcotics and barbiturates with these drugs
Adrenergics	Epinephrine Norepinephrine		Cardiac arrhythmias Tissue slough when used with local anesthetics	Avoid use with anesthetics that sensitize myocardium to catecholamines, (halothane, cyclopropane)
Antibiotics (parenteral)	Neomycin Kanamycin Streptomycin		Enhancement of neuromuscular blockade Muscle paralysis, apnea, bradycardia, hypotension	
Adrenal steroids	Cortisone Cortisol		Adrenal insufficiency and hypotension during stress of surgery after prolonged use Circulatory collapse	Administer steroids preoperatively and if necessary during surgery and postoperatively
Tranquilizers (phenothiazines)	Chlorpromazine Promazine	Thorazine Sparine	Potentiation of action of narcotics, hypnotics Central nervous system depression Hypotension Respiratory depression	Use minor tranquilizers with no adrenergic blocking effect Reduce dosages of drugs and anesthetics
Pituitary hormones	Oxytocin Vasopressin	Pitocin Syntocinon Pitressin	Coronary vasoconstriction Myocardial ischemia Hypotension	
Ergot alkaloids	Ergonovine Methylergonovine	Ergotrate Methergine	Potentiation of effects of vasopressors used to overcome hypotension caused by spinal anesthesia Severe hypertension during third stage of labor	Use pressor drugs sparingly in obstetric patient

hypotension may also occur. Severe arrhythmias occur rarely.

Respiratory. Although respirations are usually not depressed by ketamine, severe respiratory depression and apnea may occur with high doses given rapidly by intravenous injection.

Neurologic. Ketamine enhances skeletal muscle tone, and this may cause fasciculations and tremors. Convulsions have also been reported. Ketamine also increases cerebrospinal fluid pressure. It should not be used in patients with convulsive disorders or in those in whom an increase in cerebrospinal fluid pressure could be disastrous.

Gastrointestinal. Nausea and vomiting may occur but is usually not severe; patients are able to take liquids shortly after regaining consciousness.

General. Local pain and redness at injection site have been reported.

Drug interactions. Ketamine is formulated in slightly acid solutions and should not be injected in the same syringe with a barbiturate. The latter is alkaline and the mixture will form a precipitate.

Ketamine appears to be clinically compatible with commonly used general and local anesthetics.

DRUG-INDUCED REACTIONS TO ANESTHETICS

Treatment of disease with a variety of drugs having varying degrees of potency and diverse effects on body systems establishes a propensity for drug-induced reactions to anesthetics. Interactions between drugs and anesthetics may be responsible for anesthetic morbidity and mortality. Certain drugs and anesthetic agents are hepatotoxic, and their administration to the same patient can result in severe and even fatal liver damage. Drugs that have depressant effects on cardiac function in conjunction with the depressant action of anesthetics can cause decreased cardiac output and hypotension, which may result in ventricular fibrillation or cardiac arrest. Drug-induced reactions to anesthesia are not uncommon and not decreasing; indeed, this problem appears to be rapidly increasing. Not all drug interactions occur during anesthesia; some reactions are delayed or latent. The nurse needs to closely observe postoperative patients for undesirable signs and symptoms. Early detection and treatment of drug interactions may be vital.

POSTOPERATIVE COMPLICATIONS AND NURSING CARE AFTER GENERAL ANESTHESIA

Common postoperative complications. A wide variety of signs and symptoms may be observable in the postoperative patient. Nurses should be aware of the more common postoperative complications and the possible causative factors to enable them to determine effective modes of intervention.

Hypotension may result from an excess of nonvolatile drugs that depress the vasomotor center. Avoid use of narcotics; these may increase the hypotension. However, severe pain can cause hypotension; in these cases a narcotic may both alleviate pain and increase the blood pressure.

Nausea and vomiting may be caused by stimulation of the vomiting center as a result of anoxia during anesthesia.

Hypoventilation may result from excess or cumulative effects of drugs administered during anesthesia. It may be a lingering effect of neuromuscular blocking agents.

Oliguria caused by anesthesia is very common, as are *atony and urinary retention* after perineal and genital operations.

Nerve injury may follow spinal anesthesia or malpositioning during general anesthesia. Brachial, radial, ulnar, and perineal nerves are most likely to be injured.

Intestinal distention and at times paralytic ileus may occur from the anesthetic agent, postoperative sedation, or a combination of both. *Thrombosis* may also be observed.

Important in the postoperative period are protection of the patient from injury until he has fully responded and maintenance of a patent airway. Patients should be closely observed for signs and symptoms of shock, a not uncommon postoperative complication. Early detection of impending shock with institution of proper therapy may prevent or at least modify its severity. Rate, volume, and rhythm of the pulse should be noted as well as the patient's color and skin temperature. A rapid, thready, weak pulse, cyanosis or extreme pallor, cold and clammy skin, and low blood pressure are characterisitic signs of shock. The patient should be checked for bleeding at the operative site; if he continues to lose blood postoperatively, hemorrhagic shock may occur. Postoperative shock may also result from extensive surgical trauma, prolonged operating time, prolonged deep anesthesia, or even inadequate anesthesia. Patients should be adequately ventilated postoperatively to prevent atelectasis. Heavy smokers in particular are likely to have postoperative chest complications.

Other important factors to keep in mind are the following:

1. Patients on steroid therapy in the immediate postoperative period have an increased risk of infection and possible delay in wound healing. Asepsis is important with these patients.

2. Antihypertensive drugs can cause the blood pressure to be erratic when certain other drugs are given. For example, an overshoot can occur with vasopressors, and a precipitous fall may occur with narcotics or depressants. If antihypertensive therapy was discontinued preoperatively, hypertensive crisis might occur postoperatively.

3. Phenothiazine drugs given in large doses over a long period of time prior to surgery may cause the patient in the immediate postoperative period to have a prolonged recovery.

4. Antibiotics (neomycin, polymyxin) in large doses can have a curariform effect.

5. Patients who were on long-term anticoagulant therapy have a high hemorrhage risk when surgical procedures are performed on them. Blood and vitamin K should be available and the patient closely observed for any bleeding tendency.

6. Patients who have had ketamine anesthesia should be protected from unnecessary visual, tactile, and auditory stimuli to help prevent excitement and psychic reactions during emergence from anesthesia.

7. If droperidol is given to control nausea and vomiting, the nurse should remember that it has *no analgesic effect.* An analgesic will be needed to control pain. However, since droperidol po-

tentiates the action of narcotics, the narcotic dose should be reduced. The nurse's judgment in these cases is important.

8. Succinylcholine may cause muscle pains postoperatively. This pain is more likely to occur if the patient is ambulated within 24 hours after the drug has been administered. Several studies indicate that confining the patient to bed for the first 24 hours postoperatively decreases the incidence of muscle pains. This pain is believed to be caused by the initial muscle fasciculations.

9. Succinylcholine can cause prolonged muscle weakness, particularly in the respiratory muscles.

LOCAL ANESTHETICS

Local anesthetics are drugs used to abolish pain sensation in a particular part of the body. Basic mechanism of action of these drugs is unknown, but most of these drugs act by stabilizing or elevating the threshold of excitation of the nerve cell membrane without affecting resting potential. This action is a result of reduction of membrane permeability to all ions; thus depolarization and transmission of nerve impulses are prevented. Local anesthetics are capable of abolishing all sensation, but pain fibers are affected first, probably since they are thinner, unmyelinated, and more easily penetrated by these drugs. Loss of pain is followed in sequence by loss of response to cold, warmth, touch, and pressure. Most motor fibers can also be anesthetized when there is sufficient concentration of the drug over a long enough period of time.

The concentration of local anesthetic needed to block conduction of nerve impulses is much less than the concentration of local anesthetic in the blood that would cause death, but even relatively small doses of local anesthetics reaching the heart or brain may cause serious reactions. For this reason, effort is made to confine the local anesthetic to a limited region or small area near a nerve or among nerve endings. The action of the local anesthetic is reversible; it is followed by complete recovery and, as a rule, produces no damage to the nerve cells.

REACTIONS TO LOCAL ANESTHETICS

Local anesthetics produce vasodilation by direct action on blood vessels and by anesthetizing sympathetic vasoconstrictor fibers. This action can cause rapid absorption of the drug; when rate of absorption exceeds rate of elimination, toxic effects can occur. To decrease rate of absorption and incidence of toxic effects by allowing more time for metabolic degradation and to prolong local anesthetic effects, epinephrine or other vasoconstrictor drugs are used. Dosage of the latter drugs must be carefully determined to prevent ischemic necrosis at the injection site. Since local anesthetics are potentially toxic drugs, a patient's age, weight, physical condition, and liver function must be taken into account in determining drug dosage.

Most reactions to local anesthetics result from overdosage, rapid absorption into systemic circulation, and individual hypersensitivity or allergic response.

Central nervous system. At first the central nervous system may be stimulated and cause anxiety, restlessness, confusion, dizziness, tremors, and even convulsions. Then depression may occur and unconsciousness and death may ensue.

Cardiovascular system. Myocardial depression, bradycardia, and hypotension can occur because of smooth muscle relaxation and inhibition of neuromuscular conduction. The patient suddenly becomes pale, feels faint, and has a drop in blood pressure. Cardiac arrest can be the end result of a cardiovascular reaction.

Allergic reaction. True allergic reactions are said to be uncommon. Sometimes a reaction is thought to be allergic when it is really caused by overdosage. However, allergic reactions can occur. They may be relatively mild (hives, itching, skin rash) or they may be of an acute anaphylactic nature. Small test doses are frequently given by the physician to gauge the extent of the patient's sensitivity to the anesthetic agent. The anesthetic agent chosen, its concentration, the rate of injection, and physical and emotional factors in the patient all influence reactions to local anesthetics.

PREPARATION OF THE PATIENT

Preliminary medication is frequently prescribed prior to the use of a local anesthetic, much the same as before a general anesthetic. The use of a barbiturate is believed to prevent or decrease toxic reactions.

Table 14-6 Local anesthetics—administration and use

Method	Tissue affected	Preparation used	Examples of drugs used	Therapeutic use
Topical	Sensory nerve of mucous membranes and dermis	Solution Ointment Cream Powder	Cocaine Benzocaine Butacaine	Relieve pain or itching Examination of conjunctiva
Infiltration	Sensory nerve endings in subcutaneous tissues or dermis	Injection	Procaine Lidocaine	Minor operations
Block	Nerve trunk	Injection	Procaine Lidocaine	Dental and limb operations Muscle relaxation
Spinal	Spinal roots	Injection	Pontocaine Dibucaine	Abdominal operations Muscle relaxation

METHODS OF ADMINISTRATION OF LOCAL ANESTHETICS

Some local anesthetics are suited only for surface anesthesia, some must be injected, and some are suitable for both topical administration and injection. See Table 14-6. To minimize toxicity from local anesthetics, the smallest amount of the lowest effective concentration should be used.

Surface or topical anesthesia. Surface or topical anesthesia is restricted to mucous membranes, damaged skin surfaces, wounds, or burns. The local anesthetic is applied in the form of a solution, ointment, cream, or powder to produce loss of sensation by paralyzing afferent nerve endings. Local anesthetics do not penetrate unbroken skin. Topical anesthesia is used to relieve pain and itching and to anesthetize mucous membranes of the eye, nose, throat, or urethra for minor surgical procedures. Cocaine in a 4% to 10% solution continues to be one of the most widely used agents for topical anesthesia.

Anesthesia by injection. Anesthesia by injection is accomplished by infiltration, conduction, spinal, caudal, and saddle block.

Infiltration anesthesia is produced by injecting dilute solutions (0.1%) of the agent into the skin and then subcutaneously into the region to be anesthetized. Epinephrine is often added to the solution to intensify the anesthesia in a limited region and to prevent excessive bleeding and systemic effects. Repeated injection will prolong the anesthesia as long as it may be needed. The sensory nerve endings are anesthetized. This method of administration is used for minor operations such as incision and drainage or excision of a cyst.

Conduction or block anesthesia means that the anesthetic is injected into the vicinity of a nerve trunk that supplies the region of the operative site. The injection may be made at some distance from the site of surgical procedure. A single nerve may be blocked or the anesthetic may be injected in a location where several nerve trunks emerge from the spinal cord (paravertebral block). A more concentrated solution (2%) is required because of the thickness of nerve trunk fibers. This method of anesthesia is often used for operations on the foot and hand.

Spinal anesthesia is a type of extensive nerve block, sometimes called a subarachnoid block. The anesthetic solution is injected into the subarachnoid space and affects the lower part of the spinal cord and nerve roots.

Spinal anesthesia. For *low spinal anesthesia* the patient is placed in a flat or Fowler's position. A solution with a specific gravity greater than that of spinal fluid is used, since it tends to diffuse downward. For high spinal anesthesia the Trendelenburg position with the head sharply flexed is used in conjunction with an anesthetic solution of lower specific gravity than that of spinal fluid (which tends to diffuse upward) or a solution with the same specific gravity as spinal fluid (may diffuse upward or downward, depending upon position used). Solutions with the same specific gravity as spinal fluid act primarily at the site of injection.

Onset of anesthesia usually occurs within 1 to 2 minutes after injection. Duration of anesthesia is 60 to 180 minutes, depending upon the anesthetic used. Spinal anesthesia is used for surgical procedures on the lower abdomen, inguinal area, or lower extremities; it may be the method of choice for patients with severe respiratory problems or with liver, kidney, or metabolic disease. Marked hypotension, decreased cardiac output, and respiratory inadequacy tend to occur during anesthesia and are considered to be disadvantages of this method of anesthesia.

Postoperatively, headache is the most common complaint; this may be accompanied by difficulty in hearing or seeing. Headache may be postural and occur only in the head-up or sitting or standing position. This symptom is the result of the opening in the dura made by the large spinal needle, which may persist for days or weeks, permitting loss of cerebrospinal fluid. Headache and auditory and visual problems following lumbar puncture result from decreased intracranial pressure. These symptoms are usually alleviated when spinal fluid pressure returns to normal. Paresthesias, such as numbness and tingling, may occur after spinal anesthesia; these are usually located in the lumbar or sacral areas and disappear within a relatively short period of time. The success and safety of spinal anesthesia depend primarily upon the anesthetist's skill and knowledge.

Caudal anesthesia is produced by injecting an anesthetic solution into the caudal canal, the sacral part of the vertebral canal containing the cauda equina, or bundle of spinal nerves that innervates the pelvic viscera. It is used in obstetrics and for operations on pelvic or genital organs. Its advantage over spinal anesthesia is that the anesthetic does not have direct access to the spinal cord and medullary centers. Thus the respiratory muscles and blood pressure are not directly affected, and undesirable effects are less likely to occur.

Saddle block is sometimes used in obstetrics and for surgery involving the perineum, rectum, genitalia, and upper parts of the thighs. The patient sits upright while the anesthetic is injected, after a lumbar puncture has been done. The patient remains upright for a short time until the anesthetic has had a chance to be effective. The parts that would have been in contact with a saddle when riding become anesthetized, hence the name.

LOCAL ANESTHETICS
Cocaine, N.F., B.P.; cocaine hydrochloride, U.S.P., B.P.

Cocaine is one of the oldest local anesthetics and the prototype of all local anesthetics. It is an alkaloid derived from the leaves of the coca shrub, which grows in Peru, other parts of South America, and the Far East. The native people have been known to chew the leaves to give them added energy and ability to endure fatigue. In medicine, cocaine is used chiefly in the form of cocaine hydrochloride, which occurs as a white crystalline powder that is freely soluble in water and alcohol.

Action and result. Cocaine has both local and systemic actions.

Local action. Cocaine is unrivaled in its power to penetrate mucous membranes to produce surface anesthesia of the eye, nose, and throat. It is two to three times more potent than procaine. Onset of action is immediate, occurring within 60 seconds; duration of action is about 1 hour. It also causes local vasoconstrictor actions. Applied to the eye it causes pupil dilation; applied to the tongue it removes the taste of bitter substances; applied to nasal mucosa the sense of smell is paralyzed. It is usually not used with epinephrine since cocaine possesses vasoconstrictor action.

Systemic action. Today it is not recommended that cocaine be injected for anesthetic effects because of its toxicity. However, its systemic effects are of interest since it is one of the drugs often abused. Cocaine potentiates the effects of norepinephrine by inhibiting its uptake into the sympathetic nerve terminals from which it is liberated. This effect causes a higher concentration of norepinephrine and increased sympathetic stimulation. Cocaine may also inhibit monoamine oxidase, the enzyme that inactivates catecholamines. In addition, cocaine has a direct stimulant action on the central nervous system and autonomic centers in the brain.

As a result of its stimulant action, there is a feeling of euphoria, increased mental and muscular power, and increased resistance to fatigue. The individual is more talkative and active. The pulse is stronger and faster, blood pressure is elevated, respirations are faster and deeper, and vomiting may occur.

Toxic effects. Toxic doses of cocaine cause hyperexcitability and convulsions. Depression of the central and autonomic nervous systems follows stimulation.

Body temperature may increase 3° to 5° C. as a result of increased muscular activity, decreased heat loss as a result of vasoconstriction, and direct action of cocaine on the temperature-regulating center. Death is usually caused by respiratory failure but circulatory failure may also occur.

Treatment includes the control of convulsions by the administration of a muscle relaxant such as succinylcholine, evacuation of the stomach if the drug has been taken orally, and artificial respiration.

Uses. Cocaine is used chiefly for surface anesthesia of the nose and throat. Since cocaine causes opacity of the cornea and retards corneal epithelial regeneration, its use in ophthalmology has been virtually abandoned.

It is also injected in low concentrations for the removal of tonsils and similar procedures, although some authorities do not recommend its administration by injection.

Preparation and dosage. Concentrations of 1% to 4% are used for surface anesthesia of the eye and 5% to 10% for mucous membranes of the nose and throat. Cocaine crystals moistened in epinephrine hydrochloride solution for placement on the nasal mucosa prior to surgical operation in the nose is considered a dangerous procedure. A 0.2% concentration is the strength usually used for injection.

Cocaine dependence. Dependence on cocaine evidently occurs as a result of its ability to produce euphoria and an illusion of power and superiority that enables an individual to forget the inadequacies and drabness of his life.

A difference exists between dependence on cocaine and dependence on morphine or opium derivatives. Cocaine users tend to be gregarious and euphoric; drug taking tends to be intermittent; there is minimal or no abstinence syndrome, since tolerance or physical dependence does not occur with the use of cocaine. However, cocaine dependence leads to more rapid mental, moral, and physical deterioration than morphine dependence. Cocaine dependence can produce a strong paranoid psychosis along with heightened excitement and energy that cause the cocaine user to not only see enemies everywhere but also to physically attack them. Traditionally, cocaine has been taken in the form of snuff ("snow") which may cause ulceration, gangrene, or perforation of the nasal septum because of prolonged vasoconstriction. It is now more common for users to inject the drug intravenously and to mix it with heroin. Continued use of the drug results in chronic poisoning. The earliest effects may be digestive disturbances and loss of appetite and weight, but the nervous system suffers most, and gradual degeneration of mind and morals usually results. Sleeplessness, tremors, spasm, delirium, and psychoses are some of the consequences of long-continued use. To help combat the danger of dependence, cocaine and all its derivatives are classified as Schedule II drugs under the Controlled Substances Act. (See chapter on drug abuse.)

Procaine hydrochloride (Novocain)

$$NH_2$$

$$O=C-O-\overset{\overset{\displaystyle H}{|}}{\underset{\underset{\displaystyle H}{|}}{C}}-\overset{\overset{\displaystyle H}{|}}{\underset{\underset{\displaystyle H}{|}}{C}}-N\overset{\displaystyle C_2H_5}{\underset{\displaystyle C_2H_5}{}}$$

Procaine is a synthetic local anesthetic. Many synthetic local anesthetics have points of similarity in their chemical structure; they are amino esters of aromatic acids. Procaine is a white powder that is readily soluble in water. In solution it withstands sterilization with heat, although a precipitate may form when the solution stands for a long time.

Procaine is less potent than cocaine but also less toxic. It is rapidly destroyed by enzymes in the blood and other tissues. It does not constrict blood vessels and does not dilate the pupil of the eye. It produces no particular central action like cocaine, and it is not dependence producing.

Uses. Procaine is the best known of the local anesthetics and it is said to be the safest for both nerve block and infiltration. It is probably used more than any other single local anesthetic. Reactions occur comparatively seldom and tend to be mild; elimination is rapid and tissue damage is seldom produced. Procaine is not well absorbed from mucous membranes; hence, it is not suited for topical administration. It is useful for many types of local anesthesia when given by injection. Procaine hydrochloride has been used to overcome cardiac arrhythmias, although procainamide is used more often for this purpose.

D.E.S.I. rating for procaine is: *effective* for local anesthesia by infiltration injection, nerve block, caudal or epidural block, and for spinal anesthesia; *possibly effective* for analgesia by intravenous injection and for antispasmodic, antipruritic, and antiarrhythmic action.

Preparation and dosage. The following are the procaine preparations available.

Procaine hydrochloride, U.S.P., B.P. This is available as a white crystalline powder intended for parenteral solutions.

Procaine hydrochloride injection, U.S.P.; *procaine and adrenaline injection,* B.P. The U.S.P. preparation is available in concentrations of 1%, 2%, and 10% procaine hydrochloride. It may or may not contain epinephrine.

The dosage of procaine used for anesthesia varies with the technique of administration employed. Concentrations of 1% or 2% are adequate for most purposes, although concentrations of 0.25% to 0.5% may be used for infiltration. The duration of anesthesia for a nerve block is about 45 minutes and for spinal anesthesia about 1 hour. The 10% solution is used for spinal anesthesia.

Lidocaine hydrochloride, U.S.P. (Xylocaine Hydrochloride); lignocaine hydrochloride, B.P.

Lidocaine hydrochloride is another synthetic local anesthetic. It is said to produce effects more promptly and with greater intensity than those produced by an equal amount of procaine. Lidocaine is suited for surface anesthesia as well as for infiltration and block anesthesia. Common side effects are sleepiness and dizziness.

D.E.S.I. rating is *effective* for the following: (1) spinal anesthesia, (2) peripheral or caudal anesthesia, (3) nerve block, (4) infiltration anesthesia, (5) dental block, and (6) topical anesthesia of the nose, mouth, and upper digestive tract.

Preparation and dosage. Solutions are available in 0.5% to 4% concentration for injection, with or without epinephrine hydrochloride. A 2% jelly is used for mucous membranes of the urethra, and a 5% ointment is available for application to burns and skin lesions. The jelly has a D.E.S.I. rating of *possibly effective.*

Toxic effects. In low concentrations its toxicity is thought to be about the same as that of procaine. It has an advantage of being effective in small amounts of low concentrations. Overdosage may result in many of the toxic symptoms associated with local anesthetics, such as drop in blood pressure, nausea, vomiting, pallor, apprehension, muscular twitching, and convulsions. Lidocaine is contraindicated in patients with blood dyscrasias.

Drug interactions. Lidocaine enhances the neuromuscular blocking action of succinylcholine, decamethonium, and tubocurarine. The reason for this interaction is not known.

Chloroprocaine hydrochloride, N.F. (Nesacaine Hydrochloride)

Chloroprocaine is more potent and rapid than procaine. It has relatively low toxicity.

Preparation and administration. Solutions of chloroprocaine for injection in 1%, 2%, and 3% concentrations are available.

The drug is not a potent surface anesthetic.

It apparently can be given in all the ways that procaine can be given by injection, although its use for spinal anesthesia has not been fully evaluated.

Toxic effects. Its toxic effects are said to be similar to those produced by procaine. Several cases of thrombophlebitis have been reported after intravenous injection of chloroprocaine. Since it does not produce vasoconstriction, its toxicity can be decreased by giving it with epinephrine to delay absorption.

Cyclomethycaine sulfate, B.P. (Surfacaine)

Cyclomethycaine sulfate is used as a topical anesthetic for certain types of skin lesions and abrasions in which discomfort is caused by pain and itching. It is also used on vaginal, urethral, and rectal mucous membranes to reduce pain from fissures and ulcerations.

Preparation and administration. Cyclomethycaine sulfate is available in preparations that include a topical cream and ointment, a urethral jelly, topical solutions, and suppositories. The concentration of the drug in various preparations varies from 0.25% to 1%. Suppositories contain 10 mg. of the drug.

Tetracaine hydrochloride, U.S.P. (Pontocaine Hydrochloride); amethocaine hydrochloride, B.P.

Tetracaine hydrochloride is a synthetic local anesthetic, the effects of which are said to be more potent and more prolonged than those of procaine. It is also more toxic. Its ability to penetrate mucous membranes far exceeds that of procaine; it approaches that of cocaine. It can be employed in dilute concentrations and serves as a useful anesthetic for a number of purposes. It can be used to produce surface anesthesia of the eye, nose, and throat, as well as for infiltration and spinal and caudal anesthesia. Effects are believed to be more prolonged than those with procaine.

Preparation and dosage. Tetracaine hydrochloride is available in solutions of various concentrations and also in tablets. An official ophthalmic ointment, 0.5% in white petrolatum, is also available. The concentration used varies with the part to be anesthetized; a 0.5% solution is commonly employed for the eye, a 1% or 2%

Table 14-7 Properties of commonly used local anesthetics

	Cocaine	Procaine	Benzocaine
Trade names	–	Novocain	Benzocaine Anesthesin
Potency	Two to three times more potent than procaine		Very low
Onset of action	1 min.	2 to 5 min.	Immediate
Duration of action	1 hr.	1 hr.	During contact only
Dose	1% to 4% topically 5% to 10% for anesthesia of nose and throat	0.25% to 2%, depending upon method of administration 10% for spinal anesthesia Not used topically	Variable 5% to 10% ointment topically
Toxicity	Four times more toxic than procaine when injected subcutaneously	Least toxic of all local anesthetics	Relatively nontoxic
Precautions	Not recommended for infiltration, nerve block, or spinal anesthesia Repeated use causes psychic dependence Repeated use in eye may cause clouding, pitting, and ulceration of cornea	Overdose or rapid injection may cause stimulation	Suitable for topical use only Sensitization may develop

solution for mucous membranes of the nose and throat, 0.5% is used for spinal anesthesia, and 0.15% to 0.25% is used for caudal anesthesia. It can be given with epinephrine.

Butacaine sulfate, N.F. (Butyn Sulfate)

Butacaine sulfate acts rapidly and produces a prolonged effect. It does not produce constriction of blood vessels. Butacaine is used for surface anesthesia particularly of the eye, nose, and throat and has, to some extent, replaced cocaine. This drug is usually used in a 1% or 2% solution.

Toxic effects. Its toxicity is similar to that of cocaine, and its administration by injection is not recommended.

Dibucaine hydrochloride, N.F. (Nupercaine Hydrochloride); cinchocaine hydrochloride, B.P.

Dibucaine hydrochloride is not only one of the more potent local anesthetics but also one of the most toxic. It is 15 to 20 times more potent than procaine when injected and 10 to 15 times more potent than cocaine when applied topically. Onset of action is slow and may be delayed for

Lidocaine	Tetracaine	Mepivacaine	Dibucaine
Xylocaine Lignocaine	Pontocaine	Carbocaine	Nupercaine
Two times more potent than procaine	Ten times that of procaine	Two times that of procaine	Ten to twenty times that of procaine
Immediate 1 to 2 hr.	5 to 10 min. 1½ to 2 hr.	Less rapid than procaine More prolonged than procaine or lidocaine	10 min. 2½ to 3 hr.
0.5% to 4% for injection 2% and 5% topically	0.5% to 2% topically 0.15% to 0.25% for injection	1% to 2% solution	0.25% to 2% for injection or topical application
Like that of procaine	More toxic than procaine, but toxic effects rare because of low dosage used	Two times that of procaine—less than lidocaine	Ten to twenty times that of procaine
When administered rapidly or in large doses may cause convulsions and hypotension	May cause vasodepressor effects	Has vasoconstrictor action	Tissue sloughs when injected subcutaneously

15 minutes, but its effects may last 2½ to 3 hours.

It is used to produce surface anesthesia but can be used for all types of local anesthesia. Its D.E.S.I. rating is *effective* for spinal anesthesia. It can be given with epinephrine.

Preparation and dosage. Dibucaine hydrochloride is marketed in ampules and vials containing various amounts of the drug. The drug is used in concentrations of 0.25% to 2% solution for injection and topical application. It is a constituent of certain ointments used to relieve the discomfort of burns and hemorrhoids. It is also available in suppository form.

Toxic effects. Caution in its use is recommended because of its potential toxicity.

Hexylcaine hydrochloride, N.F. (Cyclaine Hydrochloride)

Hexylcaine hydrochloride is used in concentrations up to 5% for surface anesthesia, 1% for infiltration and nerve block, and 2% to 2.5% for spinal anesthesia. For surface anesthesia it is said to be as effective as cocaine, and for infiltration and nerve block it is thought to be faster and longer acting than equal amounts of procaine. It has a D.E.S.I. rating of *effective* for spinal anesthesia, caudal or epidural block, infiltration anesthesia, topical anesthesia of mucous membranes, and for dental procedures.

Toxic effects. It exhibits toxic effects similar to other local anesthetics and must be employed with the same precautions.

Piperocaine hydrochloride (Metycaine Hydrochloride)

Piperocaine hydrochloride is chemically related to cocaine but produces effects similar to procaine. It differs from procaine in that it is suited to topical application for surface anesthesia as well as for injection. It is slightly more potent and more toxic than procaine and effects last about the same length of time. It is compatible with epinephrine and is used for anything for which procaine can be used unless the patient is hypersensitive to the agent. It is *not* used for spinal anesthesia.

Preparation, dosage, and administration. Solutions of various concentrations are available for injection, as well as 150-mg. tablets and a 4% or 5% ointment. The drug is used in concentrations that vary from 0.25% to 10%, depending on the route of administration.

Butethamine hydrochloride (Monocaine Hydrochloride)

Butethamine hydrochloride is a local anesthetic similar to procaine. It has about one third more anesthetic and toxic potency than procaine but is inferior to cocaine or butacaine. It is used for surface anesthesia and for nerve block anesthesia in dentistry. It is a stable compound. It must be used with the same precautions as with other local anesthetics.

Mepivacaine hydrochloride, U.S.P. (Carbocaine Hydrochloride)

Mepivacaine is a nonirritating, potent local anesthetic similar in action to lidocaine. Its action is less rapid and more prolonged than that of lidocaine. It can be used for infiltration, regional nerve block, caudal, and peridural anesthesia. It is not effective topically except in large doses and thus should not be used topically. It exerts its effect without the use of a vasoconstrictor, thereby eliminating the necessity to use agents such as epinephrine. Thus, mepivacaine has a definite advantage over other local anesthetics for use with elderly patients or patients with cardiovascular disease, diabetes mellitus, or thyrotoxicosis. Mepivacaine may cause adverse reactions similar to those noted for lidocaine, but the drowsiness, lassitude, and amnesia observed with lidocaine do not occur. It is available in solutions of 1%, 1.5%, and 2%. It has a D.E.S.I. rating similar to that for lidocaine with the exception of topical application.

Bupivacaine, B.P. (Marcaine)

Bupivacaine is related chemically to mepivacaine, but it is four times more potent than that drug. Onset of action is comparable to that of mepivacaine and lidocaine. Duration of anesthesia with bupivacaine is two to three times longer than that of mepivacaine or lidocaine and 20 to 30% longer than that of tetracaine. The addition of epinephrine increases its duration of action; some nerve blocks may last 12 hours or more. Its long duration of anesthesia makes it a desirable drug for nerve block, epidural or caudal anesthesia for long surgical or obstetrical procedures, and relief of pain during labor.

Preparation and dosage. Bupivacaine is available as a 0.25%, 0.5%, and 0.75% solution for injection with or without epinephrine. Maximal single dose for adults should not exceed 200 mg. without epinephrine and 250 mg. with epinephrine. Dose should not be repeated at intervals of less than 3 hours, and a total dose of 400 mg. in 24 hours should not be exceeded.

Toxic effects. Bupivacaine may cause hypotension, tremors, fainting, bradycardia, nausea and vomiting, headache, and paresthesias. The same precautions should be followed as for other local anesthetics.

LOCAL ANESTHESIA BY FREEZING

Low temperatures in living tissues produce diminished sensation. This form of anesthesia is sometimes employed for minor operative procedures. Packing an extremity in ice may be used for the major operative procedure of amputation of part of an extremity, particularly in elderly and debilitated persons or in patients considered to be "high risk" patients if given a general anesthetic. Tissues that are frozen too intensely and over too long a period of time may be destroyed.

Ethyl chloride is a local anesthetic that can be used to produce this effect, although it is not employed extensively (see p. 346).

TOPICAL ANESTHETICS

A number of local anesthetic agents cannot be injected. Because they are absorbed slowly they can be used safely on open wounds, ulcers, and mucous surfaces. They occasionally cause dermatitis, which necessitates discontinuation of their use.

Benzocaine, N.F., B.P. (Anesthesin); benzocaine ointment, N.F.

Benzocaine acts as a local anesthetic when applied to painful wounds and ulcers of the skin and mucous membranes. It is widely used for relief of sunburn and pruritus. It may be applied as a dusting powder or as an ointment to denuded areas of the skin and to mucous membranes. It is used to relieve itching and discomfort associated with hemorrhoids and rectal fissures. It is also available in the form of rectal and vaginal suppositories.

Benzocaine ointment is a 5% preparation of the drug in white ointment.

Butyl aminobenzoate, N.F. (Butesin)

This preparation is used with or without a diluent as an anesthetic dusting powder. It is also marketed in the form of troches, suppositories, and ointments.

Dimethisoquin hydrochloride, N.F. (Quotane)

Dimethisoquin is a local anesthetic applied topically to the skin to relieve itching, irritation, burning, or pain of various dermatoses. It may also be used to relieve pain of sutured surgical wounds. It is available as a 0.5% lotion or ointment. Onset of action occurs in a few minutes and duration of effect lasts from 2 to 4 hours.

Diperodon, N.F. (Diothane)

Diperodon is used for surface anesthesia of the skin and mucous membranes. It is as potent as cocaine with a longer duration of action. It can be irritating, and it can cause allergic reactions. It is available as a 1% cream, ointment, or suppository.

Dyclonine hydrochloride, N.F. (Dyclone)

Dyclonine is a ketone. It does not contain the esters or amides of other local anesthetics. Thus cross sensitization with other local anesthetics does not occur, making it useful for patients hypersensitive to other agents. Its potency is like that of cocaine and its toxicity is low. It is applied topically to the skin or mucous membranes as a 0.5% or 1% solution; it is not injected. Onset of action occurs in 10 minutes; duration of effect is 45 to 60 minutes.

Pramoxine hydrochloride, N.F. (Tronothane)

Pramoxine is used primarily to relieve itching and pain of skin conditions, to anesthetize laryngopharyngeal surfaces prior to instrumentation, and to facilitate sigmoidoscopic examination. Pramoxine should not be injected or applied to the eye or nasal mucosa since it may irritate these tissues. It is used in a 1% solution, cream, or jelly.

Butacaine, N.F. (Butyn)

Butacaine has a rapid action and prolonged effect. It is used for surface anesthesia of the nose and throat but particularly of the eye. Anesthesia is produced in 1 minute with a single application; repeated instillation permits ocular surgery. Since it does not cause vasoconstriction, pupil dilation, or drying, it has largely replaced cocaine in ophthalmic surgery. It is more powerful than cocaine and, when injected, is more toxic than cocaine. Thus, butacaine is unsuitable for injection. It is used principally in the form of a 2% solution.

Eugenol, U.S.P., B.P.

Eugenol is a pale yellow liquid obtained from clove oil. It is applied topically to the skin and mucous membrane and is used especially by dentists for the relief of pain caused by dental caries.

QUESTIONS

For study and review

1 Explain the role of preliminary medications in the production of a satisfactory anesthetic state.
2 What is the difference between a volatile anesthetic and a nonvolatile anesthetic?
3 Discuss the difference between the various stages of anesthesia.
   a. between analgesia and excitement
   b. between the various planes of surgical anesthesia
4 Explain the use of a vasoconstrictor with a local anesthetic.
5 What are some important nursing care aspects for the postanesthetic patient?
6 What is meant by "dissociative anesthesia"?

Multiple choice questions

7 Which of the following statements about preanesthetic medications are correct?
   a. Preanesthesia is used to reduce apprehension.
   b. Preanesthesia decreases the amount of anesthetic required.
   c. Preanesthesia promotes smoother induction and emergence from general anesthesia.
   d. Preanesthesia may have the undesirable action of prolonging awakening from anesthesia.
8 Which of the following are *incorrect* statements?
   a. Cyclopropane is the most potent of the anesthetic gases.
   b. Vinyl ether is preferable for surgical procedures of short duration since it requires continuous administration to maintain anesthesia.
   c. Although ether (diethyl ether) is volatile and highly flammable, it continues to be widely used because of its nonirritating effects.
   d. Nitrous oxide is a highly desirable anesthetic because of its nonexplosiveness and its ability to promote optimum muscular relaxation without the use of other drugs or gases.
9 Choose the *incorrect* answer. Ethylene:
   a. is a more potent anesthetic than ether
   b. has a rapid induction
   c. does not irritate the respiratory mucosa
   d. is not noted as a good muscle relaxant
10 Choose the *incorrect* answer. Halothane:
   a. tends to cause hypotension
   b. has a low incidence of postoperative nausea and vomiting
   c. is not as potent as ether
   d. depresses salivary and mucous secretions
11 Ether has continued to be one of the widely used anesthetics because:
   a. muscular relaxation can be secured
   b. induction is easy and safe
   c. it has a wide safety range

   d. it is readily transported and used in a variety of circumstances
12 Indicate which of the following constitutes the chief disadvantage in the use of cyclopropane.
   a. cost   c. explosiveness
   b. availability   d. narrow safety range
13 Choose the correct statements about open-drop anesthesia.
   a. It does not permit controlled concentration of anesthetic.
   b. It is inexpensive and does not require elaborate equipment.
   c. It is used with liquid anesthetics.
   d. It can be safely administered without anesthesia education.
14 Select the *incorrect* answer.
   a. Ethyl chloride produces local anesthesia by freezing.
   b. Procaine is an effective topical anesthetic.
   c. Local anesthetics are potentially hazardous drugs and should be used in low concentrations.
   d. Thiopental sodium is a basal anesthetic.

REFERENCES

Aviado, D. M.: Krantz and Carr's pharmacologic principles of medical practice, ed. 8, Baltimore, 1972, The Williams & Wilkins Co.

Adriani, J.: The pharmacology of anesthetic drugs: A syllabus for students and clinicians, Springfield, Ill., 1970, Charles C Thomas, Publisher.

Covino, B. G.: Local anesthesia, New Eng. J. Med. **286:**975, 1035, 1972.

Cullen, S. C., and Larson, C. P., Jr.: Essentials of anesthetic practice, Chicago, 1974, Year Book Medical Publishers, Inc.

Dundee, J. W., Knox, J. W., and Black, G. W.: Ketamine as an induction agent in anesthetics, Lancet **1:**1370, 1970.

Dykes, M. H. M., and Bunker, J. P.: Hepatotoxicity and anesthetics, Pharmacol. Phys. **4**(11):1, 1970.

Eger, E. I., and others: A comparison of the cardiovascular effects of halothane, fluroxene, ether and cyclopropane in man: A resume, Anesthesiology **34:**25, 1971.

Goldstein, A., and Keats, A. S.: The risk of anesthesia, Anesthesiology **33:**130, 1970.

Goth, A.: Medical pharmacology, ed. 7, St. Louis, 1974, The C. V. Mosby Co.

Ngai, S. H., Mark, L. C., and Papper, E. M.: Pharmacologic and physiologic aspects of anesthesiology, New Eng. J. Med. **282:**479, 541, 1970.

Ostlere, G., and Bryce-Smith, R.: Anaesthetics for medical students, ed. 7, London, 1974, Churchill Livingstone.

Smith, B. J.: After anesthesia, Nursing 1974 **4:**28, 1974.

Tweed, W. A., Mimick, M., and Mymin, D.: Circulatory responses to ketamine anesthesia, Anesthesiology **37:**613, 1972.

Way, W. L., and Trevor, A. J.: Sedative-hypnotics: A review, Anesthesiology **34:**170, 1971.

CHAPTER 15

Skeletal muscle relaxants and their antagonists

Neuromuscular blocking agents
Centrally acting skeletal muscle relaxants
Direct acting skeletal muscle relaxant
Antagonists of curariform drugs
Antiparkinsonism drugs

Skeletal muscles are striated or striped muscles attached to the skeleton that are usually under voluntary control. These muscles function to produce body movements, maintain body position against the force of gravity, and counteract environmental stresses such as wind. An anatomic muscle is composed of numerous muscle cells or muscle fibers. Each muscle cell is connected to only one motor nerve fiber, but each of the nerve fibers is connected to several muscle cells. Therefore, stimulation of one nerve fiber will cause stimulation and activation of a group of muscle cells.

Motor nerves originate in the anterior horn cells in the gray matter of the spinal cord. Each anterior horn cell has a single axon that leaves the horn cell by way of the spinal nerve root. When this axon, or motor neuron, reaches the muscle it innervates, it branches to innervate a group of muscle fibers. The motor neuron and all the muscle fibers innervated by the same anterior horn cell constitute a motor unit. A particular muscle may contain thousands of these units. When the motor nerve is stimulated, every muscle fiber in the motor unit contracts. Individual fibers do not react on their own unless the motor nerve is nonfunctional; then individual fibers may twitch and cause *fasciculation.*

Muscle cells or fibers are long and thin with cross striations (Figure 15-1). When nerve impulses pass along motor nerves, the muscle fibers shorten and the muscle contracts; in the absence of nerve impulses the muscle relaxes. This relaxed state is called *flaccidity.*

The region where a motor nerve fiber makes functional contact with a skeletal muscle fiber (synaptic contact) is known as the neuromuscular junction (Figure 15-2). The end-plate of the muscle cell is chemically excitable; the

Figure 15-1

Striated muscle fiber with a single excitatory nerve supply.

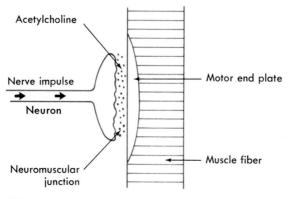

Figure 15-2

Neuromuscular junction where the motor nerve makes functional contact with a muscle fiber. Acetylcholine bridges the gap between the neuron and muscle fiber until it is destroyed.

rest of the muscle fiber is not but is electrically excitable. Acetylcholine (ACh) is the neurohormonal transmitter that chemically excites the muscle fibers. ACh is formed in the motor nerve cell or in the axon of the motor nerve and stored in vesicles in the motor nerve. Depolarization of the presynaptic membrane is followed by re-

lease of ACh, which is taken up by receptors on the motor end-plate of the muscle fiber. ACh alters the membrane permeability of the motor end-plate, allowing sodium to diffuse, thereby producing a change in voltage known as an end-plate potential. Depolarization spreads from the motor end-plate to the whole of the muscle fiber, a propagated action potential; calcium ions are released and the muscle contracts. ACh is destroyed shortly after its release by the enzyme cholinesterase; this enables the next nerve impulse to be effective (Figure 15-3).

NEUROMUSCULAR BLOCKING AGENTS

Neuromuscular blocking agents are important skeletal muscle relaxants. These drugs can be classified as: (1) *nondepolarizing*, or *competitive*, *neuromuscular blocking agents* (they may also be referred to as *stabilizing agents*), and (2) *depolarizing blocking agents*.

These drugs are used to: (1) produce adequate muscle relaxation during anesthesia and reduce excessive use of general anesthetics; (2) facilitate endotracheal intubation and prevent laryn-

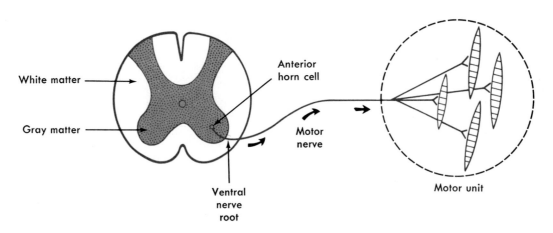

Figure 15-3 Anterior cell and motor unit.

Motor nerves originate in anterior horn cells and leave via the ventral or spinal nerve root. When the axon of the nerve reaches the muscle supplied, it branches to supply a group of striated muscle fibers. The motor nerve and all the muscle fibers supplied by the same anterior horn cell are a *motor unit*.

gospasm; (3) aid in the management of tetanus; and (4) decrease muscular activity in electroshock therapy. They do not affect pain or other sensory perception.

Neuromuscular blocking agents are usually given intravenously but may be given intramuscularly. The intravenous route is preferred, since onset of action is faster and more predictable than with the intramuscular route. All neuromuscular blocking drugs are poorly absorbed from the gastrointestinal tract.

Side effects shared by all neuromuscular blocking agents are: (1) interference with respiratory function, even progressing to respiratory paralysis; (2) residual muscle weakness, and (3) hypersensitivity reactions. Many, but not all, neuromuscular blocking agents can cause hypotension, bronchospasm, and cardiac disturbances. The hypotension is believed to be caused by sympathetic ganglionic blockade and histamine release, both of which cause peripheral vasodilation. Bronchospasm is probably caused by the histamine release.

Since these are potent drugs, not without danger, it is recommended that they be used only by persons thoroughly familiar with their effects and under conditions where the patient can receive constant, close attention for signs of respiratory embarassment. Adequate equipment for artificial respiration, antidotes, and other measures for prompt treatment of toxicity must be readily available.

In addition, there are muscle relaxants that exert their effects by action on the central nervous system, thereby decreasing voluntary muscle hyperactivity. These drugs exert a selective action on internuncial neurons of the spinal cord and reduce multisynaptic but not monosynaptic spinal reflexes. Actually, these drugs can be classified as sedatives. In large doses these drugs cause depression similar to that of the sedative-hypnotics.

Muscle spasm is a symptom associated with many conditions and is the result of several processes. These processes include injury to the muscle itself, presence of an inflammatory process of the tissues around the muscle that precipitates muscular contraction, and damage to the nerve fibers of the central nervous system responsible for the control of motor activity of muscles. Skeletal muscle relaxants are advocated for the management of almost every musculoskeletal and neuromuscular condition associated with muscle pain or spasticity. There appear to be as many skeletal muscle relaxants available as there are conditions for which they are prescribed.

NONDEPOLARIZING (COMPETITIVE) NEUROMUSCULAR BLOCKING AGENTS

Competitive neuromuscular blocking agents produce skeletal muscle relaxation by occupying the cholinergic receptor sites at the myoneural junction, thereby preventing acetylcholine from acting on these receptors. Consequently, depolarization of the postsynaptic membrane does not occur, the muscle fibers are not stimulated, and skeletal muscle contraction does not take place. These drugs may also interfere with the movement of potassium and sodium ions responsible for depolarization and repolarization of the membranes involved in muscle contraction.

Neuromuscular blockade by nondepolarizing drugs is: (1) antagonized by depolarizing agents, (2) reversed by anticholinesterases (physostigmine, neostigmine, edrophonium), which increase ACh concentration at the end-plate; and (3) intensified or prolonged by ether anesthesia. These drugs are also referred to as curariform blocking agents.

Curare

d-Tubocurarine chloride

Curare is a generic name for a number of arrow poisons obtained from tropical vines used by South American Indians. A number of separate alkaloids are extracted from the plant genus *Strychnos* and certain species of *Chondodendron. Chondodendron tomentosum* is a source of *d*-tubocurarine. Previously, curare was obtained from a variety of plants, resulting in variability in strength and composition, and it gained a reputation for unreliability. The isolation of *d*-tubocurarine by King in 1935, the development of an assay method, and standardization of the drug produced a pure crystalline compound with pure curare action.

Action and result. In therapeutic doses curare blocks transmission at the myoneural junctions of skeletal muscle. When an appropriate dose of curare is injected intravenously in man the first effects occur in the short muscles such as those found in the eyes, eyelids, fingers, and toes. Within 2 to 3 minutes haziness of vision, difficulty in talking and swallowing, ptosis of the eyelids, and weakness of the muscles of the jaw, neck, and legs occur; then follow relaxation, and finally

paralysis of the muscles of the neck, spine, legs, arms, and abdomen. The last muscles to be affected are the intercostals and the diaphragm. In recovery after the ordinary clinical dose the paralysis disappears in reverse order and may require 15 to 20 minutes.

An undesirable action of curare is that of blockage of transmission in the autonomic ganglia. This action may cause lowering of blood pressure.

Absorption and excretion. Because of its poor absorption, curare may be swallowed (ordinary doses) without ill effect, provided there are no wounds or abrasions along the digestive tract. It is rapidly excreted by the kidney and also rapidly destroyed by the liver.

Uses. Curare was formerly used to enhance muscular relaxation during anesthesia to permit adequate relaxation without subjecting patients to deep planes of anesthesia that border on medullary paralysis. However, the margin of safety between the dose that produced good relaxation

Table 15-1 Curare type muscle relaxants

	Tubocurarine	Dimethyl-tubocurarine (Metubine)	Pancuronium (Pavulon)
Maximal action Intravenous Intramuscular Oral	3 to 5 min. 10 to 25 min. No effect	3 to 5 min. 5 to 10 min. No effect	2 to 3 min. — No effect
Duration of action	Variable: 20 to 60 min.: with large single dose or multiple doses, action may last 24 hours	15 to 90 min.	35 to 45 min.
Mode of action	Competitive blocker of acetylcholine	Competitive blocker of acetylcholine	Competitive blocker of acetylcholine
Effects Central Cardiovascular Respiratory	None N.S.* Hypoventilation, apnea from cumulative effects	None N.S.* Hypoventilation, apnea	None Tachycardia
Antagonists	Neostigmine Edrophonium	Neostigmine Edrophonium	Neostigmine Edrophonium

*Not significant when administered slowly. Rapid induction may cause a precipitous fall in blood pressure.

of voluntary muscle and the one producing paralysis of respiratory muscles was small.

It was formerly used also to prevent trauma and excessive muscular contraction in electroshock therapy and to provide muscular relaxation during endoscopy and the reduction of fractures and dislocations. It has been replaced to a great extent by succinylcholine.

Other former uses of curare include relief of spasticity of muscles in certain convulsive states and neuromuscular conditions. It was also used as a diagnostic agent for myasthenia gravis. (An injection of one-fifeenth to one-fifth the average adult dose will produce profound exaggeration of symptoms if the patient has myasthenia gravis.)

Patients receiving curare had to be closely observed for respiratory failure. If this occurred, artificial respiration was instituted and an injection of neostigmine was given as an antidote.

The clinical use of curare from natural sources has been supplanted by use of tubocurarine and synthetic curarimimetic drugs.

Tubocurarine chloride, U.S.P., B.P. (*d*-tubocurarine, Tubarine, Tubadil)

Tubocurarine is the active principle of curare. It produces a paralytic effect on neuromuscular transmission. Its pharmacologic effects are similar to those of other nondepolarizing neuromuscular blocking agents.

A single intravenous dose of tubocurarine produces muscle relaxation in 3 to 5 minutes, which may persist for 20 to 30 minutes. Muscles are affected in the following order: (1) those innervated by the cranial nerves, e.g., facial muscles; (2) muscles of the trunk and extremities; and (3) muscles of respiration, with the diaphragm being affected last. After intramuscular injection paralysis occurs within 10 to 25 minutes. Additional doses will have longer durations of action than the initial dose. A large single dose or multiple small doses can saturate the body tissues; the drug may persist in the tissues for 24 hours after the last dose has been given. Duration of action is dependent upon the rate of urinary excretion. Thirty-three percent to 75% of the drug is eliminated unchanged in the urine; some of the drug

is eliminated through the intestinal tract via the bile. Thus its actions may be prolonged in patients with renal or liver disease, and in the elderly or debilitated due to delayed drug excretion.

Tubocurarine does not readily cross the blood-brain barrier and thus in therapeutic doses does not cause central nervous system effects. Significant amounts do not cross the placental barrier and, therefore, it can be used in obstetric anesthesia.

Uses. D.E.S.I. rating for tubocurarine is *effective:* (1) as an adjunct to anesthesia to induce skeletal muscle relaxation; (2) to decrease the intensity of muscle contraction in electroshock therapy; (3) as a diagnostic agent for myasthenia gravis when results with anticholinesterases have been inconclusive.

Side effects, toxic effects, and precautions. Tubocurarine can cause hypotension because of its sympathetic ganglionic blocking ability and its capacity to release histamine from storage sites. The resulting peripheral vasodilation produces a drop in blood pressure. The diminished venous return caused by loss of skeletal muscle tone also contributes to the hypotension. The histamine release may cause bronchospasm.

Since myasthenia gravis patients are particularly sensitive to tubocurarine blocking effects, this drug should be used with extreme caution in these patients. The blocking effect of tubocurarine is enhanced by acidosis and decreased by alkalosis.

Depression of the muscles of respiration can cause hypoxia and even death. Treatment includes establishing an open airway (endotracheal tube) and positive pressure artificial respiration with oxygen.

Neostigmine methylsulfate (Prostigmin Methylsulfate) and edrophonium chloride (Tensilon Chloride) are used as antidotes under certain conditions but only as supplements to artificial respiration with oxygen. These antidotes inactivate cholinesterase and permit acetylcholine to be built up, and unless large overdoses of curare have been given, this increased level of acetylcholine tends to overcome the paralysis. However, overdosage with the antidote can also produce untoward effects. Effective doses of neostigmine are likely to produce increased flow of saliva, slowing of the heart, hypotension, and increased motility of the intestine. Atropine is sometimes given to counteract the latter effects. The anticurare drugs are said to be most safely used when employed in small and, if necessary, repeated doses.

Drug interactions. The general anesthetics, particularly ether, potentiate the action of tubocurarine. This necessitates reduction in the dose of tubocurarine. Drugs that potentiate the neuromuscular blocking action of tubocurarine include many antibiotics (neomycin, streptomycin, polymyxin B, etc.); diuretics, particularly the thiazides; monoamine oxidase inhibitors, and quinidine. Drugs that inhibit the action of tubocurarine include the anticholinesterases (e.g., neostigmine, edrophonium) and epinephrine.

There have been reports of recurarization occurring postoperatively when patients were treated with antiarrhythmic drugs such as lidocaine or quinidine.

Preparation, dosage, and administration. The drug is available in 1-ml. ampules containing 15 mg. of tubocurarine; and in 10- and 20-ml. vials with 3 mg. of drug per milliliter.

As an adjunct to general anesthesia for adults, 6 to 9 mg. are given intravenously over 60 to 90 seconds. Depending upon the patient's response, this dose may be followed in 5 minutes by 3 to 6 mg. more of the drug. Additional doses, one fourth to one half the initial dose, may be given at 45- to 60-minute intervals as needed.

In children the initial dose is 0.1 to 0.2 mg. per kilogram of body weight; subsequent doses are 0.05 to 0.1 mg. per kilogram.

Dose during convulsive therapy is 100 to 200 μg. per kilogram of body weight given intravenously over 30 to 90 seconds.

Dimethyltubocurarine iodide, N.F. (Metubine)

This preparation is similar to the parent compound tubocurarine but it is about three times as potent. Dosage must be individualized. Maximum effect occurs in 3 to 5 minutes; duration of blockade ranges from 15 to 90 minutes depending on the dose and general anesthetic used. Side effects, toxic effects, and precautions are the same as those for tubocurarine. It has the same favorable D.E.S.I. rating as tubocurarine.

The iodide preparation should not be used in patients sensitive to iodides.

There are claims that dimethyltubocurarine produces less ganglionic block, histamine release, and respiratory depression than tubocurarine. However, these claims have not been unequivocally substantiated.

Gallamine triethiodide, U.S.P., B.P. (Flaxedil)

$$N^+(C_2H_5)_3$$
$$|$$
$$CH_2$$
$$|$$
$$CH_2$$
$$|$$
$$O$$

$$(C_2H_5)_3N^+-H_2C-H_2C-O-\langle\bigcirc\rangle-O-CH_2-CH_2-N^+(C_2H_5)_3$$

Gallamine triethiodide is a synthetic compound whose action, uses, drug interactions, and contraindications are similar to those of the curare drugs. It is about one fifth as potent as tubocurarine. Advantages claimed for this preparation include the following: (1) it has no effect on autonomic ganglia, (2) it does not cause bronchospasm from histamine release, and (3) it affords a high degree of flexibility because of rapid onset and short duration of action. Its major disadvantage is that it produces vagal blockade similar to that of atropine and thus can cause tachycardia and blood pressure elevation. It is antagonized by neostigmine and edrophonium.

D.E.S.I. rating is *effective* as an adjunct to anesthesia for muscle relaxation; it is not approved for electroshock therapy because of its side effects and short duration of action.

Preparation, dosage, and administration. Gallamine triethiodide is administered intravenously in an aqueous solution. It may be mixed with a 2.5% thiopental sodium solution. The average dose is 50 to 60 mg. or 1 mg. per kilogram of body weight. Muscular relaxation begins immediately after intravenous injection and reaches a maximum in about 3 minutes; duration of action is 15 to 35 minutes. Dosage must be individually adjusted for each patient.

Side effects and toxic effects. This drug may produce an allergic reaction in patients sensitive to iodine. It may also produce a marked tachycardia. It crosses the placental barrier, and although no perceptible effect on newborns has been reported, it should be used with extreme caution for cesarean section. It is excreted unchanged by the kidneys and should not be administered to patients with impaired renal function. It must be used with the same precautions as with other potent skeletal muscle relaxants. It is not the relaxant of choice for patients with cardiovascular disease.

Pancuronium bromide (Pavulon)

Pancuronium is a new synthetic nondepolarizing neuromuscular blocking agent. It is about five times more potent than tubocurarine, and it has a slightly more rapid onset of action. Pancuronium has some advantages over tubocurarine: (1) it does not cause ganglionic blockade and thus does not cause hypotension; and (2) it causes little or no histamine release and therefore does not cause bronchospasm. It may cause an increase in heart rate by blocking the ACh receptors of the heart, but this is minimal with usual doses and less than that produced by gallamine. Although it has a steroidal structure, the drug appears to have no hormonal activity.

Uses. Pancuronium is used primarily to produce skeletal muscle relaxation during surgery after general anesthesia has been induced. It is compatible with all currently used general anesthetics. It has been used to facilitate mechanical respiration in patients with status asthmaticus and to facilitate endotracheal intubation.

After intravenous injection, muscle relaxation takes place in 2 to 3 minutes; duration of action is 35 to 40 minutes.

Dosage and preparation. Dosage of pancuronium must be individually determined. However, usual initial dose as an adjunct to anesthesia is 0.02 to 0.1 mg. per kilogram of body weight. Additional doses of 0.01 mg. per kilogram may be administered at 25- to 60-minute intervals during prolonged surgery or assisted respiration. For children the initial dose is 0.02 to 0.1 mg. per kilogram of body weight with repeated doses being one fifth the initial dose.

It is available in 2- and 5-ml. ampules containing 2 mg. of pancuronium per milliliter and in 10-ml. vials containing 1 mg. of drug per milliliter.

Side effects, toxic effects, and precautions. Pancuronium has the same toxic potentials as other nondepolarizing neuromuscular blocking agents. It should not be used in patients with a history of tachycardia or in patients in whom an increase in heart rate is undesirable. It is contraindicated in patients sensitive to bromides.

Pancuronium has caused excessive salivation and sweating in children. Its use is not recommended for children under the age of 10. It should be used cautiously in children since only limited data on its use in this age group are available at this time.

Transient skin rashes, wheezing, and a burning sensation at the site of injection have been reported.

DEPOLARIZING NEUROMUSCULAR BLOCKING AGENTS

Depolarizing agents resemble acetylcholine in structure (see structural formulas, p. 370), have a high affinity for ACh receptor sites, and, like acetylcholine, produce depolarization of the motor end-plate at the myoneural junction. These drugs produce a more prolonged depolarization of the motor plate than ACh because of their high affinity for ACh receptors and their resistance to inactivation by cholinesterase. During depolarization the end-plate is incapable of responding to motor nerve stimulation. These drugs are associated with phase I and phase II blocks. Succinylcholine is an example of a depolarizing drug.

Phase I block is the initial depolarization block during which paralysis may be preceded by signs of stimulation (e.g., fasciculations). This type of block is potentiated by anticholinesterase drugs and reversed by nondepolarizing agents.

Phase II block, or desensitization block of the receptors, follows the use of a depolarizing drug for a prolonged period of time; that is, it is a block that develops with time. It is similar to a competitive block. Since the end-plate does not remain depolarized for an indefinite period of time, a state probably occurs whereby depolar-

Decamethonium

Acetylcholine

Succinylcholine

ization is no longer present but the neuromuscular block persists. During phase II block, drugs that antagonize competitive blocking agents (an anticholinesterase drug, such as neostigmine) are effective for reversing the block even though they are not effective for reversing phase I block.

The phase II block is not well understood and a variety of factors are probably involved. There is evidence that depolarization causes a considerable shift in ions. Muscle cells with greatly altered ionic distribution may be blocked more easily. There are reports that phase II block seems to occur sooner in patients with decreased potassium levels.

Succinylcholine chloride, U.S.P. (Anectine Chloride, Quelicin, Sucostrin, Sux-Cert); suxamethonium chloride, B.P.

Action and result. Succinylcholine is an ultrashort-acting myoneural blocking agent. Although the end result of its action is similar to that of curare, its action is the same as that of decamethonium—it intensifies the depolarizing effect to such an extent that repolarization of the end-plate, which is necessary for muscle contraction, does not occur.

Its action is of shorter duration than that of tubocurarine chloride. This is explained by the fact that succinylcholine is easily hydrolyzed by cholinesterase to form choline and succinic acid. Alkaline solutions of the drug undergo rapid hydrolysis; therefore, succinylcholine chloride should not be mixed with alkaline solutions of

anesthetics, such as thiopental sodium. The intensity of its effect can be modified readily by varying the rate of administration.

Clinical doses do not seem to produce significant effects on the circulatory system and autonomic ganglia, and they cause no significant liberation of histamine.

Uses. Some authorities are of the opinion that succinylcholine approaches the ideal muscle relaxant. It is the relaxant of choice whenever it is important to have rapid skeletal muscle relaxation.

It is used to produce muscular relaxation during anesthesia and in conjunction with electroshock therapy. Because of its short action, it is particularly well suited to procedures of short duration such as endotracheal intubation and endoscopy.

Preparation, dosage, and administration. Succinylcholine chloride is available as succinylcholine chloride injection, U.S.P., and is administered intravenously, either in repeated injections or as a continuous drip infusion. The range of dose is 10 to 30 mg. for an adult when used for short procedures. Relaxation occurs in about 1 minute with peak action in 2 minutes, after which there is rapid recovery in about 5 minutes. Sustained relaxation for prolonged procedures is obtained by continuous drip infusion in which approximately 2.5 mg. is given per minute. Administration of succinylcholine is said to require closer attention than administration of other muscle relaxants, but there is also greater ease of control.

Side effects and toxic effects. Succinylcholine exhibits a low level of toxicity. However, large doses produce respiratory depression, and facilities to combat respiratory paralysis must be at hand. There is no effective antagonist. Neostigmine and edrophonium chloride prolong the effect of succinylcholine and, therefore, are contraindicated as antidotes in case of overdosage. However, because it loses its potency rapidly when administration is discontinued, succinylcholine is a relatively safe drug. The patient must be observed closely to prevent undue respiratory depression.

Since succinylcholine can cause vagal stimulation, bradycardia, hypotension, and cardiac arrhythmias may occur with its use. Tachycardia and hypertension have also been reported; these symptoms are the result of sympathetic ganglion stimulation.

Precaution. Patients with a deficiency of cholinesterase resulting from a genetic defect, liver disease, severe anemia, severe dehydration, or nutritional disturbance should not be given succinylcholine. They tend to be highly sensitive to even small doses of the drug, and there is a risk of prolonged postoperative apnea occurring in these patients. Cholinesterase levels can also be decreased by topical administration of long-acting anticholinesterases, such as echothiophate, used in the treatment of wide-angle glaucoma. These drugs should be discontinued 2 to 4 weeks before surgery if succinylcholine is to be given. Succinylcholine causes a rise in intraocular pressure, which is hazardous to patients with glaucoma, those undergoing eye surgery, and patients with penetrating wounds of the eye. It may also increase intragastric pressure, particularly if the patient was unable to fast prior to surgery. Patients with neuromuscular disorders may have an abnormal response to depolarizing agents.

Drug interactions. The following drug interactions may occur:

1 Antibiotics (neomycin, streptomycin, etc.) may act as weak depolarizing agents and potentiate the action of succinylcholine and prolong recovery time.
2 Neostigmine and other anticholinesterase agents may prolong the action of succinylcholine.
3 Phenothiazines reduce plasma cholinesterase levels and enhance the blocking effects of succinylcholine.

4 Procaine should not be given intravenously concurrently with succinylcholine, since it competes with succinylcholine for hydrolysis by cholinesterase; prolonged apnea may result.
5 Quinidine potentiates the action of muscle relaxants.
6 Diazepam reduces the duration of paralysis caused by succinylcholine.

Hexafluorenium bromide, N.F. (Mylaxen)

Hexafluorenium is a cholinesterase inhibitor used only to prolong the action of succinylcholine. It delays the enzymatic hydrolysis of succinylcholine, thereby increasing the intensity and duration of succinylcholine action. Hexafluorenium is used to prevent the muscle fasciculations and pain associated with succinylcholine administration.

Bronchospasm has been caused by the combined use of succinylcholine and hexafluorenium; they should not be given concomitantly to patients with bronchial asthma.

Hexafluorenium has received a D.E.S.I. rating of *effective* as an adjunct to anesthesia for use with succinylcholine to prolong neuromuscular blockade and reduce muscular fasciculations.

Decamethonium bromide (Syncurine)

Action. Decamethonium bromide is a very potent relaxant of skeletal muscle with a rapid onset of action but rather short duration of effect.

Decamethonium bromide is more potent than tubocurarine, but the duration of its effect is said to be intermediate between that of tubocurarine and succinylcholine. It does not produce a ganglionic blocking action, and it does not cause bronchospasm from a liberation of histamine. It has no cumulative effect even after repeated dosage.

Uses. Decamethonium bromide has been used to produce marked but short-term relaxation in connection with procedures such as endoscopy, endotracheal intubation, and closure of the peritoneum during surgical procedure. However, the drug is seldom used because tachyphylaxis occurs frequently, a satisfactory antidote is not available, and its effects are rather unpredictable.

Preparation, dosage, and administration. The usual dose varies from 0.5 to 3 mg., depending on the response of the patient and the degree of relaxation desired. It is administered by a single intravenous injection that may be repeated as necessary. Muscle relaxation occurs in 3 to 4 minutes; muscle activity begins to return in about 10 minutes and is back to normal in about 30 minutes.

Side effects. Despite its relatively short duration of action this drug may cause respiratory depression. Neostigmine and edrophonium chloride are of no value as antagonists; therefore, facilities for controlled artificial respiration with oxygen are essential.

CENTRALLY ACTING SKELETAL MUSCLE RELAXANTS

Action and uses. The most beneficial results from the administration of centrally acting skeletal muscle relaxants seem to be associated with their ability to relieve acute muscle spasm of local origin. They are used as adjuncts to physiotherapy in the treatment of sprains, strains, or trauma to ligaments. They often accompany the administration of other drugs (salicylates, adrenal corticosteroids) in the treatment of myositis, fibrositis, spondylitis, bursitis, and arthritis. These agents have been used effectively to lessen motor activity in certain neurologic disorders (e.g., cerebral palsy) and in other dyskinesias characterized by abnormal reflex activity, increased muscle tonus, involuntary movements, and incoordination. Many physicians feel that benefits from their administration come from the sedative effects produced, rather than from actual muscle relaxation.

The exact mechanism of action of the central skeletal muscle relaxants is not known at present. They do not seem to affect muscle, myoneural junctions, monosynaptic pathways, or motor nerves. However they do affect the central pathways and neuronal systems that control tone and movement of muscles. These drugs are known to produce relaxation of striated muscle spasm by depression of the central nervous system (brainstem, thalamus, and basal ganglia).

Skeletal muscle relaxants exert a selective action on internuncial neurons of the spinal cord, thereby reducing multisynaptic spinal reflexes.

Central skeletal muscle relaxants most commonly used are mephenesin, carisoprodol, chlorphenesin carbamate, chlorzoxazone, metaxalone, methocarbamol, and styramate.

Side effects and precautions. Usually the side effects associated with the centrally acting skeletal muscle relaxants have been mild and transient. Mild symptoms such as drowsiness, dizziness, blurred vision, lightheadedness, headache, feelings of weakness, lassitude, and lethargy occur during initial phases of drug therapy. Physicians and nursing personnel should caution patients taking these agents to avoid undertaking activities that require mental alertness, judgment, and physical coordination—such as operating dangerous machinery or driving an automobile. After a sufficient period of time these activities are possible when it is known that the drug no longer causes drowsiness or vertigo. Large oral dosages have caused nausea, vomiting, heartburn, abdominal distress, constipation, and diarrhea. With the occurrence of other signs or symptoms of drug incompatibility, administration of these agents should be discontinued. Some of the centrally acting skeletal muscle relaxants (chlorzoxazone and metaxalone) have been reported to cause jaundice. Periodic liver function tests and blood counts are recommended to avoid complications. This group of muscle relaxants is contraindicated in patients with myasthenia gravis or muscular dystrophy, since their effects may reduce the strength of remaining active muscle fibers and produce further impairment and/or debilitation. Patients with a history of liver disease should not be given these drugs, and the therapeutic effect should be weighed against the possible side effects in their administration during pregnancy.

Since most of these drugs were introduced between 1938 and 1962, they have been subjected to evaluation by the National Academy of Sciences–National Research Council panel. Many of the drugs in this category received an *ineffective* rating for claims relating to organic diseases of the nervous system, and a rating of *possibly effective* for other claims. These drugs will probably be acceptable for the treatment of muscle spasticity of brief duration, such as in bursitis, myositis, and fibrositis. The F.D.A. disapproves of prolonged administration of these drugs and discourages their use for periods longer than 3 weeks. This is a precautionary stand taken because fatalities had occurred after prolonged use of one of these drugs (zoxazolamine), which is no longer available. The usefulness of these drugs appears to be the result of their sedative effect and ability to relieve anxiety.

Mephenesin

$$CH_3$$
$$-OCH_2CH(OH)CH_2OH$$

Action. Mephenesin exhibits a selective depressant action on the basal ganglia, brainstem, and synaptic connections in the spinal cord. Large doses produce a temporary paralysis of skeletal muscle, although the drug does not directly influence muscle as is true of curare. It also has a local anesthetic action, although it is too irritating to be used for this effect. Mephenesin also has a weak sedative action.

Uses. The transient action of mephenesin seriously limits its usefulness. It has been of value as an experimental tool and has also prompted an active search for drugs more effective for motor disturbances. It has been used to relieve spasticity of muscle associated with back injuries and bursitis, but its beneficial effects are brief. It has not been found effective either as an adjunct to anesthesia or in the treatment of Parkinson's disease. Since the drug received a D.E.S.I. rating of *possibly effective* for muscle relaxation and *ineffective* for spasms resulting from neurologic disorders (e.g., hemiplegia, cerebral palsy), most of the dosage forms of mephenesin have been removed from the market.

Preparation, dosage, and administration. Mephenesin was marketed in capsules containing 250 and 500 mg., and as an elixir containing 100 mg. per milliliter. The usual adult daily dose is 1 to 3 Gm. given three to five times a day. Its duration of action is about 3 hours regardless of the mode of administration.

Side effects. Side effects include muscle incoordination, mild ataxia, nystagmus, diplopia, weakness, anorexia, nausea, and vomiting. Giving the drug after meals or with milk or fruit juice may reduce or prevent the gastrointestinal disturbances. Prolonged use has caused hemoglobinuria, hemolysis, and leukopenia. Fatalities have been the result of renal impairment.

Carisoprodol (Rela, Soma)

$$H_2N-C\overset{O}{\overset{\|}{-}}O-CH_2-\underset{CH_3}{\overset{C_3H_7}{\overset{|}{C}}}-CH_2-O-\overset{O}{\overset{\|}{C}}-NH-\overset{CH_3}{\overset{|}{CH}}-CH_3$$

Carisoprodol is related to meprobamate and has approximately the same actions and limited degree of effectiveness as other centrally acting skeletal muscle relaxants. Its D.E.S.I. rating is *possibly effective* for treating acute muscle spasm associated with mild to moderate pain. Its muscle relaxant action is eight times greater than that of mephenesin.

Preparation, dosage, and administration. Carisoprodol is administered orally in capsules of 250 mg. and tablets of 350 mg. The average daily adult dose is 350 mg. given four times a day. Onset of action occurs in 30 minutes, and duration of action is about 6 hours.

Side effects. On rare occasions the initial dose has caused an idiosyncratic reaction that includes transient quadriplegia, ataxia, extreme weakness, diplopia, loss of vision, agitation, and confusion. These symptoms usually subside in a few hours. The patient should receive supportive and symptomatic therapy during this frightening experience. Drowsiness, which may occur with high dosages, indicates a need for dosage reduction.

Chlorphenesin carbamate (Maolate)

$$Cl-\text{⟨benzene ring⟩}-OCH_2\underset{OH}{\overset{|}{C}}HCH_2O\overset{O}{\overset{\|}{C}}HN_2$$

Chlorphenesin carbamate is chemically and pharmacologically related to mephenesin and produces similar actions and side effects. Since chlorphenesin was introduced in 1966 it has not received a D.E.S.I. rating. It is used to treat muscle spasms caused by sprains, strains, and trauma to tendons and ligaments. It is not effective for the treatment of spastic disorders involving the central nervous system.

Preparation, dosage, and administration. Chlorphenesin carbamate is administered orally in 400-mg. tablets. The average daily dose ranges from 1.6 to 2.4 Gm. for adults.

Side effects and precautions. Most frequently encountered side effects are drowsiness and dizziness. Other side effects include gastrointestinal disturbances, headache, insomnia, and weakness. Rash and pruritus occur rarely. Side effects will subside if dosage is reduced or stopped. Patients on chlorphenesin should not engage in hazardous activities or those requiring keen mental alertness or muscle coordination until it is known that the drug is not causing drowsiness.

Chlorphenesin should be used with caution or not at all in patients with renal or liver damage. Duration of therapy should not exceed 21 days.

Chlorzoxazone (Paraflex)

The actions and effects of chlorzoxazone are similar to those of the other centrally acting skeletal muscle relaxants. Its D.E.S.I. rating is: *ineffective* for treating spasticity in neurologic disease and spinal cord injuries; and *possibly effective* for decreasing spasticity in other conditions.

Preparation, dosage, and administration. Chlorzoxazone is administered orally in tablets of 250 mg. The average adult daily dose is 250 to 750 mg. three to four times a day. Peak action occurs within 2 to 3 hours; duration of action is about 6 hours. Dose for children is 20 mg. per kilogram of body weight daily divided into three or four doses.

Side effects and precautions. Adverse reactions include nausea, vomiting, diarrhea, abdominal distress, drowsiness, vertigo, and headache. A few cases of jaundice have been reported, and chlorzoxazone should not be given to patients with a history of liver disease. It is chemically related to zoxazolamine, which was withdrawn from the market following fatalities resulting from drug-induced liver damage. Patients on this drug should be observed closely for signs of liver damage.

Methocarbamol, N.F. (Robaxin)

Methocarbamol is chemically related to mephenesin carbamate and has similar actions and effectiveness. Its D.E.S.I. rating is: *possibly effective* for relieving muscle spasm in postoperative orthopedic conditions or that caused by trauma, and for relief of back pain due to nerve irritation; and *ineffective* for muscle hyperactivity resulting from chronic neurologic disorders such as parkinsonism and multiple sclerosis. Methocarbamol has a longer duration of action than mephenesin.

Preparation, dosage, and administration. Routes of administration of methocarbamol are oral, intramuscular, and intravenous. Initial daily dose for adults is 1.5 to 2 Gm. given four times a day for 2 or 3 days. One gram four times a day may be given as a maintenance dose. When given intramuscularly the dosage should not exceed 500 mg. Intramuscular injection should be given in divided doses in each buttock at 8-hour intervals. Oral administration should be initiated as soon as possible. Intravenous solutions are highly irritating and should be injected slowly at no more than 3 ml. per minute. Average dose per injection is 1 to 3 Gm. and should not exceed 3 Gm. daily. Solutions are available for injection in 100 mg. per milliliter with polyethylene glycol in 10-ml. containers. Tablets are available in 500- and 750-mg. strengths.

Side effects and precautions. Side effects from oral administration are similar to those of other centrally acting muscle relaxants. Side effects from parenteral administration include metallic taste, thrombophlebitis, sloughing at site of injection, anaphylactic reactions, and convulsions.

Methocarbamol is not recommended for pregnant women, children under 12 years of age, or epileptics. Parenteral administration is contraindicated in patients with renal disease since the polyethylene glycol 300 vehicle has the potential of being nephrotoxic.

Metaxalone (Skelaxin)

Metaxalone is pharmacologically related to meprobamate. It blocks neural transmission through polysynaptic pathways in the spinal cord. Its D.E.S.I. rating is: *ineffective* as a relaxant for the initial phase of acute muscle spasm resulting from sprains, strains, fractures, dislocations, and trauma to tendons and ligaments. There is some evidence that metaxalone is effective in reducing neurogenic spasticity. However, because its side effects are numerous and serious, its potential toxicity may outweigh potential benefits of therapy.

Preparation and dosage. Metaxalone is available in 400-mg. tablets. Adult dose is 800 mg., three or four times daily; dosage for children over 6 years of age is 45 mg. per kilogram of body weight in divided doses.

Side effects and precautions. Nausea and gastrointestinal disturbances are the most common side effects. Metaxalone has caused leukopenia, jaundice, hemoglobin depression, and liver damage. It is not recommended for pregnant patients, epileptics, or those with kidney or liver disease. Metaxalone should not be administered for more than 10 days.

DIRECT ACTING SKELETAL MUSCLE RELAXANT

Dantrolene (Dantrium)

Dantrolene produces skeletal muscle relaxation by acting directly on skeletal muscles. It probably acts by inhibiting the release of calcium from the sarcoplasmic reticulum resulting in decreased muscle response to the action potential and decreased muscle contraction. There is no apparent effect on peripheral nerve conduction or neuromuscular transmission. Central nervous system side effects may be caused indirectly by the decreased skeletal muscle activity. Clinical studies show that dantrolene produces general-

ized mild weakness of skeletal muscles and decreases the force of reflex muscle contractions, hyperreflexia, clonus, muscle stiffness, spasticity, and involuntary movements.

Absorption of dantrolene after oral administration is slow and incomplete, about 35% of the drug being absorbed from the gastrointestinal tract. Peak blood levels of the drug occur about 5 hours after oral administration. Biologic half-life in adults averages about 8.7 hours after a single 100-mg. dose; in children, the half-life averages about 7.3 hours. Dantrolene is metabolized in the liver and excreted mainly in urine.

Preparation and dosage. Dantrolene is available in 25- and 100-mg. capsules for oral administration. Recommended dosage for adults is 25 mg. daily initially, which may be increased to 25 mg. two, three, or four times daily at 4- to 7-day intervals and then by 25-mg. increments up to 100 mg. two, three, or four times daily. A few patients may require 200 mg. four times daily.

Dosage for children is 1 mg. per kilogram of body weight daily, which is gradually increased to 1 mg. per kilogram of body weight two, three, or four times daily up to 3 mg. per kilogram two, three, or four times daily if necessary. Dosages greater than 100 mg. four times daily should not be given to children.

Uses. Dantrolene is used for the symptomatic treatment of skeletal muscle spasm due to multiple sclerosis, spinal cord injury, cerebral palsy, and stroke. It is not indicated for the treatment of muscle spasms caused by rheumatic disorders. A therapeutic trial of the drug is necessary to determine whether or not a patient will benefit from the drug. Tolerance to dantrolene apparently does not occur. The safety of long-term treatment with dantrolene has not been established, but it is considered justifiable if the drug produces a significant reduction in painful and/or disabling spasticity, if it reduces the intensity of nursing care required, or if it relieves the patient of annoying manifestations of muscle spasm.

Side effects and toxic effects. Common side effects from dantrolene therapy include muscle weakness, drowsiness, malaise, nausea, dizziness, diarrhea, and lightheadedness. These side effects are usually transient, occur early in treatment, and may be prevented by initiating therapy with a low dose and gradual increments until the desired therapeutic effect is obtained. Side effects are usually related to the rate of increase in dosage and total daily dosage. If the diarrhea or weakness is severe, the dosage should be decreased or even discontinued. If diarrhea recurs after restarting dantrolene therapy, the drug should probably be permanently discontinued. Other side effects include anorexia, constipation, gastric irritation, and gastrointestinal bleeding.

Neurologic side effects include difficulty in swallowing, speech and visual disturbances, alteration of taste, mental depression, confusion, increased nervousness, and insomnia.

Urogenital side effects include urinary frequency, incontinence, nocturia, difficult urination, urinary retention, crystalluria, and difficult erection.

Additional side effects include tachycardia, erratic blood pressure, phlebitis, abnormal hair growth, dermatitis, backache, excessive tearing, chills and fever, and a feeling of suffocation. Alterations in laboratory tests have also been reported and include increased or decreased white cell count; increased serum uric acid, SGOT, BUN, alkaline phosphatase, and serum bilirubin; decreased serum phosphate; and proteinuria.

Precautions. Caution should be exercised when dantrolene is given to patients with impaired pulmonary function, impaired myocardial function, or preexisting liver disease. Its safe use in pregnancy or in children younger than 5 years of age has not been determined; it should not be given to nursing mothers. Its possible carcinogenic potential has not been established although one strain of female rats showed an increased incidence of tumors of the liver.

Patients on dantrolene therapy should be warned about engaging in activities requiring alertness and skill, such as operating hazardous equipment, particularly if central nervous system depression occurs. Since drug-induced photosensitivity may occur, patients on dantrolene should refrain from excessive or unneccessary exposure to sunlight. It should be used with caution in patients on tranquilizer therapy.

Contraindications. Dantrolene is contraindicated for patients whose spasticity is utilized to obtain or maintain upright posture and balance or body function.

ANTAGONISTS OF CURARIFORM DRUGS

Edrophonium chloride, U.S.P., B.P. (Tensilon)

Edrophonium is an antagonist of skeletal muscle relaxants, such as tubocurarine and similar preparations that act by competing with acetylcholine for end-plate receptors at the myoneural junction. Edrophonium is an anticholinesterase agent; it inactivates or inhibits acetylcholinesterase at sites of cholinergic transmission, permitting accumulation of ACh to overcome the curare effects. It may also have a direct excitatory effect on skeletal muscle.

Uses. Edrophonium can be used to terminate the effects of curariform agents when muscular relaxation is no longer desired or to reverse respiratory muscle paralysis produced by overdosage. It is used as a diagnostic agent for myasthenia gravis. This is based on its ability to increase muscle strength in myasthenia gravis; improvement in muscle strength occurs in 30 seconds to 5 minutes. It is also used for emergency treatment of myasthenic crises. Since its action is brief it cannot be used for maintenance therapy. It has received a D.E.S.I. rating of *effective* as a curare antagonist. It is not used as an antidote for succinylcholine or decamethonium.

Preparation, dosage, and administration. Edrophonium is administered intravenously. The dosage employed for antagonism of appropriate curariform drugs varies from 5 to 10 mg. or more. It is not recommended if apnea is present. To counteract overdosage of appropriate muscle relaxants, therefore, it is used along with artificial respiration and oxygen therapy and only when some definite sign of voluntary respiration can be observed.

Side effects and toxic effects. Side effects of edrophonium include increased flow of saliva (salivation), bronchiolar spasm (especially in asthmatic patients), slow pulse, and disturbance of cardiac rhythm (especially in elderly patients).

When edrophonium is used in large doses, it intensifies the peripheral effects of the curariform drugs instead of antagonizing them. Furthermore, it does not combat circulatory collapse that is associated with respiratory depression.

Neostigmine methylsulfate, U.S.P., B.P. (Prostigmin)

Neostigmine is capable of functioning as an antagonist to curare type drugs, such as tubocurarine, which are used for skeletal muscle relaxation during surgical anesthesia. These relaxants inhibit acetylcholine depolarization at the neuromuscular junction. Neostigmine inhibits cholinesterase and permits sufficient acetylcholine to accumulate and overcome the curare action. It does not antagonize decamethonium or succinylcholine.

The usual dose as a curare antagonist is 0.5 to 2 mg. given by slow intravenous injection; this may be repeated. Total dose should not exceed 5 mg. It is recommended that atropine sulfate, 0.6 to 1.2 mg., be given intravenously when neostigmine is given intravenously.

ANTIPARKINSONISM DRUGS

Parkinson's disease, also called paralysis agitans, is a chronic disorder of the central nervous system. It is characterized by muscle tremors, rigidity, slowness of movement, and muscle weakness with alterations in posture and equilibrium. The exact cause of parkinsonism remains unknown, but it is currently believed that it reflects an imbalance between cholinergic and dopaminergic mechanisms in the central nervous system.

Dopamine, a catecholamine, is the precursor of norepinephrine. Dopamine is normally present in the corpus striatum. However, in patients with idiopathic or postencephalitic parkinsonism there is a depletion of dopamine. It has been postulated that the cholinergic and dopaminergic mechanisms are antagonistic: the cholinergic mechanisms innervated by acetylcholine are excitatory; the dopaminergic mechanisms innervated by dopamine are inhibitory. The symptoms of parkinsonism thus reflect cholinergic dominance resulting from low levels of dopamine in the brain.

Treatment of parkinsonism remains palliative rather than curative with the goals of therapy being (1) to provide maximal relief of symptoms, and (2) to maintain some independence of movement and activity. Drug therapy consists of: (1) anticholinergic drugs to inhibit the cholinergic mechanisms; (2) antihistaminic drugs, which also have anticholinergic action; (3) levodopa to replenish dopamine levels and enhance the dopaminergic mechanisms.

Two of the newer drugs introduced for the treatment of parkinsonism are levodopa and amantadine. Levodopa is the precursor to dopamine; amantadine is an antiviral drug. The use of amantadine as an anti-parkinsonism drug is based on the fact that a patient taking the drug as a prevention against influenza experienced remission of symptoms of rigidity, tremor, and akinesia. Another drug used to treat Parkinson's disease is ethopropazine (Parsidol), a phenothiazine derivative.

Levodopa, U.S.P., B.P. (L-dopa, Dopar, Larodopa)

Levodopa is the most effective drug available for treating parkinsonism. All major symptoms of parkinsonism may be relieved by levodopa therapy. Most patients show a marked reduction in akinesia and rigidity. Tremors may increase in severity during initial therapy before improving. Improvements have occurred in balance, posture, gait, speech, and handwriting. Drooling may be completely abolished, and oculogyric crisis is reduced in both severity and frequency. There may also be improved intellectual function and an elevation in mood.

Levodopa is not effective in counteracting extrapyramidal reactions induced by antipsychotic agents, such as phenothiazines.

Preparation, dosage, and administration. Levodopa is available in 100-, 250-, and 500-mg. capsules and in 250- and 500-mg. tablets. Dosage must be individualized, and optimal dosage may not be achieved before 6 to 8 weeks of therapy. Average daily dosage appears to be 4 to 6 Gm. in three or more divided doses. Constant observation and dosage adjustment are needed.

Side effects and toxic effects. Numerous side effects occur in almost all patients receiving levodopa. *Gastrointestinal* side effects range from nausea, vomiting, and anorexia to bleeding, constipation, diarrhea, and abdominal distress.

Cardiovascular side effects include a variety of arrhythmias, orthostatic hypotension, palpitation, hypertension, and phlebitis.

Musculoskeletal side effects are numerous and include various involuntary muscular movements such as grimacing, jerky movements of the shoulders or pelvis, and rhythmic movements of the neck, hands, feet, mouth, and head. Opisthotonos may also occur.

A host of *psychologic* and *neurologic* side effects can occur. These include anxiety, confusion, depression, hallucinations, insomnia, paranoia, and suicidal tendencies. Ataxia, convulsions, headaches, tremors, weakness, and numbness also occur.

Respiratory, urinary, ocular, and *hematologic* disorders have also been reported.

While many of the side effects are dose related and disappear after reduction of dosage, neurologic and psychologic side effects may persist for several months after reduction or discontinuance of the drug.

Precautions. Levodopa should be administered only with great caution to patients with almost any physiologic disorder with an organic basis. Evaluations of most body system functions (hepatic, cardiovascular, and so on) should be performed periodically. Levodopa is *not* recommended for children under 12 years of age, pregnant women, or nursing mothers.

Drug interactions. Monoamine oxidase inhibitors and other sympathomimetic drugs will increase the adrenergic effect of levodopa. Antihypertensive and antianxiety drugs that block adrenergic receptors will decrease the therapeutic effect of levodopa. Pyridoxine also decreases the effects of levodopa.

Amantadine hydrochloride, N.F. (Symmetrel)

Amantadine is a synthetic antiviral compound, which is used in the prevention of Asian influenza and in the treatment of parkinsonism. Its exact mechanism in reducing symptoms of parkinsonism and improving functional capacity is not known. It has been postulated that amantadine releases dopamine and other catecholamines from neuronal storage sites. It may also block the re-uptake of dopamine into presynaptic neurons, thus permitting accumulation of dopamine peripherally and centrally.

Although amantadine is less effective than levodopa in the treatment of parkinsonism, it produces more rapid clinical improvement and causes fewer untoward reactions. Amantadine relieves akinesia, rigidity, tremor, salivation, gait disturbances, and functional disability. It may also give the patient a sense of well being and elevation of mood. Improvement in symptoms occurs within 4 to 48 hours after initiation of therapy; optimal results occur within 2 weeks to 3 months. Improvement may last up to 30 months. In some patients a reduction in beneficial effects occurs after 4 to 12 weeks of therapy. Amantadine is usually used along with other antiparkinsonism drugs. It is well absorbed from the gastrointestinal tract and excreted unchanged in the urine.

Dosage. Amantadine is available in 100-mg. capsules and as a syrup containing 50 mg. in 5 ml. Dosage initially is 100-mg. once daily after breakfast for 5 to 7 days. If side effects do not occur, an additional 100 mg. is given after lunch. Increasing the dosage beyond this level increases the severity of side effects without significantly increasing beneficial effects. Amantadine therapy should be discontinued gradually; abrupt cessation of the drug has been associated with exacerbations of parkinsonism symptoms within 24 hours and onset of parkinsonian crises within 3 days.

Side effects and precautions. Many of the side effects of amantadine are central nervous system disturbances, such as nervousness, mental depression, psychoses, slurred speech, blurred vision, feeling of drunkenness, inability to concentrate, detachment, insomnia, confusion, and ataxia. Reversible livedo reticularis is a common side effect. It may appear within 1 month to 1 year following institution of therapy; it disappears gradually in 2 to 12 weeks upon withdrawal of the drug. Other side effects include edema, orthostatic hypotension, skin rash, nausea, vomiting, abdominal discomfort, constipation, urinary retention, and increased frequency of urination.

Amantadine should be used cautiously (if at all) in elderly patients, epileptics, psychotics, those with liver, kidney or cardiac disease, pregnant women, and those with cerebrovascular disease. Amantadine is contraindicated in nursing mothers. There have been reports of it being embryotoxic and teratogenic in rats.

Ethopropazine hydrochloride, U.S.P., B.P. (Parsidol)

Ethopropazine is a phenothiazine derivative used to treat parkinsonism usually in conjunction with other drugs. Like some phenothiazines, ethopropazine has antihistaminic, ganglion blocking, adrenergic blocking, and local anesthetic action. It usually produces central nervous system depression. Ethopropazine helps to control tremor and rigidity and improves the patient's posture, gait, and speech. It also promotes better sleep. Its D.E.S.I. rating is *effective* for all forms of parkinsonism and for drug-induced extrapyramidal reactions.

Dosage. Ethopropazine is available in 10-, 50-, and 100-mg. tablets. Dosage is variable and dependent upon patient response. Dosage may range from 10 mg. two to four times a day initially to 100 to 400 mg. in mild or moderate cases of parkinsonism; severe cases may require 500 to 600 mg. daily.

Side effects and precautions. Ethopropazine causes numerous side effects, and many patients, particularly the elderly, cannot tolerate therapeutic dosages. Drowsiness, dizziness, inability to concentrate, and confusion are the most common side effects. Muscle cramps, paresthesia, epigastric distress, and hypotension may also occur. It should be used with caution in patients with glaucoma, cardiac disease, or prostatic hypertrophy.

SYNTHETIC ANTICHOLINERGICS AS ANTIPARKINSONISM DRUGS

The belladonna alkaloids, atropine and scopolamine, were the first centrally active anticholinergics used to treat parkinsonism and, for many years, were the only drugs available for such treatment. These drugs have been sup-planted by the synthetic anticholinergics. These anticholinergics were developed in an effort to produce drugs equally as effective as the belladonna drugs in treating parkinsonism but with fewer disturbing side effects.

The anticholinergics that readily cross the blood-brain barrier can produce slight to moderate improvement in functional capacity. The usefulness of these drugs is limited by their side effects and their tendency to be less effective with continued use. Anticholinergics are also used to control the extrapyramidal reactions (rigidity, akinesia, tremor, akathisia) caused by antipsychotic drugs (e.g., phenothiazines).

The anticholinergics are used alone or in conjunction with other antiparkinsonism drugs, such as levodopa. All produce "atropine-like" side effects, such as dryness of the mouth, blurred vision, dizziness, and dysuria. All have the potential of causing constipation, drowsiness, urinary hesitancy or retention, tachycardia, dilation of the pupil, increased intraocular tension, and intestinal obstruction.

Benztropine mesylate, U.S.P., B.P. (Cogentin)

Benztropine is a synthetic drug chemically related to atropine and diphenhydramine. Its anticholinergic activity is almost equal to that of atropine; its antihistaminic action is like that of pyrilamine maleate. It is assumed that benztropine acts by depressing synaptic transmission in cholinergic neurons in the central nervous system. It is used primarily in small doses to supplement levodopa or other antiparkinsonism drugs. In full dosage it causes intense side effects that are rarely tolerated.

Benztropine is considered by some physicians to be one of the best drugs available for treating parkinsonism, particularly for the control of rigidity, contracture, tremor, and insomnia. Other symptoms may also be relieved. The drug's effects are cumulative and may take 2 or 3 days to occur.

The D.E.S.I. rating for benztropine is *effective* for all forms of parkinsonism and for drug-induced extrapyramidal disorders.

Preparation and dosage. Benztropine is available in 0.5-, 1-, and 2-mg. tablets; and in 2-ml. ampules containing 1 mg. of drug per milliliter for intravenous or intramuscular injection. Range of total daily dose is 0.5 to 6.0 mg. orally.

Side effects and precautions. The side effects of benztropine are manifestations of its anticholinergic and antihistaminic action. Sedation, hypnosis, and dryness of the mouth are common. It may produce mydriasis and thus can produce or aggravate glaucoma. Patients sensitive to the drug may develop weakness and inability to move certain muscle groups. Contraindications are the same as for other anticholinergics.

Trihexyphenidyl hydrochloride, U.S.P. (Artane); benzhexol hydrochloride, B.P.

Trihexyphenidyl is considered the anticholinergic drug of choice for initiating therapy in patients with moderate or severe parkinsonism. It has an antispasmodic effect on smooth muscle and an inhibitory effect on the parasympathetic system. Thus it relieves smooth muscle spasm by both direct action and parasympathetic inhibition. It relieves spasticity of voluntary muscles by a cholinergic blocking action and by acting on the cerebral motor center. Trihexyphenidyl's antispasmodic action is one half that of atropine, its mydriatic effect about one third, its antisialogogic effect about one eighth, and the cardiovagal inhibitory action about one one-hundredth that of atropine.

Trihexyphenidyl has a D.E.S.I. rating of *effective* for all forms of parkinsonism and for extrapyramidal reactions to phenothiazines.

Preparation and dosage. Trihexyphenidyl is available in 2- and 5-mg. tablets; as an elixir containing 2 mg. in 5 ml., and as a sustained-release capsule containing 5 mg. Initial dosage is 1 to 2 mg. two or three times daily. Dosage is gradually increased until the therapeutic effect is obtained or severe reactions occur precluding further increase. For extrapyramidal reactions the usual daily dose is 5 to 15 mg. Onset of action occurs in 1 hour, peak action in 2 to 3 hours; duration of action is 6 to 12 hours.

Side effects and precautions. Most common side effects are dry mouth, blurred vision, dizziness, nausea, and nervousness. Overdosage causes cerebral excitement, hallucinations, and delirium. This drug should not be given to patients with glaucoma.

Biperiden, N.F. (Akineton)

Biperiden is a derivative of trihexyphenidyl and has similar actions, uses, and adverse effects. D.E.S.I. rating is *effective* for all forms of parkinsonism and for phenothiazine-induced extrapyramidal reactions and *ineffective* for muscle spasms not related to parkinsonism.

It is available in 2-mg. tablets, and is a lactate solution in 1-ml. ampules containing 5 mg. per milliliter for injection. Initial dose is 1 to 2 mg. two or three times daily. Dosage may be gradually increased to 20 mg. daily. For drug-induced extrapyramidal reactions dose for adults is 2 mg. one to three times daily; for children the dose is 0.04 mg. per kilogram of body weight, given intramuscularly and repeated in $1/2$ hour (no more than four doses should be given in 24 hours).

Cycrimine hydrochloride, N.F. (Pagitane)

Cycrimine is another derivative of trihexyphenidyl with similar actions, uses, and adverse reactions. It is slightly more potent than trihexyphenidyl. It is more effective in the treatment of rigidity, akinesia, and oculogyric crises than in the reduction of tremor. D.E.S.I. rating is *effective* for parkinsonism but *ineffective* for extrapyramidal reactions to phenothiazines. Cycrimine is available in 1.25- and 2.5-mg. tablets. Dosage must be individualized but may range from 1.25 to 5 mg. three or four times daily.

Procyclidine hydrochloride, N.F., B.P. (Kemadrin)

Procyclidine is also a derivative of trihexyphenidyl with similar actions, uses, and adverse effects. D.E.S.I. rating is *effective* for parkinsonism and drug-induced extrapyramidal reactions. It is available in 2- and 5-mg. tablets. Daily dosage initially is 2 to 2.5 mg. three times after meals and may be increased to 15 to 30 mg.

ANTIHISTAMINES AS ANTIPARKINSONISM DRUGS

Antihistamines are used primarily as adjuncts to other more potent antiparkinsonism drugs. However, they may be used alone for initial therapy in patients with mild parkinsonism or for elderly patients, since they are less likely to cause mental disturbances such as confusion and disorientation. In addition to having anticholinergic effects, antihistamines have a sedative effect that helps to counteract the insomnia that can be caused by potent anticholinergics.

Diphenhydramine hydrochloride, U.S.P., B.P. (Benadryl)

Diphenhydramine was the first antihistaminic drug available in the United States and the first antihistamine to be used in the treatment of parkinsonism. It has served as a comparison in the development of many other antihistamines. Diphenhydramine has many therapeutic effects; it is an antiemetic, anticholinergic (antispasmodic), antitussive, and it has local anesthetic and sedative actions. Its use in parkinsonism is based on its central cholinergic blocking action. It decreases rigidity and improves voluntary movement and speech. It is most commonly used with levodopa or one of the more potent anticholinergics. Its D.E.S.I. rating is *effective* for use in parkinsonism and drug-induced extrapyramidal reactions.

Preparation and dosage. Diphenhydramine is available in 25- and 50-mg. capsules; 25-mg. enteric-coated tablets; an elixir containing 2.5 mg. per milliliter; and in solutions for injection containing 10 mg. per milliliter in 10- and 30-ml. vials, and 50 mg. per milliliter in 1- and 10-ml. containers. Dose for adults is 10 to 50 mg. The maximal dose is 100 mg., and total daily dose should not exceed 400 mg. For children the usual dose is 5 mg. per kilogram of body weight divided into four doses; maximum daily dose is 300 mg. When taken orally the drug is readily absorbed from the gastrointestinal tract; peak tissue concentration occurs in 1 hour; duration of action is 4 to 6 hours.

Side effects and precautions. Diphenhydramine causes a high incidence of side effects. Fortunately, most of these are minor and most disappear with continued therapy. Sedation and drowsiness are the most common side effects. Other side effects are nausea, headache, vertigo, epigastric distress, dry mouth, blurred vision, hypotension, rash, and urticaria.

Diphenhydramine should not be given to patients with narrow-angle glaucoma, prostatic hypertrophy, or obstruction of the intestinal or urinary tract. Persons on diphenhydramine should be extremely cautious around hazardous machinery. If the drug causes drowsiness they should not drive motor vehicles.

Drug interactions. Diphenhydramine may potentiate the action of alcohol, hypnotics, sedatives, tranquilizers, and other central nervous system depressants.

Monoamine oxidase inhibitors may potentiate the action of diphenhydramine.

Diphenhydramine may enhance the action of atropine and other anticholinergic drugs.

Orphenadrine citrate, N.F.; orphenadrine hydrochloride, B.P. (Disipal)

Orphenadrine is a derivative of diphenhydramine with similar actions and uses. It is used alone or with other drugs in the treatment of parkinson's disease. It relieves muscle rigidity more than tremor, and it has a slight euphoriant action that helps to counteract depression and fatigue. Its anticholinergic action helps to control sialorrhea, diaphoresis, and oculogyria. Orphenadrine's effectiveness tends to diminish with use. Unlike diphenhydramine, it does not cause drowsiness. Side effects are relatively few and mild and similar to those caused by diphenhydramine. Orphenadrine may cause mild excitation and mental clouding in the elderly. D.E.S.I. rating is: *effective* for treatment of parkinsonism; and *possibly effective* for skeletal muscle spasm.

Orphenadrine should not be given to patients with glaucoma, obstructions, or myasthenia gravis. Extreme caution is required if given to patients with a history of tachycardia.

Preparation and dosage. Orphenadrine is available in 50-mg. tablets. Oral dosage for adults initially is 50 mg. three times daily, which may be increased to 250 mg. daily depending upon the patient's response.

Drug interactions. Use of orphenadrine with propoxyphene (Darvon) may result in mental confusion, anxiety, and tremors. Orphenadrine plus chlorpromazine has caused hypoglycemic coma. Orphenadrine may inhibit the action of griseofulvin, hexobarbital, and phenylbutazone.

Chlorphenoxamine hydrochloride, N.F. (Phenoxene)

Chlorphenoxamine is a derivative of diphenhydramine possessing antihistaminic and anticholinergic properties. Its actions and side effects are like those of diphenhydramine. Chlorphenoxamine has received a D.E.S.I. rating of *effective* for all forms of parkinsonism. It is available in 50-mg. tablets. Dosage initially is 50 mg. three times a day; this may be increased to 100 mg. two to four times daily.

QUESTIONS

For study and review

1 Explain the differences in action and uses between the centrally acting skeletal muscle relaxants and the neuromuscular blocking agents.
2 What drugs potentiate the action of tubocurarine?
3 What drugs inhibit the action of tubocurarine?
4 Name the classes of drugs used to treat parkinsonism. What precautions must be taken with these drugs?
5 Which of the following is an untrue statement?
  a. Neostigmine antagonizes the action of curare or tubocurarine.
  b. Anticurare drugs inactivate or inhibit cholinesterase, thereby permitting acetylcholine to accumulate and effect its action.
  c. Acetylcholine is important for skeletal muscle contraction.
  d. Centrally acting skeletal muscle relaxants block the liberation of acetylcholine at nerve endings.
6 Choose the *incorrect* answers. Mephenesin:
  a. has a strong neuromuscular blocking action
  b. has a depressant effect on the central nervous system
  c. exerts its primary effect on the autonomic nervous system
  d. causes skeletal muscle relaxation without loss of consciousness
7 Tubocurarine may cause a fall in blood pressure as a result of:
  a. adrenergic blockade
  b. ganglionic blockade
  c. histamine release
  d. catecholamine release
8 Choose the *incorrect* statements. Decamethonium:
  a. prolongs depolarization, which inhibits repolarization
  b. causes a flaccid muscle paralysis
  c. is easily antagonized by anticurare drugs

  d. does not cause respiratory depression because of its short duration of action
9 Of the following choose the *incorrect* statement.
  a. Skeletal muscle relaxants cause spinal cord depression.
  b. Succinylcholine is an ultrashort-acting myoneural blocking agent because it is chemically altered by cholinesterase.
  c. An overdose of tubocurarine paralyzes respirator muscles.
  d. Skeletal muscle relaxants are not known to depress the medullary respiratory center.

REFERENCES

Barbeau, A.: Long-term side effects of levodopa, Lancet **1**:395, 1971.
Feldman, S. A., and Tyrell, M. F.: A new theory of the termination of action of the muscle relaxants, Proc. Roy. Soc. Med. **63**:692, 1970.
Feldman, S. A.: Muscle relaxants, Philadelphia, 1973, W. B. Saunders Co.
Galindo, A.: Depolarizing neuromuscular block, J. Pharmacol. Exp. Therap. **178**:339, 1971.
Gissen, A. J., and Nastick, W. L.: Succinylcholine and decamethonium: Comparison of depolarization and desensitization, Anesthesiology **33**:611, 1970.
Goldstein, G.: Myasthenia gravis and the thymus, Ann. Rev. Med. **22**:119, 1971.
Greenblatt, D. J., and Shader, R. I.: Anticholinergics, New Eng. J. Med. **288**:1215, 1973.
Hannington-Kiff, J. G.: Residual postoperative paralysis, Proc. Roy. Soc. Med. **63**:73, 1970.
Karis, J. H., and Gissen, A. J.: Evaluation of new neuromuscular blocking agents, Anesthesiology **35**:149, 1971.
Katz, R. L.: Clinical neuromuscular pharmacology of pancuronium, Anesthesiology **34**:550, 1971.
Leyser, R. B., and Rowland, L. P.: Cramps, New Eng. J. Med. **285**:31, 1971.
Monks, P. S.: The reversal of non-depolarizing relaxants, Anesthesia **27**:313, 1972.
Stovner, J., and Lund, I.: The muscle relaxants and their antagonists, Br. J. Anesth. **42**:235, 1970.
Walker, J. E., and others: Amantadine and levodopa in the treatment of Parkinson's disease, Clin. Pharmacol. Therap. **13**:28, 1972.

CHAPTER 16

Respiratory system drugs

Regulation of respiration

Drugs that act on the respiratory center

Therapeutic gases
Nebulization therapy
Bronchodilators
Mucolytic agents
Direct respiratory stimulants
Reflex stimulants
Respiratory depressants or sedatives

Drugs that affect the cough center and the respiratory mucosa

Antitussives
Demulcents
Expectorants
Preparations to relieve nasal congestion and cold symptoms

Although a large number of specific substances must be supplied to maintain life, the most urgent and critical need is a continued, uninterrupted supply of oxygen. This specific need for oxygen is supplied through the process of respiration. Respiration is a term loosely used to describe three distinct but interrelated processes. These include:

1 Pulmonary ventilation, which involves the movement of air into and out of the lungs
2 Internal respiration, which involves the exchange of gases between the air in the lungs, the blood, and the cell
3 Cellular respiration, which involves the utilization of oxygen in the catabolism of energy-yielding substances for the production of energy

The process of respiration is one of the regulating systems that helps to maintain physiologic dynamic equilibrium. It also functions as a compensatory mechanism for rapid adjustment to changes in metabolic states. Anatomically, the respiratory system in man includes the nasal cavity, larynx, trachea, bronchi, lungs, bronchioles and alveolar sacs, striated and unstriated muscles of the larynx, intercostal muscles and diaphragm, respiratory centers in the upper ventral surface of the medulla, and the blood.

REGULATION OF RESPIRATION

Breathing is primarily controlled and coordinated involuntarily by the medullary rhythmicity area located beneath the lower part of the floor of the fourth ventricle in the medial half of the medulla. In this area inspiratory and expiratory

383

neurons intermingle and discharge or fire impulses alternately. Thus, it is in this area that the basic rhythm for respiration is initiated and maintained. However, signals from the spinal cord, the cerebral cortex and midbrain, the apneustic area of the pons, and the pneumotaxis area of the upper pons can enter the medullary rhythmicity area and modify the rhythm of respiration as well as contribute to the normal pattern of respiration.

Normally, the human organism is unaware of the respiratory process. However, voluntary influence and control of breathing are possible. This becomes of paramount importance in a situation in which a patient must learn to voluntarily control breathing patterns.

The medullary rhythmicity area is also influenced by various forms of sensory and peripheral stimuli, the vasomotor center, reflex mechanisms (such as the Hering-Breuer reflex), the chemoreceptors in the carotid and aortic bodies, and the baroreceptors in the carotid sinus and aortic arch. Fear, pain, stress, blood pressure, body temperature, and blood levels of oxygen and carbon dioxide can all modify the activity of the respiratory centers.

Humoral regulation of respiration is primarily achieved through changes in the concentrations of oxygen, carbon dioxide, or hydrogen ions in body fluids. In the normal well individual carbon dioxide is the chief respiratory stimulant. An increase in the carbon dioxide tension of the blood directly stimulates the inspiratory and expiratory centers, which increases both the rate and depth of breathing. This results in a blowing off of carbon dioxide to keep the carbon dioxide tension of the blood constant. The pH of the blood is determined by the ratio of bicarbonate ion (HCO_3) to carbon dioxide. When the carbon dioxide content of the blood is increased, there is a subsequent increase in the formation of carbonic acid in the blood. This alters the bicarbonate:carbonic acid ratio from the normal value of 20:1 and results in acidosis. Conversely, a decrease in the carbon dioxide content of the blood results in alkalosis. Therefore, respiration is important for regulating the pH of the blood by controlling the carbon dioxide tension of the blood.

Basically, changes in arterial oxygen concentration have little, if any, direct effect on the respiratory center. However, if the arterial oxygen concentration falls below normal, the chemoreceptors in the carotid and aortic bodies are stimulated and in turn stimulate the respiratory center to increase alveolar ventilation. This mechanism operates primarily under abnormal conditions, such as chronic obstructive pulmonary disease.

Air passages. The air passages serve the dual purpose of permitting air to flow from the external environment to pulmonary blood and of modifying the air taken in by warming and moistening it and removing noxious substances. Man's airway efficiency is determined by the following factors:

1 Shape and size of each portion of the respiratory tract (nasal cavity, pharynx, larynx, trachea, bronchi, bronchioles, alveolar sacs)
2 Presence of a ciliated, mucus-secreting, epithelial lining throughout most of the respiratory tract
3 Character and thickness of respiratory tract secretions
4 Compliance of the cartilaginous and bony supports
5 Pressure gradients
6 Traction on airway walls
7 Absence of foreign substances in the lumen of the respiratory tract

An alteration from normal of any of these factors will affect the ease with which air flows through the air passages. Congenital anomalies, injuries, allergies, or disease will cause air flow resistance if the preceding factors are abnormally affected. Resistance occurs, for example, if there is stenosis or narrowing of any portion of the respiratory tract, loss of cilia that ordinarily sweep out foreign substances, presence of thick or tenacious secretions, loss of elasticity, or presence of foreign objects.

Lungs. The lungs are elastic, membranous sacs. Air flowing to the lungs passes through the trachea, bronchi, bronchioles, and alveolar sacs. The bronchiolar musculature is regulated by bronchoconstrictor fibers in the vagi and bronchodilator fibers in the sympathetic nervous system. The walls of the alveolar sacs are dilated to form alveoli. Contained in the alveoli walls are flattened epithelial cells, a network of capillaries, and elastic connective tissue. Inhaled air mixes with the gas in the alveoli and, by simple diffusion, oxygen enters the blood in the pulmonary capillaries while carbon dioxide enters the alveoli. The total number of alveoli in the lungs of man has been estimated at 250 to 300 million.

Alveoli are lined with surfactant, a lipid surface tension–lowering agent. Surfactant produces the low surface tension when the alveoli are small. It is produced in alveolar epithelial cells and expelled onto the epithelial surface of the alveoli. The molecules of surfactant move together during expiration, thus reducing surface tension and preventing the collapse of the alveoli. If the surface tension were not reduced during expiration, the alveoli would collapse in accordance with the law of Laplace. Thus, surfactant is a stabilizer of alveolar surface forces and in normal persons contributes to the elastic properties of the lung.

A deficiency of surfactant is believed to be the cause of hyaline membrane disease in newborn infants. The lungs of these infants have a very high surface tension as well as multiple areas of atelectasis. Surfactant deficiency may also occur in patients undergoing cardiac surgery in which the pulmonary circulation is interrupted, and in those subjected to long-term inhalation of 90% to 100% oxygen. Atelectasis from lack of surfactant can also occur in cases of prolonged hypoventilation or respiratory distress. This can be counteracted to some extent by intermittent positive pressure breathing.

The efficacy of detergents (such as Tergemist and Alevaire) to liquefy and loosen thick pulmonary secretions is being questioned by the Food and Drug Administration as well as physicians. These agents may coat alveolar walls and thus interfere with the stabilizing properties of pulmonary surfactant.

Gaseous exchange in the lungs. In order to maintain normal ventilation perfusion ratios at the alveolar capillary membrane, gaseous exchange must occur. Basically, this process is concerned with the physical factors that determine alveolar concentrations of oxygen, carbon dioxide, and other gases, and factors that affect the rate at which these various gases can diffuse through the respiratory membrane. The alveolar concentration of the various gases depends upon the composition of the air inspired and upon the rate and volume of inspiration. Carbon dioxide diffusion through alveolar membranes occurs at a rate twenty times that of oxygen diffusion.

During exercise the *respiratory minute volume* (respiratory rate per minute times volume of air inspired per respiration) can increase as much as eight- to tenfold from the resting value. This difference is accounted for by an increase in respiratory rate and depth during exercise. *Tidal air* (volume of air that enters and leaves the lungs with each natural respiration) increases from about 12% of the *vital capacity* (the sum of the tidal air and inspiratory and expiratory reserves) at rest to about 50% during strenuous exercise. This increase is obtained by using portions of both the inspiratory and the expiratory reserves. Any decrease in alveolar ventilation results in interference with carbon dioxide elimination and oxygen uptake.

Dyspnea occurs when the respiratory minute volume approaches the *maximal breathing capacity* (the greatest rate of pulmonary ventilation that can be sustained for about 20 seconds). A normal individual has a maximal breathing capacity of about 160 liters per minute. If the maximal breathing capacity is reduced to 15 to 30 liters because of pulmonary abnormalities, any respiratory stimulation might raise the minute volume sufficiently to cause dyspnea.

Drugs that act on the respiratory center

THERAPEUTIC GASES
Oxygen, U.S.P., B.P.

Oxygen was discovered by Priestley in 1772. Later, Lavoisier described the role of oxygen in the respiratory process. Beddoes introduced the utilization of oxygen as a therapeutic modality in England in the eighteenth century.

Oxygen is a gas that constitutes 20.93% of inspired air and is essential for maintaining life. Oxygen, U.S.P., is a colorless, odorless, and tasteless gas. It is not flammable, but it supports combustion much more vigorously than does air.

Oxygen is compressed and marketed in steel cylinders that are fitted with reducing valves for the delivery of the gas. The cylinders are usually color coded, being green in the United States. Since the gas is under considerable pressure, the tanks must be handled carefully to prevent their falling or bumping into each other or into anything that may cause undue jarring.

Oxygen must be continuously supplied to tissue cells, for no fiber or cell can remain hypoxic for very long and survive. The adult human brain consumes from 40 to 50 ml. of oxygen per minute. The cortex consumes more than the centers in the medulla or spinal cord. Cerebral oxygen consumption proceeds without respite, and the replenishment of oxygen by the blood must be maintained continuously. Whenever any circulatory stress exists, cerebral blood flow tends to be preserved at the expense of other less vital organs. Of all the tissues affected by hypoxia, the brain is most susceptible to disruption of normal function and irreversible damage. An acute reduction of the P_{O_2} to 50 mm. Hg decreases mental functioning, emotional stability, and finer muscular coordination. Further reduction of the P_{O_2} to 40 mm. Hg produces impaired judgment, decreased pain perception, and impairment of muscular coordination. When the P_{O_2} is reduced to 32 mm. Hg or less, unconsciousness and a progressive descending depression of the central nervous system ensue.

The kidneys constitute other vital organs in which there must be considerable constancy of blood flow and oxygen supply. Oxygen consumption is greater in the renal cortex; renal medullary tissue has an oxygen consumption that is 15% less than that of the renal cortex. This difference is related to the variation in pressure gradient and the fact that cortical flow is rapid while the medullary flow is slower. The renal cortex is highly dependent on oxygen, while the medulla can function relatively independently of the oxygen supply.

The rate of oxygen consumption by the kidneys is approximately 0.06 ml. per gram per minute. They consume more oxygen than most other tissues. For each 100 ml. of blood entering the kidney, 1.4 ml. of oxygen is consumed. The oxygen consumed by the kidneys is primarily used for sodium reabsorption. When the arterial content falls to less than 55% of normal, renal vasoconstriction occurs. It is currently believed that this response is mediated by the chemoreceptors, which stimulate the vasomotor center to produce renal vasoconstriction. Renal vasoconstriction also occurs as a result of the action of ether, barbiturates, and other anesthetics. Renal blood flow is also decreased during periods of exercise. In relation to the above, it is important to note that autoregulation of renal perfusion does occur.

In skeletal muscles, oxygen consumption is related to blood flow. Oxygen consumption and blood flow are decreased when muscle is at rest, and both are significantly increased during exercise.

Reduction of oxygen supply to the intestinal tract is regarded by some investigators as a key factor for inadequate splanchnic vascular compensation (splanchnic vasoconstriction) during hypotension.

Inadequate oxygen supply impairs myocardial metabolism and function. Recent research seems to indicate that ethyl alcohol decreases myocardial oxygen consumption.

Arterial blood pressure determinations, when used alone, are unreliable indicators of the adequacy of tissue perfusion. Therefore, arterial blood gas determinations should be obtained since these results provide a more accurate and reliable indication of shifts in the partial pressures of oxygen and carbon dioxide. Severe hypoxia may produce changes in the S-T segment and T wave of the EKG, arrhythmias, ectopic beats, and myocardial infarction.

Indications for use. Oxygen is used in medicine chiefly to treat hypoxia (oxygen lack) and hypoxemia (diminished oxygen tension in the blood). There are basically four types of hypoxia described in the literature. These include the following:

1 Hypoxic hypoxia—produced by any condition causing a decrease in P_{O_2}
2 Ischemic hypoxia—inadequate blood flow to an organ or tissue in the presence of a normal P_{O_2} and hemoglobin content

3 Anemic hypoxia—inadequate hemoglobin to carry O_2 in the presence of a normal Po_2

4 Histotoxic hypoxia—adequate Po_2 and hemoglobin, but inability of tissues to utilize oxygen delivered because of a toxic agent

Clinically, hypoxic hypoxia is the most common form of hypoxia seen. There is a variety of pathologic conditions that result in hypoxic hypoxia necessitating the utilization of oxygen as a treatment modality. Some of these include: hypoventilation, increased airway resistance, pneumothorax, respiratory center depression, abnormal ventilation-perfusion ratio, congenital cyanotic heart disease, decreased pulmonary compliance, and breathing oxygen-poor air. The use of oxygen is also indicated in the following: (1) cardiac failure or decompensation, and coronary occlusion; (2) anesthesia, to increase the safety of general anesthetics; and (3) treatment of certain types of headache.

Administration of oxygen. Oxygen is administered in a number of ways, including oxygen tent, nasal catheter or cannula, face mask, hood, and oxygen chamber. Each of these methods of administering oxygen has advantages and disadvantages.

When a *nasal catheter* is used it should be lubricated with a water-soluble jelly and passed through the nose until the tip is just above the epiglottis. This distance is usually the same as the distance from the patient's external nares to the tragus of the ear, minus 1 cm. The catheter should not be inserted so far that the patient swallows oxygen, for this will cause stomach distention and abdominal discomfort. The catheter is fastened with tape to the forehead and/or nose. Flow rate varies according to patient need, but 3 to 4 liters of oxygen per minute is commonly used. Since this form of therapy is very drying to the mucous membrane, the oxygen should be humidified. In addition, nasal and oral hygiene is important to maintain cleanliness, maintain intact mucous membrane, and prevent infection and discomfort. Most patients receiving oxygen therapy are mouth breathers, and frequent mouth care is required to prevent sordes. Nasal catheters become obstructed with encrusted secretions and must be removed and cleaned or replaced several times a day.

Nasal cannulae are much more comfortable for patients than catheters. They are less likely to become obstructed with secretions. Nasal and oral mucosa still require frequent attention. A flow of 3 liters of oxygen is adequate for many patients.

Oxygen masks are the most effective means of delivering needed oxygen. Oxygen concentrations of 90% to 100% can be administered by mask. To be effective the mask must fit well over nose and mouth; high flow rates can compensate to some extent for a poor fit. Masks are better tolerated when used intermittently or when disposable plastic masks are used. Only absolutely clean and uncontaminated rubber masks should be used, since they can be a source of hospital-acquired infection.

Oxygen tents and hoods have the advantage of temperature and humidity regulation. Disadvantages include oxygen loss, carbon dioxide accumulation, and claustrophobic effect. Oxygen concentration in a tent rarely reaches 50%; in a hood the concentration may reach 90% to 100%. The tent and hood should be periodically tested with an oxygen analyzer for oxygen concentration. Oxygen should be flowing into the tent *before* it is secured over the patient. The usual rate of flow is 15 liters per minute for the first 15 to 30 minutes after the patient is in the tent, and 10 to 12 liters per minute thereafter. Tent leakage should be prevented by careful planning of care so that the tent is removed or opened as seldom as possible. The tent should also be securely tucked under the mattress and around the patient. The mattress should be covered with plastic or a rubber sheet to prevent oxygen saturation of the mattress and undue loss of oxygen. Oxygen tents and hoods are less popular today than formerly since the advent of plastic face masks and face tents.

For a child with a respiratory infection adequate oxygen concentration can be maintained in a croup tent with an open top. When indicated, the top may be covered to increase the mist.

Face tents are the most convenient, comfortable way to administer high concentrations of oxygen. A flow of 15 liters per minute can provide an oxygen concentration of 70%.

Since oxygen supports combustion and combustible material burns with greater ease and intensity, and since the patient is surrounded with combustible materials (linens, wooden furniture), smoking and the use of matches or electric equipment that may cause sparks are strictly forbidden in rooms where oxygen is being administered.

The effectiveness of oxygen administration will depend on the carbon dioxide content of the blood. Patients with chronic obstructive pulmonary disease have difficulty with carbon dioxide and oxygen exchange and are subject to hypercapnia (high carbon dioxide content). Because of the long-term presence of hypercapnia, the medullary center of these patients is relatively insensitive to stimulation of carbon dioxide; rather a low Pao_2 serves as a stimulant to respiration. Therefore, oxygen must be administered to these individuals with caution in an attempt to prevent the further accumulation of carbon dioxide with the subsequent development of toxic and narcotic levels resulting in further depression of respiration and respiratory acidosis. The nurse should be alert to the development of neurologic symptoms indicative of accumulation of carbon dioxide. Symptoms may include drowsiness, mental confusion, paresthesias, and visual disturbances. The occurrence of carbon dioxide narcosis may be prevented by gradually increasing the concentration of oxygen administered or, according to some investigators, by using intermittent positive pressure breathing. When there is no danger of accumulation of carbon dioxide, the medullary center retains its sensitivity to carbon dioxide stimulation and high concentrations of oxygen can be administered.

Oxygen administration in the premature infant. Nurses who care for premature babies in incubators must be constantly aware of the potential danger of the development of retrolental fibroplasia. This is a vascular proliferative disease of the retina that occurs in some premature infants who have been subjected to high concentrations of oxygen at birth. The oxygen concentration should be kept between 30% and 40%; however, higher concentrations can be administered to cyanotic infants without increasing the danger of retrolental fibroplasia because it is the Pao_2, not inspired Po_2, that is implicated in the development of this disease. Therefore, careful monitoring of arterial blood gases is essential. Some models of incubators are equipped with a safety valve that automatically releases any excess oxygen outside the chamber.

When orders for an infant include oxygen P.R.N., the nurse must make certain that it is administered only as needed and at low concentrations, rather than continuously. Frequently, the removal of a very small plug of mucus can clear the baby's airway, thus enabling him to breathe oxygen without assistance.

Oxygen administration in tumor therapy. Hypoxic cells are resistant to radiation damage. Therefore, if a tumor outgrows its blood supply, hyperoxygenation of the blood may increase oxygen supply to these cells and make them more sensitive to radiation. This particular therapy is still under investigation, and it will be several years before its efficacy can be accurately evaluated.

Use of hyperbaric oxygen. In recent years, hyperbaric oxygen has been used in the treatment of various conditions. In the treatment of infections caused by *Clostridium welchii*, the anaerobic bacillus producing gas gangrene, hyperbaric oxygen used intermittently has been of some value. It is felt that an increased oxygen pressure in the tissue may exert an inhibitory effect on enzyme systems of these bacteria. This same inhibitory effect may be implicated in the use of hyperbaric oxygen on other anaerobic microorganisms. Hyperbaric oxygen has been used in the treatment of tetanus, but the results are less satisfactory than those obtained in the treatment of gas gangrene.

Hyperbaric oxygen has also been used in certain circulatory disturbances. In shock, in which there is a generalized circulatory deficit, hyperbaric oxygen may be of some value. It has also been used in certain local circulatory disturbances such as various peripheral vascular diseases.

Helium-oxygen mixtures. Helium-oxygen mixtures have been used for some time to treat obstructive types of dyspnea. Helium is an inert gas and so light that a mixture of 80% helium and 20% oxygen is only one third as heavy as air. Helium is only slightly soluble in body fluids and has a high rate of diffusion. Its low specific gravity makes it possible for mixtures of this gas with oxygen to be breathed with less effort than either oxygen or air alone when there is obstruction in the air passages.

These mixtures are recommended for status asthmaticus, bronchiectasis, and emphysema, and during anesthesia for a patient with respiratory tract obstruction.

Carbon dioxide, U.S.P., B.P.

Carbon dioxide is a colorless, odorless gas that is heavier than air. It was discovered by Priestley in the eighteenth century; Lavoisier elucidated its role in the respiratory process. Its use as a pharmacologic agent has implications for respiration, circulation, and the central nervous system. Whether it affects the respiratory center directly or by increasing the hydrogen ion concentration is still a matter for debate. However, inhalation of carbon dioxide for a short period of time increases both the rate and depth of respiration unless the respiratory center is depressed by narcotics or disease.

Carbon dioxide has two opposing effects in the human body:

1 It stimulates cells of the sympathetic nervous system, the respiratory center, and the peripheral chemoreceptors.
2 It depresses the cerebral cortex, myocardium, and smooth muscle of the peripheral blood vessels.

Carbon dioxide may also interfere with nerve conduction and transmission. When carbon dioxide increases the rate and force of respiration, venous return to the heart is usually enhanced as a result of decreased peripheral resistance; there is improved rate and force of myocardial contraction and less likelihood of myocardial irritability and arrhythmias.

Too much carbon dioxide has a depressant effect and results in acidosis as well as unresponsiveness of the respiratory center to carbon dioxide. Therefore, it is important that carbon dioxide be administered with caution.

Indications for use. The following are indications for use of carbon dioxide.

Carbon monoxide poisoning. A 5% to 7% concentration of carbon dioxide in oxygen is some-times used in the treatment of carbon monoxide poisoning. Physiologically, carbon dioxide increases the rate of dissociation of carbon monoxide from carboxyhemoglobin as well as gas exchange.

General anesthesia. Most general anesthetics cause a reduction in response to carbon dioxide, which reflects central nervous system depression. The degree of depression is directly related to depth of anesthesia. The more deeply the patient is anesthetized, the greater the depression of the central nervous system. In the beginning carbon dioxide speeds up anesthesia by increasing pulmonary ventilation. By lessening the sense of asphyxiation, it reduces struggling. After anesthesia, it hastens the elimination of many anesthetics. Inhalation of 5% to 7% carbon dioxide increases cerebral blood flow by approximately 75%, primarily by dilation of cerebral vessels.

Respiratory depression. The use of carbon dioxide as a respiratory stimulant in the presence of depressed respiration is limited. When it is used, close monitoring of Pao_2 is important; if the desired results are not obtained, it should be discontinued. Usually in cases of respiratory depression, mechanical assistance to respiration plus the administration of oxygen is the treatment of choice.

Postoperative use. Occasionally, carbon dioxide is used postoperatively in an effort to increase ventilation and prevent atelectasis. Most investigators feel that the use of deep breathing exercises, coughing, frequent turning, tracheal suction, and intermittent positive pressure breathing produces better results. Carbon dioxide administration has also been used in the treatment of postoperative singultus (hiccough). Relief of singultus is apparently accomplished by stimulating the respiratory center, causing large excursions of the diaphragm that submerge spasmodic contractions of that muscle, thereby promoting regular contractions.

Administration. Carbon dioxide is kept in metal cylinders and vaporizes as it is delivered from the cylinder. When carbon dioxide is used for medical purposes it is administered in combination with oxygen. A 5% to 10% concentration of carbon dioxide is delivered through a tight-fitting face mask. The patients should inhale the mixture until the depth of respiration is definitely increased, which usually occurs within 3 minutes. For the postoperative individual, the procedure should be repeated for short periods every hour or two for the first 48 hours, and then several times a day for several days.

Another way of administering carbon dioxide is to allow the patient to hyperventilate with a paper bag held over his face. He reinhales his expired air in which the carbon dioxide content is continually increased.

Signs of carbon dioxide overdosage are dyspnea, breath-holding, markedly increased chest and abdominal movements, nausea, and increased systolic blood pressure. Administration of the gas should be discontinued when these symptoms appear. The administration should, in fact, be stopped as soon as the desired effects on respiration have been obtained.

NEBULIZATION THERAPY

Nebulization therapy is used to deposit medication in the respiratory tract in the form of droplets that have been suspended in air. The medication is inhaled as a fine mist. Nebulization therapy is used to promote:

1 Bronchodilation and pulmonary decongestion
2 Loosening of secretions
3 Topical application of antibiotics, steroids, and antifoaming agents
4 Moistening, cooling, or heating of inspired air

The effectiveness of nebulization therapy is dependent upon the number of droplets that can be suspended in an inhaled aerosol. The number of droplets that can be suspended is directly related to the size of the droplets. Small droplets can be suspended in greater numbers than large droplets. Smaller droplets (about 2 microns in diameter) are more likely to reach the periphery of the lungs—the alveolar ducts and sacs. Currently, in many institutions, ultrasonic nebulizers are utilized in the treatment of bronchial constriction and pulmonary congestion. Larger droplets (8 to 15 microns in size) will be deposited primarily in the bronchioles and bronchi.

Droplets of more than 40 microns will be deposited primarily in the upper airway (mouth, pharynx, trachea, and main bronchi).

Rate and depth of breathing are other important factors. Rapid or shallow breathing decreases the number of droplets reaching the periphery of the lungs as well as their retention. Rapid breathing permits the escape of significant amounts of fine droplets during expirations. Few droplets will escape if the breath is held long enough after deep inspiration to permit droplet deposit in the lung periphery. Small droplets are considered more effective for maximum absorption of antibiotics and bronchodilators.

Almost all large droplets will be retained somewhere in the air passage. Large droplets are used for keeping large airways moist (nose, trachea) and for loosening secretions. Slow and deep breathing is required for proper lung aeration and penetration of the mist into peripheral lung areas. The breath should be held for a few seconds after a full inspiration. Nebulizers commonly used in hospitals all produce similar mists. Droplet size can be controlled by the amount of pressure used to force oxygen or room air through the solution to produce a mist. The tubing used, its length, and number of bends affect turbulent flow and mist temperature. More precise studies are required to settle controversies and to determine how to provide more effective nebulization therapy for various respiratory disorders. With most nebulizers maximum density of the inhaled mist is achieved by making the flow of mist as smooth and direct as possible.

Drugs used for nebulization therapy include bronchodilators and mucolytic agents (see following sections), antibiotics, steroids, and antifoaming agents.

Systemic antibiotics are often the drugs of choice to combat pulmonary infection. Certain antibiotics that can be given in limited doses only when administered systemically because of their toxicity can often be given in large doses by nebulization. These antibiotics include polymyxin, colistin, neomycin, and bacitracin. Since these antibiotics are irritating and may cause bronchospasm, bronchodilators are usually given prior to, or along with, the antibiotic.

Nebulized steroids are given for their effect

on respiratory mucosa. The true effectiveness of nebulized steroids has not been established.

Antifoaming agents (ethyl alcohol or octyl alcohol) have been used to supplement therapy to reverse severe fulminating pulmonary edema. Alcohol reduces the surface tension of pulmonary edema bubbles and causes them to break, and it produces some bronchodilation. The result is better ventilation. This form of aerosol therapy must not be administered rapidly since it will cause irritation and coughing. It should be used with intermittent positive pressure breathing (IPPB) for effective oxygenation. Aerosol alcohol should be discontinued as soon as the lungs are dry to prevent ciliary damage.

BRONCHODILATORS

Indications for use. Bronchodilators are indicated in the presence of various pathophysiologic conditions resulting in intermittent and recurring bronchial constriction. Bronchial constriction, if prolonged and untreated, results in a disruption of the normal exchange of gases at the alveolar-capillary membrane. These drugs are particularly useful in the treatment of asthma and acute respiratory distress in children.

Action. Drugs that cause bronchodilation are used for their ability to relax the smooth muscle of the tracheobronchial tree. This permits an increase in lumen size of the bronchioles and alveolar ducts and decreases resistance to air flow. These drugs also decrease congestion in the respiratory tract through vasoconstriction and a decrease in mucous membrane swelling.

SYMPATHOMIMETIC DRUGS

A more detailed discussion of these agents is given in Chapter 9. The effects of this group of drugs closely resemble the response to stimulation of adrenergic nerves. In relation to the bronchial musculature, they exert a primarily peripheral inhibitory action on smooth muscle, thus decreasing bronchial constriction.

Epinephrine, U.S.P., B.P.

The main effect of epinephrine on respiration is obtained through its peripheral action of relaxing smooth muscle. It is particularly useful in the treatment of asthma because of its powerful bronchodilator action. Epinephrine also increases vital capacity by relieving congestion of the bronchial mucosa. When epinephrine is administered as an aerosol it aids in the relief of congestion by constricting bronchial vessels. In normal subjects, epinephrine increases respiratory rate and tidal volume and results in a reduction in alveolar carbon dioxide.

Epinephrine is administered parenterally and by aerosol because it is destroyed by enzymes present in the gastrointestinal tract. The subcutaneous and/or intramuscular dose for an adult is 0.1 to 1 ml. of a 1:1000 aqueous solution; the intravenous dose is 0.05 to 0.1 ml. of a 1:1000 solution injected very slowly and with caution. Epinephrine hydrochloride is available for oral inhalation as a 0.1% to 1.0% solution or suspension; epinephrine bitartrate is marketed in a 15-ml. aerosol package containing 7 mg. per milliliter. Pediatric dose for asthma is 0.01 ml. per kilogram of body weight of the 1:1000 aqueous solution given subcutaneously.

Isoproterenol hydrochloride, U.S.P. (Isuprel Hydrochloride)

Isoproterenol is another adrenergic drug frequently used for its bronchodilator effect. This drug and its various preparations are discussed in more detail in Chapter 9.

Metaproterenol sulfate (Alupent, Metaprel, Orciprenaline Sulfate)

Metaproterenol is a synthetic sympathomimetic amine with a chemical structure and pharmacologic action similar to that of isoproterenol. It has a greater stimulating effect on the beta receptors of the bronchial and vascular smooth muscles, and a lesser effect on the beta receptors of the heart, than isoproterenol.

Metaproterenol is used as a bronchodilator in the symptomatic treatment of asthma and bronchospasm. It has a longer duration of action, has a lower incidence and severity of cardiac side effects, and is more effective after oral administration than isoproterenol. Onset of action occurs 1 minute after oral inhalation and 15 minutes after oral administration. Peak effect occurs in about 1 hour with a duration of effect of about 4 hours with either route of administration. Duration of action may shorten with long-term use, but metaproterenol retains its efficacy to a greater extent than isoproterenol.

Metaproterenol is under investigation for the treatment and prophylaxis of heart block, Adams-Stokes syndrome, and arrest of premature labor.

Preparation and dosage. Metaproterenol is available in 20-mg. capsules and tablets for oral administration and as a powder, 225 mg. in metered dose vials of 15 ml. with mouthpiece. Each metered dose delivers approximately 0.65 mg. of metaproterenol; range of dose is one to three inhalations with 2 minutes between inhalations. Inhalations may be repeated every 3 to 4 hours but should not exceed twelve inhalations in 24 hours. For oral inhalation the patient should be instructed to shake the container, exhale through the nose as completely as possible, then administer the aerosol while breathing deeply through the mouth; the patient should hold his breath for a few seconds before exhaling slowly.

Oral dosage of metaproterenol is 20 mg. three to four times daily. Use of this drug for children under 12 years of age is still being investigated. This drug should be protected from light and air.

Adverse effects and precautions. Adverse effects are usually dose related and occur with high doses. Most common side effects include tachycardia, nervousness, palpitations, tremor, hypertension, headache, dizziness, nausea and vomiting, and bad taste.

Metaproterenol should be used cautiously in patients with hypertension, coronary artery disease, hyperthyroidism, congestive heart failure, or diabetes mellitus and in those sensitive to sympathomimetic drugs. It is contraindicated in patients with a history of tachycardia.

Metaproterenol should not be used concurrently with other sympathomimetic drugs (such as epinephrine) since the additive effects may induce serious arrhythmias and toxic reactions. It is not recommended for pregnant women.

Terbutaline sulfate (Brethine, Bricanyl)

Terbutaline is a sympathomimetic amine similar to isoproterenol and metaproterenol in chemical structure and pharmacologic action. It is a beta-adrenergic stimulator; its main effect is relaxation of smooth muscles of the bronchial tree and the peripheral vasculature.

Terbutaline is used as a bronchodilator in the treatment of bronchial asthma and bronchospasm. Compared to ephedrine, its bronchodilator activity is about equal, but onset and duration of action are longer. Compared to metaproterenol, terbutaline has equal or slightly greater effectiveness, a slower onset of action, and a longer duration of action.

After oral administration, onset of action occurs in 30 minutes and peak action in 2 to 3 hours, with a duration of action ranging from 4 to 8 hours. After subcutaneous injection, onset of action occurs in 15 minutes, peak effects occur in 30 to 60 minutes, and duration of action ranges from $1^1/_2$ to 4 hours.

Terbutaline is under investigation for the prevention of spontaneous and oxytocin-induced uterine activity during advanced term labor.

Preparation and dosage. Terbutaline is available in isotonic solution for injection containing 1 mg. of drug per milliliter and in 2.5- and 5-mg. tablets for oral administration. Subcutaneous dose for adults is 0.25 mg. injected into the lateral deltoid area; for children the subcutaneous dose is 3.5 to 5 µg. per kilogram of body weight. The use of the drug in children under 12 is still being investigated.

Oral dosage for adults is 5 mg. three times daily at 6-hour intervals; dosage should not exceed 15 mg. daily. For children 12 to 15 years of age, dosage is 2.5 mg. three times daily; daily dosage should not exceed 7.5 mg.

Adverse effects and precautions. Commonly observed side effects include an increase in heart rate, nervousness, tremor, palpitations, and dizziness. These effects usually occur when the subcutaneous dosage is in excess of 0.25 mg. Headache, nausea and vomiting, anxiety, restlessness, lethargy, drowsiness, sweating, and tinnitus have also been reported.

Terbutaline should be used with caution in patients with diabetes, hypertension, hyperthyroidism, or cardiac disorders associated with arrhythmias. Terbutaline should not be given concurrently with other sympathomimetic agents because of the possibility of additive cardiovascular side effects. However, it can be used with an adrenergic aerosol bronchodilator to relieve acute bronchospasm.

THE XANTHINES

This group of drugs includes caffeine, theophylline, and theobromine. Beverages from aqueous extracts of plants containing these alkaloids have been used by man since ancient times. Xanthines relax smooth muscle, particularly bronchial muscle, stimulate cardiac muscle, stimulate the central nervous system, and also produce diuresis probably through a combined action of increased renal perfusion and increased sodium and chloride ion excretion.

This group of drugs can be administered orally, rectally, or parenterally. Given orally, theophylline may cause gastric irritation, nausea, and vomiting. This constitutes a generally accepted drawback to its use in individuals with gastrointestinal conditions. The xanthines are most effective when administered intravenously; however, the preferred route is oral if appropriate blood levels can be achieved. The xanthines are readily absorbed from both gastrointestinal and intravenous administration, and readily distributed uniformly throughout the body. However, depending upon the state of the patient's gastrointestinal tract, when xanthines are given orally or rectally, absorption may be erratic and slow. These drugs are probably partially metabolized in the liver and excreted in the urine in the form of incompletely demethylated metabolites.

Of the xanthines presently marketed in the United States, the theophylline derivatives are the most useful of the xanthines for bronchodilation.

Aminophylline, U.S.P., B.P. (Theophylline Ethylenediamine)

Aminophylline, a theophylline derivative, provides a prototype for most of the other theophylline compounds. It plays an important role in the management of asthma and other disorders resulting in bronchial constriction and spasm. It is also used in the treatment of pulmonary edema. It is available for oral administration in 100- and 200-mg. tablets and is usually given T.I.D. For intravenous administration, ampules containing 250 mg. per 10 ml. and 500 mg. per 20 ml. are available. Rectal suppositories come in 125-, 250-, and 500-mg. strengths.

Side effects may include gastric irritation, nausea, vomiting, anxiety, convulsions, delirium, restlessness, hypotension, and occasionally a feeling of fullness of the head and headache. If administered intravenously too rapidly, cardiovascular distress may occur. Intramuscular injection produces local pain at injection site; therefore, it is the least desirable route.

Nursing interventions important in the administration of aminophylline include the following:

1 Vital signs, especially the quality and rate of the pulse and respirations, should be carefully monitored.
2 When administered intravenously it should be given slowly to avoid cardiovascular distress.
3 Oral preparations should be given with food to minimize gastric irritation.
4 Rectal preparations should be administered when the rectum is free of feces since this will enhance the absorption of the drug.
5 Any form of this drug given over a long period of time may have cumulative effects or may become ineffective.
6 If side effects occur, discontinue the drug and notify the physician.
7 Ephedrine given in conjunction with aminophylline has a combined central stimulant action and may necessitate the administration of a barbiturate.

Various other theophylline derivatives and other preparations used for their bronchodilating effects are the following: choline theophylline (Choledyl), theophylline (Aqualin, Elixophyllin), and pseudoephedrine hydrochloride (Sudafed).

ASTHMA PROPHYLACTIC
Cromolyn sodium (Aarane, Intal)

Cromolyn is a bronchial asthma prophylactic agent. It is not a bronchodilator, antihistaminic, or an antiinflammatory drug. Cromolyn appears to act primarily through a local effect on lung mucosa. It inhibits the release of histamine and the slow-reacting substance of anaphylaxis (SRS-A) from sensitized mast cells following exposure to various allergens. It inhibits late allergic reactions to a lesser extent.

Cromolyn has no role in the treatment of an acute attack of asthma or in status asthmaticus. Its approved use is as an adjunct to the overall management of patients with severe, perennial, bronchial asthma. A satisfactory response to cromolyn therapy is indicated by a reduction in the number of attacks, reduced cough, decreased sputum production, and/or a decreased need for other antiasthma drugs. Some patients show improvement in pulmonary function. These responses usually occur in the first 2 to 4 weeks of treatment. Only those patients showing improvement should continue to receive cromolyn.

Preparation, dosage, and administration. Cromolyn is available in 20-mg. capsules for inhalation using a special oral inhaler (Aarane Inhaler, Spinhaler). Patients must be carefully instructed in the use of the inhaler and advised that the drug's effectiveness is dependent upon administering it at regular intervals. After placing the capsule into the inhaler, the patient exhales as completely as possible, places the mouthpiece of the inhaler between his lips, tilts the inhaler upward and his head backward, and inhales rapidly and deeply through the inhaler with a steady, even breath. The patient should then remove the inhaler from his mouth, hold his breath for a few seconds, and exhale. This procedure is repeated until all the capsule has been inhaled. The patient should be cautioned not to exhale into the inhaler since moisture from his breath will interfere with proper inhaler function.

Usual dosage of cromolyn for adults and children 5 years of age and older is 20 mg. four times a day at regular intervals. The amount of drug reaching the lungs depends upon the patient's proficiency in using the inhaler, the degree of bronchoconstriction, and the presence or absence of mucous plugs. It has been estimated that 5% to 10% of a dose of cromolyn reaches the lungs after inhalation and is readily absorbed into the systemic circulation and excreted into the urine and feces. Small amounts of the drug may be exhaled. The remainder of the dose is swallowed and excreted in the feces. The absorption half-life of cromolyn from the lungs is

1 hour; the elimination half-life is 81 minutes. Cromolyn is not effective when taken orally.

Adverse effects and precautions. Common side effects from cromolyn therapy include irritation of the throat and trachea, cough, and bronchospasm. Nausea, maculopapular rash, erythema, and urticaria have been reported.

Cromolyn toxicity appears to be low, but caution is recommended when it is given to patients with impaired renal or hepatic function. It is not recommended for pregnant women or for children under 5 years of age. Caution should be used when the dosage of cromolyn is reduced or withdrawn since asthmatic symptoms may recur. Cromolyn is contraindicated in patients who show hypersensitivity to it.

MUCOLYTIC AGENTS

Mucolytic agents reduce the thickness and stickiness of purulent and nonpurulent pulmonary secretions. They are usually administered by aerosol inhalation to facilitate the removal of secretions and permit more adequate pulmonary ventilation. These drugs are used in the management of individuals with chronic bronchitis, emphysema, bronchiectasis, cystic fibrosis, pneumonia, and as an adjunct for tracheostomy care. When used appropriately few adverse effects are seen. Some patients may develop nausea and/or vomiting, but this is probably due to the odor and quantity of respiratory secretions eliminated. With the aid of these agents and postural drainage most individuals can expectorate pulmonary secretions without further assistance; however, in the elderly or debilitated, suctioning may be indicated.

Acetylcysteine, N.F. (Mucomyst, Respaire)

Acetylcysteine is an amino acid derivative that is administered by nebulization as a 10% or 20% solution. The 20% solution may be converted to a 10% solution by dilution with isotonic sodium chloride or sterile water. Range of dosage is from 1 to 10 ml. of the 20% solution, or 2 to 20 ml. of the 10% solution for about 15 minutes, three or four times daily. Since the solution tends to concentrate, it should be diluted with sterile water when three fourths of the original volume has been used. It may also be administered for a single continuous treatment by means of a closed tent or croupette. This may require up to 300 ml. of a 20% solution. It is effective within 1 minute; however, it takes 5 to 10 minutes for maximum effect to occur.

Acetylcysteine may cause stomatitis, nausea, and rhinorrhea. Bronchospasm may occur in patients with bronchial asthma. This drug has a wide margin of safety. Currently, in some institutions a 2% to 5% saline solution is being used instead of acetylcysteine to avoid side effects.

Solutions of acetylcysteine will harden rubber and become discolored on contact with certain metals. It should be used with equipment made out of glass, plastic, or stainless steel. If the vacuum seal has been broken on the bottle, it should be refrigerated to retard oxidation and used within 48 hours.

Desoxyribonuclease (Dornavac)

Desoxyribonuclease is an enzyme that degrades DNA. It is obtained from beef pancreas. It reduces the tenacity or thickness of pulmonary secretions. Desoxyribonuclease is available in powder form, 100,000 units per vial. The powder is dissolved in 1 to 2 ml. of sterile saline. The average dose is 50,000 to 100,000 units three times a day by aerosol inhalation for 2 to 6 days. It is relatively free of side effects; however, individual sensitivity to the drug should be watched for. The drug is expensive, which is one disadvantage to be considered.

DIRECT RESPIRATORY STIMULANTS

This group of drugs comes under a broader classification of central nervous system stimulants and are often referred to as *analeptics*. These agents act by blockage of inhibition at the pre- or postsynaptic area or by enhancement of synaptic excitation. These drugs act directly on the medullary center to increase rate and tidal exchange. While drugs from this category are available for stimulating depth of respiration and concomitantly, but to a lesser degree, rate of respiration, airway management and support of ventilation are more effective in the treatment of respiratory depression. Indeed, the latter is often superior to the use of drugs, since respiratory stimulants in large doses are convulsants.

Respiratory stimulants (analeptics) have in the past been advocated in the treatment of drug-induced respiratory depression, but since these drugs are not specific antagonists to sedatives or narcotics, their use in drug-induced respiratory depression is now considered obsolete. Indeed, repeated doses of an analeptic may potentiate the depressant effects of central nervous system depressants.

Analeptics have also been used to counteract respiratory depression due to anesthetics or to shorten postanesthetic recovery time. However, these methods of therapy are not recommended since decreasing the concentration of the anesthetic agent in the blood is accomplished more effectively with mechanical ventilatory measures.

Ethamivan, N.F. (Emivan)

Ethamivan is a centrally acting respiratory stimulant used for treating respiratory depression resulting from barbiturate poisoning, tranquilizers, and acute and chronic pulmonary disease or other conditions producing acute or chronic hypoventilatory states.

Preparations and dosage. Ethamivan is available for intravenous injection in a solution containing 50 mg. per milliliter in 2- and 10-ml. ampules. Onset of action occurs in 1 minute; duration of action is 10 to 30 minutes. Dosage depends on the degree of respiratory depression. In barbiturate poisoning or carbon dioxide narcosis with severe respiratory depression, 0.5 to 5 mg. per kilogram of body weight may be administered slowly over a period of several minutes, or 1 Gm. of ethamivan may be diluted in 250 ml. of dextrose or saline solution. For infants and children 0.5 to 5 mg. per kilogram of body weight is used. Rate of infusion or amount of drug administered is determined by respiratory response.

D.E.S.I. rating for the parenteral preparation

is *possibly effective;* the oral tablets used for mild respiratory stimulation for patients with chronic pulmonary disease received an *ineffective* rating.

Side effects are usually transient and include generalized pruritus, flushing, lightheadedness, muscular twitching, laryngospasm, restlessness, sneezing, and coughing.

This drug is contraindicated in epilepsy or in conjunction with other drugs that may cause convulsions.

Doxapram hydrochloride, N.F. (Dopram)

Doxapram is a centrally acting respiratory stimulant. It is particularly useful for treatment of postanesthetic respiratory depression and to hasten return of protective pharyngeal and laryngeal reflexes after anesthesia. Depth of respiration is significantly increased by doxapram, and the rate of respiration may also increase. The action of doxapram is thought to be primarily caused by stimulation of the respiratory center. It may also have some effect on the chemoreceptors. Mild vasopressor activity is noted with the use of doxapram, resulting in elevation of blood pressure and heart rate. In addition, doxapram produces an increase in salivation, body temperature, gastric secretions, and tone and motility of the gastrointestinal tract and urinary bladder.

Preparation, dosage, and administration. Doxapram is available in solution form for intravenous injection, 20 mg. per milliliter in 20-ml. vials. When administered postoperatively, a single dose of 0.5 to 1.5 mg. per kilogram of body weight may be given over a period of 30 to 90 seconds. Repeated doses may be necessary, but maximum dosage, even when multiple injections are used, should not exceed 2 mg. per kilogram of body weight. Intravenous infusion may also be used. With this method of administration the dose is usually 5 mg. per minute initially; this is reduced to 1 to 3 mg. per minute when the desired response has been obtained. Doxapram is metabolized rapidly and has a brief duration of action. During administration, the patient's blood pressure, heart rate, and other vital signs should be carefully monitored to prevent overdosage and toxic reactions.

Side effects. Doxapram can cause a wide variety of side effects as a result of its central stimulating effect. Minor side effects include singultus, nausea, vomiting, sneezing, headache, fever, spontaneous urination, confusion, dyspnea, and cough. The most serious side effects are hypertension, tachycardia, muscle rigidity, and cardiac arrhythmias.

Precautions. The adverse cardiovascular effects of doxapram may be greatly increased in individuals receiving sympathomimetic drugs or monoamine oxidase inhibitors. Doxapram is contraindicated for patients with hypertension, convulsive disorders, cardiac arrhythmias, cerebral edema, or hyperthyroidism. It is not recommended for use in patients with chronic pulmonary disease.

Nursing interventions in the administration of doxapram include:

1 Maintenance of a patent airway
2 Monitoring of vital signs continuously during administration and for 30 to 60 minutes following discontinuation of the drug
3 Availability of oxygen and equipment for mechanical ventilation
4 Periodic determination of arterial blood gases to ascertain degree of effective ventilation

Bemegride (Megimide)

Bemegride is used to treat respiratory depression resulting from drugs and anesthesia. Side effects are those of central nervous system stimulation. It is available in solution form for intravenous injection, 5 mg. per milliliter in 10-ml. ampules and 30-ml. vials. Dosage depends upon degree of respiratory depression, but 50 mg. may be injected every 3 to 5 minutes until signs of improvement or toxicity occur.

Nikethamide, B.P. (Coramine)

Nikethamide is a synthetic compound chemically related to nicotinamide, the vitamin that prevents pellagra. Apparently, nikethamide has its most pronounced effect upon the respiratory center when the center is in a state of depression. Respiratory stimulation is a result of increasing the sensitivity of the respiratory center to carbon dioxide, or possibly to action on the chemoreceptors. When used on experimental animals, the medullary centers give evidence of stimulation, resulting in increased rate and depth of respiration and inconsistent peripheral vasoconstriction.

Nikethamide may be used to treat acute respiratory depression caused by hypnotics, anesthetics, or alcohol. It has low toxicity and is considered to be a relatively safe stimulant since it is less likely to cause convulsions than other centrally acting stimulants.

Nikethamide is available in solution form for parenteral injection. It is usually given intravenously. Dose varies according to degree of respiratory depression and may range from 1 to 10 ml. of a 25% solution (250 mg. to 2.5 Gm.). Anxiety, nausea, and vomiting may occur, but side effects are usually mild.

REFLEX STIMULANTS

Camphor, ammonia, and carminatives act as mild respiratory stimulants when taken by mouth. Ammonia, however, is the only drug given by inhalation for its action as a reflex respiratory stimulant. Aromatic spirits of ammonia is administered in cases of fainting by inhaling the vapor. When given orally, 2 ml. of aromatic ammonia spirits is diluted with at least 1 fluidounce of water. Reflex stimulation of the medullary center occurs through peripheral irritation of sensory nerve receptors in the pharynx, esophagus, and stomach. The rate and depth of respiration are then increased through afferent messages to the control centers. Reflex stimulation of the vasomotor center results in a rise in blood pressure.

RESPIRATORY DEPRESSANTS OR SEDATIVES

The most important respiratory depressants are the central depressants of the opium group and those of the barbiturate group of drugs. These drugs depress the respiratory center, thereby making breathing slower and more shallow and lessening the irritability of the respiratory center. Respiratory depression, however, is seldom desirable or necessary, although it is sometimes unavoidable. It is frequently a side effect in otherwise very useful drugs. Occasionally, a cough is so painful or harmful that an opiate, such as codeine, is administered to inhibit

the rate and depth of respiration. A greater value, however, lies in its action to depress the cough reflex. Too-high concentrations of carbon dioxide in inhalation mixtures may paradoxically act to depress respiration.

Drugs that affect the cough center and the respiratory mucosa

Coughing is a protective reflex for clearing the respiratory tract of environmental irritants, foreign bodies, or accumulated secretions and thus should not be depressed indiscriminately. A cough is *productive* when irritants or secretions are removed from the respiratory tract; it is *nonproductive* when it is dry and irritating. The severity of frequent and prolonged coughing should be diminished since it can be exhausting, painful, and taxing to the circulatory system and the elastic tissue of the respiratory system, particularly in the elderly and in young children. Most coughs can be suppressed without danger to the patient and thereby foster comfort and rest. Some coughs occur primarily at night or when the patient is recumbent because of the accumulation of secretions, and some coughs occur in the morning upon arising as a result of gravitational movement of secretions. Coughing is to some extent under voluntary control; an individual can cough at will and at times can suppress coughing. However, coughing is usually initiated by respiratory tract reflexes responding to irritations by sending impulses to the cough center. The value of adequate hydration of the patient, by oral intake of fluids as well as by inhalation of fully water-saturated vapors (steam), should be stressed as one of the most important means of producing increased amounts of mucus as well as thinning such secretions.

Treatment of the cough is secondary to treatment of the underlying disorder. Antitussives should not be given in situations in which retention of respiratory secretions or exudates may be harmful. The therapeutic objective is to decrease the intensity and frequency of the cough yet permit adequate elimination of tracheobronchial secretions and exudates. Medications that may be used to relieve the cough include narcotic and nonnarcotic antitussives, demulcents, antiseptics, expectorants, and others.

ANTITUSSIVES
NARCOTIC ANTITUSSIVES

Narcotics such as morphine, dihydromorphinone, and levorphanol are potent suppressants of the cough reflex, but their clinical usefulness is limited by their side effects. They inhibit the ciliary activity of the respiratory mucous membrane, depress respiration, and may cause bronchial constriction in allergic or asthmatic patients. In addition, they can cause drug dependence.

Codeine and dihydrocodeinone exhibit less pronounced antitussive effects but they also have fewer side effects. They have been widely used. Dihydrocodeinone is more active than codeine, but its drug dependence liability is also greater. The usual dose is 5 to 10 mg. three to four times a day.

Methadone is not an opiate, but it resembles morphine in a number of respects. Its ability to suppress the cough reflex is similar to that of morphine. A dose of 1.5 to 2 mg. will effectively relieve a cough. Its main disadvantage as an antitussive agent lies in its drug dependence qualities.

NONNARCOTIC ANTITUSSIVE AGENTS

The instillation of a local anesthetic agent prior to various diagnostic techniques such as bronchoscopy has proved effective in suppressing the cough reflex. This has led to the investigation of other agents that exert a similar action. The clinical effectiveness of these drugs against pathologic cough still remains to be established. Newer nonnarcotic drugs in this group have fewer gastrointestinal side effects than do codeine and related compounds.

Nursing interventions that apply to this entire group of agents should include the following:

1 Accurate reporting of the frequency and quality of coughing and sputum production

2 Deep breathing exercises, postural drainage, frequent change of position, limitation or cessation of smoking, maintenance of adequate humidity in the environment, and adequate hydration
3 Observing for and reporting to the physician any untoward side effects to the drug
4 Proper administration of liquid antitussives (a liquid nonnarcotic antitussive agent should be administered undiluted and the individual should be instructed not to drink water for approximately 30 to 35 minutes)

Benzonatate, N.F. (Tessalon)

Benzonatate is chemically related to the local anesthetic tetracaine. It has received a D.E.S.I. rating of *effective* for symptomatic treatment of cough. It relieves cough without suppressing respiration. Benzonatate relieves cough through two mechanisms, one of which is a peripheral action involving selective anesthesia of stretch receptors in the lungs. The second mechanism involves a direct action on the sites of medullary transmission.

Preparation and dosage. Benzonatate is marketed in 50- and 100-mg. capsules, and the dosage is 100 mg. several times a day for adults and children over 10 years of age. For younger children the dose is 8 mg. per kilogram of body weight in three to six divided doses. It is also available in intravenous and intramuscular preparations. However, oral administration is the route of choice. After oral administration its effects are noticed within 15 to 20 minutes, and they last for 3 to 8 hours. Benzonatate produces temporary local anesthesia of the oral mucosa; therefore, the patient should be instructed to swallow the capsule immediately.

Side effects do not seem to be serious but may include drowsiness, nausea, tightness in the chest, skin eruptions, chilling, and nasal congestion. On occasion, benzonatate may produce constipation. Side effects like those associated with the narcotic antitussives have not been reported.

Carbetapentane citrate (Toclase)

This is a synthetic preparation said to exhibit properties similar to atropine and certain local anesthetics. Its antitussive potency seems to be similar to that of codeine phosphate. It is marketed in 25-mg. tablets and as a syrup (1.45 mg.

per milliliter) for oral administration. The proposed dosage for adults is 15 to 30 mg. three to four times a day.

Noscapine, B.P. (Nectadon)

Noscapine is one of the isoquinoline alkaloids of opium, formerly known as narcotine. It is structurally related to papaverine and resembles it in its effects on smooth muscle, but its present use is based on its ability to depress the cough reflex. Noscapine resembles codeine in potency but does not produce opiate effects such as constipation, respiratory depression, constriction of the pupils, analgesia, and psychologic or physical dependence.

Preparation and dosage. Noscapine is marketed for oral administration. The usual adult dose is 15 to 30 mg. three or four times a day. Side effects after therapeutic dosage are minimal and include drowsiness, headache, nausea, rhinitis, and conjunctivitis.

Dextromethorphan hydrobromide, B.P., N.F. (Romilar Hydrobromide)

This drug is a synthetic derivative of morphine but is employed only as an agent to relieve cough. However, it possesses no significant analgesic properties, does not depress respiration, and does not cause dependence. It is the only agent in this group whose antitussive effects have been well documented through extensive experimental and clinical studies.

Preparation and dosage. Dextromethorphan hydrobromide is available in 15-mg. tablets and in a syrup (3 mg. per milliliter). The usual adult dose is 10 to 20 mg. once to several times daily. It acts within 20 to 30 minutes and is effective for 3 to 5 hours. Adverse reactions are mild and infrequent; they include slight drowsiness, nausea, and dizziness. This drug may be purchased across the counter without a prescription.

Levopropoxyphene napsylate, N.F. (Novrad)

This drug has no analgesic properties but it does have antitussive effects. It has received a D.E.S.I. rating of *effective* for the symptomatic treatment of cough. Adverse reactions include nausea and vomiting, epigastric distress, headache, dizziness, tremors, urticaria, rash, dry mouth, and drowsiness.

Levopropoxyphene is available in 50- and 100-mg. capsules and as a suspension containing 50 mg. per 5 ml. Dosage for adults is 50 to 100 mg. every 4 hours as needed. Dose for children is 1 mg. per kilogram of body weight.

Chlophedianol hydrochloride (Ulo)

This antitussive drug has been cited as having cough suppressant potency comparable to that of the narcotics but with a slower onset of peak effect and a longer duration of action. It has mild anticholinergic properties. Dependence has not been reported. D.E.S.I. rating for chlophedianol is *effective* for the symptomatic treatment of cough.

Adverse reactions include nausea and vomiting, urticaria, dry mouth, vertigo, visual disturbances, excitability, nightmares, and hallucinations. Chlophedianol should be used with caution in patients taking drugs that stimulate or depress the central nervous system and in debilitated patients.

Chlophedianol is available as a syrup containing 25 mg. per 5 ml. Usual dosage for adults is 25 mg. three or four times daily; for children over 6 years of age, 2 mg. per kilogram of body weight in four divided doses; for children 2 to 6 years of age, 1 mg. per kilogram of body weight in divided doses.

DEMULCENTS

Demulcents are agents with a soothing effect. Respiratory demulcents are often sticky substances that protect the lining of the respiratory tract from the irritation of contact with air and in this way they check coughing. They are used as gargles, lozenges, and syrups and as vehicles for other drugs. The most common are syrups (tolu, citric acid, acacia, or glycyrrhiza).

Cough syrups are soothing partly because of their local effect in the throat; hence, they should not be diluted and the patient should not drink water immediately after their administration.

Home remedies with a soothing effect include simple syrup, honey, or hard candy. Steam inhalations have a well-known soothing effect upon irritated mucous membranes. Plain or medicated steam may be administered with a special apparatus or by placing a basin of hot water over a hot plate to increase room humidity. There is little value, however, in administering steam when the doors or windows are open. Therefore, if the patient is to have the benefit of moisture-laden air to soothe the irritated respiratory tract, it is important to keep the room warm and the doors and windows closed. The addition of some aromatic substance such as menthol or oil of pine may make the inhalation more pleasant or soothing.

EXPECTORANTS

Expectorants are drugs that increase or modify the secretion of mucus in the bronchi and reduce its viscosity, thereby facilitating the expulsion of secretions. They are used in the treatment of coughs, bronchitis, and pneumonia.

Experimentally, little is known of their mode of action, but clinical experience attests to their value. They are used empirically to modify respiratory tract physiology. The respiratory tract is lined with ciliated epithelium that normally carries secretions of the tract toward the exterior. Mucus that becomes thick and tenacious probably interferes with these ciliated movements and coughing results. It is not known whether or not expectorants modify these movements.

Atropine, although not classed as an expectorant, may be given cautiously to check secretion and excessive expectoration in certain forms of bronchitis.

Many remedies used to treat colds contain atropine. Morphine, codeine, and papaverine not only act as sedatives but also tend to dry the mucous membranes. In many cases the best treatment of a cold or inflammation of the respiratory mucous membranes consists of prescribing extra rest, forcing fluids, and simple but nutritious food.

Ammonium chloride, N.F., B.P.; ammonium carbonate, N.F.

Ammonium chloride is frequently administered in some vehicle such as wild cherry syrup, citric acid syrup, or orange syrup. The NH_4^+ ions produce local gastric irritation, which acts reflexly to stimulate respiratory tract secretory ac-

tivity. Used as an expectorant, ammonium chloride is given in doses of 250 to 500 mg. four times a day in some suitable medium. It should be accompanied by a full glass of water because increased fluid intake also plays a part in the formation of increased mucus, thus decreasing viscosity of secretions.

Ammonium carbonate acts like ammonium chloride except that it causes gastric distress more easily. It is given in much the same manner and dosage as ammonium chloride. It is an alkaline salt and cannot be given in acid syrups. The usual dose is 250 to 500 mg.

Sodium iodide, U.S.P., B.P.; potassium iodide, U.S.P., B.P.

Iodides increase bronchial secretions reflexly by causing gastric irritation. These preparations are too irritating to be used in acute inflammatory conditions of the respiratory tract. When sputum becomes particularly tenacious, they are given to liquefy the secretion or loosen the cough. The average expectorant dose for adults is 300 mg. every 4 to 6 hours; dosage for children is 0.25 to 1 ml. in two to four doses daily. The salts may be administered in a saturated solution or in a cough mixture. If use is long continued, these drugs frequently produce symptoms of iodism. These are caused by irritation of the nasal passage, bronchi, and skin and include coryza and pain in the region of the frontal sinus and various skin eruptions, generally of a papular character. When such toxic symptoms occur, the drug should be discontinued, but it may be resumed in smaller doses after the disappearance of the symptoms.

Ipecac syrup, U.S.P.

Ipecac syrup is prescribed in doses of 1 to 8 ml. with a glass of water for adults and 5 minims for infants 1 year of age. A small increase of dosage is made for each additional year. In children, it is used to increase secretions and relieve bronchitis associated with croup. Ipecac syrup is also used as an emetic, particularly in children.

Terpin hydrate, N.F.

Terpin hydrate occurs as colorless, lustrous crystals, nearly odorless, having a slightly aromatic odor and somewhat bitter taste. Terpin hydrate is antiseptic, diaphoretic, and diuretic in action, but it is used chiefly as a vehicle for other drugs. Usual dose of terpin hydrate elixir, N.F., and terpin hydrate and codeine elixir, N.F., is 4 to 5 ml. (1 fluidram) every 4 to 6 hours. When terpin hydrate is combined with codeine it is the high alcohol content of the elixir that produces its expectorant action. The amount of terpin hydrate in the combined preparation is usually too small to exert a significant effect and therefore it acts only as a vehicle for the codeine.

PREPARATIONS TO RELIEVE NASAL CONGESTION AND COLD SYMPTOMS
NASAL DECONGESTANTS

Perhaps the attribute for which vasoconstricting drugs are most commonly used is their capacity to shrink the engorged nasal mucous membranes in mild upper respiratory infections. Many drugs are used exclusively as nasal vasoconstrictors. Because of their wide popular use and lack of serious hazard (when used topically), a confusingly large number of preparations have been provided by the pharmaceutical industry for direct sale to the public. Some of the more widely used agents in this group are phenylephrine hydrochloride (Neo-Synephrine), ephedrine sulfate, mephentermine sulfate (Wyamine Sulfate), propylhexadrine (Benzedrex), tuaminoheptane (Tuamine), xylometazoline hydrochloride (Otrivin Hydrochloride), phenylpropylmethylamine hydrochloride (Vonedrine), and naphazoline hydrochloride (Privine). Students will recognize these drugs as adrenergic agents. They are used to shrink engorged mucous membranes of the nose and to relieve nasal stuffiness. However, there is a tendency on the part of patients to misuse them by using them in too large an amount and too frequently. This may result in "rebound" engorgement or swelling of the mucous membranes. Preservatives, antihistaminics, detergents, and antibiotics are sometimes added to the preparation of the decongestant. In some cases untoward reactions are believed to be caused by the additive rather than by the decongestant. Too-frequent interference with the vasomotor mechanism in the nose may do more harm than good, and there is always the possibility of spreading the infection deeper into the sinuses or to the middle ear. Sprays and nose drops are of benefit when used judiciously under the advice of a physician.

ANTIHISTAMINIC AGENTS FOR COLDS

Considerable difference of opinion exists at the present time as to the usefulness of the antihistaminic drugs for the prevention or treatment of the common cold. These drugs include diphenhydramine hydrochloride (Benadryl) and tripelennamine hydrochloride (Pyribenzamine) as well as a number of others. They are discussed in Chapter 17. Some investigators are of the opinion that if these drugs are taken early during the onset of a cold, the allergic manifestations of the disease are relieved. The patient experiences relief from the tickling sensation in the nose, sneezing, and the continuous irritating discharge from the nasal mucous membrane. The Council on Drugs warns that their indiscriminate use is not without harmful effects—people may become excessively drowsy and fall asleep while driving a car or operating machinery. It is also possible that profound effects may occur in the central nervous system and the blood-forming tissues after prolonged use of these drugs.

QUESTIONS

For study and review

1 Explain the therapeutic uses of carbon dioxide and state what precautions should be taken when carbon dioxide is administered.
2 What precautions must be taken when oxygen is administered to patients with severe respiratory disease?
3 Discuss the beneficial and harmful effects of coughing.
4 Discuss the advantages and disadvantages of "across-the-counter" preparations for coughs and nasal congestion.
5 What are the advantages of nebulization therapy?
6 Discuss the effects of the following, and give an example of each:
  a. detergent   c. antifoaming agent
  b. mucolytic agent   d. bronchodilator
7 What nursing care measures are important for the patient receiving oxygen via:
  a. nasal catheter
  b. mask
  c. tent

8 When is it advantageous to use large droplets for nebulization therapy? To use small droplets?

9 Under what conditions is it preferable to stimulate expectoration?

10 Why does increased humidity of atmosphere in itself help to relieve coughing?

11 Discuss the therapy and nursing care for a patient with an acute asthmatic attack.

12 How do drugs act to produce relief from a cough?

REFERENCES

Beeson, P. B., and McDermott, W.: Cecil-Loeb textbook of medicine, ed. 13, Philadelphia, 1971, W. B. Saunders Co.

DiPalma, Joseph R.: Drill's pharmacology in medicine, ed. 4, New York, 1971, McGraw-Hill Book Co.

Foley, Mary F.: Pulmonary function testing, Am. J. Nurs. **71:**1134, 1971.

Ganong, William F.: Review of medical physiology, ed. 5, Palo Alto, Calif., 1971, Lange Medical Publications.

Goodman, L., and Gilman, A.: The pharmacologic basis of therapeutics, ed. 4, New York, 1970, The Macmillan Co.

Goth, A.: Medical pharmacology, ed. 7, St. Louis, 1974, The C. V. Mosby Co.

Govani, L., and Hayes, J.: Drug and nursing implications, ed. 2, New York, 1971, Appleton-Century-Crofts.

Griffith, E. W.: Nursing process: A patient with respiratory difficulty, Nurs. Clin. North Am. **6:**145, 1971.

Guyton, A. C.: Textbook of medical physiology, ed. 4, Philadelphia, 1971, W. B. Saunders Co.

Marlow, D. R.: Textbook of pediatric nursing, ed. 3, Philadelphia, 1969, W. B. Saunders Co.

Modell, W., editor: Drugs of choice 1976-1977, St. Louis, 1976, The C. V. Mosby Co.

Morrison, R. J., and Boyd, R. N.: Organic chemistry, ed. 3, Boston, 1973, Allyn and Bacon, Inc.

Said, S. I.: Role of pulmonary surfactant in health and disease, Med. Clin. North Am. **51:**391, 1967.

Schwaid, M. C.: The impact of emphysema, Am. J. Nurs. **70:**1247, 1970.

Sedlock, S. A.: Detection of chronic pulmonary disease, Am. J. Nurs. **72:**1407, 1972.

Senior, R. M., and Fishman, A. P.: Disturbances in alveolar ventilation, Med. Clin. North Am. **51:**403, 1967.

Szidon, J. P., Pietra, G. G., and Fishman, A. P.: The alveolar-capillary membrane and pulmonary edema, New Eng. J. Med. **286:**1200, 1972.

Winter, P. M., and Lowenstein, E.: Acute respiratory failure, Science **221:**23, 1969.

CHAPTER 17

Histamine and antihistaminics

Histamine
Histamine-antagonizing drugs

HISTAMINE

Histamine is the enigma of pharmacology. Although it is widely distributed throughout the body with high concentrations in the lungs, skin, and stomach, its role in normal physiology remains a mystery. Histamine means "tissue amine." It was isolated from extracts of ergot in 1910 and firmly established as a natural body substance in 1927. When liberated from binding sites it causes untoward reactions that range in intensity from mild itching to angioneurotic edema, shock, and death. There is some evidence that histamine has some function in anaphylaxis, allergies, drug reactions, and inflammatory processes. It is possible that histamine is important to anabolic events such as growth and repair, for it is found wherever there is protein breakdown or putrefaction.

HISTAMINE RELEASE

Histamine release can provoke allergic responses and troublesome side effects, and health professionals should know which substances are most commonly implicated in this phenomenon. Histamine-releasing agents can be classified into seven groups.

1 Antigens and substances that combine with proteins to form antigens and provoke formation of antibodies. The antigen-antibody reaction releases histamine (and other substances) from sensitized tissue, giving rise to an "altered response" or allergic reaction—asthma, hay fever, urticaria. Antigens are also known as allergens and include pollens and food, particularly dietary protein (such as eggs, milk, shellfish, and fresh berries).
2 Proteolytic enzymes such as trypsin and penicillinase
3 Surface-active agents such as detergents and bile salts
4 Monoamines
5 High molecular weight compounds such as the plasma expanders and dextrans
6 Mechanical and chemical trauma to the skin: abrasion, laceration, wasp and bee stings, snake venom, plant poisons (poison ivy, poison oak), or toxins
7 Drugs that are histamine liberators—that "explosively" release histamine

Histamine phosphate, U.S.P., B.P.

Histidine

Histamine

Histamine, like epinephrine, norepinephrine, and 5-hydroxytryptamine, is a compound of pharmacologic and physiologic interest, since, in contrast to most drugs, it occurs naturally in the body. Like the other natural-body constituents just named it is an amine possessing the basic group NH_2. Histamine is derived from the amino acid histidine by the removal of the carboxyl group as carbon dioxide—a reaction that takes place in body cells and intestinal contents.

Histamine's interest to medicine is multiple; the compound itself can be used to produce certain pharmacologic effects employed chiefly for diagnostic tests. Much more important than this use, however, is the fact that certain compounds that prevent the pharmacologic action of histamine (histamine antagonists, antihistaminics) have very useful effects, including the prevention or relief of allergic symptoms and motion sickness.

Action and result. The principal actions of histamine are: (1) contraction of smooth muscle, (2) dilation of capillaries, and (3) promotion of gastric acid secretion. In man a noticeable dilation of the arterioles also occurs.

An intradermal injection of histamine causes a series of reactions called the "triple response." Blood vessels (capillaries) immediately affected by the histamine dilate and produce a *flush* or redness. Surrounding blood vessels then dilate to produce a *flare* or diffuse redness. This reaction is probably the result of a neural mechanism—axon reflexes stimulate sensory nerves and their branches to produce dilation of blood vessels. Widely dilated blood vessels have increased permeability. There is an increase in tissue fluid or local edema, which is termed a *wheal.* Any chemical or mechanical injury to the skin can cause this triple response of flush, flare, and wheal. Therefore, it is believed that histamine is released from injured skin. The triple response is believed to be one of the body's protective mechanisms, since increased permeability of blood vessels permits the passage of plasma proteins and white cells into the tissues.

The marked dilation of the arterioles and capillaries by histamine produces a definite flushing of the skin, a rise in skin temperature, an itching or burning sensation, and a fall in blood pressure. Vasodilation in the meningeal vessels is accompanied by an increase in intracranial pressure, which may cause headache. The fall in blood pressure after small doses of histamine is followed by rather quick recovery,

caused by the release of epinephrine and the activity of cardiovascular reflexes.

A marked fall in blood pressure may follow a large dose of histamine, and the same vascular changes that take place in surgical shock may occur. The permeability of capillary beds increases, and sufficient blood proteins are lost to the tissues so that blood volume cannot be maintained and circulation is slowed. While an increase in cardiac rate and output occur after injection of histamine, this is mainly reflexly induced by the fall in blood pressure.

Uterine and intestinal muscle is stimulated, as well as the smooth muscle of the bronchial tubes. Bronchospasm may be induced in man after large doses of the drug, especially if the patient suffers from chronic conditions of the respiratory tract, such as asthma and bronchitis.

Histamine stimulates the gastric, salivary, pancreatic, and lacrimal glands. The chief effect in man, however, is seen in the gastric glands. The resulting secretion in the normal stomach is high in acid because of the selective action on the acid-forming cells.

Some investigators maintain that histamine is liberated in the body in large amounts as a result of extensive tissue damage or of antigen-antibody reactions. Attempts to demonstrate that histamine tolerance can be achieved by desensitization of the patient have been inconclusive.

Because the symptoms of acute histamine poisoning and those of anaphylactic shock are quite similar, it was suggested long ago that acute allergic reactions (resulting from the exposure of a sensitive individual to an antigen) resulted in the release of histamine. Since then it has been found that when allergic shock is produced either in the whole animal or in an isolated organ (such as the guinea pig uterus), histamine is released. The thesis is now well accepted that abnormal release of histamine from storage sites accompanies acute allergic reactions, both mild and severe, and accounts for at least some of the changes observed in the patient. A further convincing finding has been that antihistaminics can modify and significantly lessen the picture of some acute allergic reactions.

Wasp, bee, and snake venom, gnats, and plant poisons contain histamine that can cause the triple response in man. Other agents known to release histamine are detergents and surface-active agents, trypsin and proteolytic enzymes, and basic protein substances such as amines. Many drugs are histamine liberators that may be responsible for side effects; examples are morphine and codeine. Certain foods are potent histamine releasers in allergic patients, for example, fresh berries, shellfish, and eggs.

Ordinarily, histamine is altered in the body partly by methylation and by the enzyme diamine oxidase, also known as histaminase, which converts histamine to imidazole-acetic acid. Diamine oxidase is present in greatest amounts in the intestinal mucosa and kidney. It acts slowly to inactivate histamine.

Uses. Histamine is rarely used therapeutically but has occasionally been used for diagnostic purposes.

One diagnostic use is concerned with gastric acid production. Histamine is a potent stimulus to the secretion of gastric hydrochloric acid, and there is some evidence suggesting that it may be the natural trigger that starts the secretion of hydrochloric acid. Accordingly, it can be used to reveal the absence of gastric acid (achlorhydria), a diagnostic aid for certain anemias. If a patient does not respond with a significant secretion of gastric acid to the challenge of a small dose of histamine, it is likely that he cannot make gastric acid. This is believed to be caused by a degenerative change in the gastric mucosa.

Another use is in the diagnosis of pheochromocytoma. Tumors of the medullary portion of the adrenal gland that secrete epinephrine and norepinephrine are uncommon, but their discovery is important since they represent one type of hypertension that can be permanently cured by surgery. Small doses of histamine stimulate the secretion of the adrenal medulla; in the normal individual the pressor amines secreted by the adrenal gland are insufficient to produce a marked rise in blood pressure, but in the patient with pheochromocytoma histamine may lead to a very prominent secretion of medullary amines with a resultant striking rise in blood pressure. The histamine test is one of several "pharmacologic" provocative tests for pheochromocytoma.

Histamine may also be used to test the capacity of capillaries to dilate in certain peripheral vascular diseases.

Preparation, dosage, and administration. Prior to the test for gastric acid production the patient should have fasted and rested for 12 hours. A gastric tube is inserted and the gastric contents are aspirated. The patient may then be given 300 ml. of water. The histamine is injected subcutaneously; the dose is usually 0.25 to 0.5 mg. of histamine in the form of a 1:1000 solution. Pulse and blood pressure should be taken immediately after injection; the usual response is increased pulse rate and slightly decreased blood pressure. Observations for side effects should be continued during the test. Epinephrine hydrochloride 1:1000 (0.5 to 1.0 ml.) should be readily available to treat severe reactions if they occur. After injection of histamine, gastric contents are aspirated every 10 to 15 minutes for 1 hour and tested for volume, total acidity, blood, bile, and mucus. Maximum secretory response to histamine usually occurs in 30 minutes; the effect lasts about $1^{1}/_{2}$ hours. Gastric achlorhydria after histamine injection is usually pathologic and often indicative of pernicious anemia.

In the test for pheochromocytoma, 25 to 50 μg. of histamine is injected intravenously. The patient should be at rest and his basal blood pressure level should have been determined. Following a decrease in blood pressure within 30 seconds, if a marked rise in blood pressure occurs (60 mm. Hg systolic, 30 mm. Hg diastolic) in 1 to 4 minutes associated with symptoms of pallor, fear, sweating, and so on, the test is positive for the presence of the tumor. Blood pressure usually returns to preinjection levels within 5 to 15 minutes. Pulse rate and blood pressure must be frequently determined both during and following the test. This test is contraindicated for elderly persons or for those with marked hypertension (blood pressure in excess of 150 mm. Hg systolic and 100 mm. Hg diastolic).

Side effects and toxic effects. Symptoms of overdosage include rapid drop in blood pressure, intense headache, dyspnea, flushing of the skin, vomiting, diarrhea, shock, and collapse. The toxic symptoms are rarely dangerous, although they may be alarming. If the patient goes into

Table 17-1 Histamine effects

Blood vessels	
Capillaries	Dilation, increased permeability
Arterioles	Dilation
Arteries	Dilation
Cerebral vessels	Dilation (headache)
Heart	Increased rate, indirect effect
Blood pressure	Decrease
Secretions	
Bronchial	Increase
Gastric	Definite increase
Intestinal	Slight increase
Salivary	Slight increase
Uterus	Mild contraction
Gastrointestinal tract	Contraction
Adrenal medulla	Stimulated epinephrine and norepinephrine release
Skin	Flush, flare, wheal

shock, the blood volume may need to be restored. Epinephrine is a specific physiologic antagonist and will prevent or counteract symptoms if administered promptly.

Contraindications. Histamine should not be administered to the elderly, those with cardiovascular disease, or those with bronchial asthma.

Betazole hydrochloride, U.S.P. (Histalog)

Betazole is an analogue of histamine with similar pharmacologic actions. It is also used in diagnostic tests of gastric secretion. It stimulates gastric secretion equal to that of histamine, particularly during the first hour of gastric analysis; but the amount of acid secreted during the second hour and later is usually greater with betazole. Betazole produces fewer side effects than histamine. D.E.S.I. rating is *effective* for clinical testing of gastric secretions.

Side effects. Flushing, sweating, and a feeling of warmth occur in about 20% of the patients tested with betazole. Headache occurs in about 3% of the patients, and urticaria and syncope occur rarely.

Precautions. Betazole should be used with caution in patients with bronchial asthma, recent gastrointestinal bleeding, or heart disease.

HISTAMINE-ANTAGONIZING DRUGS

Histamine can be antagonized by the use of drugs that: (1) produce pharmacologic effects opposed to those of histamine, of which the best example is epinephrine, and (2) in some way prevent histamine from showing its typical actions. The latter drugs are the group generally called antihistaminics.

Epinephrine

Epinephrine is a lifesaving drug in anaphylactic shock. The most serious effects of anaphylaxis (or severe acute allergic reactions) in man are the extensive arteriolar dilation with hypotensive shock and collapse and the marked constriction of bronchial tubes that can lead to extreme respiratory difficulty and even suffocation. By promoting vasoconstriction and by dilating the bronchial tubes epinephrine can antagonize the physiologic effects of anaphylaxis or of histamine poisoning.

ANTIHISTAMINICS

Antihistaminics are believed to act not by opposing but by preventing the physiologic action of histamine. It is postulated that the antihistaminics act by preventing histamine from reaching its site of action, that is, by competition for the receptors. The first antihistaminic was found in 1933 as a result of a conscious attempt to discover a compound with this activity. Although the initial compounds were quite toxic and therefore not very useful, hundreds of antihistaminics have been synthesized and tested. Many of these compounds have similar chemical features, represented by three typical compounds:

Diphenhydramine
(Benadryl)

Tripelennamine
(Pyribenzamine)

Chlorpheniramine
(Chlor-Trimeton)

It can be seen that a common structural feature is the short straight chain terminating in a tertiary amine, $-C-C-N\begin{smallmatrix}R'\\R''\end{smallmatrix}$ and it has been suggested that this portion of the antihistaminics is an analogue of the $-C-C-NH_2$ chain of histamine.

Pharmacologically, it is known that antihistaminics block histamine action somewhat selectively. They tend to prevent the muscular (circulatory and bronchiolar) action of histamine but are not as effective against the secretory actions of histamine. The usual antihistaminics do not block the gastric secretory and some other actions of histamine. It is now believed that the body has two different types of receptors for histamine, the H_1 and H_2 receptors. The usual antihistaminics are H_1 receptor antagonists. Recently, drugs have been synthesized in Great Britain that antagonize the H_2 receptors, such as the ones in the stomach. These new drugs, one of which is metiamide, which is undergoing clinical trial, can block histamine-induced gastric secretion.

During the past few years histamine antagonists of various types have been tried for histamine shock, anaphylactic reactions, and allergy. The antihistaminics have the greatest therapeutic effect on nasal allergies, particularly on seasonal hay fever. They relieve symptoms better at the beginning of the hay fever season than during its height but fail to relieve the asthma that frequently accompanies hay fever. These preparations are palliative and do not immunize the patient or protect him over a period of time against allergic reactions. Their benefits are therefore comparatively short lived and provide only symptomatic relief. They must be regarded only as adjuncts to more specific methods of treatment. They do not begin to replace such remedies as epinephrine, ephedrine, and aminophylline. In acute asthmatic reactions, the antihistaminic drugs serve only as supplements to these older remedies. Furthermore, relief of various symptoms of allergy is obtained only while the drug is being taken. Antihistaminics do not appear to have a cumulative action and can therefore be taken over a period of time.

Different antihistamines are either more or less effective in different individuals. If one drug provides an unsatisfactory clinical response, a different antihistaminic may provide a favorable effect. Although the use of antihistamines for treatment of the common cold is controversial, many over-the-counter cold remedies contain an antihistaminic.

One peculiar and unanticipated action of many of the antihistaminics is their ability to relieve or abolish the symptoms of motion sickness, both in animals and in man. Thus a number of anti-motion sickness agents are also potent antihistaminics. The commonly used compound dimenhydrinate (Dramamine), for example, is simply diphenhydramine with a different acid neutralizing the basic nitrogens of the antihistaminic itself.

The most common untoward effect of these preparations is drowsiness, which may become so marked that deep sleep may result. Other untoward symptoms include dizziness, dryness of the mouth and throat, nausea, disturbed coordination, lassitude, muscular weakness, and gastrointestinal disturbances. Sedation may disappear after 2 or 3 days of treatment. However, in some patients symptoms of excitation occur, such as insomnia, nervousness, and even convulsions.

Patients receiving these preparations for continuous treatment should have the benefit of periodic medical examinations since blood dyscrasias can occur.

Brompheniramine maleate, N.F. (Dimetane, Disomer)

Brompheniramine is an effective antihistaminic for treatment of allergic reactions and as an adjunct for anaphylactic reactions after the acute manifestations have been controlled. Principal side effects are drowsiness and rash. Usual oral adult dose is 4 to 8 mg. three or four times daily, or one extentab every 8 to 12 hours; parenteral dose is 5 to 20 mg. twice daily. Dose for children is 0.5 mg. per kilogram of body weight divided into three or four doses. Dimetapp is brompheniramine with phenylephrine.

Chlorcyclizine hydrochloride, N.F., B.P. (Di-Paralene Hydrochloride, Perazil)

Advantages claimed for chlorcyclizine hydrochloride are a prolonged action and low incidence of side effects. It is effective in 30 minutes; action may last for 12 hours. A dose of 50 mg. or more is given orally up to four times a day. For children dose is 1.5 mg. per kilogram of body weight divided into two doses. Chlorcyclizine hydrochloride tablets, U.S.P., are available in 25 and 50 mg. each. It is contraindicated in pregnancy because of potential harm to the fetus.

Chlorpheniramine maleate, U.S.P., B.P. (Chlor-Trimeton, Histaspan, Teldrin)

This preparation produces a low incidence of side effects but compares favorably with other antihistaminics in therapeutic usefulness and does so after comparatively low dosage. The effect of the drug is prolonged by the use of a special tablet form that contains twice the average single dose, half of which is contained in an enteric-coated core that delays absorption. The drug is available in dosage forms suited for parenteral as well as oral administration. Its action tends to be slow. The usual adult oral dose is 2 to 4 mg. every 6 to 8 hours. Tablets of 4 mg. are available. The repeat-action tablet and sustained-release capsules are available in 8 and 12 mg.; the syrup contains 2.5 mg. per milliliter; the injection solution contains 10 and 100 mg.

per milliliter. The usual parenteral dose is 5 to 40 mg. For children dose is 0.35 mg. per kilogram of body weight divided into four doses.

Diphenhydramine hydrochloride, U.S.P., B.P. (Benadryl Hydrochloride)

Diphenhydramine is similar to other members of the group. In addition to its antihistaminic activity it has a moderate antispasmodic action. This is sometimes significant in cases of bronchial asthma. When given in full therapeutic doses, it causes a high incidence of sedation, which makes it more suitable for use at night than during the day. The average oral dose for adults is 25 to 50 mg. given three or four times daily. For children under 12, dose is 5 mg. per kilogram of body weight in four divided doses over a 24-hour period. It is available in a number of dosage forms suited for topical, oral, and parenteral administration. The usual intravenous dose is 10 to 50 mg.

It is the antihistamine of choice for treatment of anaphylactic and other allergic reactions, but it is not a substitute for epinephrine. For anaphylactic reactions it is given intravenously or by deep intramuscular injection.

Diphenhydramine is also an effective antiemetic and antiparkinsonism drug.

Promethazine hydrochloride, U.S.P., B.P. (Phenergan)

Promethazine hydrochloride exhibits a number of pharmacologic effects although its pronounced sedative effect limits its use. It is a potent antihistaminic, it can be used for the relief of motion sickness, and it relieves apprehension. It potentiates the action of drugs that depress the central nervous system, making possible a reduction of their dosage. It has a relatively prolonged action, lasting up to 18 to 24 hours. Its sedative action is utilized clinically for surgical and obstetric patients. Promethazine hydrochloride is administered orally, parenterally, and rectally. The usual oral dose is 25 mg., although the range of dosage may be 6 to 75 mg. Parenterally, the dosage is up to 1 mg. per kilogram of body weight. Dose for children is 0.13 mg. per kilogram of body weight taken when necessary. It is available in 12.5- and 25-

mg. tablets, as a syrup, and as a sterile solution for injection (25 mg. per milliliter). Promethazine suppositories are available (25 mg.). Since it is a phenothiazine, precautions applicable to phenothiazines should be observed.

Pyrilamine maleate, N.F. (Neo-Antergan, Histalon); mepyramine maleate, B.P. (Anthisan)

This compound is available in 25- and 50-mg. tablets and as a syrup, 2.5 mg. per milliliter, for oral administration, after which effects last 4 to 6 hours. The usual adult dose is 25 to 50 mg. three or four times daily. The incidence of sedation is low, but it may cause gastrointestinal irritation.

Tripelennamine hydrochloride, U.S.P. (Pyribenzamine)

This drug is therapeutically effective, and the incidence of untoward reactions is low. Stimulation of the nervous system does occur as well as gastrointestinal irritation, but the latter is not severe. Sedation is moderate. This agent is available in a number of dosage forms for topical, oral, and parenteral (subcutaneous, intramuscular, and intravenous) administration. The usual oral adult dose is 25 to 75 mg. three or four times a day, although doses of 100 to 150 mg. are tolerated by most patients.

Tripelennamine citrate, U.S.P. (Pyribenzamine)

This preparation is more palatable than the hydrochloride when administered in a liquid form. It provides the same therapeutic action as does the hydrochloride. The dosage is greater for the citrate than for the hydrochloride preparation of the drug because of the difference in the molecular weights of the compounds. The usual adult dose is 50 mg. three times a day.

Other antihistaminics

There are a number of additional antihistaminic agents listed in the N.F. These include bromophenhydramine (Ambodry), carbinoxamine maleate (Clistin), methapyrilene hydrochloride (Dozar, Histadyl), cyproheptadine (Periactin),

dimethindene (Forbistal, Triten), and pyrrobutamine phosphate (Pyronil).

DRUGS USED FOR MOTION SICKNESS

Motion sickness is a reaction to certain kinds of movement, sometimes any kind if it is sufficiently severe. Most persons are well adjusted to horizontal movements, but some are unable to tolerate continuous vertical movements. Such persons are likely to become ill when traveling in cars, trains, airplanes, or ships. Disturbance of the cells in the labyrinth of the ear is believed to be the cause of motion sickness. The person usually becomes pale, perspires, feels chilly or warm, and salivates freely. If he continues to be subjected to the motion, symptoms usually progress to nausea and vomiting.

A number of drugs have been used for motion sickness, including sedatives such as barbiturates, autonomic drugs such as scopolamine, as well as a number of the tranquilizing agents. Promethazine, mentioned previously, has been widely tested and found effective. The following agents have also been found useful for prevention of motion sickness and vestibular dysfunction (disturbance of functions of the inner ear). The exact mechanism of their action is unclear, but most of them appear to depress the central nervous system and decrease sensitivity of the labyrinth of the ear. Like other antihistaminics they should be used with caution by persons who are responsible for the operation of power machines.

Cyclizine hydrochloride, U.S.P., B.P. (Marezine)

Cyclizine is an antihistaminic drug that has been found effective in a high percentage of cases in the prevention of nausea and vomiting associated with motion sickness.

Although dry mouth, drowsiness, and blurred vision can be observed after large doses, these symptoms seldom appear after ordinary therapeutic doses. Cyclizine is teratogenic in the rat. This fact should be taken into consideration before its use in pregnancy is contemplated.

Cyclizine hydrochloride is administered orally and rectally. The usual adult dose is 50 mg. 30 minutes before departure and 50 mg. three times daily before meals. Reduction of dosage may be indicated after the initial dose, depending on the duration of the trip, type of travel, and reaction of the individual person. For the relief of dizziness and associated symptoms of vestibular disorder (in conditions other than motion sickness) the usual dose is 50 mg. three times a day.

Cyclizine hydrochloride is available in 50-mg. tablets and 50- and 100-mg. suppositories. Cyclizine lactate has the same effects as cyclizine hydrochloride but is suited for intramuscular injection. The dosage is the same as that for hydrochloride.

Dimenhydrinate, U.S.P., B.P. (Dramamine)

As mentioned previously, dimenhydrinate is chemically related to diphenhydramine (Benadryl). It produces mild sedation. It is effective for a high percentage of persons who suffer from motion sickness. It is also used to control nausea, vomiting, and dizziness associated with a number of conditions such as stapedectomy operations, radiation sickness, and Meniere's disease. It has also been employed for the relief of postoperative nausea and vomiting. Its status an an antiemetic for this purpose is not well established because of the variety of factors that contribute to the illness.

Dimenhydrinate is available in a number of dosage forms for oral, rectal, or intramuscular administration. The usual oral dose is 50 mg. 30 minutes before departure to prevent motion sickness. Dosage up to 100 mg. every 4 hours may be prescribed not only for motion sickness but also for the control of nausea and vomiting associated with other conditions. The usual intramuscular dose is 50 mg.

Meclizine hydrochloride, U.S.P. (Bonine Hydrochloride)

Meclizine hydrochloride exerts a mild but prolonged antihistaminic action and is effective in the prevention of motion sickness. The duration of its effects may be as long as 24 hours. Like other members of this group of drugs, it appears to affect the central nervous system and the inner ear.

The incidence of its side effects seems to be low, although like most other antihistaminic drugs it can cause drowsiness, blurred vision, dryness of the mouth, and fatigue. Meclizine is teratogenic in the rat and thus should not be taken during pregnancy.

It is administered orally. The usual adult dose is 25 to 50 mg. once a day for the prevention of motion sickness (1 hour before departure). For the relief of nausea and vomiting from other causes the dosage is similar or the same. The drug is available in tablets of 25 mg., as well as an elixir containing 12.5 mg. in 5 ml.

NURSING ASPECTS

1 Many antihistaminics produce sedation, which causes drowsiness and even some slowing of reflexes. Patients should be cautioned about driving cars or motor bikes if drowsiness occurs and to be cautious when around hazardous machinery or tools.
2 Patients should be informed that antihistaminics can potentiate the effects of other sedatives, hypnotics, tranquilizers, and alcohol.
3 The drying effect of some antihistamines may produce a dry cough and even hoarseness. If this occurs, dosage may need to be decreased, the antihistamine stopped for a few days, or a different antihistamine prescribed.

4 Some antihistamines can cause an increase in blood pressure, particularly if overdosage occurs.

5 Patients with hypertension or cardiovascular disease should be advised not to use over-the-counter cold remedies except with the permission of their physician. The vasoconstrictor effects may be deleterious to their condition.

QUESTIONS

For study and review

1 Explain the rationale for linking histamine with allergic reactions.

2 What are the advantages and disadvantages of the various antihistaminics?

3 Explain what is meant by the "triple response."

4 Explain how histamine may be used for diagnosing achlorhydria; for diagnosing pheochromocytoma.

REFERENCES

A.M.A. drug evaluations, ed. 2, Acton, Mass., 1973, Publishing Sciences Group, Inc.

Aviado, D. M.: Krantz and Carr's pharmacologic principles of medical practice, ed. 8, Baltimore, 1972, The Williams & Wilkins Co.

Black, J. W., and others: Definitions and antagonism of histamine H_2-receptors, Nature **236**:385, 1972.

Brand, J. J.: The pharmacologic basis for the control of motion sickness by drugs, Pharmacol. Phys. **2**(3):1, 1968.

Money, K. E.: Motion sickness, Physiol. Rev. **50**:1, 1970.

Osol, A., and Pratt, R.: The United States dispensatory, ed. 27, Philadelphia, 1973, J. B. Lippincott Co.

Rodman, M. J.: Drugs for allergic disorders. Part 1. Anaphylaxis and asthma, R. N. **34**:63, 1971. Part 2. Pollinosis, perennial rhinitis, dermatitis, R. N. **34**:53, 1971.

Witiak, D. T.: Antiallergenic agents. In Burger, A., editor: Medicinal chemistry, Part II, New York, 1970, Wiley Interscience, pp. 1643-1668.

CHAPTER 18

Fluids, electrolytes, and nutrients

Fluids

Water
Water balance
Abnormal states of hydration
Intravenous fluid therapy

Electrolytes

Potassium
Calcium
Magnesium

Nutrients

Fat-soluble vitamins
Water-soluble vitamins

If the student stops to consider the place of certain drugs in the body economy, he will quickly recognize that in some instances substances given as medicaments are not foreign to the body but are provided as replacement therapy. They stand in contrast to a large number of drugs, the "foreign" compounds such as the anesthetics, antibiotics, and antihistaminics given to achieve a desirable pharmacologic effect. This "normal" group of drugs are natural constituents of the body or diet that are required in certain quantities to preserve healthy function. When absent, as in nutritional deficiency diseases, they must be replaced if the disease is to be cured. However, they may also be given when a deficiency is not present to obtain physiological actions available only at high blood levels.

Fluids

WATER

In humans water comprises from 45% to 75% of the total body weight depending upon the amount of adipose tissue present. Infants and young children have more water per unit of body weight than adults, and female adults have less water content than male adults. The greatest amount of body water (up to 45% of body weight) is to be found in the *intracellular fluid*, that is, the fluid inside the cells. It is in this fluid that the chemical reactions of all metabolism so essential to life occur. The remainder of body water is located in the *extracellular fluid*, that is, the fluid surrounding the cells. This extracellular fluid consists of plasma, interstitial fluid, and lymph, and extracellular portions of dense connective tissue, cartilage, and bone. The volume of fluid in the two body fluid compartments varies with age and differs in the two sexes. It is in this fluid that metabolic exchanges between cells and tissues and the external environment occur.

The importance of body water is highlighted by the facts that (1) it is the medium in which all metabolic reactions occur, and (2) precise regulation of volume and composition of body fluid is essential to health. In the healthy individual body water remains remarkably constant, maintained by a balance between intake and excretion —the water gained each day is equal to the water lost. If the water gained exceeds the water lost, there will be *water excess*, or *overhydration* and edema. If the water lost exceeds the water

K^+ $PO_4^=$ Protein$^-$ Intracellular fluid	Na^+ Cl^- $HCO_3^=$ Extracellular fluid

Cell

Figure 18-1

Principal ions in intracellular and extracellular fluid.

gained there will be a *water deficit*, or *dehydration*. The importance of body water is further emphasized by the fact that if 20% to 25% of body water is lost, death usually occurs.

Water is an excellent solvent that permits many substances to be dispersed through it. It also has a high dielectric constant, which permits ionization of electrolytes. These electrolytes are important in maintaining body fluid volume and distribution. They include the cations sodium (Na^+) for extracellular fluid, and potassium (K^+) and magnesium (Mg^{++}) for intracellular fluid; and the anions chloride (Cl^-) and bicarbonate (HCO_3^-) for extracellular fluid, and phosphate ($PO_4^=$) and protein for intracellular fluid. Intracellular ions also occur in the extracellular fluid but in smaller amounts.

Water is also an excellent lubricant between membranes, and it functions well as a heat insulator.

WATER BALANCE

As previously stated water balance must be maintained between the amount of water taken in and the amount of water excreted. Water intake occurs primarily by: (1) drinking fluids, (2) ingesting food containing moisture (most foods contain a high percentage of water), and (3) water formed by the oxidation of hydrogen in the food during metabolic processes. This latter method produces about $1/2$ liter of water per day.

Water is lost from the body in five principal ways: (1) via the kidneys as urine, (2) through the skin as *insensible perspiration* and sweat; (3) through expired air as water vapor, (4) through

feces, and (5) through the excretion of tears and saliva. Urine excretion accounts for 50% to 60% of the total daily water loss. Urine output, of course, varies with the amount of water ingested. In humans, some daily intake of water is essential to maintain water balance. During starvation man can go several weeks without food intake but can survive only a few days without water intake.

Thirst, the subjective desire to ingest water, helps to maintain water balance. Although thirst is complex and not well understood, it is induced by a decrease in saliva and dryness of the mouth and throat. It may be that dehydration of thirst receptors leads to their stimulation.

ABNORMAL STATES OF HYDRATION

A dynamic relationship exists in the human body between water and sodium, and abnormal states of hydration can be classified as: (1) dehydration (volume depletion); (2) overhydration (hypervolemia or volume excess); (3) loss of water in excess of sodium ("hypernatremia"); and (4) loss of sodium in excess of water ("hyponatremia").

DEHYDRATION

Isotonic dehydration, or volume depletion, is the excessive loss of water and sodium in nearly equivalent proportions. This may result from vomiting, diarrhea, or fistula drainage. An isotonic solution of sodium chloride (0.9%) is often used to correct this condition. Flow rate of intravenous isotonic solutions is usually 125 ml. per hour, or about 2 ml. per minute. However, the flow rates may vary depending upon the patient's age, body surface area, ability to assimilate fluid, and cardiac and renal function.

Sodium chloride injection, U.S.P.

Sodium chloride injection is a 0.9% solution containing 154 mEq. of sodium and 154 mEq. of chloride per liter. It is administered intravenously to replace water and electrolytes that have been depleted in isotonic, or equivalent, proportions. The infusion is continued until signs of dehydration are corrected. It is also given during and after surgery to patients with normal renal function to maintain stable circulation and to reduce the need for blood transfusions by helping to maintain adequate circulating fluid volume.

If the patient can take fluids orally, he may be given a solution to drink containing 3 to 4 Gm. of sodium chloride and 1.5 to 3 Gm. of sodium bicarbonate per liter.

Simple dehydration involving water loss without electrolyte loss, such as that caused by insufficient water intake, can be remedied by giving water by mouth or by giving a 2.5% to 5% dextrose solution intravenously.

Dextrose 5% in water, U.S.P., B.P.

Dextrose solution is almost isotonic with blood and provides about 170 calories per liter. In the body the dextrose is also oxidized to yield water. If the patient has normal renal function, he may receive from 2 to 3 liters of fluid per day. This will provide a liberal fluid intake. Exceeding 3 liters per day is not recommended and therefore rarely ordered because of the danger of circulatory overload.

Dextrose 5% or sodium chloride 0.11% to 0.45% ($^1/_2$ normal saline) with dextrose 5% in water is the preferred solution when there has been a loss of water in excess of sodium.

Subcutaneous administration of dextrose solutions is not recommended since they are irritating and may cause fluid and electrolytes to be drawn into interstitial areas causing edema and possibly necrosis.

Balanced electrolyte injection

After dehydration has been corrected and the serum sodium level is normal, the extracellular fluid is further increased by the injection of a balanced electrolyte solution which approaches that of normal blood plasma. This solution contains 140 mEq. of sodium, 5 mEq. of potassium, 3 mEq. of magnesium, 98 mEq. of chloride, 27 mEq. of acetate, and 23 mEq. of gluconate.

OVERHYDRATION

Overhydration results in increased volume of body fluid and decreased concentration, or dilution, of plasma electrolytes and protein. This condition, also known as water intoxication, produces symptoms of headache, nausea, vomiting, muscular pains, abdominal cramps, weakness, stupor, coma, and convulsions.

Water excess may also result from administering excessive amounts of fluids parenterally, impaired renal and cardiac function, or administration or excessive secretion of antidiuretic hormone. It is also seen in complex endocrine disturbances.

Basic treatment is water restriction. However, if there is also a deficit of sodium, saline solutions are usually given to promote movement of intracellular fluid into the extracellular space.

The most common form of water excess occurs after extensive losses of water and electrolytes by sweating, followed by drinking large amounts of plain water. Its prevention and treatment involve normalizing the tonicity of body water by increasing the intake of salt, often in the form of salt tablets, to balance the amount of water ingested.

HYPERNATREMIA

Increased concentration of extracellular sodium may be caused by water loss without equivalent sodium loss (simple dehydration), excessive sodium administration or intake without adequate water intake, or retention of sodium because of heart failure, cirrhosis of the liver, or nephrosis.

Treatment must be based on serum sodium levels. If hypernatremia is the result of water deficit, treatment consists of replenishing body water either orally or by giving dextrose and water intravenously. Administration of drugs containing sodium may also be withheld and the patient may be placed on a sodium-restricted diet. The natriuretic diuretics may be administered to increase sodium excretion.

HYPONATREMIA

Decreased concentration of sodium may result from loss of sodium, which can occur with vigorous diuretic therapy, prolonged or excessive sweating, renal insufficiency, Addison's disease, and loss of gastrointestinal fluid. This type of hyponatremia may be treated with 0.9% sodium chloride solution or Ringer's solution with or without lactate. If the sodium deficit is severe, a 3% or 5% sodium chloride solution may be administered.

Sodium chloride in 3% or 5% solution

These solutions are recommended for treatment of severe sodium deficits. The 3% solution contains 513 mEq. of sodium per liter; the 5% solution contains 855 mEq. of sodium per liter. These solutions must be used with caution because of the danger of increased venous pressure, which may lead to pulmonary edema. Extreme caution is required if administered to patients with cardiovascular or renal disease. These solutions should be administered slowly and in small volumes (200 to 400 ml.). The patient's central venous pressure should be monitored.

INTRAVENOUS FLUID THERAPY

Intravenous solutions are used to supply electrolytes, nutrients, and water. Electrolytes contained in intravenous solutions include sodium, potassium, calcium, ammonium chloride, bicarbonate, and phosphate. These solutions can be grouped into single salt and multiple salt solutions. Intravenous fluid therapy has become routine therapy before, during, and after surgery. Fluid loss during these times is estimated and replaced by the proper solution; the consequences of using the wrong solution can be disastrous.

SINGLE SALT SOLUTIONS

The following single salt solutions are used for replacement therapy. Sodium chloride solution has already been discussed.

Ammonium chloride injection, N.F.

Ammonium chloride injection is available as a 2% solution; 100 to 500 ml. is infused over a 3-hour period. It must be infused slowly to allow for metabolism of ammonium ions by the liver and to avoid ammonia toxicity. Its D.E.S.I. rating is *effective* for treatment of chloride loss caused by vomiting, fistula drainage, gastric suc-

tion, or excessive use of alkalinizing drugs or mercurial diuretics. When used to treat metabolic alkalosis it should be given with potassium chloride and sodium chloride to prevent potassium and sodium depletion.

Calcium gluconate, U.S.P., B.P.

Calcium gluconate solution is available for intravenous injection as a 10% solution in 10-ml. vials for rapid replacement of calcium ions. It is the drug of choice for severe hypocalcemic tetany. It must be administered slowly and care should be taken to prevent infiltration into surrounding tissues and tissue necrosis.

Potassium chloride injection, U.S.P.

Potassium chloride is available for intravenous injection in 10 to 40 mEq. solutions. It should not be administered undiluted but administered at a moderate rate in solutions containing not more than 40 to 60 mEq. per liter. Rapid administration may cause pain or burning at the infusion site or cardiac arrhythmias. Infusions should be regulated by EKG monitoring and repeated serum potassium determinations. D.E.S.I. rating is *effective* for treatment of potassium deficiency when oral therapy is not feasible.

Sodium bicarbonate injection, U.S.P.

Sodium bicarbonate injection is the drug of choice in the treatment of metabolic acidosis. It is available as a 7.5% solution in a 50-ml. ampule to be added to 1 liter of solution. It is also available as an isotonic solution (1.5%), a hypertonic solution (2 to 5%), and in a 0.15 to 0.3% solution in combination with sodium chloride (0.3 to 4%). This drug is used to restore the bicarbonate ion and elevate the pH of the blood. Giving excessive amounts of sodium bicarbonate may cause metabolic alkalosis. This drug must be used very cautiously in patients with cardiac or renal disease since large amounts of sodium can intensify the disorder.

Sodium lactate injection, U.S.P.

This drug is available in 50 ml. as a 7.5% solution to be added to 1 liter of solution and premixed as 1 liter of one-sixth molar solution,

Table 18-1 Multiple salt solutions for intravenous administration

Generic name	Trade name or common name	Cations mEq./L.					Anions mEq./L.		
		Na^+	K^+	Ca^{++}	Mg^{++}	NH_4^+	Cl^-	$HCO_3^=$	$PO_4^=$
High electrolyte content									
Ringer's solution		147	4	4			155		
Lactated Ringer's solution	Hartmann's solution	130	4	3			109	28	
Lactated potassic saline	Darrow's solution	121	35				103	53	
Sodium, potassium chloride, and sodium lactate	Duodenal solution	138	12				103	50	
	Ionosol D-CM	138	12	5	3		103	50	
	Normosol-R	140	5		3		98	50	
	Plasma-Lyte	140	10	5	3		103	55	
	Polysal	140	10	5	3		103	55	
Medium electrolyte content									
Sodium, potassium-ammonium chloride	Gastric solution	63	17			70	150		
	Ionosol B	57	25		5		49	25	13
	Normosol-M	40	13		3		40	16	
	Electrolyte-2	56	25		6		50	25	12
	Polysal-M	40	16	5	3		40	24	
Low electrolyte content									
	Ionosol MB	25	20		3		22	23	3
	Electrolyte 48	25	20		3		22	23	3
	Isolyte P	25	20		3		22	23	3

which is to be given at a rate not exceeding 300 ml. per hour. It is used in the treatment of metabolic acidosis when there is no evidence of an elevated lactic acid level. Since sodium lactate must be metabolized to sodium bicarbonate the patient with lactic acidosis should be given sodium bicarbonate solution.

MULTIPLE SALT SOLUTIONS

Ringer's lactate solution was the first multiple salt solution introduced for replacement therapy. At the present time there are fifteen additional multiple salt solutions on the market. These solutions contain two or more cations. Multiple salt solutions can be classified as high, medium, or low electrolyte content solutions based primarily on their sodium content.

Multiple salt solutions are used to replace lost salt and to help correct electrolyte balance in patients unable to ingest food and water. The composition of electrolytes in various solutions is summarized in Table 18-1.

PARENTERAL HYPERALIMENTATION

Parenteral hyperalimentation is the intravenous feeding of protein hydrolysate (Amigen), amino acid solution (FreAmine), or high calorie solutions. It is used in the treatment of patients unable to eat, digest, or absorb nutrients for prolonged periods of time (6 days or more) or to supplement oral protein intake in malnourished and burned patients. For these patients parenteral feeding provides nutritional support to help sustain life. It is recommended by the A.M.A. that patients unable to eat and drink for 1 to 3 days be provided with 100 to 150 Gm. of carbohydrate intravenously each day to minimize protein breakdown (catabolism) and possible ketosis. Patients receiving protein or amino acid solutions should receive at the same time large amounts of carbohydrate, vitamins, and minerals to prevent negative nitrogen balance and to reduce weight loss. It is claimed that it takes 100 to 150 carbohydrate calories per gram of nitrogen for the patient to effectively use amino acids administered intravenously.

Hyperalimentation fluids are unstable and good culture media. Kits are available for the preparation of these fluids. Once prepared, these solutions should be administered as soon as possible because of their instability and potential for bacterial contamination. Commercially prepared solutions must be used as soon as the seal on the container is broken. For safety, medications should not be added to these solutions. Strict aseptic technique should be used. These solutions must be administered slowly, over 8 to 24 hours, via a large vein, such as the subclavian, which permits more rapid dilution than can occur in a superficial vein.

Intravenous lipid (fat) solutions are under clinical investigation for their high caloric value. At present these preparations are not commercially available in the United States.

High caloric solutions for injection (Isolyte H 900 cal.; Normosol-M 900 cal., Polyonic M-900)

These solutions contain dextrose 20% or mixtures of carbohydrates in a multiple electrolyte solution. Two liters per day provide from 1350 to 2100 calories. Rate of utilization of dextrose varies from patient to patient. Glycosuria and diuresis occur if the patient's capacity to utilize dextrose is exceeded. High caloric solutions frequently cause thrombosis and phlebitis.

Protein hydrolysate injection, U.S.P. (Amigen, Aminosol, C.P.H., Hyprotigen); amino acid solution (FreAmine)

Protein hydrolysates may be prepared from pure proteins such as casein or lactalbumin or other sources of protein such as blood, liver, or yeast with the aid of acids, alkalis, or enzymes. Determinations are made of the amino acid con-

tent and pure amino acids are added or excesses removed so that only those amino acids considered essential to human nutrition are contained in the solution. These solutions also contain varying amounts of electrolytes. About 60% of the amino acids are free, the rest are peptides which are excreted unchanged. See Table 18-1 for electrolyte content of the various preparations available.

Amino acid solution contains synthetic amino acids but no peptides. Patients unable to tolerate protein hydrolysate may be able to tolerate amino acid solution.

Dextrose is usually administered with these solutions because of the protein-sparing action of carbohydrates. If the protein is administered without adequate calories in the form of carbohydrate, the protein will be used for the body's caloric need rather than for repair and regeneration of tissue.

Adverse effects. Protein hydrolysates may cause nausea and vomiting, headache, flushing, hypotension, abdominal pain, convulsions, thrombosis, phlebitis, and edema at the site of injection. Hyperpyrexia (fever) may occur after the solutions have been administered for a few days. These solutions must be used with caution in patients with liver or renal impairment. Solutions that are cloudy or contain a sediment should not be used. If administration of the solution is interrupted, discard the remaining solution.

THE NURSE AND INTRAVENOUS THERAPY

Intravenous therapy is such a common, everyday phenomenon in hospitalized patients that nurses are often less attentive to the problems and complications of intravenous therapy than is desirable if the therapy is to be effective and safe. Many of the complications of intravenous therapy can be avoided if the nurse is a keen observer, knowledgeable, and skillful.

Complications. Complications of intravenous therapy include the following.

Infiltration. This occurs when the needle is dislodged from the vein permitting the solution to enter the surrounding tissues causing pain and edema of the area. Patients or relatives should be informed to notify the nurse if pain or swelling occurs at the infusion site. In addition, nurses should frequently check the infusion site for signs of infiltration. The infusion should be stopped if infiltration occurs. Restarting the intravenous therapy usually requires a new infusion site.

Extravasation. This occurs when fluids in the vein escape through the vascular wall into the tissues surrounding the vein. This may occur because of (1) changes in osmotic pressures, (2) the type of fluid being infused, (3) overdistention of the vein caused by too rapid a flow rate, or (4) stretching of the venipuncture site permitting fluids to escape. In the latter case there is no longer a closed system, and microorganisms may invade the venous system. Sterile aseptic technique should be followed and the infusion restarted at a different site.

Thrombosis. An intravascular blood clot occurs when platelets agglutinate and fibrin strands and red and white blood cells adhere to the platelet mass. A thrombus may form any time a blood vessel is injured, including injury by venipuncture. A thrombus may form around the needle or catheter plugging the lumen; if this occurs the infusion stops. The infusion should be restarted at a new site with a new needle or catheter. Attempts to unplug the needle by forcing a bolus of solution through the needle into the vein is not a wise or safe practice. The thrombus may become an embolus and lodge in a vital organ causing more serious complications such as pulmonary embolus.

Thrombophlebitis. Blood clot formation and inflammation of the vein may result from a number of factors: prolonged duration of infusion, use of contaminated equipment or contaminated solutions, irritation from drugs in the infusion, toxicity and pH of the solution, site of administration, and infection. Thrombophlebitis is manifested by pain, heat, swelling, redness, and loss of motion of the affected part. When this occurs the infusion should be stopped, the needle withdrawn, and the condition reported and recorded immediately. Treatment usually consists of the application of moist heat to the affected area; anticoagulant therapy may also be ordered. Nurses should take the necessary precautions to prevent occurrence of thrombophlebitis by (1) using sterile aseptic technique with proper cleansing of skin before insertion of needle; (2) being certain equipment is not contaminated; (3) checking solutions for precipitation, debris or sediment, or change in color prior to and during intravenous therapy; (4) ascertaining that no intravenous bottle is left in place for more than 24 hours,* since some organisms proliferate at room temperature in intravenous fluids (for open intravenous therapy, 250 ml. bottles should be used); (5) changing the administration set every 24 hours to reduce the possibility of sepsis; and (6) administering irritating drugs slowly.

Pain at administration site. Pain occurs when the needle touches the venous wall, when there is too much tension on the needle or tubing, and when irritating drugs are administered too rapidly. Adjusting the needle, relieving the tension by readjusting the needle support or relaxing the pull on the tubing, and administering irritating drugs at a slow rate may alleviate the pain and discomfort.

Necrosis. Death and sloughing of tissue can occur when irritating drugs or solutions, such as levarterenol, infiltrate into the tissues. The infusion should be stopped *immediately*. If the infiltration contains levarterenol, the antidote Regitine should be injected subcutaneously in minute amounts at many sites in the edematous area immediately upon discovery.

Pulmonary edema. This occurs when the circulatory system is overloaded with fluids. Central venous pressure monitoring (particularly in cardiac patients) can help to prevent this hazardous complication.

Pyrogenic reactions. This occurs when pyrogens are introduced into the circulatory system. This condition is characterized by fever and chills, malaise, headache, nausea, and vomiting. The infusion should be stopped *at once*. The intravenous solution may contain the pyrogens. The solution should not be discarded but sent to the pharmacist. The stock number should be noted, since an entire batch of solutions may be contaminated. Pyrogenic reactions must be reported and recorded.

---

*The Communicable Disease Center recommends a 24-hour rule-of-thumb for bottle and administration set changes.

Electrolytes

POTASSIUM

Potassium is the major positively charged ion in the intracellular fluid. The amount of potassium in the intracellular fluid is 150 mEq. per liter; the amount in the plasma is 3.5 to 5 mEq. Even though this latter amount appears to be quite low, it is of great importance since serum potassium must be maintained between 3.5 and 5 mEq. per liter for survival. The diet of most individuals contains from 35 to 100 mEq. of potassium daily. Normally, any excess potassium is excreted by the kidney in the urine. Potassium plays an important part in: (1) muscle contraction, (2) conduction of nerve impulses, (3) enzyme action, and (4) cell membrane function. High and low concentrations of potassium affect these physiologic functions.

HYPOKALEMIA

Potassium deficit, or hypokalemia, can be caused by the following:

1 Reduced dietary intake (rare)
2 Poor absorption because of steatorrhea, regional enteritis, or short bowel syndrome
3 Loss of gastrointestinal secretions (which are rich in this ion) as a result of vomiting, diarrhea, gastrointestinal suction, or fistula drainage
4 Kidney disease
5 Diuretic therapy
6 Infusions of solutions containing little or no K^+
7 Extensive burns
8 Excessive amounts of adrenocortical hormone

Unlike sodium, which is reabsorbed when serum sodium level is low, potassium ions continue to be excreted in the urine when the serum potassium level is low. As potassium loss continues the patient's condition deteriorates until potassium intake is increased and normal levels are reestablished.

With hypokalemia there is impaired muscle function. Impairment of skeletal muscle function may cause profound weakness or paralysis, including paralysis of the respiratory muscles. Impaired smooth muscle function may result in ileus.

Cardiac effects of hypokalemia include increased sensitivity to digitalis and EKG changes such as S-T segment depression, U waves, and T wave flattening, depression, or inversion. Atrioventricular block and cardiac arrest may occur.

Hypokalemia also causes movement of Na^+ and H^+ from extracellular fluid, the excretion of H^+, and reabsorption of HCO_3^-. This elevates the plasma pH, which results in *metabolic alkalosis*. Other effects are decreased water reabsorption in the renal tubule resulting in polyuria, and hypochloremia.

Treatment. Hypokalemia is treated by replacing potassium orally or parenterally. A hazard of parenteral correction of potassium deficit is the production of potassium poisoning, or hyperkalemia. Administration of potassium salts intravenously must be performed cautiously to avoid reaching a concentration that can cause *asystole* or cardiac arrest. The patient should be monitored since the EKG will show changes more rapidly than will serum potassium levels. Urinary output and urinary loss of potassium should also be measured. Potassium should not be given in the immediate postoperative period until urine flow is established.

Potassium salts are contraindicated in severe renal impairment, untreated Addison's disease, acute dehydration, and hyperkalemia from any cause. They must be used with caution in cardiac patients.

Potassium acetate, potassium bicarbonate, potassium chloride, potassium citrate, and potassium gluconate are available alone or in combinations for oral administration. Potassium acetate, potassium chloride, and potassium phosphate are available as parenteral solutions. In addition, potassium chloride is a component in a number of multiple electrolyte intravenous fluids (e.g., Ringer's solution).

Liquid preparations are preferred for oral therapy and most contain 10, 20, or 40 mEq. of K^+ per 15 ml. These preparations must be diluted with fruit juice or water before ingestion and taken after meals with a full glass of water to minimize gastric irritation. Powdered preparations should be dissolved according to the manufacturer's instructions. Ingestion of potassium-rich foods may also be helpful. Uncoated tablets are not recommended by the A.M.A. because they cause gastric irritation; enteric-coated tablets are not recommended because their rate of absorption is undependable and they cause small bowel ulcerations. Potassium chloride tablets are no longer official or generally available.

Dosage of potassium supplements depends upon individual requirements. Approximate minimum daily requirement for adults is 40 to 50 mEq.; for infants it is about 2 to 3 mEq. per kilogram of body weight daily. Oral dosage is usually gradually increased over a 3- to 7-day period to avoid producing hyperkalemia.

Intravenous administration of potassium should not exceed 3 mEq. per kilogram of body weight per day; intravenous fluids should not contain more than 40 mEq. of potassium, and rate of administration should not exceed 20 mEq. of potassium per hour. The nurse should know how fast the solution is to run; rapid infusion causes pain or burning at the infusion site and may cause cardiac arrhythmias.

Preparation, dosage, and administration

Potassium chloride injection, U.S.P., B.P. Potassium chloride injection is available in sterile solutions containing 10, 20, 30, 40, 60, and 100 mEq. of K^+ and Cl^- for injection.

Potassium chloride oral solution, U.S.P. This solution contains 20 mEq. of potassium per 15 ml.

Potassium acetate. This preparation is available in 30-ml. vials containing 3 and 4 mEq. of K^+, and as a powder.

Potassium bicarbonate (K-Lyte). Potassium bicarbonate is available as effervescent tablets which, when dissolved in 3 to 4 ounces of water, produce a liquid containing 25 mEq. of K^+. It has also been used as a gastric antacid and to alkalinize the urine.

Potassium citrate, N.F., B.P. Potassium citrate is available in powder and tablet form containing varying amounts of potassium.

Potassium triplex. This is a nonofficial preparation of potassium acetate, potassium bicarbonate, and potassium citrate in an aqueous solution. There are 500 mg. of each potassium salt in 5 ml., which yields 15 mEq. of potassium.

Other trade names of this preparation are Tri-Pli, Randall's solution, and Triple Potassium.

Potassium gluconate, N.F. (KaON). This preparation is available as a powder, an elixir containing 6.7 mEq. of K^+ per 5 ml., as chewable tablets containing 1.1 mEq. of K^+, and as tablets containing 2.1 or 5 mEq. of K^+. This drug may be used for patients who cannot tolerate potassium chloride.

Potassium phosphate, dibasic. This is available as a powder and as an injection containing 2 mEq. of K^+ and 1 mEq. of HPO_4^- per milliliter in 30-ml. vials.

HYPERKALEMIA

Potassium excess, or hyperkalemia, can be caused by the following:

1 Acute or chronic renal failure; severe oliguria due to trauma whereby the kidney fails to excrete K^+
2 Release of large amounts of intracellular K^+ such as occurs in burns, crush injuries, or severe infections
3 Overtreatment with potassium salts
4 Metabolic acidosis, causing a shift of potassium from the cells into the extracellular fluid

Hyperkalemia causes interference with neuromuscular function, which can produce weakness and paralysis. Abdominal distention and diarrhea also occur. Cardiac effects caused by hyperkalemia result from impaired conduction. The EKG shows widening and slurring of the QRS complexes, peaked T waves, depressed S-T segments, and there may be a disappearance of P waves. Ventricular fibrillation and cardiac arrest may occur.

Treatment. Hyperkalemia is treated by withholding potassium and administering sodium polystyrene sulfonate, U.S.P. (Kayexalate), a cation exchange resin. The drug is usually given orally or by stomach tube. It may also be given by high retention enema, although this is not a reliable method of administration.

In the intestines, particularly the colon, the sodium of the resin is in part replaced by potassium, approximately 3.1 mEq. of potassium per gram of resin. The potassium is eliminated from the body when the resin is eliminated with the feces or enema. Laxatives must be used when the drug is given orally. Since its action is slow, up to 24 hours, other treatment is indicated if EKG changes indicate advanced potassium intoxication. Administration should be discontinued when the serum potassium level falls to 4 or 5 mEq. per liter.

Side effects of sodium polystyrene sulfonate treatment include anorexia, nausea, vomiting, hypokalemia, hypocalcemia, constipation, and fecal impaction. The latter can be prevented by the use of laxatives.

Oral dose for adults is 15 Gm. up to four times daily by mouth in 150 to 200 ml. of water. Rectal dose for adults is 30 to 80 Gm. suspended in 150 to 200 ml. of 1% methylcellulose solution, 10% dextrose solution, or water. This dose may be given one to three times daily. The solution should be retained for 4 to 10 hours if possible, followed by a cleansing enema.

CALCIUM

Calcium, a positively charged ion (Ca^{++}), is essential for:

1 Growth and ossification of bone
2 Neuromuscular transmission
3 Cell membrane permeability
4 Maintaining excitability of nerve fibers
5 Hormone secretion and action
6 Muscle contraction
7 Maintenance of cardiac and vascular tone
8 Many enzyme activities
9 Normal coagulation of blood

Almost all of the 1000 to 1200 Gm. of calcium present in the normal adult is in the skeletal tissue, and only about 1% of the total body calcium is in solution in body fluids. About half of the calcium in plasma is bound to serum proteins; a small portion is bound to complex organic anions (e.g., bicarbonate and phosphate). Almost all unbound serum calcium is ionized. Normal serum calcium concentration is 4.5 to 5.5 mEq. per liter, or 9 to 11 mg. per 100 ml.

The recommended dietary allowance of calcium for adults is 800 mg. daily. Pregnant or lactating women need 1.2 to 1.3 Gm.; children age 6 to 18 years need 0.9 to 1.4 Gm. The intake of calcium in a balanced diet is sufficient for nor-

mal body needs. Absorption of calcium depends upon how well it is kept in solution in the digestive tract. An acid medium favors calcium solubility; thus calcium is absorbed mainly in the upper intestinal tract. Absorption is decreased by the presence of alkalies and large amounts of fatty acids with which the calcium forms insoluble soaps. Adequate intake of vitamin D appears to promote calcium absorption. Calcium is excreted in the urine and feces; it is also excreted in perspiration.

Maintenance of normal concentration of serum calcium depends upon the interactions of three agents: parathyroid hormone, vitamin D, and calcitonin. Parathyroid hormone and vitamin D mobilize the removal of calcium from bone, the principal source of calcium for extracellular fluids. Parathyroid hormone also promotes renal tubular reabsorption of calcium and a slight increase in intestinal absorption of calcium. Calcitonin is synthesized in the thyroid gland; it moderates or decreases the rate of removal of calcium from the bone.

HYPOCALCEMIA

A decrease in serum calcium results from: (1) hypoparathyroidism; (2) chronic renal insufficiency; (3) rickets and osteomalacia; (4) malabsorption syndrome; and (5) deficiency of vitamin D. Hypoparathyroidism may follow thyroidectomy, since several of the parathyroid glands are frequently removed by this operation. If the function of the remaining gland(s) is impaired the result is depressed parathyroid activity.

Patients who are bedridden tend to develop a negative calcium balance because the ion is lost from bones and is excreted. This effect is likely to be serious only when long immobilization of the patient is necessary.

Hypocalcemia causes increased excitability of the nerves and neuromuscular junction, which leads to muscle cramps, muscle twitching, and tetany. Numbness and tingling of the fingers, toes, and lips occur. The hypertonicity of muscle may cause tonic contractions of the hands and feet (carpopedal spasm). The increased neural excitability may cause convulsions, abnormal behavior, and personality changes. In children, prolonged hypocalcemia has resulted in mental retardation. Other effects of hypocalcemia include dyspnea, laryngeal spasm, diplopia, abdominal cramps, and urinary frequency. Diminished cardiac contractility may occur. The EKG shows a prolonged Q-T interval and an inverted T wave. In prolonged hypocalcemia defects can occur in the nails, skin, and teeth; cataracts may appear, and calcification of the basal ganglia may occur.

Treatment. Regardless of the underlying cause, severe hypocalcemia is treated initially with the intravenous administration of rapidly available calcium ions. For latent tetany, mild symptoms of hypocalcemia, and maintenance therapy, a calcium salt is given orally. Vitamin D may be given. Parathyroid injection is now considered obsolete and is not used for therapy; its biologic activity is uncertain. Overdosage of calcium may cause hypercalcemia, which results in anorexia, nausea, vomiting, weakness, depression, polyuria, and polydipsia. Calcium must be administered cautiously to patients on digitalis therapy, since calcium potentiates the effect of digitalis and may precipitate arrhythmias. EKG monitoring of the patient is recommended.

Preparation, dosage, and administration. Calcium salts are used as a nutritional supplement, particularly during pregnancy and lactation. They are specific in the treatment of hypocalcemic tetany. They have also been used for their antispasmodic effects in cases of abdominal pain, tenesmus, and colic resulting from disease of the gallbladder or painful contractions of the ureters. The basic salts of calcium are used as antacids.

Calcium chloride, U.S.P., B.P. This is a salt of calcium irritating to tissues when given parenterally other than by intravenous injection. It is available as a 10% solution. Care must be taken that the needle does not slip out of the vein and cause serious tissue irritation. Calcium chloride may be given orally but tends to cause gastric disturbance. When administered orally, it is best given in capsules. It is an acidifying salt and for that reason promotes the absorption of calcium. It may evoke acidosis. The average adult dose for oral administration is 1 Gm. (gr. 15) four times a day.

Calcium gluconate, U.S.P., B.P. This preparation is a white, crystalline or granular powder, which is odorless and tasteless. It has an advantage over calcium chloride since it is more palatable for oral administration and can be given parenterally. It should not be administered intramuscularly, since there is danger of abscess formation and tissue slough. For severe hypocalcemic tetany, calcium gluconate injection, U.S.P., B.P., is administered slowly in a 10% solution, intravenously (5 to 30 ml.). A 0.3% solution (30 ml. of a 10% solution in 1 liter of sodium chloride injection) may be given by slow drip infusion throughout the day. For mild hypocalcemic tetany, calcium gluconate may be given orally, 5 Gm. three times a day 1 to 1½ hours after meals. Dosage for children is 500 mg. per kilogram of body weight in divided doses. It is available in tablet form for oral administration.

Calcium lactate, U.S.P., B.P. This compound is given orally. Its physical properties are similar to those of calcium gluconate. The usual adult dose is 5 Gm., which may be repeated three or four times a day. For children, dosage is 500 mg. per kilogram of body weight in divided doses. It is marketed in 300- and 600-mg. tablets. Calcium lactate is more soluble in hot water than in cold and should be dissolved in hot water before it is given to the patient. Calcium lactate is not given parenterally. Some hospital pharmacies prepare a solution of calcium lactate for oral administration (1-liter bottles containing 2 Gm. in 40 ml. of water).

Calcium gluceptate. This drug is available in a 1.8% solution (18 mg. per milliliter) in 5-ml. ampules. It is used in the treatment of severe hypocalcemia. Intravenous dosage for adults and children is 90 to 360 mg. It may also be given intramuscularly; dosage for adults and children is 36 to 90 mg. in the gluteal region or lateral aspect of the thigh; for infants, dose is 36 to 90 mg. in the lateral thigh. Mild local irritation may occur.

Calcium phosphate, dibasic, N.F.; *calcium phosphate, tribasic,* N.F. These salts are administered orally for treatment of mild and latent hypocalcemic tetany and for maintenance therapy. They are not used if the patient has renal insufficiency accompanied by hyperphosphatemia. These drugs are particularly useful for supplying calcium and phosphorus to pregnant and lactating women and to children. Oral dose is 1 to 2 Gm. three times daily with meals.

Dihydrotachysterol, U.S.P., B.P. (Hytakerol). Dihydrotachysterol is an irradiated form of vitamin D used to treat hypocalcemia. When compared to ergocalciferol, dihydrotachysterol produces almost as great phosphate excretion, less absorption of calcium from the intestine, and more rapid rise in serum calcium levels. Dihydrotachysterol has a shorter duration of action and less potential for accumulation and hypercalcemia than ergocalciferol. It may act more rapidly than vitamin D_2 or D_3. Tolerance or refractoriness does not seem to occur.

Dihydrotachysterol is effective when taken orally. Overdosage produces hypercalcemia, anorexia, nausea, vomiting, headache, renal calculi, and stupor. These symptoms disappear with withdrawal of the drug.

Dosage should be determined by frequent determinations of serum calcium levels. Initially, dosage is 0.75 to 2.5 mg. daily; maintenance dose is 0.25 to 1.75 mg. once or twice weekly.

HYPERCALCEMIA

Hypercalcemia may be caused by neoplasms with or without bone metastases. Carcinoma of the ovary, kidney, or lung can synthesize and secrete a parathyroid-like hormone causing hypercalcemia. Other common causes are hyperparathyroidism, thiazide or diuretic therapy, multiple myeloma, sarcoidosis, and vitamin D intoxication.

Clinical manifestations. Clinical manifestations of hypercalcemia are highly variable and involve many organ systems. Calcium may be deposited in various body tissues.

Gastrointestinal system. Symptoms are anorexia, nausea and vomiting, constipation, and abdominal pain. Hyperchlorhydria may occur, and 15% to 25% of the patients develop peptic ulcer. Antacids containing calcium should not be used.

Central nervous system. Symptoms include apathy, depression, amnesia, headaches, and drowsiness. In severe cases disorientation, syncope, hallucinations, and coma may occur.

Renal system. Polyuria and polydipsia occur from loss of renal concentrating ability. Kidney stones may be formed. Nephrocalcinosis may occur, seriously impairing renal function. This may lead to edema, uremia, and hypertension, which may be irreversible.

Neuromuscular system. Neural excitability is diminished causing weakness and muscle flaccidity.

Cardiovascular system. Elevated serum calcium causes increased cardiac contractility, ventricular extrasystoles, and heart block. EKG changes include a short Q-T interval and characteristic signs of heart block. In severe calcium toxicity, cardiac arrest in systole may occur.

Treatment. Treatment is variable and aimed at controlling the underlying disease. If hypercalcemia is due to thiazide diuretic therapy, the diuretic is discontinued; the serum calcium returns to normal levels in about 1 month.

Renal excretion of calcium can be promoted with a number of drugs. Infusions of sodium chloride may be given to increase sodium excretion, which in turn increases calcium excretion. Natriuretic drugs, such as furosemide (Lasix) or ethacrynic acid (Edecrin) may be used. Chelating, or binding, agents, such as disodium edetate, increase renal excretion of calcium by forming soluble complexes with the calcium that are not reabsorbed by the renal tubules. Inorganic phosphates may be given orally or intravenously to foster deposition of calcium in bone, thereby decreasing serum levels. An antineoplastic drug, mithramycin, also reduces serum calcium levels.

Phosphate salts. Monobasic or dibasic sodium or potassium phosphate may be used to treat mild to moderate hypercalcemia when other forms of therapy are ineffective. Mechanism of action of phosphate salts is not known. However, they decrease serum levels of calcium probably by depositing calcium phosphate in the tissues; if there are bone lesions these show improvement.

Oral administration for adults consists of 24 ml. of 1 molar dibasic sodium phosphate or a mixed salt solution four times daily to supply 3 Gm. of phosphorus. Oral doses may cause nausea and vomiting.

Intravenous dose is 1 liter of a 0.1 molar solution of phosphate salts (0.081 mole of dibasic sodium phosphate and 0.019 mole of monobasic potassium phosphate). This dose is administered over a period of 6 to 12 hours. Intravenous doses may cause hypotension, acute renal failure, and even myocardial infarction. Deaths have been reported. Overdosage will cause tetany.

The use of phosphate is hazardous, and patients should be carefully observed and monitored if possible.

MAGNESIUM

Magnesium (Mg^{++}) is an important activator ion for the function of many enzymes. Normal serum concentration is 1.5 to 2.5 mEq. per liter with one third bound to protein and two thirds as free cation. About 50% of the total body magnesium exists in an insoluble state in bone, 45% is intracellular cation, and 5% extracellular cation. Magnesium is excreted via the kidney. Magnesium has physiologic effects on the nervous system similar to those of calcium.

HYPOMAGNESEMIA

A deficit of magnesium may be encountered in chronic alcoholism, malabsorption, starvation, diarrhea, prolonged gastrointestinal suction, vigorous diuresis, and diseases causing hypocalcemia and hypokalemia.

Table 18-2 Minerals and human nutrition

Mineral	Source	Daily requirements in adult male	Specific functions	Deficiency clinical state
Sodium	Common salt Citrate and tartrate in fruits	0.5 to 1.0 Gm.	Control of body water Electrophysiology of nerve, muscle, gland cells Regulation of pH, isotonicity	*Hyponatremia* Lassitude, hypotension, vomiting, cramps, hemoconcentration
Potassium	Present in all plant and animal food	2.0 Gm.	Necessary for electrophysiology of cell membranes Regulation of pH, isotonicity	*Hypokalemia* Mental changes, loquacity, hallucinations Limp, soft, weak muscles EKG: prolonged QT, depressed ST, inverted T
Calcium	Milk, cheese, sardines, salmon	800 mg.	Calcification of bones and teeth, blood clotting, excitation-coupling mechanisms, cofactor in enzyme reactions	Hypocalcemia Tetany Osteomalacia
Magnesium	Fruit, peas, beans, nuts	350 mg.	Electrophysiology, enzyme reactions	Neuromuscular disorders
Iron	Meat, liver, kidney, fruits, vegetables, cereals	18 mg.	Hemoglobin	Iron-deficiency anemia
Copper	Liver, oysters, salmon, fruits	2 mg.	Hemoglobin synthesis	Anemia

Hypomagnesemia is characterized by increased irritability of the nervous system, which may lead to disorientation and convulsions. Increased neuromuscular irritability and contractility also occur. There may be jerking, coarse, and flapping tremor; athetoid movements; and nystagmus. Tetany may occur. Hypomagnesemia also causes tachycardia, hypertension, and vasomotor changes.

Treatment. Hypomagnesemia is treated with intravenous fluids containing magnesium, 10 to 40 mEq. per day for severe deficit followed by 10 mEq. per day for maintenance.

HYPERMAGNESEMIA

Hypermagnesemia occurs primarily in patients with chronic renal insufficiency. An excess of magnesium causes depression of the central nervous system, which leads to sedation and confusion. Blockade of the myoneural junction occurs by inhibiting acetylcholine (ACh) release and diminishing muscle cell excitability. This causes muscle weakness. Respiratory muscle paralysis may occur causing death. Hypermagnesemia also causes blockade of sympathetic ganglia and has a direct vasodilating effect that results in a decrease in blood pressure.

Treatment	Excess clinical state	Treatment
Ringer's solution Sodium chloride 0.9% solution	*Hypernatremia* Edema, hypertonicity	Dextrose and water intravenously
Potassium chloride oral solution or injection	*Hyperkalemia* Central nervous system stimulation and paralysis EKG: peaked T waves, prolonged QRS, PR interval Listlessness, weakness, numbness	Intravenous glucose and insulin Extracorporeal dialysis Calcium gluconate
Intravenous calcium chloride or calcium gluconate Oral calcium lactate or calcium gluconate	Hypercalcemia Renal calculi	EDTA
Magnesium ion replacement	Diminished excitability of muscle fibers Hypotension Respiratory paralysis	Intravenous injection of calcium salts Artificial respiration
Ferrous sulfate and gluconate	Hemosiderosis	Chelating agent
	—	—

Excess magnesium has a cardiac inhibitory effect. Conduction time is increased and the EKG will show lengthened P-R interval and prolonged QRS complex. If the Mg^{++} concentration continues to increase, cardiac arrest in diastole may occur. Third-degree atrioventricular block may also occur.

Treatment. An excess of Mg^{++} may require dialysis. Since calcium acts as an antagonist to Mg^{++}, calcium salts may be given parenterally.

Nutrients

Vitamins have great biochemical importance for they are essential for maintenance of normal metabolic function, growth, and health. The name *vitamin* means "vital for life." Originally the word was spelled with an "e" on the end (vitamine), since it was believed that these substances were amines; the "e" was dropped upon recognition that all vitamins were not amines.

Only a few vitamins are synthesized in the body; vitamin K is formed by bacteria in the gut and vitamin D is produced by exposure of the skin to sunlight. Thus most vitamins must be ingested in food or in their pure form as dietary supplements. Only small amounts of the vitamins are necessary for growth and health, and an adequate and varied diet will provide all the vitamins needed except during pregnancy and infancy. Restricted diets as a result of cultural or idiosyncratic beliefs, alcoholism, poverty, ignorance, or disorders of the gastrointestinal tract that interfere with absorption will lead to vitamin deficiency. In these cases, vitamin preparations are therapeutic. In the United States and Canada, mild forms of avitaminosis are more common than the pronounced deficiency states of beriberi, pellagra, rickets, or scurvy.

Vitamins are classified as being *fat soluble* or *water soluble*. Fat-soluble vitamins are A, D, E, and K. They are stored in the liver and fatty tissue in large amounts, and a deficiency in these vitamins occurs only after long deprivation from an adequate supply or disorders preventing their absorption. Water-soluble vitamins include the B group and C. These vitamins are not stored in the body in large amounts, and short periods of inadequate intake can lead to a deficiency. Vitamins are important components of enzyme systems that catalyze the reactions for protein, fat, and carbohydrate metabolism.

The sale of vitamins in the United States constitutes a multimillion-dollar business. They are widely used, and often unjustifiably, primarily because of successful advertising that vitamins will improve even normal health. The indiscriminate use of vitamins is not likely to decline in the near future.

The potency of vitamins A and D, when described on a label, must be in U.S.P. units, but the vitamin content of ascorbic acid, thiamine, riboflavin, nicotinic acid, nicotinamide, pyridoxine, and menadione and other vitamin K preparations, when expressed, must be in terms of milligrams.

Recently the F.D.A. proposed regulations dividing vitamin-mineral products into three categories:

1 *Supplement*—all ingredients are within established limits
2 *O-T-C/Proprietary*—the vitamin-mineral contents exceed the limits established for supplement use but not excessively
3 *Prescription status*—contents exceed the upper limit for O-T-C/proprietary products

Many multivitamin capsules and tablets vary in their contents. Some contain ingredients such as biotin and pantothenic acid for which evidence as to their essential role in human nutrition is inconclusive. However, the presence of such ingredients in these preparations is not contraindicated. In 1972 the F.D.A. published proposed regulations limiting the amounts of vitamins A and D in oral nonprescription vitamin preparations to not more than 10,000 I.U. of vitamin A and not more than 400 I.U. of vitamin D.

"Optional vitamins" (E, B_6, folic acid, pantothenic acid, and B_{12}) may or may not be included as ingredients in over-the-counter, multivitamin preparations. However, the most popular O-T-C multivitamin preparations are those that contain all vitamins needed by humans. Most O-T-C vitamin preparations are designed to fulfill daily body needs completely without regard for the amount of various vitamins contained in the daily diet.

Stability of vitamins is of great importance, since vitamin preparations may be on the pharmacy or grocery shelf for months before being purchased and used. Vitamins may lose as much as one third of their potency in 1 month, and 80% of their potency in 6 months. If the label is not dated concerning potency expiration, vitamins should preferably be purchased at stores with high sales volume. Patients should be instructed not to purchase a large amount of vitamin preparations at one time and to discard old vitamin preparations.

FAT-SOLUBLE VITAMINS
Vitamin A

Vitamin A, the fat-soluble, growth-promoting vitamin, is essential for growth in the young and for maintenance of health at all ages. The chemistry of this vitamin has been established and is related to the carotenoid pigments of plants, especially carotene. In fact, the term *vitamin A* may be applied to vitamin A, alpha-carotene, beta-carotene, gamma-carotene, and cryptoxanthin. The last four factors are formed in plants and are precursors of vitamin A in the body. Beta-carotene in the body is hydrolyzed to form two molecules of vitamin A.

Chemists have failed to discover vitamin A in any plant foodstuff. The carotene of plants, therefore, seems to supply the provitamin from which the body tissues prepare vitamin A. The amount of chlorophyll in the plant is a rough indication of the amount of carotene present. Animal fats, such as those found in butter, milk, eggs, and fish liver, are sources of the carotenoids; they were originally derived from plants and stored in animal tissue.

Vitamin A is essential in man to promote normal growth and development of bones and teeth and to maintain the health of epithelial tissues of the body. Its function in relation to normal vision and the prevention of night blindness has been carefully studied. Vitamin A actually makes up a portion of one of the major retinal pigments, rhodopsin, and is thus required for normal "rod vision" in the retina of man and many of the animals.

Vitamin A is also functional in conversion processes resulting in corticosterone and cholesterol.

Absorption, storage, and excretion. Vitamin A and carotene are readily absorbed from the normal gastrointestinal tract. Efficient absorption is dependent on fat absorption and, therefore, on the presence of adequate bile salts in the intestine. Certain conditions, such as obstructive jaundice, some infectious diseases, and the presence of mineral oil in the intestine, may result in vitamin A deficiency in spite of the fact that the amount ingested was normal.

Vitamin A is stored in the liver to a greater extent than elsewhere. The liver also functions in changing carotene to vitamin A; this function is inhibited in liver diseases and in diabetes. The amount of vitamin A stored depends upon the dietary intake. When intake is high or excessive, the stores formed in the liver may become sufficient to last a long time. Vitamin A is lost chiefly by destruction. Little is lost through the ordinary channels of excretion.

$(CH_3)_2$ —CH=CH—$\underset{\underset{CH_3}{|}}{C}$=CH—CH=CH—$\underset{\underset{CH_3}{|}}{C}$=CH—$CH_2OH$

Vitamin A

$(CH_3)_2$ —CH=CH—$\underset{\underset{CH_3}{|}}{C}$=CH—CH=CH—$\underset{\underset{CH_3}{|}}{C}$=CH—CH

$(CH_3)_2$ —CH=CH—$\underset{\underset{CH_3}{|}}{C}$=CH—CH=CH—$\underset{\underset{CH_3}{|}}{C}$=CH—CH

Beta-carotene (provitamin A)

Uses. Vitamin A is used to treat or relieve symptoms associated with a deficiency of vitamin A (avitaminosis), such as night blindness (nyctalopia), hyperkeratosis, retarded growth, xerophthalmia, keratomalacia, weakness, and increased susceptibility of mucous membranes to infection. It has a D.E.S.I. rating of *effective* for treating the first three conditions.

The diet low in vitamin A should be corrected with foods rather than with drugs. It appears that large doses of vitamin A may be given with no apparent harm to the adult, although excessive doses have been known to produce toxic effects in rats and in young children.

There are times when vitamin A concentrates have a legitimate use as supplements to the diet. Increased need occurs during pregnancy and lactation, in infancy, and in conditions characterized by lack of normal absorption and storage of vitamin A.

Daily requirement. It has been conclusively established that the vitamin A daily requirement is a rather large one, if optimum conditions of nutrition are to be maintained. The minimum daily requirements for vitamin A are 400 to 420 units for infants, 400 to 1000 units for children, and 800 to 1000 units for adults. During pregnancy and lactation, requirements equal 1000 to 1200 units, respectively. Therapeutic dosages may be three times these amounts. Although larger doses have been used in experimental studies, there is no evidence that justifies the use of more than 25,000 units per day. It has not been shown that excess dosage over and above the daily requirement is of value in the prevention of colds, influenza, and so on. Large dosages are injurious to infants. Symptoms of hypervitaminosis A include anorexia, altered liver function, brittle nails, cracked and bleeding lips, dry, itchy, and scaly skin, hyperirritability, and neurologic symptoms. Symptoms disappear after cessation of ingestion of the vitamin.

When the vitamin A requirement is met in the form of carotene or the provitamin A, twice as many units of the carotene are required to produce the same effect.

Preparation, dosage, and administration. The following are preparations of vitamin A and combinations of vitamins A and D.

Vitamin A, U.S.P. This is either fish liver oil, fish liver oil diluted with vegetable oil, or a solution of vitamin A concentrate in fish liver oil or vegetable oil. Vitamin A capsules are available, containing 1.5, 7.5, or 15 mg. of vitamin A (5000,

25,000, or 50,000 U.S.P. units). The usual therapeutic dose is 7.5 mg. (25,000 units) daily.

Water miscible vitamin A (Aquasol A). This is available in 25,000 and 50,000 unit capsules and in a parenteral form containing 50,000 units per milliliter. Absorption is greater for aqueous preparations. Intramuscular injections should be given deep and slow.

Oleovitamin A and D capsules, N.F. These contain 5000 units of vitamin A and 100 units of vitamin D.

Vitamin A ester concentrate, B.P. This contains not less than 485,000 units of vitamin A activity in each gram.

Cod liver oil, N.F., B.P. This is partially destearinated. The usual dosage is 4 ml. orally, which contains 3000 U.S.P. units of vitamin A and 300 U.S.P. units of vitamin D. This is one of the cheapest sources of vitamins A and D.

Halibut liver oil, B.P. Usual daily prophylactic dose for infants and adults is 0.1 ml. ($1\frac{1}{2}$ minim). Halibut liver oil contains in each gram not less than 30,000 units of vitamin A and between 2500 and 3500 units of vitamin D. In 0.1 ml. there are 5000 units of vitamin A.

Halibut-liver oil capsules, B.P. Each capsule contains 4500 units of vitamin A activity. The dose is one to three capsules daily.

A and D ointment. A and D ointment is a preparation containing both vitamins in a lanolin-petrolatum base. It is used in treatment of epithelial lesions, such as diaper rash, superficial burns, and excoriations.

Vitamin D

Vitamin D$_2$ (calciferol)

Vitamin D is a term applied to two or more substances that affect the proper utilization of calcium and phosphorus in the body. Two forms of naturally occurring vitamin D have been isolated. One of these forms is obtained as one of the products of irradiated ergosterol and is known as D_2 or calciferol. Ergosterol has therefore been shown to be a precursor of vitamin D. Further investigation has shown that there are a number of precursors that can be changed by irradiation into compounds that have vitamin D activity. Irradiation of 7-dehydrocholesterol results in the formation of vitamin D_3 (cholecalciferol) and is the form of vitamin found in irradiated milk and fish oils. It is formed also in skin exposed to sunlight. Irradiated ergosterol (calciferol) is the active constituent in various vitamin preparations such as viosterol and irradiated yeast.

Vitamin D_2 and vitamin D_3, as well as other products of irradiated ergosterol, are capable of antirachitic activity.

Although vitamin D is an essential vitamin, it is contained in only a few foods of the average American diet. Small amounts are present in herring, sardines, salmon, tuna fish, eggs, and butter. Vitamin D is found in high concentrations in a number of fish oils (cod, halibut).

At present, milk is the chief commercial food product enriched by the addition of vitamin D concentrate. By federal regulation, milk products are standardized at 400 International Units per quart, which represents a day's requirement of vitamin D.

Action and result. The exact mechanism by which vitamin D functions in the metabolism of calcium and phosphorus is not known. There is evidence that a complex relationship exists between vitamin D and parathyroid hormone, but this is not yet conclusive. The vitamin seems to be concerned directly with the absorption of calcium and phosphorus from the intestinal tract and their deposition in bone and teeth. In the absence of vitamin D the amount of these substances absorbed from the bowel is diminished to such an extent that even though the calcium and phosphate intake is adequate, rickets results in the child and osteomalacia in the adult.

An enzyme called alkaline phosphatase exists in the body and is closely related to phosphorus metabolism. It is distributed widely in the animal body and is particularly active in ossifying cartilage. When rickets is present the level of phosphatase in blood serum is high. This is thought to be caused by leakage from the diseased bone. Administration of vitamin D causes the enzyme to return to normal slowly.

Recently it has been shown that vitamin D is converted into hydroxy-vitamin D in the liver, and then to dihydroxy-vitamin D by the kidney when blood calcium is low. The dihydroxy compound is more potent than vitamin D and greatly increases the absorption of calcium from the digestive tract. When serum calcium becomes normal, this conversion ceases and calcium absorption declines.

Symptoms of deficiency. The chief indication of vitamin D deficiency is rickets, characterized by irritability, craniotabes, prominent frontal bones, delayed closing of the fontanels, soft bones, pigeon breast, rachitic rosary, flaring ribs, epiphyseal enlargement at wrists and elbows, muscular weakness, protruding abdomen, bowed legs, delayed eruption of teeth, abnormal ratio of calcium and phosphorus in the blood, and tetany.

Daily requirement. It is thought that either the human requirement of vitamin D is relatively low or else it is met by the action of sunlight on the skin. A daily intake of 400 units is considered adequate to meet the ordinary requirements of all age groups.

Older children and adults who live in a climate where they do not have access to abundant sunshine need to supplement their vitamin D intake. The amount supplied probably should be up to the minimum requirements for the infant. To prevent the development of rickets, it is important to start the administration of vitamin D early in the infant's life, and full dosage should be given by the second month.

Uses. The prevention of rickets in young children is one of the most justified uses of vitamin D. The initial dose should be about 200 units daily, with an increase in dosage up to 800 units by the second month. Premature infants or those who seem to be especially susceptible to the development of rickets need a larger intake (800 to 1200 units usually). When children already have rickets the dosage is also greater. The average daily dose usually is about 1200 to 1500 units, but in some instances it may be increased to as much as 60,000 or more units daily. Vitamin

D–resistant rickets is a condition that does not respond to usual doses of vitamin D but requires unusually large doses. If nausea or anorexia appears, the vitamin should be discontinued temporarily. Hypervitaminosis D causes hypercalcemia, which may lead to calcification of soft tissues.

In adults osteomalacia also calls for large doses of vitamin D, improved dietary and living conditions, and more exposure to sunlight.

Patients suffering from bone fractures, especially elderly individuals, may benefit from the administration of vitamin D, thus promoting optimum conditions for bone healing.

Vitamin D may be administered in a number of conditions such as arthritis, psoriasis, diarrhea, and steatorrhea, if there is good evidence that a deficiency of this vitamin exists.

Preparation, dosage, and administration

Ergocalciferol, U.S.P.; *calciferol*, B.P. (vitamin D_2, Drisdol); *cholecalciferol*, U.S.P. The preparation of this vitamin is available in capsules, each containing 50,000 U.S.P. units (1.25 mg.) and in solution, 0.25 mg. (10,000 U.S.P. units) per gram for oral administration. The average therapeutic dose for rickets is 1200 U.S.P. units (30 μg.). The normal daily intake for adults is 400 U.S.P. units (10 μg.). This preparation is especially suitable for severe or refractory rickets. Therapeutic dosage varies from 30 μg. to 5 mg. D.E.S.I. rating is *effective* for treating hypoparathyroidism and rickets.

Side effects and toxic effects. Certain pathologic changes have been noted in animals after the administration of excessive doses of vitamin D_1. This vitamin represents the exceptional case of a vitamin in which excessive dosage can cause disease. Symptoms of hypervitaminosis D include anorexia, nausea, vomiting, weakness, weight loss, diarrhea, vague aches, stiffness, and drowsiness. Doses greatly in excess of the usual therapeutic level can so increase the renal excre-

tion of phosphate and calcium that these elements are withdrawn from bone, producing demineralization and calcium deposition in soft tissues. It is curious that both a lack and an excess of vitamin D may produce softening of the bones, although by different mechanisms. Elevation of serum calcium above 12 mg. per 100 ml. is considered a danger signal, and dosage should be reduced or temporarily discontinued.

Vitamin E, N. F. (tocopherol)

Vitamin E is a fat-soluble vitamin, the richest source of which is wheat germ oil, although it occurs in other vegetable oils such as cottonseed oil and peanut oil. It is also found in green leafy vegetables.

A number of compounds have been found that exhibit vitamin E activity. The most active of these are the tocopherols, of which three are naturally occurring compounds known as alpha-, beta-, and gamma-tocopherol. The most biologically potent of these compounds is alpha-tocopherol.

In laboratory animals a lack of vitamin E manifests itself by infertility or failure of the female to carry a pregnancy to term, muscular dystrophy, paralysis of the hindquarters, and cardiac lesions. In humans a deficiency of vitamin E results in hemolysis of erythrocytes. Vitamin E plays an important role in heme synthesis. The requirement for vitamin E increases with the intake of polyunsaturated fats. Daily requirement for adults is 12 to 15 I.U.

Vitamin E in human physiology does not appear to be of value in the treatment of sterility or prevention of abortions.

Vitamin E, N.F. (Aquasol E, E-Ferol). Official capsules contain 30 to 1000 I.U. of vitamin E in the form of alpha-tocopherol. Injectable forms contain 100 or 200 I.U. per milliliter. It has been successfully used to treat anemia unresponsive to iron or other drugs.

Alpha-tocopherol

Vitamin K

Vitamin K is also a fat-soluble vitamin that has been presented in Chapter 10.

WATER-SOLUBLE VITAMINS
VITAMIN B COMPLEX

The vitamin B complex refers to a group of vitamins that are often found together in food, although they are chemically dissimilar and have different metabolic functions. Grouping them together is based largely on the historical basis of their having been discovered in a sequential order. They have little in common other than their sources and the fact that they are water soluble. There is a sensible and increasingly popular trend to discard such names as B_1 and B_2 and to refer to these vitamins as thiamine and riboflavin. Vitamin B complex includes thiamine, riboflavin, nicotinic acid, pyridoxine, pantothenic acid, biotin, choline, inositol, and para-aminobenzoic acid.

Thiamine (vitamin B_1)

Thiamine is also known as the antineuritic or antiberiberi vitamin. It was first synthesized in 1937. It is found abundantly in yeast, in whole grain cereals, and in pork and liver.

Thiamine is believed to play an essential role in the intermediate steps of carbohydrate metabolism. Specifically, thiamine is a major portion of the coenzyme decarboxylase necessary for the normal metabolism of pyruvic acid and other compounds as well. Thus it plays a part in the metabolism of all living cells.

Thiamine deficiency is recognized as being of fundamental importance in beriberi. This disease is still found in Asia but is seldom encountered in the United States and Europe except in persons whose dietary pattern is abnormal. The symptoms of thiamine deficiency are particularly related to changes in the nervous and cardiovascular systems and include the following: muscular weakness, disturbances of sensation, tenderness over nerve trunks, polyneuritis, loss of appetite, dyspnea, epigastric disorders, and irregularities of heart action. Milder symptoms may consist of muscular aches and pains, anorexia, tachycardia, irritability, and mental depression. Deficiency states in the United States are much less common since white flour has been enriched with thiamine.

Daily requirement. It has been estimated that adult females require 1 mg. of thiamine chloride daily. The recommended amount for males is from 1.2 to 1.4 mg. For the infant, 0.3 to 0.5 mg. is the optimum daily dose, increasing to 1.2 to 1.5 mg. between the ages of 10 and 18 years. Requirements are increased during pregnancy and lactation and when the metabolic rate is increased or the body is unable to absorb or utilize the vitamin. Treatment of thiamine deficiency states requires several times the amount ordinarily needed. Thiamine is found to some extent in all body tissues but, like all B vitamins, exists in high concentrations in the liver. It is absorbed from the gastrointestinal tract as well as from parenteral sites of administration.

Uses. The only therapeutic value of thiamine is in the treatment or prevention of thiamine deficiency. Since deficiency in one of the vitamin B factors may be accompanied by deficiency in others, some authorities prefer to give several components of the vitamin B complex. Treatment is best accomplished by an adequate diet or preparations rich in the B factors, such as brewers' yeast. Thiamine is indicated for treatment of beriberi and polyneuritis and for the relief of symptoms that accompany milder forms of thiamine deficiency.

Thiamine replacement is necessary for patients receiving nourishment parenterally and only in the form of dextrose. Carbohydrate metabolism is increased and, therefore, requires additional amounts of thiamine.

Preparation, dosage, and administration
Thiamine hydrochloride, U.S.P., B.P. This preparation is marketed in tablets for oral administration and in solution for injection. When injected, thiamine hydrochloride is usually administered subcutaneously, or it may be added to

Table 18-3 Vitamins and human nutrition

Vitamin	Source	Daily requirements in adult male	Specific functions	Deficiency	Therapeutic source
A	Dairy products, carrots, green vegetables, liver, kidneys, eggs	1000 I.U.*	Visual pigments Maintenance of epithelial tissue	Nightblindness Corneal softening Hyperkeratosis	Halibut liver oil Cod liver oil
C	Fruits, fresh green vegetables, corn, tomatoes, rose hips	45 mg.	Oxidation-reduction processes Maintenance of normal connective tissue Adrenal-cortical function	Scurvy Swelling, redness, and bleeding of gums Petechiae Capillary fragility Anemia	Ascorbic acid tablets and injection Decavitamins
D	Egg yolk, butter, milk, fish liver oils, shrimp, salmon	400 I.U.	Absorption of calcium from intestine Deposition of mineral in bone	Rickets in children Osteomalacia in adults	Cod liver oil Halibut liver oil Calciferol tablets Sunlight
E	Wheat germ, egg yolk, liver, vegetable oils	15 I.U.	Essential for normal hematopoiesis	Hemolytic anemia†	Multivitamins Tocopherol capsules and tablets
B complex Thiamine (B₁)	Cereal grains, yeast, meat, peas, beans	1.2 to 1.5 mg.	Carbohydrate metabolism	Central and autonomic nervous system disturbances Fatigue Neuritis Beriberi	Thiamine hydrochloride tablets or injection Multivitamins
Riboflavin (B₂)	Yeast, meat, liver, green leafy vegetables	1.5 to 1.8 mg.	Coenzymes for metabolism of respiratory proteins	Glossitis Dermatitis Stomatitis	Riboflavin tablets and injection Decavitamins
Niacin (nicotinic acid)	Yeast, lean meat, liver	16 to 20 mg.		Pellagra	B complex vitamins
Pyridoxine (B₆)	Yeast, cereal grains, egg yolk, liver, nuts, peas, potatoes, meat, fish	2 mg.	Formation of aminobutyric acid, an inhibitory transmitter substance Metabolism of amino acids, nucleic acids, protein	Convulsions Hyperirritability Neuritis Edema	Pyridocine tablets Decavitamins

*I.U., International Units, which are identical to U.S.P. units.
†Not well established.

Table 18-3 Vitamins and human nutrition—cont'd

Vitamin	Source	Daily requirements in adult male	Specific functions	Deficiency	Therapeutic source
B complex—cont'd Pantothenic acid	Liver, eggs, wheat germ, cheese	5 to 10 mg.	Component of coenzyme A	Neurologic disturbances Irritability Fatigue Muscle cramps Dry, scaly skin Adrenal hypofunction	Decavitamins
Biotin	Egg yolk, liver, nuts, cereals	—	Coenzyme for carbon dioxide fixation	Anorexia Malaise Dermatitis	Multivitamin preparations

intravenous fluids. The usual dosage of thiamine hydrochloride is 1 to 50 mg. daily. It is marketed under a number of trade names such as Berocca, Betalin, and Betaxin. D.E.S.I. rating is *effective* for treating thiamine deficiency.

Thiamine mononitrate, U.S.P. This form is available in 3-, 5-, 10-, and 25-mg. tablets.

Dried yeast, U.S.P. Dried yeast must contain in each gram not less than 0.12 mg. of thiamine hydrochloride, 0.04 mg. of riboflavin, and 0.30 mg. of niacin. The usual dose is 10 Gm. four times a day.

Side effects and toxic effects. Large doses of thiamine when given intravenously have been known to cause anaphylactic shock, probably because of allergic responses to the preparation. However, the incidence of toxicity is so low as to be almost nonexistent.

Riboflavin, U.S.P. (vitamin B₂)

$$CH_2(CHOH)_3—CH_2OH$$

Crystals of riboflavin are an orange-yellow color and are slightly soluble in water. Thiamine contains sulfur; riboflavin does not. Riboflavin was identified first in milk. Later it was identified in other substances and was called lactoflavin because of its intense yellow color. Its relationship to the vitamin B complex was not appreciated until it was observed that concentrates of vitamin B₂ had a yellow color, the intensity of which was related to the potency of the concentrate. At present, vitamin B₂ is synthesized and all doubt of its identity has been removed. It was named riboflavin because of the presence of ribose in its structure.

Metabolic function. Riboflavin seems to function in cellular respiration and is a constituent of all cells. It is slightly water soluble and heat stable. Many enzymes contain the riboflavin molecule as an essential portion of their molecule. These so-called flavo-enzymes include a number of oxidizing enzymes such as those that oxidize the common amino acids to ketoacids. In addition, flavo-enzymes form part of the chain of "electron transport" by which the energy obtained from oxidizing foodstuff is stored as chemical energy in the form of adenosine triphosphate (ATP). The flavo-enzymes can carry out their function because the riboflavin molecule can be easily iodized and reduced (loss and gain of electrons) so that it can act as a link in the bridge by which electrons are removed from organic compounds and transferred to oxygen.

The functions of flavo-enzymes are therefore so extensive and important that it becomes difficult to pinpoint single specific reactions that result from a riboflavin deficiency.

Symptoms of deficiency. Deficiency in human beings is associated with superficial fissures about the angles of the mouth (cheilosis) and nose at the junction between the mucous membrane and the skin, visual disturbances, glossitis, and a peculiar red color of the tongue. Actual tissue changes in the eye may occur. Riboflavin deficiency is likely to occur along with a deficiency of other members of the B complex.

Milk is one of the most important sources of riboflavin. Other sources include yeast, liver, kidney, eggs, lean meat, and leafy vegetables. The addition of riboflavin to white flour has helped to increase the intake of this vitamin for many persons.

Daily requirement. The requirement of riboflavin does not appear to be related to caloric intake or to muscular activity, but there does seem to be a relationship to body weight. The Food and Nutrition Board of the National Research Council in 1974 recommended 1.1 to 1.4 mg. for women and 1.5 to 1.8 mg. for men as a daily requirement for optimal nutrition. During pregnancy and lactation the recommended allowance should be increased by 0.3 to 0.5 mg. per day. For infants the recommended daily allowance is from 0.4 to 0.6 mg. and for children ages 1 to 18 the daily recommended allowance is from 0.8 to 1.5 mg.

Uses. Riboflavin is used to prevent and to treat deficiency states and is used along with niacin in the treatment of pellagra.

Preparation, dosage, and administration
Riboflavin, U.S.P., B.P.* (Lactoflavin). Riboflavin is usually administered orally because it is well absorbed from the gastrointestinal tract. Tablets of 5, 10, and 25 mg. are available for oral administration. Riboflavin injection, U.S.P., 0.5 to 50 mg. per milliliter, can be given subcutaneously. The usual therapeutic daily dose is 5 mg., although 2 to 20 mg. daily may be needed, depending upon the degree of deficiency. D.E.S.I. rating is *effective* for treatment of riboflavin deficiency. Yeast preparations are also given for their riboflavin content.

---

*Spelled riboflavine in the B.P.

Side effects and toxic effects. Riboflavin is completely nontoxic and reactions to it do not seem to occur. No side effects have been noted after relatively large doses.

Niacin (nicotinic acid)

Niacin   Niacinamide

Niacin is related chemically to nicotine but possesses none of the latter's pharmacologic properties. Niacin is converted in the body to niacinamide, a dietary essential, the lack of which is responsible for the symptoms of pellagra. Pellagra is characterized by disturbances of the gastrointestinal tract, skin, and nervous system. In a milder degree of deficiency, patients are nervous or irritable and have indigestion, diarrhea or constipation, and abnormal skin pigmentation.

Pellagra occurs among persons of low economic means and has been noted especially among peoples who eat a good deal of corn (maize) but whose total diet is limited in protein. It is also seen as a result of dietary fads and disease of the gastrointestinal tract in which there is poor intestinal absorption.

Lean meats, poultry, and fish have been found to be a better source of niacin than vegetables and fruits. Milk and eggs are good sources of the precursor substance, tryptophan. The enrichment of white flour has made an appreciable contribution to the increase of niacin in the average diet in the United States.

Unlike some of the other water-soluble vitamins, man can synthesize niacin from the essential amino acid, tryptophan. Diets low in both niacin and tryptophan are the most likely to produce clinical deficiency.

Metabolic function. As in the case of riboflavin, a large group of enzymes depends for their function on coenzymes containing niacin. The vital oxidation-reduction coenzymes, diphosphopyridine nucleotide and triphosphopyridine nucleotide, are required for the early reactions of many metabolic pathways.

Ribose-phosphate-phosphate-adenine

Both contain the nicotinamide molecule as part of their structure. No biologic role of niacin is known except for its presence in coenzymes, but so many metabolic processes are dependent on the pyridine nucleotides that this is ample to explain the widespread symptoms caused by niacin lack.

Daily requirement. The National Research Council (U.S.A.), in its 1974 revision of Recommended Dietary Allowances, states the daily niacin requirements in terms of niacin equivalents, assuming that 60 mg. of tryptophan will supply 1 mg. of niacin. Requirements are estimated on the basis of body weight and caloric intake and then increased by 50% to provide for varying physiologic needs and dietary situations. The niacin requirement for women is given as 12 to 14 mg. and is 16 to 20 mg. daily for men. For pregnancy and lactation an increase of from 2 to 4 mg. per day is recommended. For infants the daily recommended intake is 5 to 8 mg. The recommended allowance for children ages 1 to 18 is 9 to 20 mg. daily.

Uses. Both nicotinic acid and nicotinamide are used in the treatment and prophylaxis of pellagra, but since pellagra is a disease associated with multiple vitamin deficiencies, riboflavin and thiamine are also indicated. Optimal treatment of the disease must include the administration of all members of the vitamin B complex as well as a diet adequate in animal protein. Results of therapy are frequently dramatic. Some positive results have been noted when niacin has been administered to patients with a variety of diagnoses, ranging from sprue to Meniere's syndrome. It has been used to reverse some characteristics of aging, in lowering cholesterol levels, and in psychiatric contexts to differentiate between psychoses of dietary and nondietary origin.

Preparation, dosage, and administration. The following are available preparations of niacin.

Niacin, N.F.; *nicotinic acid,* B.P. Nicotinic acid is available as a powder and in tablet form of 25, 50, or 100 mg. for oral administration.

Niacin injection, N.F. This form is available in 10-ml. ampules containing 100 mg. of the drug for parenteral use.

Niacinamide, U.S.P.; *nicotinamide,* B.P. Official preparations include tablets of 25, 50, 100, and 500 mg. and ampules containing a solution for injection. The concentration of the solution is 50, 100, or 200 mg. per milliliter.

These vitamins are usually given orally but they may also be given parenterally. The dose for the treatment of pellagra may be as much as 500 mg. daily by mouth in divided doses or 100 to 200 mg. by injection. The dose must be determined by the degree of deficiency.

Side effects and toxic effects. The administration of large doses of nicotinic acid (especially when given intravenously) causes flushing of the face and neck, which may be associated with burning and pruritus. This does not occur after the administration of nicotinamide, which is therefore preferred for parenteral administration. In spite of this transient reaction, niacin is considered a nontoxic substance.

Pyridoxine hydrochloride, U.S.P., B.P. (vitamin B6)

Vitamin B6 occurs as a group of chemically related compounds—pyridoxine, pyridoxal, and pyridoxamine. In the body tissues these compounds can be converted from one form to another. Pyridoxine is changed into pyridoxal, which seems to be especially active. Pyridoxal phosphate functions as a coenzyme and is involved in changing tryptophan to the nicotinamide portion of the pyridine coenzymes. It plays an important role in the metabolism of amino acids and fatty acids and is said to participate in energy transformation in the brain and nerve tissues.

Pork and glandular meats are said to be especially rich in the vitamin B_6 group of enzymes, although these substances are found in many different foods.

Although no specific deficiency disease has been recognized in man, convulsive disorders have been observed in infants who were fed a diet deficient in vitamin B_6 and adults who have received a vitamin B_6 antagonist have developed seborrheic dermatitis, lesions on mucous membranes, and peripheral neuritis. Patients with an unusual type of hypochromic anemia have responded well to the administration of vitamin B_6.

Daily requirement. The daily recommended allowance of vitamin B_6 is from 0.3 to 0.4 mg. for infants and from 0.6 to 1.6 mg. for children ages 1 through 14. The requirement is 2 mg. for adolescents and adults. An increase of 0.5 mg. daily is recommended during pregnancy and lactation.

Uses. Pyridoxine hydrochloride is used as an adjunct in the treatment of nausea and vomiting of pregnancy and irradiation sickness.

Isoniazid, an antituberculosis drug, acts as an antagonist of vitamin B_6, and when used over a period of time it may produce a vitamin deficiency unless additional amounts of vitamin B_6 are administered.

Preparation, dosage, and administration. Official preparations are available in 5-, 10-, 25-, and 50-mg. tablets for oral administration and in solution (concentrations varying from 50 to 100 mg. per milliliter) for intramuscular or intravenous injection. The usual dosage is 5 mg. daily, although as much as 25 to 100 mg. has been administered. Pyridoxine has a D.E.S.I. rating of *effective* for treatment of pyridoxine deficiency. The combination of pyridoxine and thiamine (Gravidox) has been rated as *possibly effective* for the relief of nausea and vomiting of pregnancy.

Pantothenic acid

Pantothenic acid is widely distributed in nature. It is believed to be a constituent of coenzyme A, which plays an important role in the release of energy from carbohydrates, and in the synthesis and degradation of fatty acids, sterols, and steroid hormones. Pantothenic acid is be-

lieved to be essential for human beings, although what constitutes the daily requirement is uncertain. An average American diet is said to provide 8.7 mg. daily. It is known to prevent nutritional dermatosis in chicks and to promote normal growth in rats. Calcium pantothenate, U.S.P., is available in 10- and 30-mg. tablets. It is included in many multivitamin preparations. The usual dose is 10 mg.

Biotin

Biotin is a substance that plays a role in metabolism as a coenzyme with an important function in carbon dioxide fixation. Deficiency states have been reported in man only when fed a diet containing a large amount of raw egg white. Avidine, a protein found in egg white, binds the biotin and prevents its absorption from the intestine. This results in the development of anorexia, malaise, and dermatitis. Daily administration of 150 to 300 μg. will prevent the development of these symptoms in human beings. This amount is found in an average American diet.

Choline; inositol; para-aminobenzoic acid

These compounds have been included in the vitamin B complex, but their status is uncertain. Choline and inositol have been found to have a lipotropic (exhibiting an affinity for fat) effect. The lipotropic effect of choline was first noted in the liver, and this led to its use for the treatment of fatty infiltration of the liver and other disorders of fat metabolism. However, the evidence to support claims for clinical usefulness is questionable. Choline is a precursor of acetylcholine.

Vitamin B_{12}; folic acid

Vitamin B_{12} and folic acid (pteroylglutamic acid) were discussed in Chapter 10.

Ascorbic acid (vitamin C)

Scurvy was formerly common among sailors deprived of fresh fruits and vegetables during long voyages. The well-known effects of lemon and orange juices in curing this disease led to attempts to concentrate the active principle by chemical means. Crystalline ascorbic acid in large amounts has been prepared from Hungarian red pepper. Biologic tests show that ascorbic acid is pure vitamin C, which is now synthesized on a commercial scale. Ascorbic acid is a powerful reducing agent and is therefore sensitive to oxidation. It is relatively stable in an acid medium but quickly oxidized in an alkaline medium. It is believed to be concerned in the oxidation-reduction reactions of living cells.

However, less is known about its function than is known about many of the other water-soluble vitamins already discussed. Ascorbic acid is concerned with the formation of collagen in all fibrous tissue, including bone, and with the development of teeth, blood vessels, and blood cells. It is also involved in carbohydrate metabolism. It is believed to stimulate the fibroblasts of connective tissue and thus promote tissue repair and the healing of wounds. It is said to help maintain the integrity of the intercellular substance in the walls of blood vessels, and the capillary fragility associated with scurvy is explained on this basis.

A deficiency in the intake of vitamin C results in scurvy, the chief symptoms of which are spongy, bleeding gums; loosened teeth; hemorrhagic tendencies in regions subjected to trauma or mechanical stress; sore, swollen joints; fatigue; pallor; and anemia. Vitamin C deficiency is thought to be a contributory factor in dental caries, pyorrhea, and certain oral infections.

Foods rich in vitamin C include citrus fruits (oranges, lemons, limes, and grapefruit) as well as tomato juice, raw cabbage, broccoli, and strawberries.

Daily requirement. Vitamin C is constantly being destroyed in the body, probably through the process of oxidation. If deficiency is to be avoided, daily requirements must be met. The optimum daily intake of ascorbic acid for adults is 45 mg.; for infants, 35 mg.; and 40 mg. for children. During pregnancy and lactation the requirement is 60 to 80 mg.

Uses. The specific use of vitamin C is in the prevention and treatment of scurvy and for the subclinical manifestations of this disease. An optimum amount of ascorbic acid should be supplied for individuals of all ages to prevent the development of scurvy. In the absence of vitamin C changes occur in the collagen of fibrous tissues, in the matrix of tooth substance (dentin), in bone

and cartilage, and in the endothelium of blood vessels. Since vitamin C is not stored to any appreciable extent, deficiency can develop easily. Patients who do not eat well or who do not receive a diet adequate for their needs or those who must be fed intravenously for a long time may develop a deficiency unless they are given ascorbic acid as a dietary supplement. Vitamin C deficiency may result in delay in wound healing, or it may actually cause a breakdown in the healing process. Its prophylactic use to prevent colds is highly controversial.

The administration of vitamin C is not considered specific treatment for pyorrhea, dental caries, and certain gum infections, unless these symptoms are associated with vitamin C deficiency. In fact, bleeding gums are a rather common finding among otherwise healthy individuals. Vitamin C deficiency to the extent necessary to cause capillary bleeding is quite rare. It is therefore most unreasonable to treat bleeding gums with an increased and supernormal intake of ascorbic acid.

Nurses who instruct young parents should stress the importance of not heating orange juice or adding vitamins to formula before it is heated, because heat destroys the vitamin C.

Preparation, dosage, and administration. The following are available preparations.

Ascorbic acid, U.S.P., B.P. Ascorbic acid is available in 25-, 50-, 100-, 250-, and 500-mg. tablets. A number of multiple-vitamin preparations also contain vitamin C.

Ascorbic acid injection, U.S.P. This is a preparation of ascorbic acid, 50 to 500 mg./ml., suited for parenteral administration.

Ascorbic acid may be given orally because it is well absorbed from the intestinal tract, or the injectable form may be given intramuscularly or added to intravenous fluids. The therapeutic dose for adults is 500 mg. daily. High doses may cause diarrhea.

MULTIPLE-VITAMIN PREPARATIONS

The daily intake of principal vitamins recommended by the Food and Nutrition Board of the National Research Council (1974 revision) is as follows for adults who are normally vigorous and living in a temperate climate: vitamin A, 1000 units for men, 800 units for women; vitamin D, 400 units; thiamine (vitamin B₁), 1 to 1.5 mg.; riboflavin, 1.5 to 1.8 mg.; niacin, 12 to 20 mg.; ascorbic acid (vitamin C), 45 to 60 mg.

Many of the multiple-vitamin preparations that have come into extensive use in recent years contain amounts of the aforementioned vitamins that bear no relation to established therapeutic dosage or to normal daily requirements. In addition, many such preparations contain purified vitamins that are not yet known to be represented by any known deficiency diseases.

Certain multiple-vitamin preparations not only have excessive amounts of each vitamin but also contain vitamins whose importance in human nutrition is open to question. The cost of "overstuffed" vitamin preparations is unnecessarily high. Vitamin requirements may be abnormally high, for a time, in individuals who are acutely and severely ill, but that is another matter.

Decavitamin Capsules, U.S.P.; *Decavitamin Tablets*, U.S.P. These preparations contain in each capsule or tablet not less than 1.2 mg. (4000 U.S.P. units) of vitamin A, 10 μg. (400 U.S.P. units) of vitamin D, 70 mg. of ascorbic acid, 10 mg. of calcium pantothenate, 1 μg. of cyanocobalamin, 50 μg. of folic acid, 20 mg. of niacinamide, 2 mg. of pyridoxine hydrochloride, 2 mg. of riboflavin, and 2 mg. of thiamine hydrochloride. The usual daily dose is one capsule or one tablet. These preparations are the only official multiple-vitamin therapeutic drugs.

QUESTIONS

For study and review

1 Where is vitamin A stored?
  a. liver
  b. muscle tissue
  c. fat deposits
  d. intestine
  e. spleen
2 Of the following, which is a precursor of vitamin A?
  a. proteins
  b. tocopherols
  c. carotenes
  d. calciferols
3 Which vitamin is the most important for prevention of degenerative changes in the central nervous system?
  a. B complex
  b. A
  c. C
  d. D
4 Which of the following combinations contain all the fat-soluble vitamins?
  a. B complex, E, K
  b. A, B complex, D
  c. A, D, E, K
  d. A, B, C, D
5 Absorption of vitamin A from the gastrointestinal tract is dependent upon:
  a. acid-base balance
  b. presence of bile
  c. hydrochloric acid
  d. pancreatic enzymes
6 A rich source of vitamin A for therapeutic use is:
  a. fish liver oils
  b. liver
  c. eggs
  d. carrots
7 Which component of vitamin B complex prevents pellagra?
  a. riboflavin
  b. niacin
  c. pentothenic acid
  d. inositol
8 Night blindness can be caused by a deficiency of which vitamin?
  a. B complex
  b. E
  c. D
  d. A
9 Which vitamin is essential for prothrombin formation?
  a. B complex
  b. A
  c. K
  d. C
  e. E
10 Vitamin B₁ is most effective in the treatment of:
  a. scurvy
  b. pellagra
  c. beriberi
  d. pernicious anemia
11 Pyridoxine is which of the following vitamins?
  a. B₁
  b. niacin
  c. B₁₂
  d. B₆
  e. B₂

REFERENCES

General

A.M.A. drug evaluations, ed. 2, Acton, Mass., 1973, Publishing Sciences Group, Inc.

Aviado, D. M.: Krantz and Carr's pharmacologic principles

of medical practice, ed. 8, Baltimore, 1972, The Williams & Wilkins Co.

Di Palma, J. R., editor: Drill's pharmacology in medicine, New York, 1971, McGraw-Hill Book Co.

Goodman, L. S., and Gilman, A., editors: The pharmacological basis of therapeutics, ed. 5, New York, 1975, The Macmillan Co.

Goth, A.: Medical pharmacology, ed. 7, St. Louis, 1974, The C. V. Mosby Co.

Grollman, A., and Grollman, E. F.: Pharmacology and therapeutics, ed. 7, Philadelphia, 1970, Lea & Febiger.

Meyers, F. H., Jawetz, E., and Goldfien, A.: Review of medical pharmacology, ed. 4, Los Altos, Calif., 1974, Lange Medical Publications.

Modell, W., editor: Drugs of choice 1976-1977, St. Louis, 1976, The C. V. Mosby Co.

Osol, A., and Pratt, R.: The United States Dispensatory, ed. 27, Philadelphia, 1973, J. B. Lippincott Co.

Turner, P., and Richens, A.: Clinical pharmacology, Edinburgh, 1973, Churchill Livingstone.

Fluids and electrolytes

Dudrick, S. J.: Rational intravenous therapy, Am. J. Hosp. Pharmacol. **28:**82, 1971.

Flack, H. L., and others: The current status of parenteral hyperalimentation, Am. J. Hosp. Pharmacol. **28:**326, 1971.

Hall, R. C. W., and Joffe, J. R.: Hypomagnesemia: physical and psychiatric symptoms, J.A.M.A. **224:**1749, 1973.

Hutchin, P.: Metabolic response to surgery in relation to calorie, fluid and electrolyte intake, Curr. Probl. Surg., April 1971.

Inglott, A. S.: I.V. additive review. Part I. Drug Intell. Clin. Pharmacol. **6:**28, 1972.

Inglott, A. S.: I.V. additive review. Part II. Drug Intell. Clin. Pharmacol. **6:**69, 1972.

Kramer, W.: Precipitates found in admixtures of potassium chloride and dextrose 5% in water, Am. J. Hosp. Pharmacol. **27:**548, 1970.

Klotz, R., and Sherman, J. O.: Preparation of hyperalimentation solutions for the pediatric patient, Am. J. Hosp. Pharmacol. **28:**102, 1971.

Moore, F. D., and Brennan, M. F.: Intravenous feeding, New Eng. J. Med. **287:**862, 1972.

Rovner, D. R.: Use of pharmacologic agents in the treatment of hypokalemia and hyperkalemia, Ration. Drug Ther. **6:**1, 1972.

Share, L., and others: Regulation of body fluids, Ann. Rev. Physiol. **34:**235, 1972.

Shils, M. E.: Guidelines for total parenteral nutrition, J.A.M.A. **220:**1721, 1972.

Turco, S., and Davis, N.: Clinical significance of particulate matter: a review of the literature, Hosp. Pharmacol. **8:**137, 1970.

Turco, S., and Davis, N.: Glass particles in intravenous injections, New Eng. J. Med. **287:**1204, 1972.

Nutrients

Avioli, L. V., and Haddad, J. G.: Vitamin D: Current concepts, Metabolism **22:**507, 1973.

Axelrod, A. E.: Immune processes in vitamin deficiency states, Am. J. Clin. Nutr. **24:**265, 1971.

Bollag, W.: Vitamin A and vitamin A acid in the prophylaxis and therapy of epithelial tumours, Int. J. Vitamin Res. **40:**299, 1970.

Coulehan, J. L., and others: Vitamin C prophylaxis in a boarding school, New Eng. J. Med. **290:**6, 1974.

Deluca, H. F., and Suttie, J. W.: The fat-soluble vitamins, Madison, 1970, University of Wisconsin Press.

Di Palma, J. R.: Vitamins: Facts and fancies, R. N. **35:**57, 1972.

Editorial: Dietary osteomalacia, Lancet **1:**1037, 1969.

Hall, R. C. W., and Joffe, J. R.: Hypomagnesemia: Physical and psychiatric symptoms, J.A.M.A. **224:**1749, 1973.

Katsikas, J. L., and others: Disorders of potassium metabolism, Med. Clin. N. Am. **55:**503, 1971.

Laflamme, G. H., and Jowsey, J.: Bone and soft tissue changes with oral phosphate supplements, J. Clin. Invest. **51:**2834, 1972.

Lawson, D. E. M.: Vitamin D: new findings on its metabolism and its role in calcium nutrition, Proc. Nutr. Soc. **30:**47, 1970.

Muenter, M. D., and others: Chronic vitamin A intoxication in adults, Am. J. Med. **50:**129, 1971.

Nair, P. P., and others: The effect of vitamin E on porphyrin metabolism in man, Arch. Int. Med. **128:**411, 1971.

Olson, R. E.: The mode of action of vitamin K, Nutr. Rev. **28:**171, 1970.

Pace, H. B., and Barnes, B. A.: Vitamins. In Griffenhagen, G. B., and Hawkins, L. L., editors: Handbook of non-prescription drugs, Washington, 1973, American Pharmaceutical Association.

Pauling, L.: Vitamin C and the common cold, San Francisco, 1970, W. H. Freeman and Co.

Raisz, L. G.: A confusion of vitamin D's, New Eng. J. Med. **287:**926, 1972.

Raisz, L. G.: The pharmacology of bone, Ration. Drug Ther. **5:**1, June 1971.

Ritchie, J. H., and others: Edema and hemolytic anaemia in premature infants: A vitamin E deficiency syndrome, New Eng. J. Med. **279:**1185, 1968.

Rivlin, R. S.: Riboflavin metabolism, New Eng. J. Med. **283:**463, 1970.

Roels, O. A.: Vitamin A physiology, J.A.M.A. **214:**1097, 1970.

Rosenberg, L. E.: Vitamin-dependent genetic disease, Hosp. Pract. **5:**59, 1970.

Rovner, D. R.: Use of pharmacologic agents in the treatment of hypokalemia and hyperkalemia, Ration. Drug Ther. **6:**1, Feb. 1972.

Schwartz, P. L.: Ascorbic acid in wound healing—a review, J. Amer. Diet. Assoc. **56:**497, 1970.

CHAPTER 19

Diuretics and other urinary tract agents

The kidneys

Diuretics

Diuretics with primary action in proximal tubule or loop of Henle
Diuretics with primary action in distal tubules
Nursing measures for patients receiving diuretic therapy

Nondiuretic agents that affect diuresis

Drugs that act on the bladder

THE KIDNEYS

The kidneys are the chief organs that excrete nonvolatile, water-soluble substances from the body. These substances include products of metabolism such as urea, uric acid, and creatinine, as well as electrolytes such as sodium chloride and potassium salts. Foreign substances that may have gained entrance into the blood are also excreted by the kidneys.

The normal kidney does not excrete colloids, such as plasma proteins, or large molecular weight colloids introduced into the bloodstream, such as gelatin or gum acacia. The kidney plays an important part in maintaining the osmotic pressure of the blood. It also acts to maintain optimum concentrations of the individual constituents of the plasma. This is accomplished by the excretion of water and specific solutes in carefully regulated amounts. It is largely the responsibility of the renal tubules to effect this precise regulation of the substances excreted into the urine. The tubules accomplish this function in a number of ways. Some substances such as glucose and amino acids are completely reabsorbed from the tubular urine and are returned to the blood quantitatively. Others, such as sodium and chloride, are partially reabsorbed. Substances such as inulin and creatinine are not reabsorbed at all and are excreted quantitatively. The renal tubules also add some substances to the urine by a process of secretion. Potassium and hydrogen ions are secreted by the cells of the renal tubule.

HISTOLOGY OF THE KIDNEYS

The kidneys are composed of many functional units called nephrons (Figure 19-1), each of which begins as a dilated ovoid-shaped structure known as Bowman's capsule. Into Bowman's capsule is invaginated a tuft of capillary vessels, the glomerulus, through which flows blood that originally came from the renal arteries.

The glomerulus is connected to a long tortuous tubule that is divided into several segments. The first part is called the proximal convoluted tubule. This is followed by a narrowed hairpin-shaped structure called Henle's loop. The initial part of Henle's loop descends toward the pelvis of the kidney and is called the descending limb. This is lined with flattened squamous cells. This descending limb is followed by the ascending limb, which is lined with cuboidal

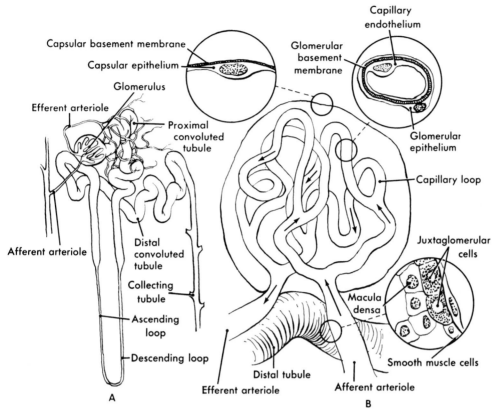

Figure 19-1

A, Diagram of a nephron. The nephron consists of the glomerulus, the ball of capillaries at upper left; the tubule, which twists from the glomerulus to the urine-collecting duct at right; and the bed of capillaries around the tubule. The water of the blood containing small molecules such as urea and sodium chloride is filtered out of the glomerulus into the tubule where virtually all of the water and other useful substances are reabsorbed. Blood enters the glomerulus via the afferent arteriole and leaves it via the efferent arteriole. **B,** Diagram of a glomerulus showing cross sections of its various component parts.

epithelium. The next part of the tubule is the distal convoluted tubule, which is also lined with cuboidal epithelium. The distal part of the tubule empties into the collecting tubule, which eventually terminates in the renal pyramid and pelvis of the kidney. The collecting tubule is also lined with cuboidal epithelium. The number of glomeruli in the kidney of man is estimated to be 1 million in each kidney. The total tubule length of both kidneys is estimated to be approximately 75 miles.

In general, the excretion of urine is attuned to the needs of the body. For most substances the kidney serves to maintain constant amounts and concentrations in the body fluids. This is accomplished by excreting the same amounts of solutes and water as are acquired each day (minus the amounts lost through sweat, feces, and other extrarenal routes). In physiologic terms, the kidney acts to preserve balance of most major constituents of body fluids.

VOLUME AND COMPOSITION OF URINE

Factors that most affect the formation of urine include glomerular filtration, tubular reabsorption, and tubular secretion.

Glomerular filtration. The force needed for filtration through the glomerular capillaries and into the glomerular capsule is derived from the force of the blood (blood pressure). It is sometimes referred to as hydrostatic pressure. The osmotic pressure of the plasma proteins represents an opposing force to hold fluid in the blood. Various constituents dissolved in the plasma filter through the glomerulus and are found in the filtrate in about the same concentration as they are found in the blood. Blood cells, plasma proteins, and lipids do not diffuse through the capillary walls and are not found in the glomerular filtrate if the kidney is functioning normally. Increased glomerular filtration caused by dilution of the plasma or by increased intraglomerular pressure usually achieves a moderately increased formation of urine.

Tubular reabsorption. The cells lining the renal tubules exhibit a high level of metabolic activity and expend considerable energy in recovering and transporting electrolytes and water back into the extracellular fluid (blood, lymph, and interstitial fluid) of the body. Because they tend to be active cells they are also the cells that are most easily injured when renal damage occurs. For every 100 ml. of fluid filtered through the glomerulus, approximately 99 ml. are reabsorbed in the tubule. Most diuretics used clinically act by interference with tubular reabsorption (water and electrolyte reabsorption). The activity of the tubule cells is greatly affected by the pituitary hormone, antidiuretic hormone (ADH), and certain adrenal hormones. Reabsorption of water is also affected by the amount of nonreabsorbable substances in the blood, which in turn enter the tubule and obligate the excretion of water.

Tubular secretion. It has been found that the tubule cells actively secrete certain substances into the urine as well as absorb certain other substances from the urine. Penicillin is an example of a drug that is excreted this way.

The secretion of hydrogen ions by the tubule cells is an effective way whereby the kidney helps to maintain acid-base equilibrium. The hydrogen ions in the tubular cells are exchanged for the sodium ions in the urine. The rate of this exchange can be greatly affected by drugs and this constitutes a basis of diuresis.

Diuretics

Diuretics are drugs that increase the flow of urine. The purpose of a diuretic is to increase the net loss of water, and to achieve this there must also be a loss of sodium. Diuretics are not all equally effective in removing fluid of edema.

Diuretics act in one of the following ways. (1) Some increase glomerular filtration of sodium. Examples of these drugs are the acidifying salts, plasma expanders and xanthines. (2) Some inhibit reabsorption of sodium by a direct action on the kidney tubules. These agents include the mercurials, carbonic anhydrase inhibitors, benzothiazides, furosemide, and ethacrynic acid. (3) Others inhibit tubular reabsorption of sodium by an indirect mechanism. Included in this group are the osmotic diuretics (such as potassium salts, urea, glucose, and sucrose) and inhibitors of aldosterone action. Inhibiting the secretion of antidiuretic hormone from the posterior pituitary will also increase urine output. Water and ethyl alcohol produce this effect. However, because they do not increase the excretion of electrolytes they do not relieve edema. The cause of a patient's edema is an important factor in determining which diuretic should be used. See Figure 19-2 for a schematic representation of diuretic action sites. It is important to remember that the effectiveness of diuretics is dependent upon the presence of functionally active kidneys.

SITES OF DIURETIC ACTION OF VARIOUS AGENTS

Site 1—renal vasculature. Agents effecting renal vasodilation will increase renal blood flow, promoting diuresis. While the diuretic effect is often desirable, drugs are not usually administered solely for this renal effect.

Site 2—proximal tubule. Mercurial diuretics appear to exert their primary diuretic effect on the proximal tubule, although they probably also act at other sites. Agents acting at this site inhibit

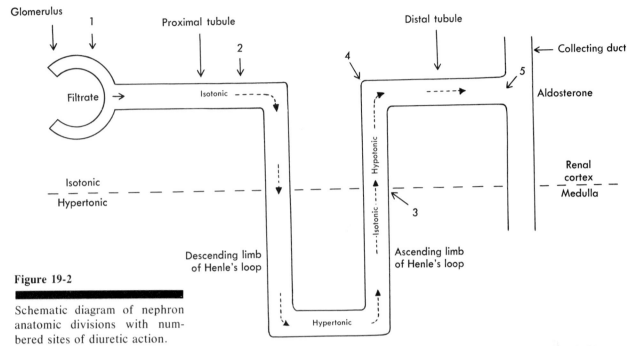

Figure 19-2

Schematic diagram of nephron anatomic divisions with numbered sites of diuretic action.

sodium and chloride ion reabsorption. A large volume of isosmotic filtrate is thus presented to the distal tubule, where some sodium is reabsorbed and a large volume of free water is generated. The urine becomes more alkaline and contains increased amounts of sodium, potassium, bicarbonate, and chloride.

Site 3—ascending limb of Henle's loop. Furosemide and ethacrynic acid appear to exert their major effect at this site. These drugs probably act at other sites also.

Site 4—renal cortical diluting site and distal tubule. Triamterene apparently blocks sodium reabsorption in the distal tubule. The result is increased sodium excretion accompanied primarily by chloride. There may be no increase in potassium excretion because the drug blocks the sodium-potassium exchange. Thiazides inhibit the reabsorption of sodium and chloride from the distal tubule and augment the secretion of potassium from the distal tubule. Triamterene acts at this site also but not as a pharmacologic antagonist of aldosterone.

Site 5—distal segment of the distal tubule and collecting duct site. Spironolactone, the aldosterone antagonist, probably exerts its major effect at this site. In the distal portions of the tubule sodium is reabsorbed from tubular fluid in exchange for potassium and hydrogen ions. Blocking the action of aldosterone results in increased sodium and chloride excretion and decreased potassium and ammonium excretion.

An inadequate or poor response to diuretic therapy, particularly when treatment consists of a single drug, may result from:

1 Unrestricted or liberal salt or sodium intake
2 Low glomerular filtration rate, which occurs in patients with renal insufficiency
3 Increased tubular reabsorption of sodium and water, which may be caused by:
   a. Hyperaldosteronism, nephrosis, or cirrhosis
   b. Heart failure, which results in low cardiac output and reduced renal blood flow
   c. Impaired venous or lymphatic drainage, which traps fluid in various tissues

The most frequent side effects of diuretic therapy include:

1 Hypokalemia
2 Hyperuricemia (especially with thiazides)
3 Impaired glucose tolerance
4 Hyponatremia
5 Reduced glomerular filtration rate
6 A transient decrease in plasma volume, cardiac output, blood pressure, and renal function

DIURETICS WITH PRIMARY ACTION IN PROXIMAL TUBULE OR LOOP OF HENLE

MERCURIAL DIURETICS

Mersalyl

The organic mercurial diuretics are considered to be among the more potent drugs for increasing the output of urine. Development of newer and orally effective diuretics has limited their use. While the mercurials, under optimal conditions, are four times as effective as thiazides in increasing sodium excretion, they have the disadvantages of requiring repeated parenteral administration and causing nephrotoxicity. Table 19-1 lists some of the mercurial diuretics.

Action. Mercurials do not alter filtration rate and do not affect renal blood flow. Their diuretic effect appears to be that of inhibiting active reabsorption of sodium chloride and water from the proximal tubule and the loop of Henle. The loss of sodium decreases the body's capacity to retain water, which relieves edema. Loss of chloride and water is a passive action. Mercurials also increase calcium and magnesium excretion with prolonged use; potassium excretion may also increase but not to the same extent as with thiazides (this is a distal effect).

Uses. The organic mercurial diuretics are used chiefly to relieve cardiac edema or the edema associated with nephroses, cirrhotic conditions of the liver, or portal obstruction and for patients resistant to less potent diuretics.

Preparation, dosage, and administration. The preferred route of administration is intramuscular. Although the subcutaneous route can be used, it can cause local irritation. Oral administration may cause gastric distress. In addition, absorption after oral administration is highly variable, and loss of edema is less dramatic than that obtained from parenteral administration. Chlormerodrin is the only mercurial diuretic that is not injectable.

Certain preparations may be administered intravenously, but they should be given slowly and only under the most carefully controlled condi-

Table 19-1 Some mercurial diuretics

Name		Route of administration	Range and frequency of dosage	Remarks
Generic	Trade			
Mersalyl	Salyrgan	Intramuscular	0.5 to 2 ml. (40 mg. per ml.)	Most widely used of all mercurials
Meralluride	Mercuhydrin	Intramuscular, intravenous	1 to 2 ml. (40 mg. per ml.) one or two times per week	Each milliliter may also contain 48 mg. of theophylline
Mercaptomerin	Thiomerin	Intramuscular or subcutaneous Rectal suppositories	0.2 to 2 ml. of 13% solution 500 mg. suppository daily	Requires refrigeration, destroyed by heat May cause local irritation
Chlormerodrin	Neohydrin	Oral	10-mg. tablets	
Mercumatilin	Cumertilin	Intramuscular, intravenous	0.5 to 2 ml. (39 mg. per ml.)	

tions. Injections, as a rule, are not repeated more often than every 3 or 4 days, since a small amount of mercury remains in the body for 1 to 3 days. The dose must be determined individually. Initial parenteral dose for adults varies from 0.2 to 2.0 ml., depending on the specific drug. The drug is preferably given in the morning so that the major effects occur during the day.

After parenteral administration of an average dose, the diuretic effect of the organic mercurials can be expected to begin within 1 to 3 hours and to reach a peak effect in 6 to 9 hours. The diuretic effect can be expected to end within 12 to 24 hours. As much as 8 or 9 liters of urine may be excreted the first day by an edematous patient.

The addition of theophylline to the mercurial preparations increases their diuretic effects by improving absorption, and it also decreases irritation at the site of injection. At present, most mercurial preparations are available in combination with theophylline. Mercaptomerin is the only injectable mercurial diuretic that is not combined with theophylline to promote absorption when given intramuscularly. Administration may be preceded by large doses of an acidifying salt such as ammonium chloride to enhance the diuretic effect.

Side effects and toxic effects. The signs of toxic reactions of mercurial diuretics include stomatitis, gingivitis, increased salivation, diarrhea, albuminuria, hematuria, circulatory collapse, flushing, febrile reactions, and skin eruptions. Severe reactions are characterized by sudden fall in blood pressure, cardiac irregularity, cyanosis, and severe dyspnea. Renal damage may result from prolonged usage.

Contraindications and precautions. Mercurials are contraindicated in acute nephritis and in advanced chronic kidney disease. Patients who are sensitive to one mercurial may, however, tolerate another satisfactorily. Caution needs to be exercised when mercurials are given intravenously because sudden fatalities, thought to be caused by ventricular arrhythmia, have occurred. Patients who have frequent ventricular beats or myocardial infarction or who have been heavily digitalized may react to mercurials unfavorably. Patients who receive mercurials are

carefully selected and initial tests for sensitivity are given. When it is necessary to give these drugs repeatedly, the urine is examined periodically for blood cells, albumin, and casts.

Intense chloride diuresis after the administration of these drugs may produce hypochloremic alkalosis, which may be treated by the administration of potassium chloride.

FUROSEMIDE AND ETHACRYNIC ACID
Furosemide, U.S.P. (Lasix); frusemide, B.P.

Furosemide is a powerful diuretic. While its use is likely to be more limited than the previously discussed thiazides, it may be very important in selected cases.

Furosemide is rapidly absorbed. Diuresis begins in 20 to 60 minutes, maximum effect occurs 2 to 4 hours after oral ingestion, and its action lasts for 6 to 8 hours. After intravenous injection, diuresis begins in 5 minutes, reaches a peak in $1/2$ hour, and lasts 2 to 4 hours. The ascending limb of Henle's loop appears to be the principal site for the action of furosemide. In maximum effective doses it is probably eight to ten times as powerful as the thiazides. Its potency is unaltered by the acid-base balance. Since it causes a high rate of chloride excretion, hypochloremic alkalosis may occur.

Uses. Furosemide finds its greatest application in congestive heart failure, cirrhosis of the liver, and nephrosis whenever a diuretic of very great potency is required.

Preparation, dosage, and administration. Furosemide is supplied in tablets of 40 mg. The usual dose is one to two tablets, preferably given as a single dose in the morning. In some cases additional doses may be required. Usual parenteral dose is 20 to 40 mg. intramuscularly or by slow intravenous injection. A second dose can be given 2 hours or more after the first dose if necessary.

Antihypertensive dose is 40 mg. twice daily.

Side effects and toxic effects. The great potency of furosemide makes careful medical supervision mandatory. Dehydration and reduction of blood volume can lead to vascular collapse, thrombosis, and embolism. Hepatic coma may occur in cirrhotic patients who receive the drug. Potassium supplementation may be necessary when furosemide is used.

Side effects are primarily the result of marked diuresis and electrolyte imbalance. Side effects include nausea and vomiting, diarrhea, dermatitis, pruritus, blurring of vision, and postural hypotension. Weakness, fatigue, dizziness, muscle cramps, thirst, and urinary bladder spasm may occur. Rare cases of blood dyscrasias have been reported.

Contraindications. Furosemide is contraindicated in pregnancy and nursing mothers; it is known to cause fetal abnormalities in animals. The drug, like other diuretics, is contraindicated in states of anuria, hepatic coma, and electrolyte depletion. Children should not receive this drug since there has been little experience with its pediatric use.

Drug interactions. The following interactions can occur with furosemide:

1. Furosemide potentiates the hypotensive effect of antihypertensive agents. Dosage of these drugs should be reduced.
2. Competitive renal excretion between furosemide and salicylates may cause salicylate toxicity (e.g., tinnitus, hyperpnea, confusion, acid-base disturbance) in patients on high doses of salicylates.
3. Furosemide causes decreased response to catecholamines and enhanced response to curare derivatives. Oral furosemide therapy should be discontinued for 1 week and parenteral therapy for 2 days prior to elective surgery.
4. Excessive loss of K in patients on digitalis therapy may precipitate digitalis toxicity.
5. Monoamine oxidase inhibitors may potentiate the hypotensive effect of furosemide.

Ethacrynic acid, U.S.P., B.P. (Edecrin)

$$CH_3-CH_2-\underset{\underset{CH_2}{\parallel}}{\overset{\overset{O}{\parallel}}{C}}-C-\underset{}{\overset{Cl\quad Cl}{\bigcirc}}-OCH_2COOH$$

Ethacrynic acid is a powerful diuretic and saluretic. Like furosemide, it is more powerful than the thiazides, but its usefulness will probably be more limited. The action of ethacrynic acid is of short duration. However, it is so powerful that excessive diuresis with marked loss of water and salt can result from its use.

Uses. Patients with congestive heart failure who are unresponsive to other diuretics may respond to ethacrynic acid. Acute pulmonary edema caused by heart failure may also respond to the intravenous administration of the drug. The drug has also been used successfully in renal edema in patients with nephrotic syndrome and for the removal of ascites in hepatic cirrhosis.

Preparation, dosage, and administration. Ethacrynic acid is supplied in capsule-shaped tablets of 25 and 50 mg. Injectable Lyovac Sodium Edecrin is available in vials containing sodium ethacrynate equivalent to 50 mg. of ethacrynic acid for intravenous use.

Dosage must be regulated carefully to prevent an excessive loss of water and electrolytes. The smallest effective dose is determined by administering 50 mg. after a meal the first day, 50 mg. twice daily the second day, and 100 mg. in the morning and 50 to 100 mg. in the evening the third day. Onset of diuresis usually occurs with an oral dose of 50 to 100 mg. for adults. Maximum effect occurs in 2 hours and diuresis persists for 6 to 8 hours. Dose for children initially is 25 mg. Optimum loss of water is 1 to 2 lb. per day until desired diuresis is achieved. Maintenance dose varies from 50 to 200 mg. daily on a continuous or intermittent dosage schedule.

When intravenous use is indicated, Lyovac Sodium Edecrin is injected in the average adult dose of 50 mg. The drug should not be given subcutaneously or intramuscularly because of local pain and irritation.

Side effects and toxic effects. Ethacrynic acid is contraindicated in anuria or increasing oliguria and azotemia. Severe diarrhea may be produced in some patients, in which case the administration of the drug should be stopped. Vertigo, tennitus, and permanent or temporary hearing loss have been reported, usually after intravenous administration of ethacrynic acid. Severe loss of water and electrolytes, hepatic coma in cirrhotic patients, weakness, loss of appetite, tetany, hyperuricemia, dizziness, skin rash, and hypokalemia constitute some of the additional reasons why ethacrynic acid should be used only under very close medical supervision. A few deaths have occurred following its use. These deaths were probably caused by acute hypokalemia in cardiac patients who had been taking digitalis at the same time or in cirrhotic patients who developed hepatic coma.

Contraindications. These are the same as for furosemide.

Drug interactions. The following are in addition to those listed under furosemide:

1 It may potentiate the activity of the anticoagulant warfarin. Anticoagulant dose may need to be decreased, prothrombin level should be tested, and patients observed for bleeding tendencies.
2 Ethacrynic acid antagonizes the uricosuric action of probenecid, and the latter antagonizes the diuretic action of ethacrynic acid.

DIURETICS WITH PRIMARY ACTION IN DISTAL TUBULES
POTASSIUM-EXCRETING DIURETICS— THE THIAZIDES

All thiazides are carbonic anhydrase inhibitors, but this is not the main mechanism for their diuretic action. Thiazides appear to act directly on the distal tubule, although some studies indicate that their ability to depress proximal tubular resorption of sodium and chloride may also be of major importance to their diuretic activity. Thiazide diuretics have the following characteristic effects:

1 They decrease reabsorption of sodium, potassium, chloride, bicarbonate, and water.
2 They decrease urinary diluting capacity. This property accounts for thiazide effectiveness in the treatment of diabetes insipidus.
3 Thiazides have an antihypertensive effect. This effect remains obscure but may result from decreased body sodium and a reduction of potassium from vascular walls. There is also indication that thiazides decrease pressor effects of catecholamines (epinephrine and norepinephrine).
4 They have no marked effect on acid-base balance, and their diuretic effectiveness is not influenced by changes in acid-base balance. They remain effective in both acidosis and alkalosis.

5 They cause less elimination of bicarbonate than acetazolamide and related carbonic anhydrase inhibitors.
6 They potentiate mercurial diuretics and antihypertensive drugs.
7 Resistance to their effects is slow to develop.
8 They have no serious effects on diseased kidneys.

The thiazides are synthetic drugs chemically related to the sulfonamides. They are the result of studies that began with the observation that sulfonamides inhibit carbonic anhydrase. The development of the thiazides marked a major breakthrough in the search for potent nonmercurial diuretics. Chlorothiazide is considered the prototype of this class of drugs. All thiazides are equally effective as diuretics and antihypertensive agents. Although dosage and duration of action vary, as well as their differing ability to cause chloride loss, their mode of action and precautions for use are similar.

Chlorothiazide

Hydrochlorothiazide

Thiazides are potent drugs capable of seriously disturbing the fluid and electrolyte balance. Hypokalemia (less than normal amount of potassium in the blood) may precipitate digitalis toxicity. This is of significance in the patient who is receiving digitalis as well as chlorothiazide or a related compound. Chlorothiazide and related drugs have been known to promote the retention of urea, and particularly uric acid, which in turn has been known to cause an attack of gouty arthritis. This effect, however, is considered an unusual response. The drugs may also aggravate diabetes mellitus. The reason for this is not known.

Chlorothiazide was the first of the benzothia-

Table 19-2 Comparison of various thiazide compounds

Generic name	Trade name	Daily adult dosage range (mg.)	Peak action (hours)	Duration of action*(hours)
Chlorothiazide	Diuril	500 to 2000	4	6 to 12
Chlorothiazide sodium†	Lyovac Diuril	1000	4	6 to 12
Hydrochlorothiazide	HydroDiuril	50 to 100	3 to 4	6 to 12
	Esidrix			
	Oretic			
Hydroflumethiazide	Saluron	50 to 100	2 to 4	18 to 24
Benzthiazide	NaClex	50 to 200	4 to 6	12 to 18
Methychlothiazide	Enduron	2.5 to 10	6	24†
Bendroflumethiazide	Naturetin	5 to 20	4 to 6	10 to 18†
Trichlormethiazide	Naqua	2 to 4	6	24
Polythiazide	Renese	1 to 4	6	24 to 48
Cyclothiazide	Anhydron	1 to 2	—	18 to 24
Chlorothalidone‡	Hygroton	50 to 200	6 to 18	24 to 72
Quinethazone‡	Hydromox	50 to 200	6	18 to 24

*Onset of action of all thiazides is approximately 2 hours.
†Suitable for parenteral administration.
‡Not a thiazide but resembles one.

diazine group of drugs, and since then a number of compounds have been made available. They all resemble chlorothiazide, both as diuretics and as antihypertensive agents. Some of these compounds are indicated in Table 19-2. These drugs offer certain advantages over older diuretics.

1 They are convenient to use since they can be taken orally and are relatively inexpensive.
2 They are effective over long periods of time.
3 On the whole, they are regarded as drugs of low toxicity and seem to have a low incidence of side effects (although these do occur).
4 Their effectiveness is comparable to the organic mercurial diuretics, and in some instances they have the advantage of being more effective than the oral forms of the mercurial diuretics.
5 Although they produce electrolyte imbalance, this reaction can be kept to a minimum when proper precautions are taken.

Their main pharmacologic effect as diuretics seems to be the excretion of sodium and chloride and secondarily of water. They are useful for the relief of practically all kind of fluid retention in the body. The increased load of sodium ions causes increased secretions of potassium ions. This accounts for the hypokalemic effect of the thiazides.

Thiazides are used for management of edema resulting from congestive heart failure, certain forms of renal disease, portal cirrhosis, pregnancy, and the use of certain drugs such as cortisone. These drugs may also be used to relieve fluid retention during premenstrual tension. Their use as antihypertensive agents is discussed in Chapter 10.

Thiazides do not penetrate the blood-brain barrier or the blood-ocular barrier and therefore have no effect in glaucoma. Side effects produced by these preparations are similar to those of chlorothiazide.

The introduction of new derivatives is based on the hope of obtaining a compound that is (1) more potent, (2) less likely to produce loss of potassium, and (3) less likely to cause other side effects. The search for a compound of greater potency has been successful, since some of the thiazides now available are many times more potent than the parent substance, chlorothiazide. Potency alone, however, is not a meaningful advantage. If a smaller dose produces the same amount of diuresis with decreased incidence and severity of side effects, then a real advantage has been achieved. The loss of potassium can be prevented to a great extent by the oral administration of potassium. Furthermore, some pharmaceutical houses sell their products in fixed combination with a potassium salt, such as bendroflumethiazide with potassium chloride.

Drug interactions with thiazides. Nurses should know the drug interactions that can occur with the thiazides and take the necessary precautions to avoid hazardous interactions. These interactions include the following:

1 Alcohol, barbiturates, and narcotics may potentiate the orthostatic hypotensive effects of the thiazides.
2 Insulin requirements in diabetics may be increased, decreased, or unchanged. Thiazides can cause hyperglycemia and glycosuria necessitating an increase in insulin dosage.
3 Thiazide-induced hypokalemia in patients on digitalis therapy may render the maintenance dose of digitalis toxic to the patient and lead to arrhythmias.
4 Thiazides decrease arterial response to catecholamines (norepinephrine); thiazides should be discontinued 48 hours before elective surgery.
5 Thiazides may increase the effects of tubocurarine.
6 Used with steroids or corticotropin, thiazides potentiate the likelihood of hypokalemia.

Chlorothiazide (Diuril)

Chlorothiazide is a synthetic drug chemically related to the sulfonamides. It first became available for clinical use in 1958.

Action and result. Chlorothiazide was the first member of the thiazide group to be synthesized. Diuretic doses of chlorothiazide bring about diminished reabsorption of sodium and chloride ions, which result in an increased urine output. Potassium is also excreted after diuretic doses of the drug. This may necessitate the administration of potassium chloride or a food rich in potassium such as orange juice (8 oz.) to avoid serious depletion of potassium (hypokalemia). At higher dose levels, inhibition of carbonic anhydrase causes excretion of bicarbonate. Chlorothiazide potentiates the action of a number of antihypertensive agents.

Uses. Chlorothiazide is effective in relieving edema associated with congestive heart failure and cirrhosis of the liver. It is said to be much less effective when there is a reduction of glomerular filtration in the kidney. It is also used to diminish fluid retention in toxemia of pregnancy, in the management of hypertension, and for the relief of premenstrual tension and dysmenorrhea associated with the retention of fluid. Its diuretic effectiveness is said to be only slightly less than that of the parenterally administered mercurials.

Preparation, dosage, and administration

Chlorothiazide, U.S.P., B.P. (Diuril). This drug is available in 250- and 500-mg. tablets for oral administration. The usual diuretic dose for adults is from 500 mg. to 1 Gm. daily or twice daily. Diuretic effects occur within 2 hours after oral administration and last over a period of 6 to 12 hours. To avoid disturbing the patient at night, it is better to give the drug early in the day.

It is also available as a syrup, 250 mg. per 5 ml. Oral dosage range for children is from 20 to 40 mg. per kilogram of body weight per day in two divided doses. Infants under 6 months may require 30 mg. per kilogram of body weight in two divided doses.

As an antihypertensive, usual initial dose is 500 mg. twice daily; dosage is increased or decreased according to the patient's blood pressure response. Some patients may require 2 Gm. daily. If used with another antihypertensive drug, dosage of one or both drugs may be reduced. As blood pressure decreases, dosage may need to be further reduced and one of the drugs may be discontinued.

Chlorothiazide sodium (Lyovac Diuril). This is the sodium salt of chlorothiazide; it is more soluble than chlorothiazide and is therefore better suited to parenteral administration. It is available in vials that contain 500 mg. of the drug in the form of a powder.

Side effects and toxic effects. Side effects include allergic reactions, skin eruptions, nausea, epigastric discomfort, weakness, dizziness, paresthesias, and muscle cramps. A lowering of the number of leukocytes and thrombocytes, as well as agranulocytosis, has occurred, but the incidence is said to be low. Bicarbonate is excreted when large doses are administered, and this can cause acidosis.

Chlorothiazide may be contraindicated for patients with severe hepatic or renal dysfunction.

Thiazides may cause hyperglycemia and glycosuria in patients with latent diabetes. These drugs should be used with caution in diabetic patients.

Hydrochlorothiazide, U.S.P., B.P. (HydroDiuril, Oretic, Esidrix)

Hydrochlorothiazide is ten times more effective than chlorothiazide; thus its dosage is about one tenth that for chlorothiazide. It is available for oral administration in tablets, capsules, and extended-release forms and in combination with other drugs such as hydralazine, reserpine, and potassium chloride. The usual adult diuretic dose is 25 to 100 mg. once or twice daily. The recommended daily dosage for children is 2 mg. per kilogram of body weight, and for infants under 6 months, the dosage is 3 mg. per kilogram of body weight daily in divided doses. Infants apparently are more resistant to the effects of the drug.

POTASSIUM-SPARING DIURETICS
Spironolactone, U.S.P., B.P. (Aldactone)

Spironolactone is a diuretic that acts by blocking certain effects of the adrenocortical hormone, aldosterone, a hormone known to promote the retention of sodium and the excretion of potassium. Spironolactone, by blocking the effects of aldosterone competitively, brings about the excretion of sodium and chloride and the retention of potassium. Excretion of water, of course, accompanies the excretion of sodium and chloride. Thus, this agent promotes diuresis and also helps to counteract the loss of potassium when administered with other diuretics such as chlorothiazide or one of the mercurials.

Spironolactone is said to be particularly effective in promoting diuresis in patients who are resistant to the usual diuretics. Spironolactone is employed in the management of edema associated with cirrhosis of the liver (ascites), congestive heart failure, and the nephrotic syndrome. Edematous conditions that do not respond to the administration of spironolactone or to a combination of this drug and another diuretic sometimes respond favorably when one of the glucocorticoids is added to the therapeutic regimen. This response occurs because certain glucocorticoids are capable of diuretic effects in certain patients. Their action is believed to be either a direct one on the kidney or an indirect action on the pituitary gland, where they inhibit the secretion of antidiuretic hormone. In treatment of patients with nephrotic syndrome the physician may try one of the glucocorticoids first, and if the response is not satisfactory, he will prescribe spironolactone alone or in combination with another diuretic.

Spironolactone is said to have an antihypertensive effect similar to that produced by chlorothiazide, but its value in the treatment of hypertension has not been well established.

One of the disadvantages of spironolactone is that it is poorly absorbed from the gastrointestinal tract; furthermore, it is expensive.

Preparation, dosage, and administration. Spironolactone is administered orally. It is marketed in 25-mg. tablets, and the initial dose is usually 100 mg. in four divided doses daily. Dose for children is 1.5 mg. per pound of body weight. Its full effect cannot be evaluated for 2 to 3 days because of its slow onset of action. Its effects subside gradually over 2 to 3 days after the drug is discontinued.

Side effects and toxic effects. Although spironolactone is not considered a toxic drug, serious electrolyte imbalance (hyperkalemia and hyponatremia) has been known to occur. Skin rash, drowsiness, and ataxia have been reported. Serum electrolytes should be monitored. The drug is not thought to be toxic to the normal liver and kidney, but stupor and coma have been known to develop in persons with severe disease of the liver. It is not recommended for patients with severe renal disorder or hyperkalemia.

Drug interactions. Spironolactone action is potentiated by other diuretics, and spironolactone may potentiate the action of antihypertensive drugs. Its potassium-conserving action may increase the hyperkalemic action of potassium salts and of triamterene.

Table 19-3 Action and effects of urinary excretion of various diuretics

Diuretic agent	Onset of diuresis (hours)	Peak action (hours)	Duration of action (hours)	Effects on excretion*			
				Na^+	K^+	Cl^-	HCO_3^-
Mercurials	1 to 3	6 to 9	12 to 24	↑	↓	↑	—
Chlorothiazide	2	4 to 6	6 to 12	↑	↑	↑	↑
Ethacrynic acid	½ to 1	2 to 4	6 to 8	↑	↑	↑	—
Furosemide	½ to 1	2 to 4	6 to 8	↑	↑	↑	↑
Acetazolamide	½	2	8 to 12	↑	↑	—	↑
Spironolactone	Gradual	72	48 to 72	↑	↓	—	↑
Triamterene	2	4 to 8	12 to 24	↑	↓	—	↑

* ↑, Increased; ↓, decreased; —, no change.

Triamterene, U.S.P., B.P. (Dyrenium)

Although triamterene is not a very powerful diuretic and not a competitive aldosterone antagonist, it is used for purposes similar to spironolactone. The drug potentiates other diuretics and causes the increased elimination of sodium but does not cause a loss of potassium. For that reason triamterene is used sometimes in combination with the thiazides. The usual dose is 100 to 200 mg. by mouth daily. Diuretic effect begins in 2 hours and reaches a peak in 4 to 8 hours.

Side effects and precautions. Diarrhea, nausea and vomiting, weakness, headache, dry mouth, and rash may occur. Since hyperkalemia may occur, serum potassium levels should be determined. Because blood dyscrasias have been reported, periodic blood tests should be performed.

Drug interactions. Triamterene potentiates the action of antihypertensive drugs and the cytotoxic drug methotrexate. It inhibits the action of oral antidiabetic drugs.

XANTHINES

Xanthine diuretics include caffeine, theobromine, and theophylline, all of which exert similar actions in the body but differ in degree of effect upon various tissues and organs. Caffeine exerts a marked action on the central nervous system but is relatively weak in its action on the kidney. Theobromine and theophylline are weak in their action on the nervous system but have a somewhat greater effect on the kidney and cardiovascular system.

Xanthines produce their diuretic effect by: (1) improving glomerular function by increasing renal blood flow (caffeine and theobromine have this effect), (2) improving renal blood flow as a result of their ability to stimulate heart action and improve cardiac output, which enhances their slight direct action on the kidneys; and (3) inhibiting tubular reabsorption of sodium and chloride (most pronounced with theophylline).

Theophylline

The effects of the xanthine diuretics are inferior to those that can be obtained from the organic mercurials. For the patient with cardiac edema, especially the patient who has become refractory to other forms of treatment, xanthines are sometimes used to supplement therapy with digitalis and the mercurials. The oral forms of the xanthines are little used as diuretics since more effective oral drugs are available. At present, aminophylline is used more commonly in the treatment of asthma than as a diuretic.

Tolerance to these drugs develops with repeated dosages. Xanthines are contraindicated in patients with renal insufficiency.

ACID-FORMING SALTS

Agents that increase renal excretion of sodium include the acid-forming salts and the plasma expanders. The latter act by increasing plasma colloid osmotic pressure, which mobilizes edema fluid and promotes diuresis. Only the acid-forming salts will be discussed here.

Diuretics that produce acidosis exert only transient action. The acidifying diuretics are chiefly ammonium chloride, ammonium nitrate, and calcium chloride. Of these, only ammonium chloride continues to be used with any regularity.

Ammonium chloride, N.F., B.P.

Action. After absorption, the ammonium portion of the compound is converted in the liver to urea with the liberation of hydrogen ions and chloride ions. Neutralization of the hydrogen ions is accomplished by a shift in the buffer system $\frac{H_2CO_3}{BHCO_3}$, with a compensatory loss of carbon dioxide via the lungs and a loss of available base to the excess of chloride ions. A state of acidosis results.

The number of chloride ions reaching the renal tubules is greatly increased, causing an increase in the urinary loss of chloride with an equivalent amount of cation (chiefly sodium) and water. By achieving a net loss of water and electrolytes (sodium chloride), ammonium chloride promotes the movement and excretion of edema fluid.

The action of ammonium chloride would soon deplete the body of sodium were it not for several compensatory mechanisms that effect a return to a state of equilibrium. The diuretic effect of this compound is therefore greatest during the first day or two of administration. The principal compensatory mechanisms include increased renal excretion of cations (hydrogen and potas-

sium) and the formation of ammonia by the renal cells with the recovery of corresponding amounts of sodium ions.

Preparation, dosage, and administration. Ammonium chloride is available in 0.5-Gm. enteric-coated tablets or capsules for oral administration. The dose varies, although 4 to 12 Gm. is sometimes given daily in divided doses. It may cause gastric irritation, nausea, and vomiting. It should not be used if renal function is seriously impaired because of the danger of causing uncompensated acidosis. The chief value of ammonium chloride as a diuretic is observed when it is used in combination with the mercurial diuretics.

OSMOTIC DIURETICS

Substances exerting an osmotic pressure that is additive to that of the solutes already present in tubular fluid cause a reduction in sodium chloride and water reabsorption and increased water excretion. When the amount of any solute delivered to the tubules exceeds tubular reabsorptive capacity, diuresis will occur. The body attempts to compensate for high concentrations of solute through dilution so that equal concentrations of solute will exist on both sides of the cell membrane. It is a physiologic principle that fluids flow from areas of less concentration to areas of higher concentrations. Potassium, urea, glucose, and sucrose have been used for osmotic diuresis.

Osmotic diuretics are rarely used today. They are not very effective agents for increasing sodium excretion and must often be given in very large amounts.

Potassium salts

The diuretic action of potassium salts is the result of competition in the distal tubule to exchange potassium ions for sodium ions, resulting in increased excretion of sodium and water. Potassium salts also appear to dilate renal blood vessels, which increases renal blood flow.

They should be administered only when renal function is normal. Potassium salts can produce toxic effects if the function of the kidney is impaired and the daily urinary volume is low (less than 500 ml.).

These preparations, however, have fallen into disuse with the advent of newer and better diuretics. The current use of potassium salts is to restore electrolyte balance.

Urea, U.S.P., B.P. (Carbamide)

Urea, though normally present in body fluids, serves as an osmotic diuretic when given in sufficiently large amounts. In a person with normal kidneys it is rapidly eliminated and is not toxic. It should not be administered when there is renal disease characterized by retention of nitrogen. Since a large amount of it is not reabsorbed by the tubular cells it prevents the reabsorption of a proportional amount of water.

At present, urea is not widely used because of the large dosage, bitter taste, and its ineffectiveness in terms of net sodium removal.

Sterile preparations are available, from which solutions can be prepared for intravenous administration. The dosage is 0.1 to 1 Gm. per kilogram of body weight.

Glucose and sucrose

Glucose, when given in quantity sufficient to exceed the renal threshold for this substance, is excreted into the urine and results in increased excretion of water and, to a lesser degree, sodium and chloride. To bring about this effect the glucose in the blood must be increased significantly and, in general, the route of administration must be intravenous. The usual dose is 50 ml. of a 50% solution.

Sucrose solution also acts as an osmotic diuretic, and in some ways it is more efficient than glucose. It is little used, however, because it can cause severe renal damage (sucrose nephrosis). When given directly into the bloodstream its form is too complex to be utilized by the tissues and the kidney excretes it as a foreign substance with little or no reabsorption in the tubule. It exerts osmotic effects similar to those produced by glucose. Since so little is reabsorbed in the tubule, its effects are greater than those of glucose.

Mannitol, U.S.P., B.P. (Osmitrol)

Mannitol is a sugar alcohol that occurs naturally in a number of plants and fungi. It is also synthesized. Since mannitol is not reabsorbed by the tubules, it is excreted along with the water that is bound to it. It is considered to be the most effective osmotic diuretic. Mannitol is also used to test kidney function.

Mannitol is used for its diuretic action to relieve cerebral edema and to reduce elevated intraocular pressure, for treatment of oliguria resulting from transfusion reactions and accidents, and to promote excretion of toxic substances resulting from overdosage of sedatives.

Preparation, dosage, and administration. Mannitol is available in 5%, 10%, 15%, and 20% solutions in bottle of 150, 250, 500, and 1000 ml. and as a 25% solution in 50 ml. for intravenous injection. A preparation of mannitol and sodium chloride injection is available in various concentrations. The adult dosage is 50 to 200 Gm. infused over 24 hours. Dosage must be regulated according to the patient's fluid and electrolyte balance, urinary output, and clinical signs.

Side effects. Side effects include headache, nausea, chills, mild chest pain, and low sodium and chloride blood levels. Fatal convulsions and anaphylaxis have also been reported.

Precautions. Mannitol should not be given to patients with severe congestive heart failure or to patients with chronic edema regardless of cause. Its use in patients with impaired renal function should be preceded by administration of a test dose of 200 mg. per kilogram of body weight over a period of 3 to 5 minutes. Mannitol may be given if the patient produces 40 ml. or more of urine within 1 hour for 2 to 3 hours.

CARBONIC ANHYDRASE INHIBITORS

Agents that inhibit carbonic anhydrase, such as acetazolamide (Diamox), are no longer used clinically as diuretics. They are used, however, for other clinical conditions such as glaucoma.

NURSING MEASURES FOR PATIENTS RECEIVING DIURETIC THERAPY

It is important that patients receiving diuretic therapy be placed on recorded intake and output.

If the patient is ambulatory or has bathroom privileges, he can be instructed in maintaining daily records of his intake and output.

A weight record should also be maintained on these patients if at all possible. Weight should be recorded prior to and during therapy. Daily weight may be required during the first few days of therapy. Thereafter it may be sufficient to record the weight only once or twice weekly.

When giving care to patients who tend to develop edema, the nurse should examine those areas most susceptible to edema formation because of gravitational forces and dependency (sacral, ankle, and pedal tissue) for increase in tissue fluid (swelling or pitting). Signs of increased tissue fluid and gain in weight may indicate the development of refractoriness or tolerance to therapy. Diuretics should be administered early in the day to avoid nocturnal diuresis and disturbance of sleep patterns.

Nurses should remember that the most common toxic response to diuretic therapy is systemic acidosis, which results from excessive elimination of sodium and potassium. To avoid undue potassium loss, patients on diuretic therapy may be instructed to increase dietary intake of potassium. Foods high in potassium include oranges, tomatoes, grapefruit juice, and whole milk. Many other foods are high in potassium and are listed in most hospital or clinic diet manuals.

Nurses should be alert to the signs and symptoms of drug interactions and electrolyte imbalance and exert the necessary precautions to prevent or modify their occurrence.

Nondiuretic agents that affect diuresis

CATION EXCHANGE RESINS

Cation exchange resins are occasionally used in the management of sodium retention associated with chronic heart failure, cirrhosis of the liver, and nephrosis. They are used to remove sodium from food, and they cause sodium to be eliminated from the gastrointestinal tract, which prevents its absorption. Use of these exchange resins appeals to patients whose diet must be low in salt or salt free. Prevention of absorption of sodium can result in considerable loss of edema fluid. Unfortunately, potassium and calcium ions may be removed as well as sodium. This effect can result in potassium and calcium deficiencies unless suitable precautions are taken. The patients who receive these drugs should be watched for constipation. Some will object to the disagreeable texture of these substances or to the gastric distress that may follow the taking of large doses. These resins may supplement the action of mercurial diuretics in the treatment of recurring edema, but they are not intended to supplant the use of them.

WATER

Water is a physiologic diuretic. Fluid intake is frequently forced to increase urine output. The barrier to water reabsorption presented by the tubule cells appears to be related to the concentration of the posterior pituitary secretions in the blood. When fluid intake is increased, posterior pituitary activity is decreased, less water is removed from the urine, and diuresis results. Water is not a diuretic in the sense that it causes the excretion of edema fluid from the tissues. It frequently is considered unnecessary to restrict fluids for edematous patients, provided there is a restriction placed on intake of sodium.

Drugs that act on the bladder

Disturbance of bladder function as seen in hospitalized patients frequently results from one of two causes. Either the patient's bladder has too much muscle tone or too little. If the bladder is hypertonic and irritable, the emptying reflex is stimulated very easily and the bladder feels full although it really has not filled to anywhere near its normal capacity. The patient then has symptoms of frequency of urination, and voiding may be accompanied by painful contractions. In such instances derivatives of belladonna are more effective than the opiates. Hyoscyamus tincture is sometimes the preparation of choice. It acts like other belladonna derivatives to relax the hypertonic muscle of the bladder. When the bladder is lacking in muscle tone, the patient is often unable to empty the organ completely, and this condition may predispose the patient to the development of infection, particularly when he is catheterized. Neostigmine and bethanechol chloride have been used to improve atonic condition, encourage micturition, and eliminate the need for catheterization.

QUESTIONS

For study and review

1 Explain the important nursing care aspects for patients on diuretic therapy.
2 How do plasma expanders mobilize edema fluid and promote diuresis?
3 What aspects of nursing intervention can be used by the nurse to prevent or inhibit urinary tract infections?
4 Explain how antialdosterone compounds promote diuresis.
5 Explain the need for caution when diuretics are administered to patients receiving digitalis preparations.

Multiple choice

6 As much as 90% of the glomerular filtrate is reabsorbed in the:
  a. loop of Henle
  b. proximal convoluted tubule
  c. distal convoluted tubule
  d. collecting tubule
7 Which of the following statements about diuretics are *incorrect*?
  a. Mercurial diuretics are more potent than the thiazides in increasing sodium excretion.
  b. Tolerance to xanthine diuretics develops with repeated dosages.
  c. The combined use of diuretics and digitalis may precipitate digitalis toxicity.
  d. Mannitol exerts its diuretic effects by being reabsorbed by the kidney tubules and attracting fluid from the tissues.
8 Which of the following statements about mercurial diuretics are correct?
  a. Their diuretic effect is the result of inhibiting proximal tubular reabsorption.
  b. During mercurial diuresis the urine contains more chloride than sodium, which may cause alkalosis.
  c. They increase the flow of urine by increasing filtration pressure.

  d. Most mercurials are combined with theophylline to promote absorption of injectable mercurials.
9 Toxic reactions to mercurials do not include which of the following?
  a. renal damage   c. stomatitis
  b. hypertension   d. ventricular arrhythmias
10 After parenteral administration of an organic mercurial diuretic to an edematous patient, peak effects can be expected in:
  a. 1 to 2 hours   c. 6 to 8 hours
  b. 3 to 4 hours   d. 12 to 18 hours
11 Xanthine diuretics:
  a. increase renal blood flow
  b. improve urine output by a stimulating effect on the heart, which improves cardiac output
  c. cause diuresis by inhibiting tubular reabsorption
  d. are more effective than mercurial diuretics
12 The diuretic action of the thiazides:
  a. is not influenced by changes in the acid-base balance
  b. is not primarily the result of carbonic anhydrase inhibition
  c. does not account for their antihypertensive effects
  d. promotes the excretion of equal amounts of sodium and chloride
13 The antidiuretic hormone exerts its action on the:
  a. bladder   c. glomerulus
  b. proximal tubule   d. distal tubule

REFERENCES

Anderton, J. L., and Kincaid-Smith, P.: Diuretics. I. Physiological and pharmacological considerations, Drugs **1**:54, 1971.

Cannon, P. J.: Use of diuretics in liver disease with ascites, Mod. Treatm. **7**:420, 1970.

David, D. S., and Hitzig, P.: Diuretics and ototoxicity, New Eng. J. Med. **284**:1328, 1971.

Gantt, C. L.: Diuretic therapy, Rational Drug Ther. **6**:1, 1972.

Giebisch, G.: Coupled ion and fluid transport in the kidney, New Eng. J. Med. **287**:913, 1972.

Giebisch, G., Boulaep, E. L., and Whittembury, G.: Electrolyte transport in kidney tubule cells, Trans. Roy. Soc. London (Biol.) **262**:175, 1971.

Gottschalk, C. W.: Function of the chronically diseased kidney. The adaptive nephron, Circ. Res. **29**(Suppl. 2):1, 1971.

Guyton, A. C., Granger, H. J., and Taylor, A. E.: Interstitial fluid pressure, Physiol. Rev. **51**:527, 1971.

Heinemann, H. O.: Use of diuretics in congestive heart failure, pulmonary edema, and cor pulmonale, Mod. Treatm. **7**:380, 1970.

Kim, K. E., and others: Ethacrynic acid and furosemide. Diuretic and hemodynamic effects and clinical uses, Am. J. Cardiol. **27**:407, 1971.

Kleit, S. A., and others: Diuretic therapy—current status, Am. Heart J. **79**:700, 1970.

Orloff, J., and Burg, M.: Kidney, Ann. Rev. Physiol. **33**:83, 1971.

Perez-Stable, E. C., and Materson, B. J.: Diuretic drug therapy of edema, Med. Clin. North Am. **55**:359, 1971.

Reiderberg, M. M.: Renal function and drug action, Philadelphia, 1971, W. B. Saunders Co.

Spencer, R.: Problems of drug therapy in congestive heart failure, R.N. **35**:46, 1972.

Welt, L. G., Black, H. R., and Krueger, K. K.: Symposium on uremic toxins, Arch. Intern. Med. **126**:773, 1970.

CHAPTER 20

Antimicrobial agents

General considerations

Mechanisms of action
General adverse reactions to antimicrobial agents
General principles of antimicrobial therapy
Nursing management in antimicrobial therapy

Specific antimicrobial drug categories

Penicillins and cephalosporins
Sulfonamides
Urinary tract antiseptics
Tetracyclines
Aminoglycosides
Nonaminoglycoside tuberculostatic drugs
The macrolides
Polymyxins
Chloramphenicol
Specialized antimicrobial drugs against gram-positive bacteria

Antiviral chemotherapy

Antifungal chemotherapy

General considerations

The "antibiotic era" as we know it today began with the therapeutic evaluation of penicillin by Florey in 1938. The advent of many effective antimicrobial agents since that time has completely altered medical practice. The first antimicrobial agents were *antibiotics* in strict definition. That is, they were substances derived from living organisms, usually microorganisms, that destroyed or inhibited the growth of other microorganisms. There are now also many synthetic and semisynthetic chemical compounds (called *antibacterial or antimicrobial agents*) capable of exerting the same effects through selective toxicity to the invading microorganisms. The goal of chemotherapy of infectious diseases is to destroy or to suppress the growth of infecting microorganisms so that normal host defense mechanisms can gain control in their efforts to eliminate the infecting organisms. Among the microorganisms that can be controlled by these drugs today are most bacteria, many fungi, a few viruses, and parasitic invaders such as protozoa and worms.

MECHANISMS OF ACTION

In order to exert their effects, antimicrobial agents must first gain access to target sites. Usually this can be accomplished by absorption of the drug into and distribution via the circulatory system. Sometimes, as in the case of infections of the skin and eyes, local application to the infected area may be necessary. Once the drug has reached its site of action, it can have bacteriostatic or bactericidal effects, depending on its mechanism of action.

Bacteriostatic agents inhibit bacterial growth, allowing host defense mechanisms additional time to remove the invading microorganisms. *Bactericidal agents*, on the other hand, cause bacterial cell death and lysis, superimposing the killing effect of the drug on the effects of host defenses. Antimicrobial agents may be divided into bacteriostatic and bactericidal categories, with the sulfonamides as an example of the former and the penicillins exemplifying the latter. Such categorization is not always valid or reliable, however, since the same antimicrobial agent may have either effect depending on the dose administered and the concentration achieved at its site of action. Tetracycline, for example, is generally bacteriostatic but may be bactericidal in high concentrations.

Antimicrobial agents may exert their bacteriostatic or bactericidal effects in one of four major ways:

1 Inhibition of cell wall synthesis in bacteria. Unlike host cells, bacteria are not isotonic with body fluids. Their contents are under high osmotic pressure and their viability depends on the integrity of the cell walls. Any compound that inhibits any step in the synthesis of this cell wall causes it to be weakened and the cell to lyse. Antimicrobial agents having this mechanism of action are bactericidal.
2 Disruption or alteration of membrane permeability, resulting in leakage of essential bacterial metabolic substrates. Agents causing these effects can be either bacteriostatic or bactericidal.
3 Inhibition of translation of genetic information and

Table 20-1 Classification of antimicrobial agents by mechanism of action

Inhibit cell wall synthesis	
Penicillins	Bacitracin
Cephalosporins	Cycloserine
Vancomycin	

Alter membrane permeability	
Amphotericin B	Polymyxin B
Nystatin	Colistin

Inhibit protein synthesis	
Impede replication of genetic information	*Impair translation of genetic information*
Nalidixic acid	Chloramphenicol
Griseofulvin	Tetracycline
	Erythromycin
	Aminoglycoside antibiotics
	Rifampin

Antimetabolites	
Sulfonamides	Ethambutol
Sulfones	Trimethoprim
PAS	
INH	

Adapted from Kagan, B. M., editor: Antimicrobial therapy, ed. 2, Philadelphia, 1974, W. B. Saunders Co., p. 4.

of protein synthesis. The antimicrobial agents inhibiting translation and actual synthesis of a protein induce the formation of defective protein molecules and are bactericidal in their action. The antimicrobial agents inhibiting specific steps in synthesis are bacteriostatic.
4 Inhibition of synthesis of essential metabolites. These antimicrobial agents structurally resemble physiologic compounds and act as competitive inhibitors in a metabolic sequence. With the exception of isoniazid, they are bacteriostatic.

GENERAL ADVERSE REACTIONS TO ANTIMICROBIAL AGENTS

While the development of antimicrobial agents represents one of the most important advances in drug therapy, these drugs are not free of adverse and toxic effects. The list of side effects and toxic effects of each specific drug group is long and varied, but all antimicrobial agents are capable of producing three general types of adverse reactions of which the nurse must be aware.

1. Allergic or hypersensitivity reactions. These reactions occur in response to all presently available antimicrobial agents. Allergic reactions may range from mild responses, such as rash, fever, or urticaria with pruritus, to the extreme of anaphylactic shock, simultaneously or in some sequence. When untoward effects are more severe than a rash, therapy with the drug is usually discontinued. Allergic reactions have become more of a serious problem in antimicrobial therapy because sensitization to antimicrobial agents may occur without any history of previous administration of the drug in question. Sensitization has been known to occur through exposure to a drug that is not obvious, such as through drinking milk from cows treated for mastitis with penicillin.

Treatment of allergic reactions includes use of antihistamines and epinephrine, which serve to block or to counteract the effects of the vasoactive mediators of allergy, and the use of corticosteroids, which may reduce tissue injury and edema in the inflammatory response.

2. Resistance. Resistance is defined as the ability of a microorganism previously sensitive to an antimicrobial agent to withstand the effects of that drug. Resistance can develop either gradually or suddenly in response to high drug concentrations. Bacterial resistance is suspected when the infectious process becomes less responsive and/or the patient's condition regresses. It is generally the result of genetic events leading to the development of mutants of the microorganism that are drug resistant and that proliferate in the presence of the drug, becoming the predominant bacterial form. Mutants resist the activity of an antimicrobial agent by (1) elaboration of specific inactivating enzymes; (2) restriction of uptake of the drug; or (3) alteration or elimination of binding of the drug to its target site. As a rule, microorganisms resistant to a certain drug will tend to be resistant to all other chemically related antimicrobial agents, a phenomenon known as *cross-resistance.* For example, bacteria unresponsive to tetracycline will also be resistant to oxytetracycline and chlortetracycline.

3. Superinfection. Superinfection may occur when the normal microbial flora of the body is disturbed, thereby allowing entry to an organism that normally would be unable to penetrate. Superinfection may be defined as the appearance of bacteriologic and clinical evidence of a new infection during the chemotherapy of a primary one. It is relatively common and potentially very dangerous because the microorganisms responsible for the new disease are often *Proteus* strains, drug-resistant staphylococci, *Pseudomonas, Candida,* and the true fungi, which may be very difficult to eradicate with presently available antimicrobial agents. The proper management of superinfections includes (1) discontinuation of the drug being given, (2) culture of the suspected infected area, and (3) administration of an antimicrobial agent effective against the new offending organism.

GENERAL PRINCIPLES OF ANTIMICROBIAL THERAPY

Several important principles guide the judicious and optimal use of the antimicrobial agents and help to minimize adverse effects. Causes of adverse reactions to antimicrobial agents and of therapeutic failures are often related to lack of adherence to the following principles of antimicrobial therapy.

DETERMINATION OF INFECTING ORGANISM

Because most antimicrobial agents have a specific effect on a very limited range of types of microorganisms, the physician must attempt to formulate a specific diagnosis about the organism most likely to be causing a given infectious process. The drug most likely to be specifically toxic against the suspected microorganism can then be selected. This is most validly and reliably accomplished by obtaining specimens from the infected area if possible (e.g., urine, sputum, wound drainage) or by obtaining venous blood specimens and sending them to the laboratory for culture and identification of the causative organism. The recovery of a specific microorganism from appropriate specimens is always a significant factor in determining choice of antimicrobial therapy. When a significant microorganism is isolated, laboratory tests for antimicrobial susceptibility (sensitivity) to different antimicrobial agents are often also requested.

It is always desirable to receive culture and sensitivity reports before initiating antimicrobial therapy. In some situations, however, it is not practical to await these laboratory results. For example, antimicrobial therapy must be initiated without delay in acute, life-threatening situations such as peritonitis, septicemia, or pneumonia. In such situations, the choice of antimicrobial agent for initial use must be based on tentative identification of the pathogen. It is known, for example, that microorganisms commonly isolated in acute adult infections of the lung include pneumococci, streptococci, and staphylococci. Antimicrobial agents specifically toxic to those organisms may be administered temporarily. The choice of drug can then be changed, if necessary, pending laboratory reports. When even tentative identification is difficult, *broad-spectrum* antibiotics that are effective against a wide range of microorganisms can be prescribed or several antimicrobial agents may be prescribed for simultaneous administration.

It must be noted here that some infections are most effectively treated with the use of only one antibiotic. In other situations, such as the one described above, *combined antimicrobial drug therapy* may be indicated. Other indications for the simultaneous use of two or more antimicrobial agents include (1) the treatment of mixed infections in which the drugs may each act on a separate portion of a complex microbial flora; (2) need to delay the rapid emergence of bacteria resistant to one drug; and (3) need to reduce the incidence or intensity of adverse effects by decreasing the dose of a potentially toxic drug. Indiscriminate use of multiple antimicrobial drugs is avoided because of expense, toxicity, and higher incidence of superinfections and resistance.

ASSESSMENT OF HOST DEFENSE MECHANISMS

No antimicrobial agent will effect cure of an infectious process if host defense mechanisms are inadequate. These drugs act only upon the causative organisms of infectious disease and have no effect on the defense mechanisms of the body, which need to be assessed and supported. Many infections do not require drug therapy and are adequately combatted by individual defense mechanisms such as antibody production, phagocytosis, interferon production, fibrosis, or gastrointestinal rejection (vomiting, diarrhea). However, host defense mechanisms may be diminished, as, for example, in diabetes mellitus, neoplastic disease, and immunologic suppression. The therapeutic problem may be complicated, requiring therapy of preexisting disease conditions as well as supportive care in adequate oxygenation, fluid and electrolyte balance, etc., before antimicrobial therapy can be optimally effective. In some situations surgical intervention is also necessary. In general, in the presence of a substantial amount of pus, necrotic tissue, or a foreign body, the most effective treatment is a combination of an antimicrobial agent plus an appropriate surgical procedure.

The status of the host's defense mechanisms will also influence choice of therapy, route of administration, and dosage. If an infection is fulminating, for example, parenteral (preferably intravenous) administration of a bactericidal drug will be selected rather than oral administration of a bacteriostatic drug. Large "loading" doses of antimicrobial agents are often administered at the beginning of treatment of severe infections to achieve maximum blood concentrations rapidly. However, factors influencing drug dosage are also related to the status of a patient's renal function. Because many antimicrobial agents are metabolized and/or excreted by the kidneys, a major management problem exists in regard to patients with compromised renal function. Drug doses are then generally reduced in parallel with the patient's creatinine clearance levels. Hemodialysis may further alter the therapeutic regimen.

In short, the administration of an antimicrobial agent specifically toxic to the isolated microorganism is not the only important measure in antimicrobial therapy. An additional and very important determinant of the effectiveness of an antimicrobial agent is the functional state of the host's defense mechanisms.

PROPER DOSAGE AND DURATION OF THERAPY

Administering antimicrobial drugs in adequate dosage and for long enough periods of time is an important principle of infectious disease therapy. Failures in antimicrobial therapy are not infrequently created by administration of drug doses that are too small or are given for too short a period of time. Generally, antimicrobial therapy should not be discontinued until the patient has been afebrile and clinically well for 48 to 72 hours. Follow-up cultures should be obtained to assess the effectiveness of therapy. Abbreviation of treatment as soon as the patient is asymptomatic usually promotes development of resistance and/or results in a disease process characterized by repeated remissions and exacerbations.

ASSESSMENT OF POTENTIAL DRUG INTERACTIONS

Because the patient receiving more than one drug is now the rule rather than the exception in current hospital practice, the possibility of drug interactions must be taken into account if antimicrobial therapy is to be optimally effective. Table 20-2 notes some common drugs interacting with some antimicrobial agents. Table

Table 20-2 Drug interactions

Antibiotic	Interfering agent	Effect
Polymyxins	Aminoglycosides Muscle relaxants	Potentiate the competitive neuromuscular blockade
Tetracyclines	Antacids Divalent cations Coumarins	Form complex with the antibiotic and prevent absorption May potentiate anticoagulant by depressing GI flora and decreasing vitamin K synthesis
Sulfonamides	Sulfonylureas Coumarins Phenylbutazone Antacids Acidifiers	Enhance action of the interfering agent by displacement from binding site and conversely Decreased absorption at alkaline pH May cause crystallization of sulfas in the urine
Aminoglycosides	Polymyxins Muscle relaxants Alkalinizing agents	Potentiate the competitive neuromuscular blockade Enhance antibacterial activity
Nitrofurantoin	Antacids	Decreased absorption at alkaline pH
Furazolidone	MAO inhibitors Catecholamines Phenothiazines	Antibiotic potentiates all of these agents
Griseofulvin	Coumarins	Enzyme induction to cause more rapid metabolism of anticoagulant

From Rosenfeld, M. G., editor: Manual of medical therapeutics, ed. 20, Boston, 1971, Little, Brown & Co., p. 219.

Table 20-3 Incompatibilities between antimicrobial drugs and other agents when mixed for intravenous administration

Antimicrobial drug	Other agent	Results
Amphotericin B	Benzylpenicillin, tetracyclines, aminoglycosides	Precipitate
Cephalosporins	Calcium gluconate or calcium chloride, polymyxin B, erythromycin, tetracyclines	Precipitate
Chloramphenicol	Polymyxin B, tetracyclines, vancomycin, hydrocortisone, B complex vitamins	Precipitate
Gentamicin	Carbenicillin	Inactivation
Methicillin	Any acidic solution, tetracyclines	Inactivation in 6 hours
Nafcillin	Any acidic solution, B complex vitamins	Inactivation in 12 hours
Novobiocin	Aminoglycosides, erythromycins	Insoluble precipitate
Oxacillin	Any acidic solution, B complex vitamins	Inactivation in 12 hours
Penicillin G	Any acidic solution, B complex vitamins, amphotericin B, chloramphenicol, tetracyclines, vancomycin, metaraminol, phenylephrine, carbohydrate at pH > 8.0	Inactivation in 12 hours, precipitate
Polymyxin B	Cephalothin	Precipitate
Tetracyclines	Calcium-containing solutions, amphotericin B, cephalosporins, heparin, hydrocortisone, polymyxin B, chloramphenicol, any divalent cations, iron	Chelation, inactivation, precipitate
Vancomycin	Heparin, penicillins, hydrocortisone, chloramphenicol	Precipitate

From Meyers, F. H., Jawetz, E., and Goldfien, A.: Review of medical pharmacology, ed. 4, Los Altos, California, 1972, Lange Medical Publications, p. 518.

20-3 notes incompatibilities between antimicrobial drugs and other agents when these are mixed for intravenous administration.

NURSING MANAGEMENT IN ANTIMICROBIAL THERAPY

Hundreds of antimicrobial agents are marketed currently and it is impossible for the nurse to be finitely knowledgeable about each drug. However, in spite of the numerous and varied drugs available, there are still only a few categories of drugs among them. Knowledge of general characteristics of each drug category and knowledge of general principles of antimicrobial drug therapy should enable the nurse to function effectively.

General principles of nursing management common to all antimicrobial drugs derive from principles of antimicrobial therapy described above. More specific nursing measures will be identified in context of individual drugs and drug categories.

Nursing interventions in antimicrobial drug therapy generally relate to (1) assisting to identify the infecting organism; (2) actual administration of the drug; (3) assessment of the patient's response to the drug; (4) patient teaching; and (5) the prevention and treatment of adverse responses.

ASSISTING TO IDENTIFY THE INFECTING ORGANISM

Obtaining cultures of the infected areas is frequently the nurse's responsibility and should be performed quickly so that antimicrobial therapy could be instituted without delay. It is very rare that the nurse cannot take the few minutes necessary to obtain cultures. In the event that antimicrobial agent orders have been given, the nurse should obtain cultures before administering the first dose of the drug ordered. Specimens obtained for culture should be taken directly to the laboratory and not allowed to stand. Delay may cause the death of fastidious organisms and allow contaminating organisms to overgrow the pathogen.

ADMINISTRATION OF ANTIMICROBIAL DRUGS

The consistent administration of an antimicrobial drug at prescribed dosage intervals is necessary to prevent the emergence of resistance, and the nurse should administer these drugs according to prescribed times as accurately as possible. This may mean awakening sleeping patients and assuring that patient tests or therapies do not interrupt this schedule.

When antimicrobial agents are administered intravenously, the nurse must observe additional precautions: (1) the drugs should be administered in neutral solutions (pH 7.0 to 7.2) of isotonic sodium chloride (0.9%) or 5% dextrose in water; (2) these drugs should be administered without the admixture of any other drug in order to avoid chemical or physical incompatibilities; (3) the drugs should be administered by intermittent addition to intravenous infusions to avoid inactivation (e.g., by temperature) and prolonged vein irritation from high drug concentration, and (4) the infusion site must be changed every 48 hours to reduce chances of superinfection.

ASSESSMENT OF PATIENT RESPONSE TO DRUG

Assessment of the patient for therapeutic responses to antimicrobial agents is also the nurse's responsibility. The nurse should observe the patient for signs and symptoms such as decreased fever, decreased purulence of drainage (if appropriate), decreased white blood cell count, and a subjective feeling of increased well-being.

PATIENT-TEACHING

Patients should be taught principles of antimicrobial therapy clearly enough to understand that these drugs should never be taken without medical supervision and should be taken in strict accordance to physicians' prescriptions. This is especially important because many patients receiving antimicrobial drugs are not hospitalized and are responsible for self-medication. Patients should be taught, for example, not to take "leftover" antimicrobial drugs for new illnesses, even if symptoms appear similar; not to stop taking these drugs as soon as symptoms abate; and not to share these drugs with family and friends.

Patients who are allergic to an antimicrobial agent should be taught clearly how to protect themselves from future treatment with the drug in question.

PREVENTION AND TREATMENT OF ADVERSE RESPONSES

Allergic responses. Assessment of a patient's previous reactions to drugs and to antimicrobial agents in particular is especially important in avoiding allergic reactions to drugs. Careful questioning of the patient regarding drugs previously taken and his responses to them is an important part of the patient's history. Once drug allergy is known, warnings should be prominently displayed in the patient's record or hospital chart. As additional precautions, the nurse should (1) tell the patient what drug he is receiving; (2) observe the patient for at least one-half hour after administration of the drug (penicillin in particular), especially if it is administered parenterally and the patient has never taken the drug previously; and (3) know what drugs are used for the treatment of allergic responses and where they are kept.

Resistance. The emergence of resistance may be suspected if the infectious process becomes less responsive to drug therapy and/or the patient's condition regresses. The nurse should be vigilant to signs and symptoms indicative of lack of progress or regression.

Superinfection. The emergence of superinfection may be suspected in the presence of new fevers or other new problems, such as vaginal discharge in females or diarrhea. Children, elderly patients, and other patients whose normal host defense mechanisms may be weakened should be especially observed for signs of superinfection. In the course of prolonged antimicrobial drug therapy, periodic cultures of the upper respiratory tract and of feces may be indicated to determine changes in bacterial flora that subsequently may be responsible for secondary infection. The nurse should be careful not to introduce new microorganisms and should emphasize asepsis in contacts with patients on antimicrobial therapy.

Stop and renewal orders. The establishment of automatic stop and renewal orders in many hospitals is another precaution against adverse reactions. Such orders restrict the administration of a prescribed antimicrobial agent to a definite time period (e.g., 7 days) and its continued use past that time requires a new prescription from the physician.

Specific antimicrobial drug categories

Antimicrobial agents currently used will be discussed as chemically related groups of drugs in order to help the nurse and nursing student think of them in an organized manner. The nurse should be familiar with the general characteristics of each drug group or category and with one or two prototype drugs in each group.

PENICILLINS AND CEPHALOSPORINS
Penicillin

The penicillins are antibiotics derived from a number of strains of *Penicillium notatum* and *Penicillium chrysogenum*, common molds often seen on bread or fruit. They were introduced into clinical practice in 1941 and comprise a large group of antimicrobial agents that remain the most effective and least toxic of all available antimicrobial drugs. The penicillins encompass both true antibiotics as well as many newer semisynthetic compounds that share a common chemical nucleus and a common mechanism of action.

Figure 20-1

Typical penicillus of *Penicillium notatum;* Fleming's strain. (From Raper, K. B., and Alexander, D. F.: J. Elisha Mitchell Sc. Soc. **61:**74, 1945.)

Mechanism of action. The penicillins specifically inhibit synthesis of bacterial cell walls, probably by interfering with the biosynthesis of mucopeptides and preventing linkage of structural components of the cell wall. They are bactericidal for a wide variety of gram-positive and some gram-negative organisms. Bacterial species considered highly susceptible to the penicillins include *Diplococcus pneumoniae,* group A β-hemolytic streptococcus, *Neisseria meningitidis, Neisseria gonorrhea,* nonpenicillinase-producing *Staphylococcus aureus, Clostridium tetani, Clostridium perfringens, Corynebacterium diphtheriae, Actinomyces,* and *Treponema pallidum* and other spirochetes. Most penicillins are much more active against gram-positive than gram-

Basic formula for penicillins

Formula for penicillin G or benzylpenicillin

negative bacteria. There are exceptions, however. Gram-negative gonococci, for example, are penicillin susceptible.

Absorption, distribution, metabolism, and excretion. Absorption of the penicillins after oral administration is incomplete, being limited by gastric acidity and binding to food. The penicillins are completely and rapidly absorbed after parenteral administration and achieve wide distribution throughout the body. They do not readily enter cerebrospinal fluid when meninges are normal, but do achieve therapeutically effective levels in CSF when meninges are inflamed. The penicillins cross the placenta. They are excreted primarily by the kidneys, although some excretion occurs into sputum and milk. Their renal excretion is rapid and can be therapeutically delayed by concurrent administration of probenecid (Benemid), which partially blocks tubular transport of penicillin, resulting in higher and more prolonged blood levels following a given dose.

Clinical uses. The penicillins remain by far the most effective and most widely used antibiotics. Their clinical effectiveness encompasses the treatment of pneumococcal pneumonia; streptococcal infections such as pharyngitis, tonsilitis, scarlet fever, otitis media, rheumatic fever, and bacterial endocarditis; meningococcal meningitis, gonorrhea, syphilis, and salmonella infections. The penicillins are not useful in the presence of bacteria producing enzymes capable of destroying penicillins, such as penicillinase-producing *Staphylococcus aureus*, *Escherichia coli*, indole-positive *Proteus*, or *Pseudomonas aeruginosa*.

The prophylactic use of penicillin has been studied with evidence of proved value in (1) treatment of persons exposed to group A *Streptococcus pyogenes*, (2) prevention of rheumatic fever recurrences, (3) prevention of gonorrhea and syphilis, and (4) prevention of subacute bacterial endocarditis in patients with valvular heart disease who must undergo surgical procedures.

Adverse effects and toxic effects. The penicillins are virtually nontoxic for mammalian cells, and their use has been attended only by minor cases of skin rashes, mild gastrointestinal disturbances, and local irritation following parenteral administration. It must be noted, however, that all penicillins have potential central nervous system toxicity and are capable of producing CNS excitation and convulsions when administered in very high doses, especially to patients with preexisting renal disease.

There is some evidence that the semisynthetic penicillins may have inherent toxicity not found in the parent compound, benzylpenicillin.

Despite their unquestioned value, the penicillins have three distinct disadvantages that are not direct toxic effects: (1) they are readily destroyed by gastric acid, rendering their oral absorption unpredictable; (2) they are rendered inactive by penicillinase,* making them useless against microorganisms that elaborate this substance; (3) their use is characterized by a relatively high incidence of allergic reactions; and (4) they have a somewhat "limited" antibacterial spectrum, especially in relation to gram-negative bacteria.

Allergic reactions to penicillin are thought to be the most common type of drug allergy and are a significant problem. Acute anaphylactic reactions constitute the most important immediate danger associated with the use of these agents. Among all the antimicrobial drugs, the penicillins are most often responsible for anaphylaxis. In more mild allergic reactions to penicillin, skin rashes, contact dermatitis (especially among physicians, nurses, and pharmacists), oral lesions, fever, and eosinophilia have been observed.

Production of semisynthetic penicillin derivatives has attempted to overcome these serious disadvantages. Consequently, many preparations of both natural penicillins and semisynthetic penicillins are available. The various preparations of penicillins are obtained by chemical or biologic modification of the 6-aminopenicillanic acid nucleus. The semisynthetic preparations are characterized either by increased stability in gastric acid, increased penicillinase resistance, or extended bacterial spec-

---

*Penicillinase is an enzyme secreted by a number of bacteria that hydrolyzes a portion of the penicillin molecule and produces a derivative (penicilloic acid) that is inactive against bacteria. It is believed to have little or no antigenic or allergenic activity.

Figure 20-2

Urticaria such as may be seen in patients who are sensitive to penicillin.

trum properties. Only the most widely used preparations will be discussed.

Preparation and dosage of natural penicillins

Penicillin G potassium, U.S.P.; *benzylpenicillin*, B.P. This is one of the most potent of all antimicrobial agents on a weight-for-weight basis and the prototype form of all penicillins. It is unpredictably absorbed from the gastrointestinal tract; therefore, the dose administered must be from three to five times that which would be given parenterally. It is available in tablets and liquid form in doses ranging from 50,000 to 500,000 units and as aqueous penicillin G for parenteral administration for subcutaneous, intramuscular, intravenous, or intrathecal injection.

Penicillin G procaine, U.S.P., B.P. This form of penicillin G can be used only by the intramuscular route. It has the advantage of slow absorption with prolonged effectiveness and needs to be administered only every 12 hours. Blood levels of the drug are somewhat lower than those obtained following intramuscular injection of aqueous penicillin. Usual adult dose is 300,000 units every 12 to 24 hours.

Penicillin G benzathine, U.S.P., B.P. (Bicillin). This is the longest lasting form of penicillin. Oral tablets contain 200,000 units. A single injection of 1.2 million units is absorbed so slowly that it can provide therapeutic effects for as long as 1 month. Disadvantages of this drug form include very low blood levels of the drug, local pain attendant to the injection, and the risk of severe and sometimes prolonged allergic reactions.

Preparation and dosage of semisynthetic penicillins

Acid-resistant penicillins. Acid-stable penicillins are relatively resistant to hydrolysis by gastric acids and may be given orally in most instances.

Penicillin V potassium, U.S.P.; *phenoxymethylpenicillin*, B.P. The antibacterial spectrum of this drug is identical to that of penicillin G. Its advantage is that it is both insoluble and stable at a low pH, escaping destruction in gastric juice. It is available for oral use in tablet and liquid forms. It is more expensive and less active against some bacteria than penicillin G. The usual adult dose is 250 mg. every 6 hours.

Phenethicillin potassium, N.F. This drug shares with penicillin V the property of stability in acid and better absorption from the gastrointestinal tract. In other ways it is comparable to penicillin G. It is available in tablet form and as a powder for pediatric use. The usual adult dose is 125 or 250 mg. three times a day.

Penicillinase-resistant penicillins. An increasing number of penicillin cogeners have been developed that resist hydrolysis by penicillinase and, by virtue of their resistance to this enzyme, exert remarkable antistaphylococcal activity.

Methicillin sodium, U.S.P. (Staphcillin, Celbenin). This drug is inactivated by gastric acid and must be administered parenterally. It is more expensive than penicillin G, but has the advantage of having bactericidal activity against nearly all strains of *Staphylococcus aureus*, including penicillinase-producing strains. It is not as effective as penicillin G against other gram-positive organisms. It has been recommended that its use be reserved for treatment of patients hospitalized with severe staphylococcal infections. Usual adult dose is 6 to 12 Gm. daily.

Acid- and penicillinase-resistant penicillins. These semisynthetic penicillins possess greater stability in gastric acid as well as resistance to penicillinase.

Oxacillin sodium, U.S.P. (Prostaphlin). This drug is stable in acid media as well as resistant to destruction by penicillinase. Its advantages over methicillin include oral administration and greater effectiveness against gram-positive organisms other than staphylococci. The usual adult dose is 500 mg. every 6 hours.

Cloxacillin sodium, U.S.P. (Tegopen). This analogue of oxacillin is identical in its pharmacologic and therapeutic properties to the parent compound. Its advantages over oxacillin are said to be more uniform gastrointestinal absorption with achievement of higher blood levels and more sustained action. The usual adult dose is 250 to 500 mg. every 6 hours.

Dicloxacillin sodium, U.S.P. (Dynapen). Dicloxacillin is appreciably more active against penicillinase-producing *Staphylococcus aureus* than either oxacillin or cloxacillin. It is well absorbed from the gastrointestinal tract and is available for oral use in capsule and suspension form. The usual adult dose is 250 mg. every 6 hours.

Nafcillin sodium, U.S.P. (Unipen). This semisynthetic penicillin is highly resistant to penicillinase and is more effective than methicillin against penicillin G–resistant *Staphylococcus aureus*. It is inactivated to a variable degree in gastric acids and its absorption after oral administration is somewhat irregular. It is available for oral and parenteral use and the usual adult dose is 250 mg. to 1 Gm. every 6 hours.

Extended spectrum penicillins. The following are broad-spectrum penicillins.

Ampicillin, U.S.P., B.P. (Omnipen, Polycillin). Ampicillin differs from other semisynthetic penicillins by virtue of its broad-spectrum antimicrobial effects. It was the first of the semisynthetic penicillins to provide increased activity against some of the gram-negative bacilli including *Hemophilus influenzae, Salmonella, Shigella, Escherichia coli,* and *Proteus mirabilis.* It is not penicillinase resistant. It is available in both oral and parenteral forms. The average dose for gram-negative infections in adults is 2 to 4 Gm. daily, given in divided doses. Ampicillin has been popular in pediatric practice, especially in the treatment of otitis media and meningitis.

Ampicillin

Hetacillin (Versapen). This new drug is a cogener of ampicillin and has a similar antibacterial spectrum.

Amoxicillin. This new drug is also a cogener of ampicillin and produces consistently higher blood levels of antibiotic than do comparable doses of ampicillin, probably because of better gastrointestinal absorption. Usual adult dosage is 125 to 250 mg. every 6 hours.

Carbenicillin, U.S.P., B.P. This drug is a semisynthetic penicillin that has attracted attention because of its bactericidal activity against a number of gram-negative bacteria, especially *Pseudomonas aeruginosa* and some strains of *Proteus* resistant to ampicillin. It is less active than penicillin G and ampicillin against gram-positive organisms and is less active than ampicillin against many of the gram-negative bacilli. It is not absorbed from the gastrointestinal tract and must be administered parenterally. Its major usefulness is in the treatment of urinary tract infections. Usual adult dose is 1 to 2 Gm. every 6 hours.

Table 20-4 The penicillins

Approved name	Other name	Resistant to gastric acid	Resistant to penicillinase	Antibacterial spectrum	Remarks
Natural penicillins Benzylpenicillin (penicillin G)	Penicillin G	No	No	High activity against gram-positive bacteria Low activity against gram-negative bacteria	Only one-third oral dose absorbed, so oral dose must be three to five times that given parenterally For maximum absorption give oral dose 1 hour before or 2 to 3 hours after meal
Semisynthetic penicillins Penicillin V (phenoxymethyl penicillin; Compocillin V)	Pen-Vee	Yes	No	Like penicillin G but less potent	Yields a serum peak level two to five times greater than penicillin G Can be given orally
Phenethicillin	Syncillin Chemipen Darcil	Yes	No	Like penicillin G but slightly less active against gram-positive cocci More active against penicillinase-producing *Staphylococcus aureus*	Give between meals since food delays absorption
Methicillin	Staphcillin	No	Yes	Like penicillin G but with lower activity; only 1/150 as potent	Use only for penicillinase-producing staphylococci Intramuscular injections quite painful
Oxacillin	Prostaphlin Resistopen	Yes	Yes	Less active than penicillin G, more active than methicillin	Give between meals since food delays absorption
Cloxacillin	Tegopen	Yes	Yes	Effective against staphylococci resistant to penicillin G Like methicillin	Yields a serum peak level two times that of oxacillin Available only for oral use
Dicloxacillin	Dynapen Pathocil Veracillin	Yes	Yes	More active against penicillinase-producing *Staphylococcus aureus* than oxacillin or cloxacillin	Yields a serum peak level four times that of oxacillin
Nafcillin	Unipen	—	Yes	Staphylococci, pneumococci, group A beta-hemolytic streptococci More active than methicillin	Irregular absorption when given orally
Ampicillin	Polycillin Penbriten	Yes	No	Like penicillin G but more active against gram-negative bacteria; broad spectrum	
Amoxicillin		—	No	Like ampicillin	Produces higher blood levels of antibiotic than ampicillin
Carbenicillin		No	—	Like ampicillin High activity against some *Proteus* species Moderate activity against *Pseudomonas aeruginosa*	Not absorbed when given orally Under clinical investigation

Cephalosporins

The cephalosporin antimicrobial agents were introduced in the early 1960's and are a group of semisynthetic derivatives of cephalosporin C, an antibiotic produced by the fungus *Cephalosporium acremonium.* This group of antimicrobial drugs has many similarities to the penicillins: (1) they have similar, but not identical, chemical structures, (2) they have the same mechanism of action, and (3) they exhibit a similar bacterial spectrum. Their advantage over the penicillins lies in the fact that they are resistant to hydrolysis by the penicillinases. It was also claimed that the cephalosporins could be administered to persons allergic to penicillin without fear of reaction. At present, however, this is controversial, and it is not clear whether or not the cephalosporins have cross-sensitivity with the penicillins.

7-Aminocephalosporanic acid
The nucleus of the cephalosporins

There appears to be no universally agreed upon, single, firm indication for the use of cephalosporins. There are numerous situations in which they are effective, but in no case are they the outstanding drug of choice at present. Diseases produced by *Staphylococcus aureus*, group A *Streptococcus pyogenes*, some non–group A streptococci, *D. pneumoniae*, and *Clostridium welchii* respond very favorably to proper doses of these agents. Infections caused by a number of gram-negative bacilli, such as *E. coli*, *Klebsiella*, and *Proteus*, also respond to cephalosporins.

Adverse effects and toxic effects. Toxic reactions to the cephalosporins include the development of a positive Coombs test when large doses are administered, reversible renal tubular necrosis, and pain and sterile abscesses at injection sites.

Preparation, dosage, and administration

Cephalothin sodium (Keflin). This drug is not absorbed after oral administration and must be given parenterally. It is usually injected intravenously after being dissolved in 25 to 50 ml. of 5% dextrose in water and is administered over a 30-minute period. Usual adult doses range between 4 and 12 Gm. per day. Because of its rapid excretion, requiring repeated doses at 4- to 6-hour intervals, and the necessity for parenteral administration, cephalothin is used mainly in treatment of hospitalized patients.

Cephaloridine, N.F., B.P. (Loridine). Cephaloridine, like cephalothin, is not well absorbed from the gastrointestinal tract and must be administered parenterally. It appears to be more soluble and less irritating than cephalothin, rendering it more appropriate for intramuscular injection. It differs from other members of the penicillin-cephalosporin family by having the potential to cause serious nephrotoxicity. The usual adult dose is 0.5 to 1 Gm. three times daily. When larger doses are necessary, cephalothin is preferred in order to avoid nephrotoxicity.

Cephalexin, U.S.P., B.P. (Keflex). This cephalosporin is well absorbed from the gastrointestinal tract although it appears somewhat less active than the parent compound cephalothin. The usual adult dosage is 1 to 4 Gm. daily in four divided doses.

NURSING MANAGEMENT SPECIFIC TO ANTIMICROBIAL THERAPY WITH PENICILLINS AND CEPHALOSPORINS

In addition to performing nursing measures common to all types of antimicrobial drug therapy, the nurse must be especially cognizant of several factors when penicillins or cephalosporins are prescribed.

Because allergic reactions are a significant problem in the use of penicillins, the nurse must meticulously assess the patient's previous drug experiences. For infants less than 3 months old, a history of penicillin allergy in the mother should be sought. If at all possible, no penicillin preparation of any kind should be prescribed for or administered to a patient with a previous history of allergic reaction to the drug. Because of possible cross-sensitization, it also seems wise to avoid the use of cephalosporins in patients with severe or immediate allergic reactions to penicillins.

In administering penicillins, the nurse should

remember that oral penicillins are bound to food and are poorly absorbed in acid media. Their administration, therefore, should not be preceded or followed by food for at least 1 hour in order to minimize binding. It is also recommended that penicillins not be taken with acidic fruit juices because these may facilitate decomposition of penicillins.

In administering penicillins intravenously, the nurse should note that most penicillins in clinical use are sodium or potassium salts. Significant amounts of cation may be administered when these drugs are given intravenously in massive dosage. For example, 20 million units of potassium penicillin G contain 33 mEq. of potassium ion. Fatalities have occurred because of the toxic effect of potassium on the heart following administration of such large doses in the presence of renal insufficiency. Signs and symptoms of hyperkalemia and hypernatremia should be duly noted and reported.

SULFONAMIDES

The sulfonamides were the first effective non-antibiotic antibacterial agents in safe therapeutic dosage ranges and were the mainstay of antimicrobial therapy before the penicillins were introduced. At present, many other antimicrobial agents have replaced the sulfonamides, but they are still among the most widely used antimicrobial agents in the world, chiefly because of their low cost and effectiveness in treating common bacterial infections. All the sulfonamides used therapeutically are synthetically produced and contain the para-amino-benzene-sulfonamide group which gives them their common characteristics.

NH$_2$	NH$_2$
SO$_2$—NH—R	COOH
The sulfonamide drugs	Para-aminobenzoic acid (PABA)

R = a variety of nitrogen-containing groups

Mechanism of action. The sulfonamides are primarily bacteriostatic in concentrations that are normally useful in controlling infections in the human being. They act as antimetabolites of para-aminobenzoic acid (PABA), which is required by susceptible microorganisms in order to form folic acid, an essential step in the production of purines. Sulfonamides can enter into the reaction in place of PABA, compete for the enzyme involved, and form nonfunctional analogues of folic acid. Consequently, further growth of the microorganisms is prevented. The presence of pus, necrotic tissue, and serum interferes with the activities of the sulfonamides, since PABA is present in such materials. Among the microorganisms highly susceptible to sulfonamides are group A streptococci, pneumococci, *Neisseria meningitidis, Neisseria gonorrhea, Escherichia coli, Pasteurella pestis, Bacillus anthracis, Shigella* species, *Hemophilus influenzae,* and those causing granuloma inguinale, lymphogranuloma venereum, psittacosis, and actinomycosis.

Absorption, distribution, metabolism, and excretion. All of the sulfonamides are absorbed from the gastrointestinal tract, although some are more readily absorbed than others. They are distributed widely to tissues and body fluids, including the central nervous system and cerebrospinal fluid, placenta, and fetus.

Acetylation is the major process by which the sulfonamides are metabolically inactivated. This change is probably caused by the action of the liver. Acetylation is important to the physician when choosing a drug because the acetylated forms are believed to be nontherapeutic, but they may produce toxic symptoms. A sulfonamide with a low percentage of acetylation in the tissues could be given in smaller doses than one that undergoes greater acetylation, other factors being equal.

Excretion of the sulfonamides occurs chiefly by way of the kidney, where both the free and the acetylated forms of the drug are filtered through the glomerulus. Most sulfonamides are reabsorbed to some extent in the kidney. Some of the sulfonamides, and especially their acetyl derivatives, are relatively insoluble in neutral or acid media, and as the kidney concentrates the urine and it becomes acid in reaction, there is some danger that the sulfonamide will precipitate out of solution causing crystalluria, hematuria, and even renal shutdown. The forcing of fluids to keep the urine dilute and the administration of an alkaline substance such as sodium bicarbonate help to keep a number of the sulfonamides in solution in the urine. However, sulfonamide precipitation is no longer a great clinical problem. Newer sulfonamides, such as sulfisoxazole and sulfacetamide, are quite soluble even in acid urine. The problem of solubility in the urine can also be dealt with by combinations of small doses of two or three different sulfonamides. The saturation point of each is not reached in this way and each drug remains in solution. The "insoluble" sulfonamides are poorly absorbed from the gastrointestinal tract and are excreted largely in the feces. Their action is mainly on intestinal flora and they are used to inhibit bacterial growth in the colon.

Clinical uses. The therapeutic importance of the sulfonamides has been continually modified with the introduction of new antimicrobial agents. Many infections that were formerly treated with sulfonamides are now being treated with other agents which offer special advantages. There are, however, some infectious processes that are more susceptible to the sulfonamides or sulfonamides plus an antibiotic than to antibiotics alone. Among these are acute urinary tract infections caused by *E. coli, Proteus,* or *Klebsiella;* chancroid; nocardiosis; toxoplasmosis; falciparum malaria; trachoma; inclusion conjunctivitis; lymphogranuloma venereum; ulcerative colitis; and dermatitis herpetiformis. The sulfonamides are also therapeutically effective in rheumatic fever prophylaxis, preoperative intestinal "antisepsis," in the prevention and treatment of *Pseudomonas* infections of burns, and in topical form for ophthalmic and vaginal infections. In general, the application of sulfonamides to the skin, in wounds, or on mucous membranes is undesirable because of their low activity and high risk of allergic sensitization. Exceptions to this rule may be the use of sulfonamides in the treatment of conjunctival infections and burns.

Adverse effects and toxic effects. The sulfonamides can produce a wide variety of side effects, the most common being gastrointestinal and urinary tract disturbances. Anorexia, nausea, and vomiting are the commonest manifestations of gastrointestinal disturbances. Urinary tract disturbances, such as crystalluria, hematuria, and obstruction may be due to the insolubility of many sulfonamides in acid urine. Other toxic effects include hematologic effects (anemia, granulocytopenia, thrombocytopenia), dermatologic effects (such as rashes, photosensitivity, contact dermatitis, Stevens-Johnson syndrome, erythema multiforme), and hypersensitivity effects. Long-term treatment with "insoluble" sulfonamides is capable of greatly reducing the bacterial population of the bowel and may lead to vitamin K deficiency. This should be considered in patients who exhibit any bleeding tendency while taking these drugs.

Preparation and dosage of short-acting sulfonamides. These agents are rapidly absorbed after oral administration, and therapeutic blood levels are maintained by administering these drugs every 4 to 8 hours. Short-acting sulfonamides are the preparations of choice for treatment of systemic and urinary tract infections. Several commonly used preparations are described. In the B.P. the sulfa prefix is "sulpha."

Sulfisoxazole, U.S.P., B.P. (Gantrisin). Sulfisoxazole is the most popular agent for the treatment of urinary tract infections. Compared to other sulfonamides it is relatively more soluble in urine and only infrequently produces crystalluria or hematuria. It is available for oral, topical, and parenteral use. The usual adult dose (oral) is 1 to 2 Gm. every 4 to 6 hours.

Sulfisoxazole with phenazopyridine hydrochloride, N.F. (Azo-Gantrisin). This drug combines the bacteriostatic properties of the sulfonamide with the mucosal analgesic properties of phenazopyridine. It is specifically used for urinary tract infections accompanied by urgency, frequency, and dysuria. It gives the urine an orange-red color that should not be mistaken for blood.

Sulfadiazine, U.S.P., B.P. Sulfadiazine is rapidly absorbed from the gastrointestinal tract and is preferred for general use in systemic infections. Because therapeutic levels are attained in the cerebrospinal fluid within 4 hours, it is particularly recommended for treatment of meningitis caused by susceptible organisms. It is available for oral and parenteral administration. Dosage depends on the severity of the infectious process.

Trisulfapyrimidines, U.S.P. This is a sulfonamide mixture designed to minimize or prevent renal damage from the systemic use of this class of drugs. The combination takes advantage of the fact that each drug behaves as though it were alone in solution as far as solubility is concerned. Antibacterial effects of the three drugs contained in the mixture (sulfadiazine, sulfamerazine, and sulfamethazine) are additive. These mixtures may also be made up of sulfadiazine in combination with any other short-acting sulfonamide. They are available for oral administration only.

Preparation and dosage of intermediate-acting sulfonamides. These sulfonamides are excreted more slowly than the short-acting drugs, and it may be necessary to administer them only twice daily. They are particularly useful when prolonged therapy is necessary, as in chronic urinary tract infections.

Sulfamethoxazole, N.F., B.P. (Gantanol). This drug is a close cogener of sulfisoxazole, but it is absorbed and excreted more slowly. It is employed for both systemic and urinary tract infections. Precautions must be observed because it has a greater tendency to cause crystalluria.

Trimethoprim and sulfamethoxazole (Bactrim, Septra). This recently introduced synthetic antimicrobial agent produces its effects by virtue of two consecutive steps blocking protein synthesis in susceptible bacteria. One step is blocked by sulfamethoxazole and the other by trimethoprim. Thus, this drug exerts synergistic bacteriostatic effects. It is rapidly absorbed, but slowly excreted, necessitating administration only twice daily. Its only approved use in the United States currently is in the treatment of urinary tract infections. Its administration to pregnant women, nursing mothers, and neonates is not advised.

Preparation and dosage of long-acting sulfonamides. These agents are absorbed relatively rapidly, but their excretion is so slow that therapeutic blood levels may be maintained for several days.

Sulfamethoxypyridazine, B.P. (Kynex, Midicel). This is a very toxic drug that should not be employed without special indication. Its greatest value is in prophylactic therapy or in long-term suppressive therapy, as in chronic urinary tract infections. Great care must be taken not to exceed safe dosage range, and the patient must be closely observed for toxic reactions. Most reactions are not serious and subside with discontinuation of the drug. However, severe episodes of Stevens-Johnson syndrome have resulted from its use, and deaths have resulted from severe allergic responses.

Sulfamethoxydiazine, B.P. (Sulfameter, Sulla). This is a relatively new drug that has had only limited clinical trial in the United States. It is used in treatment of urinary tract infections, but has much toxic potential.

Preparation and dosage of poorly absorbed sulfonamides. The following sulfonamide is poorly absorbed from the gastrointestinal tract and achieves high concentrations in the bowel, where it suppresses bacterial growth. It is commonly used to "sterilize" the bowel prior to intestinal surgery.

Phthalylsulfathiazole, N.F., B.P. (Sulfathalidine). This drug is employed only as a bowel "sterilizing" agent and is probably the drug of choice if a sulfonamide is administered preoperatively. The drug tends to produce soft stools. It is available in 500-mg. tablets.

Preparation and dosage of topical sulfonamides. Topical sulfonamides are used in the treatment of burns and ophthalmic infections. The following are suitable for topical application.

Mafenide acetate, U.S.P. (Sulfamylon). This drug is one sulfonamide that presently can be recommended for application to the skin and that is effective in the presence of pus and necrotic tissue. It is an agent of choice in the treatment of burns for prevention and eradication of *Pseudomonas* infections. The hydrochloride was initially used and sometimes resulted in hyperchloremic alkalosis because of some systemic absorption. The current preparation is the acetate, which seems to be more effective and less toxic. A major disadvantage of mafenide is the severe pain that may follow topical application. It is available as 8.5% cream, to be applied to the skin twice daily 1 mm. thick.

Silver sulfadiazine (Silvadene). This silver salt of sulfadiazine has been recently introduced and appears to be comparable to mafenide in the treatment of burns. It does not cause pain on application and it is less toxic than mafenide.

Sulfacetamide sodium, U.S.P. (Sulamyd). This drug is used primarily in the treatment of ophthalmic infections. It is also marketed as a lotion in combination with hydrocortisone and sulfur for the treatment of acne.

NURSING MANAGEMENT SPECIFIC TO ANTIMICROBIAL THERAPY WITH SULFONAMIDES

In addition to nursing measures common to all types of antimicrobial therapy, the nurse should observe the following precautions when patients are receiving sulfonamides:

1 Because renal toxicity may still present a potentially serious problem, the nurse should monitor the hospitalized patient's urinary output and assure that it amounts to at least 1200 ml. in 24 hours. Maintenance of urinary output at this level decreases the tendency for crystals to form. Patients who are not hospitalized should be instructed to drink large amounts of liquids. The urine should be visually examined for the presence of crystals, and in long-term sulfonamide therapy periodic urinalysis should be done to determine if crystal accumulation and renal irritation are present.
2 The patient should be carefully observed for toxic effects, such as rash, sore throat, or purpura. Non-hospitalized patients should be instructed to report these symptoms to their physician and to discontinue taking the drug. In prolonged sulfonamide therapy, periodic blood counts should be performed to assess the occurrence of hematologic side effects.
3 Administration of sulfonamides is contradindicated during the last trimester of pregnancy, to nursing mothers, and in infants.
4 Although cross-sensitization is not as severe as among penicillins, it is safer to avoid all sulfonamides in patients who develop hypersensitivity to any one agent.
5 Sulfonamides should not be administered with antacids because the latter inhibit their action by decreasing absorption. Sulfasuxidine and sulfathalidine should not be administered with mineral oil because the oil prevents drug absorption.

SULFONES USED IN THE TREATMENT OF LEPROSY

A number of drugs closely related to the sulfonamides have been used effectively in the long-term treatment of leprosy. Although these drugs, the sulfones, have an antibacterial spectrum similar to that of the sulfonamides, their chief usefulness is in the treatment of leprosy. Their action is probably similar to the sulfonamides; that is, they interfere with the nutrition of bacteria. They exert a bacteriostatic effect on *Mycobacterium leprae*, evidenced by the slow disappearance of the organisms from leprous lesions. The drugs bring about a suppression of the disease, prevent new lesions from appearing, promote the healing of many lesions, and allow the defense mechanisms of the body to keep the disease inactive. Their action is slow, and improvement may not be seen for several months. The clinical manifestations of leprosy can be suppressed by treatment extending over several years.

The sulfones in current use are synthetic compounds chemically related to the parent drug, diaminodiphenylsulfone. The latter substance was found to be an effective antibacterial agent, but because the effective dose produced toxic reactions, it was soon replaced by less toxic sulfones. The members of this group of drugs that have been studied most extensively are sulfoxone sodium, glucosulfone sodium, and thiazosulfone.

Absorption, distribution, metabolism, and excretion. All of the sulfones are well absorbed from the intestinal tract and are distributed widely in all tissues. These drugs tend to be retained in skin, muscle, liver, and kidney. Skin involved in leprosy contains ten times more of the drug than normal skin. The sulfones are excreted into the bile and reabsorbed by the intestine.

Preparation, dosage, and administration. The following are the preparations and dosages of sulfones.

Sulfoxone sodium, N.F. (Diasone). This compound is available in 330-mg. enteric-coated tablets for oral administration. The usual adult dose is 300 mg. daily, which is gradually increased to 900 mg. unless toxic symptoms occur.

Periodic rest periods are advocated. At least 6 months of treatment are required to evaluate therapeutic effects.

Sodium glucosulfone injection (Promin). This drug is available as a solution for intravenous injection (5 Gm. in 12.5 ml.). The intravenous dose is 2 to 5 Gm. given 6 days of each week. Periodic rest periods are recommended, but the treatment may continue over many months.

Dapsone, U.S.P., B.P. (Avlosulfon, DDS). This drug is the most widely used and least expensive sulfone. The initial dosage is 25 to 50 mg. twice weekly, increasing by 50 to 100 mg. every month until 200 to 400 mg. are given twice weekly.

Solapsone (Sulfetrone). This drug is a derivative of dapsone. It is administered initially in oral doses of 0.5 Gm. three times daily, the dose then being increased until a total daily dose of 6 to 10 Gm. is attained.

Side effects and toxic effects. Toxic reactions are related to the toxic reactions to the sulfonamides. Anorexia, nausea, and vomiting are common, and blood dyscrasias may occur.

URINARY TRACT ANTISEPTICS

Urinary tract antiseptics are drugs that exert antibacterial activity in the urine but have little or no systemic antibacterial effects. Their usefulness is limited to the treatment of urinary tract infections.

NITROFURANS

The nitrofurans are synthetic compounds that are bacteriostatic and bactericidal against a wide variety of gram-positive and gram-negative organisms, protozoa, and fungi. Other drugs used as urinary tract antiseptics are nalidixic acid, methenamine mandelate, and phenazopyridine hydrochloride.

Nitrofurantoin, U.S.P., B.P. (Furadantin, Macrodantin)

This is the main urinary antiseptic among the nitrofurans. It is rapidly and completely absorbed from the intestine. Blood concentrations achieved are low, but bactericidal concentrations are attained in the urine. Most organisms are sensitive to levels attained in the urine, with the exception of *Pseudomonas*. It is therapeutically used in pyelonephritis, pyelitis, and cystitis. While it is not the drug of first choice in the treatment of urinary tract infections, it is often valuable if other agents fail.

Hypersensitivity and gastrointestinal disturbances occur in a number of patients receiving nitrofurantoin. This drug will produce yellow-brown discoloration of the urine because of formation of inactive metabolites. It is available for oral and intravenous administration. The usual adult dose is 100 to 150 mg. four times daily.

Nitrofurazone, N.F. (Furacin)

This nitrofuran, which is related to nitrofurantoin, is an excellent agent for topical treatment of skin and wound infections. It has a broad bactericidal spectrum, but has little effect on *Pseudomonas*. It is effective in the presence of blood and pus, but is nontoxic to surface tissues and does not interfere with healing. It may produce sensitization in some patients. It is available as an ointment, powder, solution, cream, and as an impregnated gauze dressing.

OTHER URINARY TRACT ANTISEPTICS
Nalidixic acid, N.F. (NegGram)

Nalidixic acid is a urinary antiseptic chemically unrelated to other antimicrobial agents. It is a naphthyridine derivative that is active primarily against gram-negative organisms, except for *Pseudomonas*. Unlike many other drugs, it is active against infections caused by *Proteus* species. It is useful in treating acute and chronic urinary tract infections caused by sensitive bacteria. However, resistance develops frequently and rapidly. The incidence of toxicity is low, with nausea, vomiting, rashes, and urticaria most frequently reported. Occasional central nervous system disturbances have been reported, including headache, drowsiness, vertigo, visual disturbances, and convulsions in patients with preexisting convulsive disorders. Nalidixic acid is available in 250- and 500-mg. tablets. The recommended dosage is 4 Gm. daily in divided doses for 10 to 14 days. Nalidixic acid potentiates the anticoagulant effect of coumarin drugs, leading to an increase in prothrombin time.

Methenamine mandelate, U.S.P. (Mandelamine)

Methenamine mandelate combines the action of methenamine and mandelic acid and is used for treatment of urinary tract infections. Its effectiveness depends on the release of formaldehyde, which requires an acid medium. Thus it is ineffective if the urine is alkaline. Because of its fairly wide bacterial spectrum, its low toxicity, and low incidence of resistance, it is often the drug of choice in long-term suppression of infections. It is available for oral administration and is given four times daily in the average dose of 1 Gm. It should not be used with sulfona-

mides, since an insoluble precipitate forms in the urine.

Phenazopyridine hydrochloride, N.F. (Pyridium)

This drug is a synthetic azo dye that was once used as a urinary antiseptic, but is now used more frequently as a urinary tract analgesic. It is used in the treatment of cystitis accompanied by burning, urgency, and frequency. It is also useful in producing surface analgesia in urologic surgical procedures and after diagnostic tests necessitating instrumentation. It causes the urine to be orange or red in color, and patients should be informed of this so they do not become alarmed. It is available in 100-mg. tablets; 600 mg. is administered daily in divided doses.

TETRACYCLINES

The tetracyclines were introduced in 1948 and were the first truly broad-spectrum antibiotics. They include a large group of drugs with a common basic structure and chemical activity.

Mechanism of action. The most important mechanism of action of the tetracyclines is their blocking of the binding of the transfer RNA–amino acid complex to the ribosome. Thus no amino acid is available to the messenger RNA

Chlortetracycline

Oxytetracycline

Tetracycline

Demeclocycline

Formulas for the tetracyclines

and no polypeptides can be produced, thereby preventing protein synthesis. The tetracyclines are bacteriostatic for many gram-negative and gram-positive organisms, including anaerobes, and are strongly inhibitory for the growth of mycobacteria, rickettsiae, mycoplasmas, agents of the psittacosis–lymphogranuloma venereum–trachoma group, and some protozoa. *Proteus* and *Pseudomonas* are generally resistant. Complete cross-sensitivity and cross-resistance among all tetracyclines is the rule.

Absorption, distribution, metabolism, and excretion. The tetracyclines are readily but incompletely absorbed from the gastrointestinal tract. Their absorption is inhibited by food, milk, milk products, and by concurrent administration of antacids with aluminum, magnesium, or calcium bases. The tetracyclines are well distributed throughout the body with the exception of cerebrospinal fluid. They diffuse into brain, saliva, synovial tissues, placenta, and fetal tissues. They are readily bound to calcium deposited in newly forming bone and to certain malignant tissues. Because of their binding to newly formed bone and teeth, these drugs should not be administered during pregnancy or to small children. They are excreted in both urine and feces and also appear in the milk of lactating patients. Patients with impaired renal function require dose reduction in order to avoid serious side effects.

Clinical uses. Because of their broad spectrum, tetracyclines are most valuable in the treatment of mixed infections, such as chronic bronchitis and peritonitis. They are drugs of choice, however, for only a few bacterial infections: cholera, granuloma inguinale, chancroid, and gastrointestinal infection with *Bacteroides*. They are the best drugs for treatment of rickettsial disease such as Rocky Mountain spotted fever, Q fever, and typhus and are also effective in the treatment of psittacosis, lymphogranuloma venereum, trachoma, and inclusion conjunctivitis. Long-term therapy with the tetracyclines has been effective in decreasing the severity and frequency of febrile episodes in chronic bronchitis and bronchiectasis and in the treatment of acne vulgaris. In the latter, it is used in low doses daily for periods of months to years. It acts by excretion into the sebum, resulting in the reduction of the number and frequency of skin lesions.

Adverse effects and toxic effects. The tetracyclines are relatively nontoxic, the most common side effects being gastrointestinal disturbances, which are manifested by epigastric burning, nausea, vomiting, and diarrhea. Allergic reactions may be manifested as rash, urticaria, anaphylaxis, angioneurotic edema or simulated lupus erythematosus, but they are relatively rare. Phototoxicity may occur with the administration of demeclocycline. Large doses of these drugs (over 2 Gm. per day parenterally) may produce liver damage. Administration during pregnancy and in children under age 7 may produce discoloration of teeth and depression of bone growth. Superimposed infections, especially caused by *Monilia* and staphylococci, represent a serious hazard to patients receiving long-term therapy. The tetracyclines are also irritative when given intravenously and can cause thrombophlebitis.

Preparations available. The tetracycline family is represented by so many dosage forms for each member that a detailed description is not possible here. In general, when a tetracycline is indicated, an oral preparation should be used. Parenteral tetracyclines are available and should be used only for initial treatment of severe infections. Besides these major dosage forms, there are ophthalmic and otic solutions and ointments, powders, tablets, troches, vaginal tablets, and dental paste.

The tetracyclines may vary somewhat in the intensity of their action on different strains of bacteria, frequency of dose, absorption, and rate of excretion. Aside from these variations, the different tetracycline preparations do not vary significantly in clinical effectiveness.

Chlortetracycline and oxytetracycline were the first drugs of this class to be introduced. Newer drugs, such as demeclocycline, doxycycline, and minocycline, produce longer lasting antimicrobial activity and can be administered in lower and less frequent doses.

Tetracycline hydrochloride, U.S.P., B.P. (Achromycin, Panmycin, Tetracin). This drug is primarily excreted by the kidneys. The usual adult dose is 250 mg. every 6 hours.

Chlortetracycline hydrochloride, N.F., B.P. (Aureomycin). The usual adult dose is 250 mg. every 6 hours.

Oxytetracycline hydrochloride, U.S.P., B.P. (Terramycin). The usual adult dose is 250 mg. every 6 hours.

Demeclocycline, N.F., B.P. (Declomycin). The antibacterial potency of this drug is about twice that of the others. It produces blood levels of drug that are higher and more sustained than equal doses of the preceding tetracyclines. The usual adult dose is 100 to 300 mg. every 6 to 12 hours. This drug demonstrates a phototoxic effect that is much less common with other tetracyclines.

Doxycycline, U.S.P., B.P. (Vibramycin). Doxycycline is better absorbed than other tetracyclines when administered orally, and blood levels are sustained longer. This drug is excreted by the kidneys to a much lesser extent than are other tetracyclines and should be the drug of choice when it is necessary to administer a tetracycline to a patient with renal insufficiency. The usual adult dose is 50 to 100 mg. every 12 to 24 hours.

Minocycline, U.S.P. (Minocin). Minocycline, like doxycycline, is a long-lasting form of tetracycline. This drug is also excreted by the kidneys to a much lesser extent than other tetracyclines. The usual adult dosage is 50 to 100 mg. every 12 hours.

NURSING MANAGEMENT SPECIFIC TO ANTIMICROBIAL THERAPY WITH TETRACYCLINES

In addition to nursing measures common to all types of antimicrobial drug therapy, the nurse should observe the following measures when patients are receiving drugs of the tetracycline family:

1 The tetracyclines should not be administered together with milk, milk products, antacids, or iron preparations because they combine with metal ions to form nonabsorbable compounds.
2 Gastrointestinal side effects may be controlled by concurrent administration of food (not milk products).
3 The tetracyclines should not be administered to pregnant women or children under age 7 because

they can delay bone growth and produce discoloration of teeth.
4 Because the potential of superinfections is greater in tetracycline therapy than in therapy with other antimicrobial agents, patients should be observed carefully for signs and symptoms of secondary infections, especially monilial infections. Meticulous oral and perineal hygiene is helpful in preventing monilial superinfections.
5 Tetracyclines decompose with age, exposure to light, and when stored in extreme heat and humidity. Because the resulting products may be toxic, the nurse should store (or instruct the patient to store) these drugs properly. Manufacturers' expiration dates on tetracycline containers should be duly noted and outdated drugs discarded.
6 Patients receiving tetracyclines should be instructed to avoid intense exposure to sunlight or to artificial ultraviolet light.
7 Tetracyclines will delay blood coagulation.

AMINOGLYCOSIDES

The aminoglycosides are a group of drugs sharing chemical, antimicrobial, pharmacologic, and toxic characteristics. The drugs presently included in this category are streptomycin, kanamycin, gentamicin, neomycin, paromomycin, tobramycin, and spectinomycin. They especially share a common mechanism of action, metabolism, and toxicity. They differ in clinical uses.

Mechanism of action. The aminoglycosides act upon the bacterial ribosome to induce specific misreading of the genetic code. They are bactericidal against a wide range of gram-positive and gram-negative species and mycobacteria. Their widespread clinical use has resulted in some resistant strains, and these drugs manifest a high degree of cross-resistance.

Absorption, distribution, metabolism, and excretion. The aminoglycosides are generally poorly absorbed after oral administration, but are well absorbed following intramuscular injection. They are moderately well distributed except for the central nervous system. They do cross the placenta. Excretion is primarily by glomerular filtration. In the presence of renal damage, cumulation of the aminoglycosides to toxic levels can occur.

Adverse effects and toxic effects. All of the aminoglycosides have dose-related toxic effects and are ototoxic and nephrotoxic. They all damage both the vestibular and auditory branches of the eighth cranial nerve, resulting in deafness, vertigo, and loss of balance. Vestibular damage may be partially reversed after the drugs are discontinued, but auditory damage is often permanent and may progress even after discontinuation of the drug. Ototoxicity is more frequent in older patients and in patients with renal failure.

The nephrotoxicity of the aminoglycosides varies in degree according to the particular drug used. Neomycin is the most toxic; kanamycin is intermediate; streptomycin and gentamicin are generally mild. Nephrotoxicity is usually manifested by proteinuria and nonprotein nitrogen retention. Because of this nephrotoxic tendency, these drugs are not administered in combination and, if administered to patients with renal insufficiency, only in greatly modified doses.

Neuromuscular blockade leading to respiratory arrest has been observed with use of the aminoglycosides. It is particularly likely to occur in the presence of renal failure; when these drugs are used concurrently with neuromuscular blocking agents or anesthetic agents, such as ether, tubocurarine, succinylcholine, and decamethonium; and when these drugs are administered to patients with myasthenia gravis, rapidly injected intravenously, or applied directly to serosal surfaces. It can be reversed with neostigmine. Peripheral neuritis and allergic reactions are less common but do occur.

Streptomycin sulfate, U.S.P., B.P.

The isolation of streptomycin from *Streptomyces griseus* was reported in 1944. It was the first useful agent against a broad spectrum of gram-negative bacteria and mycobacteria, and it revolutionized the treatment of tuberculosis. Because of the rapid emergence of resistant bacterial strains, the use of streptomycin alone is rarely indicated. The majority of strains of certain gram-negative pathogens, such as *Proteus vulgaris*, *Pseudomonas aeruginosa*, and *Aerobacter aerogenes*, now being isolated in infections are streptomycin-resistant. In addition, many organisms, with the exception of the tubercle bacillus, that are sensitive to streptomycin are also sensitive to the tetracyclines. The latter are safer to use, and organisms usually do not acquire resistance to the tetracyclines as rapidly as they do to streptomycin. Therefore, it is recommended by many authorities that streptomycin be limited to the treatment of tuberculosis and to infections in which the bacteria are resistant to other, safer antibiotics but susceptible to streptomycin.

In the treatment of tuberculosis, streptomycin is used in combination with other tuberculostatic drugs such as para-aminosalicylic acid (PAS), isoniazid (INH), ethambutol, or rifampin. It is believed best not to give streptomycin and isoniazid together except in extreme need, so that resistance to both drugs will not develop at the same time, depriving the patient of the two most powerful antituberculosis drugs. To prevent toxicity during treatment of tuberculosis, the dosage of streptomycin is carefully regulated. The dosage schedule is adjusted according to the severity of the disease and the other drugs given.

One other important use of streptomycin has been as an adjunct to penicillin G in the treatment of subacute bacterial endocarditis caused by *Streptococcus faecalis*. Tularemia and the plague are among the few diseases for which the drug may be used alone with a high degree of specificity and effectiveness. Generally, the need for streptomycin in the therapy of other nontuberculous infections has decreased as other less toxic drugs have emerged, but for systemic infections, streptomycin may be given in doses of 0.5 to 1.0 Gm. two to four times daily.

Although streptomycin is usually administered by intermittent, deep intramuscular injection, it can be administered intravenously, and the intrathecal route may be used in patients with meningitis caused by organisms susceptible to streptomycin. Intramuscular administration of streptomycin commonly produces pain at the site of injection and may produce sterile abscesses.

Neomycin sulfate, U.S.P., B.P. (Myciguent)

Neomycin is an aminoglycoside antibiotic obtained from *Streptomyces fradiae*. It is severely toxic and rarely used parenterally. It has been used widely for topical therapy of skin infections, including burns, wounds, ulcers, and infected dermatoses, in the form of 0.5% ointment or solution. Oral administration of neomycin has been used in preoperative preparation of the bowel and in the treatment of hepatic coma for reduction of intestinal flora and subsequent decrease in blood ammonia levels. In the treatment of hepatic coma, a daily dosage of 4 to 8 Gm. can be administered in divided doses. When used as a bowel preparatory agent, the administration of neomycin in doses of 1 Gm. every 4 to 6 hours is combined with a low residue diet and cleansing enemas for 2 or 3 days preoperatively. Following oral administration, intestinal malabsorption with a sprue-like syndrome may occur. Absorption of neomycin into the blood stream may be facilitated in the presence of impaired gastrointestinal motility or mucosal ulceration, and prolonged topical application of the drug has also resulted in toxic effects.

Paromomycin sulfate, N.F. (Humatin)

Paromomycin has been used in place of neomycin in the treatment of hepatic coma and for preparation of the bowel preoperatively. It has also been effective in the treatment of bacillary dysentery. It is available in 250-mg. capsules and as a pediatric syrup.

Kanamycin sulfate, U.S.P., B.P. (Kantrex)

Kanamycin is an antibiotic derived from *Streptomyces kanamyceticus* that was first iso-

lated in 1957. It resembles neomycin and paromomycin but is slightly less toxic than neomycin. Presently it is the preferred drug for parenteral administration. It is of greatest usefulness in the treatment of systemic infections caused by gram-negative bacilli, except for *Salmonella typhosa* and *Pseudomonas*. It has been used in "sterilization" of the bowel prior to surgery. Like other aminoglycosides, kanamycin is quite toxic and it should not be used for treatment of infections known to be sensitive to less toxic drugs.

Gentamicin sulfate, U.S.P., B.P. (Garamycin)

Gentamicin is an aminoglycoside antibiotic derived from *Micromonospora purpura*. It was introduced in the early 1960s and possesses rapid bactericidal activity for many gram-positive and gram-negative bacteria.

Gentamicin has been very effective treatment for bacteremia with species of *Klebsiella*, *Enterobacter*, *E. coli*, and *Serratia*, and it has found great clinical usefulness in the treatment of infections caused by *Proteus* species and by *Pseudomonas*. In these severe infections, gentamicin is employed in doses of 2 to 3 mg. per kilogram per day intramuscularly in divided doses for 7 to 10 days. While it is effective against penicillin-resistant staphylococci, the semisynthetic penicillins and the cephalosporins are less toxic and remain the drugs of choice for these organisms. Gentamicin is available for intramuscular injection or as cream, ointment, or solution containing 0.1% to 0.3% gentamicin sulfate for treatment of infected burns, wounds, or skin lesions.

Tobramycin (Nebcin)

Tobramycin is a recently licensed aminoglycoside antibiotic that is similar to gentamicin but appears to have more marked anti-*Pseudomonas* activity.

Spectinomycin (Trobicin)

Spectinomycin is an aminoglycoside antibiotic elaborated by *Streptomyces spectabilis* and *Streptomyces flavopersicus*. It was marketed in 1971 with the sole therapeutic indication being the treatment of infections caused by *Neisseria gonorrhea*. It is largely bacteriostatic and quite effective in the treatment of uncomplicated gonorrhea, acute gonorrheal urethritis, and proctitis. It is given intramuscularly and offers the advantage over most other agents in that it is a single-dose treatment administered at the time of diagnosis. Spectinomycin has been used successfully in patients allergic or unresponsive to penicillin. The dose is 2 Gm. for males and 4 Gm. for females.

Cycloserine, U.S.P., B.P. (Oxamycin, Seromycin)

Cycloserine is an aminoglycoside antibiotic produced by *Streptomyces orchidaceus* that was isolated in 1955. It has been employed in the treatment of tuberculosis in conjunction with other tuberculostatic agents, but it is not as effective as INH or streptomycin. It is slowly but completely absorbed from the gastrointestinal tract and widely distributed throughout the body. It penetrates well into cerebrospinal fluid, passes through the placenta, and is secreted in the milk of lactating women. It is excreted in the urine. It is more toxic than other drugs used in the treatment of tuberculosis and may produce serious central nervous system toxicity manifested by somnolence, headache, tremor, vertigo, acute psychosis, and convulsions. Seizure precautions are advisable. Resistance to the drug develops rapidly. The usual adult dose is 10 mg. per kilogram of body weight given in two or three divided doses orally. It is supplied in 250-mg. capsules.

Viomycin sulfate, U.S.P., B.P.

Viomycin was isolated from *Streptomyces puniceus* in 1951. It inhibits the growth of a number of bacteria, but its use is confined to the treatment of tuberculosis when streptomycin and isoniazid resistance has occurred. Because absorption of viomycin from the gastrointestinal tract is limited, the drug is administered intramuscularly. Distribution to cerebrospinal fluid is poor. Viomycin toxicity is greater than that of streptomycin, manifesting itself in renal damage, electrolyte disturbances, and impaired vestibular function.

NURSING MEASURES SPECIFIC TO ANTIMICROBIAL THERAPY WITH THE AMINOGLYCOSIDES

Because the aminoglycosides exhibit characteristic toxicity, the nurse should make the following assessments of patients receiving these drugs:

1 Observe carefully for beginning signs and symptoms of toxicity to the eighth cranial nerve, such as tinnitus, vertigo, hearing loss, and ataxia.
2 Observe carefully for beginning signs and symptoms of nephrotoxicity. Intake and output should be monitored, and periodic urinalyses and renal function tests (e.g., creatinine clearance) may be necessary in long-term treatment.
3 The nurse should be alert to the neuromuscular blocking potential of the aminoglycosides, especially when these drugs are:
   a. Used concurrently with other neuromuscular blocking agents, such as muscle relaxants or sedatives
   b. Administered to patients with myasthenia gravis
   c. Injected rapidly into the venous system
   d. Applied to serosal surfaces
4 The toxic potential of the aminoglycosides is greater in the presence of renal impairment, prematurity, old age, and dehydration, and with simultaneous use of potent diuretics. Patients characterized by any of these factors should be observed carefully.

NONAMINOGLYCOSIDE TUBERCULOSTATIC DRUGS

The chemotherapy of tuberculosis requires a long course of treatment (12 to 36 months). This prolonged treatment presents several problems: (1) Drugs that are effective against the tubercle bacillus may produce serious toxic effects after prolonged administration. (2) The chance of emergence of drug-resistant organisms increases with the length of treatment. (3) Tubercle bacilli multiply in poorly vascularized caseous lesions that do not always receive high levels of the drugs. As a consequence, drug therapy may be complex. Drugs are often given initially in the highest tolerated dosages and in combination with other drugs in efforts to delay the emergence of resistance and to increase tuberculostatic effects. Dosage and time intervals between doses must be carefully regulated.

Streptomycin (p. 478) was the first antimicrobial drug to exhibit striking action against tubercle bacilli. It remains an important agent in the management of servere tuberculosis. Other important antituberculosis drugs include para-aminosalicylic acid, isoniazid, and ethambutol. In some instances, the use of a single drug is sufficient therapy; the drug then employed is usually isoniazid. Combination therapy is significantly more effective than the use of any single drug. For example, concurrent use of streptomycin, isoniazid, and ethambutol is more tuberculostatic than either agent alone and also decreases the emergence of resistance. Rifampin is a drug new to the United States market that also has been used successfully for primary treatment of tuberculosis.

If these drugs do not produce an effective therapeutic response, less common and generally more toxic drugs must be employed. These include the previously mentioned aminoglycosides, such as cycloserine, kanamycin, and viomycin.

Appropriate chemotherapy is the most important aspect of treatment in tuberculosis, but surgery and adjunctive measures may be necessary. Progress is evaluated by periodic examinations, x-rays, and sputum cultures.

Aminosalicylic acid, N.F. (para-aminosalicylic acid, PAS)

Para-aminosalicylic acid has some bacteriostatic activity against the tubercle bacillus, but is less potent than either streptomycin or isoniazid. The chief value of PAS lies in the fact that it apparently competes with isoniazid for acetylation in the liver, thereby establishing higher blood levels of isoniazid. It also acts to delay the emergence of bacterial resistance to both streptomycin and isoniazid, making it an important ancillary agent in the treatment of tuberculosis.

PAS is well absorbed from the gastrointestinal tract and diffuses rapidly into pleural fluids and into various tissues. It is excreted chiefly by way of the kidneys, although it is not effective in the treatment of tuberculosis of the urinary tract since it is subject to change in the liver, and the resulting metabolic products are therapeutically inactive.

Gastrointestinal intolerance to PAS with nausea, vomiting, anorexia, gaseous distention, and diarrhea occurs frequently and constitutes the principal toxic effect. It may be diminished by administering the drug with meals or antacids or by reducing drug dose. Allergic reactions often occur during PAS therapy, necessitating discontinuation of the drug either temporarily or permanently. Allergic reactions appear to be most common between the second and seventh weeks of treatment. Hematologic disturbances that have occurred during PAS treatment include leukopenia, agranulocytosis, eosinophilia, lymphocytosis, and thrombocytopenia.

PAS is available in 0.5-Gm. capsules, tablets, enteric-coated pills, as a syrup, and as a powder from which solutions can be made for use in cavities and sinuses. The drug should be used only when freshly prepared, and discolored preparations should be discarded. Solutions are stable for only 24 hours and only if stored in a dark place or in light-resistant containers and refrigerated. Usual adult dosage is 8 to 12 Gm. daily in divided doses.

Isoniazid, U.S.P., B.P. (INH, isonicotinic acid hydrazide)

Isoniazid, introduced in 1952, is the most potent tuberculostatic drug available presently, being superior to streptomycin. The mechanism of action of INH is not known. Isoniazid is readily absorbed after either oral or parenteral administration. It penetrates freely into cerebrospinal fluid and into caseous tissue. Metabolism of the drug varies, and two groups of people ("metabolizers") have been identified—the "slow" and the "rapid" inactivators of the drug. Isoniazid is excreted chiefly by the kidneys.

The most common and important toxic effects of isoniazid are manifested by disturbances of the peripheral and central nervous systems. Peripheral neuritis is probably a result of pyridoxine deficiency, since it can be controlled by daily administration of the vitamin. "Slow" metabolizers tend to develop polyneuritis more often that "rapid" metabolizers. Headache and vertigo have been reported and large doses of isoniazid have been known to provoke convulsions in patients with preexisting seizure disorders. Other side effects include gastrointestinal dysfunction, allergic reactions, and hepatic dysfunction.

The present trend in the treatment of tuberculosis is the simultaneous use of INH with either PAS, ethambutol, or streptomycin.

Isoniazid is available for oral and parenteral administration. Usually 2 to 8 mg. per kilogram of body weight is administered twice daily, but higher doses are necessary for the treatment of miliary tuberculosis and tuberculous meningitis. The dose should be determined by 6-hour serum drug levels and adjusted accordingly. Pyridoxine in doses of 50 to 100 mg. also may be administered daily to prevent peripheral neuritis.

Ethambutol, U.S.P., B.P. (Myambutol)

$$H-\underset{\underset{C_2H_5}{|}}{\overset{\overset{CH_2OH}{|}}{C}}-NH-(CH_2)_2-HN-\underset{\underset{CH_2OH}{|}}{\overset{\overset{C_2H_5}{|}}{C}}-H$$

Ethambutol is a tuberculostatic drug introduced in the early 1960's that has been used with considerable success in the management of treatment failures. It has been so successful that it is now also being used for primary treatment.

Ethambutol is well absorbed from the gastrointestinal tract. It is better tolerated than PAS and causes less toxicity. Like PAS, when given in conjunction with other tuberculostatic agents, it acts to delay the emergence of resistance. Mycobacterial resistance to ethambutol emerges fairly rapidly when the drug is used alone, and the drug is best administered in combination with other drugs, most commonly INH. The chief toxic effect of ethambutol is retrobulbar neuritis with loss of visual acuity and disturbances in color discrimination. A decrease in the ability to perceive red and green colors is an early sign of toxicity. Discontinuation of the drug usually results in complete recovery. Ethambutol is available in 100- and 400-mg. tablets. The usual adult dose is 15 to 25 mg. per kilogram of body weight, administered once a day.

Pyrazinamide, U.S.P., B.P. (PZA)

This is a synthetic drug made from nicotinamide. It is less effective than streptomycin and isoniazid but more effective than cycloserine and viomycin. It is considered an effective drug, especially when given with isoniazid for short-term therapy, such as that which precedes surgery of patients in whom the causative organism is resistant to other drugs. Tubercle bacilli develop resistance to the drug relatively quickly. It is available in 500-mg. tablets for oral administration. A dose of 1.5 to 2 Gm. daily (after meals) in two or three equally divided portions is recommended.

Hepatic toxicity is the most common untoward effect. All patients being treated with pyrazinamide should have hepatic function studies performed prior to and periodically during treatment. If hepatic dysfunction becomes apparent, the drug must be discontinued.

Rifampin, U.S.P.

Rifampin is a semisynthetic derivative of rifomycin, an antibiotic produced by *Streptomyces mediterranei*. It is the most important of the rifomycins and has been available in the United States since 1971. Rifampin is active against many gram-negative and gram-positive bacteria, as well as *Mycobacterium tuberculosis* and other mycobacteria. It acts by inhibiting RNA synthesis in bacteria and chlamydiae. It has been used mainly in the treatment of tuberculosis. It is administered in conjunction with other tuberculostatic drugs and has given results comparable to those obtained with INH and streptomycin. A number of patients in whom other therapy has failed have been treated successfully with rifampin and ethambutol.

Rifampin is well absorbed from the gastrointestinal tract although the presence of food in the stomach appears to delay its absorption. It is well distributed throughout the body. It has been found in cerebrospinal fluid and diffuses into milk and saliva. It is eliminated primarily in the bile. Toxic effects of rifampin are unusual. Some gastrointestinal disturbances have been reported, as well as liver dysfunction, blood abnormalities, and a "flu-like" syndrome that occurs when administration of the drug is stopped and then resumed. Rifampin may produce a harmless reddish color of the urine, sputum, and lacrimal fluid. Administration during pregnancy and in infancy is not recommended.

Rifampin must be used in combination with other tuberculostatic drugs. It is administered orally in a single daily dose of 8 to 12 mg. per kilogram of body weight.

CHEMOPROPHYLAXIS OF TUBERCULOSIS

Some patients require antituberculosis drug therapy despite the absence of clinical symptoms or positive sputum cultures. Patients who have a positive tuberculin test or have recently converted to PPD-positive and who are under 20 years of age, in contact with patients with active tuberculosis, or have diseases such as leukemia, silicosis, measles, or diabetes mellitus should receive prophylactic treatment. The drug most commonly used in chemoprophylaxis of tuberculosis is isoniazid.

NURSING MEASURES SPECIFIC TO ANTIMICROBIAL THERAPY WITH NONAMINOGLYCOSIDE TUBERCULOSTATIC AGENTS

1 The nurse should attempt to administer these drugs with consideration of the patient's comfort. For example, gastrointestinal disturbances following administration of PAS can be reduced by concurrent administration of food or antacids.

2 It is imperative that patients take prescribed medications regularly and without interruption. If the patient is responsible for self-medication, he should be instructed about the necessity to take these drugs according to the prescribed regimen, and not to discontinue them when he feels better.

3 Patients responsible for self-medication also should be instructed about the necessity for periodic medical evaluations.

4 Because of the long-term nature of drug therapy in tuberculosis, patients may need support in maintaining the therapeutic regimen and in tolerating side effects of the tuberculostatic drugs.

THE MACROLIDES

The macrolide antibiotics are a large group of substances that were introduced in the early 1950's. They are bacteriostatic by virtue of inhibiting protein synthesis, but they may also be bactericidal in high concentrations. The macrolides are effective against gram-positive cocci, especially pneumococci, streptococci, staphylococci, and *Corynebacteria. Neisseriae, Hemophilus*, and *Mycoplasma* are also susceptible to the macrolides.

The most important of the macrolide antimicrobial drugs is erythromycin. Others that are available for clinical use are oleandomycin, spiramycin, and carbomycin. Only erythromycin, oleandomycin, and troleandomycin will be considered here.

Erythromycin, U.S.P., B.P. (Ilotycin, Erythrocin); erythromycin estolate, N.F., B.P. (Ilosone); erythromycin stearate, U.S.P., B.P. (Erythrocin); erythromycin lactobionate, U.S.P.

Erythromycin is an antibiotic obtained from *Streptomyces erythreus*.

Absorption, distribution, metabolism, and excretion. Erythromycin is readily absorbed from the gastrointestinal tract. Because it has a bitter taste and is destroyed by gastric acid, it is administered in enteric-coated tablets or in the form of insoluble preparations that are slowly hydrolyzed. It diffuses through most of the body but is not found in appreciable amounts in the cerebrospinal fluid. It passes from the maternal blood to the fetus in amounts sufficient to be antibacterial. It is concentrated in the liver and excreted in the bile and urine.

Clinical uses. Erythromycin is probably the drug of choice in some *Corynebacteria* infections, such as erythrasma and diphtheria, and in disease caused by *Mycoplasma pneumoniae.* The effectiveness of erythromycin in the treatment of infections caused by group A, beta-hemolytic streptococcus also has been firmly established. Otherwise, it is most useful as a penicillin substitute in persons allergic to penicillin. Unfortunately, staphylococci develop resistance to erythromycin rapidly and penicillin-resistant strains also are often erythromycin resistant.

Adverse effects and toxic effects. Erythromycin administration is accompanied by relatively few adverse reactions. The most frequently encountered adverse effect is gastrointestinal disturbance with nausea, vomiting, and diarrhea. Allergic reactions may occur. Hepatotoxicity in the form of cholestatic hepatitis has occurred with erythromycin estolate and with troleandomycin.

Preparations. Erythromycin is available for oral, topical, intramuscular, and intravenous use in a wide variety of commercial preparations. The usual adult dose of any of the forms of erythromycin is 250 to 500 mg. every 6 hours.

Oleandomycin phosphate (Matromycin); troleandomycin (Cyclamycin, TAO)

Oleandomycin is a macrolide antibiotic produced by *Streptomyces antibioticus.* It has been shown to be effective against much the same spectrum of organisms as erythromycin. Troleandomycin is a derivative of oleandomycin, differing from the parent compound in that it is more active after oral administration because of better absorption from the gastrointestinal tract. Adverse reactions to these drugs include hepatic changes. The most common adverse reactions are hypersensitivity and gastrointestinal upset. In clinical practice, the oleandomycins have limited usefulness. Indications for their use are essentially the same as for erythromycin and they seem to offer no special advantages. Usual adult doses are 250 to 500 mg. four times daily.

POLYMYXINS

The polymyxins are a small group of antimicrobial agents discovered in 1947. All but two of the original polymyxins have been discarded from clinical use because of excessive nephrotoxicity. Polymyxin B sulfate and polymyxin E sulfate (colistin) are the agents currently available for clinical use.

Mechanism of action. Polymyxins act by disrupting the cytoplasmic membrane by a detergent-like effect, thereby causing immediate cell death. They are bactericidal for many gram-negative bacteria including most *Pseudomonas* species and *E. coli*, as well as many *Klebsiella, Enterobacter, Salmonella, Shigella,* and *Hemophilus* species.

Absorption, distribution, metabolism, and excretion. The polymyxins are not absorbed after oral administration. If administered orally, the drugs exert their antibacterial effects in the lumen of the bowel and are then excreted in the feces. Parenterally injected polymyxins do not diffuse into cerebrospinal fluid. The polymyxins are strongly protein-bound and also strongly bound by cell debris, acid phospholipids, and purulent exudates. The drugs are excreted by the kidneys.

Clinical uses. Since other antibiotics have been developed that are either more potent or less toxic than the polymyxins, these drugs are not drugs of choice now for the treatment of any systemic infection. The polymyxins are often used in the treatment of *Pseudomonas* infections resistant to other antimicrobial drugs. They have also been effective in the treatment of urinary tract infections caused by *Pseudomonas* or other gramnegative bacilli. Infections of the skin, mucous membranes, eye, and ear due to polymyxin-sensitive organisms have responded well. The drugs have been used to suppress *Shigella* in bacillary dysentery and other gram-negative members of bacterial flora.

Adverse effects and toxic effects. The most serious toxic effects of the polymyxins include renal damage, peripheral neuropathy, and respiratory arrest. Nephrotoxicity is manifest in proteinuria and hematuria. Neurotoxic effects include paresthesias, vertigo, flushing, and incoordination. All of these signs and symptoms usually disappear when the drugs are discontinued and are excreted. Respiratory arrest has occurred after administration of polymyxins to patients receiving anesthetics or muscle relaxants and to patients with myasthenia gravis. The drugs should be administered parenterally only to hospitalized patients.

Preparation, dosage, and administration

Polymyxin B sulfate, U.S.P., B.P. (Aerosporin Sulfate). This drug is available as a topical powder, an otic solution, as tablets, and in vials for parenteral use. When given intramuscularly, the drug is routinely mixed with procaine hydrochloride to decrease pain accompanying the injection. The total daily intramuscular dosage is 1.5 to 2.5 mg. per kilogram of body weight injected in divided doses.

Colistin sulfate, U.S.P. (Coly-Mycin Sulfate); *colistimethate sodium*, U.S.P. (Coly-Mycin Injectable). This drug is marketed for oral and parenteral use. Unlike polymyxin B, colistin cannot be administered intraspinally or intravenously unless special preparations are used. It may be given in doses varying from 2 to 5 mg. per kilogram per day for adults.

CHLORAMPHENICOL
Chloramphenicol, U.S.P., B.P. (Chloromycetin)

$$O_2N - \left\langle \bigcirc \right\rangle - \underset{\underset{H}{|}}{\overset{\overset{OH}{|}}{C}} - \underset{\underset{H}{|}}{\overset{\overset{CH_2OH}{|}}{C}} - \underset{\underset{H}{|}}{\overset{}{N}} - \overset{\overset{O}{\|}}{C} - CHCl_2$$

Chloramphenicol is an antimicrobial agent derived from *Streptomyces venezuelae* in 1947. It is a potent inhibitor of protein synthesis and is bacteriostatic for a wide variety of gram-negative and gram-positive organisms as well as rickettsiae.

Absorption, distribution, metabolism, and excretion. Chloramphenicol is readily absorbed from the gastrointestinal tract. It is widely distributed throughout the body, diffusing into cerebrospinal fluid and passing the placental barrier. It is bound to plasma albumin and rapidly excreted by the liver and kidneys.

Clinical uses. Because of its broad spectrum and apparent lack of toxicity, chloramphenicol

was widely used between 1948 and 1951 before its serious toxicity was documented. In spite of its significant therapeutic effectiveness, controversy now exists regarding the use of chloramphenicol because of its infrequent but severe hematologic side effects. It is now possibly the drug of choice for only a few types of infections: (1) typhoid fever and other salmonelloses, (2) occasional bacteremia caused by gram-negative bacteria expected to be resistant to other drugs, and (3) severe rickettsial infections. The drug should be used primarily for hospitalized patients, and therapy must be stopped at the first sign of adverse reaction.

Adverse effects and toxic effects. The most important toxic effect of chloramphenicol is the occurrence of blood dyscrasias, most notably bone marrow depression, anemia, and leukopenia. Aplastic anemia that may be irreversible and fatal has been known to occur with the use of this drug. Frequent periodic blood counts must be performed during chloramphenicol therapy, and the drug must be discontinued if agranulocytosis, leukopenia, or thrombocytopenia appear. In newborn infants, chloramphenicol toxicity may be manifest as the "gray baby" syndrome. This often fatal syndrome consists of vasomotor collapse, hypothermia, rapid and irregular respirations, diarrhea, and an ashen gray color. Other toxic effects include gastrointestinal disturbances and optic neuritis.

Preparation and dosage. Chloramphenicol may be administered orally, intramuscularly, intravenously, as an ophthalmic ointment, and as an otic solution. The usual adult dose is 2 to 4 Gm. daily.

SPECIALIZED ANTIMICROBIAL DRUGS AGAINST GRAM-POSITIVE BACTERIA
Bacitracin, U.S.P., B.P. (Baciguent)

Bacitracin is produced by culture of *Bacillus subtilis* and is bactericidal against gram-positive cocci, corynebacteria, neisseriae, *Treponema pallidum*, and clostridia. It exerts its bactericidal effects by interference with cell wall synthesis.

This drug was once an important agent in the systemic treatment of penicillin-resistant staphylococcal infections but is now primarily used for the topical treatment of infections of the skin and wounds and of suppurative conjunctivitis. Systemic use of bacitracin is associated with marked nephrotoxicity.

Bacitracin is not absorbed from the gastrointestinal tract and must be administered topically or intramuscularly. For topical administration, it is frequently combined with polymyxin, neomycin, or both. The drug is available as an ointment in doses of 500 units per gram or as a sterile powder in doses of 10,000 units per vial.

Lincomycin hydrochloride, U.S.P., B.P. (Lincocin); clindamycin hydrochloride, U.S.P. (Cleocin)

Lincomycin

Lincomycin is an antibiotic produced by *Streptomyces lincolnensis* that was made available in the early 1960's. It is principally bacteriostatic and exerts its action by inhibiting protein synthesis in sensitive bacteria. Its antibacterial spectrum and pharmacologic properties are similar to those of erythromycin, but its chemical structure is different. The antibacterial spectrum of this drug includes most gram-positive cocci.

Clindamycin is a derivative of lincomycin that offers the advantage of more complete and predictable absorption from the gastrointestinal tract and is said to cause severe diarrhea less frequently.

Lincomycin has been used successfully in the treatment of a variety of ear, nose, throat, respiratory, dental, skin and soft tissue, bone and joint, and septicemic infections caused by streptococci, staphylococci, and pneumococci. It is useful primarily as an alternative antibiotic choice to the penicillins and cephalosporins.

Lincomycin produces few adverse effects, with diarrhea appearing to be the most frequent

after oral dosage. Allergy is not common. Superinfections in the intestinal tract may occur. Cardiopulmonary arrest after rapid intravenous injection has been reported.

The recommended adult oral dose of lincomycin is 500 mg. every 6 or 8 hours. Lincomycin may also be administered intramuscularly or intravenously. Clindamycin is available for oral administration; recommended dosage is 0.15 to 0.3 Gm. every 6 hours.

Sterile vancomycin hydrochloride, U.S.P., B.P. (Vancocin)

Vancomycin, discovered in 1956, is produced by *Streptomyces orientalis*. It is not related to any other antimicrobial agent and its exact structural formula is not known. Vancomycin is bactericidal for many gram-positive bacteria by virtue of inhibiting bacterial cell wall synthesis. It is not absorbed from the gastrointestinal tract and must be administered intravenously because intramuscular injection is painful. It is widely distributed in the tissues and excreted primarily through the kidneys. If renal function is impaired, vancomycin may accumulate, with increased risk of toxicity.

The drug possesses significant ototoxicity and nephrotoxicity and may also produce allergic reactions. It is highly irritating to tissues and may result in pain and thrombophlebitis after intravenous injection. Because other less toxic drugs are available, the principal clinical indication for the use of vancomycin is in treatment of serious gram-positive infections in which other drugs cannot be given. Vancomycin can be very useful in the treatment of serious staphylococcal infection or enterococcal endocarditis not responding to other treatment. For staphylococcal enterocolitis, 3 to 4 Gm. are administered orally daily. For staphylococcal septicemia, 0.5 Gm. is injected intravenously over a period of 20 to 30 minutes every 6 to 8 hours in adults.

Fusidic acid

Fusidic acid was isolated in 1962 from *Fusidium coccineum.* It is mainly bactericidal, exerting its effects by inhibition of bacterial protein synthesis.

The main importance of fusidic acid is in its

Table 20-5 Summary of some major allergic and toxic effects of antimicrobial agents

Anaphylaxis	Hematologic effects	Nephrotoxicity	Injury to eighth cranial nerve	Potential of neuromuscular blockade
Penicillin	Chloramphenicol (low incidence but high mortality) Sulfonamides (low incidence)	Polymyxins Aminoglycosides Sulfonamides (low incidence with newer drugs)	Aminoglycosides	Polymyxins Aminoglycosides

use against *Staphylococcus aureus,* and its chief clinical use is in the treatment of severe or fulminating staphylococcal infections or in persistent infections in which other treatment has failed. The therapeutic response to fusidic acid is dramatic and the drug should be reserved for such use.

Fusidic acid produces irritation and necrosis of tissue when administered intramuscularly or subcutaneously. It also may cause hemolysis, venous spasm, and thrombosis when administered intravenously. It is normally administered orally in recommended daily doses of 1.5 to 3 Gm. for adults. To date, few side effects have been reported, especially when the drug is used orally.

Antiviral chemotherapy

The chemotherapy of viral diseases has been more limited than the chemotherapy of bacterial diseases, with only two antiviral agents licensed for clinical use in 1974.

Development and clinical application of antiviral drugs is difficult. In many viral infections, the replication of the virus in the body reaches its peak before any clinical symptoms appear. By the time signs and symptoms of illness appear, the multiplication of the virus is ending and the subsequent course of the illness has been determined already. In order to be clinically effective, therefore, antiviral drugs would have to be administered in a chemoprophylactic manner, that is, prior to the appearance of disease. A second factor limiting the development of antiviral drugs is that viruses are true parasites; they replicate within the mammalian cell and utilize the host cell's enzyme systems. Thus drugs that would inhibit virus replication would also disturb the host cells and, therefore, would be too toxic for use.

Amantadine hydrochloride, N.F. (Symmetrel)

Amantadine is a synthetic agent introduced in the middle 1960's that is the only antiviral drug in common use. It exerts a prophylactic action on certain myxoviruses (influenza A, rubella, and some tumor viruses) by inhibiting their penetration into susceptible host cells. The drug is well absorbed from the gastrointestinal tract and is excreted in the urine. The only clinical use of amantadine is for the prevention of A2 influenza. Its use is recommended in the presence of a documented influenza A2 epidemic, especially to high risk patients.

The most marked untoward side effects are central nervous system disturbances and include hyperexcitability, insomnia, slurred speech, vertigo, and ataxia. Doses higher than those recommended may produce convulsions. The drug should be administered cautiously to patients with any disease affecting the central nervous system and should not be administered to pregnant women. The recommended daily dosage for adults is 200 mg. in divided doses.

Idoxuridine, U.S.P., B.P. (Dendrid, Herplex, Stoxil)

Idoxuridine inhibits the replication of certain viruses, probably by inhibiting synthesis of DNA. It has been used primarily in the treatment of herpes simplex keratitis and is available as a 0.1% solution or ointment. One drop should be instilled into the conjunctival sac every hour during the day and every 2 hours during the night, until definite improvement is noted, after which the dose can be decreased. The ointment should be applied every 4 hours during the day.

Immune human serum globulin, U.S.P. (gamma globulin)

When gamma globulin contains specific antibodies directed at antigens of a specific virus, it can interfere with viral penetration into the host cell. The intramuscular injection of pooled gamma globulin, if administered during the early incubation period, may modify infections caused by the viruses of measles, hepatitis, rabies, and poliomyelitis. The usual dose is 0.02 to 0.1 ml per pound of body weight. The prophylactic effect of a gamma globulin injection lasts 2 to 3 weeks, and injection may have to be repeated for infections with prolonged incubation periods.

Antifungal chemotherapy

Antifungal chemotherapy, like antiviral chemotherapy, has not developed to the same degree as has antibacterial chemotherapy. Most fungi are completely resistant to the action of chemicals at concentrations that can be tolerated by the host, and only a few antifungal compounds are currently available for use.

Amphotericin B, U.S.P., B.P. (Fungizone)

Amphotericin B is an antibiotic agent derived from *Streptomyces nodosus* in 1956. It is used in the treatment of disseminated mycotic infections, including coccidioidomycosis, cryptococcosis, disseminated moniliasis, histoplasmosis, and North American blastomycosis. The antibiotic is both fungistatic and fungicidal and has no effect on bacteria or viruses. It is the only effective drug for the treatment of deep fungal disease.

Very little amphotericin B is absorbed following oral, subcutaneous, or intramuscular administration. An oral tablet containing 250 mg. of amphotericin B is designed for treatment of candidal enteritis and as concurrent therapy in the local treatment of vaginal candidiasis. The drug is usually administered by the intravenous route and the dose increased in small increments until a total daily dose of 1 mg. per kilogram of body weight is attained. Intravenous injection usually produces chills, fever, vomiting, and headache. These side effects may be minimized by reducing dosage temporarily, administering corticosteroids, or discontinuing the drug for several days.

Therapeutic doses of amphotericin B also produce hepatic and renal dysfunction and may result in anemia. Shock-like hypotension, electrolyte disturbances, and a variety of neurologic symptoms may also occur.

All patients receiving amphotericin B must be hospitalized, and renal and hepatic function tests must be performed frequently during therapy with the drug.

Nursing measures. Amphotericin B should not be used if there is any evidence of precipitate or foreign matter in the vial. It should not be mixed with any other drug unless absolutely necessary. Administration of the drug on alternate days may reduce the incidence of some side effects. Frequent renal function tests, blood counts, and electrolyte levels are necessary during therapy.

Griseofulvin, U.S.P., B.P. (Fulvicin, Grifulvin)

Griseofulvin is a fungistatic agent obtained from *Penicillium griseofulvum.* It inhibits the growth of dermatophytes, including *Epidermophyton, Microsporum,* and *Trichophyton.* It is used in the treatment of mycotic disease of the skin, hair, and nails.

After absorption following oral administration, griseofulvin is bound to keratin and deposited in diseased epidermis, hair, and nails. The infected fungus is not killed, but its growth into new cells is prevented. As the keratinized structures are shed, they tend to be replaced by normal, uninfected ones. The drug is absorbed when taken with a high-fat meal and when taken in the ultra-fine particle form. It is poorly distributed to other tissues, and the bulk of orally ingested griseofulvin is eliminated unchanged in the feces. The drug is more effective for chronic fungal infections. It is not recommended for deep or systemic fungal infections.

The incidence of toxic effects associated with the administration of griseofulvin is relatively low. Hepatotoxicity, photosensitivity, and mental and neurologic difficulties have been reported. Headache may be severe at the beginning of therapy, but usually abates. Leukopenia may occur, but reverses itself as therapy is continued.

Griseofulvin is administered in dosages of 1 to 2 Gm. per day for the regular preparation or 0.75 Gm. per day for the micronized preparation. Its absorption is enhanced by concurrent administration of milk and other fatty foods. The duration of treatment is determined by the rate of complete turnover of the cells in the infected area.

Concurrent administration of phenobarbital reduces the effectiveness of griseofulvin. Griseofulvin interferes with the effectiveness of coumarin anticoagulant therapy and may precipitate acute porphyria.

Nursing measures. Because treatment with griseofulvin may last several months, and because symptoms may abate soon, the patient needs to be taught the importance of adhering to the prescribed dosage schedule. Frequent shampoos and clipping of the hair and nails will support the therapeutic effect of the drug. Frequent blood counts during therapy may be necessary to monitor leukopenia, periodic renal and hepatic function tests also may be ordered.

Nystatin, U.S.P., B.P. (Mycostatin)

Nystatin is an antibiotic obtained from *Streptomyces noursei* that is primarily useful in the treatment of infections caused by the monilial organism *Candida albicans.* It is administered topically in creams, powders, and ointments that contain 100,000 units of nystatin per gram and is also available in suppository form. Nystatin may be administered orally for the suppression of *Candida* of the bowel, especially during tetracycline administration. Untoward effects of nystatin are not common. Mild gastrointestinal discomfort may occur after oral administration.

Nursing measures. Unused portions of nystatin should be preserved in light-resistant containers.

Flucytosine, U.S.P. (5-fluorocytosine)

Flucytosine is a recently introduced antifungal substance that is effective against a number of yeasts and yeast-like organisms, especially *Cryptococcus neoformans* and *Candida albicans.* It is fungistatic and slowly fungicidal. It has been used in the treatment of meningitis caused by *Cryptococcus* and of systemic infections caused by *Candida.*

Flucytosine is well absorbed from the gastrointestinal tract and diffuses into cerebrospinal fluid. It is generally well tolerated, although abdominal bloating and diarrhea have been noted. Other side effects need more documentation. The recommended daily adult dose is 150 mg. per kilogram of body weight in four equally divided doses.

QUESTIONS

For study and review

1 Identify the goal of chemotherapy of infectious diseases.
2 Differentiate between "antibiotic" and "antimicrobial" agent.
3 Differentiate between "bacteriostatic" and "bactericidal" drug effects.

4 Describe the four major ways in which antimicrobial drugs act.

5 Identify and describe the three major adverse effects common to all types of antimicrobial drug therapy.

6 Identify the four major principles of antimicrobial therapy.

7 Why should the nurse assure that specimens for culture and sensitivity testing are taken before the patient receives his first dose of an antimicrobial drug?

8 Describe several nursing measures that may be taken to prevent allergic reactions to antimicrobial drugs.

9 Identify the seven major categories of antibacterial drugs discussed in this chapter.

10 What is the antibacterial spectrum of the penicillins?

11 What is the role of probenecid (Benemid) in drug therapy with the penicillins?

12 Identify the major clinical uses of the penicillins.

13 Identify the three major disadvantages of the penicillins that are not direct toxic effects of the drugs.

14 What are the advantages of the newer semisynthetic penicillins?

15 What is the major clinical use of methicillin?

16 What are the advantages and disadvantages of penicillin G benzathine (Bicillin)?

17 What advantage do the cephalosporins offer over the penicillins?

18 Name the cephalosporins currently in use.

19 Why should the nurse administer the penicillins at a time when they are not preceded or followed by food for at least one hour?

20 How do the sulfonamides differ from the penicillins in regard to their origin and to their antibacterial effects?

21 Describe the mechanism of action of the sulfonamides.

22 What are the major clinical uses of the sulfonamides?

23 What are the major adverse effects and toxic effects of the sulfonamides?

24 Why are patients who are going to have intestinal surgery sometimes treated with sulfonamides preoperatively and postoperatively? Why might vitamin K be administered together with these drugs?

25 What is the advantage of the trisulfapyrimidines?

26 What precautions should the nurse take in regard to the potential renal toxicity of the sulfonamides?

27 Name a specific sulfa preparation used for each of the following conditions:
a. urinary tract infection
b. preoperative bowel preparation
c. meningitis
d. bacillary dysentery

28 Define the term "urinary antiseptic" and name several drugs belonging to this category.

29 What is the anti-bacterial spectrum of the tetracyclines?

30 For what clinical conditions are the tetracyclines currently drugs of choice?

31 Why is the administration of tetracyclines contraindicated during pregnancy and for children under the age of 7?

32 What are the major adverse effects and toxic effects of the tetracyclines?

33 Why should the nurse remember not to administer the tetracyclines together with milk or antacids?

34 Identify the seven drugs included in the aminoglycoside antimicrobial drug category.

35 What are the three major toxic effects of the aminoglycosides?

36 Identify the major clinical uses of the aminoglycosides.

37 What is the major clinical use of spectinomycin?

38 Describe the three major problems attendant to chemotherapy of tuberculosis.

39 Name several nonaminoglycoside drugs used in the therapy of tuberculosis.

40 What is the major function of PAS in the chemotherapy of tuberculosis?

41 What is the major function of INH in the chemotherapy of tuberculosis?

42 What are the most common toxic effects of INH and how are they treated?

43 Why is the chemotherapy of tuberculosis characterized by the concurrent use of several drugs?

44 What is the major function of ethambutol in the chemotherapy of tuberculosis?

45 What is the chief toxic effect of ethambutol?

46 In what kinds of situations should the nurse be especially alert for the neuromuscular blockade potential of the aminoglycosides?

47 Identify the major clinical indications for the use of the macrolide antimicrobial drugs.

48 Identify the two drugs of the polymyxin category that are currently in clinical use.

49 What are the principal toxic effects of the polymyxins?

50 What are the current clinical uses of the polymyxins?

51 Why is chloramphenicol no longer a widely used antibiotic?

52 For what clinical conditions does chloramphenicol remain a drug of choice?

53 Describe the major factors that have limited the development of antiviral chemotherapy.

54 Identify the two antiviral drugs currently available and name their therapeutic uses.

55 What are the clinical uses of amphotericin B?

56 What are the primary clinical uses of griseofulvin?

57 What is the primary clinical indication for the use of nystatin?

REFERENCES

General references

Barker, B. M. and Prescott, F.: Antimicrobial agents in medicine, Oxford, 1973, Blackwell Scientific Publications.

Caldwell, J. R., and Cluff, L. E.: The real and present danger of antibiotics, Rational Drug Ther. 7:1, 1973.

DiPalma, J. R., editor: Drill's pharmacology in medicine, ed. 4, New York, 1971, The McGraw-Hill Book Company.

Garrod, L. P., and O'Grady, F.: Antibiotic and chemotherapy, ed. 3, Baltimore, 1971, The Williams & Wilkins Company.

Goodman, L. S., and Gilman, A.: The pharmacological basis

of therapeutics, ed. 5, New York, 1975, The Macmillan Company.

Kagan, B. M., editor: Antimicrobial therapy, ed. 2, Philadelphia, 1974, W. B. Saunders Co.

Melmon, K. L., and Morelli, H. F., editors: Clinical pharmacology: Basic principles in therapeutics, New York, 1972, The Macmillan Company.

Meyers, F. H., Jawetz, E., and Goldfein, A.: Review of medical pharmacology, ed. 3, Los Altos, Calif., 1972, Lange Medical Publications.

Pittinger, C. B., and Adamson, R.: Antibiotic blockade of neuromuscular function, Ann. Rev. Pharmacol. **12:**169, 1972.

Pratt, W. B.: Fundamentals of chemotherapy, New York, 1973, Oxford University Press.

Rosenfeld, M. G., editor: Manual of medical therapeutics, ed. 20, Boston, 1971, Little, Brown & Co.

Seneca, H.: Biological basis of chemotherapy of infections and infestations, Philadelphia, 1971, F. A. Davis Co.

Tolhurst, J. C., Buckle, G., and Williams, S. W.: Chemotherapy with antibiotics and allied drugs, Canberra, 1972, Australian Government Publishing Service.

Penicillins and cephalosporins

Benner, E. J., Lewis, A. A. G., and Waife, S. O., editors: Cephalosporin antibiotics, Postgrad. Med. J. **47**(Suppl.):5, 1971.

Dillon, M. L., Bowling, K. A., and Postlethwait, R. W.: Cephaloridine therapy in patients with surgical infections, Surg. Gynecol. Obstet. **134:**83, 1972.

Fishman, L. S., and Hewitt, W. L.: The natural penicillins, Med. Clin. North Am. **54:**1081, 1970.

Gilbert, D. N., and Sanford, J. P.: Methicillin: critical appraisal after a decade of experience, Med. Clin. North Am. **54:**1113, 1970.

Griffith, R. S., and Black, H. R.: Cephalexin, Med. Clin. North Am. **54:**1229, 1970.

Marcy, S. M., and Klein, J. O.: The isoxazolyl penicillins: Oxacillin, cloxacillin, and dicloxacillin, Med. Clin. North Am. **54:**1127, 1970.

Sabath, L. D.: Phenoxymethylpenicillin (penicillin V) and phenethicillin, Med. Clin. North Am. **54:**1101, 1970.

Sidell, S., Burdick, R. E., Brodie, J., Bulger, R., and Kirby, W. M. M.: New antistaphylococcal antibiotics. Comparative in vivo and in vitro activity cephalothin, nafcillin, cloxacillin, oxacillin, and methicillin, Arch. Intern. Med. **112:**21, 1973.

Speight, T. M., Brodgen, R. N., and Avery, G. S.: Cephalexin, a review. Australian Drug Information Services, Drugs **3:**9, 1972.

Sulfonamides; urinary tract antiseptics

Brumfitt, W., Hamilton-Miller, J. M., and Kosmidis, J.: Trimethoprimsulfamethoxazole: The present position, J. Infect. Dis. **128**(Suppl):778, 1973.

Kunin, C. M.: Detection, prevention and management of urinary tract infections, Philadelphia, 1972, Lea & Febiger.

Mafenide acetate cream: A review, Drugs **1:**434, 1971.

Nichols, R. L., and Condon, R. E.: Antibiotic preparation of the colon: Failure of commonly used regimens, Surg. Clin. North Am. **51:**223, 1971.

Tetracyclines

Ory, E. M.: The tetracyclines, Med. Clin. North Am. **54:**1173, 1970.

Medical Letter: The choice and uses of tetracycline drugs, Med. Letter Drugs Ther. **11:**62, 1969.

Aminoglycosides

Bodey, J. P., and Stewart, D.: In vitro studies of tobramycin, Antimicrob. Agents Chemother. **2:**109, 1972.

Bunn, P. A.: Kanamycin, Med. Clin. North Am. **54:**1245, 1970.

Burger, L. M., Sanford, J. P., and Zweighaft, T.: Tobramycin: Bacteriological evaluation, Am. J. Med. Sci. **265:**135, 1973.

Clark, J., and Wallace, A.: The susceptibility of mycobacteria to rifamide and rifampicin, Tubercle **48:**144, 1967.

Cox, C. E.: Gentamicin, a new aminoglycoside antibiotic: Clinical and laboratory studies in urinary tract infection, J. Infect. Dis. **119:**486, 1969.

Cox, C. E.: Gentamicin, Med. Clin. North Am. **54:**1305, 1970.

Hobby, G. L.: Summation of experimental studies on the action of rifampin, Chest **61:**550, 1972.

Hyams, P. J., Simberkoff, M. S., and Rahal, J. J., Jr.: In vitro bactericidal effectiveness of four aminoglycoside antibiotics, Antimicrob. Agents Chemother. **3:**87, 1973.

Mann, C. H., editor: Kanamycin: Appraisal after 8 years of clinical application, Ann. New York Acad. Sci. **132:**771-1090, 1966.

Martin, W. J.: The present status of streptomycin in antimicrobial therapy, Med. Clin. North Am. **54:**1161, 1970.

Pyle, M. M.: Ethambutol and viomycin, Med. Clin. North Am. **54:**1317, 1970.

Simon, V. K., Mosinger, E. U., and Malerczy, V.: Pharmacokinetic studies of tobramycin and gentamicin, Antimicrob. Agents Chemother. **3:**445, 1973.

Sinanian, R., Panzer, J. D., and Atkinson, W. H.: Time of eradication of Gonococcus following spectinomycin therapy, Clin. Med. **79:**15, 1972.

Sunahara, S., and Nakagawa, H.: Metabolic study and controlled clinical trials of rifampin, Chest **61:**526, 1972.

Wagner, J. G., Novak, E., Leslie, L. G., and Metzler, C. M.: Absorption, distribution, and elimination of spectinomycin dihyrochloride in man, Int. J. Clin. Pharmacol. **4:**261, 1968.

Macrolides

Anderson, R. C., Harris, P. N., and Chen, K. K.: Toxicity and distribution of ilotycin, J. Am. Pharm. Assoc. **41:**55, 1972.

Griffith, R. S., and Black, H. R.: Erythromycin, Med. Clin. North Am. **54:**1119, 1970.

Ross, S.: Erythromycin, oleandomycin, and triacetyloleandomycin, Ped. Clin. North Am. **15:**119, 1968.

Polymyxins

Hoeprich, P. H.: The polymyxins, Med. Clin. North Am. **54**:1257-1265, 1970.

Price, D. J. E., and Graham, D. I.: Effects of large doses of colistin sulfphomethate sodium on renal function, Br. Med. J. **4**:525, 1970.

Chloramphenicol

Snyder, M. J., and Woodword, T. E.: The clinical use of chloramphenicol, Med. Clin. North Am. **54**:1187, 1970.

Specialized antimicrobial drugs

Sanders, E.: Lincomycin: Fact, fancy, and future, Med. Clin. North Am. **54**:1295, 1970.

Antiviral chemotherapy

Eggers, H. J., and Tamm, I.: Antiviral chemotherapy, Ann. Rev. Pharmacol. **6**:231-250, 1966.

Goz, G., and Prusoff, W. H.: Pharmacology of viruses, Ann. Rev. Pharmacol. **10**:143, 1970.

Kaufman, H. E.: Virus chemotherapy. In Cluff, L. E., and Johnson, J. E., editors: Clinical concepts of infectious diseases, Baltimore, 1972, The Williams & Wilkins Company.

Merigan, T. C., editor: Symposium on interferon and host response to viral infections, Arch. Intern. Med. **126**:49, 1970.

Antifungal chemotherapy

Butler, W. T.: Pharmacology, toxicity, and therapeutic usefulness of amphotericin B, J.A.M.A. **195**:127, 1966.

Fass, R. J., and Perkins, R. L.: 5-Fluorocytosine in the treatment of cryptococcal and candida mycoses, Ann. Intern. Med. **74**:535, 1971.

Goldman, L.: Griseofulvin, Med. Clin. North Am. **54**:1339-1345, 1970.

CHAPTER 21

Chemotherapy of parasitic diseases

Antiprotozoan agents
Anthelmintics
Amebicides

ANTIPROTOZOAN AGENTS
ANTIMALARIAL DRUGS

Protozoan infections, with the exception of toxoplasmosis, are relatively uncommon in the United States, but are of vast importance in developing countries that have been made accessible by the ease of travel.

Malaria is one of the most prevalent of all diseases in spite of efforts to control the causative organisms and their insect vectors. Human malaria can be caused by four species of protozoal parasites: *Plasmodium vivax*, *Plasmodium malariae*, *Plasmodium ovale*, and *Plasmodium falciparum*. The first three parasites cause what is termed "relapsing" malarias, because they have a secondary, or persisting, stage of their life cycle. This secondary stage of development provides a reservoir of parasites for the reinfection of erythrocytes that can cause symptoms months or years after clinical cure has been obtained. Treatment for the relapsing malarias must be continued for several weeks after an individual's last exposure to infection. *Plasmodium falciparum* is the most lethal form of malaria and has no secondary stages. If the strain is not resistant, it responds readily to treatment, and cure can be achieved.

Malarial parasites undergo two phases of development: the sexual cycle, which takes place in the mosquito, and the asexual cycle, which occurs in the human body. The mosquito that bites an infected human being ingests the asexual forms, known as schizonts, and the sexual forms, known as gametocytes. In the mosquito the asexual forms are destroyed, but the female gametocytes are fertilized by the male gametocytes and development into asexual forms results. These are introduced into the blood of human beings by the bite of the anopheles mosquito.

The parasites, when injected into man by the mosquito bite, are known as sporozoites. Shortly after their introduction into the blood they disappear and enter fixed tissue cells (reticuloendothelial cells of liver) and possibly certain other organs where development and multiplication take place. For a period of time, which varies with the different plasmodia (6 to 14 days or longer), the patient exhibits no symptoms, no parasites are found in erythrocytes, and the blood is noninfective. This phase is known as the *prepatent* period or *tissue phase*. The parasites are called primary tissue schizonts or preerythrocytic forms. After the prepatent period the parasites burst from the tissue cells as merozoites, enter the bloodstream, penetrate erythrocytes, and begin the *erythrocytic phase* of their existence. In the case of *P. vivax* (but not *P. falciparum*) some of the merozoites invade other tissue cells to form secondary exoerythrocytic forms. The relapses in *P. vivax* malaria are believed to be caused by the successive formations of merozoites produced by various

493

secondary exoerythrocytic forms of the parasite. Drugs that affect malarial parasites in the blood-stream do not necessarily destroy those in the exoerythrocytic or tissue stage.

The erythrocytic phase of development refers to the activity of the parasite within the red blood cell. The merozoites bore into the cell, undergo development and multiplication, and finally cause rupture of the red cell to set free many more merozoites. Some of the merozoites may be destroyed in the plasma of the blood by leukocytes and other agents, but many more enter other erythrocytes to repeat the cycle. The recurring chills, fever, and prostration that are prominent clinical symptoms of malaria occur when the red cells rupture and release the young parasites. This process takes place in malaria caused by *P. falciparum*, particularly in the capillaries of internal organs, and explains the pernicious nature of this kind of malaria; for example, in the comatose type the parasites accumulate in capillaries of the brain.

After a few cycles some of the asexual forms of the malarial parasites develop into sexual forms called gametocytes (the female form is called a macrogamete and the male is a microgamete). When the mosquito bites a person infected with malarial parasites and ingests the sexual forms, a rather complicated phase of sexual development takes place in the stomach of the mosquito. The female parasite is fertilized by the male, enters the wall of the stomach of the mosquito, where it becomes encysted, and forms many spindle-shaped forms known as sporozoites. After a time the cyst ruptures and the sporozoites find their way into the saliva of the mosquito and are thus transferred to the next victim of its bite.

Persons who harbor the sexual forms of the plasmodia are called carriers, since it is from carriers that mosquitos receive the forms of the parasite that perpetuate the disease. The asexual forms cause the clinical symptoms of malaria.

Different antimalarial drugs exert their effects at different stages of the parasite's life cycle. Treatment may be aimed at the preerythrocytic stages, the erythrocytic stages, or the exoerythrocytic or secondary tissue stages of the relapsing malarias. The goals of chemotherapy include chemoprophylaxis (the chief way for travelers to protect themselves); clinical cure with relief of symptoms; and radical cure (that is, the complete elimination of infection so that relapses cannot occur after treatment has been terminated). Existing chemoprophylactic drugs act by suppression; they destroy most erythrocytic parasites as soon as they enter the bloodstream but permit the continued existence of exoerythrocytic forms.

Antimalarial drugs are sometimes classified as follows:

1 Primary tissue schizonticides—drugs that destroy preerythrocytic tissue schizonts in the liver soon after infection (e.g., primaquine)
2 Blood schizonticides—drugs that suppress symptoms by destroying the schizonts and merozoites in the erythrocytes (e.g., quinine)
3 Gametocides—drugs that prevent infection of mosquitoes and therefore prevent the spread of infection by mosquitoes by destroying gametocytes in the blood (e.g., primaquine)
4 Secondary tissue schizonticides—drugs used to cure the chronic relapsing fevers resulting from infection by *P. vivax*, *P. malariae*, and *P. ovale* by destroying the secondary tissue schizonts developing in the liver (e.g., primaquine)

Characteristics of a good antimalarial drug. The ideal antimalarial drug should be effective in the treatment of all forms of malaria, effective both as a prophylactic agent to destroy the exoerythrocytic forms and as a suppressive agent to prevent the development of clinical symptoms. It should also bring about a rapid curative action, and it should not create parasitic resistance. It should be excreted slowly so that the drug need not be given often. It should be palatable, inexpensive, and readily available. No drug is known that combines all these qualities, but research continues. Quinine is of historic importance and will be presented first, although it is now one of the least important drugs used for malaria. It is sometimes used for strains of *P. falciparum* that are resistant to newer drugs.

Quinine sulfate, U.S.P., B.P.

Cinchona bark is the source of quinine, the alkaloid that was long considered a specific in the treatment of malaria. The cinchona trees are indigenous to South America, but because of the great demand for quinine they were introduced into the East Indies, Jamaica, Java, and other countries.

The most important alkaloids belonging to the cinchona group are quinine and quinidine. The latter is discussed in Chapter 10.

Action and result. Quinine acts as a selective parasiticide, although its exact mechanism of action is uncertain. In sufficient concentration it is fatal to all cells and has been called a "general protoplasmic poison." It affects protozoa more than it affects bacteria. In therapeutic doses it is effective against the plasmodia that cause malaria. Adequate doses promptly suppress the symptoms of the disease, killing the asexual forms of all types of malaria. It kills the sexual forms of both *P. vivax* and *P. malariae* but not of *P. falciparum*. It is not effective against the preerythrocytic forms of the parasite; hence, relapse is likely to occur when treatment is discontinued for infection caused by *P. vivax* or *P. malariae*.

Quinine has:

1 Analgesic and antipyretic action similar to salicylates
2 A distinct curare-like action (It decreases response of the motor end-plate to tetanic stimulation and to acetylcholine and is a competitive inhibitor of cholinesterase.)
3 Cardiovascular effects identical to those of quinidine
4 A powerful local anesthetic effect when injected near a peripheral nerve
5 A slight oxytocic effect on the pregnant uterus during the third trimester of pregnancy
6 A peripheral vascular dilating effect

These numerous actions account for the wide diversity of side and toxic effects resulting from administration of quinine.

Uses. Quinine is used in some parts of the world when other antimalarials are not available or are too expensive. It has a number of disadvantages, among which are the following: the inconvenience of daily administration (doses should not be missed), bitter taste, and the likelihood of side effects associated with therapeutic dosage. However, it can be used to cure vivax malaria with a drug such as primaquine. Quinine

has been used against strains of *P. falciparum* resistant to newer drugs.

It has been used alone or in combination with other drugs to lower fever. Occasionally, it is used as an analgesic for relief of headache and pain in muscles and joints.

Preparation, dosage, and administration. When used in the treatment of malaria, the oral route of administration is preferred. When oral administration is not feasible, quinine hydrochloride may be given intravenously; this method is recommended only for emergencies, and the injection should be made slowly, for a dangerous lowering of blood pressure usually occurs. EKG monitoring is also important to detect cardiac arrhythmias.

Quinine sulfate, U.S.P., B.P. Quinine sulfate is available in 120-, 200-, and 300-mg. tablets and capsules. The antimalarial dose of quinine sulfate varies widely. The A.M.A. Drug Evaluations, 1973, recommends 650 mg. every 8 hours for 10 to 12 days; for children the dose is 15 mg. per kilogram of body weight three times daily for 10 days.

Side effects and toxic effects. When taken orally, large doses cause nausea, vomiting, and diarrhea. When injected intramuscularly, it is likely to cause abscesses. When injected intravenously, it causes irritation of the intima, which may result in thrombosis. Quinine has the disadvantage of a bitter taste. It must be taken daily when used for malaria. When the maximum therapeutic dosage is administered, symptoms of cinchonism are likely to occur. Such symptoms include ringing in the ears, headache, nausea, dizziness, and disturbance of vision. More severe poisoning may be indicated by the following: renal damage; acute hemolytic anemia; and involvement of the central nervous system, which includes stimulation of the respiratory center and eventual respiratory arrest.

Quinacrine hydrochloride, U.S.P. (Atabrine); mepacrine, B.P.

Quinacrine is a synthetic drug of the acridine dye series that is used in treatment of malaria. It is yellow in color. Although quinacrine was the drug of choice for prophylaxis of malaria between 1940 and 1945, it has been replaced by chloroquine and amodiaquine. Quinacrine is also used as an anthelmintic (500 mg. with 500 mg. sodium bicarbonate).

Preparation, dosage, and administration. Quinacrine hydrochloride is available in 100-mg. tablets for oral administration. To suppress symptoms the dose for adults and children over 8 years of age is 100 mg. daily for 6 days a week. For treatment of a clinical attack, 200 mg. of quinacrine with 1 Gm. of sodium bicarbonate is administered every 6 hours for five doses and then 100 mg. three times daily for 6 days. All doses of the drug should be accompanied by a full glass of water or sweetened fruit juice and taken after meals. Quinacrine hydrochloride can also be administered intramuscularly.

Side effects and toxic effects. The untoward effects are usually mild and consist of nausea, headache, vomiting, and diarrhea. Discoloration (yellow color) of the skin occurs, and the urine becomes yellow. This color change usually disappears a few weeks after the drug is discontinued. The drug is not toxic to the liver and kidneys. Toxic psychosis and aplastic anemia have been known to occur after long periods of suppressive therapy.

The treatment must suit the symptoms. Mild poisoning usually subsides when the medication is discontinued. In the more severe forms body temperature must be maintained and respirations supported.

Chloroquine; amodiaquine; primaquine; pyrimethamine

More important than quinine or quinacrine is a series of synthetic drugs that are active antimalarials and that share certain chemical features with the naturally occurring cinchona alkaloids. These synthetic drugs include chloroquine, amodiaquine, primaquine, and pyrimethamine. The structural similarities can be seen by studying the accompanying formulas. It should be noted that many of these drugs contain the quinoline nucleus and also share certain general types of side chains.

Chloroquine, amodiaquine, pyrimethamine, and primaquine are among the drugs most often employed in programs for eradication of malaria. At the present time no drug is available that will act with equal effectiveness on all species and all developmental stages of the malarial parasites.

Chloroquine and amodiaquine are especially useful in the treatment of acute malaria. They are also effective for suppressive therapy for all kinds of human malaria. However, since they

Quinine

Primaquine

Chloroquine

Quinacrine

Pyrimethamine

do not affect the primary or secondary tissue forms of the parasites, they do not prevent infection or relapse.

Pyrimethamine is said to be the most effective single suppressive agent. Single weekly doses will prevent clinical attacks of malaria associated with all species of human malarial parasites so that the mosquito is unable to transmit the disease after feeding on persons taking this drug. Primaquine and related members of this group of drugs also have the advantage of destroying persistent exoerythrocytic parasites in the liver that are known to cause relapses of malarial infections.

In some parts of the world antimalarial drugs such as chloroquine are added to salt in much the same way that iodine is added to salt to prevent goiter. This would appear to be a useful way of dealing with malaria in places where difficulties are encountered in using other methods of eradication.

Chloroquine phosphate, U.S.P., B.P. (Aralen). Chloroquine is a synthetic antimalarial drug. It was synthesized in Germany in 1934 and introduced in the U.S. for the treatment of malaria in 1944. It is the most effective and least toxic antimalarial drug. The mechanism of its action is to block the enzymatic synthesis of DNA and RNA. It is effective against the asexual forms of all plasmodia causing human malaria. It abolishes acute attacks of falciparum malaria and brings about complete cure of the infection (suppressive cure). However, it does not kill the sexual forms, and therefore patients continue to be infective to mosquitoes for a period of time. It does not cure malaria caused by *P. vivax*, but it is an effective suppressive agent, terminates attacks, and delays relapse. Chloroquine is not effective against the preerythrocytic forms of the plasmodia (tissue phase). Only falciparum infections, in which there are no persistent tissue forms, are radically cured by this drug. Some falciparum strains have become resistant to chloroquine. Chloroquine also possesses amebicidal properties. D.E.S.I. rating is *effective* for treatment of malaria and extraintestinal amebiasis.

Chloroquine is rapidly and almost completely absorbed from the gastrointestinal tract, with maximum plasma concentrations occurring 1 to 2 hours after administration. A portion of it is slowly eliminated in the urine.

Chloroquine phosphate is available in 125- and 250-mg. tablets for oral administration before or after meals. For acute attacks, an initial dose of 1 Gm. is followed by 500 mg. after 6 or 8 hours and by 500 mg. on each of 2 successive days. This dosage is sufficient to eradicate most infections caused by *P. falciparum* and to terminate an acute attack caused by *P. vivax*. Suppressive doses of 500 mg. every 7 days prevent clinical attacks of vivax malaria. Dosage for children is 16.66 mg. per kilogram of body weight initially, then 8.33 mg. per kilogram in 6 hours and then daily for the next 2 days.

Chloroquine phosphate injection, B.P., is available for parenteral (intramuscular or intravenous) use. The B.P. also lists chloroquine sulfate and chloroquine sulfate injection for oral and parenteral administration, respectively.

Chloroquine toxicity resembles mild cinchonism, but high doses of the drug can have severely toxic effects, such as dermatologic problems, toxic psychoses, and peripheral neuropathies. Permanent nerve deafness in adults has followed high-dose chloroquine therapy, and congenital deafness and mental retardation have been reported in children born to mothers taking high doses of chloroquine during pregnancy. Severe and often permanent eye damage also may be caused by prolonged administration of chloroquine in high doses. Corneal changes and retinal changes can occur; the latter are often permanent. Vision tests and retinal examinations must be done at least every 3 months on patients receiving chloroquine in high dosage. This drug should be used with caution in patients with a history of liver damage, neurologic disorders, or hematologic disorders.

Amodiaquine hydrochloride, U.S.P., B.P. (Camoquin). Amodiaquine is a synthetic antimalarial drug that greatly resembles chloroquine both in its effectiveness for treatment of malaria and in its level of toxicity. Like chloroquine, it is effective only in the erythrocytic stages of malaria. It is capable of producing a radical cure only when the infection is caused by *P. falciparum*. It does not effect a similar cure for other forms of malaria, but it is effective in the treatment of an acute attack, relieves symptoms, and delays relapse. It is therefore an effective suppressive agent in areas of the world where malaria is endemic.

Like chloroquine, amodiaquine is rapidly absorbed from the gastrointestinal tract and concentrated in the liver, spleen, kidney, and blood cells. It is said to be concentrated slightly less than chloroquine.

Amodiaquine hydrochloride is available in 200-mg. tablets for oral administration. The usual single dose for adults in an acute attack of the disease (in term of the base) is 400 to 600 mg. For suppression of endemic malaria the usual dose is 400 to 600 mg. administered once every 2 weeks. The dosage for children is reduced in accordance with the age of the child.

Side effects include nausea and vomiting, increased flow of saliva, and diarrhea. Large doses may produce spasticity, incoordination of movement, and convulsions, but these are seldom encountered. Amodiaquine does not discolor the skin. Prolonged usage in high doses may also result in corneal and retinal damage, blood dyscrasias, and hepatitis.

Primaquine phosphate, U.S.P., B.P. Primaquine, pamaquine, and pentaquine are all synthetic antimalarial drugs that belong to the same chemical group of drug (8-aminoquinolines). The latter two members are more toxic and less potent than primaquine and hence will be omitted from this edition. D.E.S.I. rating of primaquine is *effective* for the cure and prevention of vivax malaria.

Primaquine exerts a distinctive action on all gametocytes (sexual forms), especially those of *P. falciparum.* The gametocytes cause no clinical symptoms, but they are responsible for the transmission of malaria to the mosquito and thus keep the mosquito effective in the malarial cycle. The drug is ineffective or only slightly effective against asexual forms of the parasites *(P. falciparum);* hence, effective treatment of acute attacks of malaria is dependent on simultaneous administration of another antimalarial such as chloroquine. Its greatest value lies in its ability to destroy the late tissue forms (which can cause secondary erythrocytic parasites) and thus treat relapses of vivax malaria. If it is administered during the latent period (period between the time the person is bitten by an infected mosquito and the time that the parasites enter the red blood cells), radical cure of vivax malaria can be secured by this drug alone.

Primaquine phosphate, U.S.P., is available in tablets containing 26.3 mg. of the drug for oral administration. For the treatment of relapsing vivax infections, one tablet each day for 14 days is considered adequate to produce a radical cure. If the patient has symptoms of an attack or a relapse, primaquine phosphate is supplemented with chloroquine or amodiaquine.

When given in the dosage recommended, primaquine exhibits a low level of toxicity, but it can cause depression of the bone marrow, hemolytic anemia, and agranulocytosis. Epigastric distress, nausea and vomiting, and abdominal pains occur occasionally. Large doses result in hemolytic effects, particularly in persons belonging to the deeply pigmented races, and the drug should be stopped immediately on any sign of darkening of the urine or a sudden drop in hemoglobin concentration or leukocyte count. Its main disadvantages are its narrow margin of safety between therapeutic and toxic dose and ineffectiveness against asexual forms of *P. falciparum.*

Pyrimethamine, U.S.P., B.P. (Daraprim). Pyrimethamine is a potent antimalarial agent especially valuable as a suppressive agent. It therefore prevents the clinical attacks of all forms of malaria, and it interrupts the malarial cycle by preventing the formation of sporozoites in the mosquito. If suppressive therapy is continued long enough, suppressive cure of vivax infections may occur. Its use as a suppressive agent for falciparum infections results in a radical cure in most cases. This cure occurs because the gametocytes eventually disappear spontaneously after the asexual blood forms are eliminated by the suppressive drug. Pyrimethamine acts slowly and should not be used in the treatment of acute primary attacks.

Pyrimethamine is available in 25-mg. tablets for oral administration. The usual suppressive dose is 25 mg. per week. It is recommended that this dosage be continued indefinitely in areas where malaria is endemic. The dosage is 12.5

mg. for children under the age of 15 years. Therapeutic dosage (adults) is 25 mg. daily for 2 days.

Pyrimethamine has a wide margin of safety, and toxic effects are seldom encountered, although overdosage can result in anemia and leukopenia. Plasmodia that are resistant to chloroguanide, an antimalarial drug used in some countries, may develop resistance to pyrimethamine. Therefore its use is not recommended in areas of the world where it is known that the plasmodia have developed resistance to chloroguanide.

Drugs of choice in treatment of malaria. According to current concepts the following are the drugs of choice for various forms of malaria:

1 Uncomplicated attacks by any plasmodia—chloroquine phosphate, amodiaquine hydrochloride, injections of chloroquine hydrochloride (if infection is severe)
2 Malaria caused by resistant strains of *P. falciparum*—quinine sulfate plus pyrimethamine and sulfadiazine
3 Prevention of disease in endemic area—chloroquine phosphate, 500 mg. once a week (The individual may develop the disease when discontinuing the medication upon leaving the area.)

OTHER ANTIPROTOZOAN AGENTS
Pentamidine, B.P. (Lomidine)

Pentamidine, a trypanocidal drug, is the drug of choice for the prevention and treatment of *Trypanosoma gambiense* and *Trypanosoma rhodesiense* forms of trypanosomiasis (sleeping sickness). It is not effective for treating late stages of African sleeping sickness. It is also used for treatment of leishmaniasis. The basic mechanism of action of pentamidine is unknown but the organisms are known to accumulate high concentrations of the drug. *In vitro* experiments have shown that pentamidine inhibits no fewer than twenty enzyme systems. Pentamidine has both bactericidal and fungicidal action.

Pentamidine is poorly absorbed from the gastrointestinal tract and must be given intramuscularly or intravenously. After injection the drug is quickly taken up by the liver, kidney, and adrenal gland. Very little of the drug penetrates the central nervous system. Signs of a trypanocidal effect are evidenced by disappearance of organisms from the blood and lymph.

Side effects and toxic effects. The most common side effect is itching. Intravenous injection causes peripheral vasodilation and a sharp fall in blood pressure that is only partially blocked by atropine. This may be caused by release of tissue-bound histamine and peripheral adrenergic blockade.

Pentamidine may cause central nervous system depression, which may produce a rise of blood urea nitrogen and nonprotein nitrogen. Toxic effects are rare but tremor, convulsions, nystagmus, ataxia, vomiting, and death have been reported.

Preparation, dosage, and administration. Pentamidine is available as a dry powder in ampules of 200 mg. It is available in the United States only from the Parasitic Disease Drug Service, U.S. Public Health Service. Average dose is 4 mg. per kilogram of body weight intramuscularly daily or on alternate days. In the early stages of trypanosomiasis, pentamidine is given in dosages of 1.5 to 4 mg. intramuscularly every 1 to 2 days for 10 days. For chemoprophylaxis, 4 mg. per kilogram of body weight is given intramuscularly every 3 to 6 months.

Suramin (Antrypol, Germanin, Naphuride)

Suramin is a nonmetallic dye that is used both as a prophylactic and as a therapeutic agent for trypanosomiasis. This disease, which is caused by a parasitic protozoan organism that is spread by the bite of the tsetse fly, is also known as African sleeping sickness. There is more than one species of the parasite, and they are not equally virulent. Therapy in which suramin is given with an arsenical (tryparsamide) or alternated with it is particularly successful. This drug is excreted slowly and tends to persist in the tissues for some time after administration is discontinued.

Preparation, dosage, and administration. Suramin is not manufactured in the United States because it is used very little in this part of the world. The usual single dose is 1 Gm. weekly for 5 weeks given intravenously. Dosage for children is 10 to 15 mg. per kilogram of body weight weekly for 5 weeks. A course of treatment consists of five to ten weekly injections.

Side effects and toxic effects. Side effects of suramin include nausea, vomiting, low-grade fever, headache, joint pains, myalgia, ocular symptoms, edema of the face or limbs, and cutaneous hyperesthesia of the soles and palms. Protein, casts, and occult blood may appear in the urine, and "allergic" reactions due to release of foreign protein from dying parasites may occur. Rare and sometimes fatal reactions such as circulatory collapse, loss of consciousness, and severe prostration, have been reported. Patients receiving suramin should be hospitalized during the course of treatment, and therapy should be discontinued if intolerance to an initial test dose is manifested.

ANTHELMINTICS

Anthelmintics are drugs used to rid the body of worms (helminths). The use of anthelmintics (*anti*, against; Gr. *helmins*, worms) is among the most primitive types of chemotherapy. It has been estimated that over 800 million people, or one third the world's population, are infested with these parasites.

Helminths may be present in the gastrointestinal tract, but several types also penetrate the tissues and some undergo developmental changes, during which they wander extensively in the host. Because most anthelmintics used today are highly effective against specific parasites, the organism must be accurately identified before treatment is started, usually by finding the parasite ova or larvae in the feces, urine, blood, sputum, or tissues of the host.

Undesirable effects that may result from helminthiasis. Parasitic infestations do not necessarily cause clinical manifestations, although they may be injurious for a number of reasons:

1 Worms may cause mechanical injury to the tissues and organs. Roundworms in large numbers may cause obstruction in the intestine; filariae may block lymphatic channels and cause massive edema; and hookworms often cause extensive damage to the wall of the intestine and considerable loss of blood.
2 Toxic substances made by the parasite may be absorbed by the host.

3 The tissues of the host may be traumatized by the presence of the parasite and made more susceptible to bacterial infections.
4 Heavy infestation with worms will rob the host of food. This is particularly significant in children.

Classification of helminths. Worms that are parasitic to man may be classified as cestodes, nematodes, and trematodes. The *cestodes* are the tapeworms, of which there are four varieties: (1) *Taenia saginata* (beef tapeworm), (2) *Taenia solium* (pork tapeworm), (3) *Diphyllobothrium latum* (fishworm), and (4) *Hymenolepis nana* (dwarf tapeworm). As indicated by the name of the worm, the parasite enters the intestine by way of improperly cooked beef, pork, or fish or from contaminated food, as in the case of the dwarf tapeworm.

The cestodes are segmented flatworms with a head and a number of segments, or proglottids, which in some cases may extend for 20 or 30 feet in the bowel. The tapeworms, with the exception of the dwarf tapeworm, spend part of their life cycle in a host other than man—pigs, fish, or cattle. The dwarf tapeworm does not require an intermediate host.

The nematodes are round, unsegmented worms that vary in length from a fraction of an inch to a foot or more. They include *Ascaris lumbricoides* (roundworm), *Necator americanus* and *Ancylostoma duodenale* (two species of hookworms), *Trichuris trichiura* (whipworm), *Trichinella spiralis* (which produces trichinosis and for which there is no effective anthelmintic), *Oxyuris (Enterobius) vermicularis* (pinworm), *Wuchereria bancrofti* (causing filariasis), and *Strongyloides stercoralis* (infestation with which is known as strongyloidiasis).

The trematodes are flukes, among which are several blood flukes—*Schistosoma mansoni, S. japonicum,* and *S. hematobium*. There are other flukes parasitic to man. Schistosomiasis is a disease caused by blood flukes. They penetrate the skin of persons who bathe in contaminated waters or in some other way come in contact with the infected water in which snails serve as the intermediate host. The adult blood flukes live in the veins of the mesentery and pelvis of man and accumulate in the portal tube. The liver and spleen are the organs mainly involved.

Properties of a good anthelmintic. Anthelmintics should be relatively safe and at the same time sufficiently potent to achieve their purpose. Many anthelmintics are toxic to man as well as to the parasite. A good anthelmintic has a minimal toxic effect on the host and a maximal toxic effect on the parasite. Other desirable properties include easy administration and low cost.

Effective treatment of the patient demands knowledge of the type of worm or worms, determination of the best anthelmintic to use, and a method for determining success of treatment. Although the technique of treatment necessarily varies with the drug used, maximum effects are sometimes related to how well the intestinal tract is emptied before the drug is administered and how well it is evacuated afterward. Some of the newer anthelmintics do not require that the patient be purged and starved to promote effectiveness of the drug.

DRUGS USED AGAINST CESTODES AND NEMATODES
Quinacrine hydrochloride, U.S.P. (Atabrine); mepacrine, B.P.

Quinacrine hydrochloride is usually effective against the beef tapeworm after a single dose. It is also effective against pork and fish tapeworm. A saline purgative is given the evening before the administration of the drug. The next morning no food is allowed, but quinacrine hydrochloride may be given orally in divided doses along with sodium bicarbonate, or it may be given in solution through a duodenal tube. It is available in 100-mg. tablets. The usual adult dose is 800 mg. in divided doses together with 1 Gm. of sodium bicarbonate. The latter agent helps to prevent gastric irritation and vomiting. A saline cathartic is again given 2 hours after administration of the drug. Dosage for children weighing 18 to 34 kg. is 400 mg. in divided doses, and 600 mg. in divided doses for children weighing 34 to 45.5 kg.

Quinacrine hydrochloride is also an antimalarial agent (see p. 495).

Piperazine salts

Piperazine compounds were introduced into medicine as agents for the treatment of gout. Although they proved to be ineffective for this condition, they have come to be considered drugs of choice for the treatment of roundworms and pinworms. They seem to induce a state of narcosis and paralysis in the worms, and they are then expelled by intestinal peristalsis in the patient. The drug appears to have a selective action on the myoneural junction of the worms. Since the worms may revive after expulsion from the body, general hygienic measures should be used.

Piperazine is more effective on the mature than on the immature forms of the worm; therefore, an interrupted treatment schedule is advisable. These drugs have the advantage of being low in toxicity. Furthermore, fasting and purgation need not accompany their administration.

Adverse reactions to the piperazine salts are manifest in a wide range of symptoms. Mild symptoms usually consist of nausea and vomiting, diarrhea, abdominal pain, and headache. Rarely reported are transitory vertigo, incoordination, difficulty in focusing, muscular weakness, erythema multiforme, urticaria, and lethargy. The piperazine drugs should be administered cautiously in the presence of renal disease, since the drugs may be cumulative when impaired renal function is present. Their use in the presence of epilepsy is not recommended.

Preparation, dosage, and administration

Piperazine citrate, U.S.P., B.P. (Antepar). This agent is available in 250- and 500-mg. tablets and as a syrup, 100 mg. per milliliter, for oral administration. The daily dose for pinworm infection is calculated on a basis of 65 mg. per kilogram of body weight, but a daily dose of 2.5 Gm. should not be exceeded. For pinworms, a single course of treatment for 7 days is recommended. For roundworms (ascaris), the usual dose is 75 mg. per kilogram of body weight with a maximum dose of 3.5 Gm. daily. A single course of treatment of 5 to 7 days is usually satisfactory. In severe infections treatment may be repeated after a 1 week rest period.

Piperazine tartrate (Piperat). This form is available in 250- and 500-mg. tablets and as an oral solution, 100 mg. per milliliter. Administration and dosage are the same as for piperazine citrate.

Piperazine calcium edetate (Perin). This form is available in 500-mg. wafers and as a syrup, 100 mg. per milliliter, for oral administration.

For pinworms, the proposed dosage is 75 mg. per kilogram of body weight per day (children and adults), administered at one time or in two divided doses for a period of 15 days; for round-worms, 100 mg. per kilogram of body weight is administered.

Piperazine adipate and piperazine phosphate, N.F. These preparations are official in B.P.

Side effects and toxic effects. As mentioned previously, these drugs are among the least toxic of the anthelmintics. Excessively large doses may produce urticaria, muscular weakness, blurred vision, and vomiting. The symptoms dis-appear when the drug is discontinued.

Diethylcarbamazine citrate, U.S.P., B.P. (Hetrazan)

Diethylcarbamazine is a piperazine derivative that has been used for a number of years in the treatment of filariasis. It is the drug of choice for infections with the following parasites: *Wuchereria bancrofti, Brugia malayi,* and *Loa loa,* and is preferable to older antifilarial drugs containing antimony or arsenic. Like the piperazine preparations, its use need not be accompanied by purgation and starvation. It appears to offer no advantage over salts of piperazine in the treatment of ascariasis.

Preparation, dosage, and administration. Diethylcarbamazine citrate is available in 50-mg. tablets. For the treatment of filariasis in adults and children, the dose is 2 mg. per kilogram of body weight three times daily after meals for 7 to 21 days.

Side effects and toxic effects. Diethylcarbamazine citrate is a safe drug at therapeutic levels. Adverse responses may manifest themselves as headache, lassitude, malaise, anorexia, and nausea and vomiting. Mild to severe allergic reactions are frequent as a result of the release of foreign protein from dying microfilariae or adult worms. If allergic reactions become severe, drug dosage should be reduced or treatment inter-rupted.

Hexylresorcinol, N.F., B.P.

Hexylresorcinol is a phenol derivative that is less effective against specific parasites than several newer anthelmintics. However, its broad spectrum of antiparasitic activity, together with its low toxicity, make it an effective alternative preparation.

Hexylresorcinol is effective against round-worm, hookworm, pinworm, and the dwarf tape-worm. It exerts a paralyzing effect on the muscle of the parasite. It is less potent than some of the other anthelmintics, but it has the advantages of low toxicity and mildness that permit it to be used for children and debilitated individuals, for whom some of the other anthelmintics are con-traindicated. It is useful when mixed infestations are present.

Preparation, dosage, and administration. Hexylresorcinol is available in pills containing 100 and 200 mg. of the drug. They are coated with a tough gelatin covering. A single oral dose of 1 Gm. for adults, 600 mg. for children 6 to 8 years of age, and 800 mg. for children 8 to 12 years of age may prove effective in a large number of infections. A saline purgative the eve-ning before and also 2 to 4 hours after adminis-tration of the drug is recommended. Food is withheld during the treatment. The procedure may need to be repeated after 3 to 4 days.

When the capsules of hexylresorcinol are ad-ministered, it is important that they be swal-lowed intact. If broken in the mouth, extensive irritation may result.

Side effects and toxic effects. The main un-toward effect of hexylresorcinol is that of local irritation. Therapeutic doses do not seem to cause systemic toxicity. Topically, it is corrosive to oral mucosa and to perianal skin. When given orally, hexylresorcinol may cause mucosal ulcer-ations unless the crystals are incorporated into hard, gelatin-coated pills.

Tetrachloroethylene, U.S.P., B.P.

Tetrachloroethylene is a drug that has been used against hookworm. It is especially effective against *Necator americanus.* It is not particularly effective against other intestinal parasites. It has, to a great extent, replaced carbon tetrachloride as an anthelmintic because of the toxic effect of the latter on the liver. It is relatively insoluble in water, and in the absence of alcohol and fat in the intestine, very little drug is absorbed after oral administration. This probably explains its low level of toxicity.

Tetrachloroethylene should not be used for

ascariasis because it irritates the worms, and in their attempt to escape the drug they may migrate into the bile ducts and liver or cause intestinal obstruction and perforation. In mixed infestations of both hookworm and ascaris (which often occurs), hexylresorcinol or piperazine should be administered first. Tetrachloroethylene has to some extent been supplanted by bephenium hydroxynaphthoate.

Preparation, dosage, and administration. Gelatin capsules containing 0.2, 0.5, 1, 2.5, or 5 ml. of tetrachloroethylene are available for oral administration. The adult dose is 5 ml., and the dose for children is 0.12 ml. per kilogram of body weight to a maximum of 5 ml.

The drug should be stored in a cool place to avoid formation of the poisonous substance phosgene. A light low fat diet should be given the evening before treatment. Food is withheld the morning of treatment, and fats, oils, and alcohol should be avoided throughout the treatment and for the next 24 hours. Patients should be kept at bed rest and under observation for 2 to 4 hours after administration of the drug. A purgative should not be given since this increases toxicity to the drug and decreases effectiveness of the drug. One dose of the drug may prove sufficient unless ova are found in the stools after a period of 1 week.

Use of the drug is contraindicated in debilitated patients, small and seriously ill children, patients with liver disease, pregnant women, and alcoholism patients.

Side effects and toxic effects. Dizziness, drowsiness, giddiness, nausea, and vomiting occur occasionally.

Pyrvinium pamoate, U.S.P. (Povan)

Pyrvinium is a cyanine dye effective in the treatment of pinworm infections; both the worm and its ova are eliminated. About 90% or more of patients treated with pyrvinium are cured when a single adequate dose is given. Pyrvinium interferes with the respiratory enzyme of the parasite and inhibits its oxygen uptake and carbohydrate metabolism.

Preparation, dosage, and administration. Pyrvinium is available in 50-mg. tablets and as an oral suspension containing 50 mg. in 5 ml. The usual dose for children and adults is 5 mg.

per kilogram of body weight. Periodic treatment at intervals of 2 or 3 weeks is recommended because of repeated recurrence of the parasite.

This dye colors the stools bright red. Clothing may become stained a bright red; vomitus may also stain clothing or furniture.

Side effects. Pyrvinium is essentially nontoxic. Nausea, vomiting, and cramping have occurred. A case of photosensitization has been reported.

Bephenium hydroxynaphthoate, U.S.P. (Alcopar)

Bephenium hydroxynaphthoate is the drug of choice for the treatment of human hookworm and ascaris infections. The recommended dose is 5 Gm. for adults and children over 22.5 kg. given as a suspension on an empty stomach twice daily for 1 day. For children under 22.5 kg., dosage is 2.5 Gm. twice daily for 1 to 3 days. For whipworm treatment may be extended to 5 days. Nausea, vomiting, and abdominal pain have been reported as side effects. However, it is a safe, well-tolerated drug with low toxicity.

The drug is available in 5-Gm. packets. The dose should be mixed with milk, orange juice, or carbonated beverages just prior to administration. Food should be withheld for 2 hours after ingestion of the drug. Children are usually given half the adult dose.

Thiabendazole, U.S.P. (Mintezol)

Thiabendazole has a wide spectrum of anthelmintic activity. It is effective in the treatment of threadworms, cutaneous larva migrans, pinworms, and other worm infestations.

Preparation, dosage, and administration. The drug is available as a suspension of 500 mg. per 5 ml. and in 500-mg. tablets. Average dose is 25 mg. per kilogram of body weight twice a day after meals for 2 days; for pinworms the dosage is 25 mg. per kilogram of body weight twice a day for 1 day with dosage repeated in 1 week.

Side effects. Side effects are common but usually mild and transient. They occur 3 to 4 hours after ingestion of the drug and last 2 to 8 hours. Side effects are decreased if the drug is given after meals. Most common side effects are dizziness, anorexia, nausea and vomiting, abdominal cramping, diarrhea, headache, drowsiness, lethargy, and pruritus.

DRUGS USED IN THE TREATMENT OF SCHISTOSOMIASIS

Schistosomiasis is a disease caused by a parasite that burrows through the skin. The antimony compounds are the principal and most widely used drugs in the treatment of individual and mass schistosomiasis. They are not ideal drugs, since every one possesses one or more major limitation, including severe toxicity, difficulty of administration, length of treatment, or low effectiveness.

Mechanism of action. The antimony compounds appear to damage intrauterine eggs and inhibit phosphofructokinase, an enzyme necessary for glycolysis, a major source of energy for the parasites. In addition, the drugs paralyze schistosome adults.

Absorption, distribution, and excretion. These drugs are irritating to the gastrointestinal tract and are poorly absorbed. They are therefore administered parenterally. Little is known about their distribution. They are excreted mainly through the kidneys, although small amounts appear in the feces.

Antimony potassium tartrate, U.S.P., B.P. (Tartar Emetic)

Antimony potassium tartrate is administered intravenously as a 0.5% solution. The initial dose recommended is 30 mg. Dosage thereafter is gradually increased. The total dosage for a course of treatment is 1.5 to 2 Gm. Every injection must be administered scrupulously since phlebitis is common and leakage of the drug causes severe necrosis. Injection should be very slow to decrease the incidence of immediate side effects such as cough, dyspnea, tachycardia, a sense of chest constriction, vomiting, vertigo, and hypotension. Epinephrine should be readily accessible when tartar emetic is administered. Nausea, vomiting, and arthralgia are other frequent side effects. Electrocardiogram changes may occur, as with other antimony preparations.

Patients should be hospitalized during treatment and remain recumbent for several hours after the drug is administered.

Stibophen, B.P. (Fuadin)

Stibophen is a compound of antimony that is considered the drug of choice for treating schistosomiasis. It is administered intramuscularly. It is available in a 6.3% solution in 5 ml. (300 mg. in 5 ml.). Small doses are given initially and gradually increased. Therapy is interspersed with rest periods. The initial dose is 100 mg., and this is increased to as much as 300 mg., up to a total dose of 6.3 Gm. This drug may cause nausea and vomiting, and occasionally muscle and joint pains may occur. Stibophen is contraindicated in the presence of renal and cardiac disease. During repeated courses of treatment patients should be observed closely for the development of hemolytic anemia, which may be preceded by a marked febrile reaction. A course of therapy with stibophen may be repeated after 2 months if live schistosome eggs are detected on reexamination of stool or urine or muscle biopsy.

Stibocaptate

This drug is not yet licensed for use in the United States but can be obtained for investigational use. It is effective in the treatment of schistosomiasis and is administered in a dose of 40 mg. per kilogram of body weight in five divided doses; for children over 6 years of age dose is 50 mg. per kilogram in five divided doses. Adverse reactions to stibocaptate are more common in adults than in children and are manifest by pain at the injection site, vomiting, headache, dizziness, fatigue, myalgia, arthralgia, and fever. Most side effects are not severe and disappear within several days of the last injection. Administration of the drug should be discontinued in the event of severe vomiting, progressive proteinuria, substernal pain, or purpura. Most patients can be treated on an ambulatory basis if their cardiac and renal status is carefully followed.

Lucanthone hydrochloride

Lucanthone hydrochloride is an oral preparation used for the treatment of schistosomiasis that is no longer marketed in the United States.

Its precise mode of action is unknown, but it interferes with the reproductive function of the parasite (egg production) and eventually causes its death. It can be administered orally in enteric-coated tablets. Dosage is calculated on the basis of 10 to 20 mg. per kilogram of body weight. It is given in divided doses daily for approximately 10 days. Nausea, vomiting, and gastric distress are sometimes experienced. The skin may turn yellow or orange with treatment, but this usually disappears in about 4 weeks. Insomnia, headache, convulsions, psychosis, and hepatic and renal damage have been reported. Toxic dosage is said to border closely on therapeutic dosage. The drug is used more frequently in children under age 16 since side effects in adults occur more frequently and are more severe.

THERAPEUTIC RÉSUMÉ

The drugs of choice for the treatment of helminthiasis include the following:

1 Against tapeworms—quinacrine, aspidium, and hexylresorcinol
2 Against roundworms—piperazine salts and diethylcarbamazine
3 Against whipworms—hexylresorcinol
4 Against pinworms—piperazine salts and hexylresorcinol. Pinworms do not cling to the intestinal wall and may also be expelled by the use of a cathartic or enema. The anal region must be kept clean, and scratching of the anal region must be avoided if reinfection is to be prevented. Underclothing, washcloths, and so on must be boiled to kill the eggs of the parasite. Reinfection is a major problem.
5 Against hookworms—tetrachloroethylene, hexylresorcinol, and bephenium
6 For strongyloidiasis—thiabendazole
7 For schistosomiasis—antimony compounds (antimony potassium tartrate and stibophen)
8 For filariasis—diethylcarbamazine, especially for the removal of the microfilariae, although the adult form of the worm is not much affected

AMEBICIDES

Although a number of nonpathogenic amebas may be found in the human bowel, amebiasis, or amebic dysentery, is a disease caused by the *Entamoeba histolytica*. It may be manifest as a severe intestinal infection, a mild symptomatic intestinal infection, an asymptomatic intestinal infection, or as a liver abscess or other extraintestinal infection. The disease is worldwide and not limited to tropical regions. The parasite occurs in two forms: the active motile form, known as a trophozoite, and the cystic form, which is inactive, resistant to drugs, and present in the intestinal excretions. In the lumen of the intestine, the ameba forms a cyst when living conditions, for some reason, become unfavorable. Outside the body the cyst becomes the source of infection to others when transmitted by flies or contaminated food and water. Only the cystic forms of the parasite can cause amebiasis because the motile forms are killed by gastric acid.

The initial infection of the bowel is known as intestinal amebiasis and is associated with diarrhea and the presence of motile parasite forms in the stools.

Secondary amebiasis means that the parasites have migrated to other parts of the body, such as the liver (where an amebic abscess may develop), spleen, and lungs. Only motile forms of the parasite invade the tissues. The amebas live at the expense of the host and always produce areas of tissue destruction in the bowel, although in certain individuals few symptoms of the disease may be noted. Apparently in these persons tissue repair keeps up with the tissue destruction.

Complete cure of the disease is difficult to attain because it is necessary to kill all of the parasites if relapse is to be avoided.

Drugs available for the treatment of amebiasis can be classified according to the site of their antiamebic action. The tissue amebicides, or drugs used for extraintestinal amebiasis, are drugs that act primarily in the bowel wall, liver, and other extraintestinal tissues. They include emetine and chloroquine. Luminal amebicides, or drugs used for the treatment of intestinal amebiasis, act primarily in the bowel lumen and are ineffective against parasites in the bowel wall or tissues. The luminal amebicides include the iodohydroxyquinoline compounds. Treatment may require the concomitant or sequential use of several drugs. No drugs are recommended as safe or effective for chemoprophylaxis.

DRUGS USED FOR EXTRAINTESTINAL AMEBIASIS
Ipecac and emetine hydrochloride, U.S.P., B.P.

Ipecac is the dried root of the *Caphaelis ipeca-cuanha*, a perennial shrub that grows in Brazil and other South American countries. It was long used by native people in the treatment of diarrhea. It contains two alkaloids, emetine and cephaeline, both of which are amebicidal, although emetine is the more potent agent. Emetine apparently has a direct lethal action on the *Entamoeba histolytica* when it is in a motile form, but it has little effect on amebic cysts. When used for the treatment of amebiasis, emetine is not administered orally because it is absorbed erratically and may induce emesis as a result of its local irritant effect on the intestinal mucosa. It is readily absorbed from parenteral sites of administration but is excreted rather slowly. It may therefore produce cumulative effects in the tissues.

Uses. The chief use of emetine is to control the symptoms of acute amebic dysentery or the symptoms that may suddenly develop during chronic phases of the disease. It has come to be regarded as second only to chloroquine for the treatment of amebic hepatitis and amebic abscess in the liver. It should not be used for the relief of mild symptoms or for the treatment of carriers. The full therapeutic regimen for severe intestinal amebiasis includes concurrent administration of a full course of oxytetracycline, followed by a course of diiodohydroxyquin plus chloroquine.

Preparation, dosage, and administration. Emetine hydrochloride is available in 1-ml. ampules containing 65 mg. of the drug in solution. The usual daily adult dose is 1 mg. per kilogram of body weight but should not exceed 65 mg. given daily. The dosage range for adults may be from 30 to 65 mg. For children, the dose is 10 to 20 mg., depending on their weight and age. The drug is given both by deep subcutaneous and deep intramuscular injection over a period of 5 to 10 days; for children, one or two injections are given daily for not more than 4 to 6 days. Enteric-coated tablets have been given orally, but they are prone to cause irritation of the digestive tract.

Side effects and toxic effects. Emetine is a general protoplasmic poison and causes a variety of toxic reactions. Degenerative changes in the liver, heart, kidney, and muscles may occur. Cardiac changes may vary from disturbance in rhythm to acute myocarditis and heart failure. Other symptoms of poisoning include dizziness, nausea and vomiting, severe diarrhea, and albuminuria. Pain is often experienced at the site of injection. Emetine is contraindicated for patients with organic disease of the heart and kidneys. It is not used for pregnant, aged, or debilitated persons. Emetine is potentially a very dangerous drug and should be administered only to hospitalized patients. Great care must be taken not to inject it intravenously.

From 6 weeks to 2 months should intervene between courses of treatment.

Chloroquine phosphate, U.S.P., B.P. (Aralen)

Chloroquine is one of the antimalarial drugs that also exhibits amebicidal activity. Because it reaches many parts of the body and localizes in organs such as the liver, it is highly effective for the treatment of extraintestinal amebiasis, particularly amebic hepatitis and amebic abscess. It is not recommended for intestinal forms of amebiasis, partly because it is well absorbed from the small bowel and partly because the tissue in the wall of the bowel fails to concentrate the drug as well as does the liver. Since hepatic involvement may occur early in amebiasis with few if any clinical signs, some physicians recommend early use of chloroquine or emetine along with a drug that is effective against the intestinal forms of the disease, such as one of the arsenicals or one of the oxyquinoline drugs.

Preparation, dosage, and administration. Chloroquine phosphate is available in 250- and 500-mg. tablets and in solution for injection containing 50 mg. per milliliter in 5-ml. ampules. For extraintestinal amebiasis the usual oral dose for adults is 500 mg. two times daily for 2 days, followed by 250 mg. two times a day for 2 weeks or more. For children dosage is 20 mg. per kilogram of body weight daily in two doses for 2 days, then 10 mg. per kilogram daily for 2 to 3 weeks. The course of treatment may be repeated or alternated with emetine therapy. To effect a cure it is necessary to administer this drug along with another drug known to be effective for intestinal amebiasis.

Side effects and toxic effects. Severe side effects or toxic effects are not associated with therapeutic doses of chloroquine phosphate. However, patients may complain of headache, itching, visual disturbances, and gastrointestinal upsets. These symptoms subside when the administration of the drug is stopped. However, retinal damage can be very serious.

Metronidazole, U.S.P., B.P. (Flagyl)

Metronidazole is a potent amebicide for the luminal and hepatic forms of *Entamoeba histolytica.*

Metronidazole is rapidly and almost completely absorbed from the gastrointestinal tract. About 70% of the drug is excreted in the urine unchanged. It crosses the placenta and is excreted in the saliva, milk, semen, and vaginal secretions. It colors the urine a dark brown.

Metronidazole can cause numerous adverse effects.

When used for the treatment of amebiasis, metronidazole is administered in doses of 750 mg. three times daily for 5 to 10 days. The drug is also effective in the treatment of urogenital trichomoniasis, Mexican cutaneous leishmaniasis, Chagas' disease, and giardiasis.

DRUGS USED FOR INTESTINAL AMEBIASIS

Organic arsenicals

Pentavalent arsenic compounds such as acetarsone and carbarsone, as well as trivalent compounds such as thioarsenites, are amebicidal. Some arsenicals first used for syphilis have been found effective for amebic dysentery.

Carbarsone, N.F.

Carbarsone is one of the organic arsenicals and contains 28.5% arsenic. It is absorbed after oral or rectal administration and excreted rather slowly by the kidney.

It is especially effective for chronic intestinal amebiasis uncomplicated by hepatic involvement. It is not effective against amebas in abscesses of the liver or other organs. It is also used in treatment of trichomonal infections of the vagina.

Preparation, dosage, and administration. Carbarsone is available in 250-mg. tablets for oral administration and in suppositories containing 2 grains of the drug. The adult oral dose for amebiasis is 250 mg. two or three times daily for 7 to 10 days. Dose for children is 7.5 mg. per kilogram of body weight daily in three divided doses for 10 days. For acute amebiasis, a retention enema (for adults) may be prepared by dissolving 2 Gm. of the drug in 200 ml. of a warm 2% sodium bicarbonate solution. The enema may be repeated every other night for five times. A cleansing enema should preferably precede the treatment. For trichomonal infections the dose is one suppository daily.

Side effects and toxic effects. Although carbarsone is considered one of the least toxic of the arsenicals, overdosage can produce damage to the liver and kidneys. Serious toxic effects rarely occur, however, although cutaneous rash, loss of weight, abdominal distress, and diarrhea have been noted. Exfoliative dermatitis, encephalitis, and damage of the optic nerve are almost unknown, but such effects must be kept in mind when an arsenical drug is being administered. Since excretion of the drug is rather slow there is a tendency to develop cumulative effects. BAL is effective in the treatment of arsenical poisoning.

Carbarsone is contraindicated for patients who have renal or hepatic pathology, abnormalities of visual fields, and in patients with a history of arsenic sensitivity.

Glycobiarsol, N.F. (Milibis)

Glycobiarsol is a pentavalent arsenical combined with bismuth (15% arsenic and 42% bismuth). It is recommended for the treatment of intestinal amebiasis only. It exhibits low toxicity because it is not very soluble and is poorly absorbed. It needs to be supplemented with other therapy when amebic hepatitis or deep-seated infestation is present. This drug has also been used for monilial and trichomonal infections of the vagina. D.E.S.I. rating is *effective* for the treatment of amebiasis in adults and children over 80 lb., but it is not considered the drug of choice.

Preparation, dosage, and administration. Glycobiarsol is available in 250- and 500-mg. tablets and in vaginal suppositories, 250 mg. The usual adult dose for amebiasis is 500 mg. three times daily for 7 to 10 days. Larger doses are sometimes necessary when diarrhea is severe. Additional course of treatment is indicated if pathogenic amebas continue to be found in the stool. This drug turns the stools black.

Side effects and toxic effects. This drug is not very toxic, but the presence of arsenic in the compound necessitates caution in its use.

Arsthinol (Balarsen)

Arsthinol is an organic thioarsenical compound. D.E.S.I. rating is *possibly effective* for intestinal amebiasis and also for yaws.

Preparation, dosage, and administration. This compound is available in 100-mg. tablets for oral administration. The daily oral dose is 10 mg. per kilogram of body weight, not to exceed 500 mg. daily. It is given over a period of 5 days.

Side effects and toxic effects. The side effects are said to be minor, but the possibility of arsenic poisoning should not be overlooked. Rest periods between courses of treatment are recommended.

Iodohydroxyquinoline compounds

Included in this group of compounds are diiodohydroxyquin and iodochlorhydroxyquin. The following formulas indicate why these compounds are also called halogenated hydroxyquinolines.

Diiodohydroxyquin (Diodoquin)

Iodochlorhydroxyquin (Vioform)

Diiodohydroxyquin, U.S.P. (Diodoquin); di-iodohydroxyquinoline, B.P.

Diiodohydroxyquin is an oxyquinoline derivative that contains about 64% iodine. It is directly amebicidal, although the mechanism of its action is not known. It is useful for intestinal amebiasis but not for amebic abscess or amebic hepatitis. It is the drug of choice for the treatment of mild or asymptomatic amebiasis, but is not indicated for chemoprophylaxis.

It is also used in the treatment of trichomonal infections of the vagina.

Preparation, dosage, and administration. Diiodohydroxyquin is available as a bulky powder and in tablets, containing 210 and 650 mg. (300 mg., B.P.). It is administered orally as an amebicide and by insufflation for vaginitis. The adult dose is 650 mg. three times a day for 20 days and is given preferably between meals. Dosage for children is 40 mg. per kilogram of body weight daily in two or three doses for 20 days. Treatment may be repeated after a 2 or 3 week interval.

Side effects and toxic effects. Diiodohydroxyquin exhibits a low level of toxicity, which is probably explained by the fact that it is not very soluble. Symptoms of iodism may develop (itching, dermatitis, abdominal discomfort, diarrhea, and headache). It produces less diarrhea and gastric irritation than iodochlorhydroxyquin and is preferred over that drug in the United States. It is contraindicated for patients who have liver damage and for those who are hypersensitive to iodine.

Iodochlorhydroxyquin, N.F., B.P. (Vioform)

Iodochlorhydroxyquin has an iodine content of approximately 40%. It is poorly soluble, although some intestinal absorption does occur. Like the other drugs of this group of compounds, it is most effective for intestinal amebiasis and is ineffective for amebic abscesses or amebic hepatitis. It is expensive, and its administration does not require bed rest for the patient. It stains clothing and linens a yellow color. Some authorities consider this least effective of the iodohydroxyquinolines, but differences of opinion exist about their relative values. It is also employed in treatment of trichomonal infections of the vagina and for various types of dermatitis.

Preparation, dosage, and administration. Iodochlorhydroxyquin is available as a powder, as 250-mg. tablets, and as an ointment. The powder is suitably buffered for use as a vaginal insufflate. The usual adult dose is 500 to 750 mg. three times a day for 10 days. Treatment may be repeated after an interval of 8 days. Only two courses of treatment should be given. The drug may be used alternately with carbarsone—courses of treatment with one drug may follow the use of the other drug.

Side effects and toxic effects. Toxic reactions are seldom encountered. Mild symptoms of iodism may occur, and some patients may experience a severe gastritis.

Antibiotics for amebiasis

A number of antibiotics have been used in the treatment of amebiasis but only a few such as paromomycin have been found to be directly amebicidal. Other antibiotics, such as erythromycin and oxytetracycline, are effective indirectly by decreasing the number of intestinal bacteria on which the *Entamoeba histolytica* depends for some essential factor or factors.

Intestinal amebiasis appears to be controlled only as long as the associated bacteria are held in check. The tetracyclines and erythromycin are discussed elsewhere. One of the disadvantages of drugs such as oxytetracycline is that, while it may be effective for mild amebiasis, it may produce gastrointestinal symptoms (diarrhea) more troublesome than the mild amebiasis.

Since antibiotics are not effective for extraintestinal amebiasis, the concomitant administration of a drug such as chloroquine is advocated.

Paromomycin, N.F. (Humatin)

Paromomycin is an antibiotic obtained from *Streptomyces rimosus.* It is said to have a direct amebicidal action and also an antibacterial action on both normal and pathogenic microorganisms found in the bowel. Its range of antibacterial action is said to resemble that of neomycin. Little of the drug is absorbed into the systemic circulation.

Uses. Paromomycin appears to be effective for both acute and chronic forms of amebiasis, but it does not seem to be effective for extraintestinal forms of the disease.

Preparation, dosage, and administration. Paromomycin sulfate is available in capsules (250 mg. of the base) and as a syrup (125 mg. in 5 ml.) for oral administration. The dosage recommended for adults and children is 25 to 35 mg. per kilogram of body weight daily. It is ad-ministered in divided doses at mealtime for 5 to 10 days.

Side effects. Paromomycin is nephrotoxic when administered parenterally but not when given orally. The chief side effect is diarrhea. Other side effects include nausea, vomiting, abdominal cramps, headache, pyrosis, and skin rash. Paromomycin is contraindicated for patients with intestinal obstruction.

QUESTIONS

For study and review

1 Suppressive treatment of malaria refers to:
 a. radical cure of the malarial infection
 b. eradication of malarial mosquitos
 c. prophylactic therapy
 d. prevention of clinical symptoms
2 Which of the following antimalarial drugs is capable of completely eradicating the infection when it is caused by *Plasmodium vivax?*
 a. quinine
 b. primaquine
 c. quinacrine
 d. chloroquine
3 Describe the symptoms of cinchonism that may occur with the use of quinine sulfate.
4 Describe the symptoms of chloroquine toxicity that may occur with the use of high doses of this drug.
5 Explain how the various anthelmintics exert their therapeutic effect.
6 What precautions must be taken when patients are treated with the following drugs?
 a. hexylresorcinol
 b. quinacrine
 c. tetrachloroethylene
 d. emetine
7 What instructions should patients receive to prevent reinfection or the spread of infection to others?
8 Explain why aspidium is no longer the drug of choice to treat tapeworm infections.
9 Which of the anthelmintic drugs can cause allergic reactions because of the release of foreign protein from dying parasites?

REFERENCES

General

A.M.A. drug evaluations, ed. 2, Acton, Mass., 1973, Publishing Sciences Group, Inc.

Aviado, D. M.: Krantz and Carr's pharmacologic principles of medical practice, ed. 8, Baltimore, 1972, The Williams & Wilkins Co.

Di Palma, J. R., editor: Drill's pharmacology in medicine, New York, 1971, McGraw-Hill Book Co.

Goodman, L. S., and Gilman, A., editors: The pharmacological basis of therapeutics, ed. 4, New York, 1970, The Macmillan Co.

Goth, A.: Medical pharmacology, ed. 7, St. Louis, 1974, The C. V. Mosby Co.

Grollman, A., and Grollman, E. F.: Pharmacology and therapeutics, ed. 7, Philadelphia, 1970, Lea & Febiger.

Meyers, F. H., Jawetz, E., and Goldfien, A.: Review of medical pharmacology, ed. 4, Los Altos, Calif., 1974, Lange Medical Publications.

Modell, W., editor: Drugs of choice 1976-1977, St. Louis, 1976, The C. V. Mosby Co.

Osol, A., and Pratt, R.: The United States dispensatory, ed. 27, Philadelphia, 1973, J. B. Lippincott Co.

Turner, P., and Richens, A.: Clinical pharmacology, Edinburgh, 1973, Churchill Livingstone.

Antimalarial drugs

Aviado, D. M., and others: Cardiopulmonary effect of antimalarial drugs, Toxicol. Appl. Pharmacol. **17**:107, 1970.

Brown, I. N.: Immunological aspects of malaria infection, Adv. Immunol. **11**:267, 1969.

Catchpool, J. F.: Antiprotozoal drugs. In Meyers, F. H., Jawetz, E., and Goldfien, A.: Review of medical pharmacology, Los Altos, Calif., 1972, Lange Medical Publications.

Clyde, D. F.: The problem of drug resistant malaria, Am. J. Trop. Med. Hyg. **21**:736, 1972.

Clyde, D. F., and others: Treatment of falciparum malaria caused by strain resistant to quinine, J.A.M.A. **213**:2041, 1970.

Fisher, G. U., and others: Malaria in soldiers returning from Vietnam: Epidemiologic, therapeutic and clinical studies, Am. J. Trop. Med. **19**:27, 1970.

Hunsicker, L. G.: The pharmacology of antimalarials, Arch. Intern. Med. **123**:645, 1969.

Malaria eradication in 1970, WHO Chronicle **25**:298, 1971.

Neva, F. A., and others: Malaria: Host defense mechanisms and complications, Ann. Intern. Med. **73**:295, 1970.

Peters, W.: Chemotherapy and drug resistance in malaria, New York, 1970, Academic Press.

Powell, R. D.: Development of new antimalarial drugs, Am. J. Trop. Med. Hyg. **21**:744, 1972.

Rieckmann, K. H.: Determination of the drug sensitivity of *Plasmodium falciparum*, J.A.M.A. **217**:573, 1971.

Schmitt, L. H.: Chemotherapy of the drug-resistant malarias, Ann. Rev. Microbiol. **23**:427, 1969.

Sheehy, T. W., and Dempsey, H.: Methotrexate therapy for *Plasmodium vivax* malaria, J.A.M.A. **214**:109, 1970.

Sitprija, V.: Renal involvement in malaria, Tr. Roy. Soc. Trop. Med. Hyg. **64**:695, 1970.

Smitskamp, H., and Walthus, F. H.: New concepts in treatment of malignant tertian malaria with cerebral involvement, Br. Med. J. **1**:714, 1971.

Tigrett, W. D.: The malaria problem, Arch. Intern. Med. **129**:604, 1972.

VanDyke, K., and others: Quinacrine: Mechanisms of antimalarial action, Science **169**:492, 1970.

Anthelmintics

Brown, H. W.: The treatment of four common parasitic infections, Pharmacol. Phys. **3**(1):1969.

Bueding, E.: Some biochemical effects of anthelmintic drugs, Biochem. Pharmacol. **18**:1541, 1969.

Desowitz, R. S.: Antiparasite chemotherapy, Ann. Rev. Pharmacol. **11**:351, 1971.

Goldsmith, R. S.: Antihelmintic drugs. In Meyers, F. H., Jawetz, E., and Goldfien, A.: Review of medical pharmacology, Los Altos, Calif., 1972, Lange Medical Publications.

Klein, N. C., and Dennis, D. T.: Parasitic problems in practice: Therapeutic guidelines, Postgrad. Med. **47**(6):120; **48**(1):150, 1970.

Marsden, P. D., and Schultz, M. G.: Intestinal parasites, Gastroenterology **57**:724, 1969.

Most, H.: Treatment of common parasitic infections of man encountered in the United States, New Eng. J. Med. **287**:495; **287**:698, 1972.

Neva, F. A.: Parasitic diseases of the GI tract in the United States, DM (Disease-a-month), Chicago, 1972, Year Book Medical Publishers, p. 44.

Waalkes, T. P., and others: Pentamidine: Clinical pharmacologic correlations in man and mice, Clin. Pharm. Ther. **11**:505, 1970.

Treatment of schistosomiasis

Bueding, E., and Fisher, J.: Biochemical effects of schistosomicides, Ann. N.Y. Acad. Sci. **160**:536, 1969.

Kanani, S. R., and others: The treatment of schistosomiasis with niridazole in Britain, J. Trop. Med. Hyg. **73**:162, 1970.

Symposium: The pharmacological and chemotherapeutic properties of niridazole and other antischistosomal compounds, Ann. N.Y. Acad. Sci. **160**:423, 1969.

Amebicides

Pittman, F. E., and Pittman, J. C.: Amebic liver abscess following metronidazole therapy for amebic colitis, Am. J. Trop. Med. **23**:146, 1974.

Powell, S. J., and others: Single and low dosage regimen of metronidazole in amoebic dysentery and amoebic liver abscess, Ann. Trop. Med. Parasitol. **61**:26, 1969.

Powell, S. J.: Therapy of ambiasis, Bull. N.Y. Acad. Sci. **47**:469, 1971.

Powell, S. J., and others: Further trials of metronidazole in amoebic dysentery and amoebic liver abscess, Ann. Trop. Med. Parasitol. **61**:511, 1969.

Rubidge, C. J., and others: Treatment of children with acute amoebic dysentery, Arch. Dis. Child. **45**:196, 1970.

Scott, F., and Miller, M. J.: Trials with metranidazole in amebic dysentery, J.A.M.A. **211**:118, 1970.

Weber, D. M.: Amebic abscess of liver following metronidazole therapy, J.A.M.A. **216**:1339, 1971.

World Health Organization Expert Committee: Amoebiasis, Technical Report Series No. 421, 1969.

CHAPTER 22

Antiseptics and disinfectants

Early in the history of mankind it was found that certain gums, balsams, and resins had the power to prevent decay in the bodies of the dead, and today the Egyptian mummy is evidence of the efficiency of the materials used. Some of these substances were also used for healing wounds, but it was not until the latter part of the nineteenth century, when Pasteur made his astounding discoveries regarding the germ theory and Lister, in consequence, began the systematic use of carbolic acid in his surgical work, that antiseptics came into general use.

Local antiinfectives now include a wide variety of agents used for many purposes. A number of the older agents continue to be used for such purposes as the preparation of the skin prior to surgical incision or parenteral administration of drugs, the disinfection of thermometers, and the treatment of contaminated clothing and infected human excreta. Local antiinfectives are used in the home for the treatment of minor wounds and abrasions, and in the community at large they play a role in the safe handling of sewage, in the purification of water supplies, and in the preservation of food supplies.

DEFINITIONS

There continues to be some misunderstanding about the terms used when speaking about groups of antiinfective agents. An *antiseptic* is a chemical agent that inhibits the growth and development of microorganisms but does not necessarily kill them. It is synonymous with the term *bacteriostatic*. It means against sepsis or, more literally, "against putrefaction or decay." This term was used long before bacteria were known to exist. It is now used especially to mean agents applied to living tissues, such as an antiseptic for the skin.

Disinfectants, germicides, or *bactericides* are agents that produce rapid death of harmful microorganisms, and the terms are used synonymously. There is a trend to use the word *disinfectant* to refer to germicides used on inanimate objects. Whether a given agent kills microorganisms or inhibits their growth may depend upon a number of factors, such as the mechanism of action, the length of time the organisms are subjected to the agent, the number of micro-

511

organisms present, the concentration of the chemical agent, the temperature, and the presence and amount of organic matter.

The older disinfectants were used for killing harmful microorganisms on dishes, instruments, or the surface of the skin, but they were generally found to be too poisonous to be used internally. The introduction of antibiotics, however, changed this concept of bactericidal agents, since antibiotics include many effective bactericidal agents that are quite nontoxic for man. Although in theory antibiotics could also be used topically like the older disinfectants, they are generally too costly to be used for instruments, and their topical use on the skin is often objectionable because of their capacity to induce allergic reactions in the individual. Exceptions are found in the use of bacitracin and neomycin, which exhibit a low incidence of hypersensitivity reactions when applied topically or when they act locally. Agents used to treat local fungal, viral, or parasitic infections may also be thought of as local antiinfectives.

MECHANISMS OF ACTION

Antiinfectives may act in three ways. (1) They may bring about a change in the structure of the protein of the microbial cell (denaturation), which often proceeds to coagulation of protein with increased concentration of the chemical agent. (2) They may lower the surface tension of the aqueous medium of the parasitic cell. This increases the permeability of the plasma membrane, and the cellular constituents are destroyed by lysis. The cell is unable to maintain its equilibrium in its environment. (The surface-active agents are thought to act this way.) (3) They may interfere with some metabolic processes of the microbial cells in such ways as to interfere with the cell's ability to survive and multiply.

Concern about the effectiveness of disinfectants has been heightened by the problem of hospital-acquired infections caused by antibiotic-resistant staphylococci. On the other hand, these microorganisms are apparently no more resistant to the usual chemical disinfectants than

they ever were. A good antiinfective must be more effective against the parasitic cells than against the cells of the host. Many good antiinfectives are so toxic to all cells that they cannot be used except on inanimate objects, and they constitute a hazard around a home or anywhere human beings may be accidentally poisoned. Both physical and chemical agents are used in disinfection, but in this chapter emphasis is given to chemical agents. There is no ideal chemical agent suitable for all purposes for which these agents are needed.

CRITERIA FOR EVALUATING DISINFECTANTS

An ideal disinfectant may never be found. It should be able to destroy all forms of infectious agents without being toxic to the cells of human tissues, and it should not induce sensitization. In present-day practice, what constitutes a satisfactory germicide for a given article depends on whether only vegetative organisms must be destroyed or whether fungi, tubercle bacilli, viruses, and spores also must be killed, since the latter are generally more resistant to germicides. It is important to select the best antiinfective to accomplish the results desired. All germicides and disinfectants recommended for hospital use must be effective against gram-negative enteric organisms and gram-positive pyogenic organisms, when used as directed. The demands made of a good disinfectant have gradually become greater as better disinfectants have been developed. Some authorities now say that a solution of a disinfectant should be expected to kill within 10 minutes all vegetative bacteria and fungi, tubercle bacilli, animal parasites, and viruses with the possible exception of the viruses causing hepatitis. (The disinfectant cannot be expected to kill spores.) Not all disinfectants in present-day use will do this, at least not in a few minutes. Some may do so when several hours of exposure to the disinfectant are provided. The ideal disinfectant should not only kill all the organisms mentioned but should also act in the presence of organic material and be stable, noncorrosive, and inexpensive.

It should never be overlooked that heat, and particularly moist heat under pressure (autoclaving), is the method of choice for killing all forms of living organisms, but since not all things that require disinfection can be autoclaved, there continues to be a need for satisfactory chemical disinfectants.

PHENOL AND RELATED COMPOUNDS

Within the phenol group of compounds a relationship between chemical structure and antimicrobial activity has been noted. For this reason the chemical formulas have been included. This relationship has not been observed for all chemical agents.

Phenol, U.S.P., B.P. (carbolic acid)

OH

Phenol is a crystalline compound with a characteristic odor. The needle-shaped crystals may become pinkish upon standing. Phenol was introduced into medicine as an antiseptic by Sir Joseph Lister in 1867. Its use was so firmly established that it has been employed as a standard against which the antibacterial activity of other similar compounds (particularly other phenols) is measured. The relative power of a disinfectant as compared to phenol is known as the phenol coefficient (P/C). A disinfectant thirty times as efficient as phenol (producing the same killing effect at one thirtieth the concentration) is said to have a phenol coefficient of 30.

Solutions of phenol are antiseptic, germicidal, or escharotic (scarring to tissue), depending upon the concentration used. Antiseptic solutions are irritating or toxic to tissues, and concentrated solutions may produce death when taken internally or when applied topically to abraded surfaces of the skin. When applied locally, phenol penetrates the skin and exerts a local anesthetic effect on sensory nerve endings. This explains its presence in certain lotions or ointments used to relieve itching (antipruritics).

Phenol is believed to exert its germicidal action by altering the structure of the protein in the parasitic cells (denaturation). In high concentrations it precipitates cellular protein. It is not affected much by the presence of organic matter or by high concentrations of bacteria. The use of phenol has declined because better disinfectants have been found that are less irritating, less toxic to human tissues, and more efficient in killing microorganisms. Bacterial spores and viruses tend to be resistant to phenol. Phenol is occasionally used in full strength (89% aqueous solution) to cauterize small wounds such as snake bites, in 5% strength to disinfect sinks, toilets, and excreta, and in dilute solution (0.5% to 1%) to relieve itching.

Liquified phenol, U.S.P., B.P. This is an 89% aqueous solution of phenol (80%, B.P.).

Cresol, B.P.

Cresol is available as a mixture of the ortho-, meta-, and para-methyl phenols and is derived from coal tar. Cresols are phenols in which one of the hydrogen atoms in the benzene ring has been replaced by a methyl group (CH_3).

OH	OH	OH
—CH_3	—CH_3	—CH_3
o-cresol	*m*-cresol	*p*-cresol

Cresol is a thick, heavy, straw-colored liquid with a phenol-like odor. It is two to five times as active as phenol but no more toxic. It is only slightly soluble in water but is soluble in liquid soap. Preparations of cresol are used for disinfecting excreta, sinks, bedpans, toilets, and the like. All are poisonous and should be used for external purposes only or as mentioned. If accidentally spilled on the skin, a burning sensation will be noted. The area should be washed with copious amounts of water to prevent a painful burn.

Saponated cresol solution. This is a 50% solution of cresol in vegetable oil (saponified). This solution is also known as Lysol.

Lysol forms a milky emulsion in water, but it is more soluble than pure cresol. Its action is not hampered by the presence of organic material. It is used in 2% to 5% strength to disinfect excreta, sinks, toilets, bedpans, and similar utensils. It is like the other cresols and phenol in that it is poisonous.

Hexachlorophene, U.S.P. (Gamophen, pHisoHex, Surgi-Cen, Surofene); hexachlorophane, B.P.

Hexachlorophene is a chlorinated diphenol. It is a white to light tan powder, relatively insoluble in water but soluble in alcohol, fats, and soaps. It is incorporated into detergent creams, oils, soaps, lotions, ointments, shampoos, and other media for topical application to reduce numbers of pathogenic bacteria on the skin and to reduce the incidence of pyogenic skin infections. It is much more effective against gram-positive than gram-negative bacteria. Optimum effects are secured only when regular and repeated applications are made. If other cleansing agents are substituted, a rapid increase of organisms normally found on the skin may be observed.

Regularly repeated scrubs leave a residual film on the skin that causes a steady decrease in bacterial flora. This antiseptic property permits a 2-minute preoperative scrub.

Antibacterial detergents have been used to prevent and control staphylococcal infections spread by hospital personnel. To control hospital nursery infections a 1% to 3% hexachlorophene preparation can be used for short-term, once daily bathing followed by rinsing.

Hexachlorophene should not be looked upon as a substitute for mechanical cleansing of the skin, although products containing this substance are used for preoperative preparation of the skin. It is also used by food handlers and dentists. Its activity is reduced by the presence of organic material and blood serum. Alcohol and other organic solvents should be avoided when hexachlorophene is used.

Precautions. According to the A.M.A., hexachlorophene should not be used routinely to bathe infants, particularly premature infants, since it can be absorbed and cause neurotoxic effects. In animals it has caused degeneration of the brain. Its use on the skin of any age group should be followed by thorough rinsing.

Cardiovascular disturbances, convulsions, and respiratory arrest have been reported following accidental ingestion or applications of high concentrations (6%) to children.

Hexachlorophene liquid soap, U.S.P. The soap contains between 225 and 260 mg. of hexachlorophene in each 100 ml. of 10% to 13% potassium soap base.

Resorcinol, U.S.P., B.P.

Resorcinol resembles phenol in effectiveness, but it is less toxic, irritating, and caustic. It is used chiefly as an antiseptic and keratolytic (softening or dissolving the keratin-containing epidermis) in the treatment of various diseases of the skin. It is used in strengths that vary from 2% to 20%. It acts by precipitating cell proteins.

This compound occurs as colorless needle-shaped crystals with a faint odor. It is applied topically as an ointment, lotion, or paste.

Compound resorcinol ointment, N.F., contains 6% resorcinol in a number of media to make a suitable ointment.

Hexylresorcinol, N.F., B.P.

Hexylresorcinol was first introduced as a urinary antiseptic. Much of its efficiency is the result of its low surface tension. This accounts for the name "ST 37" that is used for a 1:1000 solution of hexylresorcinol in glycerin and water.

Hexylresorcinol is stainless and odorless, but

it may be irritating to tissues. Persons who become hypersensitive to it may exhibit allergic reactions. One of its more important uses is the treatment of patients with worm infestations (see Chapter 21).

Thymol, U.S.P., B.P.

Thymol is a colorless crystalline solid with an aromatic odor and taste. Chemically, it is related to one of the cresols and is more effective than phenol. It possesses fungicidal properties, and it is an effective anthelmintic for hookworm. Because of its pleasant odor and taste it is an ingredient of many gargles and mouthwashes.

O-syl and Amphyl

O-syl and Amphyl are both phenol derivatives.

A combination of *o*-phenyl phenol and potassium resinoleate furnishes the active ingredient of O-syl. A similar compound is marketed under the name of Amphyl. These compounds do not have the typical odor of phenolic compounds. When used in 3% concentrations they are said to be effective against vegetative forms of microorganisms, but they do not kill spores. They are moderately active against tubercle bacilli and viruses. They are suitable as germicidal solutions to be used for cleaning of walls, furniture, and floors.

DYES

Certain dyes are used as antiseptics and antiprotozoal agents as well as to promote the healing of wounds. Because they are rapidly adsorbed on proteins, they exhibit limited ability to penetrate tissues, and their germicidal action tends to be slow.

Triphenylmethane dyes (rosaniline dyes)

Triphenylmethane dyes are a group of basic dyes that include crystal violet, gentian violet,

methyl violet, brilliant green, and fuchsin. Solutions of these dyes are used in the form of antiseptic dressings on wounds, serous surfaces, and mucous membranes, or they are applied topically for the treatment of superficial fungous or gram-positive infections of the skin and mucous membranes. Gentian violet is also used in the treatment of certain types of worm infestation. Concentrations of 1:1000 to 1:5000 are used for direct application to tissues. For instillation into body cavities the concentration is decreased to 1:10,000.

Gentian violet, U.S.P.; *crystal violet*, B.P. This dye is available in bulk powder and in tablet form, 10, 15, and 30 mg.

Gentian violet solution, U.S.P. The solution consists mainly of gentian violet with some admixture of the other two violet compounds. It is a 1% solution of the dyes in 10% alcohol.

Carbol-fuchsin solution (Castellani's paint). This preparation contains fuchsin, phenol, resorcinol, and boric acid in an acetone-alcohol-water solution. It is used in the treatment of fungous infections. Fuchsin is para-rosaniline chloride and is a red dye.

Azo dyes

The azo dyes are more effective as agents that promote the healing of wounds than they are as antiseptics. They appear to stimulate the growth of epithelium and are sometimes used in the treatment of burns, chronic ulcers, and bedsores. Difference of opinion, however, exists regarding their effectiveness.

Scarlet red ointment. This preparation contains 5% scarlet red in olive oil, wool fat, and petrolatum.

Pyridium (phenyl-azo-diamino pyridine hydrochloride). Pyridium is used for its analgesic action on irritated mucous membrane of the urinary tract. It is for this reason that it is found in combination with urinary antiseptics, such as Azo Gantrisin.

Acridine dyes

Acridine dyes have been called "flavines" because of their yellow color. They are applied to open wounds in 0.1% to 1% solutions or ointments. In this strength they are relatively nonirritating and they do not retard the healing of wounds. They are bactericidal and bacteriostatic upon a variety of microorganisms, with greatest activity against gram-positive bacteria in an alkaline medium.

HEAVY METALS
Mercury compounds

Inorganic compounds. Inorganic compounds of mercury were among the earliest antiseptics to be used, and they long were regarded as potent germicides. Investigation has shown that their action, in many instances, is bacteriostatic rather than bactericidal, since their effects can be reversed under some conditions and microorganisms have been revived that were previously considered dead. Although the mercuric ion brings about the precipitation of cellular proteins, its bacteriostatic action is said to be the result of inhibition of specific enzymes of bacterial cells. Mercurial antiseptics may also exert toxic effects on the tissue cells of the host when taken internally. The mercurials fall far short of being ideal antiseptics or germicides. The inorganic compounds are irritating to tissues, penetrate poorly, are toxic systemically, are adversely affected by the presence of organic materials, have little or no action on spores, and are corrosive to metals. However, they are effective bacteriostatic agents for certain uses. Some of the organic compounds are more potent than the inorganic ones, especially if they are in alcoholic solution. Some authorities believe that certain organic mercurials are useful antiseptics if they are used appropriately in proper concentration.

Mercury bichloride; mercuric chloride, B.P. (Corrosive Sublimate). This is the oldest of the mercurial antiseptics. Tablets of mercury bichloride are coffin shaped and are stamped with a skull and crossbones and the word "Poison." They are colored blue to prevent their solutions from being mistaken for water. Mercuric chloride is availabe in 0.5- and 0.12-Gm. tablets. It is occasionally used in a 1:1000 concentration to disinfect objects that would be harmed by heat or to disinfect hands that have previously been scrubbed with soap and water.

Mercurial ointments. A number of compounds of mercury and metallic mercury are incorporated into ointments for use as antiseptics. The drug slowly dissolves in the tissues to release a low concentration of mercuric ions and thus exerts a prolonged effect. A number of such ointments are listed in *The National Formulary.* Two official ointments are included in this discussion.

Ammoniated mercury ointment, U.S.P., B.P. (White Precipitate Ointment). The U.S.P. preparation contains 5% ammoniated mercury; the B.P. preparation contains 2.5%. The U.S.P. preparation has a base of white ointment and liquid petrolatum. The B.P. preparation is made with simple ointment. Ammoniated mercury is also used in ointments of 2% to 10% concentrations as antiseptics and local stimulants in cases of suppurating dermatitis, eczematous and parasitic skin diseases, and particularly impetigo.

Ammoniated mercury ophthalmic ointment. This contains 3% ammoniated mercury and is applied as an antiseptic to the eyelids.

Organic mercurial preparations. Organic mercurial compounds are less toxic and less irritating than the inorganic mercurial antiseptics.

Merbromin (Mercurochrome). Although widely used at one time, merbromin has been supplanted by more effective agents since it is primarily bacteriostatic. It was the first organic mercurial to be used.

Thimerosal, N.F., B.P. (Merthiolate). Thimerosal is a light cream-colored, crystalline powder. It contains about 50% mercury. It can be used safely as a skin antiseptic on abraded skin in concentrations of 1:1000, and aqueous solutions can be used on mucous membranes. Thimerosal solution, N.F., is an aqueous solution that has been colored red by a suitable coaltar color. Thimerosal solutions are incompatible with acids, salts of other heavy metals, and iodine. Thimerosal tincture (an acetone-alcohol solution) and thimerosal ointment are also listed in *The National Formulary.*

Nitromersol, N.F. (Metaphen); *nitromersol tincture,* N.F. This is a 0.5% solution of nitromersol in acetone, alcohol, and water. It is used chiefly as a skin disinfectant. Nitromersol solution, N.F., is an aqueous solution sometimes used to disinfect instruments in concentrations of 1:1000 to 1:5000; to disinfect the skin it is used in a concentration of 1:1000 to 1:5000; and for irrigation of mucous membranes (eye and urethra) it is used in a concentration of 1:5000 to 1:10,000.

Acetomeroctol (Merbak). This is an organic mercurial applied topically as an antiseptic. Its activity and effectiveness are similar to those of other organic mercurials. A 1:1000 concentration contains 50% alcohol and 10% acetone, which contribute to its effectiveness.

Phenylmercuric compounds. Phenylmercuric compounds are active against a variety of pathogenic bacteria and exhibit a low level of toxicity in human tissue. Like other mercurial antiseptics, they cannot be depended upon to kill spores. These compounds occasionally cause irritation and poisoning in persons of undue sensitivity. Buffered solutions are odorless, colorless, and stainless and do not react with body proteins. They are noncorrosive to metals with the exception of aluminum, and they do not destroy rubber.

Phenylmercuric nitrate, U.S.P., B.P. (Merphenyl Nitrate Basic). This drug is applied topically in 1:1500 solutions for prophylactic disinfection of intact skin and minor injuries and in 1:1500 to 1:24,000 solutions for mucous membranes and wet dressings.

Silver compounds

Inorganic salts. Silver compounds are used in medicine for their antiseptic, caustic, and astringent effects, which are caused by the release of free silver ions. The soluble salts of silver ionize readily in solution, whereas the colloidal silver compounds dissociate only slightly. Silver ions will precipitate cellular protein; inorganic salts of silver are germicidal in solution but colloidal preparations are bacteriostatic. It is thought that silver, like mercury, is capable of interfering with important metabolic activities of microbial cells.

Silver nitrate, U.S.P., B.P. Silver nitrate occurs as flat, transparent crystals that become grayish black on exposure to light and in the presence of organic material. It is odorless and has a bitter strongly metallic taste. It is freely soluble in water, ionizes readily, and is germicidal. Silver nitrate reacts with soluble chloride, iodides, and bromides to form insoluble salts; therefore, the action of silver salts can be stopped by contact with a solution of sodium chloride. This chemical property also explains why solutions of silver salts penetrate tissues slowly as a result of the precipitation of silver ions in the tissues by chlorides or phosphates. A 1:1000 solution is antiseptic. Weak solutions are astringent on mucous membranes, and strong solutions are caustic when applied to mucous membranes or the skin. Silver salts stain tissues black because of the deposit of silver. This discoloration slowly disappears.

Silver nitrate is used on inflamed mucous membranes and ulcerated surfaces. For diseases of the conjunctiva, solutions varying in strength from 0.2% to 2% may be used. To prevent the development of gonorrheal conjunctivitis in the newborn infant, a drop or two of 1% solution is instilled into each eye as soon as possible after delivery. A stronger solution has been used, but it is dangerous, because strong solutions will kill tissue in a short time and may permit the gonococcus to enter and spread into deeper tissues. Blindness has been caused in this way. To stop the action if too much has been used, the eye should be washed with physiologic saline solution. Even a 1% silver nitrate solution produces a chemical conjunctivitis in a rather large number of cases. For this reason, some physicians have advocated the use of penicillin ointment. Silver nitrate is also used as a wet dressing for treatment of burns in a 0.5% solution. Solutions of silver nitrate that vary in concentration from 1:1000 to 1:10,000 are used for irrigation of the bladder and urethra. A 1:1000 solution is germicidal but irritating. Long-continued use of any silver preparation may produce permanent discoloration of the skin and mucous membranes, a condition known as argyria.

Toughened silver nitrate, U.S.P., B.P. (Lunar Caustic). This form is a white solid generally used in the form of pencils or cones. It is applied as a mild caustic to wounds, ulcers, warts, and granulation tissue. It should be moistened before use and, to avoid blackening the fingers, should be held with forceps. It may be fused on a probe for application to parts with difficult access. The mucous membranes to which solutions of silver nitrate are applied should receive a preliminary cleansing to remove mucus, pus, and food that would interfere with drug action.

Colloidal silver preparations. Colloidal preparations do not ionize readily and do not act as corrosives, irritants, or astringents. They penetrate tissue more readily than do the solutions of simple salts of silver. They exert a bacteriostatic effect because of the concentration of silver ions that is gradually produced.

The colloidal preparations of silver are used as antiseptics, particularly on mucous membranes of the nose and throat, the urinary bladder, the urethra, and the conjunctiva. Gonococci are particularly susceptible to the action of silver compounds.

The terms *strong* and *mild* refer to the relative antiseptic values and not to the amount of silver they contain, for the strong preparation contains about 8% silver and the weak contains about 20%. The antiseptic value depends on the extent of ionization in any given liquid. Mild silver protein preparations should be freshly made and dispensed in amber-colored bottles.

Strong silver protein (Protargol). This compound contains not less than 7.5% and not more than 8.5% of silver.

Mild silver protein (Argyrol, Silvol). The mild form contains from 19% to 23% silver. It is entirely nonirritating but it also has less antiseptic action than the strong silver protein. It is usually employed in concentrations of 5% to 25%. A concentration of 5% is commonly used for bladder irrigation, 10% to 15% in the nose, and 20% to 25% in the eye.

HALOGENS
Chlorine

Chlorine is a nonmetallic element that occurs in the form of a greenish-yellow gas. It has an intensely disagreeable odor. One part of chlorine in 10,000 parts of air causes irritation of the respiratory tract, and exposure to a 1:1000 concentration is fatal after 5 minutes. It causes spasm and pain of the muscles of the larynx and bronchial tubes, coughing, a burning sensation, fainting, unconsciousness, and death. Its extensive use for the purification of water, however, makes it one of the most widely used disinfectants. One part of chlorine in 1 million parts of water will destroy most bacteria in a few minutes. Acid-fast organisms such as *Mycobacterium tuberculosis* are unusually resistant to it. Chlorine is effective against amebas, viruses, organisms of the colon-typhoid group, and many of the spore-forming pathogens. The antibacterial action of chlorine is said to be caused by the formation of hypochlorous acid, which results when chlorine reacts with water. Hypochlorous acid is a rapidly acting bactericidal agent. Its effect is partly the result of its oxidizing action and partly of its effect on microbial enzymes that are concerned with the metabolism of glucose.

The activity of chlorine and chlorine-releasing compounds is influenced by a number of factors, such as the presence of organic material, the pH of the solution, and the temperature. Chlorine is more effective when there is a minimum of organic matter, when the medium is acid in reaction, and when the temperature is elevated. Chlorine is an efficient deodorant and a strong bleaching agent, and it corrodes many metals.

Gaseous chlorine has limited usefulness because it is difficult to handle. There are a number of compounds that yield hypochlorous acid and that are useful for certain kinds of disinfection.

Sodium hypochlorite solution, N.F., B.P. This is a 5% solution of sodium hypochlorite. This concentration is too great to be used on living tissues. It is used to disinfect utensils and swimming pools.

Diluted sodium hypochlorite solution, modified Dakin's solution, N.F. This preparation is a 0.5% aqueous solution of sodium hypochlorite. It was once used extensively in the treatment of suppurating wounds. Although it is useful in cleansing wounds, it also interferes with the formation of thrombin, delays clotting of blood, and is irritating to the skin. Dilute solutions have been used to prevent the development of athlete's foot (epidermophytosis). A 0.5% solution of sodium hypochlorite is also used to disinfect walls, furniture, and especially floors. Preparations of sodium hypochlorite are unstable and need to be freshly prepared.

Chloramines. Several compounds are available in which chlorine is linked with nitrogen. The chloramines exert their effects by the release of chlorine to form hypochlorous acid and also by direct action of the parent compound. The chloramines are more stable, less irritating, and slower acting than the hypochlorites. Their action is more prolonged and they are less readily affected by the presence of organic material.

Chloramine-T, U.S.P.; *chloramine*, B.P. This compound is used in 0.1% to 2% aqueous solutions for irrigations of wounds or for dressings.

Halazone. Halazone is available in 4-mg. tablets and is employed for the sterilization of drinking water. All pathogens usually found in water will be killed in 30 to 60 minutes by the addition of one to two tablets (4 to 8 mg.) per liter of water.

Iodine

Iodine is a heavy, bluish-black, crystalline solid that has a metallic luster and a characteristic odor. It is slightly soluble in water but is soluble in alcohol and in aqueous solutions of sodium and potassium iodide. Iodine is volatile, and its solutions should not be exposed to air except during use. The mechanism of disinfectant action is not entirely known. The concentration at which iodine acts as a disinfectant is similar for all bacteria. Iodine is thought to be one of the more efficient chemical disinfectants in present-day usage. Its activity does not vary greatly for vegetative pathogens; it is effective over a wide range of pH, and it is effective against spores, viruses, and fungi. It is not affected by the presence of organic material found in body fluids and exudates. In combination with alcohol, iodine in 0.5% to 1% solution will kill tubercle bacilli. However, iodine does not kill spores readily, and it has the disadvantage of staining skin and clothing. In rare instances, individuals exhibit hypersensitivity reactions to iodine when it is applied to the skin. Iodine is used chiefly for disinfection of small wounds and abraded surfaces and in the preoperative preparation of skin surfaces. A fact often overlooked is that aqueous solutions as well as alcoholic solutions of iodine are germicidal. Aqueous solutions are less irritating and are best used on abraded areas of the skin. Iodine penetrates the skin and slight amounts are absorbed.

Another use that may be made of iodine tincture is the emergency disinfection of water that is suspected of harboring pathogenic amebas. Three drops of iodine tincture to a quart of water will kill amebas and bacteria in 15 minutes without making the water unpalatable.

Iodine stains the skin and linens a brown color. These stains can be removed from the skin with alcohol or ammonia and from fabrics with boiling water.

Iodine tincture, U.S.P., B.P. This preparation contains 2% iodine and 2.4% sodium iodide in 46% ethyl alcohol. It has to a great extent replaced the strong iodine tincture. Weak iodine solution, B.P., contains approximately the same amount of iodine along with potassium iodide and 90% ethyl alcohol.

Strong iodine tincture. This form is an alcoholic solution containing 7% iodine and 5% potassium iodide in 83% ethyl alcohol.

Strong iodine solution, U.S.P. (Lugol's Solution). Strong iodine solution is similar in preparation to strong iodine tincture. The aqueous solution contains 5% iodine and 10% potassium iodide. It is given orally for the treatment of goiter rather than for its antiseptic effect.

Iodine solution. This aqueous solution contains 2% iodine and 2.4% sodium iodide.

Iodophors. Iodophors are complex combinations of iodine and a carrier or agent that increases the water solubility of iodine. The word literally means "iodine carrier." The combination contains and slowly releases iodine as it is needed but does not stain as aqueous solutions of iodine do. As used today, it frequently means a combination of iodine and a detergent. *Wesco-dyne* is one that is said to kill tubercle bacilli as well as other organisms sensitive to iodine. Undecoylium chloride-iodine (Virac) is a combination of iodine and a cationic detergent that is said to make a useful surface-acting agent.

Povidone-iodine solution, U.S.P. (Betadine, PVP, Isodine). Povidone-iodine is an organic iodine and polyvinylpyrrolidone complex. It is water soluble, and when the solution is used as an antiseptic, the complex breaks down on contact with the skin or mucous membranes and free iodine is slowly released. This preparation has the advantage of combining the desirable properties of iodine as a potent germicide with a highly antibacterial, surface-acting agent. It is thought to be superior to soap, hexachlorophene scrubs, and cationic agents as a skin disinfectant, but somewhat less effective than aqueous or alcoholic solutions of iodine. It is relatively nonirritating, nontoxic, and nonsensitizing to the skin except in those persons sensitive to iodine.

Povidone-iodine is used as an antiseptic on the skin, mucous membranes, and scalp, and for surgical preparation of the skin. Available solutions contain 0.75%, 1%, or 1.5% of available iodine.

OXIDIZING AGENTS

Certain oxidizing agents are destructive to pathogenic organisms but mild enough to be used on living tissues. Their activity is caused by the oxygen that they liberate. Oxygen combines readily with organic matter and, once combined, it is inert. Oxygen is especially harmful to anaerobic organisms. On the whole, microorganisms vary considerably in their sensitivity to oxygen.

Hydrogen peroxide solution, U.S.P., B.P.

The U.S.P. preparation of hydrogen peroxide solution is a 3% solution of hydrogen peroxide in water.* It is a colorless, odorless liquid that deteriorates upon standing. It should be kept in a cool, dark place and should be well stoppered. Hydrogen peroxide decomposes to water and oxygen. This reaction occurs rapidly when the solution is in contact with organic matter. It is an active germicide only while it is actively releasing oxygen. Solutions have a high surface tension and do not penetrate readily. The effervescence (caused by rapid formation of oxygen bubbles) that accompanies decomposition helps to clean suppurating wounds, but it should not be injected into closed body cavities or into abscesses from which the newly formed gas cannot easily escape. The official solution is usually diluted with 1 to 4 parts of water before it is used. It is used for the cleansing of wounds, for repair of cleft lip, and for the treatment of Vincent's infection (trench mouth). In the latter case it is employed full strength for a limited period of

*The preparation described in B.P. is approximately a 6% solution.

time. Nurses use it frequently to remove collections of mucus from the inner cannula of a tracheostomy tube.

Medicinal zinc peroxide

Medicinal zinc peroxide consists of zinc peroxide, zinc carbonate, and zinc hydroxide. Upon hydrolysis it yields hydrogen peroxide. It has some value in the disinfection and deodorization of wounds, especially those infected with anaerobic organisms. It leaves a residue of zinc oxide that is slightly astringent in effect.

Potassium permanganate, U.S.P., B.P.

Potassium permanganate occurs as dark purple crystals that are soluble in water (1:15). It decomposes on contact with organic matter and liberates oxygen, which combines with bacteria and inhibits their growth or destroys them. The bactericidal efficiency of solutions of potassium permanganate vary with the type of organism and the amount of organic material present. Solutions stronger than 1:5000 may be irritating to tissues. It is used in vaginal douches in concentrations of 1:1000 to 1:5000 and is applied topically in concentrations of 1:500 to 1:10,000. After potassium permanganate solutions have lost oxygen they appear brown and are inert. Stains may be removed with dilute acids (lemon juice, oxalic acid, or dilute hydrochloric acid).

Potassium permanganate solutions produce irritant, astringent, and deodorant, as well as germicidal effects. It is used much less now than formerly.

Sodium perborate. This is a white powder soluble in water. In solution it forms hydrogen peroxide. It is used as a dusting powder or in 2% solution as an oral antiseptic. Its chief use is in the treatment of Vincent's infection.

SURFACE-ACTIVE AGENTS

Surface-active agents are also known as wetting agents, emulsifiers, and detergents. In some respects, certain of these agents are considered superior to ordinary soap because they can be used in hard water, are stable in both acid and alkaline solutions, decrease surface tension more effectively, and are less irritating to the skin than ordinary soaps. They all lower surface tensions and aid in the mechanical removal of bacteria and soil. Many also exert a bactericidal action. Many are believed to depress metabolic activities of bacteria, but how they do it is not fully known. They have a weak action against fungi, acid-fast organisms, spores, and viruses. Their activity is reduced greatly by the presence of organic matter. If the active portion of the surface-active agent (surfactant) carries a negative electric charge, it is known as an anionic compound; if the active portion carries a positive charge, it is known as a cationic surfactant or surface-active agent.

Cationic agents. The most effective cationic agents have been the quaternary ammonium compounds (sometimes referred to as "quats"). These compounds combine detergent and antiseptic action. In general, they are more effective antiseptics than the anionic group of compounds. They inhibit both gram-positive and gram-negative organisms. Soap inactivates cationic detergents and therefore it must be removed before the detergent is used. Hard water also inactivates these agents and causes precipitation. Although they are recommended in the final rinse of laundry materials, they are often ineffective because traces of soap or hard water remain. Cationic detergents cannot be relied upon to sterilize instruments and articles that cannot be subjected to heat, but they are sometimes used to preserve sterility of stored materials. They have also been used in aerosols to increase the penetrating power of antibiotics.

Benzalkonium chloride, U.S.P., B.P. (Zephiran Chloride). When employed in proper concentration, benzalkonium chloride is an effective, relatively noninjurious surface disinfectant. It is germicidal for a number of pathogenic nonspore-forming pathogens, including fungi after several minutes of exposure. However, it has no effect on tubercle bacilli. Its viricidal activity is said to be limited. Benzalkonium chloride solutions have a low surface tension and possess keratolytic, detergent, and emulsifying properties. Solutions of soap reduce its germicidal activity unless well rinsed from the area to be disinfected. Seventy percent alcohol serves to diminish the reaction of both the soap and disinfectant. Alcohol can be used *after* the skin

has been prepared with soap and water and *before* the disinfectant is applied.

Solutions of benzalkonium chloride have a relatively low level of toxicity when used as recommended.

It is suitable for prophylactic disinfection of the intact skin and in the treatment of superficial injuries when used in 1:1000 concentration (tincture).

Solutions of 1:1000 are used for preservation of metallic instruments and rubber articles. For disinfection of operating room equipment, solutions of 1:5000 may be used.

Benzethonium chloride, N.F. (Phemerol Chloride). This is a detergent that exerts an inhibitory effect on the growth activities of commonly occurring bacteria and fungi. Tincture of phemerol chloride, 1:500, and benzethonium chloride solution, N.F., 1:1000, are used full strength as general germicides and antiseptics except for use in the nose and eye. For the latter, the aqueous solution is used and diluted with 4 parts of water.

Cetylpyridinium chloride, N.F., B.P. (Ceepryn Chloride). This agent is used for preoperative disinfection of intact skin, in the treatment of minor wounds, and for the therapeutic disinfection of mucous membranes. Its effectiveness is reduced by detergents, ordinary soap, and serums and tissue fluids, and it is ineffective against clostridial spores. Strengths used vary from 1:100 for skin preparations and 1:1000 for minor abrasions to 1:5000 and 1:10,000 for mucous membranes.

Methylbenzethonium chloride, N.F. (Diaparene Chloride). This preparation produces bacteriostasis of urea-splitting organisms. It is used for disinfecting babies' diapers and linen and clothing of incontinent adults; the articles should be free of soap, however, before being rinsed in this disinfectant. It is available in 0.09-Gm. tablets, and the solution is made by dissolving one tablet in 2000 ml. of warm water. This amount is sufficient for rinsing six diapers. They should remain immersed in disinfectant for 3 minutes.

Anionic surface agents. Anionic surface agents are the neutral or faintly alkaline salts of acids of high molecular weights. Common soaps and a number of other compounds belong to this group. They are incompatible with cationic compounds. They act best in an acid medium and are most effective against gram-positive organisms.

Tincture of green soap, N.F. This preparation is an alcoholic solution containing about 65% soft soap perfumed with oil of lavender. It is called green because it was first made from oils that contains chlorophyl-like coloring matter. Modern "green soap" may be colorless.

Green soap, N.F.; *soft soap*, B.P. This is a potassium soap made by the saponification of vegetable oils without the removal of glycerin. Soft soap has little antiseptic value but is used as a cleansing agent.

Hexachlorophene liquid soap, U.S.P. This is a potassium soap to which hexachlorophene has been added.

Sodium tetradecyl sulfate (Sodium Sotradecol). This is an anionic surface-acting agent that lowers surface tension of certain antiseptic solutions to which it may be added. It is also used as a sclerosing agent in the treatment of varicose veins and internal hemorrhoids.

Other anionic surface agents include pHisoderm, which is a synthetic compound sometimes used as a substitute for soap. It is available as a cream or creamy emulsion. It is sometimes used for certain dermatologic conditions when soap is contraindicated. pHisoHex is pHisoderm to which 3% hexachlorophene has been added. It exerts a prolonged antiseptic as well as emollient effect when used routinely. pHisoHex is used frequently for preoperative preparation of patients' skin.

MISCELLANEOUS AGENTS
Alcohol

Alcohol, ethanol, ethyl alcohol, U.S.P., B.P. Alcohol is one of the oldest and most widely used of the skin disinfectants. Both ethyl alcohol and isopropyl alcohol are used as disinfectants, and their germicidal power is said to be underrated. They are used extensively to prepare the skin prior to venipuncture, subcutaneous and intramuscular injection, and ear or finger pricks for samples of blood. Ethyl alcohol is reported to be most effective in concentrations of 50% to 70%. The growth of some organisms is said to be inhibited by a 1% solution, although the

bactericidal action is unreliable when the concentration falls below 20% or is above 95%.

Isopropyl alcohol, N.F. This form is slightly more antiseptic than ethyl alcohol. It is employed full strength (99%) or as *isopropyl rubbing alcohol*, N.F., which is a 70% aqueous solution. It is also used extensively as a 75% aqueous solution for the disinfection and storage of oral thermometers. It can be combined with other disinfectants, such as formaldehyde solution, to make an effective germicide.

Formaldehyde solution, U.S.P., B.P.

Formaldehyde in a gaseous form is a powerful parasiticide because of its penetrating power, but it is active only in the presence of abundant moisture. It was used formerly for the fumigation of rooms.

Formaldehyde solution is a 37% solution of formaldehyde (by weight) known as formalin. It is a clear, colorless liquid that, on exposure to air, liberates a pungent, irritating gas. In proper concentration formaldehyde solution is germicidal against all forms of microorganisms. A 0.5% solution will kill all organisms, including spores, in 6 to 12 hours. Higher concentrations are effective in less time. It is not affected by organic matter, and it is effective against viruses. It acts as a precipitant of protein.

Formaldehyde solution hardens tissues, and for this reason it is used as a preservative for specimens and as an astringent. When it is combined with isopropyl alcohol or hexachlorophene, it is probably the most powerful germicidal solution available at the present time. Various modifications of the Bard-Parker germicidal solution are made with formaldehyde solution, isopropyl alcohol, and antirust agents for the disinfection of instruments and articles that cannot be subjected to heat. These solutions are sometimes called "cold sterilization solutions."

The chief disadvantage encountered in using solutions of formaldehyde is that it is irritating to tissues and mucous membranes and has an unpleasant odor.

Boric acid, B.P.

Boric acid is a mild antiseptic and astringent. Dilute solutions of boric acid are nonirritating and therefore suitable for use on delicate structures such as the eye. Boric acid is an ingredient of many antiseptic solutions used as washes and gargles. It is still widely used for conditions of the skin in the form of wet dressings, dusting powders, and ointments.

Although boric acid is not customarily considered a toxic substance since it is used externally, serious poisoning and deaths have resulted from its ingestion. Solutions of boric acid should be colored to help prevent accidents. Toxic reactions have occurred from topical application to large denuded areas because of the absorption that took place.

Boric acid solution is a 5% aqueous solution of boric acid.

Ethylene oxide

Ethylene oxide has come to be used for gaseous sterilization of materials that cannot be subjected to heat or pressure, such as certain plastic parts of machines and optical instruments.

Ethylene oxide is a colorless gas at ordinary temperatures; it has a rather pleasant ethereal odor, and its toxicity when inhaled is said to compare with ammonia gas. It is flammable and when confined is capable of explosive violence. This agent is used in a mixture of ethylene oxide with carbon dioxide to reduce its flammability. A preparation of 10% ethylene oxide and 90% carbon dioxide is on the market under the name Carboxide.

Ethylene oxide is apparently effective against all types of microorganisms, including viruses and tubercle bacilli. It is also effective against spores. Its action is bactericidal rather than bacteriostatic. It is a more expensive form of sterilization than that achieved with heat or other chemical agents, but it has good penetrating power and can be used for many things that would be injured by heat.

QUESTIONS

For study and review

1 Explain how antiseptics and disinfectants exert their bacteriostatic or bactericidal action.
2 Make a list of the preparations of heavy metals used as antiseptics or disinfectants in the hospital in which you obtain your clinical experience. For what particular purposes are these substances used?
3 An antiseptic is a substance that:
  a. inhibits all microorganisms
  b. kills bacteria
  c. does not sterilize the surface being treated
  d. inhibits growth of infectious agents
4 Which of the following statements are correct?
  a. Increasing the concentration of an antiseptic at the site of action increases its effectiveness.
  b. Phenol antiseptics are not used to disinfect skin or tissue because they precipitate or coagulate proteins.
  c. Phenol antiseptics are effective against bacterial spores.
  d. The development of phenol-resistant organisms is not a problem.
5 The disinfectant activity of ethyl alcohol is:
  a. inferior to that of isopropyl alcohol 70%
  b. greatest at a concentration of 95%
  c. most effective at a concentration of 50% to 70%
  d. very limited
6 Select the *incorrect* answer.
  Anionic surface agents:
  a. are incompatible with cationic surface agents
  b. have a selective action against gram-negative bacteria
  c. act best in an acid medium
  d. have reduced effectiveness in the presence of organic matter (such as blood)
7 Iodine as a chemical disinfectant:
  a. is effective against spores, viruses, and fungi
  b. does not have reduced effectiveness in the presence of organic matter
  c. will kill tubercle bacilli when used in combination with alcohol as a 1% solution
  d. is nonirritating to human tissue

REFERENCES

A.M.A. drug evaluations, ed. 2, Acton, Mass., 1973, Publishing Sciences Group, Inc.

Aviado, D. M.: Krantz and Carr's pharmacologic principles of medical practice, ed. 8, Baltimore, 1972, The Williams & Wilkins Co.

Dineen, P.: Local antiseptics. In Modell, W., editor: Drugs of choice 1974-1975, St. Louis, 1974, The C. V. Mosby Co.

Dineen, P.: Prevention of infection in the operating room, Bull. Am. Coll. Surg. Vol. 55, No. 10, Dec. 1970.

Kimbrough, R. D.: Review of evidence of toxic effects of hexachlorophene, Pediatrics **51:**391, 1973.

Kimbrough, R. D.: Review of the toxicity of hexachlorophene, Arch. Environ. Health **23:**119, 1971.

Lawrence, C. A., and Block, S. S.: Disinfection, sterilization, and preservation, Philadelphia, 1968, Lea & Febiger.

Perkins, J. J.: Principles and methods of sterilization in health sciences, ed. 2, Springfield, Ill., 1969, Charles C Thomas, Publisher.

CHAPTER 23

Serums and vaccines

Agents containing antibodies: immune serums
Antigenic agents used to produce active immunity
Agents for cutaneous immunity tests
Nursing aspects

Immunity is of two kinds, natural and acquired. If an individual is so constituted that the microbes causing a disease will not grow in his tissues or the toxins of those microbes are harmless to him, he is immune to that particular disease. Such immunity is called *natural immunity.*

When natural immunity is not effective and organisms attack the tissues and live and grow at their expense, the body protects itself by preparing substances destructive to the particular organism making the attack. These substances are called antibodies. They are present in the blood and other body fluids and are carried to the point of infection by the blood and lymph. The antibodies gradually disappear from the blood, but the body cells have seemingly acquired the ability to continue to resist the same organisms. Immunity resulting from these antibodies and the special ability to produce them is known as *acquired immunity.* Since the individual himself developed the antibodies, the immunity is known as *active immunity.* It is usually present after an attack of an infectious disease such as smallpox or typhoid fever and may be induced artificially by the injection of substances known as antigens. The antigen may be a suspension of living microorganisms, such as the vaccinia virus, or a suspension of dead microorganisms, such as typhoid vaccine. It may be an extract of the bodies of bacteria, as tuberculosis

vaccine, or a soluble toxin produced by bacteria, of which diphtheria toxin is an example.

Passive acquired immunity against certain diseases is secured by transferring to a person the blood serum of an animal that has been actively immunized by injections with the specific organisms or toxins of those diseases; it may also be secured by injection of the blood serum from an immune person. Immunity acquired in this way is called passive immunity because the body plays no part in the preparation of the antibodies. The body cells are not prepared to resist infection as they are in active immunity, and as the blood is renewed the antibodies are lost and the patient is in the same condition as if no antibodies had been administered.

Biological preparations are regulated by the Bureau of Biologics of the F.D.A. The Public Health Service's Advisory Committee on Immunization Practices of the Center for Disease Control, Atlanta, Georgia, makes recommendations for the use of preparations for the control of infectious diseases. Many diseases that once were dreaded have been almost eradicated by the use of biologic preparations. Today these preparations can be used in the prevention of eighteen diseases.

A number of these products may cause untoward reactions when they are administered as therapeutic or prophylactic agents. Individual sensitivities to animal products, especially horse serum and egg, are primarily responsible for adverse symptoms, and idiosyncrasies toward the products of bacterial metabolism are responsible for the others.

AGENTS CONTAINING ANTIBODIES: IMMUNE SERUMS

An immune serum is the serum of a human being or an animal that has antibodies in the bloodstream.

Serum treatment consists of the transfer of the immune serum into the circulation of the patient. This immune serum contains specific antibodies that act upon disease germs.

There are two kinds of immune serums: the naturally produced and the antitoxic.

NATURALLY PRODUCED HUMAN SERUMS

Naturally produced human serums are preparations obtained from normal blood, such as plasma, serum, or globulins or serum from patients who have recovered from a disease and retain the immune bodies in their blood serum.

Immune human serum globulin, U.S.P.; gamma globulin

This is a sterile solution of globulins, primarily gamma globulin, that contains those antibodies normally present in adult human blood. Each lot of the preparation is derived from an original plasma or serum pool that represents at least 1000 individuals. It is thought to be as useful as convalescent serum and is more readily available. It is useful in the prevention of measles as well as in the treatment of that disease and for the prevention of infectious hepatitis. The dosage varies. It is administered intramuscularly.

Immune human serum globulin is used in the following:

1 *Hypogammaglobulinemia.* Children with recurrent bacterial infections, predominantly of the respiratory tract, may have deficient antibody production or enhanced catabolism of immunoglobulins. Giving them an injection of 150 mg. per kilogram of body weight of immune serum globulin once each month usually prevents these infections.
2 *Viral hepatitis.* Immune globulin serum can prevent

or minimize infectious hepatitis. Its use is recommended for: (a) persons intending to travel to an area where the disease is endemic; 0.02 ml. per kilogram of body weight every 4 to 6 weeks will provide partial passive protection; (b) nonimmune persons living in an area where the disease is highly endemic; 0.1 ml. per kilogram of body weight is given every 4 to 6 months; and (c) persons exposed to the disease. They should receive as promptly as possible an injection of 0.02 ml. per kilogram of body weight, which is repeated 3 weeks later to prevent or modify the disease.
3 *Measles.* Immune globulin serum can be used to minimize untoward reactions in patients vaccinated with the attenuated live strain of measles virus (0.02 ml. per kilogram). It can also be used to modify clinical measles if given within 8 days after exposure. No effect is obtained if given after the development of rash.
4 *Rubella.* Serum immune globulin may be given to pregnant women after exposure to rubella to modify or prevent the disease (0.2 to 0.5 ml. per kilogram).

Reactions are mild and infrequent. Fever, malaise, and headache may occur.

Measles immune globulin, U.S.P.

Measles immune globulin is a sterile standardized preparation with a known measles antibody titer. For prevention of measles the drug must be given within 6 days after exposure; dose is 0.25 ml. per kilogram of body weight. For modification of measles, globulin is given during the first week of exposure or later in the incubation period; dose is 0.05 ml. per kilogram. Modification usually imparts permanent immunity.

Prevention is recommended for infants and chronically ill children. They should then be given active immunization with live vaccine 8 or more weeks later.

Pertussis human immune globulin, U.S.P.

This is the liquid or dried serum of blood obtained from donors who have recovered from pertussis (whooping cough) and who for the preceding 7 or more days have been without active clinical manifestations of the disease, or from donors immunized with pertussis vaccine. The usual intramuscular dose is 1.25 to 2.5 ml. repeated one or two times at 1-week intervals. Therapeutic dose is the same but injections are repeated at 1-day intervals.

Poliomyelitis immune globulin (human)

Poliomyelitis immune globulin is a sterile solution of globulins derived from pooled adult human blood. It is also obtained from placental blood.

It is used for the attenuation or prevention of poliomyelitis, measles, and infectious hepatitis. It is administered only by intramuscular injections, preferably in the buttock, using care to avoid accidental intravenous injection. The dosage varies considerably, depending on the purpose of the injection; for protection against paralytic poliomyelitis, the average dose to be injected is calculated on the basis of 0.31 ml. per kilogram of body weight.

Rh$_o$ (D) immune human globulin, U.S.P. (Gamulin Rh, Rh$_o$ GAM, Rho-Immune)

This is a sterile concentrated solution of gamma globulins prepared from plasma of donors with high Rh antibody titers. It is used to suppress formation of active antibodies in Rh negative mothers after delivery of an Rh positive infant or abortion of an Rh positive fetus. This effect provides protection against hemolytic disease (erythroblastosis fetalis) in the next pregnancy.

If an Rh negative mother is found to be D$_u$ positive, the immune globulin is not needed since such individuals do not develop Rh antibodies.

To be effective the immune globulin must be given to the *mother within 72 hours after delivery or abortion.* It must not be given to the infant.

Dose. The entire contents of one vial is given intramuscularly.

Adverse reactions. Adverse effects are uncommon. Pain and tenderness may occur at the injection site. Malaise, headache, and low grade fever may occur. Angioneurotic edema and anaphylactic shock have been reported.

Contraindications. Rh$_o$ (D) immune globulin is contraindicated in Rh positive patients, and Rh negative patients who have developed Rh antibodies due to previous delivery, abortion, or transfusion with Rh positive blood.

ANTITOXIC SERUMS OF ANIMAL ORIGIN

Antitoxic serums are formed in the bodies of animals that have been actively immunized by a specific toxin. The animal is then bled and the serum separated from the blood. The serum is purified in most instances to remove inactive substances and to concentrate the antibodies. Antitoxins are given to neutralize the toxins produced in certain diseases.

Horses and rabbits are the animals most often utilized for artificial production of immune serums. One inoculation with the animal product may sensitize a patient to the blood components of that species, and subsequent inoculations of products from the same species may cause serum sickness or anaphylactoid shock. Tests for sensitivity to horse serum or other suspected antigens should be made on patients before injection of serums.

Diphtheria antitoxin, B.P.

Diphtheria antitoxin is a sterile solution of antitoxic substances obtained from the blood serum or plasma of a healthy animal immunized against diphtheria toxin. It contains not less than 500 antitoxic units per milliliter. It is used to confer passive immunity to the individual exposed to diphtheria or ill with the disease. The usual prophylactic dose is 1000 to 10,000 units and the therapeutic dose is 20,000 units, although it may range from 10,000 to 100,000 units. It is administered intramuscularly or intravenously.

Mixed gas gangrene antitoxin, B.P.

Mixed gas gangrene antitoxin is a sterile solution of antitoxic substances obtained from the blood of healthy animals that have been immunized against the toxins of *Clostridium perfringens, Clostridium septicum,* and *Clostridium oedematiens.* The usual initial therapeutic or prophylactic dose is the contents of one or more packages, given parenterally.

Tetanus antitoxin, U.S.P., B.P.

Tetanus antitoxin is prepared from blood of horses in much the same way as diphtheria antitoxin; the animal has been immunized with tetanus toxin or toxoid. The usual therapeutic dose is 10,000 to 100,000 units; the prophylactic dose range is 1500 to 10,000 units given subcutaneously or intravenously. Active immunization with tetanus toxoid should be given at the same time in a different site with a different syringe.

The use of tetanus antitoxin is recommended only when human tetanus immune globulin is not available.

Because tetanus antitoxin is obtained from horse serum, sensitivity tests are done prior to administration. Hospital policies may vary regarding who administers the serum. Nurses should administer horse serum under the supervision of a physician, and the patient should be observed closely for any untoward reaction.

Tetanus immune human globulin, U.S.P.

Tetanus immune globulin (TIG) is a sterile solution of globulins derived from the blood plasma of adult human donors who have been immunized with tetanus toxoid. It is used to provide passive immunity to tetanus in patients with tetanus-prone injuries who are not known to be immune to tetanus and to treat active tetanus infections. In comparison to tetanus antitoxin, tetanus immune globulin has a lower risk for hypersensitivity reactions and longer lasting protective levels of circulating antibodies with lower doses. It provides protective levels of antibodies for 3 to 4 weeks, which is the incubation period for most cases of tetanus.

Prophylactic dose for adults is 250 units; for children it is 4 units per kilogram of body weight given intramuscularly. Optimal treatment dose for tetanus has not been established, but 3000 to 10,000 units have been recommended. The drug may be given as a single dose or in 500 units daily until 3000 to 6000 units have been given.

Passive immunization with this agent should not be a substitute for active immunization with tetanus toxoid. Active immunization should begin immediately (or within 1 month after administration of tetanus immune human globulin) using a different syringe and a different injection site. Adverse effects include low grade fever, erythema, and pain at the injection site.

Tetanus and gas gangrene antitoxins, N.F.

This antitoxin is made by mixing the serums of horses individually immunized to the toxins of tetanus and gas gangrene. Each package of the antitoxins contains not less than 1500 units of tetanus antitoxin and not less than 2000 units of each of the other component antitoxins (*Clostridium perfringens* and *Clostridium septicum*). The usual dose is the contents of one or more packages, given parenterally, as a prophylactic measure.

Botulism antitoxin, U.S.P.; botulinum antitoxin, B.P.

Botulism antitoxin is obtained from the serum of animals immunized with the toxin of *Clostridium botulinium*, type A, B, or E. It is available as pooled polyvalent antitoxin. Prompt injection of the antitoxin as soon as the diagnosis of botulism is made is essential to neutralize the toxins before they are *irreversibly bound* to receptor sites. Hypersensitivity tests should be made before injection. Usual dose is 10,000 units intravenously every 4 hours until the toxic condition is alleviated.

ANTIGENIC AGENTS USED TO PRODUCE ACTIVE IMMUNITY
VACCINES

Vaccines are suspensions of either attenuated or killed microorganisms that are administered for the prevention or treatment of infectious diseases. The viruses for vaccines are commonly grown in living tissues, such as chick embryos; this type of vaccine is absolutely contraindicated in persons with a history of hypersensitivity to egg, chicken, or chicken feathers. Vaccines do not afford immediate protection. An interval of days or several weeks elapses between inoculation and the production of antibodies. Because of this, if there is danger of immediate infection and there is a serum available, a prophylactic dose of serum is first given to afford immediate protection, followed later by the vaccine injection to ensure a prolonged immunity.

Cholera vaccine, U.S.P., B.P.

Cholera vaccine is a sterile suspension of killed cholera vibrios *(Vibrio cholerae)* in isotonic sodium chloride solution or other suitable diluent. At the time of manufacture, cholera vaccine contains 8 billion cholera organisms in each milliliter of suspension. The usual subcutaneous dose is 0.5 ml., followed by another dose of 1 ml. 4 weeks later, making a total of two injections. If necessary, a 0.5-ml. dose may be repeated every 6 months. It is only 50% effective for 3 to 6 months.

Influenza virus vaccine, monovalent, type A (Asian strain)

This vaccine is a sterile suspension of formaldehyde-killed influenza virus, type A, grown in chick embryos. It is administered subcutaneously in doses of 1 ml. for adults and 0.5 ml. for children from 5 to 12 years of age. For children between 3 months and 5 years, the dose of 0.1 ml. given subcutaneously or intracutaneously is suggested. It is also suggested that these doses for infants and children be repeated within 1 or 2 weeks.

Influenza virus vaccine, U.S.P.; influenza vaccine, B.P.

This vaccine is a suspension of inactivated influenza virus cultivated in chick embryos. Influenza virus vaccine is used prophylactically to produce active immunization against influenza. The maximum amount of antibody formation occurs during the second week after vaccination, and the titer remains constant for about 1 month, after which there is a gradual decline. The vaccine should not be given to persons sensitive to material derived from chick or egg protein. Dosage for prophylactic active immunization is 0.5 to 1 ml. given subcutaneously, followed by 0.5 to 1 ml. in 2 months.

Prophylactic value is limited since (1) the disease can occur in spite of high serum antibody levels, (2) the vaccine may not contain antigens prepared from the offending strains of virus, and (3) protection lasts only a few months. However, flu vaccine does reduce the incidence and severity of influenza, and it is recommended for high risk groups (elderly and chronically ill).

Mumps vaccine

Mumps vaccine is a sterile suspension of mumps virus grown in chick embryos, inacti-vated by ultraviolet light or formaldehyde. It is administered subcutaneously in two doses of 1 ml. each, given at an interval of 1 to 4 weeks. A booster injection 6 to 12 months later may be given.

Live mumps virus vaccine, attenuated, U.S.P. (Mumpsvax)

This is a preparation of live organisms of the Jeryl Lynn (B level) strain of mumps virus that has been grown in chick embryo tissue culture. It should be refrigerated at 2° to 8° C. and used within 8 hours after its reconstitution. Unused portions should be discarded. The vaccine should be protected from bright light and sunlight.

Duration of immunity has not been determined, but evidence indicates that good protection exists for about 6 years after vaccination. It is not recommended for use in children under 1 year of age or in pregnant women or for those allergic to eggs, chicken, or neomycin.

Dosage is 0.5 ml. of vaccine given subcutaneously into the upper arm. Antibodies develop in about 28 days. Serious reactions are rare. Fever, redness, and soreness at the injection site may occur.

Pertussis vaccine, B.P. (whooping cough vaccine)

Pertussis vaccine is a sterile suspension of killed pertussis bacilli. Field studies show that this vaccine possesses sufficient antigenic value to afford considerable protection against whooping cough. It does not always prevent attacks of the disease, but it lowers the death rate from the disease. The usual dose is three injections of 0.5 to 1 ml. 4 to 6 weeks apart. Pertussis vaccine is given subcutaneously or intramuscularly.

Recommended age for prophylactic immunization is 3 months. In epidemics infants as young as 1 month may be injected; these infants should be given a fourth dose. Older children may also be immunized. However, since 80% of the cases of whooping cough occur in the first 5 years of life, and since the incidence and severity of adverse reactions increase with age, it is not advisable to give this vaccine to children over the age of 6.

Side effects. Side effects to pertussis vaccine

include fever, malaise, and myalgia. Severe central nervous system reactions and even death have occurred, but rarely. This vaccine should not be given to children with central nervous system disease.

Adsorbed pertussis vaccine

Adsorbed pertussis vaccine is a sterile suspension of the killed pertussis bacilli of a strain or strains selected for high antigenic efficiency and adsorbed or precipitated by the addition of alum, aluminum phosphate, or aluminum hydroxide and resuspended. Because of the adsorption, there is a delay in absorption. The dose is the same as that for pertussis vaccine and is given intramuscularly. Local irritation is greater but systemic reaction less than that caused by pertussis vaccine.

Poliomyelitis vaccine, U.S.P. (Salk Vaccine)

Poliomyelitis vaccine is a sterile solution of inactivated poliomyelitis virus of types 1, 2, and

Table 23-1 Immunization recommendations*

Disease	Immunizing agent	Preferred age for initial dose	Dosage	Number of doses	Interval for doses	Booster
Diphtheria Tetanus Pertussis	Diphtheria toxoid, tetanus toxoid, and pertussis vaccine combined (DPT)	3 months†	0.5 ml. IM	3	4-6 weeks	0.5 ml. 1 year later and 4 to 5 years later DT every 10 years thereafter
Tetanus Diphtheria	Tetanus and diphtheria toxoid (TD)	6 years and older	0.5 ml. IM	2	4-6 weeks	0.5 ml. 1 year later and every 10 years thereafter
Poliomyelitis	Live oral poliovirus vaccine, trivalent	2-3 months	See package insert	4	6-8 weeks, for second and third; 15-18 third; 15-18 months for fourth	1 dose at entry into school
Measles (rubeola)	Live measles vaccine	1 year	0.5 ml. Sub-Q	1		
Rubella	Live rubella vaccine	Between 1 year and puberty	0.5 ml. Sub-Q	1		
Mumps	Live mumps vaccine	Between 1 year and puberty	0.5 ml. Sub-Q	1		
Smallpox‡	Smallpox vaccine			1		3-year intervals for high risk groups

*From A.M.A. drug evaluations, A.M.A. Department of Drugs, ed. 2. With permission of Publishing Sciences Group, Acton, Mass. © 1973.
†When given over the age of 6, use DT.
‡Routine vaccination no longer recommended.

3, grown separately on cultures of renal tissue of monkeys. It is administered by subcutaneous or intramuscular injection. It is given in four doses of 1 ml. each; three injections are given at 1-month intervals, the fourth 6 to 12 months later.

Adverse effects. Reactions to Salk vaccine are infrequent and usually mild. Side effects include headache, low grade fever, sore throat, vomiting, pain at injection site, erythema, and stiffness of the neck, arms, and legs. Reactions may also occur to the small amount of antibiotic used to inhibit bacterial growth during production.

Live oral poliovirus vaccine, U.S.P. (Sabin vaccine); poliomyelitis vaccine (oral), B.P.

Attenuated live virus strains 1, 2, and 3 were introduced by Dr. Albert Sabin. This vaccine can be cultured in renal tissue cells of monkeys. Strains 1, 2, and 3 represent the three separate monovalent vaccines for the prevention of poliomyelitis caused by types 1, 2, or 3 of the poliovirus. This liquid vaccine is intended for oral administration only, not for injection. It is stored in the frozen state. When thawed for use, it is stored at refrigeration temperatures up to 50° F. and must be used within 7 days. The dosage varies with the potency of the pharmaceutical preparation used. Preparations of higher potency may be dropped on a lump of sugar before ingestion. Preparations of lower potency may be taken from a cup or teaspoon. For some infants it may be desirable to administer the drug by dropper. Each of the three types administered separately at intervals of 6 to 8 weeks and a fourth reinforcing dose 8 to 12 months later will ordinarily be expected to induce immunity. It is an active immunizing agent.

When the trivalent vaccine is used, three doses are given: the second one 6 to 8 weeks after the first dose; the third dose 8 to 12 months after the second. A rise in antibody titer begins 7 days after administration, reaching a peak in about 21 days.

On rare occasions paralytic disease has occurred within 2 months after ingestion of live oral poliovirus vaccine.

This vaccine is preferred over the Salk vaccine since it provides longer lasting immunity, is easier to administer, and produces an immune response like that induced by natural poliovirus infection. Immunization should start at 6 to 12 months of age; a booster dose should be given when the child enters school. Persons traveling to a foreign country where polio occurs frequently should be immunized against polio.

Immunization should be done during the period of November to May when incidence of enterovirus infection is lowest, since the occurrence of such an infection may result in failure of immunization.

Rabies vaccine, U.S.P., B.P.

This vaccine is a sterile freeze-dried suspension of killed rabies virus prepared from duck embryo or from brain tissue of rabbits infected with this virus. The virus obtained from the brain tissue is either attenuated or killed.

The administration of rabies vaccine may rarely result in paralysis of one or more extremities. Because paralysis is more likely to occur following undue exertion, it is suggested that activity be reduced during the vaccination period.

Rabies vaccine is injected subcutaneously for 14 to 21 days. When the killed virus vaccine is administered, 2 ml. of 5% suspension is given daily. When the attenuated virus vaccine is given, 1 ml. of the 5% suspension is administered.

Vaccine prepared from duck embryo is preferred to that prepared from brain tissue of rabbits. The latter causes a high incidence of central nervous system reactions, of which 25% are fatal.

Vaccine from duck embryo can cause abdominal pain, nausea and vomiting, dizziness, diaphoresis, and urticaria. These can occur immediately after injection. Local erythematous reactions at injection site occurs in about one third of the patients given either type of vaccine.

Persons with a high risk of exposure to rabies, such as veterinarians, should be immunized with rabies vaccine.

Smallpox vaccine, U.S.P., B.P.

Smallpox vaccine was the first vaccine prepared. It consists of a glycerinated suspension of vaccinia viruses that have been grown in healthy vaccinated animals of the bovine family or in membranes of the chick embryo. It loses its potency if kept at a temperature above 8° C. Failure of vaccination is often caused by inactive virus and indicates that the vaccination should be repeated. The usual dose is the contents of one container, administered by multiple puncture of the skin. No bleeding or pain should occur with properly administered vaccine. Protection lasts from 3 to 10 years.

In 1971, the U.S. Public Health Service recommended discontinuing routine smallpox vaccination, and this was supported by the Committee on Infectious Diseases of the American Academy of Pediatrics. In the United States the hazard of smallpox vaccination now exceeds the risk of contracting the disease. Encephalitis and deaths have occurred from smallpox vaccine. The last documented case of smallpox in the U.S. occurred in 1949, and that was by importation. In 1972, there were only six countries in which smallpox was still a problem.

Smallpox vaccination is recommended for international travel and for health personnel. Persons with eczema or chronic dermatitis should not be vaccinated.

Typhoid vaccine, U.S.P.

Typhoid vaccine is a sterile suspension of killed typhoid bacilli in physiologic saline solution or other suitable diluent. The usual prophylactic subcutaneous dose is 0.5 ml., to be repeated two to three times at intervals of 28 days, or three doses given at weekly intervals.

Routine immunization is not required. It is recommended for travelers to countries where typhoid is endemic, for persons exposed to a typhoid carrier, and for those in a community where there is an outbreak of typhoid fever.

Typhus vaccine, U.S.P., B.P.

Typhus vaccine is a sterile suspension of the killed rickettsial organism of a strain or strains of epidemic typhus rickettsiae cultured in chick embryos. The usual dose, subcutaneously, for active immunization is 0.5 to 1 ml., to be repeated once 4 weeks later. A booster dose is given every 6 to 12 months as long as exposure exists. The typhus vaccine listed in B.P. contains the killed murine typhus rickettsiae as well as the epidemic rickettsiae.

Tuberculosis vaccine, BCG vaccine, N.F.; bacillus Calmette-Guérin vaccine, B.P.

This is a freeze-dried preparation of the culture of an attenuated strain of the bovine tubercle bacillus.

The vaccine is used only in individuals who are negative in their reaction to the tuberculin test. Conversion of negative tuberculin-tested subjects to positive reactors after vaccination is usually considered presumptive evidence that immunity has developed similar to that which follows a naturally resisted or healed primary sensitizing infection. Physicians have a choice either of using the vaccine to reduce the risk of clinical disease or of not using the vaccine and having the tuberculin skin test for early diagnosis and as a guide to the need for further study and treatment.

Tuberculosis vaccine is usually administered by multiple puncture or by intradermal injection. The dose in drops varies, depending on the gauge of the needle or other openings from which the vaccine is deposited on the skin. For example, using the resuspended vaccine (50 mg. per milliliter) 4 drops from a 22-gauge needle would be used for the multiple-puncture method. For intradermal injection 0.1 ml. (equivalent to 0.2 mg.) is further diluted and injected as superficially as possible with a tuberculin syringe and a 26-gauge needle so that a wheal of 8 to 10 mm. is produced.

Yellow fever vaccine, U.S.P., B.P.

The U.S.P. preparation of yellow fever vaccine is the living virus of an attenuated strain of the yellow fever virus, prepared by culturing the microorganism in the chick embryo. It is dried from the frozen state; the powder is rehydrated immediately before use. It is administered subcutaneously, and the usual dose is 0.5 ml. A single dose provides protection for about 10 years. For international travel vaccination must be obtained at WHO-approved yellow fever vaccination centers, and an International Certificate of Vaccination must be validated.

Live attenuated measles virus vaccine, U.S.P., B.P. (Lyovac Rubeovax)

Live, attenuated measles virus vaccine is prepared from measles virus grown in chick embryo tissue culture. It also contains streptomycin, penicillin, and neomycin. The vaccine is lyophilized and must be reconstituted with the diluent before use. It is used for immunization against rubeola.

Following a single dose, the vaccine induces an active form of immunity to rubeola in 99% of recipients that lasts at least 4 years. Most children experience a febrile response following vaccination, which is generally mild but may be moderately severe. Vaccination should be delayed for 8 weeks if the patient has received immune serum globulin (human), blood, or plasma, since the measles antibody titer of these may neutralize the vaccine virus.

This vaccine is available as an injectable suspension of 0.5 ml., which is administered subcutaneously in the upper arm. At the same time immune serum may be given intramuscularly in the other arm to reduce the severity of reaction to the live vaccine. The best age to vaccinate children is at 1 year.

Adverse effects and contraindications. The live vaccine can reproduce most of the symptoms of measles, although it is a noncommunicable form of the disease. Rash and/or fever may occur 5 to 12 days after injection. The simultaneous administration of measles immune globulin tends to reduce the incidence and severity of the reaction. The live vaccine should not be given to pregnant women or to those patients who suffer from severe or debilitating illnesses or whose resistance is lowered by steroids, irradiation, or toxic antineoplastic drugs. It is also contraindicated in patients who are allergic to some of the constituents of the vaccine preparation, such as egg proteins or the antibiotics that are present in the preparation.

Live measles and rubella virus vaccine, U.S.P.

This is a combination of live, attenuated measles and rubella viruses for active immunization of children from 1 year of age to puberty. Usual dose is 0.5 ml. of constituted vaccine given subcutaneously.

TOXOIDS

A toxoid is a toxin modified so that it is nontoxic but still antigenic. Formaldehyde is the agent generally used for the detoxification of toxins. Toxoids are supplied in the plain form and as precipitated and adsorbed preparations. Alum is used for the precipitated products, and aluminum hydroxide and aluminum phosphate are employed to provide an adsorption surface for toxoids. The precipitated and adsorbed products are absorbed more slowly by the circulating and tissue fluids of the body and excreted slowly; therefore, they provide higher immunizing titers than does plain toxoid.

Diphtheria toxoid, U.S.P.

Diphtheria toxoid is an aqueous solution of the products of the growth of *Corynebacterium diphtheriae,* so modified by formaldehyde that it has lost its toxic effects for guinea pigs but not its power to produce active immunity. From 0.5 to 1 ml. is administered subcutaneously to produce active immunity in three doses with 4-week intervals between doses. A fourth reinforcing dose is given 6 to 12 months later. Since some general as well as local reactions are observed in adults and older children, a test dose should be given to determine sensitivity. Tenderness at injection site, fever, and malaise may occur.

Adsorbed diphtheria toxoid, U.S.P.

Adsorbed diphtheria toxoid is a sterile suspension of diphtheria toxoid precipitated or adsorbed by the addition of aluminum hydroxide, aluminum phosphate, or alum. For active immunization it is given subcutaneously, 0.5 or 1 ml., two injections 4 to 6 weeks apart, and a third reinforcing dose 6 to 12 months later.

Diphtheria vaccine, B.P.

Diphtheria vaccine is prepared from diphtheria toxin and is indicated as alum-precipitated toxoid, purified toxoid aluminum phosphate, formol toxoid, and toxoid-antitoxin floccules. It is given subcutaneously or intramuscularly.

Tetanus toxoid, U.S.P.; tetanus vaccine, B.P.

Tetanus toxoid is a sterile solution of the products of growth of *Clostridium tetani,* so modified by formaldehyde that it has lost the ability to cause toxic effects in guinea pigs but retains the property of inducing active immunity. Usual subcutaneous dose is 0.5 or 1 ml. according to label specifications, repeated three times at intervals of 3 to 4 weeks, followed by 0.5 ml. 1 year later and every 5 to 10 years thereafter. If possible exposure to tetanus occurs, 0.5 ml. should be given as soon as possible.

Prior to the development of tetanus toxoid, passive immunization with tetanus antitoxin was the only effective method of tetanus prevention. Although there is an increasing number of actively immunized persons, the majority of our population still does not have this protection.

Adsorbed tetanus toxoid, U.S.P.

This is tetanus toxoid precipitated or adsorbed by the addition of alum, aluminum hydroxide, or aluminum phosphate. Dosage for active immunization is two injections of 0.5 or 1 ml. at intervals of 4 to 6 weeks, given intramuscularly, followed by 0.5 ml. 1 year later and every 10 years thereafter. This toxoid preparation is used as a booster for the actively immunized person who sustains superficial puncture wounds or lacerations that are potentially infected. For adequate protection the actively immunized person needs booster doses every 4 years.

Adsorbed diphtheria and tetanus toxoids and pertussis vaccine, U.S.P. (DPT)

This preparation is a sterile mixture of diphtheria toxoid, tetanus toxoid, and pertussis vaccine adsorbed on aluminum hydroxide, aluminum phosphate, or alum. The antigens are combined in such proportion as to yield a mixture containing one immunizing dose of each in the total dosage prescribed on the label. The dosage is three injections of 0.5 or 1 ml., as specified on the label, 3 to 4 weeks apart, and a fourth reinforcing dose 12 months later. It is administered subcutaneously.

Adsorbed tetanus and diphtheria toxoids for adult dose, U.S.P. (DT)

This preparation is a sterile suspension prepared by mixing suitable quantities of the adsorbed forms of diphtheria and tetanus toxoids.

Two injections of 0.5 or 1 ml., as specified on the label, are given intramuscularly, 4 to 6 weeks apart, and a third reinforcing dose is given 6 to 12 months later. Thereafter reinforcing doses should be given every 5 to 10 years. This combination is used for adults for whom the triple vaccine including pertussis is not recommended.

Diphtheria and tetanus toxoids; pertussis vaccine, U.S.P., B.P.

This preparation is administered subcutaneously or intramuscularly in doses of 0.5 or 1 ml. three times at intervals of 4 to 6 weeks, with a fourth reinforcing dose 12 months later.

Preparations of tetanus toxoid, diphtheria toxoid, and pertussis vaccine are available for separate administration. However, "triple toxoid" (a combination of the three) is preferred for childhood immunization.

AGENTS FOR CUTANEOUS IMMUNITY TESTS
Diphtheria toxin, U.S.P.

Diphtheria toxin for the Schick test is used to determine the susceptibility of an individual to diphtheria. The toxin that is used is carefully standardized on human beings. The usual dose is 0.1 ml. This is injected intracutaneously, usually on the forearm. If the person is susceptible to diphtheria (if his blood does not contain a sufficient amount of antitoxin to protect him from the disease), a small area of redness, usually with some infiltration, will occur at the point of injection in 24 to 48 hours. This is known as a positive reaction. It persists about 7 to 10 days and then fades slowly.

Old tuberculin, U.S.P., B.P. (Koch's tuberculin)

Old tuberculin is prepared by filtering a glycerin bouillon culture of the tubercle bacillus through a Berkefeld filter. It contains the toxins of the tubercle bacilli and is used largely in diagnosing tuberculosis. It is given by intracutaneous injection. If the patient has been infected with tuberculosis at some time, there is an area of redness, usually with a papule at the point of application of the tuberculin. The usual dose for diagnostic purposes is 0.1 ml. of a 1:1000 dilution. A reaction indicates that the patient has at some time been infected with tuberculosis but not necessarily that he has clinical tuberculosis.

PPD (purified protein derivative of tuberculin), U.S.P., B.P.

This preparation is a sterile soluble purified product of the growth of the *Mycobacterium tuberculosis*, which is prepared in a special liquid medium free from protein. It is standardized to be clinically equivalent to PPD-S, the international standard of the World Health Organization. It is used as a diagnostic aid. Dosage is 5 tuberculin units given intracutaneously.

NURSING ASPECTS

When serums and vaccines are used, nurses should take into consideration the following:

1 Expiration dates of preparations should always be noted. Fresh preparations are the most reliable.
2 Check for contraindications for using these substances by obtaining a patient history, particularly history of allergy or asthma, sensitivity to protein substances, and whether or not the patient has a chronic or recurring skin condition.
3 Instruct the patient not to scratch or irritate the injection site. In smallpox vaccination, autoinoculation can occur.
4 For some preparations tests for sensitivity should precede administration. Check the package insert.
5 Epinephrine 1:1000 solution should be immediately available.
6 Observe the patient for systemic reactions (fever, malaise) and report them immediately if they occur. If patient is an outpatient inform him of side effects and instruct him to consult his physician if they occur.

QUESTIONS

For study and review

1 Differentiate between an immune serum, a toxoid, and a vaccine. Give an example of each.
2 Differentiate between active and passive immunity.
3 Explain the difference between a toxoid and an antitoxin.
4 What precautions are necessary when immunization or vaccination is contemplated?

REFERENCES

A.M.A. drug evaluations, ed. 2, Acton, Mass., 1973, Publishing Sciences Group, Inc.

Cockburn, W. C.: World problems in viral vaccines, Br. Med. Bull. **25:**121, 1969.

DiPalma, J. R.: Status report on immunizations, R.N. **33:**69, 1970.

Francis, B. J.: Current concepts in immunization, Am. J. Nurs. **73:**646, 1973.

Goz, G., and Prusoff, W. H.: Pharmacology of viruses, Ann. Rev. Pharmacol. **10:**143, 1970.

Kaufman, H. E.: Virus chemotherapy. In Cluff, L. E., and Johnson, J. E., III, editors: Clinical concepts of infectious diseases, Baltimore, 1972, The Williams & Wilkins Co.

Lane, J. A., and others: Complications of smallpox vaccination, New Eng. J. Med. **281:**1201, 1969.

Osol, A., and Pratt, R.: The United States dispensatory, ed. 27, Philadelphia, 1973, J. B. Lippincott Co.

Pampiglione, G., Griffith, A. H., and Bramwell, E. C.: Transient cerebral changes after vaccination against measles, Lancet **2:**5, 1971.

Stokes, J., Jr.: Recent advances in immunization against viral diseases, Ann. Intern. Med. **73:**829, 1970.

CHAPTER 24

Antineoplastic agents

Classification of antineoplastic agents
Alkylating agents
Antimetabolites
Antibiotics
Plant alkaloids
Radioactive isotopes
Miscellaneous antineoplastic agents
Nursing functions in antineoplastic chemotherapy

Human cancer encompasses a group of over 100 related diseases that constitute the second greatest cause of death in the United States and in Western Europe. While surgery and x-ray therapy are still the most effective treatments for cancer, great advances have been achieved in antineoplastic drug therapy since the 1940's. There is now a variety of drugs that can be used, either alone or in conjunction with surgery and x-ray therapy, to produce palliation of symptoms, regression of the neoplastic process, and prolongation of life.

It must be clearly stated that no antineoplastic drugs have been discovered that effect total cure of malignant processes. Likewise, no antineoplastic drugs have been discovered that are free of severe limitations in their therapeutic application. One major factor limiting the effectiveness of these drugs is their lack of selective toxicity. No antineoplastic drug possesses the same selective toxicity for cancer cells that some antibiotics have for bacteria. Most antineoplastic drugs, when used in therapeutically effective doses, are likely to be nonselective, highly toxic, and produce many undesirable side effects. A second major factor limiting the effectiveness of these drugs is the potential emergence of resistance

that is probably analogous to the resistance that develops in antimicrobial therapy.

Antineoplastic drugs lack selective toxicity because they are not able to destroy malignant cells without appreciably damaging normal host cells. Many effective antineoplastic agents are active because they influence the structural and functional aspects of proliferating cells. Because malignant cells proliferate rapidly, they are highly dependent upon critical building blocks such as amino acids, purines, and pyrimidines, as well as intact DNA for their replication. In order to be effective, antineoplastic agents must interfere with the supply and utilization of building blocks or disrupt nuclear materials. When antineoplastic drugs are employed in doses sufficient to accomplish this, they also affect normal cells that have high rates of proliferation. This effect on rapidly dividing normal cells accounts for the toxic symptoms attendant to the use of almost all antineoplastic drugs, for example, bone marrow depression, alopecia, and ulceration of oral and intestinal mucosa. These drugs, therefore, are used for short periods of time in small doses and with frequent intermissions in the dosage schedule.

The types of neoplastic processes in which

535

"cure" (or long-term remission) can be achieved include gestational choriocarcinoma in women, Hodgkin's disease, childhood acute lymphocytic leukemia, Burkitt's lymphoma, embryonal carcinoma of the testicle, Wilms' tumor, Ewing's sarcoma, lymphocytic leukemia, rhabdomyosarcoma, and retinoblastoma.

CLASSIFICATION OF ANTINEOPLASTIC AGENTS

The antineoplastic drugs can be divided into several categories on the basis of their probable mechanisms of action.

Alkylating agents. This group of antineoplastic drugs was developed from a sulfur mustard vesicant gas used in World Wars I and II. In addition to their vesicant effect on the skin, these agents were found to produce atrophy of the lymphoid tissue and bone marrow, discoveries that led to their use in the treatment of malignancies. The alkylating agents act in a number of ways, but their primary mechanism of action is probably the alkylation of the nucleic acids, resulting in inactivation of DNA. These agents are also referred to as radiomimetic drugs, since they affect cells in much the same way as irradiation. Since the initial use of the parent compound of this group, nitrogen mustard, other alkylating agents have been developed in the search for more effective and less toxic drugs. Many of the alkylating agents are practically interchangeable except for dose, route of administration, and the rapidity and duration of the effect desired. They are primarily used in the treatment of malignancies of the hematopoietic tissues, neuroblastoma, and disseminated carcinomas of the lungs, ovaries, testes, and breasts. They are curative only in the treatment of Burkitt's lymphoma.

Antimetabolites. Antimetabolites are compounds whose chemical structures resemble chemical structures of substances normally used by cells for growth and metabolism. They interfere with the synthesis of nucleic acids by interfering with the function of the normally occurring physiologic substance. When it became apparent that compounds structurally related to folic acid could inhibit white cell production, the folic acid antagonists were among the first antimetabolites developed. Eventually, several purine, pyrimidine, and amino acid antagonists were discovered. The antimetabolites appear to be most effective in the treatment of malignancies that are metabolically very active.

Plant alkaloids. This group of drugs derived from various plants has demonstrated ability to block cell division in metaphase. The most important drugs in this group are vincristine and vinblastine, derived from the periwinkle plant, *Vinca rosea.*

Antibiotics. Several antibiotics have found usefulness in cancer chemotherapy, exerting their cytotoxic effects by blocking the transcription of new DNA or RNA.

Radioisotopes. These agents are used in the treatment of cancer because they liberate highly penetrating beta and gamma rays that destroy cells. Tissues vary in sensitivity to ionizing radiation; cells with a short life and high rate of reproduction are especially vulnerable. Examples are germinal cells of the ovaries and testes, bone marrow, lymphocytes, and the epithelial cells of the gastrointestinal tract. The radioactive isotopes are therefore most useful in hematologic malignancies, Hodgkin's disease, and for control of localized tumor masses.

Hormones. The rationale underlying the use of hormones as antineoplastic agents is based on the assumption that malignancies arising from sexual organs have hormonal requirements similar to those of nonmalignant sexual organs. By changing the hormonal environment, therefore, it is possible to alter, to some degree, the course of the neoplastic process. In contrast to other antineoplastic agents, the hormones have greater selective toxicity, each hormone acting on specific tissue. Androgens, for example, are used in the treatment of metastatic breast cancer in premenopausal women. Estrogens are used in the treatment of metastatic breast cancer in postmenopausal women, and progestational agents have been used effectively in the treatment of advanced endometrial carcinoma. Because of their lymphocytic effects, the adrenocorticosteroids find their greatest value in the treatment of acute leukemia in children. They are also used in conjunction with x-ray therapy to decrease the

Table 24-1 Classification of antineoplastic agents

Alkylating agents	Antimetabolites
Nitrogen mustard	Methotrexate
Chlorambucil	Mercaptopurine
Busulfan	Fluorouracil
Melphalan	Thioguanine
Thiotepa	Cytosine
Triethylenemelamine	arabinoside
(TEM)	
Cyclophosphamide	Antibiotics
	Actinomycin D
Plant alkaloids	Mithramycin
Vincristine	Bleomycin
Vinblastine	Adriamycin
	Daunomycin
Hormones	
Adrenocorticosteroids	Radioisotopes
(prednisone)	Phosphorus (^{32}P)
Androgens	Gold (^{198}Au)
(testosterone	Iodine (^{131}I)
propionate)	Cobalt 60
Estrogens	
(stilbestrol)	
Progestins	
(progesterone)	

occurrence of radiation edema in critical areas such as the superior mediastinum, brain, and spinal cord.

Individual drugs belonging to this category are discussed in Chapters 25 and 26.

ALKYLATING AGENTS
Mechlorethamine hydrochloride, U.S.P. (Mustargen Hydrochloride); mustine hydrochloride, B.P.

The nitrogen mustard that has been used most extensively is mechlorethamine, which is the prototype of the alkylating agents.

Absorption, distribution, metabolism, and excretion. Mechlorethamine can be absorbed from either the gastrointestinal tract or parenteral routes of administration, but severe local reactions limit its administration to the intravenous route. Within minutes after administration, the drug undergoes chemical transformation and

combines with body tissues. Less than 0.01% of the drug is excreted in the urine.

Toxicity. Profound nausea and vomiting occur following the administration of mechlorethamine and last for 12 to 24 hours. This side effect may be minimized by administering the drug late in the day and sedating the patient for the night and/or by concurrently administering phenothiazines and barbiturates. Mechlorethamine also produces depression of the bone marrow, with leukopenia and thrombocytopenia being the principal effects. Bone marrow cell necrosis and disintegration appear within 12 hours of administration and continue for 4 to 6 days; return to normal cellularity takes 3 to 4 weeks. Mechlorethamine is a potent vesicant and a sclerosing agent. Great care must be exercised to avoid contact of this drug with the skin of the nurse or patient, and care should be exercised in avoiding extravasation of the drug into the tissues at the injection site. Amenorrhea of several months' duration follows a course of therapy. When used in high doses, the alkylating agents can also produce central nervous system stimulation and convulsions. The drug is contraindicated during pregnancy.

Clinical uses. D.E.S.I. rating for mechlorethamine is *effective* when given intravenously for the palliative treatment of disseminated Hodgkin's disease, lymphosarcoma, bronchogenic carcinoma, certain types of chronic leukemia, polycythemia vera, and mycosis fungoides; *effective* when given intracavitarily for palliative treatment of pleural, peritoneal, or pericardial effusion due to metastatic carcinoma; and *possibly effective* by intra-arterial administration. It is a drug of choice for hospitalized patients when prompt treatment is indicated. Remissions induced by mechlorethamine tend to become progressively shorter with each course of drug therapy. For this reason, this drug is sometimes used in conjunction with other antineoplastic agents.

Preparation, dosage, and administration
Mechlorethamine hydrochloride for injection, U.S.P. (Mustargen Hydrochloride); *mustine injection,* B.P. (nitrogen mustard). This drug is available in vials containing 10 mg. of the powder and 90 mg. of sodium chloride. Prior to injection, the drug is dissolved in 10-ml. of distilled water.

The drug must be prepared immediately before use because it rapidly reacts with water and undergoes chemical transformation.

It is administered intravenously by injecting the solution into the tubing of an intravenous infusion. The total dose administered is 0.4 mg. per kilogram of body weight in single or divided doses; range of dose is 0.2 to 0.6 mg. per kilogram of body weight. Because of the depressant effects on bone marrow, the subsequent dose of mechlorethamine is not administered until an interval of 3 to 4 weeks has passed or until satisfactory recovery of bone marrow has occurred. Direct injection of mechlorethamine into body cavities in cases of malignant effusions also has been effective.

Chlorambucil, U.S.P., B.P. (Leukeran)

$$CH_3-\underset{\underset{O_2}{\|}}{S}-O-(CH_2)_4-O-\underset{\underset{O_2}{\|}}{S}-CH_3$$

Chlorambucil is a derivative of nitrogen mustard and its action and uses are similar to those of mechlorethamine hydrochloride. At recommended doses, chlorambucil is the slowest acting and least toxic nitrogen mustard in use.

Absorption, distribution, metabolism, and excretion. Oral absorption of chlorambucil is adequate and reliable. Information regarding the distribution, metabolism, and excretion of this drug is incomplete.

Toxicity. This drug is usually well tolerated and few side effects are noted when chlorambucil is administered in therapeutic doses. With large doses, anorexia, nausea, and vomiting occur. Excessive dosage or prolonged administration may cause severe depression of bone marrow, and weekly blood counts are recommended.

Clinical uses. Chlorambucil has received a D.E.S.I. rating of *effective* in the palliative treatment of chronic lymphocytic leukemia, lymphomas, some forms of Hodgkin's disease, and reticulum cell sarcoma. Chlorambucil is also sometimes used in maintenance therapy to prolong the more immediate efforts of mechlorethamine.

Preparation, dosage, and administration. Chlorambucil is available in 2-mg. tablets for oral administration. The initial dosage is 0.1 to 0.2 mg. per kilogram of body weight for 3 to 6 weeks, usually administered in a single daily dose 1 hour before breakfast or 2 hours after the evening meal. The usual dosage is 2 to 4 mg. per day.

Busulfan, U.S.P., B.P. (Myleran)

The cytotoxic action of busulfan is restricted chiefly to the cells of the bone marrow. It has received a D.E.S.I. rating of *effective* in the palliative treatment of chronic granulocytic leukemia. This drug is unique in that its cytotoxic effects do not appear to extend to other tissues.

Absorption, distribution, metabolism, and excretion. Busulfan is well absorbed after oral administration. It is metabolized to methanesulfonic acid, which is then excreted by the kidneys.

Toxicity. Because busulfan has a low incidence of side effects, it can be used in maintenance of therapy of ambulatory patients. It causes little nausea and vomiting, but it is a bone marrow depressant like the other alkylating agents. Blood counts should be done weekly, and monthly during remission. Its use should be avoided during the first trimester of pregnancy.

Preparation, dosage, and administration. Busulfan is available in 2-mg. tablets for oral administration. The usual dosage is 4 to 8 mg. per day until the leukocyte count falls below 10,000 per cubic millimeter. During remission therapy is resumed when the leukocyte count reaches 50,000 per cubic millimeter. Initial dose for children is 0.06 mg. per kilogram of body weight daily; this dose is then adjusted to provide a leukocyte count of 20,000 per cubic millimeter.

Cyclophosphamide, U.S.P., B.P. (Cytoxan)

Cyclophosphamide was developed in a search for greater selective toxicity and is similar in its antineoplastic activity to mechlorethamine hydrochloride.

Absorption, distribution, metabolism, and excretion. This drug is well absorbed after oral administration and is probably activated in the liver. It seems to accumulate preferentially in neoplastic tissue.

Toxicity. The toxicity attendant to the use of cyclophosphamide is primarily hematologic; the drug is capable of producing severe bone marrow depression. Alopecia and hemorrhagic cystitis are common, and hepatotoxicity also occurs. Hematuria can be avoided by maintaining high urine output. Nausea and vomiting after the administration of cyclophosphamide are not as violent as that following administration of mechlorethamine but are more prolonged. Unlike other alkylating agents, this drug is not a vesicant or tissue irritant, seems to produce thrombocytopenia less commonly, and does not seem to possess the CNS toxicity characteristic of other nitrogen mustards. Sterility commonly follows the use of this drug.

Clinical uses. Cyclophosphamide has received a D.E.S.I. rating of *effective* for treatment of lymphoma, lymphosarcoma, Hodgkin's disease, leukemias, multiple myeloma, mycosis fungoides, and malignancy of the ovary, breast, and lung; and *possibly effective* for other forms of malignancies. Complete remissions for more than 5 years have been reported when this drug is used in conjunction with other agents to treat Burkitt's lymphoma. Cyclophosphamide can also be used as an immunosuppressive agent.

Preparation, dosage, and administration. Cyclophosphamide may be administered orally, parenterally, and by intrapleural, intraperitoneal, and intratumor injection. The injectable form is unstable and must be used soon after it is prepared. It is available in 25- and 50-mg. tablets and as a powder for injection in doses of 100, 200, and 500 mg. Initial dose is 30 to 40 mg. per kilogram of body weight given orally or intravenously over a period of 1 to 4 days. Oral maintenance therapy is 1.5 to 2.0 mg. per kilogram of body weight, which is started when the leukocyte count returns to 3000 to 5000 per cubic milli-

meter. Leukocyte count should be maintained between 2500 and 4000 per cubic millimeter. Intravenous maintenance therapy is 10 to 15 mg. per kilogram of body weight every 7 to 10 days or at 3- to 4-week intervals. Children tolerate larger amounts of drug than adults.

Melphalan, U.S.P., B.P. (Alkeran)

Melphalan is also known as phenylalanine nitrogen mustard and is used in the treatment of multiple myeloma. Its toxic effects are similar to those of other alkylating agents, but thrombocytopenia seems to be more common. Nausea and vomiting are infrequent.

Preparation, dosage, and administration. Melphalan is well absorbed orally and is available in 2-mg. tablets. The dosage range is 2 to 6 mg. per day and can be administered in an intermittent high-dose schedule or in a low-dose continuous regime.

Triethylenemelamine, N.F. (TEM)

The discovery that nitrogen mustards undergo conversion into ethyleneimmonium compounds that are highly reactive led to the synthesis of several compounds to be used as antineoplastic agents. Two of these are triethylenemelamine and thiotepa. While these drugs remain official drugs, they have been replaced by nitrogen mustards and seldom are used clinically.

Triethylenemelamine produces nuclear changes in cells and shatters chromosomes. It has received a D.E.S.I. rating of *effective* for the treatment of lymphomas and chronic leukemias and *ineffective* for polycythemia vera, carcinomas of the lung, and mycosis fungoides. Toxic effects on the bone marrow are unpredictable and severe. Other alkylating agents are considered safer and equally effective.

Preparation, dosage, and administration. Triethylenemelamine is available in 5-mg. tablets for oral administration. The drug is inactivated by the presence of acid and food and therefore should be given an hour or more before breakfast along with 2 Gm. of sodium bicarbonate. The latter substance enhances both absorption and activity of the drug. During initial therapy, 2.5 mg. is given on two successive mornings. If adverse effects do not develop, 2.5 to 5 mg. is given biweekly for 4 weeks. Whether or not administration is continued depends upon the condition being treated and the response of the patient (condition of the appetite and the blood cell count).

Thiotepa, N.F., B.P.

$$CH_2{-}{-}CH_2$$
$$CH_2 \quad N$$
$$N{-}P{=}S$$
$$CH_2 \quad N$$
$$CH_2{-}{-}CH_2$$

Thiotepa is a less toxic alkylating agent than TEM. Thiotepa has a D.E.S.I. rating of *effective* for treating a wide variety of neoplastic diseases including treatment of advanced cancer of the ovary, cancer of the breast, lymphomas, and cancers of the lung; it is *possibly effective* against neoplasms of the genitourinary, gastrointestinal, and central nervous systems. Thiotepa has a slow onset of action, and immediate side effects such as nausea and vomiting are minimal, although they do occur. It is capable of producing cumulative toxic effects in the blood-forming tissues and, therefore, caution in its use is recommended. Irreversible aplastic anemia has been known to develop.

Preparation, dosage, and administration. Thiotepa is available in vials containing 15 mg. of powdered drug. For intrapericardial, intraperitoneal, and intrapleural infiltration, dosage for adults and children over 12 years of age is 45 to 60 mg. weekly depending on the patient's physical state. If the leukocyte count is below 3000 per cubic millimeter, therapy should be postponed. For intravenous therapy dosage is 0.8 mg. per kilogram of body weight given at 1- to 4-week intervals. The dosage for maintenance therapy is determined by the clinical response of the patient and changes in the patient's blood. The powder should be refrigerated, and when solutions are prepared they should be used immediately or discarded. Because this preparation has no vesicant action and because solutions can be prepared at a pH that produces no irritation of tissues, it is suitable for all routes of parenteral administration.

REGIONAL CHEMOTHERAPY

Because vascular supply to tumor areas is often poor, adequate drug concentrations are sometimes not achieved. Regional chemotherapy can be helpful in such situations. In carefully selected patients, for example, the intracavitary injection of alkylating agents can provide palliation of recurrent pleural and peritoneal effusions. Regional perfusion of certain parts of the body (e.g., an extremity) is also possible, with the achievement of higher drug concentrations than could be used by parenteral injection. In the use of regional chemotherapy, care must be exercised to avoid escape of the drugs into general circulation.

ANTIMETABOLITES

Antimetabolites include the folic acid antagonists, purine antagonists, and pyrimidine antagonists.

FOLIC ACID ANALOGUES
Methotrexate, U.S.P., B.P. (Amethopterin)

Methotrexate is the most widely used of the folic acid antagonists.

Mechanism of action. Methotrexate inhibits folic acid reductase, thereby interfering with the synthesis of a coenzyme necessary for DNA synthesis.

Absorption, distribution, metabolism, and excretion. Methotrexate is absorbed from both the gastrointestinal tract and from parenteral sites of administration. About 50% is bound to plasma proteins, and the drug is retained in human tissues for long periods of time. Of the drug absorbed, a substantial portion is excreted unchanged by the kidneys within 48 hours. Because so much of the drug is rapidly excreted by the kidneys with more excretion to occur over a long period, special caution must be exercised when methotrexate is administered to patients with impaired renal function. The drug is transported poorly across the blood-brain barrier and must be administered by the intrathecal route for neoplasms involving the central nervous system.

Toxicity. Methotrexate toxicity consists primarily of bone marrow depression, which sometimes can be avoided by the concurrent administration of folinic acid. The drug should be used only in facilities where abundant platelet transfusions and measures for preventing and treating infections are available. Oral and gastrointestinal mucosal ulceration, hemorrhage, alopecia, and hepatotoxicity are also common. Mouth lesions develop as necrotic patches on the lips, gums, buccal surfaces, palate, or uvula and are painful. Treatment should be interrupted at their appearance.

Clinical uses. The principal use of methotrexate is in the treatment of acute lymphoblastic leukemia in children. It is also effective in the treatment of choriocarcinoma in women, mycosis fungoides, and carcinomas of the breast, tongue, pharynx, and testes. D.E.S.I. rating for these conditions is *effective.* Temporary benefits also have been obtained after intraarterial perfusion of localized, surgically incurable solid tumors, especially melanoma and tumors of the head, neck, and pelvis. D.E.S.I. rating for these conditions is *possibly effective.* Methotrexate also has been used in the treatment of severe psoriasis and as an immunosuppressive agent.

Preparation, dosage, and administration. Methotrexate can be administered by a wide variety of routes: oral, parenteral, intrathecal, and by intraarterial perfusion. It is available in 2.5-mg. tablets and in powder form consisting of 5 or 50 mg. in sterile vials. Dosages vary according to the route of administration, individual tolerance, and the condition being treated. Oral dosage ranges are 2.5 to 10 mg. daily; intravenous doses are highly variable.

PURINE ANALOGUES
Mercaptopurine, U.S.P., B.P.
(6-mercaptopurine, Purinethol)

Mercaptopurine is the most important and most widely used purine antagonist.

Mechanism of action. Mercaptopurine probably exerts its effects by inhibiting DNA synthesis either by preventing incorporation of purine into DNA or by the utilization of mercaptopurine to form unnatural DNA.

Absorption, distribution, metabolism, and excretion. This drug is well absorbed from the gastrointestinal tract without any damage to the intestinal mucosa and is distributed widely in body tissues. It is rapidly metabolized and excreted by the kidneys. Degradation of the drug may be inhibited by concurrent administration of allopurinol.

Toxicity. Mercaptopurine toxicity consists primarily of bone marrow depression, although this generally develops more slowly than with folic acid antagonists. Anorexia, nausea, vomiting, and jaundice are common. Resistance to mercaptopurine is said to develop fairly rapidly.

Clinical uses. This drug is primarily effective in the treatment of acute lymphocytic leukemia, but may be used in the treatment of other acute leukemias. It may be used alone to maintain remissions in acute lymphoblastic and acute myeloblastic leukemia and in combination with other drugs to induce remission. It has a D.E.S.I. rating of *effective* for the treatment of leukemias, but *less effective* for the acute blastic phase. Mercaptopurine and other purine analogues also have immunosuppressive effects and have been used in the treatment of autoimmune diseases, such as systemic lupus erythematosus.

Preparation, dosage, and administration. Mercaptopurine is marketed in 50-mg. tablets for oral administration. The average daily dose is 2.5 mg. per kilogram of body weight orally and the dosage range is 50 to 250 mg. per day. When hematologic and clinical improvement occur, the dose is diminished for maintenance therapy. Dosage should be decreased for patients receiving allopurinol concurrently.

Thioguanine, U.S.P.

This drug is similar in its cytotoxic action and dosage requirements to mercaptopurine. It has been used in the treatment of acute leukemia and as an immunosuppressive agent. Its activity is not influenced by allopurinol. Thioguanine is available in 40-mg. tablets for oral administration. The average daily dose is 2.0 mg. per kilogram of body weight.

Azathioprine, U.S.P., B.P. (Imuran)

This drug is a derivative of mercaptopurine that has found clinical application as an immunosuppressive agent in the treatment of rejection reactions, idiopathic thrombocytopenic purpura, autoimmune hemolytic anemia, and systemic lupus erythematosus. The initial oral dosage for immunosuppressive therapy is 3 to 5 mg. per kilogram of body weight daily, which later may be reduced to 1 or 2 mg. per kilogram of body weight daily.

Allopurinol, U.S.P., B.P. (Zyloprim)

Although it is not a cytotoxic drug, allopurinol is frequently used in antineoplastic chemotherapy. It is a potent inhibitor of the enzyme xanthine oxidase, which is responsible for the conversion of hypoxanthine to xanthic to uric acid. This property has led to the therapeutic use of allopurinol in diseases characterized by excess production of uric acid such as gout, leukemia, and lymphoma, especially during treatment which causes rapid dissolution of neoplastic cells with consequent production of uric acid.

PYRIMIDINE ANALOGUES
Fluorouracil, U.S.P.

Mechanism of action. This drug is believed to affect specific steps in pyrimidine metabolism in such a way as to interfere with the synthesis of thymine, an essential part of deoxyribonucleic acid. It also inhibits the synthesis of ribonucleic acid (RNA) and is incorporated into the latter to form a fraudulent molecule of RNA. As a result, synthesis of proteins and proliferation of cancer cells are inhibited.

Absorption, distribution, metabolism, and excretion. Fluorouracil is absorbed irregularly from the gastrointestinal tract and is therefore administered intravenously. Most of the drug is converted into carbon dioxide and urea in the liver and about 10% of the injected dose is excreted by the kidneys.

Toxicity. The earliest signs of toxicity resulting from fluorouracil are stomatitis, diarrhea, and decreased leukocyte and platelet counts. Therapy should be discontinued at the appearance of these signs, since continued administration of fluorouracil beyond this point can cause severe and sometimes fatal gastrointestinal ulcerations and bone marrow aplasia. Alopecia is also common. This drug should not be administered without extremely close supervision of the patient and his hematologic status.

Clinical uses. Fluorouracil has a D.E.S.I. rating of *effective* for the palliative treatment of breast, colon, or rectal cancer. Other tumors responsive to this drug include gastrointestinal malignancies and ovarian, bladder, prostatic, and pancreatic carcinomas.

Preparation, dosage, and administration. Fluorouracil is available in 10-ml. ampules containing 500 mg. of the drug for intravenous administration. The recommended dose for an average patient is 12 to 15 mg. per kilogram of body weight per day for 4 days, then weekly doses of 15 mg. per kilogram of body weight as long as there is evidence of clinical improvement.

Cytarabine, U.S.P. (Cytosar, Ara-C)

Cytarabine is an antimetabolite which profoundly inhibits biosynthesis of DNA.

Absorption, distribution, metabolism, and excretion. Cytarabine is not active orally and is administered intravenously or subcutaneously. It is rapidly metabolized by the liver and possibly by the kidney.

Toxicity. The primary toxicity of this drug is manifested by leukopenia and thrombocytopenia. Other toxic manifestations include gastrointestinal disturbances, stomatitis, hepatic dysfunction, and thrombophlebitis at injection sites.

Clinical uses. Cytarabine is primarily indicated for the induction of remissions in acute granulocytic leukemia.

Preparation, dosage, and administration. The drug is supplied in vials containing 100 or 500 mg. to be reconstituted for injection. Various dosage schedules have been studied. The recommended dosage is 2 mg. per kilogram of body weight by rapid injection daily for 10 days or 0.5 to 1 mg. per kilogram by infusion over several hours daily for 10 days.

ANTIBIOTICS

Dactinomycin, U.S.P. (actinomycin D, Cosmegen)

Dactinomycin is an actinomycin antibiotic isolated from a *Streptomyces* culture that has been found to inhibit synthesis of RNA.

Absorption, distribution, metabolism, and excretion. This drug can be administered both orally and parenterally, but is much less potent when given orally. About 50% of the drug is excreted unchanged in the bile.

Toxicity. Dactinomycin severely depresses bone marrow and causes gastrointestinal ulceration. It is extremely irritating to the tissues. Irradiation effects are potentiated by this drug.

Clinical uses. Dactinomycin appears to be the most effective drug in the treatment of Wilms' tumor. It is also useful in the treatment of methotrexate-resistant carcinoma in women, neuro-

blastomas, soft-tissue sarcomas, and testicular tumors.

Preparation, dosage, and administration. This drug is supplied in vials containing 0.5 mg. The usual dose for children is 15 µg. per kilogram of body weight per day intravenously for 5 days. The dose for adults is 0.01 mg. per kilogram of body weight daily for 5 days. Courses of therapy are repeated at 6-week to 3-month intervals. Because of its irritant properties, dactinomycin should be given by injection into the tubing of a rapidly flowing intravenous infusion, and great care should be taken to avoid extravasation. Any unused portion must be discarded.

Mithramycin, U.S.P. (Mithracin)

This antibiotic also inhibits RNA synthesis and is employed in the treatment of embryonal cell carcinoma of the testes. One commonly used dosage is 25 to 30 µg. per kilogram of body weight per day by intravenous injection for 8 to 10 days. An important toxic effect is hemorrhagic diathesis, and the drug should be discontinued when signs of vasculitis occur (e.g., flushing, conjunctivitis). Myelosuppression, hypocalcemia, and hepatotoxicity also occur.

Mitomycin (Mutamycin)

Mitomycin is a cytotoxic antibiotic with activity similar to alkylating agents. It is used as an adjunct to surgery and radiation therapy and to treat advanced metastatic disease in patients resistant to other antineoplastic drugs. Hematologic toxicity occurs frequently.

ANTHRACYCLINES
Daunorubicin (Daunomycin); doxorubicin hydrochloride (Adriamycin)

Daunorubicine is an experimental antibiotic agent that has demonstrated significant activity in the treatment of acute myelocytic leukemia. It is also active in acute lymphocytic leukemia, especially when used together with vincristine and prednisone. Severe bone marrow depression is very common, and life-threatening cardiotoxicity (congestive heart failure and arrhythmias) also has been reported.

Doxorubicin is similar to daunorubicine and appears to be active in the treatment of many solid tumors, cancers of the lung and bladder, lymphomas, many sarcomas, and metastatic tumors. Complete alopecia usually occurs with doxorubicin therapy. It appears to possess less cardiotoxic potential than daunorubicin; both drugs are given intravenously.

Bleomycin (Blenoxane)

Bleomycin inhibits cell mitosis and DNA synthesis. It is extremely active in squamous cell skin cancer, testicular tumors, and most lymphomas. Its toxicity is considerable and is manifested by fever, skin ulceration (especially of the fingers and toes), anorexia, nausea, stomatitis, pulmonary fibrosis, and severe hypotension. Recommended doses are 30 to 50 mg. per square meter administered once weekly.

PLANT ALKALOIDS

Vinblastine and vincristine are two alkaloids derived from the periwinkle plant, *Vinca rosea.* The mechanisms of action of these drugs are not well understood currently, but appear to relate to metaphase arrest. The drugs are not absorbed well after oral administration and must be given intravenously. They may bind preferentially to neoplastic tissues and appear to be excreted primarily by the liver into the biliary system. Despite their similarities in structure and in mechanism of action, the drugs differ in toxicity and in therapeutic application. Doses of both drugs should be decreased for patients with biliary obstruction.

Vinblastine sulfate, U.S.P., B.P. (Velban)

The principal use of vinblastine is in the treatment of Hodgkin's disease, in which it produces results that are equal or superior to those of the alkylating agents. Vinblastine also may be effective in the treatment of lymphomas, choriocarcinoma, and embryonal carcinoma of the testis.

Toxicity occurs primarily to the bone marrow, but other toxic manifestations include gastrointestinal disturbances, neurologic disturbances, and alopecia.

Vinblastine is available as a dry powder in ampules containing 10 mg. of drug. Reconstituted solutions may be stored under refrigeration for a month without loss of potency. Recommended dosage is 0.1 to 0.2 mg. per kilogram of body weight intravenously weekly.

Vincristine sulfate, U.S.P., B.P. (Oncovin)

Vincristine, in contrast with vinblastine, is very effective in inducing remissions in acute leukemias in children. It is also less toxic to the bone marrow, but highly neurotoxic. The neurotoxicity consists of manifestations such as paresthesias, muscle weakness, loss of deep tendon reflexes, headache, vocal cord paralysis, ptosis, diplopia, and paralytic ileus. The neurotoxicity is usually reversed when the drug is withdrawn. Gastrointestinal disturbances and alopecia may also occur.

Vincristine is available as a dry powder in vials containing either 1 or 5 mg. of the drug, which can be stored under refrigeration for 2 weeks after being reconstituted. Commonly employed doses are 1.5 to 2.0 mg. per square meter of body surface for children and adults, given weekly.

RADIOACTIVE ISOTOPES

Radioactive isotopes have the advantage of greater selective toxicity than other antineoplastic agents. Tumor cells may be more susceptible to radiation than normal cells and, because the tumor is usually small, high concentrations can be used in a small space, exerting great toxicity to the tumor, but sparing normal host cells.

The mechanism of action for the cytotoxic effects of ionizing radiation is not yet well understood. Toxic effects of radioactive materials affect rapidly proliferating cells such as hematopoietic, skin, intestinal, and germinal cells, in much the same way as do other antineoplastic agents. Skin reactions occur frequently with the use of external and implanted sources of radiation and are known as "radiation burns." The skin becomes erythematous, temporary epilation occurs, and hyperpigmentation may follow. Symptoms of toxicity to the gastrointestinal tract include vomiting, diarrhea, ulceration, and bleeding. Hematopoietic toxicity is manifest as leukopenia and thrombocytopenia.

It must be noted that both the patient and the nurse caring for him are susceptible to the toxic effects of radiation therapy when an implanted source is used. Precautions to protect the nurse, other health care personnel, and visitors must be exercised, which will vary according to the type of radiation emitted, the half-life of the isotope, the amount of isotope used, the method of administration, and the method of excretion. General principles of precautionary measures relate to (1) *time* of allowable exposure to patients being treated with radioactive materials, (2) the permissible *distance* between nurse (or visitors) and patient, and (3) appropriate *shielding* of the nurse (or visitors) from the radioactive material. For more specific information regarding precautionary measures, the nurse should receive instructions from the radioisotope laboratory of the hospital. (Special precautions are not necessary for patients who receive radiation therapy from external sources because they carry no source of radioactivity.)

Some of the most common radioactive isotopes used therapeutically are ^{131}I, ^{32}P, ^{198}Au, ^{125}I, ^{226}Ra, ^{222}Rn, ^{137}Cs, ^{90}Sr, ^{90}Y, and ^{60}Co. Of these, cobalt 60 is a most useful source of gamma radiation. ^{131}I has been useful in treating thyroid diseases, because the thyroid gland readily concentrates it, as it does all body iodine. ^{32}P has been useful in treating chronic granulocytic leukemia, lymphocytic leukemia, and polycythemia vera. Radiogold 198 is most generally employed in body cavities to treat effusions.

MISCELLANEOUS ANTINEOPLASTIC AGENTS
Procarbazine hydrochloride, U.S.P. (Matulane)

The greatest effectiveness of procarbazine is in the treatment of Hodgkin's disease. This drug is well absorbed orally but can also be administered parenterally. It seems to lack cross-resistance with other antineoplastic agents. It is supplied in 50-mg. capsules and administered in a dosage range of 100 to 300 mg. per day. Its principal toxic effects are nausea and vomiting, leukopenia, and thrombocytopenia, but CNS toxicity has also occurred.

Hydroxyurea (Hydrea)

The primary role of this drug seems to be in the treatment of chronic granulocytic leukemia, but other therapeutic uses are being explored. It is available in 500-mg. capsules. Hematopoietic depression is its major toxic effect. Dosage for solid tumors is 80 mg. per kilogram of body weight as a single dose every third day; continuous dose is 20 to 30 mg. per kilogram of body weight daily as a single dose.

L-asparaginase

Knowledge regarding this drug is still limited, but it produces temporary, brief remissions in a substantial percentage of patients with acute lymphoblastic leukemia. It is administered in a dosage range of 200 to 1000 I.U. per kilogram of body weight three to seven times weekly for 28 days. Toxicity takes the form of nausea and vomiting, fever, allergy, confusion, hepatic dysfunction, and blood dyscrasias.

NURSING FUNCTIONS IN ANTINEOPLASTIC CHEMOTHERAPY

Nursing functions related to drug therapy with antineoplastic agents are complex and inseparably related to nursing care of the total patient as well as his family. The patient may be at any stage of adaptation to his disease process and to the possibility of impending death and will inevitably be under stress. The nurse must recognize this and adapt the approach to the patient in a sensitive and appropriate manner.

In caring for patients receiving cancer chemotherapy, nurses have several responsibilities in relation to the assessment aspect of the nursing process. They should assess each patient's degree of acceptance of chemotherapy and may need to assist the patient to deal with ambivalent feelings. The patient's and family's knowledge regarding chemotherapy and their expectations should also be assessed. Teaching the patient about drug administration and drug effects may help to ameliorate future anxieties. Assessment may reveal that expectations are unrealistic, and the patient and his family may need assistance in accepting a more realistic view of the results of chemotherapy. Expectations of total cure are usually unrealistic and should not be reinforced, while expectations of remissions are usually more achievable.

In the management of patients receiving antineoplastic agents, the nurse has many responsibilities in dealing with the inevitable side effects and toxic effects of these drugs. Bone marrow depression, for example, greatly increases the patient's vulnerability to infection. The nurse should use strict aseptic techniques in contacts with the patient and should protect the patient from individuals harboring harmful microorganisms. Frequent blood counts are necessary, and it is often the nurse's responsibility to ensure that they are done. Special prophylactic care should be given to patients with thrombocytopenia, including the administration of stool softeners, use of soft toothbrushes, and use of side rails on beds. Intramuscular injections and any soft tissue injury should be avoided. Venipunctures should be done by experienced personnel utilizing strict sterile technique. Platelet transfusions may be necessary in thrombocytopenic patients. Patients with granulocytopenia should also receive stool softeners prophylactically, maintain scrupulous oral hygiene, and receive local antibiotics for abrasions or scratches.

Alopecia is a side effect extremely distressing to women, even when they have been prepared for it and have cosmetic aids available. These patients will need assistance in coping with body image problems. The vesicant properties of the alkylating agents and the irritant properties of most antineoplastic agents necessitate careful handling of these drugs by both nurse and patient. Alkylating agents should not come in contact with the skin or with mucous membranes. It is recommended that personnel reconstituting these drugs use protective gloves and glasses. If contact should occur, the affected areas should be washed immediately with copious amounts of water for at least 15 minutes. A 2% sodium thiocyanate solution may also be used locally to neutralize the drug's alkylating activity. Extravasation of drugs can best be avoided by injecting them into rapidly flowing intravenous infusions. Subcutaneous extravasation may be treated by local infiltration with normal saline.

Other side effects and toxic effects will also require the nurse's interventions. Nausea and vomiting attendant to the use of these drugs can be ameliorated by prior administration of antiemetics and sedatives. Stomatitis resulting from these drugs can be very uncomfortable and can interfere with the patient's nutrition. A topical anesthetic mouth rinse and bland, nonirritating foods may enable the patient to eat in greater comfort. Treatment with some radioactive isotopes will necessitate precautions, and treatment with hormones may necessitate support for the patient in the event of side effects such as masculinization in female patients and feminization in male patients.

Undoubtedly, one of the most important nursing interventions is that of providing emotional support to the patient with a destructive disease who is receiving therapy that is both physically and psychologically distressing. The long period of therapy, with frequent interruptions and sometimes slow progress, may compound the patient's stress.

Evaluation of drug effects is another integral aspect of nursing function in antineoplastic chemotherapy. The nurse should observe for and report both therapeutic and toxic effects of the antineoplastic agents. This is especially important because with antineoplastic agents there is often no predetermined dosage schedule for the drug used that is universally therapeutic. Dosage will change according to the patient's response, and the nurse's evaluation and communication of that response are essential. In evaluating for toxic drug effects, the nurse should be vigilant for very early signs of toxicity, since their progression may have severe and irreversible consequences. Early signs of irritation of the oral mucous membranes, for example, can be noted by frequent examinations of the patient's mouth during which time the nurse observes for erythema, white patchy membranes, and ulceration. Early signs of bone marrow depression may be identified from frequent blood counts, and the nurse should monitor these carefully.

QUESTIONS

For study and review

1 Identify the types of malignancies that have been cured with antineoplastic agents. *Hodgkins ALL Ewings Wilms Burkitts chorio & embryo*

2 What are the goals of cancer chemotherapy when cure cannot be accomplished? *pallention regression, regression of process, prolongation of life*

3 Identify the six major categories of antineoplastic agents, naming one drug from each category. *Alkylating, Antibiotic Radioactive Isotopes, Antimetabolite Hormones, Plant Alkaloids*

4 What does it mean to say that most antineoplastic agents lack selective toxicity? *destroy all proliferative cells*

5 Describe the major toxic effects that occur in therapy with almost all antineoplastic agents. *nausea, vomiting, alopecia thrombocytopenia, hematologic*

6 How can the sclerosing effects of the antineoplastic drugs be avoided when these agents need to be administered intravenously? *quick inj. tubing*

7 How can the severe nausea and vomiting accompanying the use of these drugs be ameliorated? *antiemetics, sedatives 1 hr. before + night*

8 What is the rationale for the use of hormones in the treatment of malignancies of the reproductive organs? *change environ.*

9 Why must a course of therapy with the alkylating agents be interrupted? *toxicity*

10 What is the primary advantage of regional chemotherapy? *[ ]*

11 Explain why allopurinol is frequently used as an adjunct to antineoplastic chemotherapy. *↑ effectiveness*

12 What is the primary indication for the therapeutic use of cytosine arabinoside? *AGLeukemia*

13 How can nurses protect themselves from the vesicant action of the alkylating agents? Describe what measures must be taken if these drugs come in contact with the skin or mucous membranes. *gloves, glasses water +++ 0-15 min. 2% Na thiocynate soln*

REFERENCES

Bergel, F.: Today's carcinochemotherapy: some of its achievements, failures and prospects, Ergebn. Physiol. 62:91, 1970.

Clarkson, B. D., and Fried, J.: Changing concepts of treatment in acute leukemia, Med. Clin. North Am. 55:561, 1971.

DiPalma, J. R., editor: Drill's pharmacology in medicine, ed. 4, New York, 1971, The McGraw-Hill Book Co.

DeVita, V. T., and Schein, P. S.: The use of drugs in combination for the treatment of cancer, New Eng. J. Med. 288:998, 1973.

DeVita, V. T., Serpick, A., and Carbone, P. C.: Combination chemotherapy with treatment of advanced Hodgkin's disease, Ann. Intern. Med. 73:881, 1970.

Folkman, J.: Tumor angiogenesis: Therapeutic implications, New Eng. J. Med. 285:1182, 1971.

Goodman, L. S., and Gilman, A.: The pharmacological basis of therapeutics, ed. 5, London, 1975, The Macmillan Co.

Gordon, G. S., Wessler, S., and Avioli, L. V.: Calusterone in the therapy for advanced breast cancer, J.A.M.A. 219:483, 1972.

Goth, A.: Medical pharmacology, ed. 7, St. Louis, 1974, The C. V. Mosby Co.

Greenwald, E. S.: Cancer chemotherapy, New York J. Med. 66:2532, 2670, 1966.

Handschumacher, R. E.: L-Asparaginase, Ann. Rev. Med. 21:433, 1970.

Hersh, E. M., and others: Chemotherapy, immunocompetence, immunosuppression and prognosis in acute leukemia, New Eng. J. Med. 285:1211, 1971.

Hiatt, H. H.: Cancer chemotherapy—present status and prospects, New Eng. J. Med. 276:157, 1967.

Isler, C.: Care of the pediatric patient with leukemia, R.N. 35:30, 1972.

Isler, C.: The cancer nurses—how the specialists are doing it, R.N. 35:28, 1972.

Knock, F. E.: Anticancer agents, Springfield, Ill., 1967, Charles C Thomas, Publisher.

Krakoff, I. H.: Cancer chemotherapeutic agents, C. A. 23:208, 1973.

Krakoff, I. H.: The present status of cancer chemotherapy, Med. Clin. North Am. 55:683, 1971.

Meyers, F. H., Jawetz, E., and Goldfein, A.: Review of medical pharmacology, ed. 3, Los Altos, Calif., 1972, Lange Medical Publications.

Pinkel, D.: Five year follow-up of "total therapy" of childhood lymphocytic leukemia, J.A.M.A. 216:648, 1971.

Pratt, W. B.: Fundamentals of chemotherapy, New York, 1973, Oxford University Press.

Rodman, M. J.: Anticancer chemotherapy: Part 1. The kinds of drugs and what they do, R.N. 35:45, 1972. Part 2. Against solid malignant tumors, R.N. 35:61, 1972. Part 3. Against the leukemias and lymphomas, R.N. 35:49, 1972.

Rosenfeld, M. G., editor: Manual of medical therapeutics, ed. 20, Boston, 1971, Little, Brown, & Co.

Silverstein, M., and Morton, D.: Cancer immunotherapy, Am. J. Nurs. 73:1178, 1973.

Teitelbaum, A. C.: Intra-arterial drug therapy, Am. J. Nurs. 72:1634, 1972.

CHAPTER 25

Endocrine hormones

Pituitary
Parathyroid hormone
Thyroid hormones and drugs
Hormones of the adrenal gland
Hormones from the pancreas

The hormones are natural chemical substances that act after being secreted into the bloostream from the ductless, or endocrine, glands. The word "hormone" is derived from the Greek word *hormaein*, which means "to excite." The word "endocrine" is from the Greek word *endon*, meaning "within."

Hormones have physiologic interrelationships. Hormones from various endocrine glands work in concert to obtain physiologic control of vital processes. Their relationship may be synergistic or antagonistic, this allows for flexibility and control. There are six major areas in which hormones play a crucial regulatory role:

1 Control and coordination of the secretory and motor activities of the digestive tract
2 Control of energy production
3 Control of composition and volume of extracellular fluid
4 Adaptation, such as acclimatization and immunity
5 Growth and development
6 Reproduction and lactation

To maintain the internal environment there must also be control of hormone secretion. This is achieved by a self-regulating series of events known as "negative feedback"; that is, a hormone produces a physiologic effect that, on attaining sufficient magnitude, inhibits further secretion of that hormone, thereby inhibiting the physiologic effect. Increased hormonal secretions may be evoked in response to stimuli from the external environment; cessation of external stimuli terminates the internal secretion response.

Hormones are not "used up" in exerting their physiologic effects but must be inactivated or excreted if the internal environment is to be in dynamic equilibrium. Inactivation occurs enzymatically in the blood or intercellular spaces, in the liver or kidney, or in the target tissues. Excretion of hormones is primarily via the urine and to a lesser extent the bile.

Most hormones are rapidly destroyed, having a half-life in blood of 10 to 30 minutes. However, some, like the catecholamines, have a half-life of seconds, while thyroid hormones have a half-life measured in days. Some hormones exert their physiologic effects almost instantaneously while others require minutes or hours before their effects occur. In addition, some physiologic effects disappear immediately upon the hormone's disappearance from the circulation, while other physiologic responses may persist for hours after hormone concentrations have returned to basal levels. This wide range of onset and duration of hormonal activity contributes to the flexibility of the endocrine system.

Hormones may exert their effects by:

1 Controlling the formation or destruction of some intracellular regulator, such as cyclic AMP

548

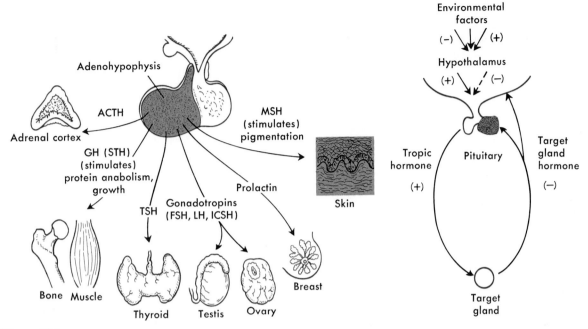

Figure 25-1

Various internal and external environmental factors may inhibit or stimulate the hypothalamus to secrete inhibitory (−) or releasing (+) factors to control output of hormones from the anterior pituitary and ultimate hormone release from target glands. Hormone secretion from target glands (adrenal cortex, thyroid, etc.), upon reaching a critical level, have an inhibitory effect on the secretion of tropic hormones by the anterior pituitary and releasing factors (RF) by the hypothalamus. *ACTH*, Adrenocorticotropic hormone; *GH*, growth hormone; *STH*, somatotropin hormone; *TSH*, thyroid-stimulating hormone; *FSH*, follicle-stimulating hormone; *LH*, luteinizing hormone; *ICSH*, interstitial cell-stimulating hormone; *MSH*, melanocyte-stimulating hormone.

2 Controlling protein synthesis
3 Controlling membrane permeability and the movement of ions and other substances

One of the major developments of this century in the fields of biology and medicine has been the recognition and then the isolation, purification, and chemical understanding of most of the hormones we now know. In addition, once their chemical structure is known, it becomes hypothetically possible to duplicate them by chemical synthesis. This has been accomplished for some hormones, although not for all.

Exactly what should be called a hormone and what should not is not well defined. A broad definition could be any chemical substance released by one tissue, circulated by the blood, and having characteristic effects on other tissues. This

would include many substances not ordinarily classed as hormones, such as carbon dioxide. In common usage, hormones are confined to those well-recognized and chemically specific products of the various endocrine glands that are released in small amounts and that have specific well-defined physiologic effects on metabolism. The list of major hormones includes the products of the secretions of the anterior and posterior pituitary, the thyroid hormone, insulin and glucogen from the pancreas, epinephrine and norepinephrine from the adrenal medulla, several potent steroids from the adrenal cortex, and the gonadal hormones of both sexes.

In medicine these substances are generally used in two ways: (1) for replacement when a patient lacks sufficient endogenous hormone, exemplified by the use of insulin in diabetes or the use of adrenal steroids in Addison's disease, and (2) for pharmacologic effects beyond those of replacement, exemplified by the use of large doses of the adrenal steroids for their anti-inflammatory effects.

PITUITARY

Because the hormones of the pituitary gland exert an important effect in regulating the secretion of other hormones, it is fitting that they be considered first.

The pituitary body is about the size of a pea and occupies a niche in the sella turcica of the sphenoid bone. It consists of an anterior lobe, a posterior lobe, and a smaller pars intermedia composed of secreting cells. The anterior part is particularly important in sustaining life. The function of the pars intermedia is not well known. It should be noted that the oral administration of any part of the whole gland is without visible effect because it is destroyed by proteolytic enzymes and the pituitary hormones are protein or peptide in nature.

Regulation of anterior pituitary function. The pituitary and target glands have a negative feedback relationship. A tropic hormone from the pituitary stimulates the target gland to secrete a hormone that inhibits further secretion of the tropic hormone by the pituitary. When the serum concentration of the target gland hormone falls below a certain level, the pituitary again secretes the tropic hormone until the target gland produces enough hormone to inhibit the pituitary secretion. However, the negative feedback concept alone is not enough to account for changes in serum levels of target gland hormones, especially those due to changes in the external environment—thus the theorizing that the central nervous system plays a decisive role in regulating pituitary function to meet environmental demands.

Of great research interest is the discovery of various hypothalamic releasing factors (also called hypophysiotropic hormones), which cause the release or inhibition of the various hormones from the anterior pituitary. Just where these releasing factors are synthesized in the central nervous system and what controls their secretion is not known at the present time. An additional factor under consideration is the possibility that the anterior pituitary hormones themselves contain releasing-inhibiting factors.

ANTERIOR PITUITARY HORMONES

Present evidence indicates that a number of factors are concerned in the action of extracts of the anterior lobe of the pituitary gland. How many hormones are secreted by the gland is unknown, but at least seven extracts have been prepared in a relatively pure state, and they have definite specific action.

1 A growth factor influences the development of the body. It promotes skeletal, visceral, and general growth of the body. Acromegaly, gigantism, and dwarfism are connected with pathology of the anterior lobe of the pituitary gland.

   The growth hormone or somatotropin has been obtained as a small crystalline protein, but thus far the growth hormone has found no established place in medicine, and its use in various clinical conditions is largely experimental. It tends to increase the blood sugar and antagonize insulin, and it may be the "diabetogenic" hormone postulated some years ago.

2 The follicle-stimulating hormone (FSH) stimulates the growth and maturation of the ovarian follicle, which in turn brings on the characteristic changes of estrus (menstruation in women). This hormone also stimulates spermatogenesis in the male. FSH appears to be a protein or is associated with a protein, but it has not yet been obtained in a highly purified form.

3 Luteinizing hormone (LH), also known as the interstitial cell-stimulating hormone (ICSH), together with FSH causes maturation of the graafian follicles, ovulation, and the secretion of estrogen in the female. It causes spermatogenesis, androgen formation, and growth of interstitial tissue in the male. The luteinizing hormone also promotes the formation of the corpora lutea in the female.

4 Thyrotropic hormone (TSH) is necessary for normal development and function of the thyroid gland and, if present in excess, is known to produce hyperthyroidism and an increased size of the gland in laboratory animals.

5 A lactogenic factor (prolactin or mammotropin) plays a part in proliferation and secretion of the

mammary glands of mammals. This may be identical with the hormone responsible for the development of the corpus luteum. In its absence the corpus luteum fails to produce progesterone.

6 The adrenocorticotropic hormone (corticotropin or ACTH) stimulates the cortex of the adrenal gland.

7 Melanocyte-stimulating hormone (intermedin) is probably produced in the intermediate lobe. Its physiologic role is unknown but when injected in man it will darken the skin.

Although the hormones produced by the anterior lobe of the pituitary gland are important physiologically, a number of reasons explain their limited usefulness. Only in relatively recent times have purified preparations been available, at least for clinical study, and such preparations are both expensive and limited in supply. Increased application of their effects may be expected in the future, however, as chemically defined preparations become available.

Corticotropin

The adrenocorticotropic hormone (corticotropin or ACTH), exerts its action primarily on the cells of the adrenal cortex and causes it to secrete its entire spectrum of hormones.

The ultimate effects in the body, therefore, are the effects of the various adrenocortical steroids and, in general, these effects are similar to those of cortisone. Corticotropin is effective only if a functioning adrenal gland is present. The present source of corticotropin is from the pituitary glands of domesticated mammals such as hogs and cattle. The labor involved in the removal of the glands is such that this source is an expensive one.

During conditions of stress and strain the activity of the adrenal cortex is increased. This is thought to be the result of an increased secretion of corticotropin. One explanation for the regulation of corticotropic activity is that during stress the tissues of the body utilize more of the adrenal hormones than usual, which results in a decreased concentration of the adrenocortical hormones in the blood. This in turn brings about stimulation of cells in the anterior pituitary gland and the production of more corticotropin. On the other hand, when stress has subsided, the tissues use less of the adrenocortical hormones, their concentration in the blood increases, and this causes activity of the pituitary gland as well as the adrenal cortex to be decreased.

Absorption. Corticotropin is destroyed by enzymes in the gastrointestinal tract and therefore cannot be given orally. It is absorbed readily from sites of injection when given intramuscularly or intravenously. It is said to disappear from the blood rapidly after intravenous injection. Its effects rarely last longer than 6 hours. This necessitates frequent intramuscular injections, administration by slow intravenous drip, or the use of a preparation that is absorbed slowly. Its effectiveness depends upon the presence of normal adrenal glands capable of responding to the stimulant made by the pituitary gland.

Uses. Corticotropin is used for many of the same conditions for which cortisone and hydrocortisone are used, such as rheumatic diseases, skin diseases, ocular diseases, and allergic manifestations. It is also used to treat chronic ulcerative colitis and multiple sclerosis. It has the advantage of rapid absorption and rapid utilization, but it is more expensive than the cortical steroids. For maintenance therapy the smallest effective dose and the longest possible interval between doses should be used.

Preparation, dosage, and administration. The following are preparations of corticotropin.

Corticotropin injection, U.S.P., B.P. (Acthar). Corticotropin injection is used for definitive diagnosis of adrenal insufficiency and to establish if the disease is primary or secondary (e.g., due to pituitary disease). Corticotropin is administered intravenously for 2 or 3 consecutive days (over an 8-hour period; 8 A.M. to 4 P.M.) and 24-hour urine collections are made to determine the amount of 17-hydroxycorticoids secreted. Patients with normal adrenal function will show a threefold increase in baseline values; patients with primary adrenal cortical deficiency will show a very small increase on the first day with no further increase on remaining days; and patients with secondary insufficiency will show a stepwise increase over the 3-day period.

Corticotropin is also used to manage severe myasthenia gravis. The hormone is given in doses of 100 I.U. daily until a total of 1000 to

2000 units has been given (1 mg. of the International Unit is equal to the activity contained in 1 U.S.P. unit). Marked deterioration of muscle strength occurs 2 to 3 days after initiation of therapy; equipment for assisting respiration should be available. Two days to 1 week after completion of treatment muscle strength improves and lasts for an average of 3 months. A second course of treatment may then be given, or a weekly dose of the drug may be given.

When corticotropin is given to diabetics, insulin requirements might be increased.

Corticotropin injection is marketed as a powder in 10, 25, or 40 U.S.P. units and in solution of 10 to 40 U.S.P. units per milliliter. The average dose of corticotropin for adults is 20 U.S.P. units four times daily when given intramuscularly. When the drug is administered intravenously, 5 to 20 U.S.P. units are dissolved in 500 ml. of 5% glucose solution, and the solution is administered slowly over an 8-hour period (once daily).

Repository corticotropin injection, U.S.P. (Corticotropin Gel); *corticotrophin gelatin injection*, B.P. This is corticotropin dissolved in a gelatin solution, which results in slow absorption and more satisfactory clinical effect per unit of activity. Repository corticotropin is administered intramuscularly. Maximum effect occurs in 15 to 18 hours; duration of effect may be as long as 72 hours. A daily injection exerts a prolonged and continuous effect. The usual intramuscular dose is 40 U.S.P. units. The maintenance dose is 20 U.S.P. units two or three times a week.

Sterile corticotropin–zinc hydroxide suspension, U.S.P.; *corticotrophin zinc injection*, B.P. This is purified corticotropin adsorbed on zinc hydroxide. Absorption after parenteral administration is delayed, and thus its action is prolonged. Action of one dose may persist for 3 days. It is administered intramuscularly and is available as a suspension containing 100 and 200 U.S.P. units in 5 ml. The usual initial dose is 40 U.S.P. units; the maintenance dose is 20 U.S.P. units two or three times a week.

Side effects and toxic effects. Effects are much the same as those noted after administration of cortisone or hydrocortisone (see pp. 568-569).

Cosyntropin (Cortrosyn)

Cosyntropin is a synthetic peptide subunit of natural corticotropin. A dose of 0.25 mg. of cosyntropin has the biologic activity of 25 units of natural corticotropin. Cosyntropin is not used as a therapeutic substitute for corticotropin but as a diagnostic agent for adrenal insufficiency. After its administration, if the adrenal cortex is able to function, there is an increase in plasma cortisol levels; if no increase occurs 1 hour after 0.25 mg. is given intramuscularly, adrenal insufficiency is present. If the latter occurs, 0.25 mg. of cosyntropin is diluted in saline and injected intravenously over 8 hours on 2 to 3 consecutive days. If no increase in plasma cortisol level occurs the patient has primary adrenal insufficiency. If pituitary disease is suspected, pituitary functioning can be tested. Urinary excretion of steroids may be used to determine response in place of plasma cortisol levels.

Patients on hydrocortisone or estrogens may have abnormally high plasma cortisol levels.

Thyrotropin

Thyrotropin is an extract of the thyroid-stimulating hormone obtained from bovine anterior pituitary glands. It is not used as a therapeutic agent but to evaluate thyroid function. D.E.S.I. rating is *effective* for determining low thyroid reserve, for differentiating primary and secondary hypothyroidism, and for evaluating the need for thyroid medication in patients receiving thyroid therapy. Ten units of thyrotropin are injected intramuscularly followed by a tracer dose of radioiodine 18 to 24 hours later. After 24 hours the uptake of iodine by the thyroid increases in a patient with hypopituitarism but does not increase in a patient with primary hypothyroidism.

PITUITARY GONADOTROPIC HORMONES

The pituitary gonadotropic hormones are discussed in Chapter 26.

POSTERIOR PITUITARY HORMONES

When solutions of extracts of the posterior lobes of the pituitary glands of animals (domestic) are administered parenterally, a number of effects have been observed: (1) stimulation of the uterine muscle (oxytocic effect), (2) promotion of the absorption of water in the renal tubules (antidiuretic effect), and (3) stimulation of the muscle of the superficial blood vessels (pressor effect) and of the intestine.

A great advance in the pharmacology of the posterior lobe has been the identification and chemical analysis of two major hormones obtained from the gland in pure form. These compounds, oxytocin and vasopressin (antidiuretic hormone, ADH), are both peptides, each containing eight amino acids. After their isolation and determination it proved possible to synthesize them chemically. Availability of the oxytocic and vasopressor pituitary hormones in pure form has clarified a number of uncertainties about their action and has also encouraged their better-controlled therapeutic use. It is known, for example, that there is a certain overlap of pharmacologic action even in the pure preparation; pure oxytocin has some vasopressor activity, and vice versa. Vasopressin is also the antidiuretic hormone, its antidiuretic potency being much more marked than its pressor potency. Although the cruder preparations of oxytocic and vasopressor activity are still used, it may be expected that eventually the pure compounds will replace the older extracts.

Oxytocin

Oxytocin is discussed in Chapter 26, Sex hormones.

Vasopressin

Vasopressin functions as an antidiuretic hormone (ADH) by enhancing water permeability of the tubular epithelial membranes of the distal convolution and collecting ducts so that water can be absorbed by osmotic flow. Secretion of ADH is influenced by body hydration; if the body is hydrated no ADH can be detected in the urine or plasma, but if the body is dehydrated it is present in both fluids.

Vasopressin is used as an antidiuretic for the symptomatic treatment of polyuria accompanying diabetes insipidus (a condition in which the patient excretes a large amount of urine due to lack of ADH). It is also used to relieve intestinal gaseous distention since it markedly increases bowel motility.

Vasopressin can be used for rapid testing of renal function. Five to 10 units are given intramuscularly, and the specific gravity of urine is determined 1 and 2 hours later. In normal renal function the specific gravity rises to 1.018 or more. No special preparation is required for this test, and it can be used in place of the test in which patients are deprived of water for 18 hours. Vasopressin is not used for its oxytocic or pressor action because of the danger of myocardial depression and ischemia and because better drugs are available for these actions.

Vasopressin is ineffective if given by the oral route. It may be applied topically or given by subcutaneous or intramuscular injection.

Vasopressin injection causes oliguria in 1 to 2 hours, which reaches a peak in 3 hours; duration of action may be as long as 10 hours.

Preparation, dosage, and administration. The following are available preparations of vasopressin.

Vasopressin injection, U.S.P., B.P. (Pitressin). This is a purified preparation of antidiuretic and pressor hormone separated from the oxytocic hormone. The usual dose is 0.25 to 0.5 ml. (5 to 10 U.S.P. units) three or four times daily; for children, dose is 2.5 to 10 units three or four times daily. It is given subcutaneously or intramuscularly.

Vasopressin tannate (Pitressin). This compound is marketed in solution for intramuscular injection 0.5 to 1 ml. (2.5 to 5 units) is injected at intervals of 36 to 48 hours. For children the dose is 1.25 to 2.5 units. Its effect is more prolonged than that of vasopressin. It cannot be given intravenously. Prolonged rotation of the ampule is necessary in order that all of the particles be included in the suspension. Failure to shake the ampule thoroughly can result in inaccurate dosage and inadequate therapeutic response. Vasopressin tannate has received a D.E.S.I. rating of *effective* for the control or prevention of symptoms and complications of diabetes insipidus due to deficiency of the antidiuretic hormone.

Lypressin (Diapid). Lypressin is a synthetic polypeptide structurally identical to the antidiuretic hormone found in man. It is applied as a nasal spray; it is rapidly absorbed from the nasal mucosa. It is effective as sole therapy in controlling the polyuria of diabetes insipidus in mild or moderate cases. Lypressin can be used as adjunctive therapy between injections in more severe cases. It is less likely to cause rhinopharyngitis than posterior pituitary powder. No significant systemic or local allergic reactions have been reported.

One or more sprays are applied to one or both nostrils, one or more times daily. Each spray contains about 2 U.S.P. posterior pituitary pressor units. Four sprays in each nostril is the maximal amount that can be absorbed at one time. Lypressin is available in 5-ml. containers, which contain 50 pressor units per milliliter.

Posterior pituitary powder, B.P. This powder is dried pituitary gland, which can be snuffed into the nose. Absorption from the nasal mucous membrane makes it possible to use it for the relief of symptoms of diabetes insipidus. It is less expensive than the injectable forms. It must be applied several times daily. Irritation of the nasal mucosa limits its use. It may cause sneezing, wheezing, dyspnea, asthmatic attacks, and other hypersensitivity reactions.

Side effects and toxic effects. Vasopressin can cause spasm of coronary arteries, and caution is recommended when it is administered to patients with inadequate coronary circulation. Water retention and occasionally water intoxication have been known to occur. The patient with diabetes insipidus will probably have to take the drug the remainder of his life. Large doses may cause intestinal and uterine cramps.

PARATHYROID HORMONE

Lying just above the thyroid, or, in some animals, embodied in it, are a variable number of bean-shaped glands (two pairs in man) known as the parathyroids. The primary function of the parathyroids is the maintenance of adequate levels of calcium in the extracellular fluid. The most significant function of parathyroid hormone is mobilization of calcium from bone. It also reduces phosphate concentration, permitting more calcium to be mobilized. Hypoparathyroidism leads to manifestations of hypocalcemia and tet-

any, the symptoms of which include muscle spasms, convulsions, gradual paralysis with dyspnea, and death from exhaustion. Before death gastrointestinal hemorrhages and hematemesis frequently occur. At death the intestinal mucosa is congested and the calcium content of the heart, kidney, and other tissues is increased.

The symptoms of tetany are relieved by administration of calcium salts. It is usually necessary to administer calcium salts intravenously for rapid relief. Large doses of vitamin D are also useful to relieve tetany and to restore the normal level of calcium in the blood. The patient is hospitalized because a frequent check on the blood calcium and phosphate levels is essential. Although parathyroid injection, U.S.P. was formerly used to treat tetany, its use is now considered to be obsolete.

THYROID HORMONES AND DRUGS

The thyroid gland secretes thyroxin and other closely related hormones that are essential for proper regulation of metabolism. The thyroid gland is one of the most richly vascularized tissues in the body; only the lungs and carotid body have a greater blood supply. Blood flow to the thyroid is normally about 5 ml. per minute per gram, while that for the kidney is about 3 ml. per minute per gram. Blood flow may increase to as much as 1 liter per minute with extreme stimulation. Blood is supplied to the thyroid via the superior and inferior thyroid arteries, which arise from the external carotids and subclavian arteries. Venous drainage is via superior and middle thyroid veins into the internal jugular veins and via the inferior thyroid vein into the innominate veins. The thyroid also has a rich lymphatic system, which may also serve to distribute hormone to the general circulation. Both sympathetic and parasympathetic fibers from the cervical sympathetic ganglia and the vagus nerve innervate the thyroid gland.

Three hormones are known to be produced by the thyroid gland: thyroxine, triiodothyronine, and thyrocalcitonin. Thyrocalcitonin helps to regulate calcium metabolism (see p. 421).

Thyroxine (tetraiodothyronine) and triiodothyronine contain four and three atoms of iodine, respectively, and because of this are abbreviated as T_4 and T_3. Thyroxine was isolated by Kendall on Christmas day in 1914. He erroneously thought the hormone was an iodinated oxyindole and proposed the name "thyroxin" for "thyroid oxyindole." The correct structure was identified by Harrington and Barger in 1929, which then permitted them to synthesize thyroxine. Although the name thyroxine is incorrect for identifying the structural formula, it has been retained. Kendall later won the Nobel Prize for his work on adrenal hormones. The large amount of iodine in thyroid hormones and the availability of radioactive iodine has led to farily detailed knowledge about thyroid physiology and its role in metabolism.

Thyroxine (tetraiodothyronine)

Liothyronine (triiodothyronine)

BIOSYNTHESIS OF THYROID HORMONES

Iodine is essential for thyroid hormone synthesis. About 1 mg. of iodine per week is required, most of which is ingested in food, water, and iodized table salt. About two thirds of the iodine ingested is excreted into the urine with the remaining one third being taken up by the thyroid gland for hormone synthesis. This process is aided by the "iodide pump," which takes up the iodide from the extracellular fluid, traps it, and concentrates it to many times that found in plasma. The ratio of iodide in the thyroid gland to that in the serum is expressed as the T/S ratio; normally this ratio is 25:1. In

hypoactivity the ratio may be 10:1; in hyperactivity it may be as great as 250:1.

Thyroglobulin is synthesized first. It contains thyrosine, an amino acid which reacts with iodine to form thyroid hormones. The thyroglobulin–thyroid hormone complex is stored in the follicles of the thyroid gland and is termed "colloid"; about 30% of the thyroid mass is stored thyroglobulin, which contains enough thyroid hormone to meet normal requirements for 2 to 3 months without any further synthesis.

Normally, thyroglobulin is not released into the circulation but undergoes proteolytic digestion, which releases the thyroid hormones T_3 and T_4. Hormone synthesis—iodine trapping, iodination and proteolysis of thyroglobulin, and hormone release—is controlled by the thyroid-stimulating hormone (TSH) from the anterior pituitary.

About 95% of the hormone in plasma is thyroxine; the remainder is triiodothyronine. In the plasma, about 99% of the hormones are bound to proteins and may be expressed as iodide; thus the term protein-bound iodine (PBI). Normal PBI is 4 to 8 mg./100 ml. of plasma. T_4 is bound more firmly than T_3; this permits a more rapid entry of T_3 into the cells.

Thyroid hormones are primarily metabolized in the liver, excreted into the bile and then into the intestine. The hormone can be reabsorbed from the intestine; that which is not is excreted in the feces. Metabolism of thyroid hormone can also occur in the kidneys and to a small extent in other tissues.

PHYSIOLOGIC EFFECTS OF THYROID HORMONES

The precise physiologic role of the thyroid hormones is not yet known, although a number of hormonal actions have been identified and studied. Three generalizations can be made about thyroid hormones:

1 They have a diffuse effect and do not seem to have any discrete target organ effect; no special cells or tissues appear to be particularly affected by the thyroid hormones.
2 Their long delay in onset of action and their prolonged action rule them out as minute-to-minute regulators of physiologic function. Instead, their

role is more likely to be that of establishing and maintaining long-term functions such as growth, maturation, and adaptation.

3 They are not necessary for survival, although quality of life is affected.

Thyroxine and triiodothyronine appear to have the same physiologic actions, although T_3 is far more potent than T_4. Their primary action is to increase the metabolic rate.

Thyroid hormones have the following physiologic effects:

1 *Growth and maturation.* A normal, functioning thyroid is essential for normal growth. The hormones must be present in the right amounts for growth to occur at the normal rate. In children who are hypothyroid, rate of growth is retarded, which may lead to shortness of stature. Conversely, children who are hyperthyroid may have excessive skeletal growth and become taller than they otherwise would. However, if there is premature closing of the epiphyses because of accelerated bone maturation, stunting of growth results. In the adult, excess thyroid hormone causes increased demineralization of bone and increased loss of calcium and phosphate.

2 *Central nervous system function.* At time of birth through the first year of life thyroid hormone must be present for normal development of the cerebrum; if the hormone is not present, irreversible mental retardation occurs. In the adult, hypothyroidism causes listlessness, a general dulling of mental capacity, decreased sensory capacity, slow speech, impaired memory, and somnolence. Hyperthyroidism in the adult results in hyperexcitability, irritability, restlessness, exaggerated responses to environmental stimuli, and emotional instability. Psychosis can occur in either hypo- or hyperthyroidism.

3 *Basal metabolic rate.* Thyroid hormones increase oxygen consumption in most cells of the body with the exception of the lungs, spleen, gastric smooth muscle, the gonads, and accessory sex organs. In hypothyroidism the basal metabolic rate is subnormal; in hyperthyroidism it may be 40% to 60% above normal.

4 *Carbohydrate and lipid metabolism.* Thyroid hormones accelerate glucose catabolism, increase cholesterol synthesis, and enhance the liver's ability to excrete cholesterol in the bile. Since the effect on cholesterol excretion is greater than that on cholesterol synthesis, the result is a decrease in plasma cholesterol level. The hormones also stimulate the mobilization of fatty acids from adipose tissue. The hypothyroid individual will have an elevated serum cholesterol level and increased blood levels of phospholipids and triglycerides.

5 *Protein metabolism.* Thyroid hormones are essential for the development of protein mass. In hypothyroidism both the synthesis and breakdown of protein are diminished, but the effect on protein synthesis is more profound. In addition, there is deposition of mucoproteins in subcutaneous spaces, which osmotically attracts water causing "puffiness." In hyperthyroidism there is increased catabolism of protein, or breakdown of muscle mass, and increased nitrogen excretion.

6 *Gastrointestinal function.* Thyroid hormones increase gastrointestinal motility, absorption of food, and secretion of digestive juices. Hypothyroidism decreases both intestinal absorption and secretion of pancreatic enzymes. Constipation may also occur.

7 *Water and electrolyte balance.* In thyroid hormone deficiency water and electrolytes accumulate in subcutaneous spaces; administering a thyroid hormone results in diuresis and a loss of fluid and electrolytes from the subcutaneous spaces.

8 *Cardiovascular function.* Since the thyroid hormones increase metabolism, there is increased need in the tissues for oxygen and nutrients and this in turn necessitates increased blood flow. In hyperthyroidism these effects bring about increased cardiac output, increased pulse pressure, and tachycardia. If these effects are prolonged, cardiac hypertrophy, and even high-output myocardial failure, may occur. Opposite effects occur in hypothyroidism.

9 *Muscle function.* Moderate increases in thyroid hormone makes muscle react with vigor; large increases result in muscle weakness because of excess protein catabolism. A characteristic sign of hyperthyroidism is a fine muscle tremor. Hypothyroidism causes the muscles to be sluggish.

10 *Temperature regulation.* Thyroid hormones must be present for an increase in heat production or a decrease in heat loss to occur. Although the hormones do not initiate the physiologic response to cold, they appear to magnify the body's response to catecholamine effects, which innervate the sympathetic system during cold exposure. In hypothyroidism there is decreased tolerance to cold.

11 *Lactation.* Thyroid hormone is necessary for normal milk production; without it, fat content of

milk and total milk production are greatly reduced.

12 *Reproduction.* Thyroid hormone is required for normal rhythmicity in the reproductive cycle.

REGULATION OF THYROID HORMONE SECRETION

Recently, a hypothalamic hormone known as "thyroid-releasing hormone" (TRH) was isolated and synthesized. It is believed that TRH has an effect on the pituitary gland and, when released, stimulates the pituitary to release the thyroid-stimulating hormone (TSH), which in turn stimulates the thyroid to release its hormones T_3 and T_4.

IODINE DEFICIENCY AND ITS EFFECT ON THE THYROID GLAND

The synthesis of the thyroid hormones and their maintenance in the blood in adequate amounts depend in large part upon an adequate intake of iodine. Iodine ingested by way of food or water is changed into iodide and is stored in the thyroid gland before reaching the circulation. Prolonged iodine deficiency in the diet results in an enlargement of the thyroid gland, known as a simple goiter. When thyroid hormones fail to be synthesized because of a lack of iodine, the anterior lobe of the pituitary is stimulated to increase the secretion of thyrotropic hormone, which in turn causes hypertrophy and hyperplasia of the gland. The enlarged thyroid then mobilizes to remove residual traces of iodine from the blood. This type of goiter (simple or nontoxic) can be prevented by providing an adequate supply of iodine for the young. Iodine is not abundant in most dietary items except fish and seafoods, and iodized salt is frequently the primary resource for iodine in areas where seafood is expensive or not readily available.

HYPOTHYROID STATES

Cretinism. Hypothyroidism in the young child is known as cretinism and is characterized by cessation of physical and mental development, which leads to dwarfism and idiocy. Patients with cretinism usually have thick, coarse skin, a thick tongue, gaping mouth, protruding abdomen, thick, short legs, poorly developed hands and feet, and weak musculature. This condition may result from faulty development or atrophy of the thyroid gland during fetal life. Failure of development of the gland may be caused by lack of iodine in the mother.

Myxedema (Gull's disease). Hypothyroidism in the adult is called myxedema. Its development is usually insidious and causes a gradual retardation of physical and mental functions. There is a gradual infiltration of the skin and loss of facial lines and facial expression. The formation of a subcutaneous connective tissue causes the hands and face to appear puffy and swollen. The basal metabolic rate becomes subnormal, the hair becomes scanty and coarse, movements become sluggish, and the patient becomes hypersensitive to cold.

THYROID PREPARATIONS

There is agreement that hypothyroid patients need thyroid replacement therapy. However, considerable controversy has developed over which preparation is the best for substitution therapy. For many years desiccated thyroid served admirably for replacement therapy, and it is still considered to be satisfactory for many patients. A major problem with desiccated thyroid is variation in potency resulting from differences in glands from which it is obtained, variability of preparation, and variability in the rate at which it loses its potency. There is no requirement for metabolic potency, and preparations may not contain enough metabolically active substance to produce desired therapeutic effects even though the drug meets U.S.P. requirements. This has led to the present lack of popularity for desiccated thyroid.

Another factor contributing to the thyroid replacement controversy is the recent availability of synthetic thyroid preparations, such as levothyroxine (Synthroid), liothyronine (Cytomel), and combinations of these two drugs (Liotrix, Euthroid). These are chemically pure preparations. The question as to which preparation is superior has not yet been answered.

Treatment of the patient with hypothyroidism or myxedema is aimed at eliminating his symptoms and restoring him to a normal mental and physical state. Clinical response is more important than blood hormone level. However, laboratory assessments of T_3, T_4, and serum cholesterol and TSH levels are used as criteria for adequacy of therapy.

In children, normal skeletal growth is used as evidence of adequate therapy; an increase in serum alkaline phosphatase indicates that growth will occur. In cretinism, thyroid hormone levels equal to or above those required for the adult must be quickly established (right after birth) to prevent permanent mental and physical retardation. Treatment of the older cretin will not reverse the mental retardation that has already occurred.

Hypothyroid patients need to be informed of their life-long need for replacement therapy. Since hypothyroid individuals respond rapidly to replacement doses, therapy begins with a small dose, which is gradually increased over a period of several weeks until optimal clinical response is obtained. The dose required to maintain this response (maintenance dose) is then taken or given daily.

Other uses. Thyroid hormone is also used to treat nontoxic or nodular goiter. Therapy is aimed at decreasing the goiter or nodules by giving sufficient thyroid hormone to prevent pituitary TSH secretion. In chronic lymphocytic thyroiditis, thyroid hormones are used as replacement therapy and to suppress TSH secretion.

Thyroid may be used to lower serum cholesterol levels in euthyroid (normal thyroid) persons. However, the increased metabolic activity may cause attacks of angina pectoris or congestive heart failure in patients with cardiac disease or hypertension.

Thyroid preparations have been used extensively in the treatment of obesity. This is not an approved use, since (1) most obesity is not due to hypothyroidism but to overeating, and (2) a state of hyperthyroidism must be induced to achieve weight loss. Thyroid hormone should be regarded as a potent drug and should never be used indiscriminately.

Sterility and habitual abortion resulting from hypothyroidism are sometimes successfully treated with thyroid hormone. However, there is no evidence that thyroid hormone is effective in treating most abnormalities of reproductive function.

Side effects and toxic effects. The symptoms of overdosage are, in general, those of hyperthyroidism: palpitation, tachycardia, pain over the heart, dyspnea, nervousness, insomnia, tremor, hyperglycemia, sweating, and loss of weight.

It should be remembered that symptoms come on slowly and may last a long time. It is best, therefore, that a small dose be used at first and the patient be watched closely. One of the first symptoms of overdosage that the nurse may have occasion to note is an increase in the pulse rate. The pulse should always be counted before the next dose of the drug is given. In some hospitals it is the rule to withhold the drug if the pulse rate has reached 100 beats per minute. For younger children the pulse rate may be higher, yet within the range of safety. The rate will vary with the age of the child. In mild cases withdrawal of the drug will result in return to the normal metabolic level. In severe cases it is important to allow the patient to rest in a comfortable position. A sedative also may be indicated.

Thyroid, U.S.P., B.P.

Thyroid is a yellowish powder obtained from the thyroid glands of domesticated animals used for food by man. Thyroid is available in tablets containing 15, 30, 60, 125, 200, 250, or 300 mg. each for oral administration. After administration there is a lag of 24 to 36 hours before effects are manifested. The usual oral dose is 60 to 100 mg. daily, although the dose must be determined by the response desired and the needs of the patient. Range of dosage for 1 day may be 15 to 180 mg. or more. Initial dose for children is 30 mg. or less daily, which is increased by 15 to 30 mg. at 1- to 3-week intervals to a total of 60 mg. daily. Dose may then be increased by 30 to 60 mg. at 1- to 3-week intervals until the desired clinical response is maintained. This is the cheapest preparation of thyroid.

Levothyroxine sodium, U.S.P. (Synthroid, Letter, Titroid); thyroxine sodium, B.P.

This is the sodium salt of the levo isomer of thyroxine. It is given orally. Usual doses range from 100 to 400 μg. daily. Dose for children is quite variable, but it may be 6 μg. per kilogram of body weight daily. This may be increased gradually to 100 μg. daily. Increase in dosage is made on the basis of patient's response. Official tablets are available containing 25, 50, 100, 150, 200, 300, or 500 μg.

It is contraindicated in patients with heart disease, especially coronary insufficiency.

It enhances the effect of oral anticoagulants.

Liothyronine sodium, U.S.P., B.P. (Cytomel)

This is the active isomer of triiodothyronine. It exhibits a rapid onset of action, but after administration is stopped the duration of effect is correspondingly brief. From 5 to 100 μg. is given daily for adults being treated for hypothyroid states. Some patients will require higher dosage levels. Initial dose for children is 5 μg. daily, which is increased by 5 μg. at weekly intervals to a total daily dose of 25 μg.; further increase depends on the patient's response. It is available in 5-, 25-, and 50-μg. tablets for oral administration.

Liothyronine is more potent than desiccated thyroid and has a more rapid onset of action. It is about four times more costly than thyroid. It is used intravenously to treat myxedema coma because of its rapid onset and short duration of action. Powder for injection can be obtained from the manufacturer upon request. D.E.S.I. rating is *effective* in conditions resulting from inadequate thyroid hormone production.

Thyroglobulin, N.F. (Proloid)

Thyroglobulin is obtained from a purified extract of hog thyroid. It contains thyroxine and triiodothyronine in peptide linkage. Its potency is equal to that of thyroid, but it is twice as costly. Dosage should be started in small amounts and increased gradually. Oral maintenance dose is 30 to 180 mg. daily. It is available in oral tablets containing 15, 30, 60, 100, 120, 200, or 300 mg. D.E.S.I. rating is *effective* for treatment of inadequate thyroid hormone production.

Liotrix (Euthroid, Thyrolar)

Liotrix is a synthetic mixture of levothyroxine and liothyronine in a ratio of 4:1, respectively. This combination is preferred by some endocrinologists because of the standardized content of the two hormones, which produces more consistent laboratory test results that are more in agreement with the patient's clinical response.

Liotrix is given orally, usually as a single daily dose before breakfast. The two commercially available liotrix preparations contain different amounts of each ingredient, and patients on one brand should not be changed to the other brand before considering the differences in potency. Dosage range is 60 to 180 μg. of levothyroxine and 15 to 45 μg. of liothyronine.

HYPERTHYROID STATES (THYROTOXICOSIS) AND ANTITHYROID DRUGS

Excessive formation of the thyroid hormones and their escape into the circulation result in a state of toxicity called thyrotoxicosis. This occurs in the condition known as exophthalmic goiter (Graves' disease) or in some forms of adenomatous goiters.

Hyperthyroidism leads to symptoms quite different from those seen in myxedema. The metabolic rate is increased, sometimes as much as a plus 60 or more. The body temperature frequently is above normal, the pulse rate is fast, and the patient complains of feeling too warm. Other symptoms include restlessness, anxiety, emotional instability, muscle tremor and weakness, sweating, and exophthalmos.

Prior to the advent of antithyroid drugs treatment was more or less limited to a subtotal resection of the hyperactive gland. Since these patients usually are poor operative risks, they may be hospitalized for a time and prepared for surgery by giving them as much mental and physical rest as possible, a diet particularly rich in carbohydrate, vitamins, and iodine. Thyroidectomy is indicated when the pulse has been slowed and the basal metabolic rate lowered to a somewhat stationary level. Antithyroid drugs provide less rapid control of hyperthyroidism than do surgical measures. Radioactive iodine is one of the more effective antithyroid drugs.

An antithyroid drug is regarded as a chemical agent that lowers the basal metabolic rate by interfering with the formation, release, or action of the hormones made by the thyroid gland.

Those that interfere with the synthesis of the thyroid hormones are known as goitrogens. A wide variety of compounds might be included in this category of antithyroid drugs, but only iodine (iodide ion), radioactive iodine, and certain derivatives of thiouracil will be included.

Iodine; iodide

Iodine that has pharmacologic or biochemical significance is either inorganic iodine (iodine ion) or iodine that is bound in an organic compound such as thyroxine. There is thought to be little in common between the physiologic effects of elemental iodine (the iodide ion) and organic compounds that contain iodine in their structure. Confusion seems to have arisen from the incorrect or loose usage of the word *iodine.*

When elemental iodine is administered locally, a certain proportion of it is converted to iodide and is absorbed. This brings about general systemic effects of iodide. Lugol's Solution contains elemental iodine, but it is changed into iodide before absorption. As a result, significant amounts of iodide reach the bloodstream and are effective in the treatment of toxic goiter.

Action and result. Iodide is the oldest of the antithyroid drugs. The response of the thyrotoxic patient frequently is remarkable. The metabolic rate falls at about the same rate as after surgical removal of the gland and many of the symptoms of hyperthyroidism are relieved. Maximum effects usually are attained after 10 to 15 days of continuous administration of iodide. Enlargement of the gland and hyperplasia are reduced, and the gland rapidly stores colloid, which contains highly potent thyroid hormone. During the time when the metabolic rate is somewhere near the normal range, the surgeon may be able to operate upon a patient who is nearly normal instead of on a very sick individual.

The mechanism by which iodide accomplishes its beneficial effect is not fully understood. It probably inhibits the organic binding of iodine and the degradation of thyroglobulin. Unfortunately, the beneficial effects from iodine therapy are not prolonged indefinitely. In a few weeks the symptoms are likely to reappear and may be intensified. The thyroid gland has been filled with active hormone that, when released, may plunge the patient into a critical state. Thus patients cannot be maintained on iodine solution therapy.

Uses. The chief use of iodide in the treatment of thyrotoxicosis is in preparation of the patient for thyroidectomy. Patient with severe hyperthyroidism are frequently prepared first with propylthiouracil or a related compound, and during the last part of the treatment iodide is given to prevent the development of a friable, highly vascular gland, which would increase the hazards of surgery. A certain number of patients, however, may be controlled and prepared for surgery with iodide alone. It is also used to treat "thyroid crisis."

Preparation, dosage, and administration. Convenient preparations are Lugol's Solution and saturated solutions of sodium or potassium iodide; 0.3 ml. (0.1 to 1 ml.) of these preparations can be given orally three times a day after meals for 2 or 3 weeks prior to operation. They should be well diluted in one-third to one-half glass of milk or another vehicle that may be preferred by the patient.

Strong iodine solution, U.S.P. (Compound Iodine Solution, Lugol's Solution); *aqueous iodine solution,* B.P. This preparation contains 5% iodine and 10% potassium iodide.

Sodium iodide, U.S.P., B.P. Sodium iodide may be given for severe thyroid crisis; the intravenous route is usually used and the range of dose is 1 to 3 Gm. daily. This drug may be given as an expectorant; dosage ranges from 300 mg. to 2 Gm. daily.

Potassium iodide solution, U.S.P.: *potassium iodide,* B.P. (Saturated Potassium Iodide Solution). Nurses may see this preparation ordered as SSKI, which means "Saturated Solution of Potassium Iodide." It is available in 300-mg. enteric coated tablets and as a liquid, 500 mg. per 15 ml., and in unit-dose patient cups of 15 ml. Daily dosage is usually 500 mg. The liquid is usually administered diluted with fruit juice, water, or milk. Since the medication evaporates rapidly, it should not stand open to air for long periods before administration.

Disadvantages of iodine therapy. It has been recommended that iodine solution be used only after very careful consideration because of the following disadvantages:

1 A patient who has received iodine solution cannot be treated immediately with radioactive iodine, since the gland is saturated with iodide and, therefore, will have no affinity for radioactive iodine.
2 Stopping the iodine solution and giving radioactive iodine later may induce an exacerbation of hyperthyroidism. Since iodide causes the gland to store its hormone, destroying the gland by radiation releases the hormone into the circulation, and this may produce severe thyrotoxicosis.
3 Giving iodine solution first and propylthiouracil or another antithyroid drug later may also result in an exacerbation of hyperthyroidism.

Radioactive iodine

Iodine 131 is a radioactive isotope of iodine. It is the most commonly used drug for treating hyperthyroidism. It has a half-life of 8.08 days, which means that at the end of about 8 days 50% of its atoms have undergone disintegration and in another 8 days 50% of the remaining amount has disappeared, and so on until an inappreciable amount remains. The radioactivity of this material is therefore dissipated in a relatively short time. The energy liberated during the period of radioactivity is in the form of beta particles and gamma rays. This radiation brings about the same tissue changes as are secured from radium emanations or from roentgen rays.

Radioiodine is absorbed rapidly from the stomach, and most of the dose is in the blood within the first hour. The cells of the thyroid gland have an unusual affinity for iodine and will concentrate the element to a marked degree. Radioiodine is useful because it may be located even when present in extraordinarily small amounts. Radioiodine behaves exactly as does ordinary nonradioactive iodine; hence, an infinitesimal quantity of it can be used to trace or follow the behavior of any amount of ordinary iodine with which it is mixed. Such tiny doses, appropriately called "tracers," when given to a patient are used to tag all of the ordinary iodine in the patient's body and to permit the observers to trace the behavior of the radioiodine. It has become a useful tool with which to study problems of physiology and disease of the thyroid gland. It is also of value in diagnosing functional states of the thyroid gland and in treating se-

lected cases of cancer of the thyroid gland. Some physicians believe that radioiodine is most effective as a therapeutic agent when used in treatment of patients more than 50 years of age, those who have severe complicating disease, those who have recurrent hyperthyroidism after previous resection of the thyroid, and those who have extremely small glands.

After the oral ingestion of a tracer dose of iodine 131, the following determinations are made: (1) the rate and amount of urinary excretion, (2) the rate and amount of uptake of the radioiodine by the gland, and (3) the rate and degree of incorporation of the radioiodine into the hormonal iodine of the blood. These determinations can be of value because they can be used to help differentiate the patient with a normally functioning thyroid gland from the one with hyperthyroidism or hypothyroidism.

Because radioiodine can be taken by mouth and is collected and concentrated by the thyroid tissue, a much greater degree of irradiation can be secured than is possible with radium or roentgen rays. With the latter there is danger of damaging normal tissue, particularly the skin, when large doses are used. The theoretical danger of radiation injury has limited treatment with radioiodine largely to older patients (beyond the child-bearing period) and to those who are considered poor surgical risks. For the latter type of patient this treatment is thought to be superior to the use of other antithyroid drugs. The chief disadvantage of use of radioiodine is that it may promote the formation of carcinoma or leukemia. At present this is thought possible but unlikely.

When cancer is present in the thyroid gland, the tissue exhibits a variable degree of capacity to collect iodine, depending on the degree of function of the tissue in the tumor. Therefore, the possibility of treating cancer of the thyroid gland with radioiodine appears to be somewhat limited. Metastasis from a malignant tumor of the thyroid gland sometimes can be traced with the use of the Geiger-Müller counter and definite locations of metastatic lesions found. Prolonged treatment with radioiodine may arrest metastatic spread.

D.E.S.I. rating is *effective* for treatment of

hyperthyroidism and thyroid carcinoma, and for diagnosis of thyroid function.

Preparation, dosage, and administration. The following are available radioiodine preparations.

Sodium iodide I¹³¹ solution, U.S.P., B.P. This is a solution containing iodine 131 suitable for either oral or intravenous administration. Tracer doses range from 1 to 100 microcuries (μc.); therapeutic doses range from 1 to 200 millicuries (mc.). When diagnostic tracer tests are done for evaluation of thyroid function, 1 to 100 μc. of iodine 131 given along with 100 μg. of nonradioactive sodium iodide as a recommended dosage. This may be given in the morning before breakfast. The test will be invalidated, however, if the patient has been receiving thiouracil or iodine in any form during the preceding week or potassium thiocyanate during the preceding month. Therapeutic dosage is determined by the size of the gland, the severity of the condition being treated, and the results of the preliminary study of the excretion of tracer amounts or the percentage of the tracer dose observed in the thyroid gland.

Sodium iodide I¹³¹ capsules, U.S.P. These are gelatin capsules that contain a radioactive isotope of iodine.

Precautions. Although administration of this substance is in one sense very simple, since it can be added to water and given to the patient to swallow as he would a drink of water (for it has no color or taste), the radiation from this substance is dangerous in the same way and to the same extent as are the effects from radium and roentgen rays. It follows that exposure to radioiodine, like exposure to radium or roentgen rays, should be avoided or minimized as much as possible. Special precautions must be observed, because the drug is frequently in a form that can be spilled on persons or property. The contamination that results from spilling a dose of radioiodine or the urine or other excreta from patients who have received the radioactive substance means that surroundings must be checked and measured with special monitoring instruments, usually by small portable Geiger counters. Nurses and technicians should wear rubber gloves whenever giving radioiodine

to patients and during the disposal of their excreta.

Side effects and toxic effects. Radioactive iodine can induce several temporary but potentially serious reactions during the first few days or weeks after therapy. Radioactive thyroiditis may occur causing soreness over the thyroid area. Although incidence of recurrence of hyperthyroidism is low after treatment with radioactive iodine, it may occur and be particularly hazardous in the patient with severe thyrotoxic heart disease. Occasionally, an acute swelling of the thyroid gland can occur; in patients with huge goiters asphyxiation is a possibility.

Follow-up studies on patients who received radioactive iodine reveal that many of them developed hypothyroidism requiring replacement therapy from the first year of treatment to as long as 10 years later (the duration of the study). Thus, long-term follow-up is needed to avoid the injurious effects of unrecognized and untreated hypothyroidism.

Radioactive iodine should not be given to pregnant women or nursing mothers.

Propylthiouracil and related compounds

Propylthiouracil

Propylthiouracil and related compounds interfere with the synthesis of the hormone produced by the thyroid gland. As a result the gland is depleted of hormone, less hormone reaches the tissues of the body, and the rate of metabolism is lowered. Because of the creation of a thyroid hormone deficiency, the thyrotropic hormone made by the anterior lobe of the pituitary gland is increased, and hyperplasia of the thyroid gland occurs. The inhibition of hormone synthesis is sufficiently effective to make these compounds useful in bringing about relief of symptoms of hyperthyroidism. The exact manner in which these drugs prevent synthesis of the thyroid hormone is not known, but it may be by preventing the iodination of tyrosine. However, after administration of these compounds is stopped, the thyroid gland rapidly regains its ability to synthesize the hormone as well as to store colloid, which contains thyroxin.

Propylthiouracil and related compounds are used chiefly to control the signs and symptoms of hyperthyroidism in Graves' disease and in toxic nodular goiter and to prepare the patient who must undergo surgery of the thyroid gland. It is true that the gland is made more friable and vascular with their use, but this is overcome with the simultaneous administration of iodide 10 to 15 days prior to the operation.

Propylthiouracil does not interfere with the action of thyroid hormone previously formed and stored in the gland. Because its effects do not appear until this supply of hormone has been used up, it may take several days or weeks before signs of decreased thyroid activity are noted. Patients with severe hyperthyroidism dissipate their stored hormone more rapidly than those with mild hyperthyroidism and thus may respond to therapy more quickly. Duration of treatment necessary to obtain a prolonged remission varies from 6 months to 3 years, with 1 year being the average. It has been reported that prolonged remission occurs in about 50% of patients on long-term antithyroid therapy. If gland enlargement does not stabilize or decrease during therapy, the possibility for prolonged remission is considered to be poor.

Propylthiouracil does not have a permanent effect on the thyroid gland, but it is hoped that long-term antithyroid therapy will foster a spontaneous remission of the disease. D.E.S.I. rating is *effective* for treatment of hyperthyroidism, and for preparation of patients undergoing subtotal thyroidectomy or radioactive iodine therapy.

Preparation, dosage, and administration. Propylthiouracil and related compounds are readily absorbed from the gastrointestinal tract and are administered by mouth only. Since all have the same mechanism of action, the choice depends on the incidence of side effects and on the duration of action. To ensure adequate and effective therapy these drugs should be administered at evenly spaced intervals during the day.

Maintenance doses are determined in accordance with the metabolic rate.

Methylthiouracil, N.F., B.P. (Methiacil, Muracil, Thimecil). This drug is marketed in 50-mg. tablets. The usual daily dose is 200 mg. given in divided doses. It may prove useful for patients who are refractory to other antithyroid drugs. It is slightly more potent and toxic than propylthiouracil. It is popular in Great Britain but not widely used in the United States.

Propylthiouracil, U.S.P., B.P. This preparation is similar to methylthiouracil and is marketed in 50-mg. tablets. The usual daily dose is 50 mg. every 8 hours. In severe hyperthyroidism, initial doses of 100 mg. every 8 hours may be required. In some instances much larger doses are given. Range of dose is 50 to 450 mg. Dose for children 10 years of age and older is 150 to 300 mg. daily in divided doses every 8 hours; maintenance dose is usually 100 mg. daily divided into two doses every 12 hours. For children ages 6 to 10 the dose initially is 50 to 150 mg. daily in divided doses every 8 hours.

Iothiouracil sodium (Itrumil). This drug is said to exert the combined effects of a thiouracil derivative and an iodide. It was developed to achieve gland change prior to surgery without need for additional iodide therapy. It is available in 50-mg. tablets. The usual daily dose is 150 to 200 mg. in divided doses.

Methimazole, U.S.P. (Tapazole). This is one of the most active of the thyroid-inhibiting drugs and its antithyroid activity is ten times stronger than that of propylthiouracil. It is marketed in 5- and 10-mg. tablets. Initial dose is 15 mg. for mild hyperthyroidism, 30 to 40 mg. for moderately severe hyperthyroidism, and 60 mg. or more for severe cases. These amounts are given in divided doses every 8 hours. Maintenance dose is 5 to 15 mg. daily. For children the dose initially is 0.4 mg. per kilogram of body weight divided into three doses; maintenance dose is one half the initial dose.

Methimazole

D.E.S.I. rating is *effective* for treatment of hyperthyroidism in preparation for subtotal thyroidectomy or radioactive iodine therapy.

Carbimazole, B.P. This compound is available in 5-mg. tablets. The maintenance dosage is 2.5 to 20 mg. daily given in divided doses. Claims have been made that this preparation causes less hyperplasia of the thyroid gland than certain of the other preparations of this group of drugs.

Side effects and toxic effects. Drugs of this group vary in their capacity to cause toxic reactions. Incidence of adverse effects is dose related; the higher the dose the greater the incidence of side effects and toxic effects. Thiouracil is most likely to cause toxic effects and has been discarded in favor of propylthiouracil and other less toxic substitutes. However, they are all capable of casuing serious untoward effects, which may include leukopenia, skin rash, drug fever, enlargement of the salivary glands and lymph nodes in the neck, hepatitis, loss of the sense of taste, and edema of the lower extremities. The most grave complication is agranulocytosis. Many of the aforementioned reactions necessitate discontinuing administration of the drug and giving appropriate supportive treatment. Patients should be instructed that if they develop sore throat, a head cold, fever, or malaise they should report the symptoms immediately to their physician, for these symptoms signal the onset of agranulocytosis. The nurse should be alert to note warning symptoms as well. The incidence of untoward reactions is said to be between 3% and 5%. The incidence of agranulocytosis is said to approach 0.5%. The need for close medical supervision of patients receiving these drugs is obvious.

Precautions. When given to pregnant women, the smallest effective dose should be used (less than 300 mg. daily). Since propylthiouracil crosses the placental barrier, large doses can lead to goiter in the newborn. Because the drug is excreted in breast milk, mothers who are on the drug should not nurse their babies.

Drug interactions. Propylthiouracil can cause prothrombin deficiency, thus increasing the effects of anticoagulants such as coumadin and warfarin. Dosage of anticoagulants should be reduced when the patient is also receiving propylthiouracil. Vitamin K can be administered to prevent bleeding.

HORMONES OF THE ADRENAL GLAND

The adrenal glands are located just above the kidneys and consist of two parts, the inner medulla and the outer cortex. Epinephrine, a secretion of the medullary portion, is discussed in Chapter 9. The secretion of the cells of the adrenal cortex is distinctly different from epinephrine. Adrenalectomized animals die within a few days unless they are given injections of adrenal cortex or adrenocortical hormones, whereas removal of the medullary portion of the gland does not necessarily result in death.

Adrenal corticosteroids

The first effective adrenocortical extracts were prepared between 1928 and 1930. During the 1930's there was intensive research to identify and isolate the active principles responsible for the life-sustaining role of the adrenal glands. In 1937, Reichstein prepared deoxycorticosterone synthetically and later demonstrated that it indeed was a substance normally found in the adrenal gland. In 1938, Kendall at the Mayo Clinic, isolated the glucocorticoids—a brilliant achievement, which won for him the Nobel Prize. The last physiologically important corticosteroid to be discovered was aldosterone in 1953. World War II spurred interest in the glucocorticoids, since it was suspected that they might be of great value in the treatment of shock. By 1948 several corticosteroids were available for clinical trials. Hench, also of the Mayo Clinic, made the dramatic discovery that patients severely crippled with rheumatoid arthritis, when treated with a corticosteroid, underwent a remission of the disease and could move joints that had been stiff for years. Later it was found that adrenocortical hormones could effect symptomatic improvement in a wide variety of disease conditions. In 1951, the first sensitive and relatively specific measurements of corticosteroid levels in blood were made.

Today all of the adrenocortical hormones are

commercially available as are synthetic analogues of even higher potency. The generic name for these hormones and analogues is *corticosteroids.*

During experimental and clinical investigation it was found that some corticosteroids, such as cortisol, had a profound effect on carbohydrate metabolism, while aldosterone primarily affected mineral (or electrolyte) and water metabolism. Consequently, the corticosteroids were divided into two classes, *glucocorticoids* and *mineralocorticoids.*

Biosynthesis of corticosteroids. Cholesterol is used for the biosynthesis of corticosteroids. Cholesterol is synthesized and stored in the adrenal cortex. The adrenal cortex also obtains cholesterol from the blood. This cholesterol may be from dietary sources or synthesized by the liver.

Synthesis of corticosteroids is dependent upon the adrenocorticotropic hormone (ACTH) secreted by the pituitary. The predominant action of ACTH on the adrenal cortex is synthesis of corticosteroids and secretion of glucocorticoids. The exact mechanism for these events is not known.

The release of ACTH by the pituitary is believed to be stimulated by the corticotropin-releasing hormone (CRH) from the hypothalamus, although CRH has not yet been chemically identified. There is some evidence that the corticosteroids can inhibit the adrenal glucocorticoid system by inhibiting the release of CRH from the hypothalamus and by inhibiting the release of ACTH from the pituitary.

GLUCOCORTICOIDS

Glucocorticoid rhythms. Two rhythms appear to influence glucocorticoid function—*circadian* (daily) rhythm and *ultradian* rhythm. Circadian rhythm appears to be entrained by the dark/light and sleep/wakefulness cycles. It has been found that normal subjects sleeping in the dark at night will begin to have an increase in their plasma cortisol levels in the early morning hours and reach a peak after they are awake. These levels then slowly fall to very low levels in the evening and during the early phase of sleep. The importance of this rhythm is emphasized by the finding that corticosteroid therapy is more potent when given at midnight than when given at noon. Given at midnight, corticosteroids suppress ACTH release for hours; given at noon the effect is relatively brief.

Ultradian rhythms are periodic or intermittent functions with frequencies higher than once every 24 hours. In man, from four to eight adrenal glucocorticoid bursts occur in each 24 hour period, which may follow bursts in CRH and ACTH releases. These bursts are clustered closer together and are more pronounced during the circadian rise in plasma glucocorticoid levels in the early hours of the morning than at other times when they may be so widely spaced that adrenal secretion is zero. Consequently, the adrenal cortex secretes glucocorticoids only about 25% of the time in unstressed individuals.

Cortisone; hydrocortisone

Cortisone was isolated from the adrenal gland in 1935 and for a time was known simply as Compound E. Hydrocortisone has been known as Compound F. The activity of these two adrenal steroids is similar, although hydrocortisone is more potent in its physiologic and antirheumatic effects and is less irritating to synovial membranes when injected into joint cavities. However, it is less soluble in body fluids than cortisone; hence, it is less suited to intramuscular injection.

Sources. Cortisone and hydrocortisone are white, crystalline odorless powders that are produced synthetically. Cortisone is used in medicine in the form of the acetate ester; the ester enhances stability and may prolong pharmacologic activity. Hydrocortisone differs from cortisone by having the ketone group at carbon 11 reduced to an alcohol group, thereby adding two atoms of hydrogen, hence the name hydrocortisone. Cortisol, however, is a more logical name for hydrocortisone.

Action and result. Cortisone and hydrocortisone affect carbohydrate, protein, and fat metabolism. Large doses over a period of time produce an increased excretion of potassium and retention of sodium. The patient, therefore, must be watched closely to prevent imbalance of electrolytes. Therapeutic doses of cortisone and hydrocortisone depress the function of cells in the adrenal cortex as well as cells of the anterior lobe of the pituitary gland, which produce corticotropin. If administration is prolonged and large amounts of these hormones are given, atrophy of the adrenal cortex will develop. The gland usually recovers, but it must be kept in mind that permanent damage is always a possibility.

Administration of the hormones should be withdrawn gradually rather than abruptly, for while termination of their use does not necessarily bring about symptoms of acute adrenal insufficiency, patients are known to experience muscular weakness, lethargy, and exhaustion after administration has been discontinued. Such symptoms are interpreted to mean that there is depression of cortical function.

Most patients respond to these medications with an elevated mood, which is a result of remission of symptoms or a direct result of central nervous system effects. However, neurosis and psychosis have been noted in patients with Cushing's syndrome.

Both cortisone and hydrocortisone are potent substances that exert widespread physiologic as well as pharmacologic effects in the human body. There is evidence that some of the effects are therapeutically beneficial, others are of no apparent therapeutic significance, and still others are likely to be hazardous to the patient. Although the exact mode of action is unknown, Hench and his associates were of the opinion that in diseases influenced by cortisone and corticotropin, these hormones act as buffer substances against the known or unknown irritant to which the tissues of the body are reacting. These hormones do not remove the cause of the disease or repair damaged tissues.

In other words, cortisone and the closely related hydrocortisone permit the patient to have certain diseases without having the characteristic symptoms. In spite of the fact that they do not cure the disease, glucocorticoids bring about relief of symptoms in many patients, and in addition they have provided a remarkable research tool for medical science.

Specifically, the glucocorticoids have the following actions:

1 *Antiinflammatory action.* Glucocorticoids can stabilize lysosomal membranes and thus inhibit release of proteolytic enzymes during inflammation. They can also potentiate vasoconstrictor effects.

2 *Maintenance of normal blood pressure.* Glucocorticoids potentiate the vasoconstrictor action of norepinephrine. When glucocorticoids are absent, the vasoconstricting action of the catecholamines is diminished and blood pressure falls. It has recently been found that glucocorticoids inhibit the enzyme catecholamine-O-methyltransferase (COMT), which inactivates the catecholamines. When this enzyme is not inhibited the catecholamines are rapidly metabolized.

3 *Carbohydrate and protein metabolism.* Glucocorticoids help to maintain blood sugar and liver and muscle glycogen content. They facilitate breakdown of protein in muscle and extrahepatic tissues, which leads to increased plasma amino acid levels. Glucocorticoids increase the trapping of amino acids by the liver and stimulate the deamination of amino acids. In addition, they increase the activity of enzymes important to gluconeogenesis and inhibit glycolytic enzymes. This can produce hyperglycemia and glycosuria. These effects can aggravate diabetes, bring on latent diabetes, and cause insulin resistance. Inhibition of protein synthesis can delay wound healing, cause muscle wasting and osteoporosis, and in the young can inhibit growth.

4 *Fat metabolism.* Glucocorticoids promote mobilization of fatty acids from adipose tissue. This increases the concentration of fatty acids in the plasma and their utilization for energy. In spite of this effect, patients on glucocorticoids may accumulate fat stores (rounded face, buffalo hump). The effect of glucocorticoids on fat metabolism is complex and little is known about it.

5 *Thymolytic, lympholytic, and eosinopenic actions.* Glucocorticoids can cause atrophy of the thymus and decrease the number of lymphocytes, plasma cells, and eosinophils in blood. In addition, they decrease the rate of conversion of lymphocytes into antibodies. These effects can ultimately interfere with the immune and allergic responses. This in turn, along with their antiinflammatory action, makes them useful *immunosuppressants* for delaying rejection in patients with organ or tissue transplants, and useful *antiallergenics* for the treatment of acute allergic reactions such as urticaria, bronchial asthma, and anaphylactic shock. However, steroids can be a source of danger in infections by limiting useful protective inflammation. These hormones also inhibit activity of the lymphatic system, causing lymphopenia and reduction in size of enlarged lymph nodes.

6 *Stress effects.* During stress situations (fight or flight

phenomena) an acute release of corticosteroids occurs, which is believed to be a protective mechanism. The corticosteroids support blood pressure and increase blood sugar to provide energy for emergency physiologic actions (e.g., running). Patients with decreased adrenal function require increased amounts of steroids during stress periods such as surgery; without steroid administration, hypotension and shock tend to occur.

During stress, epinephrine and norepinephrine are also released from the adrenal medulla, and these catecholamines have a synergistic action with the corticosteroids. However, controversy exists about the physiologic usefulness of the steroids during stress.

Desoxycorticosterone

Hydrocortisone

Cortisone

Aldosterone

Uses. Cortisone and hydrocortisone are indicated chiefly for replacement therapy in conditions of adrenal insufficiency, such as may be found after adrenalectomy, in Addison's disease, and hypopituitarism. For these conditions these hormones are lifesaving.

These hormones and their synthetic derivatives may also be used therapeutically for a variety of nonendocrine conditions. It is believed that, by virtue of their antipyretic, antiinflammatory, and mood-elevating properties, they can do more good than harm.

In acute rheumatoid arthritis or arthritic conditions unresponsive to other therapeutic measures, many experts advise glucocorticoid therapy. Intraarticular injection of cortisone has been practiced but with inconclusive results.

In patients with rheumatoid arthritis, there is rapid and marked reduction in the symptoms and signs of the disease. Muscle and joint stiffness, muscle tenderness and weakness, and joint swelling and soreness are diminished. The patient getting the drug for the first time usually notices distinct improvement within a few days. Appetite and weight increase; fever, if present, disappears; and the patient feels more energetic. Sedimentation rates are reduced or become normal and remain so as long as adequate doses of the hormone are given. Anemic patients usually have a rise in hemoglobin and in the number of red blood cells.

However, anatomic changes that have taken place prior to the administration of the hormones are unaffected, and joint deformities that have resulted from damage to bone and cartilage do not improve. After the withdrawal of the hormones symptoms generally reappear within a varying period of time, frequently within a short time.

Nephrotic syndrome has been effectively treated with glucocorticoids, as have cerebral edema and chronic ulcerative colitis. Glucocorticoids are also among the most useful therapeutic agents in the treatment of leukemias.

These hormones are used to relieve allergic manifestations such as may be seen in patients with serum sickness, severe hay fever, status asthmaticus, and exfoliative dermatitis. The tissue response to the allergic reaction is somehow modified by the hormones, but the precise mode of action is not understood.

Inflammatory conditions of the eye, such as uveitis, iritis, acute choroiditis, purulent conjunctivitis, allergic blepharitis, and keratitis, are also controlled. Prednisone or prednisolone is considered the steroid of choice in treatment of severe ocular inflammation requiring therapy.

Cortisone and hydrocortisone have been used extensively for the so-called collagen or mesenchymal diseases, such as lupus erythematosus, dermatomyositis, and periarteritis nodosa. In these diseases, particularly lupus erythematosus, a sensitivity seems to have been developed after some acute infection, and the brunt of the sensitivity is borne by the connective tissues of the body. Apparently, the response of connective tissues to mechanical or chemical injury as well as to states of hypersensitivity such as may be produced by disease or by drugs is somehow altered. The reactivity of the connective tissue is suppressed regardless of the cause. This effect of cortisone or hydrocortisone seems to explain their capacity to relieve symptoms in a variety of conditions.

In acute rheumatic fever the muscle tissue of the heart and the connective tissue of the heart valves respond a good deal like other muscle and connective tissues of the body of the patient with rheumatoid arthritis. These hormones suppress the signs and symptoms of the disease, but they neither shorten the natural duration of the disease process nor cure the disease. They do nothing to modify preexisting valvular damage or hypertrophy of the heart. When given especially for antirheumatic effects, the daily dose of the glucocorticoids should be given in approximately equal amounts throughout the 24-hour period. When a dose is due, it should be given promptly so intervals between doses are neither too long nor too short.

Glucocorticoids are also presently being used in shock, specifically shock with gram-negative bacteremia, but also shock from other causes. It has been postulated that the cortisones sometimes lead to "hemodynamic restoration" in circulatory shock when other measures have been futile, although the exact mechanism of action is not clear.

It must be remembered that in all of these conditions the administration of corticosteroids is primarily symptomatic, not curative, therapy.

All of the adrenal steroids used clinically have distinctive and individual qualities. Cortisone is still useful and in some cases is thought to be preferable to other steroids. It is the least costly to synthesize. Hydrocortisone is superior to cortisone, especially for local injection into joints. For prolonged systemic administration, when it is important to avoid disturbances produced by loss of potassium or retention of sodium and to minimize the amount of steroid used, some authorities consider prednisone or prednisolone the steroid of choice.

The production of synthetic compounds has demonstrated that the steroid molecule can be altered to produce compounds with more selective effects and has paved the way for the synthesis of compounds with even greater selectivity of effects.

Absorption. Cortisone acetate is absorbed effectively after both oral and intramuscular administration. Cortisone and hydrocortisone are deactivated in the liver; after degradation 75% of the hormones are excreted in the urine, the remainder being excreted in the feces. The response after oral administration is often more rapid than after intramuscular injection, but the effect is less sustained. Since a constant level of the hormone in the tissues is highly desirable, several doses of intramuscular cortisone may be given during the first days of therapy, after which the size of the maintenance dose is determined. After oral administration the absorption of hydrocortisone is highly similar to that of cortisone. Absorption of hydrocortisone from an intramuscular site of injection, however, takes place much more slowly.

Side effects and toxic effects. Toxic effects resulting from the therapeutic use of corticosteroids fall into two categories: those resulting from withdrawal and those resulting from prolonged administration in large doses. Side effects do not often constitute a problem when cortisone or hydrocortisone is given for conditions that are benefited after a short period of administration. This is also true of corticotropin. When large doses or prolonged therapy is necessary, the altered reactions of tissue cells to infections, toxins, and mechanical or chemical injury may bring about serious untoward effects. Healing of wounds may be delayed because of interference with the formation of fibroblasts and their activity in forming ground substance and granulation tissue. Growth of blood vessels into new tissue is also impaired.

Since peptic ulcers may result from therapy, corticosteroids should be administered with meals or milk. In patients who already have peptic ulcer and have been receiving cortisone, neither fever nor abdominal rigidity occurs when perforation of the ulcer and peritonitis develop. Perforation of the bowel has been reported in patients with chronic ulcerative colitis during treatment with cortisone or corticotropin. Because of the lack of symptoms the diagnosis may be missed, and healing may be impaired seriously because of the effect on new scar-forming tissue. This failure of tissue response also explains a breakdown and active manifestation of tuberculosis in persons in whom the infection has been quiescent.

Other side effects that have been noted include amenorrhea, which presumably is caused by inhibition of the anterior lobe of the pituitary gland; disorders of calcium metabolism, seen particularly after the menopause in women who have developed osteoporosis and spontaneous fractures; and increased incidence of thrombosis and embolic formations. Still other symptoms include those associated with Cushing's syndrome —a rounded contour of the face, hirsutism, purplish or reddish striae of the skin, transient retention of salt and water, cervicothoracic hump, and the appearance of edema. Psychic phenomena have also been observed in the form of restlessness, insomnia, euphoria, and even manic states. The psychic status of a patient is, therefore, considered before these hormones are administered.

Administration of the glucocorticoids may reduce the resistance of the patient to certain infectious processes and to some viral diseases. It is thought, therefore, that acute or subacute infections should be brought under control before starting the administration of these drugs if at all feasible. On the other hand, should an infection occur during the course of treatment with these hormones, it may be necessary to increase the dosage to help cope with the added stress occasioned by the infection.

It is important to remember that any patient who has received a significant amount of cortisone or related glucocorticoids is likely to have a certain amount of atrophy of the adrenal cortex. The amount of hormone that will produce atrophy is not known, nor is it known how long the atrophy will persist, but acute adrenal insufficiency results from too rapid withdrawal of therapy. Withdrawal syndrome symptoms include weakness, lethargy, restlessness, anorexia, and nausea. Muscle tenderness is common. Withdrawal should be carried out slowly and under close supervision.

A patient who must undergo surgery and who has received treatment with cortisone should be prepared preoperatively with the administration of cortisone. Its administration should be continued postoperatively in decreasing doses for several days. The nurse should be alert to obtain this type of information. It should be noted whether or not a patient has received treatment with cortisone, and if so, such information should be reported to the physician. It is just possible that it might be overlooked. If patients go to surgery with atrophy of the adrenal gland, it is altogether possible that they will be unable to cope with the stress of such procedure and death may result.

Some physicians recommend that patients who receive cortisone, related adrenocortical steroids, or corticotropin be given cards similar to those carried by diabetic patients, so that in the event of an accident the physician giving emergency treatment may be aware of this fact.

Contraindications. Glucocorticoids are contraindicated for patients with psychoses, peptic ulcer, acute glomerulonephritis, vaccinia or varicella, herpes simplex of the eye, and infections uncontrolled by antibiotics. Myasthenic crisis may be induced if these drugs are administered to patients with myasthenia gravis. Pregnancy is an indication for cautious use, if at all, since adrenal insufficiency in both mother and child is a possibility at the time of delivery. Moreover, abnormalities in the fetus are possible. Cautious use is recommended in the presence of hypertension, congestive heart failure, diabetes mellitus, thrombophlebitis, convulsive disorders, renal insufficiency, osteoporosis, and diverticulitis.

Preparation, dosage, and administration. The following are preparations available of cortisone and hydrocortisone.

Hydrocortisone sodium succinate, U.S.P., B.P. (Solu-Cortef). This is a highly soluble salt of hydrocortisone, which lends itself to parenteral therapy in smaller volumes of diluent. It is recommended for short-term emergency therapy. Dosage is 100 to 250 mg. intravenously or intramuscularly. It is available in vials containing 100, 250, and 500 mg. and 1 Gm. of the powder for injection.

Cortisone acetate, U.S.P., B.P. (Cortone Acetate, Cortogen Acetate). Cortisone has received a D.E.S.I. rating of *effective* for a wide variety of disorders. Official preparations are available in 5-, 10-, and 25-mg. tablets for oral administration and as a suspension for injection, 25 or 50 mg. per milliliter. There are also available an ophthalmic suspension (0.5% and 2.5%) and an ophthalmic ointment (1.5%). Cortisone acetate is administered parenterally, orally, or topically. Dosage varies greatly with the nature and severity of the disease being treated and with the responsiveness of the patient. In severe disorders as much as 300 mg. may be ordered the first day, 200 mg. the second day, and 100 mg. daily thereafter, reducing the dosage gradually to the minimum amount that will bring about the desired effects. Its use in the treatment of acute self-limiting conditions is usually discontinued as soon as feasible. To avoid undesirable side effects dosage must be carefully regulated when used for chronic conditions. For rheumatoid arthritis tolerable doses are frequently less than was considered satisfactory at one time. The patient's age and sex greatly affect the dose. Women, and particularly postmenopausal women, are especially sensitive to adrenocortical steroids. The average maximal daily dose for long-term therapy is 25 to 30 mg. for women and 40 to 45 mg. for men. Usual dose is 25 mg. orally four times daily or 100 mg. intramuscularly once daily. For children, the oral dose is 0.7 mg. per kilogram of body weight divided into three doses; intramuscular dose is one third to one half the oral dose.

Hydrocortisone, U.S.P., B.P. (Cortef, Cortril, Hydrocortone). Hydrocortisone is available in .5-, 10-, and 20-mg. tablets, as a suspension (2 mg. per milliliter) for oral administration, as a 1% lotion for topical application, and as a solution for injection (5 to 25 mg. per milliliter). Additional preparations include a cream (1% and 2.5%) and an ointment (1% and 2.5%) for topical application. Hydrocortisone is administered orally, intramuscularly, intravenously, and topically. The usual oral dose is 10 to 20 mg. three or four times daily; range of dose is usually 10 to 300 mg. daily. The dosage of hydrocortisone is said to be about two thirds that of cortisone. Adjustments in dosage are made to meet changes in the needs of the patient. Withdrawal of therapy is sometimes necessary but is avoided when the patient is subjected to additional stress and strain. Hydrocortisone has received a D.E.S.I. rating of *effective* for a wide variety of disorders.

Hydrocortisone acetate, U.S.P., B.P. (Cortef Acetate, Cortril Acetate, Hydrocortone Acetate). This drug is available as a suspension for injection (25 to 50 mg. per milliliter); as an ophthalmic suspension (0.5% and 2.5%); as an ointment (0.5%, 1.5%, and 2.5%); and as an ointment for topical application. The dose for intraarticular injection varies greatly with the degree of inflammation, size of the joint, and response of the patient. Doses vary from 5 to 50 mg. Ophthalmic applications of this drug also vary but may be used freely since there is no systemic reaction.

MINERALOCORTICOIDS
Aldosterone

For some years desoxycorticosterone was the only potent steroid available that had selective action in favoring water and salt retention in the patient with Addison's disease. This hormone was lifesaving in the treatment of persons with low or absent adrenal cortical function. Desoxycorticosterone was originally obtained by chemical synthesis and has been found in adrenal glands in only trace levels.

Aldosterone is the only physiologically important steroid synthesized in the adrenal cortex. Its action is to stimulate sodium reabsorption, particularly in the kidney. Aldosterone restricts the loss of sodium and its accompanying anions, chloride and bicarbonate, and thereby helps maintain extracellular fluid volume. It also maintains acid-base and potassium balance.

In adrenal insufficiency, aldosterone deficit occurs, sodium reabsorption is inhibited, and potassium excretion decreases. Hyperkalemia and mild acidosis occur. In adrenalectomy, the loss of aldosterone leads to an overall reduction of sodium reabsorption and a powerful and uncontrolled loss of extracellular fluid. Plasma volume drops and a state of hypovolemic shock may ensue. This may cause death unless a mineralocorticoid, salt, and water are administered. In excessive doses, aldosterone increases potassium excretion, and unless dietary intake compensates for the loss, hypokalemia results, and acidification of the urine occurs leading to metabolic alkalosis.

Aldosterone is much more potent in its electrolyte effects than desoxycorticosterone. Aldosterone has not yet established a therapeutic status comparable to that of desoxycorticosterone. Its use has been limited because of its cost and relative unavailability and because it must be administered intramuscularly.

The amount of aldosterone secreted by the adrenal cortex is apparently affected by the concentration of sodium in body fluids rather than by the stimulation of the adrenal cortex by ACTH.

Desoxycorticosterone acetate (Doca Acetate)

Desoxycorticosterone acetate is a white, crystalline powder, insoluble in water and slightly soluble in vegetable oils. In small amounts it has been isolated from the adrenal cortex and is synthesized as the acetate.

The activity of desoxycorticosterone acetate appears to be limited to the metabolism of sodium, potassium, and water. It is particularly effective in correcting defects in the sodium-potassium balance. It promotes the retention of the sodium ions and water and the excretion of potassium. The site of action is seemingly the renal tubule of the kidney, where reabsorption is modified. It has no noticeable effect on carbohydrate and protein metabolism.

Patients with chronic adrenal insufficiency,

such as patients with Addison's disease, may progress satisfactorily with the administration of desoxycorticosterone and sodium chloride. Some physicians prefer to use cortisone and hydrocortisone with sodium chloride along with maintenance doses of desoxycorticosterone. In acute adrenal insufficiency adrenocortical extract, cortisone, hydrocortisone, and desoxycorticosterone as well as other adrenal steroids may be used. Patients treated only with desoxycorticosterone are highly affected by states of stress or infections, and an addisonian crisis may be precipitated.

Since the advent of newer drugs, desoxycorticosterone acetate is not used as widely as in the past. Desoxycorticosterone acetate and pivalate have received a D.E.S.I. rating of *effective* in partial replacement therapy for adrenocortical insufficiency due to Addison's disease and for treatment of the salt-losing adrenogenital syndrome and *ineffective* for acute pemphigus. The buccal tablets have received a *probably effective* rating.

Preparation, dosage, and administration. The following are preparations available of desoxycorticosterone acetate.

Desoxycorticosterone acetate, U.S.P. (Doca Acetate, Percorten, Decortin, Decosterone); *deoxycortone acetate,* B.P. This is available as a solution for injection (5 mg. per milliliter) and in 2- and 5-mg. buccal tablets. The tablets should be held in the buccal cavity or under the tongue. The solution is given by intramuscular injection.

The oral and intramuscular maintenance dose of desoxycorticosterone acetate varies from 1 to 5 mg. daily, depending on the response of the patient and the intake of sodium chloride (the higher the intake of salt, the lower the requirement of adrenal steroid). In the management of an acute crisis 5 to 15 mg. once or twice a day may be needed along with cortisone or other adrenal steroids.

Sterile desoxycorticosterone pivalate suspension, N.F. This is a microcrystalline suspension of the drug. One injection lasts approximately 4 weeks for the patient with Addison's disease. It is administered intramuscularly. The usual dose is 50 mg.

Side effects and toxic effects. When large doses of desoxycorticosterone are given, patients may develop edema, pulmonary congestion, or congestive heart failure, and even death may result. A fair number of patients develop hypertension after several months or years of receiving this drug. The blood pressure should be taken periodically, and if hypertension develops, the dosage of the steroid and probably also the salt intake should be carefully adjusted. Excessive loss of potassium may account for electrocardiographic changes and sudden attacks of weakness.

Fludrocortisone acetate, B.P. (Florinef, F-Cortef)

This preparation is a derivative of hydrocortisone acetate and is marketed as a lotion and as an ointment for topical application and as a tablet for oral administration. It has intense sodium-retaining effects. For the management of allergic dermatoses, a small quantity is applied to the area of involvement several times a day. Vigorous rubbing at the time of application should be avoided. The part being treated should be carefully cleansed before the application is made. Usual oral dose for Addison's disease is 0.1 to 0.3 mg. daily; for adrenal hyperplasia the usual dose is 1 to 2 mg. daily.

Synthetic antiinflammatory glucocorticoids

Hydrocortisone is considered to be the main steroid found in the bloodstream with corticoid activity. In recent years chemical modifications of the basic steroid structure of the glucocorticoids have been made, with the aim of producing more potent and more selectively acting compounds. If an additional double bond is inserted on ring A of cortisone or hydrocortisone, the compounds called prednisone or prednisolone result (see structural formulas—ring A is the one at lower left of formula).

Prednisone and prednisolone are considerably more active in their antiinflammatory effect but have less salt-retaining action as compared to the parent compounds on a weight basis. Hence, there is less risk of undesirable side actions related to the retention of salt, hypertension, and formation of edema when the newer compounds are used for their antirheumatic activity. The addition of a methyl group in the 6 position of ring

B of prednisolone produces an even greater effect (see methylprednisolone).

Prednisone, U.S.P., B.P. (Meticorten, Deltasone, Deltra). This is available in 1-, 2.5-, and 50-mg. tablets for oral administration. Dosage varies with the severity of the disease and patient response. There is wide variation in the dosage for children. A dose of 30 to 50 mg. may be required to suppress severe symptoms, although some physicians prefer to start therapy with a relatively small dose. After 2 to 7 days, dosage is gradually reduced and a maintenance dose established. A dose of 5 to 10 mg. (or less) daily may suffice for milder conditions. The range of dose is 5 to 80 mg. daily. The daily allotment should be divided into installment doses and should be given on a regular 6- or 8-hour schedule. Not only the total daily dose but frequently individual doses in the course of the day must be adjusted to meet the needs of the patient. Patients vary in their need and tolerance to all antirheumatic steroids. The nurse should exert great care that the correct dose is given at the right time. When administration of the drug is to be discontinued, it is usually withdrawn gradually, and in the event of a medical or surgical emergency or period of unusual stress the drug

Prednisone (synthetic analogue of cortisone)

9-Alpha-fluorohydrocortisone (fludrocortisone)

Prednisolone (synthetic analogue of
hydrocortisone)

Methylprednisolone

is given again to prevent the possibility of acute adrenal insufficiency. This applies to all cortical steroids given for systemic effects.

Prednisolone, U.S.P., B.P. (Meticortelone, Delta-Cortef). Prednisolone is available in 1-, 2.5-, and 5-mg. tablets for oral administration; in addition, many dosage forms are available. It has about the same potency as prednisone, and the dosage is approximately the same.

Prednisolone acetate, U.S.P. (Sterane). This is marketed as an aqueous suspension, 125 mg. in 5 ml., for intramuscular injection. Dosage is 10 to 30 mg. daily. Prednisolone acetate, B.P., is available in 5-mg. tablets.

Prednisolone butylacetate (Hydeltra-T.B.A.). This compound is marketed as a suspension, 20 mg. per milliliter, for injection into joints, bursae, or synovial sheaths. Dosage varies from 5 to 30 mg. Relief of symptoms may not occur for a day or two because the drug is not very soluble.

Methylprednisolone, N.F., B.P. (Medrol). This is available in 2-, 4-, and 16-mg. tablets and sustained-release capsules containing 2 and 4 mg. for oral administration. Dosage is individually determined, but in general, it is about two thirds that of either prednisone or prednisolone. Sup-

pressive doses for severe conditions range from 20 to 60 mg. daily; for less severe conditions the initial daily dosage may be from 6 to 20 mg. The daily dose is divided into four parts and is given after meals and at bedtime with food. The daily maintenance dose is frequently about half the initial dose. This drug is also available for injection.

Prednisolone sodium phosphate, U.S.P., B.P. (Hydeltrasol). This drug is more soluble than prednisolone or its acetate or butylacetate. After parenteral administration it has a rapid onset and short duration of action. It is administered parenterally and topically to the skin, eye, or external ear.

Dexamethasone, U.S.P., B.P. (Decadron, Deronil, Gammacorten). This preparation is a fluorinated synthetic glucocorticoid structurally similar to hydrocortisone. It is a particularly potent antiinflammatory agent. In contrast to cortisone and hydrocortisone, it may exhibit diuretic effects in patients made edematous by the administration of other adrenocortical hormones. Dexamethasone lacks mineralocorticoid activity and hence is not suited to replacement therapy for adrenal insufficiency. It is used primarily for its antiinflammatory and antiallergic effects.

Dexamethasone is administered orally or topically. As is true for other adrenal steroids, the dosage varies considerably, depending upon the severity of the symptoms to be controlled and the response of the patient. Usual dose ranges from 0.5 to 10 mg. daily. The drug is marketed in 0.25-, 0.5-, 0.75-mg., and 1.5-Gm. tablets, as an elixir, 0.1 mg. per milliliter, and as an aerosol and cream.

Dexamethasone sodium phosphate, U.S.P. This drug is a derivative of dexamethasone, is more soluble than dexamethasone, and is suited for injection (intramuscular, intravenous, and intrasynovial).

Betamethasone, N.F., B.P. (Celestone). This drug is structurally similar to dexamethasone and has an approximately equal level of potency. It is administered orally and is available in 600-μg. tablets. A suspension containing betamethasone sodium phosphate and betamethasone acetate is available for intramuscular or local injection.

Table 25-1 Relative potency of corticoids in treatment of nonendocrine disease

Corticoid	Potency (relative to cortisone)	Trade name	Equivalent dose
Cortisone	1	Cortogen Acetate Cortone Acetate	25 mg.
Hydrocortisone	1.2	Cortril Cortef Hydrocortone	20 mg.
Prednisone	4 to 5	Meticorten Paracort Deltasone	5 mg.
Prednisolone	4 to 5	Delta-Cortef Hydeltra Meticortelone Paracortol Sterane	5 mg.
6-Methylprednisolone	5 to 6	Medrol	4 mg.
Triamcinolone	4 to 8	Aristocort Kenacort	4 mg.
Dexamethasone	16 to 30	Decadron Deronil Dexameth Gammacorten Hexadrol	0.75 mg.
Betamethasone	16 to 30	Celestone	0.6 mg.

Triamcinolone (Aristocort, Kenacort). This drug is a potent glucocorticoid that is said to produce effects comparable to prednisolone but with lower dosage. It apparently is less likely to produce retention of sodium and water than many of the related compounds and seemingly does not affect excretion of potassium except after large doses. Prolonged use and large doses, however, bring about negative protein anad calcium balance and impaired carbohydrate metabolism as well as symptoms of hyperadrenalism. It is administered orally and is available in 1-, 2-, 4-, 8-, and 16-mg. tablets. The usual initial dose varies from 8 to 20 mg. daily, given in divided portions. Maintenance dosage is determined in relation to each patient.

Triamcinolone acetonide, U.S.P., B.P. (Aristocort, Acetonide, Kenalog). This is a derivative of triamcinolone. It is available as a suspension for injection containing 10 mg. and 40 mg. per milliliter in 5-ml. vials. It is available as a cream, a lotion, an ointment, and a spray for the treatment of acute and chronic dermatoses.

Hydrocortamate hydrochloride (Magnacort). This drug is marketed as an ointment for topical application. It is a derivative of hydrocortisone and is used in treatment of dermatoses with an allergic or inflammatory basis. The ointment is applied to the infected areas two or three times a day.

Fluprednisolone (Alphadrol). This synthetic drug differs from prednisolone by having a fluorine atom, which increases its antiinflammatory activity to 2.5 times that of prednisolone. Range of dose is 1.5 to 18 mg. daily. It is available in 0.75- and 1.5-mg. tablets.

Meprednisone, N.F. (Betapar). This synthetic drug differs from prednisolone by the substitution of a methyl group for a hydrogen group. Its actions are similar to those of dexamethasone. It is available in 4-mg. tablets. Range of dose is 4 to 60 mg. daily, depending on the underlying disease and its severity.

Side effects and toxic effects. Although prednisone, prednisolone, and closely related compounds may achieve their effects with lower dosage, their capacity to produce many of the same side effects as cortisone and hydrocortisone continues to pose problems. A gain in weight, abnormal growth of hair on the face (hypertrichosis), the development of supraclavicular fat pads, increase in blood pressure, euphoria, emotional instability, undue fatigability, and menstrual irregularities are symptoms of a developing hypercortisonism that are more difficult to treat than to prevent. Postmenopausal women and young children are especially susceptible to the adrenal steroids and are more likely to develop hypercortisonism than younger women or men. Many physicians recommend that the patient be kept on doses that can be tolerated even though all symptoms may not be completely relieved. The patient should also have the benefit of other therapy.

Androgenic steroids

The chemical structure of the cortical steroids is similar to that of the sex hormones. Some of the adrenocortical steroids exhibit androgenic and some exhibit estrogenic properties. They are not of great consequence under normal conditions. Adrenal tumors, on the other hand, can cause increased formation of estrogen or androgen, which helps to explain abnormal feminization or masculinization in patients.

HORMONES FROM THE PANCREAS

Secretions from the pancreas that have an effect on blood sugar levels are glucagon and insulin. These hormones have an important role in the therapy of patients with diabetes mellitus.

Glucagon, U.S.P.

Glucagon, like insulin, is a pancreatic extract and is thought to oppose the action of insulin. Glucagon is a product of the alpha cells of the islands of Langerhans; insulin is from the beta cells. Glucagon acts primarily by mobilizing hepatic glycogen, which produces an elevation of the concentration of glucose in the blood. It has received a D.E.S.I. rating of *effective* in the treatment of hypoglycemic reactions in patients who are receiving insulin therapy for diabetes or psychiatric disorders. A patient in hypoglycemic coma will usually respond within 5 to 20 minutes after he has been given an injection of glucagon. However, in most patients, after the initial rise in the concentration of glucose in the blood, it will fall to normal or hypoglycemic levels within $1\frac{1}{2}$ hours. In order to prevent the patient from relapsing into coma after he has been aroused by glucagon, dextrose or another readily absorbable sugar is administered. Because patients who receive glucagon require close medical supervision, the drug is not recommended for home use or self-administration.

Preparation, dosage, and administration. Glucagon is available in vials containing powder suitable for injection. One milliliter of diluent is used for each milligram of glucagon. The usual dosage for the diabetic patient is 0.5 to 1 mg. If the patient does not respond in 20 minutes, additional doses may be given. The drug may be given by intravenous, intramuscular, or subcutaneous injection.

Side effects and toxic effects. Nausea and vomiting are the most frequent side effects observed in patients who have received glucagon, but these effects may be caused by hypoglycemia rather than the drug. Hypotensive reactions immediately after the administration of glucagon have also been reported. Because glucagon is an agent of protein derivation with unknown potential toxicity, nurses need to be alert to detect early signs of hypersensitivity. Glucagon has a positive inotropic effect on the heart.

Insulin

The discovery of insulin began with Johann Conrad Brunner (1653-1727), the discoverer of Brunner's glands in the duodenum. In 1683 he made incisions in the pancreas of a dog, after which the dog had extreme thirst and polyuria. Brunner suggested that there is a connection between the pancreas and diabetes. This was a pioneer experiment on the internal secretions of the pancreas.

In 1889 von Mering and Minkowski showed that removal of the pancreas from dogs produced symptoms identical with diabetes mellitus. In 1906 Minkowski showed that this experimental diabetes could be prevented by pancreatic grafts. This work practically proved that the pancreas produces an internal secretion or hormone that controls carbohydrate metabolism. Corroborative findings soon followed. Partial removal of the pancreas produced a mild diabetes in animals, and transfusion of normal blood ameliorated the symptoms. In autopsy of many diabetic patients, changes in the islets of Langerhans were found. This indicated that the hormone was produced in the islets.

Repeated attempts to isolate the hormone failed until Banting and Best, in 1921, isolated it in a sufficiently pure state to permit its use in diabetic patients. Extracts from fetal pancreata were found to cause a great reduction of blood sugar. Repeated daily injections permitted animals with the pancreas removed to live beyond the span of life usual under such conditions. Later, methods were developed for the extraction of insulin from an adult pancreas, and continuous improvement in the method of extraction has been made. Insulin is now prepared from mammalian pancreata (sheep, hogs, cattle).

Chemistry of insulin. Insulin is a protein that, upon hydrolysis, yields a number of amino acids. In its crystalline state it appears to be chemically linked with certain metals (zinc, nickel, cadmium, or cobalt). Normal pancreatic tissue is rich in zinc, a fact that may be of significance in the natural storage of the hormone. Insulin keeps rather well in a slightly acidified state but is unstable in dilute alkali. Slight changes in its chemical structure greatly change its behavior, and for this reason it cannot be given by mouth.

One of the major advances in the knowledge of insulin came when an English group headed by Frederick Sanger determined the complete amino acid sequence of insulin (for which

Sanger received the Nobel Prize). Insulin consists of two polypeptide chains and contains 48 amino acids, the exact sequence of which is known. There are slight differences in the order of amino acids in insulin from different species of animals.

Action and result. Since relatively small amounts of insulin are necessary in the body tissues, it is thought that insulin acts as a catalyst in cellular metabolism.

Carbohydrate metabolism is controlled by a finely balanced interaction of a number of endocrine factors (adrenal, anterior pituitary, thyroid, and insulin), but the particular phase of carbohydrate metabolism that is affected by insulin is not entirely known. When insulin is injected subcutaneously, however, it produces a rapid lowering of the blood sugar. This effect is produced in both diabetic and nondiabetic persons. Moderate amounts of insulin in the diabetic animal promote the storage of carbohydrate in the liver and also in the muscle cells, particularly after the feeding of carbohydrate. In the normal animal there is also an increase in the deposit of muscle glycogen but apparently no increase in the level of liver glycogen. In both diabetic and nondiabetic individuals the oxygen consumption increases and the respiratory quotient rises.

Diabetes mellitus. Diabetes mellitus is a disease of metabolism characterized particularly by an inability to utilize carbohydrate. The blood sugar becomes elevated, and when it exceeds a certain amount, the excess is secreted by the kidney (glycosuria). Symptoms include increased appetite, thirst, weight loss, increased urine output, weakness, and itching such as pruritus vulvae.

There are two types of diabetes mellitus—growth onset and maturity onset. Growth-onset diabetes seems to be the result of reduced or absent secretion of insulin and generally has its onset before age 20. This type of diabetes generally requires conscientious therapy, including administration of insulin. Maturity-onset diabetes, however, is the result of inability to utilize the insulin that is secreted. It generally occurs after the age of 30 and can frequently be controlled by oral hypoglycemic agents and/or diet.

In diabetes mellitus there is a failure to store glycogen in the liver, although the conversion of glycogen back to glucose or the formation of glucose from other substances (gluconeogenesis) is not necessarily impaired. As a result, the level of blood sugar rapidly rises. This derangement of carbohydrate metabolism results in an abnormally high metabolism of proteins and fats. The normal short-chain fatty acids, which result from oxidation of fatty acids, accumulate faster than the muscle cells can oxidize them, resulting in the development of ketosis and acidosis. The course of untreated diabetes mellitus is progressive. The symptoms of diabetic coma and acidosis are directly or indirectly the result of the accumulation of acetone, beta-hydroxybutyric acid, and diacetic acid. Respirations become rapid and deep, the breath has an odor of acetone, the blood sugar is elevated, the patient becomes dehydrated, and stupor and coma develop unless treatment is promptly started.

Therapeutic uses of insulin. Insulin is a specific in the treatment of diabetic coma and acidosis. The administration of glucose intravenously often accompanies the administration of the insulin, although not all physicians advocate that glucose be used early in the treatment of acidosis. Glucose and insulin promote the formation and retention of glycogen in the liver, and the oxidation of fat in the liver is arrested. Therefore, the rate of formation of acetone bodies is slowed and the acidosis is checked. Other supportive measures such as the restoration of the fluid and electrolyte balance of the body are exceedingly important.

Insulin has its principal use in the control of symptoms of diabetes mellitus when this disease cannot be satisfactorily controlled by diet alone. Certain mild cases of the disease can be treated by diet alone, but many patients require insulin in order to live active and useful lives. The dosage must be determined for each individual patient and can best be done when the patient is under the direct observation of the physician for a period of time. A number of factors determine the amount of insulin needed by the patient, and a patient's needs are not always constant. Adjustments in dosage may be necessary if infection is present, if the patient has an anesthetic, if

emotional strain and stress are prominent, or if his activity is increased or decreased.

It is important that the symptoms of diabetes be adequately controlled. The more nearly the blood chemistry of the diabetic patient is restored to normal, the more normal his metabolism and nutrition will be and less degenerative damage will occur in organs such as the eye and heart.

Insulin has been used also in some hospitals for the purpose of producing hypoglycemic shock for its effect on the patient with schizophrenia. It is a dangerous treatment with a relatively high mortality rate and should be used only by those who are well equipped, qualified, and familiar with the procedure. It has been replaced, to a great extent, by electroshock therapy and other drugs.

Preparation, dosage, and administration. A number of different types of insulin preparations are used in medicine. All preparations have the same fundamental pharmacologic action. Differences are those related to the time and duration of absorption of the injected insulin into the circulation, providing faster or slower, shorter or more prolonged effects.

All insulin preparations should be refrigerated. Vials of insoluble preparations (all except regular insulin) should be rotated between the hands and inverted end to end several times before a dose is withdrawn. A vial should not be shaken vigorously or the suspension made to foam.

Insulin is given subcutaneously into the loose connective tissues of the body, usually into the arms or thighs. It cannot be given by mouth because it is destroyed by digestive enzymes. Regular insulin is usually given about 20 minutes before meals. It is somewhat irritating, and since the tissues of the diabetic patient are likely to be less resistant to the invasion of pathogenic organisms than normal tissue, the technique used in administration of insulin should be flawless. The same site of injection should not be used repeatedly, but a plan of rotation should be followed so that the same site is not used more often than once a month.

There is no average dose of insulin for the diabetic; each patient's needs must be determined individually. These needs are frequently determined by testing for glycosuria and ketonuria.

U-40 1 cc. (red)

U-80 1 cc. (green)

U-80 2 cc. (green)

Figure 25-2

Insulin syringes. The first or uppermost syringe is used only for U-40 insulin (40 units of insulin in 1 cc. [ml.]). It is scaled in red. The next syringe is used for U-80 only and is scaled in green. The third syringe is also scaled in green and is used only for U-80 insulin. The last syringe is suited for use when unusually large doses of insulin must be given.

Unless complications are present, insulin is not used if the patient's glucose tolerance is sufficiently high to permit him to have a diet sufficient for light work.

Dosage of insulin is expressed in units rather than in milliliters or minims. Insulin injection is so standardized that each milliliter contains 20, 40, 80, or 100 U.S.P. units. One insulin unit will, on the average, promote the metabolism of approximately 1.5 Gm. of dextrose. To estimate the necessary insulin dosage for the patient the physician must know how much dextrose will be obtained from the diet and what the patient's glucose tolerance is—how much insulin the patient is able to make for himself. Insulin must be regularly administered and must be accompanied by carefully estimated diets of known composition.

Insulin injection, U.S.P., B.P. This is an acidified aqueous solution of the active principle of the pancreas that affects the metabolism of glucose. This preparation is marketed in 10-ml. vials in strengths of 40, 80, 100, and 500 U.S.P. units per milliliter of the injection. The maximum degree of lowering of the blood sugar occurs in 2 or 3 hours. The onset of its activity is 1 hour, and the duration of activity is 6 to 8 hours.

Protamine zinc insulin suspension, U.S.P.; *protamine zinc insulin injection*, B.P. This is a preparation of insulin to which has been added an appropriate amount of protamine and a zinc salt, which has the effect of slowing absorption.

The effects produced by protamine zinc insulin are the same as those of insulin, except that the blood sugar–lowering action is much more prolonged. It may be used in place of unmodified insulin or in combination with it. The chief indications for its use are in those cases where the unmodified insulin does not provide control of symptoms unless it is given in several daily doses or in cases where lack of control is evidenced by frequent hypoglycemic reaction, ketosis, or pronounced fluctuations in levels of blood sugar. Usually protamine zinc insulin is administered either in the morning, 30 minutes to $1\frac{1}{2}$ hours before breakfast, or in the evening, 1 hour before supper or before retiring. Its maximum blood sugar–lowering action is about 16 to 24 hours after administration. Its onset of action is 4 to 6 hours, and its duration of action is 24 to 36 hours or longer.

Hypoglycemic reactions from this drug are recognized less easily than those that occur with regular insulin. Sometimes the main symptom is a feeling of pronounced fatigue out of proportion to the degree of activity. Treatment consists of giving a combination of a rapidly absorbed and a slowly absorbed carbohydrate, something like bread and honey. Many patients carry hard candy. Protamine insulin is of no value in emergencies such as diabetic coma. A combination of protamine insulin and rapid-acting insulin is frequently necessary if adequate control of symptoms is to be maintained. It is administered subcutaneously, never intravenously. It should be mixed well (but not made to foam) before withdrawal from container in order to obtain a uniform suspension. The vial is rotated, not shaken. It is available in concentrations of 40, 80, or 100 U.S.P. units of insulin per milliliter of injection.

Globin zinc insulin injection, U.S.P., B.P. This is a preparation of insulin modified by the addition of globin and zinc chloride. The globin is obtained from globin hydrochloride prepared from beef blood. Each milliliter of the finished product contains 40, 80, or 100 units of insulin. The action of this preparation is between that of regular insulin and protamine zinc insulin. The period of maximum effect extends from 8 to 16 hours after injection. It is beneficial for those patients who require more than a single injection of regular insulin, for those who are sensitive to protamine, and for those whose levels of blood sugar are not satisfactorily controlled by other forms of insulin. It is said to produce fewer local reactions than regular insulin. It is not given when rapid effects are desired, and it should never be given intravenously or intramuscularly. It should be administered only by deep subcutaneous injection. The dosage must be regulated according to the patient's needs. The initial dose may be two thirds to three fourths of the daily dose of regular insulin and then increased gradually as needed.

Isophane insulin suspension, U.S.P., B.P. (NPH Insulin). This drug is a modified protamine zinc insulin. N indicates that it is a neutral solution; P stands for protamine zinc insulin; and H means that it originated in Hagedorn's laboratory. It is marketed in concentrations of 40, 80, or 100 U.S.P. units per milliliter of suspension. Its action places it between globin insulin and protamine zinc insulin. Its onset of action is within 2 hours, while peak effect is reached in 10 to 20 hours, and the duration of its action is 28 to 30 hours. Isophane insulin may be mixed with regular insulin. It is an intermediate-acting insulin preparation and should not be used when a quick-acting insulin is needed. It is given only by subcutaneous injection.

Lente insulins. Lente insulins consist of insulin precipitated with zinc and resuspended in an acetate buffer rather than a phosphate buffer, which is usually used in insulin preparations. By varying the way the insulin is prepared it is possible to obtain suspensions that contain particles of different size and form. It has been found that the larger crystals produce a longer but less intense effect, and this preparation is known as ultralente insulin; its action resembles that of protamine zinc insulin. Semilente insulin contains smaller particles, and its action falls between that of NPH and crystalline insulin. It is officially known as prompt insulin zinc suspension, U.S.P. Insulin zinc suspension, U.S.P., B.P. (Lente Insulin), contains a mixture of ultralente and semilente insulins. Lente insulins are available in quantities of 40, 80, or 100 units per milliliter of suspension. The duration of lente insulin is much like that of NPH insulin, and the two can be used interchangeably. Its characteristics of action place it between regular insulin and protamine zinc insulin.

The principal advantage of the lente insulins is their lack of sensitizing substances such as protamine or globin. They are useful for the treatment of diabetic patients who are allergic to other types of insulin or for those whose disease is difficult to control.

The injection should be made deep into subcutaneous tissue but not into muscle, and it should never be given intravenously. The usual time of administration is in the morning before breakfast. The dosage must be individualized for each patient. It is not used in the treatment of acidosis or for conditions that demand a rapid-acting insulin.

Symptoms of overdosage. The symptoms of hypoglycemia develop in the patient who is given an overdose of insulin or in the patient with hyperinsulinism as a result of certain changes in the pancreas. When caused by an overdose of insulin, the fall in blood sugar is in proportion to the amount of insulin given. In man, toxic symptoms occur when the blood sugar falls below 79 mg. per 100 ml. The point at which the symptoms become noticeable varies greatly, however. For each person there is a level at which severe symptoms or the convulsive stage of hypoglycemia is reached. The symptoms of hypoglycemia depend on the speed with which it develops.

Table 25-2 Tabulation of commercially available insulins*

Type of insulin	Time and route of administration	Time of onset (hours after administration)	Peak action (hours after administration)	Duration of action (hours)	Time when glycosuria most likely to occur	Time when hypoglycemia most likely to occur
Crystalline zinc† (pH 3-3.5; Zn. 0.02-0.04 mg./100 units) (regular)	Intravenously (emergency); 15 to 20 min. before meals; subcutaneously	Rapid—within 1 hr.	2 to 4	5 to 8	During night	10 A.M. to lunch
Semilente† (amorphous zinc) (pH 7.2; Zn. 0.2-0.25 mg./100 units)	30 to 45 min. before breakfast; deep subcutaneously; never intravenously	Rapid—within 1 hr.	6 to 10	12 to 16	During night	Before lunch
Globin zinc (pH 3.4-3.8; Zn. 0.25-0.35 mg./100 units)	30 min. to 1 hr. before breakfast; subcutaneously	Intermediate—rapidity of onset increases with dose—within 2 to 4 hr.	6 to 10	18 to 24; also increases with dose	Before breakfast and before lunch	3 P.M. to dinner
Lente† (combination of 30% semilente and 70% ultralente) (pH 7.1-7.4; Zn. 0.2-0.25 mg./100 units)	1 hr. before breakfast; deep subcutaneously; never intravenously	Intermediate—within 2 to 4 hr.	8 to 12	28 to 32	Before lunch	3 P.M. to dinner
NPH (neutral-protamine-Hagedorn) or Isophane (pH 7.1-7.4; Zn. 0.016-0.04 mg./100 units)	1 hr. before breakfast; subcutaneously	Intermediate—within 2 to 4 hr.	8 to 12	28 to 30	Before lunch	3 P.M. to dinner
Protamine zinc (ZPI) (pH 7.4; Zn. 0.2-0.25 mg./100 units)	1 hr. before breakfast; subcutaneously	Slow-acting—within 4 to 6 hr.	16 to 24	24 to 36+	Before lunch and at bedtime	2 A.M. to breakfast
Ultralente† (pH 4.8-5.7; Zn. 0.2-0.25 mg./100 units)	1 hr. before breakfast; deep subcutaneously; never intravenously	Very slow—8 hr.	16 to 24	36+		During night; early morning

*From a monograph on diabetes mellitus by the Upjohn Company, Kalamazoo, Mich., 1960, p. 65.

†Contains no modifying protein (protamine or globin).

Symptoms resulting from protamine zinc insulin are especially insidious.

Early symptoms include a feeling of weakness, sweating, nervousness and anxiety, pallor or flushing, and a vague feeling of apprehension. If the patient does not receive treatment, the symptoms may be intensified with the development of aphasia, convulsive seizures, coma, and even death. When the first mild symptoms are noted, the patient should receive treatment at once. Prolonged hypoglycemia is associated with diminished oxygen consumption and irreparable injury of the nervous system. Symptoms of hypoglycemia are quickly relieved by the administration of a soluble carbohydrate in the form of orange juice or two or three lumps of sugar by mouth or a soluble carbohydrate intravenously if the patient is comatose.

Ambulatory patients learn to recognize sudden hunger, sweating, and nervousness as subjective signs of insulin overdosage and carry a few lumps of sugar with them. A night nurse may find a diabetic patient asleep but in a pool of perspiration, which would indicate that he was having an insulin reaction and he should be awakened and given a soluble carbohydrate.

Other untoward effects. Repeated injections of insulin at the same site may cause local reactions of the subcutaneous tissues. These can be avoided by changing the site of injection.

Some patients experience a disturbance of vision thought to result from a change in the crystalline lens of the eye. This disappears after a few weeks. Edema of the face and sometimes of the extremities is observed occasionally, especially in young women. This, too, tends to disappear, but if troublesome it may necessitate restriction of sodium chloride and the use of a mild diuretic.

A few patients exhibit allergic reactions in the form of urticaria, redness, and itching in the region where the insulin has been injected. These symptoms can usually be controlled by changing to a different brand of insulin.

An occasional diabetic patient fails to respond to an ordinary therapeutic dose of insulin. In these cases, there has developed what is known as insulin resistance. Enormous doses (200 units or more daily) may be required to lower the blood-sugar level and to prevent acidosis. The cause of this condition is not entirely understood. In some instances it appears to be caused by the formation of antibodies, and in other cases it is thought to result from disturbance of the pituitary, adrenal, or thyroid glands. Most patients respond to large doses of insulin.

ORAL HYPOGLYCEMIC AGENTS

$$CH_3 - \bigcirc - SO_2 - NH - CO - NH - (CH_2)_3 - CH_3$$

Tolbutamide (Orinase)

$$NH_2 - \bigcirc - SO_2 - NH - CO - NH - (CH_2)_3 - CH_3$$

Carbutamide

$$Cl - \bigcirc - SO_2 - NH - CO - NH - (CH_2)_2 - CH_3$$

Chlorpropamide (Diabinese)

In the early days of insulin therapy many attempts were made to obtain a preparation or modification of insulin active after oral administration. None was successful, and it is unlikely that any can be, since polypeptides and proteins are both susceptible to destruction in the gastrointestinal tract and are poorly absorbed in an intact state.

In recent years certain drugs have been found which do have blood sugar–lowering or "insulin-like" action when given by mouth. They are principally the group of sulfonylureas. These compounds were originally discovered after observing that some of the antibacterial sulfonamides had hypoglycemic effects. These drugs are sometimes called "oral insulins," although this definitely is incorrect, since, chemically, they are completely different from insulin. They also differ from insulin in origin and mode of action.

The sulfonylureas are thought to act by increasing the pancreas' own ability to secrete insulin. They are most effective, therefore, in relatively mild diabetes when there is still some reserve islet capacity, such as the adult patient in whom the diabetes is recognized after the age of 30 years and who can be controlled with less than 40 units of insulin per day. They are less effective or ineffective in severe diabetes or juvenile diabetes in which it is presumed that no functional islet tissue is left to respond. It has also been noted that long-continued high doses of the sulfonylureas administered to normal animals can produce diabetes, apparently by permanently exhausting the capacity of the islet cells to make insulin.

Although much interest and enthusiasm have greeted this development and although these drugs have considerable scientific importance, they cannot be said to have fully replaced insulin in the treatment of diabetes. Nurses should recognize that the need for instruction that stresses dietary restrictions is even greater for patients receiving oral hypoglycemic agents than for those taking insulin, and it must be remembered that these patients, too, must be taught how and when to test for glycosuria and ketonuria, to maintain diet and personal hygiene, and to recognize dangerous symptoms. Since insulin is indispensable for management of complications, the patient must also be instructed in the use of insulin.

It must be noted that sulfonylurea drugs depress radioactive iodide uptake and may cause misleading results in diagnostic tests.

Preparation, dosage, and administration. The following are preparations of oral hypoglycemic drugs.

Tolbutamide, U.S.P., B.P. (Orinase). Tolbutamide has received a D.E.S.I. rating of *effective* for the treatment of diabetes mellitus of the stable type without acute complications such as acidosis or ketosis. This drug, a sulfonylurea derivative, is marketed in 500-mg. tablets for oral administration. Therapeutic trial with this drug is initiated with 3 Gm. on the first day and 2 Gm. on the second day; then dosage is gradually reduced until the minimum dose for satisfactory control of blood sugar has been determined. Maintenance dosage may vary from 0.5 to 2 Gm. per day. The drug is preferably given in divided doses and after meals. Traces of the drug have been found in plasma 1 hour after administration and the drug has a half-life of about 4 to 6 hours. Diabetic patients require close medical supervision, especially when the drug is first tried.

When tolbutamide therapy is begun, it will frequently be effected with a concurrent, gradual reduction of insulin dosage. During this conversion period, the nurse must be alert to the occurrence of hypoglycemic reactions that might indicate a need for modification of the dosage schedules.

Carbutamide. This drug causes allergic reactions in human beings and has not been released for use in the United States.

Tolazamide, U.S.P. (Tolinase). Tolazamide is a sulfonylurea compound pharmacologically related to tolbutamide, but it is absorbed more slowly. The average half-life of tolazamide is 7 hours, with maximal effects persisting for about 10 hours. Tolazamide is administered orally in doses ranging from 100 mg. to 1 Gm. daily. Dosage in excess of 1 Gm. is not recommended. Side effects are similar to those of other sulfonylurea drugs.

Chlorpropamide, U.S.P., B.P. (Diabinese). Chlorpropamide belongs to the sulfonylurea group and has a biologic half-life of 30 to 36 hours. The drug is available in 100- and 250-mg. scored tablets for oral administration. A dosage in excess of 750 mg. daily is not recommended. Side effects are similar to those of other sulfonylurea drugs but may be more severe. The patient must be observed closely during the first 6 weeks of therapy. Hypersensitivity reactions may occur and are an indication for discontinuation of the drug. The drug may also prolong the action of sedatives and hypnotics. It is contraindicated in pregnancy, severe hepatic or renal dysfunction, other endocrine dysfunction, and Raynaud's disease.

Phenformin hydrochloride, U.S.P., B.P. (DBI). This is not a sulfonylurea compound but a biguanide derivative. D.E.S.I. rating is *effective* for stable adult diabetes mellitus and in unstable adult and juvenile diabetes in conjunction with insulin. Its exact mode of action has not been clearly defined, but it seems to act by supplementing insulin effects in peripheral utilization of glucose. Its effectiveness requires the presence of some insulin, either exogenous or endogenous. It has been used in combination therapy with sulfonylureas when either drug alone does not produce maximal results. Side effects may include an unpleasant, metallic or bitter taste, anorexia, cramps, nausea, and sometimes vomiting and diarrhea. Phenformin should be withdrawn if vomiting occurs. Phenformin is available for oral administration in 25-mg. tablets and in 50- and 100-mg. extended-release capsules (DBI-TD). Maintenance doses are 50 to 150 mg. daily.

Acetohexamide, U.S.P. (Dymelar). This is a sulfonylurea compound closely related to tolbutamide but about twice as potent. It is available in 250- and 500-mg. scored tablets, and its usual dosage range is from 250 mg. to 1.5 Gm. Dosage in excess of 1.5 Gm. is not recommended. Side effects resemble those of other sulfonylureas.

Side effects and toxic effects. Side effects that have been reported include gastrointestinal upsets, weakness, paresthesia, headache, ringing in the ears, and intolerance to alcohol. A mild type of leukopenia has been reported. Oral hypoglycemic agents may interfere with some enzymatic reactions in the liver, and therefore their use for patients with hepatic damage is not recommended. The incidence of toxicity seems to be low. It is important that the diabetic patient observe dietary restrictions as carefully as when taking insulin. The drugs do not cure diabetes. Some patients develop allergic reactions that may require that administration of the hypoglycemic agent be stopped and that therapy with insulin be resumed. Patients should be carefully instructed concerning the limitations of tolbutamide and other sulfonylureas. Controversy has developed about these drugs since findings from studies indicate that diet and oral hypoglycemic therapy was no more effective than diet alone, and perhaps even less effective, for the prevention of complications and reduction of cardiovascular mortality. Overdosage produces characteristic hypoglycemic reactions.

QUESTIONS

For study and review

1 Name the various tropic hormones produced by the pituitary gland and their target organs.
2 What is meant by "negative feedback"?
3 How are thyroid hormones biosynthesized? How does this knowledge help you to understand thyroid therapy?
4 Explain the physiologic effects of thyroid hormones.
5 What advantage do the synthetic thyroid preparations have over desiccated thyroid?

6 What adverse effects can occur with radioactive iodine?
7 Explain the difference in physiologic action of glucocorticoids and the mineralocorticoids.
8 What adverse effects can occur with the use of hydrocortisone or cortisone?
9 What side effects occur with insulin preparations; when are they most likely to appear?
10 Prepare a teaching plan for the patient who must be maintained on steroid therapy.
11 Explain why some patients with diabetes mellitus require insulin injections while others are controlled with oral hypoglycemic agents.
12 Why would administration of corticosteroids be contraindicated during pregnancy?

Multiple choice

13 Which of the following preparations would you expect to see prescribed for a patient with myxedema?
   a. iodized salt
   b. Lugol's Solution
   c. radioactive iodine
   d. thyroid tablets
14 Effective therapy with ACTH is dependent upon a normal state of function of which of the following?
   a. thyroid gland
   b. adrenal gland
   c. islands of Langerhans
   d. anterior lobe of pituitary gland
15 Insulin must be administered parenterally for which of the following reasons?
   a. it acts more promptly when given parenterally
   b. oral administration of insulin is most likely to cause gastrointestinal irritation
   c. insulin is subject to destruction by proteolytic enzymes in the digestive tract
   d. insulin is not well absorbed from the gastrointestinal tract
16 A patient receiving insulin for diabetes mellitus is receiving a form of therapy that can be compared to which of the following?
   a. thyroid for cretinism
   b. streptomycin for tuberculosis
   c. cortisone for rheumatoid arthritis
   d. morphine for severe pain
17 Which of the following constitutes a significant side effect in a patient receiving cortisone?
   a. emotional instability
   b. polyuria
   c. increased appetite
   d. pigmentation of the skin
18 Prednisone differs from cortisone in which of the following respects? It is less likely to:
   a. cause retention of water and salt
   b. inhibit healing of tissues
   c. produce symptoms of hypercortisonism
   d. bring about depression of the adrenal cortex
19 One of your patients has rheumatoid arthritis for which her doctor has prescribed daily doses of aspirin. If she

says to you: "I don't understand why my doctor only gives me aspirin; why can't I have a medicine like cortisone?" which of the following statements would you consider most appropriate and helpful?

a. Cortisone is prescribed by many physicians, but your physician probably wants to take a conservative approach to your problem.

b. Cortisone can be a dangerous drug and can produce many undesirable side effects.

c. For the pain associated with rheumatism and arthritis, aspirin is considered one of the safest and best drugs on the market.

d. Cortisone is a relatively expensive drug whereas aspirin is inexpensive.

REFERENCES

Cope, C. L.: Adrenal steroids and disease, Philadelphia, 1972, J. B. Lippincott Co.

David, D. S., Grieco, M. H., and Cushman, P.: Adrenal glucocorticoids after twenty years, J. Chronic Dis. **22:**637, 1970.

Editorial: Treatment of acute hypercalcemia, Lancet **2:**314, 1972.

Editorial: Somatotrophin and somatomedin, Lancet **2:**469, 1972.

Editorial: Thyrotoxicosis in pregnancy, Lancet **1:**886, 1972.

Editorial: Thyrotropin-releasing hormone and depression, Lancet **2:**1015, 1972.

Editorial: Iodide-induced thyrotoxicosis, Lancet **2:**1072, 1972.

F. Raymond Keating Jr. Memorial Symposium: Hyperparathyroidism 1970, Am. J. Med. **50:**557, 1971.

Fleischer, N., and Guillemin, R.: Clinical applications of hypothalamic releasing factors, Adv. Intern. Med. **18:**303, 1972.

Fries, J. F., and McDevitt, H. O.: Systemic corticosteroid therapy in rheumatic diseases, Rational Drug. Ther. **6:**1, 1972.

Frohman, L. A.: Clinical neuropharmacology of hypothalamic releasing factors, New Eng. J. Med. **286:**1391, 1972.

Fulmer, D. H., and others: Treatment of hypercalcemia, Arch. Intern. Med. **129:**923, 1972.

Glorieux, F. H., and others: Prevention of dwarfism and rickets in X-linked hypophosphatemia, New Eng. J. Med. **287:**481, 1972.

Greaves, M. W.: The pharmacological basis for the rational use of typically applied corticosteroids, Pharmacol. Physicians **3**(10):1, 1969.

Grunt, J. Q., and others: Acute and long-term responses to human growth hormone in children with idiopathic small-for-dates dwarfish, J. Clin. Endocrinol. **35:**157, 1972.

Heller, H., and Pickering, B. T., editors: Pharmacology of the endocrine system and related drugs, New York, 1970, Pergamon Press.

Hoch, F. L.: The pharmacologic basis for the clinical use of thyroid hormones, Pharmacol. Physicians **4**(4):1, 1970.

Kadowitz, P. J., and Yard, A. C.: Influence of hydrocortisone on cardiovascular responses to epinephrine, Europ. J. Pharmacol. **13:**281, 1971.

Larsen, P. R.: Triiodothyronine: Review of recent studies of its physiology and pathophysiology in man, Metabolism **21:**1073, 1972.

Levy, G. S.: Catecholamine sensitivity, thyroid hormone and the heart, Am. J. Med. **50:**413, 1971.

Liberti, P., and Stanbury, J. B.: The pharmacology of substances affecting the thyroid gland, Am. Rev. Pharmacol. **11:**113, 1971.

McCann, S. M., and Porter, J. C.: Hypothalamic pituitary stimulating and inhibiting hormones, Physiol. Rev. **49:**240, 1969.

Melby, J. C.: Assessment of adrenocortical function, New Eng. J. Med. **285:**735, 1971.

Mills, L. C.: Corticosteroids in endotoxic shock, Proc. Soc. Exp. Biol. Med. **138:**507, 1971.

O'Malley, B. W.: Mechanisms of action of steroid hormones, New Eng. J. Med. **284:**370, 1971.

Prange, A. J., and others: Effect of thyrotropin-releasing hormone in depression, Lancet **2:**999, 1972.

Raisz, L. G.: Parathyroid gland metabolism, Arch. Intern. Med. **124:**389, 1969.

Reichlin, S.: Anterior pituitary—six glands and one, New Eng. J. Med. **287:**1351, 1972.

Rosenberg, I. N.: Evaluation of thyroid function, New. Eng. J. Med. **286:**924, 1972.

Senior, R. M., and Birge, S. J.: The recognition and management of myxedema coma, J.A.M.A. **217:**61, 1971.

Sutherland, E. W.: Studies on the mechanism of hormone action, Science **177:**401, 1972.

Talmage, R. V., and Munson, P. L., editors: Calcium, parathyroid hormone and the calcitonins, Amsterdam, 1972, Excerpta Medica.

Tashjian, A. H.: Soft bones, hard facts and calcitonin therapy, New Eng. J. Med. **283:**593, 1970.

Thorn, G. W., and Lauler, D. P.: Clinical therapeutics of adrenal disorders, Am. J. Med. **53:**673, 1972.

Utiger, R. D.: The diverse effects of iodide on thyroid function, New Eng. J. Med. **287:**562, 1972.

Vagenakis, A. G., and others: Iodide-induced thyrotoxicosis in Boston, New Eng. J. Med. **287:**523, 1972.

Volpe, R.: The immunologic basis of Grave's disease, New Eng. J. Med. **287:**463, 1972.

Walton, J., Watson, B. S., and Ney, R. L.: Alternate-day vs shorter interval steroid administration, Arch. Int. Med. **126:**601, 1970.

Wartofsky, L., Rausil, B. J., and Ingbar, S. H.: Inhibition by iodine of the release of thyroxine from the thyroid glands of patients with thyrotoxicosis, J. Clin. Invest. **49:**78, 1970.

Werner, S. C., editor: The thyroid: A fundamental and clinical text, ed. 3, New York, 1971, Harper & Row, Publishers.

Wilson, I. C., and others: Thyroid hormone enhancement of imipramine in nonretarded depressions, New Eng. J. Med. **282:**1063, 1970.

Zellman, H. E.: Hyperthyroidism, Med. Clin. N. Am. **56:**717, 1972.

CHAPTER 26

Sex hormones

Drugs that affect the myometrium

Drugs that increase uterine motility
Drugs that decrease uterine motility

Sex hormones that affect the ovaries

Pituitary gonadotropic hormones
Gonadotropic hormones of placental origin
Ovarian hormones

Male sex hormones

The reproductive system of the female consists of the ovaries, uterine (fallopian) tubes, uterus, and the vagina; in the male, it consists of the testes, seminal vesicles, prostate gland, the bulbourethral glands, and the penis. The reproductive organs of both the male and the female are largely under the control of the endocrine glands, especially the pituitary gland. The ovaries and testes are known as gonads and not only produce ova and sperm cells but also form endocrine secretions that initiate and maintain the secondary sexual characteristics in men and women. When gonadal function diminishes and finally ceases, the secondary sexual characteristics gradually change and reproductive function ceases. The period of change is marked in women by the cessation of menses and is known as the menopause. In men, diminution of output of the sex hormone also occurs in later life, but it is less clearly definable and is sometimes called the male climacteric.

Drugs that affect the myometrium

The uterus is a highly muscular organ that exhibits a number of characteristic properties and activities. The smooth muscle fibers extend longitudinally, circularly, and obliquely in the organ. The uterus has a rich blood supply, but when the uterine muscle contracts, blood flow is diminished. Profound changes occur in the uterus during pregnancy. The human uterus increases in weight during pregnancy from about 50 Gm. to approximately 1000 Gm. Its capacity increases tenfold in length, and new muscle fibers may be formed. These changes are accompanied by changes in response to drugs. Since the uterine smooth muscle responds sensitively to many drugs, the uterus of virgin guinea pigs or rabbits is used in standardizing a number of drugs that have a stimulating action on smooth muscle.

The uterus, both in situ and when excised, contracts rhythmically. Both pendular and peri-

585

staltic movements may be seen. In nongravid animals, peristaltic movements are relatively slight and, just as in the intestine, pauses occur between peristaltic contractions. These peristaltic movements vary greatly with the condition of sexual activity. Movements are depressed early in pregnancy but increase later. Parturition is accomplished by powerful peristaltic waves, which cause labor pains.

Drugs that act upon the uterus include (1) those that increase the motility of the uterus and (2) those that decrease uterine motility.

DRUGS THAT INCREASE UTERINE MOTILITY
OXYTOCICS

In the human being, stimulation of either the sympathetic or the parasympathetic division of the autonomic nervous system may bring about increased uterine contractions. However, the response of the human uterus to cholinergic or adrenergic drugs is not dependable. There are drugs that exert a selective action on the smooth muscle of the uterus; these drugs are known as oxytocics. The ones used most are alkaloids of ergot and synthetic oxytocin, although there are many other drugs that may exhibit some effect on uterine motility.

Oxytocin

Oxytocin is one of two hormones secreted by the posterior pituitary; the other hormone is vasopressin (antidiuretic hormone, ADH). Both are peptides containing eight amino acids. Because of the similarity in their structures, oxytocin has some vasopressor activity and vasopressin some oxytocic activity.

Oxytocin means "rapid birth," derived from its ability to contract the pregnant uterus. It also facilitates milk ejection during lactation.

The nonpregnant uterus is relatively insensitive to oxytocin but during pregnancy uterine sensitivity to oxytocin gradually increases, with the uterus being most sensitive at the termination of pregnancy. Oxytocin secretion may precede and possibly trigger delivery of the fetus. Large amounts of oxytocin have been detected in the blood during the expulsive phase of delivery. It is believed that oxytocin is released in response to stretching of the uterine cervix and vagina. A positive feedback mechanism may be operant; that is, more forceful contractions of uterine muscle and greater stretching of the cervix and vagina resulting in more oxytocin release. Oxytocin acts directly on the myometrium, having a stronger effect on the fundus than on the cervix.

Suckling and auditory or visual stimuli related to suckling, such as the mother seeing her baby or hearing it cry, causes release of oxytocin, which in turn causes contraction of the smooth muscle of the mammary gland and milk ejection (a conditioned reflex).

Oxytocin is also released during coitus, and it has been suggested that this may facilitate the transport of sperm from the vagina into the fallopian tubes for fertilization. The role of oxytocin in the male is not known.

Preparation, dosage, and administration. *Oxytocin injection, synthetic,* U.S.P., B.P. (Pitocin, Syntocinon, Uteracon) is used to induce active labor or to increase the force and rate of existing contractions during delivery when they are not strong enough to bring about expulsion of the fetus. It is also used to contract uterine muscle and decrease hemorrhage after delivery of the placenta. Occasionally it is used to promote milk ejection when ineffective ejection is believed to be a cause of inadequacy of breast feeding.

Oxytocin injection is available in ampules containing 5 U.S.P. units of oxytocin in 0.5 ml., and 10 units in 1 ml. It is also available as buccal tablets containing 200 units of oxytocin citrate, and as a nasal spray containing 40 units of synthetic oxytocin per milliliter.

Oxytocin can be given by intravenous, intramuscular, subcutaneous, intranasal, or sublingual routes. Intravenous infusion dose is 1 ml. of oxytocin added to 500 or 1000 ml. of 5% dextrose or normal saline and infused at a rate initially of 0.5 to 0.75 ml. per minute. Rate is carefully increased until an optimal uterine response is obtained (three or four contractions of good quality in 10 minutes). The infusion should be stopped or the rate of flow decreased if change in fetal heart tones occurs, contractions become excessive, or there is poor relaxation of the uterus.

For intravenous injection for emergency treatment of postpartum bleeding, 0.6 to 1.8 units (0.06 to 0.18 ml.) of oxytocin is diluted with 3 to 5 ml. of sodium chloride and slowly injected. Effects occur in 15 to 60 seconds.

For intramuscular injection to control postpartum bleeding dose is 3 to 10 units (0.3 to 1 ml.). Effects by this route appear in 3 to 7 minutes and persist for 30 to 60 minutes.

Buccal administration consists of placing one or more tablets in the buccal space (inner cheek) every 30 minutes until the desired uterine response is obtained or a total of 15 tablets (3,000 units) has been given. This method of administration is less precise and less reliable than intravenous administration, since rate of absorption is unpredictable. However, continuous, careful supervision is vital.

The nasal spray is used to promote milk ejection for breast feeding. Dose is one spray into one or both nostrils 2 to 3 minutes before nursing.

Contraindications. Oxytocin is usually contraindicated during the first stage of labor. If used when the cervix is undilated and rigid, severe laceration and excessive trauma are likely to occur. It is contraindicated in malpresentation of the fetus, severe toxemia, fetal distress, severe medical conditions (e.g., cardiovascular disease), and predisposition to uterine rupture (multiparas, previous cesarean section, or uterine surgery).

Side effects and toxic effects. Synthetic oxytocin produces fewer side effects and is less toxic than the older (now obsolete) preparation from the posterior pituitary of domesticated animals. The synthetic preparation lacks the vasopressin and protein components.

Water intoxication may occur when large doses of oxytocin have been infused for long periods. Allergic reactions may occur. When used injudiciously, oxytocin can cause maternal death due to uterine rupture, hypertensive crisis, and cerebral hemorrhage. Pelvic hematomas, bradycardia, and arrhythmias also occur. Arrhythmias may also occur in the fetus, and fetal deaths have been reported.

Oxytocin and related drugs should be used only in the hospital and only with continuous medical supervision.

Constant observation is required. This means the blood pressure should be taken frequently, careful and periodic check of the fetal heart tones should be made, and the strength and duration of uterine contractions should be noted. Prolonged contractions of the uterus result in diminished blood flow and decreased oxygen for the fetus.

Ergot

Ergot is the dried sclerotium (mycelium) of the parasitic fungus *Claviceps purpurea*, which grows on many species of grain but especially on rye, where it forms long black bodies on the ears of the rye. It is especially prevalent when the weather is moist and warm. It grows in the grain fields of North America and Europe. Ergot was known as an obstetric herb to midwives long before it was recognized by the medical profession. Today ergot growth is carried out in fermentation vats in factories.

Lysergic acid

Active constituents. Both levorotatory and dextrorotatory alkaloids have been isolated from ergot, but only the levorotatory compounds are pharmacologically significant. These are derivatives of lysergic acid and their basic structure is that of lysergic acid. The individual ergot alkaloids are all compounds in which substitutions have been made at the carboxyl group.

The entire large group of individual alkaloids derived from ergot can be further divided into three groups: the ergotamine group, the ergotoxine group, and the ergobasine group. Members of each group have certain common chemical features and certain common pharmacologic actions. The first two have a peptide chain substituted at the carboxyl group of lysergic acid, whereas alkaloids of the ergobasine group are chemically simpler and contain a relatively small side chain, that of an amino alcohol. In ergonovine, alaninol is linked to lysergic acid (see structural formula).

Ergonovine

Pharmacologic actions. Ergot alkaloids have three major actions in the body: smooth muscle stimulation (particularly of blood vessels and the uterus), adrenergic blockade, and central nervous system effects.

1 *Smooth muscle stimulation.* All smooth muscle is stimulated by the ergot alkaloids. The action is a direct one. This action is pronounced in the natural alkaloids but reduced in the hydrogenated derivatives.

   a. *Oxytocic effect.* Like oxytocin, the ergot alkaloids stimulate contractions of the uterine muscle in the pregnant uterus. In early stages of pregnancy the uterus is not very sensitive to the alkaloids, therefore, they cannot be used as abortifacients. During the third trimester uterine sensitivity increases. Oxytocin is used for induction and stimulation of labor. Ergonovine and methylergonovine are drugs of choice for the prevention of postpartum bleeding. Reduction of bleeding results from contraction of the uterine wall around the bleeding vessels at the placental site. Very high doses cause sustained uterine contracture.

   b. *Vasoconstriction.* All blood vessels are constricted by ergot alkaloids with the larger arteries being the most sensitive. Arteries may show localized narrowings and even occlusions, which may lead to thrombosis and gangrene. Ergotamine is used in the treatment of migraine head-ache for its vasoconstricting effect on cerebral vessels, but decreased flow in peripheral, mesenteric, and coronary arteries can result in ischemia of the respective tissues.

   In large doses, ergot alkaloids cause a definite rise in blood pressure. This is more likely to be evoked in hypertensive women than in those with normal blood pressure.

2 *Adrenergic blockade.* In high doses the ergot alkaloids block the vasoconstricting action of the catecholamines (norepinephrine) in laboratory animals. However, this effect does not occur with therapeutic doses in humans.

3 *Central nervous system effects.* The dehydrogenated alkaloids inhibit sympathetic activity and produce a slight fall in blood pressure and bradycardia. These alkaloids also have a tranquilizing action similar to that of reserpine. At one time they were used to treat agitated psychotics before the advent of the tranquilizers.

Preparation, dosage, and administration

Ergonovine maleate, N.F. (Ergotrate); *ergometrine maleate,* B.P.; *methylergonovine maleate,* N.F. (Methergine); *methylergometrine maleate,* B.P. These preparations are used primarily after delivery of the placenta to produce firm uterine contractions and to decrease uterine bleeding. They are also used for postabortal hemorrhage and during the puerperium to hasten involution of the uterus. They can be given orally since they are readily absorbed from the gastrointestinal tract. Effects occur 2 to 5 minutes after intramuscular injection and 3 to 5 minutes after oral administration.

Both preparations are available in 1-ml. ampules containing 0.2 mg. per milliliter and as tablets containing 0.2 mg. Usual intramuscular dose is 0.2 mg., which may be repeated in 2 to 4 hours. Usual oral dose is 0.2 mg. three or four times a day usually for 2 days (maximum, 1 week). Intravenous route may be used in emergency situations, but this carries a high risk and the patient should be monitored.

Side effects. These are uncommon but may include nausea and vomiting, dizziness, headache, cramps, dyspnea, and chest pain. Allergic reactions have been reported. Elevated blood pressure and bradycardia may occur; these are less frequent and less pronounced with methylergonovine than with ergonovine. Increased sensitivity to ergot alkaloids is seen in hepatic disease (the liver probably metabolizes the drug), and febrile and septic states.

Contraindications. These drugs are contraindicated in obliterative vascular disease, liver disease, kidney disease, toxemia, and hypertension. They are also contraindicated for induction of labor and threatened spontaneous abortion.

Prolonged use is not recommended since ergotism may develop, although authenticated reports of its occurrence have not been published.

PROSTAGLANDINS

Prostaglandins evidently play a key role in regulating intracellular processes, and clinical studies indicate that prostaglandins are important in the physiology of labor. In some animals, such as sheep, prostaglandins appear prior to the onset of labor and not as a consequence of it. Karim, in 1968, successfully induced term labor with prostaglandins using PGF_2 or PGE_2. Additional studies have shown conflicting results, which may have been due to study design. More refined studies using an inducibility score indicate prostaglandin F_2 is just as effective as synthetic oxytocin for inducing term labor in women with similar degrees of inducibility. No significant effects on maternal vital signs occurred; there were no gastrointestinal symptoms or blood loss, and no adverse effects were noted in the infant. However, uterine hyperstimulation can occur following prostaglandin administration.

Prostaglandins are also being investigated as abortifacients with mixed results. A major drawback is the occurrence of undesirable side effects.

Inhibition of ovulation with prostaglandins is also under investigation at the present time.

Dinoprost tromethamine ($PGF_2\alpha$-THAM, Prostaglandin F_2 Alpha Tromethamine, Prostin F2 alpha)

Dinoprost is the tromethamine salt of the naturally occurring compound, prostaglandin F_2 alpha ($PGF_2\alpha$). It produces contraction of the gravid uterus similar to that of the term uterus during labor. Contractions are usually adequate for delivery; however, dinoprost-induced abortion may be incomplete. It is believed that the drug acts directly on the myometrium. Dinoprost also stimulates gastrointestinal smooth muscle; large doses cause bronchoconstriction, hypertension, and alteration in heart beat.

After administration, dinoprost is widely distributed in the maternal and fetal bodies. It is rapidly metabolized in the maternal lungs and liver. Metabolites of the drug are excreted within 24 hours, primarily via the urine.

Investigationally, dinoprost has been administered intravenously and orally for induction of term labor; for evacuation of the uterus in missed abortion, fetal death in late pregnancy, and hydatidiform mole; and as a contraceptive agent.

Preparation, dosage, and administration. Dinoprost is available for injection in 4- and 8-ml. ampules containing 5 mg. of drug per milliliter. Dinoprost is approved by the F.D.A. for intraamniotic instillation to terminate pregnancy during the second trimester. Before injecting the drug, 1 ml. of amniotic fluid should be withdrawn by transabdominal tap. If the amniotic fluid contains blood, dinoprost should not be administered.

After intraamniotic instillation of 40 mg. of dinoprost, maximum plasma level of the drug occurs in about 2 hours. Half-life of the drug in amniotic fluid is 3 to 6 hours, while its plasma half-life is reported to be less than 1 minute. Abortion usually occurs in about 20 hours in 50% of patients, with most patients aborting within 48 hours following an initial dose of 40 mg. of dinoprost and 10 to 40 mg. 24 hours later.

Side effects. Vomiting occurs in more than one half of patients; nausea, abdominal cramps, or uterine pain occurs in about one fourth of patients. Diarrhea and lactation, which may last several days, may also occur. Bronchoconstriction, tachycardia, and hypertension can occur if the drug is inadvertently administered into maternal circulation.

The following reactions have been reported: pain, which may be epigastric, substernal, or located in the leg or shoulder; headache; flushing; diaphoresis; coughing and wheezing; convulsions; paresthesias; breast tenderness; hyperventilation; and a burning sensation in the eyes or breasts. Other reactions that have been reported include uterine rupture, urinary retention, bronchospasm, hematuria, polydipsia, and second degree heart block.

Precautions. Dinoprost must be used cautiously in patients with a history of asthma, glaucoma, hypertension, epilepsy, or cardiovascular disease.

If used before the cervix is adequately dilated, cervical perforation or cervicovaginal fistulas may result. Since cervical trauma can occur without symptoms, patients should be carefully examined following uterine evacuation.

Dinoprost is contraindicated in patients with acute pelvic inflammatory disease. Animal studies indicate that dinoprost may be potentially teratogenic.

Drug interactions. Aspirin appears to increase the time interval between administration of dinoprost and abortion, and it may be advisable to avoid use of aspirin when dinoprost has been given.

DRUGS THAT DECREASE UTERINE MOTILITY

There are times when the inhibition of uterine contractions is indicated, as when a patient begins premature labor or when uterine tone is high and contractions are unusually frequent and uncoordinated. Drugs that combat these conditions include certain depressants of the central nervous system.

Ethyl alcohol given intravenously and the beta receptor stimulants metaproterenol (Alupent), ritodrine (Premar), and isoxudrine (Vasodilan) have been used as uterine relaxants with varying degrees of success. The new drug ritodrine, which is under investigation, appears to be a powerful uterine relaxant. Until drugs are clinically available which specifically relax the uterus with minimal side effects, bed rest and sedation will continue to be the most acceptable means for arresting premature labor.

ANALGESICS AND SEDATIVES

Large doses of opiates, general anesthetics, and barbiturates tend to decrease uterine motility.

Average doses of barbiturates probably have little or no effect. Morphine is effective because it not only relieves pain but also alters the patient's emotional reaction to pain, allaying fear and anxiety. Methadone is excellent to relieve pain, but it has no effect on fear and anxiety. Meperidine as compared to morphine has less effect on respiration, although this may not be so when equianalgesic doses of the two drugs are compared. Its analgesic potency is somewhere between that of morphine and codeine. Codeine, especially when combined with aspirin, is useful to relieve the discomfort associated with repair work on the perineum, but it has little use during the course of labor. Promethazine hydrochloride is utilized clinically for obstetric sedation. It relieves apprehension and potentiates the action of drugs such as morphine sulfate and meperidine hydrochloride, permitting a reduction in their dosage.

DRUGS FOR TOXEMIA OF PREGNANCY
Diazoxide, U.S.P. (Hyperstat IV)

Diazoxide, a drug used primarily in the United States for its antihypertensive action, is useful in the treatment of hypertension associated with toxemia of pregnancy. Given as an intravenous bolus of 300 mg. within 10 seconds, diazoxide produces a drastic fall in elevated blood pressure within 5 minutes. The antihypertensive effect usually lasts 4 to 12 hours. It usually does not cause excessive hypotension and does not have a sedative effect. Diazoxide is also a powerful relaxant of the gravid and nongravid uterus, and it may be useful in dysmenorrhea and to arrest premature labor. Diazoxide has a hyperglycemic effect; it acts directly on the beta cells of the pancreas and increases hepatic glucose output. Long-term administration in pregnancy is not recommended since it might be diabetogenic and may have adverse effects on the fetus.

Magnesium sulfate, U.S.P., B.P.

Many students will think of magnesium sulfate as a saline cathartic only. However, when this salt is administered parenterally it not only will depress the central nervous system but also depress all forms of muscular tissue (smooth, skeletal, and cardiac).

When magnesium is administered parenterally in doses sufficient to produce hypermagnesemia (serum magnesium levels greater than 2.5 mEq. per liter), the drug may block peripheral neuromuscular transmission producing anticonvulsant effects. The basic mechanism of action for this effect is not known, but magnesium may inhibit the amount of acetylcholine liberated by motor nerve impulses. Magnesium ions slow the rate of sinoatrial impulse formation and prolong conduction time. Magnesium also produces peripheral vasodilation. Moderate doses produce flushing and sweating; higher doses will lower blood pressure.

Uses. Magnesium sulfate injection is one of the most important drugs in the treatment of convulsive toxemia of pregnancy. It is also effective to counteract uterine tetany that may occur after large doses of oxytocin, or it may be used when the myometrium is contracting abnormally.

Preparation, dosage, and administration. Magnesium sulfate is available for intramuscular or intravenous injection in 10%, 25%, and 50% concentrations. Each gram of magnesium sulfate contains 8.1 mEq. of magnesium. Various dosage schedules have been used for preeclampsia or eclampsia. An initial dose of 4 Gm. of magnesium sulfate in 250 ml. of 5% dextrose may be given intravenously; this dose may be followed by 4 to 5 Gm. intramuscularly into each buttock. Intramuscular doses of 4 to 5 Gm. may then be given at 4-hour intervals as needed, depending on the patient's response. Usual range of dose is 1 to 10 Gm. daily. Determinations should be made of the patient's serum magnesium levels and urinary excretion of magnesium. Effective anticonvulsant serum level ranges from 2.5 to 7.5 mEq. per liter.

When magnesium sulfate is given intravenously, the effect is immediate and duration of action is about 30 minutes. When magnesium sulfate is given intramuscularly, onset of action occurs in about 1 hour and duration of action is 3 to 4 hours. For uterine tetany, 1 to 2 Gm. is usually given intravenously. Intravenous injections should be given slowly and the patient should be observed carefully for signs of magnesium toxicity. An injectable form of calcium, usually 10 to 20 ml. of 10% calcium gluconate, should be readily available for use in case severe central nervous system depression occurs. Calcium is a specific antidote for magnesium toxicity.

Adverse reactions and precautions. Premonitory symptoms of magnesium toxicity include "feeling hot all over" and extreme thirst. Disappearance of the patellar reflex is a useful clinical sign to detect the onset of magnesium toxicity. Patellar reflex loss usually occurs when the serum magnesium level exceeds 4 mEq. per liter.

Adverse effects include flushing, sweating, hypotension, depression of reflexes, flaccid paralysis, hypothermia, circulatory collapse, and depression of cardiac and central nervous system function. The most immediate danger to life is respiratory paralysis; mechanical respiratory assistance may be necessary to support life. Abrupt injection of large doses of magnesium sulfate can cause cardiac arrest. A patient receiving magnesium sulfate parenterally *should never be left alone*. If repeated doses are given, knee jerk reflexes should be tested before each dose and if absent no further magnesium should be given until reflexes return to normal. Respiration rate should be counted before each dose; a rate of sixteen per minute should be present before each dose. In addition, urine output should be 100 ml. or more during the 4 hours prior to each dose.

Intravenous magnesium should not be given during the 2 hours preceding delivery since magnesium may cause neuromuscular or respiratory depression in the infant. Intramuscular magnesium usually does not adversely affect the newborn.

Drug interactions. Additive central nervous system effects occur when narcotics, barbiturates, general anesthetics, or other central nervous system depressants are given concomitantly with magnesium sulfate; thus dosages of these drugs must be carefully adjusted. Excessive neuromuscular blockade can occur if a neuromuscular blocking agent (such as tubocurarine) is given to a patient receiving parenteral magnesium sulfate. In digitalized patients, if calcium is used to treat magnesium toxicity, heart block may occur and extreme caution is required.

Sex hormones that affect the ovaries

The hormones concerned with ovarian function include the *anterior pituitary hormones*, which are required for the normal development and function of the gonads; the *gonadotropic hormones* of placental origin; and the *ovarian hormones* themselves. The ovarian hormones include the naturally occurring steroids, the synthetic and partly synthetic steroids, and the nonsteroid compounds, such as stilbestrol, which have an ovarian hormone-like function.

A similar group of hormones plays corresponding roles in regulating gonadal growth and function in the male.

PITUITARY GONADOTROPIC HORMONES

The endocrine gland that exerts the chief gonadotropic influence in the body is the anterior lobe of the pituitary gland. How many hormones are made by this gland is uncertain, but three are believed to have an effect on the ovary. One stimulates the development of the graafian follicle and is known as the follicle-stimulating hormone (FSH). Another, the luteinizing hormone (LH) or interstitial cell-stimulating hormone (ICSH), promotes the growth of the interstitial cells in the follicle and the formation of the corpus luteum. A third hormone is known as the luteotropic hormone (LTH); it is probably identical with the lactogenic hormone. The follicle-stimulating hormone initiates the cycle of events in the ovary. Under the influence of both FSH and LH the graafian follicle grows, matures, secretes estrogen, ovulates, and forms the corpus luteum. The LTH promotes the secretory activity of the corpus luteum and the formation of

progesterone. In the absence of LTH the corpus luteum undergoes regressive changes and fails to make progesterone.

In the male, FSH acts only on the seminiferous tubules and promotes the formation of sperm cells. ICSH stimulates the interstitial cells in the testes and promotes the formation of androgen.

The clinical use of the pituitary gonadotropic hormones has been handicapped by the lack of sufficiently refined preparations. Commercial preparations often contain other proteins and inert substances that make injections painful and make allergic reactions possible.

Some degree of success has accompanied the use of these gonadotropic extracts when used in the treatment of amenorrhea, Frohlich's syndrome, sterility, undescended testicle (cryptorchidism), and hypogenitalism. Lack of success in treatment can sometimes be attributed to the fact that when a deficiency of one of the pituitary hormones exists, it is more than likely that there is a deficiency in a number of others that may not be of a direct gonadotropic nature.

There are no official gonadotropic preparations from the anterior pituitary gland.

NONPITUITARY GONADOTROPIC HORMONES

Gonadotropic substances are formed by the placenta during pregnancy in the human being and in certain animals. Human chorionic gonadotropic hormone (HCG) differs from pituitary gonadotropins, both biologically and chemically. It produces little of the follicle-stimulating effect but affects principally the growth of the interstitial cells and the secretion of luteal hormone. In women, it is capable of prolonging the luteal phase of the menstrual cycle. Its normal role seems to be to enhance and to prolong the secretion of the corpus luteum during early pregnancy. It does not initiate the formation of corpus luteum, nor does it appear to be able to restore a regressing corpus luteum.

In the male, it stimulates the interstitial cells

of the testes, causing them to increase production of androgen, which in turn promotes the growth and development of accessory sex organs.

Chorionic gonadotropin has also been found in the blood of pregnant mares, but the human chorionic gonadotropin is preferred therapeutically because, since it is of human origin, it does not induce the formation of antihormones in the patient. It is believed to be the substance that forms the basis of some pregnancy tests (Friedman and Aschheim-Zondek). This substance was originally thought to come from the anterior pituitary gland, but it is now recognized as coming from the placenta. The reason that the urine of pregnancy can be used to test for the gravid state is that the laboratory animal used for this test is usually a rodent, and in these animals the chorionic gonadotropic factor stimulates growth of the follicle as well as the corpus luteum.

Uses. Human chorionic gonadotropin (HCG) has received a D.E.S.I. rating of *effective* for treatment of cryptorchidism not due to anatomical obstruction and in selected cases of male hypogonadism secondary to pituitary failure; *possibly effective* in the treatment of sterility due to defective luteal function; and *ineffective* menstrual disorders, female hypogenitalism, and threatened and habitual abortions.

Preparation, dosage, and administration

Chorionic gonadotropin, U.S.P., B.P. (Follutein, Pregnyl, Antuitrin-S, APL). Chorionic gonadotropin is a water-soluble gonadotropic substance and placental hormone obtained from the urine of pregnant women. It is a glycoprotein containing about 12% galactose. It is available in vials containing 5000, 10,000, and 20,000 units. One unit is equal to the gonadotropic activity of 1 mg. of the international standard powder of chorionic gonadotropin.

Dosage for cryptorchidism in boys and hypogonadism in men is 4000 I.U. three times weekly for 3 weeks. Therapy in boys should be discontinued if there is evidence of precocious sexual maturity. Dosage for anovulation is 8000 to 10,000 I.U. Chorionic gonadotropin is given intramuscularly, but never intravenously.

Adverse reactions to HCG include headache, irritability, restlessness, edema, depression, tiredness, precocious puberty, gynecomastia, and pain at the injection site.

Menotropins (Pergonal)

Menotropins is a purified preparation of gonadotropic hormones extracted from the urine of postmenopausal women. It is also known as human menopausal gonadotropin (HMG). It contains both luteinizing (LH) and follicle-stimulating hormones (FSH) in a 1:1 ratio, 75 I.U. of each hormone. Menotropins is used to promote follicular growth and maturation in women with secondary anovulation. To induce ovulation, therapy with menotropins must be followed by the administration of human chorionic gonadotropin (HCG). The dose is 75 I.U. of FSH and 75 I.U. of LH given intramuscularly daily for 9 to 12 days, followed by 10,000 units of HCG 1 day after the last dose of menotropins. If there is evidence of ovulation but no pregnancy, this dosage regimen may be repeated for two more courses before the dose is increased to 150 I.U. of FSH and 150 I.U. of LH daily for 9 to 12 days followed by 10,000 I.U. of HCG 1 day later. The same dose may be repeated for two or more courses if there is evidence of ovulation but no pregnancy.

There is marked variability in individual responses to menotropins. Monitoring of urinary estrogen permits the clinician to determine the dose and duration of treatment according to the patient's response. Pregnancy occurs in 20 to 45% of patients within four to six treatment cycles. Although a higher pregnancy rate is obtained with larger doses, the degree of hyperstimulation is also greater. To prevent hyperstimulation, HCG should be withheld when the urinary estrogen level is higher than 150 µg. in 24 hours. Abortions occur in about 25% of the patients. Daily intercourse should be engaged in from the day before HCG is administered until ovulation occurs.

Adverse effects and precautions. Adverse effects include nausea and vomiting, diarrhea, and fever. Mild hyperstimulation is evidenced by ovarian enlargement, flatulence, and abdominal discomfort which usually lasts 1 to 3 weeks and requires no treatment. Severe hyperstimulation, which usually occurs within 2 weeks after therapy, is evidenced by weight gain, ascites, pleural effusion, oliguria, hypotension, and hypercoagulability, for which hospitalization is required. These patients should have daily determinations of fluid intake and output, body weight, hematocrit, serum and urinary electrolytes, and urinary specific gravity. Patients with significant ovarian enlargement following ovulation should refrain from sexual intercourse due to the danger of hemoperitoneum from ruptured ovarian cysts. Ovarian rupture with intraperitoneal hemorrhage may require surgery.

The patient and her husband should be informed about complications from menotropins and about the frequency and potential hazards of multiple births. Reports on the incidence of multiple births ranges from 17 to 53%.

Menotropins is contraindicated in patients with overt thyroid and adrenal dysfunction, infertility other than secondary ovarian failure, abnormal vaginal bleeding of undetermined cause, ovarian cysts, and pregnancy.

OVARIAN HORMONES

The ovaries are the female sex glands that are situated on either side of the uterus. They not only develop and periodically discharge the ripened ova but also secrete the ovarian hormones.

One of the ovarian hormones is made by the cells of the graafian follicle and is referred to as the follicular hormone. The other is the luteal hormone made by the cells of the corpus luteum. Normal development and activity of the reproductive organs are dependent in part on the right state of balance between these hormones. They are secreted in sequence under the influence of the gonadotropins of the anterior pituitary gland.

Estrogens

The follicular hormone is responsible for the development of the sex organs at puberty and for the secondary sex characteristics—the growth and distribution of hair, texture of skin, distribution of body fat, growth of the breasts, and character of the voice and the maintenance of

these characteristics throughout adult life. The follicular hormone apparently exists not as an entity but as a number of related polymorphic forms that differ in their activity. These substances, which exhibit similar estrogenic activity, are called estrogens. The group includes both the natural estrogens and the synthetic substances that have similar effects in the body.

Chemistry. The naturally occurring estrogens are steroids in which ring "A" (ring at the lower left of the accompanying formula) is a benzene (aromatic ring) in place of the saturated ring of the other major steroids. (Compare formulas with those of the adrenal steroids in Chapter 25.) The primary natural estrogen believed to be secreted by the follicle is estradiol (estrin), so named for the two hydroxyl groups.

Estradiol

Estrone

Both estrone (Theelin) and estradiol are naturally occurring estrogens. In the body, estrone can be converted into estradiol and vice versa. There are a number of other naturally occurring estrogens.

The synthetic estrogens include both *steroid* and *nonsteroid* forms. The steroid forms include modifications of the naturally occurring steroid estrogens so as to increase potency (ethinyl estrogens). The more important group, however, consists of the nonsteroid synthetic estrogen compounds that do not closely resemble the natural estrogens chemically yet have remarkably similar pharmacologic action. A typical member of this group is diethylstilbestrol.

$$HO-\!\!\!\bigcirc\!\!\!-\overset{\underset{|}{CH_2}}{\underset{CH_3}{C}}=\overset{\underset{|}{CH_2}}{\underset{CH_3}{C}}-\!\!\!\bigcirc\!\!\!-OH$$

Diethylstilbestrol

Natural estrogenic substances are found in a variety of places in both plants and animals. They are found in the blood of both sexes, testicular fluid, feces, bile, and the urine of pregnant women and pregnant mares. Estrogens have also been found and isolated from the adrenal gland. These substances vary somewhat chemically in accordance with the source from which they are obtained.

Pharmacologic action and result. When estrogenic substances (natural or synthetic) are injected into immature animals such as rats, they are capable of hastening sexual maturity and producing estrus. In these animals the vaginal epithelium changes after the administration of estrogens and appears as it does in mature animals. This is the basis of bioassay and standardization of preparations of these substances.

When estrogens are administered in doses that compare favorably with the amount normally secreted by the ovaries, the effect is like that produced by the natural secretion of these glands. When estrogens are administered in larger amounts than these, however, other effects may be produced.

One effect is that of inhibiting hyperactivity of the pituitary gland. Increased activity of the pituitary gland is believed to occur at menopause or after surgical removal of the ovaries. This may cause symptoms such as flushing, sweating, and hot flashes. The administration of estrogen prevents hyperactivity of the pituitary gland at least temporarily or while the estrogen continues to be given.

When estrogens are administered, the same changes occur in the myometrium and endometrium as occur naturally; the myometrium and endometrium proliferate (cells reproduce rapidly). When the estrogen is withdrawn, uterine bleeding frequently occurs. It sometimes occurs even with continued administration of the estrogen.

Estrogens naturally stimulate the development of the breasts, that is, the development of the ducts in the gland and possibly both the ducts and the alveoli. Whether this occurs as a direct action on the mammary gland or because of indirect effect on the pituitary gland is not clear. Estrogens are known to inhibit the secretion of milk.

Estrogens exhibit effects in other parts of the body, such as the skeletal system. Large doses inhibit the development of the long bones by causing premature closure of the epiphyses and by preventing the formation of bone from cartilage (endochondral bone formation). On the other hand, some aspects of the bone formation are augmented by the presence of estrogens, and when these substances are lacking osteoporosis may develop, such as is seen in women after menopause.

Estrogens resemble the hormones made in the adrenal cortex in that large doses affect water and electrolyte balance and are prone to cause retention of sodium and development of edema. Their ability to do this is much less significant than that of the adrenal steroid hormones, however. It is known that the estrogen level in the blood is high just prior to menstruation, and at this time retention of water and electrolytes is recognized as a cause of gain in weight.

Some of the responses to estrogens in the body can be antagonized by the administration of androgens (male hormones), and the reverse is also true.

Uses. Estrogens are used for a variety of conditions in which there is a deficiency of these substances, such as to relieve certain symptoms associated with menopause. At the time of menopause the normal endocrine balance is disturbed by the gradual cessation of ovarian function. The pituitary gland apparently attempts to compensate for the lack of ovarian activity by temporary hyperfunction. Symptoms caused by this compensatory reaction respond well to estrogenic therapy because large doses of ovarian hormones depress the secretion of the gonadotropic hormones of the anterior pituitary. Vasomotor disturbances and headache can often be relieved. Symptoms that are of psychic origin do not respond to this type of therapy as a rule. The estrogenic substances may be administered orally, intravaginally, or parenterally. Both the dosage and the method of administration must be decided in relation to each individual patient. Postmenopausal osteoporosis has also been treated with estrogens with symptomatic but not roentgenographically visible benefit.

Senile vaginitis and kraurosis vulvae respond well to estrogen therapy. Some lower urinary tract infections that are part of postmenopausal atrophy have also been successfully treated with estrogens.

A major use of estrogens is in contraceptive therapy. See p. 600.

Functional uterine bleeding, failure of ovarian development, and acne have been known to exhibit positive responses to estrogen therapy.

Estrogens are also used to relieve engorgement of the breasts in a postpartum patient when lactation is to be suppressed. Administration of estrogens is believed to suppress the formation of the lactogenic hormone made by the pituitary gland.

Estrogenic material may serve as a substitute for castration for the relief of discomfort associated with prostatic carcinoma and its metastasis. Limited palliative effect has also been noted in postmenopausal women who have inoperable breast cancer with metastasis to the soft tissues.

Natural estrogens—preparation, dosage, and administration

Estrone, N.F. (Theelin, Menformon). Estrone is a crystalline estrogenic substance that is marketed in 1- and 5-ml. ampules or 10- and 15-ml. vials containing estrone in oil or aqueous suspension. The concentration varies from 1 mg. per milliliter for the preparation in oil and from 1 to 5 mg. per milliliter for the aqueous suspension. Estrone is also available in vaginal suppositories containing 0.2 mg. of the drug; dose is one suppository daily. For menopausal symptoms the drug is usually administered intramuscularly in doses of 0.1 to 1.5 mg. weekly in single or divided doses. For dysfunctional uterine bleeding dose is 2 to 5 mg. daily until bleeding is controlled.

Piperazine estrone sulfate (Ogen). This preparation has the same actions and uses as estrone. It is administered orally. Tablets containing 0.75, 1.5, and 3.0 mg. are available. For the control of menopausal symptoms the dosage is usually 1.5 to 3.0 mg. daily; for the treatment of senile vaginitis and pruritus vulvae, 1.5 to 4.5 mg.; for breast engorgement, 4.5 mg. at intervals of 4 hours for five doses; for dysfunctional uterine bleeding, 3.75 to 7.5 mg. daily until flow ceases.

Estradiol, N.F. (Aquadiol, Progynon). This drug is derived from estrone and marketed as an aqueous suspension and in pellets, tablets, and suppositories. Preparations for injection contain 0.25 to 1 mg. per milliliter. Estradiol is ten times more potent than estrone except when administered intravaginally; by this route both are effective at the same dosage level. For replacement therapy dose is 0.5 to 1.5 mg. two or three times weekly.

Estradiol benzoate, N.F. (Progynon Benzoate, Ovocylin Benzoate); *oestradiol benzoate*, B.P. This form is less subject to destruction in the tissues than the parent substance and hence is suitable for parenteral administration (intramuscularly). Dosage varies from 0.5 to 1.5 mg. two or three times weekly depending on the condition for which it is given and the severity of the symptoms.

Estradiol dipropionate, N.F. (Ovocylin Dipropionate). This preparation is absorbed more slowly and excreted more slowly than estradiol, but in other respects its effects are similar to other estradiol compounds. It is administered intramuscularly as a solution in oil and is available in 10- and 30-ml. vials containing 1 mg. of drug per milliliter. Dosage ranges from 1.0 to 5 mg. given every 1 or 2 weeks.

Estradiol cypionate, U.S.P. (Depo-Estradiol Cypionate). This preparation may produce more prolonged effects than the estradiol compounds mentioned previously and injection of 5 mg. may cause effects to persist for 3 to 4 weeks. It is available as an oil solution (1 mg. or 5 mg. per milliliter). It is administered by intramuscular injection. For maintenance effects 1 to 5 mg. may be administered weekly for 2 to 3 weeks and then every 3 or 4 weeks.

Ethinyl estradiol, U.S.P. (Estinyl, Feminone, Gynetone); *ethinyloestradiol*, B.P. This is a potent estrogen made suitable for oral administration. It is available in tablets, 0.02, 0.05, or 0.5 mg. Dosage varies greatly with the condition treated. For control of menopausal symptoms 0.01 to 0.05 mg. is given one to three times a day.

Conjugated estrogens—preparation, dosage, and administration

Conjugated estrogens, U.S.P. (Premarin, Conestron, Amenestrogen). This preparation contains water-soluble, conjugated forms of mixed estrogens from the urine of pregnant mares. The principal estrogen present is sodium estrone sulfate. These preparations are available in tablets for oral administration. They are also available in the form of topical creams and lotions as well as in powder form for injection (intramuscular or intravenous). The action and uses of conjugated estrogens are similar to those of other estrogens. Dosage of 0.3 to 1.25 mg. daily cyclically is usually sufficient to control menopausal symptoms. Senile vaginitis and pruritus vulvae are usually relieved with doses of between 1.25 and 3.75 mg. For palliation of breast cancer a daily oral dose of 30 mg. is recommended. For dysfunctional uterine bleeding 3.75 to 7.5 mg. is given daily for 3 to 5 days or until bleeding stops.

Synthetic estrogens—preparation, dosage, and administration

Diethylstilbestrol, U.S.P. (DES); *stilboestrol*, B.P. This drug is a relatively inexpensive synthetic estrogenic substance that duplicates practically all known actions of the natural estrogens. It is relatively active when given by mouth as well as when given parenterally. It is not significantly more toxic than the natural estrogens. Diethylstilbestrol has received a D.E.S.I. rating of *effective* for treatment of menopausal syndrome, female hypogonadism, amenorrhea, female castration, and primary ovarian failure; *probably effective* in osteoporosis, and *possibly effective* in menstrual disturbances and suppression of lactation. It is available in plain tablets, enteric-coated tablets, and capsules for oral administration, in solution for injection, and in the form of vaginal suppositories. These dosage forms are available in a wide range of concentrations. The average oral dose for treatment of menopausal symptoms is 0.2 to 0.5 mg. daily. The dosage is reduced if discomfort results. For the suppression of lactation, 5 mg. once or twice daily for 2 to 4 days is considered sufficient; for prostatic cancer, 3 mg. daily (intramuscularly) reduced to 1 mg. daily or 0.5 mg. three times a day (orally); and for the palliation of mammary cancer, 15 mg. is the daily oral dose recommended for initial treatment; the dose is increased according to the tolerance of the patient. Dosage of all preparations should be kept at the minimum necessary for the relief of symptoms.

Side effects are relatively common after oral administration and include nausea, vomiting, and headache. Vaginal carcinoma has been associated with diethylstilbestrol given to pregnant women. This malignancy appears many years later in the daughters of such women. Thus its use is contraindicated during pregnancy.

Diethylstilbestrol dipropionate, N.F. This form is prescribed for the same conditions for which other estrogenic substances are used. It is given intramuscularly in oil and is said to have a rather prolonged effect; hence, reactions such as nausea, vomiting, headache, and dizziness occur less frequently than with free diethylstilbestrol. It is also administered orally as tablets. Dosage for the relief of menopausal symptoms is 0.5 to 2 mg. two or three times a week; larger doses are required for suppression of lactation and for the treatment of prostatic cancer.

Dienestrol, B.P. (Restrol, Synestrol). This is a nonsteroid estrogen that can be administered orally. It is said to cause fewer side effects than diethylstilbestrol and is less potent. Dosage for the relief of menopausal symptoms is 0.1 to 1.5 mg. daily. Larger doses, up to 15 mg. daily, may be ordered for the patient with mammary cancer. Dose for postpartum breast engorgement is 1.5 mg. daily for 3 days, then 0.5 mg. daily for 7 days. Dienestrol also can be given subcutaneously and intramuscularly. It is available in 0.1-, 0.5-, and 10-mg. tablets for oral administration; in a suspension for injection, 50 mg. in 10 ml.; and as a vaginal cream, 0.1 mg. per gram.

Chlorotrianisene, N.F., B.P. (Tace). This drug in general shares the actions and uses of other estrogenic substances, although it exhibits some points of difference. The compound is stored in body fat, from which it is slowly released. Therefore, its action extends beyond the time when administration of the drug has been discontinued. It is effective in the relief of mammary engorgement, but its use in large amounts is not recommended for cancer of the breast of patients beyond the age of menopause because it may induce uterine bleeding. Average oral dose for relief of menopausal symptoms is 12 to 25 mg. daily; in cases of prostatic cancer, 12 to 25 mg. daily; for relief of mammary engorgement, 50 mg. daily. The last-mentioned dosage is to be continued only for 1 week. To suppress lactation, 72 mg. is given twice daily for 2 days; the first dose should be given within 8 hours after delivery. It is available in 12-, 25-, and 72-mg. capsules.

Hexestrol. This is a compound that is less potent and less toxic than diethylstilbestrol. It is used for many of the same conditions for which the latter estrogen is used. It is available in 1- and 3-mg. tablets for oral administration. The dosage recommended for the control of menopausal symptoms is 2 to 3 mg., which is reduced as the symptoms are brought under control.

Methallenestril (Vallestril); *benzetrol* (Benzestrol); *promethestrol dipropionate* (Meprane Dipropionate). These are additional synthetic estrogens that produce effects similar to those produced by diethylstilbestrol.

The synthetic estrogens offer the advantage of ease of administration since they can be given orally, and they are also relatively inexpensive.

Side effects and toxic effects. Side effects seen in connection with estrogen therapy frequently include nausea and vomiting, diarrhea, and skin rash. The symptoms are usually mild and related to dosage, potency of the compound, and route of administration. Other symptoms include edema and an increased amount of calcium in the blood of patients who have been given prolonged therapy. Adjustment of dosage, substitutions of another estrogen, and perhaps parenteral rather than oral administration may relieve the gastrointestinal symptoms. Periodic tests of the blood and tests of renal function are recommended.

Tenderness of nipples and breast engorgement

may occur in young women, and males may manifest gynecomastia. There is some question about the relationship between estrogens and increased mortality from cardiovascular disease in men treated with estrogens for prostatic cancer. This relationship may be dose-related, since the increase in incidence was noted in men receiving 5 mg. of drug daily, but no such increase was noted in patients given 1 mg. of drug daily.

Estrogens are carcinogenic when administered experimentally in animals that have inherited sensitivity to certain types of carcinoma. Many clinicians believe that estrogens are therefore contraindicated for women who have a personal or family history of malignancy of the reproductive system. Estrogens are used, however, for inoperable breast cancer.

Drug interactions. Estrogens can influence blood coagulation, and there is evidence that they increase incidence of thrombophlebitis and thromboembolism. Thus, when given concurrently with oral anticoagulants, dosage of anticoagulants must be adjusted.

Estrogens enhance the antiinflammatory effect of corticosteroids and dose of the latter drug should be adjusted.

Luteal hormone

The secretion of progesterone by the corpus luteum is under the influence of one of the pituitary hormones, luteotropin (LTH). The chemical structure of progesterone resembles that of the estrogens and also the androgens (see formula, p. 606).

The chemistry of progesterone and related compounds differs from the estrogens in that ring "A" (ring at the lower left of the accompanying structural formula) is not aromatic and there is also a two-carbon side chain at the 17 position (upper right). Chemically, this group is closely related to the adrenal steroids (see Chapter 25).

The luteal hormone functions in the preparation and maintenance of the lining of the uterus for the implantation and nourishment of the embryo. It supplements the action of the follicular hormone in the action on the uterus and also in the mammary glands. It suppresses ovulation during pregnancy and keeps the uterus in a quiescent state by decreasing the irritability of the uterine muscle. Progesterone decreases the sensitivity of the uterus to oxytocin and ergonovine. After the third month of pregnancy its production is taken over by the placenta.

Progesterone injections cause the endometrium to convert the proliferative phase to the secretory or progestational phase. It also induces proliferation of the secretory elements of the breast, and it causes an increase in the cornified vaginal epithelium.

Progesterone was formerly obtained from the corpus luteum, but it is now prepared synthetically because the naturally occurring hormone is inactivated or extremely weak in its effect when taken orally.

Uses. Progesterone has received a D.E.S.I. rating of *effective* for use in amenorrhea and abnormal uterine bleeding due to hormonal unbalance; *probably effective* for treatment of habitual and threatened abortion; and *possibly effective* for dysmenorrhea. In the treatment of amenorrhea, responsiveness to progesterone depends on the priming of the endometrium with estrogen.

Some progestogens are components of oral contraceptives, which suppress ovulation. Norethindrone and norethynodrel are more effective in this respect than are other progestogens.

Preparation, dosage, and administration. The following are available preparations of luteal hormone.

Progesterone, U.S.P., B.P. (Gesterol, Lutocylin, Lipo-Lutin, Progestin, Proluton). This preparation is available in an oil solution or aqueous suspension for injection. It is ineffective when given orally. The solution in oil is administered intramuscularly and the suspension may be administered subcutaneously. It is given in doses up to 25 mg. or more daily. Intramuscular dose for amenorrhea is 25 mg. three times weekly during the last 2 weeks of the menstrual cycle after estrogen therapy during the first 2 weeks of the cycle. Dose for functional uterine bleeding is 5 to 10 mg. daily for 3 to 5 days, repeated every 4 weeks for 3 to 4 months. For threatened abortion dose of 5 to 50 mg. daily may be given; for dysmenorrhea, dose is 10 to 25 mg. daily for the week prior to menstruation.

Tablets of 10 and 25 mg. are available for sublingual administration up to four times a day.

Norethindrone, U.S.P. (Norlutin). This is a semisynthetic compound chemically related to ethisterone and testosterone. It produces effects similar to those produced by progesterone but is about twice as potent and it has some androgenic qualities. It has received a D.E.S.I. rating of *effective* for the treatment of amenorrhea and abnormal uterine bleeding due to hormonal imbalance and endometriosis, and *possibly effective* for dysmenorrhea. When administered at certain times during the menstrual cycle, the drug apparently inhibits ovulation, and continuous administration causes delay of menstruation for prolonged periods of time. Norethindrone has been used successfully in suppressing ovulation when given with estrogen. On the other hand, when given to women who are amenorrheic but who have received estrogen therapy, the drug will usually produce bleeding within 24 to 72 hours after administration has been stopped. It is being used chiefly for the treatment of patients who have amenorrhea, menstrual irregularity, endometriosis, and infertility. It is available in 5-mg. tablets and is administered orally in doses of 5 to 20 mg. daily. For endometriosis up to 30 mg. daily may be given.

Norethynodrel, N.F., B.P. This is a synthetic progestogen similar to norethindrone but with fewer androgenic qualities. It is available for clinical use in combination with mestranol, an estrogen, and is marketed under the name of Enovid. As such, it is used to provide cyclic control, to prevent breakthrough bleeding, and to suppress ovulation. It is available in 2.5-, 5-, and 10-mg. tablets with varying amounts of mestranol.

As an oral test for pregnancy, 10 mg. may be administered daily for 5 days. Withdrawal bleeding occurs 2 to 7 days after the last dose if the patient is not pregnant.

This drug may also be administered in cases of threatened abortion and in treatment of habitual abortion.

Medroxyprogesterone acetate, U.S.P. (Provera). This synthetic substance differs from progesterone mainly in that it is active after oral administration. It can be used for all conditions for which progesterone is indicated and is more potent than ethisterone. It is available in 2.5- and 10-mg. tablets or as a suspension for injection. It has no inherent estrogenic activity and priming with estrogen is necessary. Drowsiness has been reported as a side effect.

Hydroxyprogesterone caproate, U.S.P. (Delalutin). A synthetic derivative of progesterone, it is a great deal like progesterone except that it has a longer duration of action after parenteral administration. Duration of action is 7 to 17 days. It is available in oil solution, 250 mg. in 2 ml., for intramuscular injection. The usual single dose is 125 to 250 mg., and one dose every 4 weeks may be sufficient in treatment of menstrual disorders and ovarian and uterine dysfunction. Its D.E.S.I. rating is similar to that for progesterone. It is also effective as a presumptive test for pregnancy and as a test for endogenous estrogen. It is ineffective for treatment of postpartum afterpains, ovarian deficiency, and senile vaginitis. Priming with estrogen is necessary.

Side effects and toxic effects. Preparations of luteal hormone or related compounds appear to have a low order of toxicity. Patients occasionally have gastrointestinal symptoms, headache, dizziness, and allergic manifestations. Cases have been reported in which masculinization of female infants occurred in connection with the administration of progesterone to the mothers during pregnancy.

Prolonged high dosages of progestogens may cause gastrointestinal disturbances, edema and weight gain, headache and vertigo, oligomenorrhea, and breast congestion.

ORAL CONTRACEPTIVES
OVULATORY SUPPRESSANTS

Contraception is as old as history and has been practiced in many forms, including the use of mechanical devices and ingestion of various herbs. Not until recently, however, has there been any consistent measure of reliability in these practices. The introduction of Enovid in 1960 dramatically demonstrated the unfailing suppression of ovulation by a combination of progesterones and estrogens. This event was preceded by a decade of research, the elucida-

tion of which was largely the responsibility of Rock, Pincus, and Garcia. Evidence of the contraceptive effect of norethynodrel was published by this group in 1956 and followed by a number of controlled studies, most notably in Puerto Rico. By 1965 refined forms of this drug multiplied, and over 5 million American women were using oral contraceptives.

Few drugs have been studied as ambitiously and intensively as have the oral contraceptives because of (1) the interest aroused concerning the effects these drugs might have on the human body when hormone levels and relationships are altered for the sole purpose of preventing conception, (2) the need for a simple method of population control in densely populated countries, and (3) the desire by many couples for planned parenthood.

Pharmacologic action and result. The development of the oral contraceptives was based on the knowledge that ovulation did not occur during pregnancy and that large amounts of estrogen and progesterone were produced by the extended function of the corpus luteum and by placental secretion.

In addition, a review of physiology of the menstrual cycle reveals that:

1 Ovulation is dependent upon the anterior pituitary gland to secrete two hormones:
  a. FSH—for maturation of the ovum
  b. LH—for release of the mature ovum from the ovary
2 The hypothalamus regulates the secretion of these hormones by the anterior pituitary by secreting hormones known as releasing factors.
3 Large amounts of estrogen (secreted by the maturing follicle and, following ovulation, by the corpus luteum) inhibit the hypothalamus releasing factors, which inhibits FSH and LH release and blocks ovulation.
4 Progesterone (secreted by the corpus luteum) inhibits the hypothalamic releasing factor for the luteinizing hormone, which also interferes with ovulation.
5 Estrogen and progesterone are responsible for endometrial buildup; decreased production of estrogen and progesterone results in endometrial sloughing and menstrual bleeding.

From this information, it can be readily understood why the administration of progesterone derivatives and estrogenic substances prevents ovulation without preventing menstruation and why these substances are the ingredients of oral contraceptives.

It is generally accepted that oral contraceptives act, at least in part, by inhibiting the secretion of gonadotropins from the pituitary gland. Other possible actions may include a direct inhibitory effect on the ovary, changes in tubal motility, or changes in the endometrium that would result in failure of implantation of fertilized ova.

The combination of drugs rapidly transforms the early secretory stage of the endometrium to one resembling secretory exhaustion. The drug is therefore judged effective because the estrogen encourages proliferative change that inhibits ovulation, while progesterone ensures that withdrawal bleeding will be physiologic, prompt, and brief.

Preparation, dosage, and administration. Although the use of exogenous estrogenic substances alone will inhibit ovulation, undesirable bleeding frequently occurs during the latter phase of the cycle. If estrogen levels are increased to prevent this, severe nausea and breast tenderness occur. It is for these reasons that estrogens are combined with progesterones in oral contraceptives.

Since naturally occurring progesterone is inactivated or extremely weak in its effect when taken orally and must be given by injection to be effective, steroidal compounds related to progesterone have been developed. These are termed progestogens. The majority of the oral contraceptives contain a synthetic progestogen, which is either norethynodrel or norethindrone.

Norethynodrel

Norethindrone

Norethynodrel is a basic progestin, while norethindrone is a more androgenic progestin. The latter is sometimes recommended for patients experiencing excess side effects from estrogen, such as greater weight gain and amenorrhea. Norethynodrel, on the other hand, is good for patients with oily skin, acne, hirsutism, and breakthrough bleeding.

Four methods of oral contraception are used; one is termed "combination therapy," another is termed "sequential therapy," a third method is called low dosage progestogens (mini-pill), and a fourth method is postcoital contraception. Combination therapy consists of taking tablets containing a progestogen and an estrogen. Sequential therapy consists of taking a tablet containing only estrogen for 15 days, then taking a tablet containing a mixture of estrogen and progestogen for 5 days (this tablet is usually a different color).

In both combination and sequential therapy, 20 tablets are taken during each menstrual cycle. The first day of menstruation is day 1; on day 5 the first tablet is taken regardless of whether menstruation has ceased. One tablet is then taken each day for the next 20 days. Menstruation will occur within 2 to 7 days after the last tablet has been taken. The fifth day after the start of menstruation, the cycle begins again.

The combination and sequential methods of therapy are equally effective. Most authorities claim them to be 100% effective; failures are the result of missed dosage. It is important that patients be instructed in the following:

1 The patient should take one tablet every day for the 20-day period without fail. Eliminating one tablet may lead to ovulation or breakthrough acyclic bleeding.
2 If breakthrough bleeding occurs, administration of the drug should be continued and the physician should be consulted. What may be required is a different balance of estrogen or a different progestogen. Breakthrough bleeding may occur only in the first cycles of treatment until the patient adjusts to the hormones. Spotting or slight brownish discharge is not breakthrough bleeding, and it eventually disappears. If bleeding is similar to that of menses, the patient is usually advised to stop taking the drug and begin the medication again 5 days later beginning a new cycle.

Table 26-1 Combination therapy oral contraceptives

Trade name	Tablet composition			
	Estrogen	Dose (mg.)	Progestogen	Dose (mg.)
Enovid	Mestranol	0.15	Norethynodrel	9.85
Enovid	Mestranol	0.075	Norethynodrel	5
Enovid-E	Mestranol	0.1	Norethynodrel	2.5
Ortho-Novum	Mestranol	0.06	Norethindrone	10
Ortho-Novum	Mestranol	0.075	Norethindrone	5
Norinyl, Novulen, Noralestrin	Mestranol	0.1	Norethindrone	2
Norlestrin, Prolestrin, Orlestrin, Etalontin	Ethinyl estradiol	0.05	Norethindrone acetate	2.5
Ovulen, Metrulen-N	Mestranol	0.1	Ethyndiol diacetate	1
Provest, Proverstral Provestrol	Ethinyl estradiol	0.05	Medroxy progestrone acetate	10

Table 26-2 Sequential therapy oral contraceptives

Trade name	Estrogen component	Number of days	Estrogen and progestogen	Number of days
C-Quens	Mestranol, 0.08 mg.	15	Mestranol, 0.08 mg. and chloramadinone, 2 mg.	5
Oracon	Ethinyl estradiol, 0.1 mg.	16	Ethinyl estradiol, 0.1 mg. and dimethisterone, 25 mg.	5
Ortho-Novum SQ Tablets	Mestranol, 0.08 mg.	14	Mestranol, 0.08 mg. and norethindrone, 2 mg.	6

3 Even if menses does not occur following completion of a medication cycle, patients should be cautioned to begin another medication cycle on the seventh day and not to wait for menstruation to begin, since ovulation may occur within 9 or 10 days after stopping the medication. Ovulation can occur in the presence of a delayed or missed menstruation.

4 Women who are early ovulators or have a shortened menstrual cycle (they menstruate every 21 days or less) should be cautioned to use another method of birth control during the first medication cycle. Under steroid therapy, these women will usually convert to a 28-day cycle.

5 The patient should be instructed to establish a definite pattern for taking the tablet at the same time each day; however, anytime within a 24-hour period is adequate.

6 The patient should be examined and reevaluated for oral contraceptive therapy at least once yearly and should report any untoward symptoms to her physician.

Side effects. Analysis of the side effects of oral contraceptives is difficult because of the different drugs and drug combinations used, the different dosages and regimens, and individual patient differences. Since ovarian hormones influence all body systems either directly or by their influence on other endocrine glands and metabolism, a variety of side effects can be expected to occur. Known adverse effects on the body systems resulting from estrogen-progestogen combinations include the following. More experience with norethindrone-alone preparation is needed to determine its adverse effects.

Gastrointestinal. Nausea is a common effect particularly during the first 2 or 3 months. Vomiting, an increase or decrease in appetite, abdominal pain, diarrhea, and constipation also occur. The absorption of folate, a water-soluble vitamin, is decreased causing anemia in some women.

Alterations in liver function have been reported. Jaundice, cholestasis, and some liver cell degeneration have been noted. Patients with a history of liver disease, such as hepatitis, may be more likely to develop these latter effects.

Cardiovascular. There is general, but not universal, agreement that there is a cause-effect relationship between oral contraceptives and thromboembolic phenomena. In the United States a study of the morbidity of thrombophlebitis indicated a fourfold increase with use of oral contraceptives; in Great Britain studies show a three to tenfold increase. The British study also showed a higher death rate for users of oral contraceptives than for nonusers, and a higher death rate for older users (35 to 44) than younger users (20 to 34). Another study in Great Britain showed a three to fourfold increase in postoperative thromboembolic disease for patients on oral contraceptives.

There is some indication that thromboembolism is related to estrogen dosage, and it is recommended that the lowest effective dose be used.

Oral contraceptives increase the number of platelets, and may increase their tendency to clump; other blood clotting factors are also increased. In addition, intimal thickening of arteries and veins has been reported, as well as abnormal vein dilation, which may cause venous stasis. All of these factors may explain the increased risk of thromboembolism in users of oral contraceptives.

Migraine headache has been intensified in some patients with a previous history of migraine, and in some patients onset of migraine occurred with use of oral contraceptives. Therapy for these patients should be discontinued.

Hypertension has occurred. Estrogen-progestogen combinations increase the amount of renin produced by the kidney, which in turn increases the production of angiotensin, a potent pressor substance. Blood pressure determinations should be made prior to therapy and regularly during therapy.

A cooperative study in the United States, Sweden, and Great Britain showed that incidence of thromboembolic disease was lower in women with type O blood. The reason for this is unknown.

Endocrine. Estrogens decrease the rate of corticosteroid metabolism, but there is no evidence that they cause adrenal dysfunction. Thyroid function tests are altered but thyroid function does not seem to be affected.

Menses usually occurs 6 to 10 weeks after discontinuance of oral contraceptive therapy. In some women inhibition of ovarian function may require the use of clomiphene or gonadotropins.

Reproductive. The cervix may undergo hyperplasia and hypersecretion of the cervical glands and increased vascularity. Regression of the myometrium has been noted, and tenderness and fullness of the breasts may occur. Estrogens and progestogens have been detected in human milk but its long-range effect on the offspring is not known. There are no definitive data to prove or disprove an association between oral contraceptives and breast or uterine cancer.

Central nervous system. Mood changes are common with the use of oral contraceptives; some women experience a sense of well-being and a release of tension; for others there is increased tension, irritability, and depression. Both increase and decrease in libido have been reported.

A few rare cases of severe ophthalmic disorders have been reported. Users of oral contraceptives experience more difficulty with contact lenses than nonusers.

Cutaneous. A variety of skin reactions may occur including chloasma, acne, and pruritus.

Contraindications. Contraindications include a history of thromboembolic disease, hepatic disease, mammary or genital carcinoma, large uterine fibroids, migraine headache, asthma, epilepsy, and blood dyscrasias. Oral contraceptives should not be taken if pregnancy is suspected because of the danger of possible masculinization of the fetus.

MINI-PILL

Contraceptive tablets containing only the progestogen, norethindrone, at a very low dose level of 0.35 mg. is known as the mini-pill. Trade names for the mini-pill include Micronor and Nor-QD. Dosage is one tablet daily without interruption. These preparations probably exert their contraceptive action by reducing the penetrability of the sperm in the cervical mucus, by interfering with luteal function by suppressing the secretion of gonadotropins, and by interfering with the implantation of the ovum. The mini-pill does not prevent ovulation. The mini-pill is believed to be slightly less effective as a contraceptive than the contraceptives containing both estrogen and progestogen. The dropout rate appears to be higher for the mini-pill than for the combination tablets, which is believed to be due to a significant incidence of unpredictable bleeding patterns.

POSTCOITAL CONTRACEPTIVE
Diethylstilbestrol (DES)

Diethylstilbestrol's mechanism of action as a postcoital contraceptive is not well understood, but the drug appears to lower the level of circulating progesterone and to inhibit implantation of the fertilized ovum in the uterus when taken within 72 hours after intercourse. Diethylstilbestrol may increase tubal motility, causing the ova to arrive in the uterus sooner than usual.

Diethylstilbestrol should be used only as an emergency method and not as a routine means of birth control; repeated use should be avoided. To prevent pregnancy, diethylstilbestrol must be taken within 24 to 72 hours after sexual intercourse.

Side effects and precautions. Frequently occurring side effects from diethylstilbestrol are nausea and vomiting. Other side effects include headache, dizziness, diarrhea, abdominal cramps, breast tenderness, weight gain, increased vaginal secretions, darkening of breast areola, rash, anorexia, and leg cramps. Changes in menstrual flow or spotting may occur while taking the drug or soon after finishing the course of therapy. Thromboembolic disease (thrombophlebitis, pulmonary embolism, and cerebral thrombosis) is the most serious side effect of synthetic estrogens; although rare, this complication can be fatal.

Diethylstilbestrol is contraindicated for patients with blood clotting disorders, impaired liver function, a history of thrombophlebitis, cancer of the breast or uterus, or undiagnosed abnormal uterine bleeding.

Diethylstilbestrol must not be given to pregnant women; every effort should be made to be certain the patient is not pregnant before treatment is started. If at all possible, a pregnancy test should be performed before instituting postcoital contraceptive therapy. If it should be determined that a patient received DES while pregnant, the patient should be informed about the risk of vaginal or cervical cancer occurring in her female offspring, and she should be given the option of deciding whether or not the pregnancy should be terminated.

Preparation and dosage. Diethylstilbestrol is available in 25-mg. tablets for use as a postcoital contraceptive. It is administered orally in a dosage of 25 mg. twice a day for 5 days beginning not later than 72 hours (but preferably 24 hours) after sexual intercourse. This dosage can prevent pregnancy but it cannot terminate pregnancy. Patients must be warned that to be effective the full course of treatment must be taken regardless of the nausea that commonly occurs.

OVULATORY STIMULANTS

Anovulation is physiologic in patients who are pregnant, breast feeding, and postmenopausal. It becomes suspected pathology in situations characterized by abnormal bleeding or infertility. The incidence of anovulation is unknown and cannot be ascertained, but diagnostic tests may determine its presence.

Methods of ovulation induction include use of gonadotropins, thyroid preparations, cortisones, estrogens, and synthetic steroids.

Gonadotropins

The use of either human chorionic gonadotropin (HCG) or human menopausal gonadotropin (HMG or menotropins) has been discussed.

Thyroid preparations

Thyroid preparations are used in hypothyroid or hyperthyroid conditions, which are often associated with anovulation.

Cortisone preparations

Cortisone preparations suppress adrenal activity, thereby decreasing androgen and estrogen secretions and encouraging release of human pituitary gonadotropins. This treatment is appropriate when adrenal gland dysfunction is etiologic in anovulation, as in adrenogenital syndrome.

Estrogens

These hormones act to induce ovulation in two ways: (1) by stimulating the release of pituitary gonadotropin and increasing secretion of FSH and LH and (2) by making the ovary more responsive to the influence of gonadotropin. Short-term therapy may be stimulating to the ovary, but long-term estrogen therapy depresses gonadotropin, which results in anovulation.

Ovulation-inducing agents

Several synthetic agents have recently become available. The mode of action of these drugs in inducing ovulation is not yet well established, but they may act either directly on the enzyme systems, suppressing estrogen production and secondary stimulation of gonadotropin, or directly on the hypothalamus, pituitary gland, or both, stimulating secretion of gonadotropin.

Side effects with any of these therapies are common, including gastrointestinal disturbances similar to those in pregnancy, breakthrough bleeding, abdominal pain, and weight gain.

Clomiphene citrate, U.S.P., B.P. This drug bears a close structural relationship to the potent synthetic estrogen chlorotrianisene (Tace). Its mechanism of action is not definitely known, but it may compete with estrogen at the hypothalamic level causing an increase in secretion of the hypothalamic releasing factor and a resultant increase in the pituitary gonadotropins LH and FSH and, consequently, ovarian stimulation. It is generally suitable for patients with amenor-

rhea of pituitary origin, the Stein-Leventhal syndrome, and the Chiari-Frommel syndrome. Dosage is 50 to 100 mg. per day for 5 to 7 days. Short-term therapies have been found more effective than long-term ones. Side effects include hot flashes and the presence of ovarian enlargement with or without cyst formation. Clomiphene is teratogenic in some animals, and it should not be given to pregnant women. Visual abnormalities (e.g., blurred vision) have been reported. If these occur the drug should be stopped. Other adverse effects include nausea, cyclic ovarian pain (mittelschmerz), breast engorgement, and abnormal uterine bleeding. These effects disappear when the drug is stopped. Incidence of ovulation has been ascertained as 76% in one study, although further research is needed. Pregnancy occurs in 25% to 30% of patients treated. Multiple pregnancies may occur in 10% of patients.

Male sex hormones

Androgens

Normal development and maintenance of male sex characteristics depend on adequate amounts of the male sex hormones, called androgens. All androgenic compounds have a steroid nucleus. In fact, natural estrogens, androgens, and some of the hormones of the adrenal cortex all exhibit an interesting similarity in their structural formulas.

There are about five steroidal hormones that manifest androgenic activity, and all are derivatives of androsterone. The most potent is testosterone, which is chemically similar to progesterone. Androgens chemically similar to testosterone are excreted in the urine and are usually referred to as 17-ketosteroids because there is a ketone group attached to carbon 17 of the steroid structure (see structural formula). It should be remembered, however, that the urinary 17-ketosteroids are products of the adrenal cortex in both men and women. Androsterone is one of the 17-ketosteroids found in the urine.

Testosterone is not excreted, as such, in the urine.

Testosterone
(male sex hormone)

Progesterone
(female sex hormone)

Androsterone
(one of 17-ketosteroids found in urine of both sexes)

Action and result. The androgens function in the development and maintenance of normal states in the sex organs. Administration to immature males causes growth of the sex organs and the appearance of secondary sex characteristics. When administered for therapeutic purposes, they simply replace the missing hormone. When a high concentration of androgenic substances is maintained in the circulation, anterior pituitary secretion is inhibited and spermatogenesis is retarded.

In mammals, both sexes form male and female hormones, although they are antagonistic to each other. The administration of testosterone can suppress menstruation and cause atrophy of the endometrium.

Another effect produced by androgens is concerned with anabolism—the formation as well as the maintenance of muscular and skeletal protein. The administration of androgenic substances is associated with an increase in muscular development and weight. They bring about retention of nitrogen (essential to the formation of protein in the body) and also affect the storage of inorganic phosphorus, sulfate, sodium, and potassium.

The retention of nitrogen, prevention of atrophy in bones from disuse, and promotion of the healing of wounds are effects of testosterone and related compounds that have been reported. These effects are of particular significance in patients who are paraplegic after trauma to the spinal cord, because in these patients the maintenance of adequate nutrition, prevention of atrophy in muscles and bones, and prevention as well as treatment of decubitus ulcers constitute serious problems. Similar problems are encountered in the care of patients who are chronically ill or malnourished or who have a wasting disease such as carcinoma.

Uses. Androgens have been used in replacement therapy for patients with hypogonadism and eunuchoidism (castrates). They produce marked changes in sex organs, body contour, and voice, provided the deficiency state has not been present too long. Androgens have little effect on elderly men and on patients with psychogenic impotence. They may increase libido in women.

Alone or with gonadotropic substances, androgens have been employed in the treatment of cryptorchidism.

Androgens have also been used in the treatment of dysmenorrhea and menopausal states and for the suppression of lactation and breast engorgement. Favorable results are sometimes obtained from their use to relieve subjective symptoms associated with the male climacteric, just as estrogens are of value in relieving symptoms of similar origin in women.

Androgens have been employed for palliative relief of advanced inoperable cancer of the breast. Their mechanism of action is not clear. Subjective improvement (improved appetite, gain in weight, and relief of pain) seems to be greater than objective improvement. Improvement is temporary and seldom exceeds a period of 1 year. Androgens are preferred for patients with this condition prior to or during menopause, since estrogens may promote the development of the cancer at this time.

Preparation, dosage, and administration. The following are preparations of androgens.

Testosterone, N.F., B.P. Testosterone produces effects similar to testosterone propionate. When given in aqueous suspension its duration of androgenic effects is slightly longer than those of testosterone propionate. It is available in 75-mg. pellets, as an aqueous injectable suspension of 25, 50, and 100 mg. per milliliter, and as tablets for oral and sublingual administration. Usual dose is 10 mg. daily by the buccal route, or 25 mg. intramuscularly twice a week to once daily. Rate of absorption by the buccal route is unpredictable.

For male hypogonadism three 75-mg. testosterone pellets are implanted subcutaneously into the medial aspect of each thigh using a pellet injector. These pellets have received a D.E.S.I. rating of *effective* for the treatment of eunuchism, eunuchoidism, and the male climacteric, and *ineffective* for advanced breast cancer.

Testosterone propionate, U.S.P., B.P. (Oreton, Andronate). Testosterone propionate has received a D.E.S.I. rating of *effective* for male hypogonadism, eunuchism, eunuchoidism, male climacteric, androgen deficiency, prevention of postpartum pain and breast engorgement, and palliation of breast cancer; *probably effective* for postmenopausal osteoporosis; *possibly effective* for cryptorchidism in young boys, suppression of lactation, and anabolic effects; and *ineffective* for menopausal symptoms, endometriosis, and uterine disorders. This form is available in 10-mg. buccal tablets (these are held in the space between the teeth and cheek) and as a solution for intramuscular injection containing 50 and 100 mg. per milliliter. Usual dose is 25 mg. two to four times a week, with a usual range of dose of 25 to 150 mg. weekly, depending upon the response obtained and the effect desired. From 5 to 10 mg. daily may be sufficient as maintenance doses for therapy in men. For relief of symptoms of breast cancer, 150 to 300 mg. weekly (in several doses) may be administered. Since there is marked variation in sensitivity to testosterone, virilism may occur in females even with small doses of the drug. This preparation is synthesized from cholesterol or extracted from bull testes.

Testosterone enanthate, U.S.P. (Delatestryl). Testosterone enanthate has a D.E.S.I. rating similar to that for testosterone propionate. This preparation is administered as a solution in oil and provides a prolonged effect of 3 weeks or more. The usual intramuscular dose is 100 to 400 mg. every 2 to 4 weeks.

Methyltestosterone, U.S.P., B.P. (Oreton M, Metandren). The D.E.S.I. rating is similar to that for testosterone propionate. This preparation is available in 5-, 10-, and 25-mg. tablets for oral administration, in 5- and 10-mg. buccal tablets, and in 5- and 10-mg. tablets for sublingual administration. Absorption from the buccal membranes is more effective than from the gastrointestinal tract. The indications and actions of this compound are essentially the same as those for testosterone propionate. The usual oral dose is 10 mg. three times a day. Range of dose is 10 to 50 mg. daily. Doses for the suppression of lactation are larger. Dosage for breast cancer is 50 to 200 mg. daily. Dosage is adjusted according to the needs and response of the patient.

Testosterone cypionate, U.S.P. Although highly similar to testosterone propionate, this exhibits the advantage of more prolonged androgenic effects. It is available in solution, 50, 100, and 200 mg. per 1 ml. It is administered intramuscularly in doses from 100 to 200 mg. at intervals of 1 or 2 weeks for androgen deficiency.

Norethandrolone, B.P. (Nilevar). This is a synthetic androgen that is chemically and pharmacologically related to testosterone. It is not used as an androgen because its androgenic properties are less significant than its ability to affect protein anabolism (see action of androgens). Its major effects include: (1) retention of nitrogen, phosphorus, and potassium in amounts required for protein anabolism, (2) retention and utilization of calcium, (3) sense of well-being, and (4) improved appetite. Patients receiving anabolic hormones should be on high-calorie, high-protein diets, if possible. It is administered orally and intramuscularly in amounts that range from 30 to 50 mg. daily in divided doses. It is available as a solution, 25 mg. per milliliter, and in 10-mg. tablets for oral administration. Large doses can produce androgenic effects like those encountered with the other androgens.

Fluoxymesterone, U.S.P., B.P. (Halotestin, Ultandren). Fluoxymesterone has received a D.E.S.I. rating similar to that for testosterone propionate. This compound is a synthetic halogenated derivative of methyltestosterone. It is available in 2- and 5-mg. tablets for oral administration. It is several times more potent than methyltestosterone from the standpoint of both androgenic and anabolic activity. Dosage for androgen deficiency is 10 to 20 mg. daily. Dosage for anabolic effects ranges from 4 to 10 mg., and for palliation of breast cancer 10 to 30 mg. daily have been used. Dosage varies greatly with the condition being treated and the response of the patient. The daily dose is given at one time or divided into three or more portions.

Nandrolone phenpropionate, N.F.; *phenyl-propionate,* B.P. (Durabolin). This is a synthetic steroid hormone related to norethandrolone. Similarly, its anabolic effects are prominent while androgenicity is low. This drug is administered intramuscularly, and usual adult dosage ranges from 25 to 50 mg. once weekly.

Nandrolone decanoate, N.F., B.P. (Deca-Durabolin). Its duration of action is longer than nandrolone phenylpropionate and the usual dosage is 50 to 100 mg. once a month.

Side effects and toxic effects. Effects that are regarded as untoward in the female include deepening of the voice, hirsutism (excessive growth of hair), flushing, acne, regression of the breasts, enlargement of the clitoris, and general masculinization. In prepuberal boys, adverse reactions include pubic hair development, phallic enlargement, and increased frequency of erections. Premature epiphyseal closure may occur in children who are small but otherwise normal and healthy if given anabolic steroids to stimulate growth. Less prominent effects, but probably more serious, are the retention of sodium, potassium, water, and chloride, which can contribute to heart failure. Jaundice has occasionally been observed after the administration of methyltestosterone and norethandrolone and means that administration of the androgen will probably be discontinued. Nausea and gastrointestinal upsets occur occasionally. Patients receiving androgens should be observed carefully for hypercalcemia, acceleration of the disease being treated, and the appearance of edema. Edema is sometimes controlled with the use of diuretics and a diet low in salt.

Contraindications. Androgens are contraindicated for patients with prostatic cancer and serious cardiorenal dysfunction. They are also contraindicated in pregnant women because of possible masculinization of the female fetus.

QUESTIONS

For study and review

1 Describe the objectives of androgen therapy.
2 Differentiate between combination therapy and sequential therapy oral contraceptives.
3 Identify some common side effects and some contraindications of oral contraceptive therapy.

Multiple choice

4 Diethylstilbestrol belongs to which of the following groups?
 a. gonadotropins
 b. androgens
 c. estrogens
5 A drug that is a male sex hormone is said to be a(n):
 a. estrogen
 b. androgen
 c. gonadotropin
6 Which of the following preparations is sometimes used to relieve symptoms associated with menopause?
 a. progesterone
 b. methyltestosterone
 c. diethylstilbestrol
 d. ergonovine maleate
7 All central nervous system depressants tend to be used in small doses for the patient in labor to avoid:
 a. prolongation of labor
 b. excessive response by the mother
 c. respiratory depression in the fetus
8 Which of the following reasons may explain why estrogens are sometimes used in treatment of mammary cancer (in patients past menopause) in preference to androgens?
 a. They are less expensive.
 b. They produce relief of symptoms more quickly.
 c. They produce no side effects.
 d. They can be administered orally.
9 Which of the following preparations might you expect to see ordered for the suppression of lactation?
 a. chlorotrianisene (Tace)
 b. oxytocin (Pitocin)
 c. diethylstilbestrol
 d. methylergonovine maleate (Methergine Maleate)
10 Patients receiving oxytocin (Pitocin) to induce labor must be watched especially for:

a. tetanic contractions of the uterus
b. maternal exhaustion
c. drop in blood pressure
d. prolapse of the umbilical cord

11 What is the primary purpose of giving promethazine hydrochloride (Phenergan Hydrochloride) to a patient in labor?
   a. to relieve pain
   b. to reduce the amount of postpartum nausea
   c. to reduce the amount of narcotic needed by the mother
   d. to produce sleep

12 Which of the following preparations might you expect to see ordered for a patient who is inactive and whose muscular and osseous tissues seem to be wasting away?
   a. diethylstilbestrol
   b. chlorotrianisene (Tace)
   c. norethandrolone (Nilevar)

13 Which of the following is a synthetic estrogen that is stored in body fat from which it is slowly released?
   a. testosterone propionate
   b. chlorotrianisene
   c. estradiol benzoate
   d. relaxin

REFERENCES

Aldercreutz, H., and Tenkuven, R.: Some aspects of the interaction between natural and synthetic female sex hormones and the liver, Am. J. Med. **49:**630, 1970.

Board, J. A.: Oral contraception with estrogen and progestin combinations, Curr. Ther. Res. **13:**1, 1971.

Carter, D. E., and others: Effect of oral contraceptives on drug metabolism, Clin. Pharmacol. Therap. **15:**22, 1974.

Council on Drugs, American Medical Association: Oral contraceptives: Current status of therapy, J.A.M.A. **214:**2316, 1970.

Dugdale, M., and Mass, A. T.: Hormonal contraception and thromboembolic disease: Effects of the oral contraceptives on hemostatic mechanisms, J. Chronic Dis. **23:**775, 1971.

Federman, D. D.: Testicular deficiency, Adv. Intern. Med. **16:**81, 1970.

Garcia, C. R.: Endocrine approach in the management of dysfunctional uterine bleeding, Clin. Obstet. Gynecol. **13:**460, 1970.

Greenwald, P., and others: Vaginal cancer after maternal treatment with synthetic estrogens, New Eng. J. Med. **285:**390, 1971.

Herbst, A. L., and others: Adenocarcinoma of the vagina: Association of maternal stilbestrol therapy with tumor appearance in young women, New Eng. J. Med. **284:**878, 1971.

Kellie, A. E.: The pharmacology of the estrogens, Ann. Rev. Pharmacol. **11:**97, 1971.

Landau, R. L., and Poulos, J. T.: The metabolic influence of progestins, Adv. Metab. Disord. **5:**119, 1971.

Marshall, J. R.: Ovulation induction, Obstet. Gynecol. **35:**963, 1970.

Masi, A. T., and Dugdale, M.: Cerebrovascular diseases associated with the use of oral contraceptives, Ann. Intern. Med. **72:**65, 1970.

Rogers, J.: Estrogens in the menopause and postmenopause, New Eng. J. Med. **280:**364, 1969.

Saruta, T., and others: A possible mechanism for hypertension induced by oral contraceptives, Arch. Intern. Med. **126:**621, 1970.

Vande Wiele, R. L., and others: Mechanisms regulating the menstrual cycle in women, Recent Prog. Horm. Res. **26:**63, 1970.

Wallach, E. E.: Physiology of menstruation, Clin. Obstet. Gynecol. **13:**366, 1970.

CHAPTER 27

Effects of drugs on human sexuality, fetal development, and nursing infant

Drugs affecting sexual behavior
Drugs affecting the fetus
Effects of maternal drug ingestion on the nursing infant

An important part of human development is the attainment of a sexual identity and the ability to live as a sexual being. This concept admits of many aspects and may be thought of, in one way, as a cyclic phenomenon that begins with the formation of the germ cell, whether sperm or ovum, and progresses through procreative activity, fertilization, fetal development, infancy, puberty, and so on in the generational evolution. There is an array of sex-related roles in human life, such as the ability to be a parent, to nurture, and to attain and to give satisfaction in sexual activity.

This chapter is limited to three aspects of human sexual life—sexual response, pregnancy, and lactation. These areas have been selected as those particularly vulnerable to the influence of drugs.

There have been and there remain vast speculation and misinformation about the influence of drugs on sexual behavior; there is an increasing body of knowledge about the effects of maternal medication on the infant and newborn. It is one task of the nurse, and other health professionals as well, to gain as much reliable information as possible. In this way, the well-being of individuals may be better understood and safeguarded.

DRUGS AFFECTING SEXUAL BEHAVIOR

Drugs influence various aspects of sexual behavior. Some affect only the physiologic response of the genitals, while others affect the intensity of sexual interest and pleasure. The data on the sexually enhancing effects of androgens and the impairment of sexual functioning caused by anticholinergic and antiadrenergic drugs are quite soundly based on observation and physiologic fact. There is little actual support for the aphrodisiac qualities attributed to hallucinogens or neurotransmitters.

Awareness of the influence of drugs on human sexuality is a needed adjunct to the pharmacologic knowledge of the nurse. An adequate patient history includes data about sexual functioning. Often this information is elicited by the nurse; certainly, it must be understood by the nurse. As in the past, sex is regarded by most persons as a highly personal area. It takes the practitioner's most refined skills and sensitivity to discuss sex-related matters with a client. While few nurses, at least at present, are qualified to be sex or marriage counselors, sound information and the clinical implications for its use are an integral part of patient management.

Mechanisms of action. There are several means by which drugs can affect sexuality. Generally, this involves a chemical alteration of the nerves that regulate sexual response. Some drugs have primary action on the brain. By altering the functioning of the cerebral sex centers, these substances can enhance or diminish libido. Other substances act on peripheral nerves, thus influencing activity of the sex organs. These substances do not affect sex drive but impair either the cholinergic mechanism governing erection or the adrenergically mediated emission phase of orgasm. Other mechanisms involve alteration of the response by genital blood vessels. Drugs may differ in specific action on the sexual response; or they may cause general toxicity thus affecting sexual functioning secondarily. Also, changes in sexuality may be a by-product of a primarily psychotropic action.

Of prime importance is the fact that a drug is but one variable in a complex system that includes the individual's personality characteristics, situational forces, expectations of what the drug will do, and relationship with a partner. There are notable gender differences, for the male response is more visible and quantifiable. The effects of drugs on erection and emission are more readily studied, and there have been no comparable investigations of the effects of these substances on female sexual response. There is some evidence to suggest that drugs influencing sexual interest by acting on the brain have similar effects on both men and women.

CENTRALLY ACTING SEXUAL STIMULANTS
Alcohol and barbiturates

In its progression of effects, alcohol first depresses brain centers governing fear and inhibition. By releasing inhibitions sufficiently to allow a temporary increase in libido, alcohol is sometimes mistakenly identified as an aphrodisiac. Increased ethanol ingestion suppresses cortical function and impairs cognitive ability. At even higher doses loss of consciousness occurs as well as irregularly descending paralysis in the manner of sedatives, hypnotics, and anesthetics.

An habitual heavy alcohol intake may seriously impair sexual functioning of both genders but especially of men. This is probably brought about by neurologic damage and the generally debilitating aspects of alcoholism.

Barbiturates and other hypnotic drugs have similar sexual and behavioral effects. While limited intake may release sexual behavior temporarily from inhibition, larger doses of sedatives depress all response. It is difficult to assess in terms of sexual functioning, however, the interactional effects of the drug with the underlying need for dependency on the drug.

Hallucinogens and marihuana

The hallucinogens, especially LSD (lysergic acid diethylamide), marihuana, and MDA (methylenedioxy amphetamine) do not seem to have specific action on the sexual centers of the brain but may affect sexuality as a part of their general action on the central nervous system.

LSD is a powerful hallucinogen believed to disrupt normal neural transmissions in the limbic and centrocephalic systems of the brain. These areas are involved with integration of perceptual processes and with emotional expression. Subjective reports of users often involve awareness of vivid images and thoughts. Erotic experiences may be recounted as "different" but "interesting." While there is vast individual difference in reaction, the sexual experience tends to be more diffuse and mixed with other perceptions. Orgasm may be a more prolonged but less absorbing experience. An adverse reaction brings about diminished awareness of sexuality as the individual is caught up in his own fear or paranoia. Effects of such substances are mediated largely by the conditions under which the drugs are taken as well as the personality and current psychic state of the individual.

THC (tetrahydrocannabinol) is the active ingredient in marihuana. Although it is a much milder hallucinogen than LSD in the amount usually taken, many persons report an enhanced erotic experience with marihuana. Some claim a more prolonged and pleasurable orgasm. These phenomena have yet to be examined under controlled conditions; thus these actions, though widely acclaimed, have no scientific base as yet. The reported enhancing effects on muscular contraction and increased awareness of proprioception of muscle contraction, integral to both male and female orgasm, have yet to be investigated.

MDA is an amphetamine-related hallucinogen

that has been reported to have sexually stimulating effects. This is not an isolated phenomenon but occurs within the context of the total hallucinogenic experience.

Amphetamines

Amphetamine is a centrally acting brain stimulant, which reportedly has some sexual effects. Some persons claim that large doses of this substance increase interest in sex as well as heighten their degree of abandon, confidence, and performance. Some, having become dependent upon the drug, say that they cannot perform sexually without it. A chronic amphetamine user may experience diminution in sexual ability and interest. A severely dependent person is usually very ill and psychotic—and most likely not interested in sex.

Cocaine

There are individual claims that cocaine brings about an unusually exciting and pleasurable sexual response. Presumably, these effects are a product of the drug's action on the brain. Even though some persons may experience aphrodisiacal effects during early cocaine use, these phenomena do not occur singly but are part of a profound general toxic behavioral state that could be a prelude to psychosis.

Androgen

Androgen affects the sex centers of the brain and also acts peripherally on the genitalia. It is the only currently available substance that increases sex drive without simultaneously altering consciousness and causing other ultimately sex-inhibiting side effects. Androgen clearly restores libido and potency that have been diminished because of androgen deficiency. However, when there is no explicit deficiency, effects of androgen are more variable. Androgens have also been used to restore libido in women, especially menopausal women. Its use is limited by its side effects, which include the development of male secondary sexual characteristics (hirsutism and deepening of the voice in women), exacerbation of prostatic cancer, and an increased hematopoietic response, which could result in cerebral and cardiovascular pathology.

The possibility of controlling aggressive behavior in human beings by manipulating androgens has been discussed in the scientific literature, but because both libido and aggression in the human female and male depend upon androgens, their control would never be a popular approach to restraining aggressiveness.

EXPERIMENTAL CENTRALLY ACTING NEUROTRANSMITTERS

There is a group of substances that may act directly on the synapses of the neurones comprising the centers and circuitry governing sexual behavior. Included are cyclazocine, L-dopa, and PCPA.

Cyclazocine is a narcotic antagonist that competes with heroin and other narcotics for receptor sites, possibly in the pleasure centers of the brain. Male heroin addicts placed on maintenance doses of cyclazocine reported some increase in libido. This claim has not been substantiated in studies and may be due, at least in part, to detoxification from narcotics rather than to drug action.

L-dopa and PCPA (p-chlorophenylalanine) are both related to neurotransmitters in the brain; both are centrally acting serotonin antagonists. L-dopa has had wide acclaim because it is highly useful in the treatment of Parkinson's disease in which there is a deficiency in the dopamine-acetylcholine ratio. Male patients receiving treatment have reported an increase in sexual interest and erection. To date, this has not been consistently confirmed in human studies.

PCPA, also a serotonin antagonist, was of great theoretical interest when it was found to increase the mounting and copulatory activity of male rats. However, these findings seem species-specific and not replicable with cats, primates, or the female rat.

PERIPHERALLY ACTING SEXUAL STIMULANTS
Androgen and estrogen

The sex hormones act on genital organs to enhance size, sensitivity, and responsiveness.

The male hormone, androgen, acts directly on the cells making up male genitalia to promote growth. The clitoris is also sensitive to androgens and will respond by hypertrophy if sufficient exogenous or endogenous androgen is present. The effect is seen whether androgen is administered parenterally or locally.

Estrogen assumes a similar role in producing maturation and growth of female genitalia and breasts. These organs generally atrophy when estrogen level diminishes at menopause. These phenomena can be delayed by estrogen replacement therapy, which also maintains or restores vaginal mucosa and musculature to a functional state. Estrogen is antagonistic to both the central and peripheral action of androgen and is frequently used for its antiandrogenic effects in medical and urologic practice.

Amyl nitrite and cantharides

These two substances are claimed to enhance genital responsiveness by alteration of local vascular response and increased irritability of the genital organs. Amyl nitrite has gained a degree of popularity by reputedly increasing the intensity and pleasure of orgasm in the male. The drug is a vasodilator sometimes prescribed to relieve the pain of angina pectoris. The use of the drug for other than therapeutic reasons is dangerous. Coronary occlusion resulting in death has occurred following the use of amyl nitrite during intercourse.

Cantharides, or "Spanish fly," does not enhance sexual functioning. It is a peripherally acting toxic substance that irritates the bladder and urethra and may cause the male to experience pseudosexual excitement. This agent can cause permanent damage by increasing vulnerability to bladder and urethral infections. It may also bring about permanent penile damage subsequent to prolonged priapism.

CENTRALLY ACTING SUBSTANCES THAT MAY IMPAIR SEXUALITY

There are many substances that impair libido and general sexual responsiveness. As has been stated, all centrally acting nervous system depressants may decrease sexual interest just as they depress other brain functions. The individual dependent upon barbiturates, hypnotics, sedatives, or alcohol is likely to lose interest in sexuality as well as experience a decreased ability to function sexually. The narcotics, specifically, seem to reduce libido.

PERIPHERALLY ACTING DRUGS THAT MAY IMPAIR SEXUAL RESPONSE

Some medications alter sexual response by acting peripherally on the genital organs. Their effects are produced by blocking nerve synapses at neuroeffector junctions that control the vascular and muscular structures necessary for sexual response. Drugs may affect the adrenergic ejaculatory response or the cholinergically mediated erective reactions.

Antiadrenergics

These substances block the nerves and the structures innervated by the sympathetic division of the autonomic nervous system. This system employs catecholamines as neurotransmitters rather than the acetylcholine of the parasympathetic nerves. Antiadrenergic drugs are often utilized in the management of hypertension and may cause difficulties with ejaculation. Guanethidine, an adrenergic blocking agent used to treat hypertension, commonly inhibits ejaculation. Ganglionic blocking agents, also used as antihypertensives, may impair both the adrenergic and cholinergically controlled phases of sexual response, which can result in impotence. They block transmission in the intermediate ganglia of both components of the autonomic nervous system.

Anticholinergics

Drugs of this category inhibit action of acetylcholine and so block parasympathetically mediated visceral responses. These substances alter sexual response by interfering with the transmission of impulses mediated by the parasympathetic nervous system, which controls vasodilation of blood vessels in the penis. Anticholinergics are used in treating gastrointestinal disturbances because they inhibit intestinal spasm and the secretion of gastric hydrochloric acid. High doses of any drug in this category impede cholinergic activity and may impair erection.

In contrast to centrally acting agents, the peripherally acting substances act primarily on

Table 27-1 Drugs that may decrease libido and impair sexual response*

Drug	Presumed mechanism of action and effect	Some common medical indications
Drugs that act on the brain Sedatives		
Alcohol and barbiturates	General depression of CNS in acute dose; neurologic damage with chronic use	Hypnotics and sedatives
Narcotics Heroin Morphine Codeine Methadone	General depression of CNS plus depression of sex centers (?)	Analgesics; methadone used in treatment of narcotic addiction
Antiandrogens	Oppose stimulating action of androgen on brain and sex organs	
Estrogens		Replacement therapy in post-menopausal women and in men with prostatic cancer
Cyproterone acetate		Experimental; treatment of compulsive sexual disorders
Adrenal steroids Cortisone ACTH Spironolactone (Aldactone) Spironolactone HCl (Aldactazide)		Allergic and inflammatory disorders Edema Hypertension
Drugs that act on the genitals	With exception of some antiadrenergic drugs, these do not impair libido except as secondary reaction Block nerves controlling smooth muscles and blood vessels of genital organs involved in sexual response	
Anticholinergic drugs Methantheline (Banthine) Propantheline (Probanthine) Atropine Quaternary ammonium compounds	Inhibit action of ACh on structures innervated by postganglionic parasympathetic nerves; may cause impotence; do not affect libido	Peptic ulcer; dyskinesias; glaucoma and other opthalmologic disorders
Antiadrenergic drugs Phentolamine Ergot alkaloids Halo-alkylamines Guanethidine Methyldopa (Aldomet)	Block autonomic adrenergic nerves and structures innervated by them; may cause ejaculatory problems Some drugs may have peripheral effects impairing ejaculation; central effects may diminish libido and erection Impotence a frequent complication of methyldopa therapy	Hypertension; peripheral vascular disorders
Rauwolfia alkaloids		Psychosis, hypertension

*Adapted from Kaplan, H. S.: The new sex therapy, New York, 1974, Brunner/Mazel, Inc.

Table 27-2 Drugs that may enhance libido and sexual functioning*

Drug	Presumed mechanism of action and effect	Some common medical indications
Drugs which act on the brain Hormones	These drugs presumably stimulate the sex centers of the CNS and so increase libido and the genital response	
Androgen	Stimulates sex centers of both genders. Fetal androgen causes gender differentiation of behavior. Androgens also act on periphery to enhance the growth, development, and functioning of the male genitals and of the clitoris	Impotence replacement therapy, anabolic agent, breast cancer
Progesterone and estrogen	Do not increase libido, in fact may decrease sexual interest; act on the cells of the female genitalia to enhance their growth, development, and functioning	Replacement therapy in menopause, endometriosis, menstrual disorders, birth control, therapy for prostatic carcinoma, postgenitourinary surgery to prevent erection
Neurotransmitters L-dopa PCPA (para-chlorphenyl-alanine)	Antiserotonin effect in sex centers of the brain Increases libido (?)	Parkinsonism Experimental—no medical indications
Stimulants Amphetamines	General brain stimulation. In acute doses, reported to enhance libido; in chronic doses, diminish libido and sexual functioning as well as causing general debility	Stimulant, appetite suppressants, minimal brain damage in children
Cocaine	General brain damage, reported to enhance libido in acute doses	High dependence potential—only medical indication is topical anesthesia
Nox-vomica (strychnine)	Increases reactivity of neurons in the spinal cord which mediate orgasm and erection reflexes; may cause priapism	Deadly poison—no medical indications
Hallucinogens LSD Dimethyltryptamine Mescaline THC (marihuana)	Disrupt neurotransmission in limbic system and reticular activating system. Reported by some to enhance libido and orgasm, by others to have no effect, while some users report impaired sexuality May have some effects on muscle contractions; some reports of enhanced erotic feelings (?)	
Drugs which act on the genital organs Cantharides (Spanish fly)	Irritates genitourinary tract; causes priapism	Poisonous—no medical indications
Amyl nitrite	Enhances vascular response of genitals (?) and reported to improve orgasm (?)	Vasodilator, angina pectoris

*Adapted from Kaplan, H. S.: The new sex therapy, New York, 1974, Brunner/Mazel, Inc.

Table 27-3 Effects of psychotropic drugs on sexuality*

Drug	Presumed mechanism of action and effect	Some common medical indications
All neuroleptic drugs	Probably no direct effect on brain sex center (haloperidol may affect sexual response directly); possible indirect effect from favorable effects on psychic state Infrequent reports of erectile and ejaculatory difficulties (probably because of mild antiadrenergic and/or anticholinergic or antidopamine effects)	
Antipsychotic drugs	Mechanism of action not clearly understood; sexual response may be improved as by-product of recovery from illness	Psychosis, notably schizophrenia
Phenothiazines Chloropromazine (Thorazine) Perphenazine (Trilafon) Trifluoperazine (Stelazine) Thioridazine (Mellaril)	"Dry" ejaculation, possibly caused by effects on internal vesical sphincter paralysis causing semen to empty into bladder	
Butyrophenones Haloperidol	Reported to reduce libido and potency; retarded ejaculations occur in some patients; mechanism unknown (may involve central or peripheral antiadrenergic and/or antidopamine actions)	Gilles de la Tourette syndrome; schizophrenia
Antianxiety drugs Chlordiazepoxides (Librium, Valium) Clorazepate dipotassium (Tranxene) Meprobamate	Depress limbic system and affect synapses in spinal cord to cause muscle relaxation Probably no direct sexual effect; sexual interest may increase as anxiety lessened; decrease in libido may also occur Orgasm disturbances reported (rare); resulting from muscle-relaxing effect	Anxiety; muscle relaxant
Mood regulators Tricyclic antidepressants Amitriptyline HCl (Elavil) Imipramine HCl (Tofranil)	No direct effects; sex drive and performance may improve as depression lifts Some peripheral autonomic effects; may rarely cause impotency and ejaculatory problems Increased or decreased libido	Depression; phobic anxiety states
MAO inhibitors Phenelzine sulfate (Nardil) Iproniazid (Marsilid) Isocarboxazid (Marplan)	Changes in libido, sexual disturbances; may be due to increase in catecholamine	Depression
Lithium	No reported effects Sexual urgency may diminish with generally diminished manic activities	Manic states; possible prevention of depression in bipolar illness

*Adapted from Kaplan, H. S.: The new sex therapy, New York, 1974, Brunner/Mazel, Inc.

Table 27-4 Miscellaneous drugs that may affect sexuality*

Drug	Presumed mechanism of action and effect	Some common medical indications
Disulfiram (Antabuse)	Occasional impotence reported	Alcohol abuse
Chlorphentermine (Pre-sate)	Occasional impotence reported	Weight reduction

*Adapted from Kaplan, H. S.: The new sex therapy, New York, 1974, Brunner/Mazel, Inc.

the genitals and produce indirect effects on libido. However, sexual difficulties can occur secondarily to the patient's adverse emotional reaction to the sex-inhibiting effect of the drug. Two antihypertensive agents, reserpine and methyldopa, produce a psychomotor depression in some patients, probably by a reduction of central nervous system catecholamine. Loss of libido and potency is frequently seen in this drug-induced depressive state.

DRUGS THAT AFFECT SEXUAL BEHAVIOR INDIRECTLY

Drugs used in the treatment of psychiatric disorders may affect sexuality. Many persons having sexual difficulties are taking psychotropic medication. Generally, the sexual effects of psychotropic drugs are nonspecific, and patients on prescribed dosage of tranquilizers and antidepressants may experience improved sexual functioning. This is reflective of diminished anxiety rather than a specific sexual effect. A highly anxious patient whose mood has been calmed may feel a lessening of his urgent sexual need. Antianxiety and antipsychotic drugs may bring about improvement in sexual behavior as part of the general positive response to drug therapy.

In addition to nonspecific central and psychologic effects, some antipsychotic, antianxiety, and antidepressant drugs may have some effect on sexual response because of mild peripheral and central autonomic influence. Reserpine, as an example, acts on autonomic nervous system control of the genitals and can impair sexual response. Some individuals taking chlorpromazine, an antipsychotic agent, report orgasm devoid of ejaculate. This phenomenon is thought

to occur because of peripheral autonomic action on the internal vesical sphincter, which causes semen to be propelled into the urinary bladder rather than into the urethra.

Haloperidol may be an exception in its direct effect on the brain sex centers. Libido and potency impairment have been reported by males on high dosages of this substance, presumably caused by its central adrenergic and/or dopamine antagonism.

Tables 27-1 to 27-4 summarize the data from the preceding section.

DRUGS AFFECTING THE FETUS

There are various factors currently bringing about heightened interest in and attention to the effects of maternal medication upon the fetus and the newborn.

The nurse and health maintenance. The nurse is in a unique position for actual and potential influence in matters of general health maintenance. With the advent of extended roles for the nurse, such as pediatric nurse practitioner and family nurse practitioner, as well as increasing interest in nurse midwifery, schools of nursing are preparing the practitioner for a strong role in establishing and maintaining optimal health among client populations. Historically, nurses have been educated with emphasis on care of hospitalized, acutely and chronically ill patients —persons already in an illness state. The condition of pregnancy is not generally considered an illness or an abnormality. To safeguard against noxious influences that may endanger the well-being of the mother and infant, the nurse must be more knowledgeable about prenatal factors, one of which is drug ingestion. As a teacher, the nurse develops means of increasing public and client awareness about diet- and drug-related matters. Finally, a nurse having adequate regard for and preparation in research methodology has unparalleled opportunity for observation, speculation, testing of ideas, analysis, and application of findings. These role functions do not readily occur in isolation but, rather, in collaboration with the patient and in colleagueship with other health professionals.

The placenta. Until recently, the placental organ was considered an effective barrier against untoward influences on the developing fetus. However, it is now known that many, if not all, substances (or their metabolites), taken by the mother find their way into placental circulation and thus to the fetus. The bulk of the placenta consists of chorionic villi, which are exposed to a collection of maternal blood. Fetal and maternal bloods are separated from each other by two layers of cells at the trophoblastic endothelial junction. Substances usually pass through the junction by simple diffusion; factors favoring placental transfer include molecular size, electrical charge, and lipid solubility. The greater degree of fat solubility of the compound, the more readily it passes through the placenta. The transfer is more rapid when drugs are in their nonionized state. Also, drugs having low molecular weight appear to permeate the placenta rather readily. Knowledge of placental physiology has advanced rapidly in this decade, although it is still limited in terms of the vast array of its activities and influences.

The fetus as an intrauterine individual. The specialty of obstetrics is a very old one. It developed as a variant of general medicine into a study of the diseases of women, including gynecology and the "disease" of pregnancy. Thus, the attendant's focus was primarily on the woman rather than on the fetus she carried. Pediatrics and child psychology are of fairly recent origin and are, obviously, concerned with the child. The pediatrician's area of authority has never extended to the period of pregnancy or even, until a few years ago, to the time of delivery. Questions of prenatal and perinatal influences on fetal devel-

opment and behavior have not been prominent areas of inquiry. So, throughout the history of medicine, psychology, and nursing, no professional specialist has been the child's advocate during the 9 months of fetal life prior to birth.

Today, the need for a "fetal advocate" has become crucial because of the increase in the development and use of specialized medical therapeutics, including drugs. Research endeavors reflect a direction of attention away from studies of maternal mortality to investigation of fetal mortality and, now, to studies of the quality of intrauterine life for the fetus. This involves, in particular, indexing (1) what normal function is and (2) the level of ability to function normally. For example, it has been practical for several years to sample amniotic fluid, drawn from the pregnant uterus, to analyze many facets of genetic and general health status. Within the past decade, intrauterine transfusion has become a therapeutic actuality in conditions of maternal/fetal blood incompatibilities. The "intrauterine patient" may receive specific treatment, such as steroids, to increase likelihood of adequate pulmonary function following premature birth. In one specific instance, phenobarbital may be introduced to maternal circulation to enhance enzyme activity in the prevention of congenital nonhemolytic, nonobstructive jaundice of the newborn. However, the practice of fetal therapeutics by way of pharmaceuticals is recent and highly experimental.

EFFECTS OF DRUGS ON THE FETUS

In the past century, the number of medications administered to pregnant women has multiplied enormously. This includes physician-recommended prescription drugs as well as over-the-counter self-treatment. At present, the fetus may be potentially more at risk from maternal ingestion of medicaments than from the processes of pregnancy and delivery. This has been particularly evident since the thalidomide tragedy of 1961. Various studies have been conducted on the percentages of mothers taking drugs during pregnancy. The mean number of drugs per person was found to be 10.3. It should be noted that many of these are taken before the pregnancy is affirmed or even suspected. Incidence

Table 27-5 Drugs taken by the mother during pregnancy

Drug classification	Percentage
Analgesic	64
Diuretic	57
Antihistamine	52
Antibiotic	41
Iron	41
Antiemetic	36
Antacid	35
Vitamin supplement	25
Sedative	24
Hormone	20
Appetite suppressant	10
Hypnotic	9
Genitourinary antibiotic	6
Narcotic	5

of drug ingestion, listed from most to least frequently used, appears in Table 27-5.

Within the individual, whether maternal or fetal, there exists considerable difference in ability to metabolize or respond to drugs. This may result from an idiosyncratic variable or may be directly related to genetic inheritance or chronologic age. For instance, 10% to 15% of black males lack the enzyme glucose-6-phosphate dehydrogenase; these individuals develop hemolytic anemia after ingestion of primaquine, sulfa, or phenacetin.

To date, there is no evidence to substantiate any claim of drug effect on human chromosomal material, either before or after fertilization has occurred. However, a drug insult within the first 3 to 4 weeks following the last menstrual period usually produces an all-or-nothing reaction. Either death or reabsorption takes place or the embryo lives. During the next 4 to 8 weeks of gestation, rapid-division organogenesis occurs, and this is the time of greatest possible risk of producing a malformation (or teratogenic effect). After 8 weeks, drug-induced problems are most frequently reflected in subsequent growth retardation, respiratory difficulties, infection, or bleeding in the newborn.

Some researchers contend that there may be several factors involved in the cause of newborn defects, including the genetic makeup of the parents, current health status of the mother, and ambient hazards such as pesticides, as well as the specific intrauterine environment. It is truism to state that whatever affects human tissue is also potentially destructive of human tissue. However, a therapeutic drug should not be withheld from the pregnant woman if the risk to the mother of no treatment is greater than risk to the infant of adverse effects from the drug (as in the treatment of a maternal bacterial infection). The basic problem is not in avoiding drugs when they are indicated; it arises when drugs are given without justification, and without thorough knowledge of contraindications, possible interaction effects with other therapy, proper dosage, and adverse reactions.

It is thought by some experts in the fields of fetology, neonatology, and perinatology that drugs are not an important factor in congenital malformations in general, since the few drugs that have been identified as having some adverse potential in man may represent only a small fraction of either the drugs used or the defects occurring. This point of view, directed to an aggregate population of pregnant women, seems to minimize the impact of infant defect on the individual and his family. Three major questions are current: (1) Is it possible to devise tests and surveillance systems that will prevent another teratologic catastrophe such as thalidomide? (2) How are interactions between drugs and other environmental factors or these and unstable genetic loci to be identified? (3) What comprises adequate genetic counseling for families at high risk and how might this be accomplished? Table 27-6 presents a listing of maternal drugs in current or potential use and gives some indication of their effect on the fetus or newborn.

EFFECTS OF MATERNAL DRUG INGESTION ON THE NURSING INFANT

The nursing infant may be the unintended recipient of drugs administered to the mother. Foreign compounds are known to be excreted into the milk of nursing mothers, and these com-

Table 27-6 Effects of maternal medication on the fetus and newborn*

Agent	Effect
Anesthesia (inhalation)	
Cyclopropane	Infant depression from narcosis depending on duration drug is given
Ether	Crosses placenta rapidly; depresses infant by direct narcotic effect; does not interfere with oxygenation
Halothane (Fluothane)	No significant depression if given for short duration
Methoxyflurane	No significant depression unless mother deeply anesthetized
Nitrous oxide	No significant depression if oxygen concentration administered to mother is adequate (20% or more)
Anesthesia (local)	
Lidocaine (Xylocaine)	Crosses placenta readily; adverse effects on the fetus not established
Mepivacaine (Carbocaine)	May depress infant by direct drug effect or indirectly via maternal hypotension when used for regional anesthesia (spinal or epidural procedures)
Procaine (Novocaine)	
Tetracaine (Pontocaine)	
Antibacterials	
Ampicillin	No untoward effect; safe use in pregnancy not established
Cephalexin (Keflex)	Crosses placenta; only 50% of infants will have bacteriostatic levels in cord blood or amniotic fluid when mother has adequate serum levels
Cephalothin (Keflin)	No untoward effect; safe use during pregnancy and in infants under 1 month of age not established
Chloramphenicol	"Gray syndrome" (gastrointestinal irritability, circulatory collapse, death) in newborn treated with this drug; never proved to occur in newborn if drug given only to mother
Erythromycin	No untoward effects demonstrated; safe use during pregnancy not established
Isoniazid (INH)	Unconfirmed, retrospective, and circumstantial evidence of psychomotor retardation
Kanamycin	Ototoxicity suspected but not proved in infants born to mothers treated for extended periods
Lincomycin (Lincocin)	Crosses placenta rapidly, fetal blood levels equal ¼ maternal blood levels; no untoward effects recorded
Metronidazole (Flagyl)	No untoward effect known; crosses placental barrier readily; not recommended during first trimester
Nitrofurantoin (Furadantin)	Megaloblastic anemia in fetus with glucose-6-phosphate dehydrogenase deficiency
Novobiocin	Increase in hyperbilirubinemia if newborn treated; not proved to occur via maternal treatment
Penicillin	No untoward effect
Sulfonamides	Sulfonamides displace protein-bound bilirubin and can cause kernicterus in fetus and in newborn infants
Sulfadiazine	
Sulfadimethoxine (Madribon)	
Sulfamethoxypyridazine	
Sulfisoxazole (Gantrisin)	
Streptomycin	Hearing loss (rare) in infants of mothers having prolonged treatment in early pregnancy
Tetracycline (Achromycin)	Staining of deciduous teeth and hypoplasia of enamel, inconclusive association with congenital cataracts, potential for bone growth retardation but not proved to occur in utero
Chlortetracycline (Aureomycin)	
Oxytetracycline (Terramycin)	
Demethylchlortetracycline (Declomycin)	
Anticoagulants	
Bishydroxycoumarin (Dicumarol)	Risk of fetal hemorrhage, particularly if mother overtreated
Heparin	No untoward effect; does not cross placenta
Warfarin (Coumadin)	Risk of fetal hemorrhage, particularly if mother overtreated; reports of malformed infants with hypoplastic nasal structures
Anticonvulsants	
Phenytoin	Increased incidence of midline clefts, congenital heart disease, eye defects, and coagulation defect

*Adapted from Bowes, W. R., Conway, E., Brackbill, Y., and Steinchneider, A.: Effects of obstetrical medication on fetus and infant Soc. Res. Child Devel. **35**(137): June, 1970.

Table 27-6 Effects of maternal medication on the fetus and newborn—cont'd

Agent	Effect
Antidiabetic agents Chlorpropamide	Respiratory distress and neonatal hypoglycemia, teratogenic effects suspected but not proved, neonatal thrombocytopenia
Insulin	No proved untoward effect
Tolbutamide (Orinase)	Effects suspected but not proved; not recommended for use in diabetic women who may become pregnant; some reports of diverse multiple congenital abnormalities
Antihistamines and antiemetics Cyclizine (Merazine) Meclizine (Bonine)	No evidence of adverse effects in humans; not generally recommended for use during pregnancy
Antimalarial agents Chloroquine (Aralen)	Abnormal retinal pigmentation reported after maternal treatment for lupus erythematosus; congenital deafness has been reported when mother treated with high doses
Quinine	Early reports of ototoxicity and congenital malformations unsubstantiated by other clinicians, danger of fetal damage probably minimal
Antineoplastic agents Methotrexate (Amethopterin) Cytosine arabinoside Mercaptopurine (Purinethol)	Congenital anomalies; hypertelorism Reports of intrauterine growth retardation and fetal death Hemolytic anemia of the newborn
Antithyroid agents Methimazole (Tapazole) Sodium iodide, I^{131} Propylthiouracil	All antithyroid drugs cross placenta and can result in fetal goiters and hypothyroidism Permanent fetal thyroid suppression (I^{131})
Barbiturates Amobarbital (Amytal) Pentobarbital (Nembutal) Phenobarbital Secobarbital (Seconal) Thiamylal (Surital) Thiopental (Pentothal Sodium)	All barbiturates and thiobarbiturates cross placenta, in usual clinical doses they cause minimal fetal depression, decreased neonatal responsiveness and inhibited ability to suck, phenobarbital induces microsomal enzymes to increase conjugation of bilirubin in the newborn
Beta-blocking agents Propranolol (Inderal)	Crosses placenta, results in beta-adrenergic blocking effects in fetus depressing circulatory responses of the newborn
Cytotoxins (local) Podophyllum	Maternal absorption resulted in peripheral neuropathy and fetal death in utero (drug is antimitotic used for venereal warts and granuloma inguinale)
Digitoxin	When administered during eighth month of pregnancy may cause digitalis intoxication of fetus
Diuretics Chlorothiazide (Diuril) Hydrochlorothiazide (Hydrodiuril)	Thrombocytopenia Thrombocytopenia
Fungistatic agents Griseofulvin	No untoward effect
Intravenous fluids	Electrolyte imbalance possible, usually hyponatremia (lethargy, poor muscle tone, poor color)

Continued.

Table 27-6 Effects of maternal medication on the fetus and newborn—cont'd

Agent	Effect
Hallucinogens Lysergic acid diethylamide (LSD)	Fetal neural tube defects have been reported to be more common in users of LSD but these patients were also on other drugs such as marihuana and amphetamines (Extensive review of literature suggests no untoward chromosomal or teratogenic effects of LSD itself.)
Narcotics Alphaprodine (Nisentil) Dihydrocodeine Heroin Levophanol (Levo-Dromoran) Meperidine (Demerol) Methadone (Dolophine) Morphine	Depression of fetal respiration; decreased responsiveness of newborn. Depresses neonatal psychophysiologic functioning. Infants born to narcotic addicts develop withdrawal symptoms of hyperirritability, shrill cry, vomiting. Can be fatal. Intrauterine growth retardation and prematurity more common. No reports of fetal or infant death due to methadone treatment of mother but infant shows typical withdrawal symptoms, which can be more difficult to treat and more prolonged than with heroin
Narcotic antagonists Levallorphine (Lorfan) Nalorphine (Nalline)	Decreases neonatal depression caused by narcotic
Nicotine (smoking)	Reports of intrauterine growth retardation, conflicting reports about long-term developmental effects of maternal smoking, no definite deleterious effect demonstrated
Organic mercurial compounds	CNS malformations, including blindness in newborn (Minamata disease)
Salicylates Aspirin	Congenital defects more common in women taking salicylates in first trimester, no cause and effect relationship proved; inhibits platelet aggregation and causes hemorrhagic tendency in newborn, may predispose to prolong pegnancy by inhibiting prostaglandin biosynthesis, salicylate poisoning can occur in fetus with maternal overdose
Sedatives Chloral hydrate Ethchlorvynol (Placidyl)	No significant effect; crosses placenta; withdrawal symptoms in newborn similar to those seen with opiates
Skeletal muscle relaxants Curare Decamethonium bromide (Syncurine) Gallamine triethiodide (Flaxedil) Succinylcholine chloride (Anectine)	In usual clinical doses, drugs do not cross placenta and do not cause any noticeable effect on fetus or newborn
Steroids Betamethasone (Decadron)	Accelerates pulmonary maturation, salutary effects on fetus (or newborn) not entirely substantiated
Cortisone Dexamethasone (Decadron) Prednisolone Prednisone	Possible relationship to cleft palate and fetal death; not definitely proved in humans Some reports of placental insufficiency syndrome and fetal distress during labor and fetal death
Progestins	Masculinization of female fetus, implicated in development of multisystem anomalies and development of congenital heart defects
Diethylstilbestrol	Delayed development of adenosis and adenocarcinoma of vagina in female infant, vaginal cancer in teenage girls born to mothers on DES during pregnancy
Testosterone	Masculinization of female fetus
Thyroid compounds Desiccated thyroid extract Liothyronine (Cytomel)	Crosses the placenta but no known untoward effect on fetus or newborn

Table 27-6 Effects of maternal medication on the fetus and newborn—cont'd

Agent	Effect
Tranquilizers Chlordiazepoxide (Librium) Chlorpromazine (Thorazine)	Crosses placenta; no untoward effects demonstrated to date; No definite effect on fetus substantiated; extrapyramidal effects may appear in newborn if drug is given during last trimester; jaundice also reported; possibility of permanent neurologic damage cannot be excluded
Diazepam (Valium)	Crosses placenta; neonatal respiratory depression, hypotonia, and hypercarpnia; lowers newborn body temperature
Meprobamate (Equanil, Miltown)	No untoward effect on human fetus substantiated; crosses placental barrier; safe use in pregnancy not established
Prochlorperazine (Compazine)	Same as for chlorpromazine
Tricyclic antidepressants Imipramine (Tofranil)	Anecdotal reports of craniofacial and CNS lesions; several large studies have refuted these findings
Vitamins Vitamin D	Anecdotal reports of hypercalcemia and cardiovascular lesions resembling vitamin D intoxication; maternal intake should not be excessive

Vitamin K and analogues
  Menadione sodium bisulfite (Hykinone)
  Phytonadione (Aquamephyton)
	Administration to mother results in hyperbilirubinemia of newborn

pounds may have beneficial, detrimental, or no visible effect on the infant.

Studies of drug effects on the breastfed infant are primarily available through retrospective studies or anecdotal reports. In these instances, the population as well as the data may be limited. It is obviously not feasible to conduct in vivo research where the well-being of the subjects would be seriously compromised. Thus current information concerning pharmacologic effects is drawn largely from what has already occurred, or from animal studies in which the findings are questionable in terms of human applicability.

This portion of the chapter is directed to what has already been documented or is strongly suspected about drug effects on infants of nursing mothers. From it, some practical application may be drawn for therapy and for patient counselling and teaching.

SYNTHESIS AND COMPOSITION OF MILK

The mammary tissue, where milk is synthesized, is a compound, tubule-alveolar gland. The secretory, or alveolar, cells are surrounded by myoepithelial cells having contractile properties, which permits the transfer of milk from alveoli into the duct system. Proteins, carbohydrates, and fats are the most important natural components of milk.

The start of synthesis and secretion of milk is a highly complex hormonal interaction achieved by the combined effects of estrogens and progesterones. These hormones interact with pituitary, placental follicle stimulating hormone (FSH), and luteotropic hormone (LH) (see Figure 27-1). Milk production begins slowly; just prior to parturition the levels of estrogen and progesterone fall, and progesterone's inhibitory effect on prolactin release by the pituitary is withdrawn. Under the influence of prolactin, the alveolar cells become highly secretory. As the infant begins to stimulate the breast by sucking, a release of oxytocin occurs, which affects the contractility of the myoepithelial cells, and a flow of milk is established. This is called the "milk ejection reflex."

Lactation may be inhibited by the administration of androgens and estrogens, either

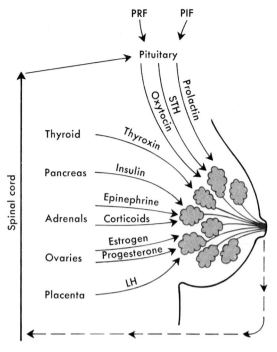

Figure 27-1

Multiple hormonal influences on human lactation. (Adapted from Catz, C. S., and Giacoia, G. P.: Drugs and breast milk, Ped. Clin. North Am. **19**:151, 1972.)

separately or in combined form. The timing and the dosage are the most important factors in eliciting response. Low dosages of progesterone or estrogen preparations, used in contraceptive therapy to suppress ovulation, may diminish lactation. If contraceptive therapy is begun after adequate milk production is established, lactation is not affected but the composition of the milk may be. For example, ethinyl estradiol augments milk protein content.

THE PRESENCE OF DRUGS IN MILK

In the maternal circulation drugs differ in their binding to plasma proteins. It is the unbound fraction that exerts the pharmacologic action and can be metabolized and excreted. Any endogenous or exogenous substance may compete with the drug and its binding to albumin, which may result in its displacement and augment its passage into the mammary duct system. In this in-

stance, the amount available for infant ingestion is increased. It is important to note that an isolated measurement of the concentration of a drug in milk is misleading unless it can be correlated to the total quantity ingested and absorbed by the infant.

The mammary gland is a *relatively* unimportant route for total drug excretion. However, this must not detract from the fact that foreign substances may appear in the milk and be ingested by the infant.

Small, water-soluble molecules (urea, antipyrine, alcohol) pass through biologic membranes by simple diffusion. Other drugs, such as sulfonamides, are bound to milk proteins. The passage of larger molecules depends on their lipid solubility and state of ionization; they pass through in a lipid-soluble, nonionized form. Drugs with low lipid solubility will diffuse rather slowly. Milk is an emulsion of fat in water, and the relative concentration of each component varies with and within each feeding. There is less fat concentration in the first milk the infant receives as compared to the last at any given feeding. Also, the time of day will determine the composition of milk, primarily in terms of fat content. Usually the fat content is higher in the morning. This becomes important when dealing with drugs like pentobarbital and secobarbital. Since they are more lipid soluble, these drugs will tend to transfer into milk as its fat content rises.

EFFECTS OF DRUGS ON NURSING INFANTS

An evaluation of present data on the effects of drugs on nursing infants results in two major categories of drugs: those causing noticeable adverse effects in the infant and those apparently not producing unfavorable consequences.

Bromides; lead. Historically, some drugs, such as bromides, have caused drowsiness and rash in breastfed infants. Lead encephalitis has been reported following the application of lead acetate ointment to the breasts of lactating women.

Pollutants. Environmental pollutants have been identified in other accidents. A severe porphyria occurred in small infants as a result of maternal exposure to the fungicide hexachlorobenzene. In Japan, waste containing mercurials contaminated the fish in Minamata Bay. The described "Minamata disease" affected the inhabitants of the area, presenting signs and symptoms of mercury intoxication. Breastfed infants were stricken as well.

Ergot. It has been known for many years that infants will develop signs of ergotism, since the active component of ergot is excreted into breast milk.

Heroin. At the beginning of the nineteenth century it was learned that heroin is present in breast milk. The infant may show signs of narcotic withdrawal when the mother is deprived of the drug or whenever the feeding is withheld. This occurs even when the dependence is subsequent to delivery.

Chloroform. Chloroform inhalation in the mother will produce anesthesia in her infant.

Alcohol. It has been reported that only small amounts of ethyl alcohol are present in breast milk; however, individual instances of alcohol intoxication of the infant have been observed.

Oral contraceptives. Controlled studies of the excretion and the effects of oral contraceptives and their metabolites are needed. Isolated reports indicate the development of gynecomastia in the infant following high maternal intake of these hormones.

Anticoagulants. Anticoagulants may be administered for the treatment of postpartum phlebitis. It is possible to alter infant prothrombin time through maternal intake of such agents as phenindione.

Types of effects. There is a lack of adverse reaction by infants to most drugs ingested with breast milk. However, this should not obscure the possibility of minimal or nondemonstrable effects, which may produce individual homeostatic complications.

Cumulative effect. An additive factor is seen with repeated administration of drugs that bind to fat tissue or to tissue proteins. These materials remain in the body for long periods of time. As an example, free chlorpromazine has been detected in tissues 18 months after discontinuation of the drug. It is not known at this time what impact this may have on the infant.

Effect on activity of drug-metabolizing enzymes. Some foreign compounds are known to increase the activity of drug-metabolizing enzymes located in the liver microsomes. Higher activity of these enzyme systems results in faster termination of drug action and also accelerates the hydroxylation of endogenous substances such as steroids. The long-term consequences of these phenomena are not known. In humans, phenobarbital and phenytoin are known accelerators of drug destruction by the liver and they are found in breast milk. It is not known, at this time, the effect of drugs on the microsomal enzymes of the infant's liver. Another possible effect of drugs is the inhibition of the activity of these enzyme systems.

Genetic defect. Persons with certain hereditary metabolic defects may react to drug doses too small to produce pharmacologic action. For example, the presence of sulfamethoxypyridazine in the breast milk has been known to cause hemolytic anemia in an infant lacking the enzyme glucose-6-phosphate dehydrogenase.

Alteration of homeostatic functions. Such alteration will facilitate effects by other agents. For example, a hypocoagulability state is likely to follow anticoagulant therapy of the mother. However, this may go unrecognized unless mechanical or surgical trauma to the infant occurs.

Interference with normal physiologic functions. Modification of infant thyroid function may result from maternal ingestion of iodides or thyroid preparations. The neonate is vulnerable to the development of goiter and hyperthyroidism.

Hypersensitivity. It is possible for the infant to develop hypersensitivity reactions following exposure to medication via breast milk. This is most likely to occur when doses are administered to both infant and mother, as in congenital syphilis, so that excessive amounts reach the infant.

Effects on normal development patterns. Infants with developmental enzymatic defects could be affected by small amounts of drugs in breast milk. Unidentified "inhibitors" are known to be responsible for breast milk jaundice in the newborn. This type of jaundice is thought to interfere with the level of maturation of gluconuryl transferase. Once full development of the enzyme is reached, these inhibitors cannot act. Ma-

Text continued on p. 635.

Table 27-7 Drugs excreted in human milk and the possible significance for nursing infants*

Drug	Excreted	Quantity excreted	Significance
Antihistamine drugs			
Diphenhydramine (Benadryl)	Yes		Not significant in therapeutic doses to affect child
Trimeprazine tartrate (Temaril)	Yes		Not significant in therapeutic doses to affect child
Tripelennamine (Pyribenzamine)	Yes		Only bovine studies reported to date; apparently not enough is excreted to be significant in therapeutic doses
Antiinfective agents			
Amantadine (Symmetrel)	Possible		Not to be administered; personal correspondence with the manufacturer suggests it will be found in maternal milk; may cause vomiting, urinary retention, skin rash
Ampicillin (Polycillin, Amcill, Omnipen, Penbritin, Principen, others)	Yes	0.07 μg./ml.	Not significant in therapeutic doses to affect child
Carbenicillin disodium (Pyopen, Geopen)	Yes	0.265 μg./ml. 1 hour after administration of 1 Gm.	Not significant in therapeutic doses to affect child
Cephalexin (Keflex)	No		
Cephalothin (Keflin)	No		
Chloramphenicol (Chloromycetin)	Yes	Half blood level 2.5 mg./100 ml.	Infants have underdeveloped enzyme system, immature liver and renal function, may not have glycuronide system adequately developed to conjugate chloramphenicol; caution advised
Chloroquine (Aralen)	No	After daily dose of 0.6 Gm. no traces could be found in milk of 105 subjects	Not significant in therapeutic doses to affect child
Demeclocycline (Declomycin)	Yes	0.2–0.3 mg./500 ml.	Not significant in therapeutic doses to affect child
Erythromycin (Ilosone, E-mycin, Erythrocin)	Yes	0.05–0.1 mg./100 ml. 3.6–6.2 μg./ml.	Higher concentrations have been reported in milk than in plasma
Isoniazid (Nydrazid)	Yes	0.6–1.2 mg./100 ml.; same concentration in milk as in maternal serum	Infant should be monitored for possible signs of isoniazid toxicity
Kanamycin (Kantrex)	Yes	1 Gm. given intramuscularly gave a concentration of 18.4 μg./ml.	Infant should be monitored for possible signs of kanamycin toxicity
Lincomycin (Lincocin)	Yes	0.5–2.4 μg./ml.	Not significant in therapeutic doses to affect child
Mandelic acid	Yes	0.3 Gm./24 hr. following maternal dose of 12 Gm./day	Not significant in therapeutic doses to affect child
Methacycline (Rondomycin)	Yes		Same precautions as with tetracyclines
Methenamine (Hexamine)	Yes		Not significant in therapeutic doses to affect child
Metronidazole (Flagyl)	Yes	Level comparable to serum	Apparently not significant in therapeutic doses; caution should

*From O'Brien, T. E.: Excretion of drugs in human milk, Nurs. Dig. **3**(4):25-31, 1975.

Table 27-7 Drugs excreted in human milk and the possible significance for nursing infants—cont'd

Drug	Excreted	Quantity excreted	Significance
Antiinfective agents—cont'd			
Metronidazole (Flagyl)—cont'd			be exercised due to its high milk concentrations
Nitrofurantoin (Furadantin)	Yes		Not significant in therapeutic doses to affect child
Nalidixic acid (NegGram)	Yes	3.9 μg./liter	Not significant in therapeutic doses; however one case of hemolytic anemia in an infant was attributed to nalidixic acid
Novobiocin (Albamycin, Cardelmycin)	Yes	0.36–0.54 mg./100 ml.	This antibiotic has been used to treat infections among infants with no untoward effects reported
Oxacillin (Prostaphlin)	No		
Paraamino salicylic acid	No		
Penethamate (Leocillin)	No	24–74 μg./100 ml.	Animal study suggests it be avoided
Penicillin G potassium	Yes	Up to 6 units/100 ml.	Controversy exists among clinicians, some feel that the risk of sensitivity symptoms must be looked for, others feel the small amount is insignificant; parent should be told to inform physician that infant has been exposed to penicillin
Penicillin, benzathine (Bicillin)	Yes	10–12 units/100 ml.	Clinical need should supersede possible allergic responses
Pyrimethamine (Daraprim)	Yes		Detected in human milk but no conclusions drawn; apparently not significant in therapeutic doses
Quinine sulfate	Yes	0–0.1 mg./100 ml. after maternal dose of 300–600 mg.	Not significant in therapeutic doses to affect child
Sodium fusidate	Yes	0.02 μg./ml.	Not significant in therapeutic doses to affect child
Streptomycin	Yes	Present for long periods in slight amounts given as dihydrostreptomycin	Risk should outweigh benefit of nursing; to be avoided
Sulfanilamide	Yes	After maternal dose of 2–4 Gm. daily 9 mg./100 ml. in milk	Not significant in therapeutic doses; may cause a rash
Sulfapyridine	Yes	3–13 mg./100 ml. after maternal dose of 3 Gm. daily	To be avoided; has caused skin rash
Sulfathiazole	Yes	0.5 mg./100 ml. after dose of 3 Gm./day	Not significant in therapeutic doses to affect child
Sulfisoxazole (Gantrisin)	Yes	Concentration similar to plasma level	To be avoided, during first 2 postpartum weeks; may cause kernicterus
Tetracycline HCl (Achromycin, Steclin, Sumycin, others)	Yes	0.5–2.6 μg./ml. after maternal dose of 500 mg. q.i.d.	Not enough to treat an infection in an infant; however, it has been hypothesized that there may be a sufficient amount to cause discoloration of the teeth in the infant; the antibiotic, however, may be largely bound to the milk calcium

Continued.

Table 27-7 Drugs excreted in human milk and the possible significance for nursing infants—cont'd

Drug	Excreted	Quantity excreted	Significance
Antineoplastics Cyclophosphamide (Cytoxan)	Yes		To be avoided, as are other antineoplastic drugs; nursing should be discontinued
Autonomic drugs Atropine sulfate[a] (ingredient in many products, both prescription and nonprescription)	Yes	Less than 0.1 mg./100 ml.	Should not be administered for two main reasons: (1) it inhibits lactation, and (2) it may cause atropine intoxication in the infant
Carisoprodol (Soma, Rela)	Yes	May be present in breast milk at concentrations four times maternal plasma	Not to be administered, based upon manufacturer's recommendation; infant may be exposed to a series of adverse reactions ranging from CNS depression to gastrointestinal upset
Ergot (Cafergot)	Yes		Avoid where possible; may cause symptoms in infants ranging from vomiting and diarrhea to weak pulse and unstable blood pressure
Hyoscine	Yes	Trace amounts	Not significant in therapeutic doses to affect child
Mepenzolate bromide (Cantil)	No		
Methocarbamol (Robaxin)	Yes	Small amounts	Not significant in therapeutic doses to affect child
Propantheline bromide (Pro-Banthine)	No		
Scopolamine	Yes		Not significant in therapeutic doses to affect child
Blood formation and coagulation Dicumarol	Yes		Therapeutic doses can be administered without deleterious effect on infant; infant should be monitored with mother
Ethyl biscoumacetate (Tromexan)	Yes	0–0.17 mg./100 ml.; no correlation with dosage	Not significant in therapeutic doses; infant should be monitored with mother
Iron	Yes		Not significant in therapeutic doses to affect child
Ferrous sulfate Iron-dextran (Feosol, Imferon)			
Phenindione (Hedulin, Dindevan)	Yes		To be avoided; may produce a prothrombin deficiency in infant; one case of massive hematoma reported in an infant receiving drug in maternal milk
Warfarin sodium (Coumadin)	Yes		Infant should be monitored with mother; benefit should outweigh possible risk

Table 27-7 Drugs excreted in human milk and the possible significance for nursing infants—cont'd

Drug	Excreted	Quantity excreted	Significance
Cardiovascular drugs			
Dextrothyroxine (Choloxin)	Yes		Not significant in therapeutic doses to affect child
Guanethidine (Ismelin)	Yes		Not significant in therapeutic doses to affect child
Methyclothiazide, deserpidine (Enduronyl)	Yes		Same precautions as with reserpine and thiazide diuretics
Methyldopa (Aldomet)	Yes		Studies performed on bovines; nothing reported in humans
Propranolol (Inderal)	No		
Reserpine (Serpasil, others)	Yes		May produce galactorrhea
Central nervous system drugs			
Alcohol	Yes	Small amounts	It appears that moderate amounts of alcohol have little, if any, effect on the nursing infant
Amitriptyline (Elavil)	No		
Aspirin	Yes	Moderate amounts	It could cause a bleeding tendency by interfering with the function of the infant's platelets or by decreasing the amount of prothrombin in the blood. Risk is minimal if mother takes aspirin just after nursing and if the infant has an adequate store of vitamin K
Barbiturates	Yes		It appears that in therapeutic doses the barbiturates have little or no effect on the infant; one case was reported where high doses had a hypnotic effect on one infant; it is best to avoid administering, since barbiturates serve as inducing agents for hepatic drug metabolizing enzymes
Barbital (Veronal)	Yes	4–5 mg. of diethylbarbituric acid/500 ml. of milk detected after a single dose of 500 mg.	Significant quantities, avoid administration; produced marked sedation in infant
Bromides (Bromo-Seltzer; many nonprescription sleeping aids)	Yes	0–6.6 mg./100 ml.	Not to be administered; reactions range from rash to drowsiness
Caffeine	Yes	1% of that ingested	Not significant in usual amounts to affect child
Chloroform	Yes		One study performed in 1908 reported that a nursing infant slept for 8 hours; not significant in therapeutic doses
Chloral hydrate (Noctec, Somnos)	Yes	0–1.5 mg./100 ml.	Not significant in therapeutic doses
Chlorazepate (Tranxene)	Yes		Not to be administered based upon manufacturer's recommendation; may cause drowsiness

Continued.

Table 27-7 Drugs excreted in human milk and the possible significance for nursing infants—cont'd

Drug	Excreted	Quantity excreted	Significance
Central nervous system drugs—cont'd			
Chlordiazepoxide (Librium)	Yes		Not significant in therapeutic doses to affect child
Chlorpromazine (Thorazine)	Yes	4.15 mg./ml. after daily dose of 200 mg. in dogs	Not significant; may cause galactorrhea
Codeine	Yes		Not significant in therapeutic doses to affect child
Cycloheptenyl ethyl barbituric acid (Medomin)	Yes		Not significant in therapeutic doses to affect child
Desipramine (Norpramin)	No		
Dextroamphetamine (Dexedrine)	No		
Diacetylmorphine (Heroin)	Yes		Not enough to prevent withdrawal in addicted infants
Diazepam (Valium)	Yes	51 ng./ml. after 4 days of diazepam; 28 ng./ml. of N-demethyldiazepam	Recent studies recommend that this drug be avoided during nursing; infant reported as lethargic and experienced weight loss; may cause hyperbilirubinemia
Diphenhydramine (Benadryl)	Yes		Not significant in therapeutic doses to affect child
Flutenamic acid (Arlef)	Yes		Excreted in small amounts; no recommendations
Hydroxyphenbutazone (Tandearil)	Yes	0 in 53 of 55 mothers	Conflicting reports; both conclude that it would have no significant effect in therapeutic doses
Imipramine (Tofranil)	No		
Indomethacin (Indocin)	Yes		Not significant in therapeutic doses to affect child
Lithium carbonate (Eskalith, Lithane, Lithonate)	Yes	Same in child's serum as in mother's milk, 0.3 mEq./liter	Infant should be monitored for possible signs of lithium toxicity
Mefenamic acid (Ponstel)	Yes		Not significant in therapeutic doses to affect child
Meperidine (Demerol)	Yes		Not significant in therapeutic doses to affect child
Meprobamate (Miltown, Equanil)	Yes	Present in milk two to four times maternal plasma level	Infant should be monitored for possible signs of meprobamate toxication if therapy is to be continued
Mesoridazine besylate (Serentil)	Yes		Not significant in therapeutic doses to affect child
Morphine	Yes	Small amounts	Not significant in therapeutic doses to affect child
Pentazocine (Talwin)	No		
Phenobarbital (Luminal, others)	Yes		To be avoided where possible; serves as an inducing agent for hepatic drug metabolizing enzymes
Phenylbutazone (Butazolidin)	No	0.63 mg./100 ml. 1½ hours after mother injected (I.M.) with 750 mg.	No side effects noted among group studied, but because of possible lethal reactions infant should be closely monitored

Table 27-7 Drugs excreted in human milk and the possible significance for nursing infants—cont'd

Drug	Excreted	Quantity excreted	Significance
Central nervous system drugs—cont'd			
Phenytoin (Dilantin)	Yes		Not significant in therapeutic doses although one case of methemoglobinemia was associated with phenytoin
Piperacetazine (Quide)	Yes		Manufacturer suggests it may have a great potential for excretion in milk
Primidone (Mysoline)	Yes		To be avoided, may cause undue somnolence and drowsiness
Prochlorperazine (Compazine)	Yes	0.4–1.5 mg./100 ml. in dogs after daily dose of 200 mg.	Not significant in therapeutic doses to affect child
Propoxyphene HCl (Darvon)	Yes	0.4% of dose to mother found in stomach of nursing rat	Not significant in therapeutic doses to affect child
Salicylates	Yes	1.0–3.0 mg./100 ml. of sodium salicylate detected 4 hours after maternal dose of 4 Gm.	Not significant in therapeutic doses; high doses (5 Gm./day) have been reported to cause a rash in infant
Thiopental sodium (Pentothal)	Yes		Not significant in therapeutic doses to affect child
Thioridazine (Mellaril)	Yes		Not significant in therapeutic doses to affect child
Tranylcypromine (Parnate)	Yes		Not significant in therapeutic doses to affect child
Trifluoperazine (Stelazine)	Yes	0.4–1.5 mg./100 ml. in dogs after daily dose of 200 mg.	Not significant in therapeutic doses to affect child
Diagnostic agents			
Carotene (natural product found in carrots)	Yes		One incident reported where infant turned yellow; mother ate 2–3 lb. of carrots per week; not significant in average quantities
Iopanoic acid (Telepaque)	Yes		Not significant in therapeutic doses to affect child
Electrolytic, caloric, and water balance			
Cyclopenthiazide (Navidrix)	No		
Cyclamate (Sucaryl)	Yes		Not significant in therapeutic doses to affect child
Furosemide (Lasix)	No		
Hydrochlorothiazide (Hydrodiuril, Esidrix, others)	Yes		To be avoided, based on manufacturer's recommendation; no specific adverse effects reported in infants to date
Spironolactone (Aldactone)	No		
Thiazides	Yes		To be avoided based on manufacturer's recommendation; no specific adverse reactions reported in infants to date

Continued.

Table 27-7 Drugs excreted in human milk and the possible significance for nursing infants—cont'd

Drug	Excreted	Quantity excreted	Significance
Expectorants and cough preparations Potassium iodide	Yes	3 mg./100 ml.	To be avoided, may affect infant's thyroid
Gastrointestinal drugs Aloe	Yes		Controversial, one author claims it may give rise to catharsis in some infants, others feel its presence is insignificant
Anthraquinone (Dorbane, Dorbantyl, Danthron, Peri-Colace, Doxidan, Dialose-Plus)	Yes		One animal study found it present in milk and in "significant" amounts; another human study did not detect it; a third human study detected it and felt it best not to administer it to nursing mothers, as it may cause catharsis in the infant
Cascara	Yes		Avoid where possible; reported to have increased gastric motility in infant
Emodin (found in cascara sagrada)	Yes		Avoid where possible; reported to have increased gastric motility in infant
Phenolphthalein (found in many nonprescription laxative products)	Yes		Not significant in therapeutic doses to affect child
Rhubarb	Yes		Not significant in therapeutic doses to affect child
Senna	Yes		Not significant in therapeutic doses; high doses may cause diarrhea in nursing infant
Hormones and synthetic substitutes Carbimazole (Neo-Mercazole)	Yes		Not to be administered; antithyroid may cause goiter in nursing infant
Chlormadione (Estalor-21)	Yes		Possible effects must be weighed against risk of pregnancy; see contraceptives (oral)
Chlorotrianisene (TACE)	Yes		Avoid where possible estrogenic substances may be in breast secretions
Contraceptives (oral)	Yes		Possible effects must be weighed against risk of pregnancy; may inhibit lactation if administered during first prenatal weeks; possible gynecomastia in male infant
Corticotropin	Yes		Destroyed during passage through gastrointestinal tract; its presence in milk is unimportant
Cortisone	Yes		No human study; among animals a 50% lower weight than control retarded sexual development, exophthalmos
Dihydrotachysterol (Hytakerol)	Yes		May cause hypercalcemia

Table 27-7 Drugs excreted in human milk and the possible significance for nursing infants—cont'd

Drug	Excreted	Quantity excreted	Significance
Hormones and synthetic substitute— cont'd			
Estrogen (oral contraceptives)	Yes	0.17 μg./100 mg.	Possible effects must be weighed against risk of pregnancy; see contraceptives (oral)
Ethisterone (Pranone)	Yes		To be avoided; may cause significant skeletal advancement
Fluoxymesterone (Halotestin, Ora-testryl, Ultandren)			Used to suppress lactation
Iodides (nonradioactive)	Yes	After a dose of 0.6 Gm. (as potassium salt) 68 mg. was recovered	To be avoided, chronic use may affect infant's thyroid gland
Liothyronine sodium (Cytomel)	No		
Lyndiol	Yes		To be avoided; caused a diminution in milk protein and milk fat
Lynestrenol (oral contraceptive under investigation)	Yes		Possible effects must be weighed against risk of pregnancy; see contraceptives (oral)
Medroxyprogesterone acetate (Provera)	No		
Mestranol (estrogenic compound found in several oral contraceptives)	Yes		Possible effects must be weighed against risk of pregnancy; see contraceptives (oral)
Norethisterone ethanate (progesterone contraceptives)	Yes		Possible effects must be weighed against risk of pregnancy; see contraceptives (oral)
Norethynodrel (Enovid)	Yes	1.1% of dose	Possible effects must be weighed against risk of pregnancy; see contraceptives (oral)
Norethindrone (Norlutin)	Yes		Possible effects must be weighed against risk of pregnancy; see contraceptives (oral)
Phenformin HCI (DBI)	Yes		Not significant; does not exert hypoglycemic effect on normal subject
Pregnane-3 (α), 20 (β)-diol	Yes		Although it may cause unconjugated hyperbilirubinemia in breastfed infants it was regarded as not being significant enough to stop nursing
Thiouracil	Yes	Higher in milk than in blood 9–12 mg./100 ml.	To be avoided; may cause goiter in nursing infant or agranulocytosis
Thyroid	Yes		Not significant in therapeutic doses to affect child
Tolbutamide (Orinase)	Yes		Not significant in therapeutic doses to affect child
Radioactive agents Gallium 67 (gallium citrate)	Yes		Avoid where possible, radionuclides are generally contraindicated during nursing; or nursing should be temporarily stopped
Iodine, radioactive (¹³¹I)	Yes	Total in 48 hours of milk; 1.3 μCi. after maternal dose of 29.5 μCi.	To be avoided; affects infant's thyroid gland

Continued.

Table 27-7 Drugs excreted in human milk and the possible significance for nursing infants—cont'd

Drug	Excreted	Quantity excreted	Significance
Radioactive agents—cont'd Sodium, radioactive, as sodium chloride	Yes	0.5-1.3% of dose per liter of milk	Not significant in therapeutic dose, although it is best to avoid the radionuclides if possible
Serums, toxoids, and vaccines Diphtheria antibodies	Yes	Less than 0.30% of dose administered	Of no value in conferring passive immunity to infant
Skin and mucous membrane preparations DDT	Yes	5 mg./100 ml.	The concentration is higher in human milk than in bovine milk; DDT poisoning
Vitamins Calciferol (vitamin D)	Yes		Caution advised; may cause hypercalcemia
Cyanocobalamin (vitamin B_{12})	Yes	0.1-0.4 μg./liter	Not significant in therapeutic doses to affect child
Folic acid	Yes	0.7 μg./liter	Not significant in therapeutic doses to affect child
Phytonadione (vitamin K_1, Aquamephyton)	Yes		Not significant in therapeutic doses to affect child
Thiamine (vitamin B_1) deficiency	Yes	10-13 μg./liter	A lack of this B vitamin in the nursing mother (beriberi) causes the excretion of a toxic substance, methylglyoxal, which has caused infant death
Miscellaneous agents Allergens (eggs, wheat flax seed, peanuts, cottonseed, etc.)	Yes		May cause allergic response in sensitive child
Colchicine	Yes		A 1929 study indicated that this drug may pass into milk; no adverse effect reported
Fluorides (found in many toothpastes)	Yes		Not significant in quantities ingested; excess could affect tooth enamel
Hexachlorobenzene[1,23]	No		Avoid use as an insecticide; has caused infant mortality
Mercury	Yes		Environmental contaminant; signs of mercury intoxication and CNS effects
Nicotine	Yes	0.4-0.5 mg./liter; 11 to 20 cigarettes/day	In moderation, no effect; not more than 20 cigarettes/day
Ribonucleic acid (RNA)	Yes		Particles from human milk contain a reverse transcriptase and high molecular weight RNA that serves as a template; these particles have two features diagnostic of known RNA tumor viruses

ternal intake of phenytoin and phenobarbital has been considered the causative factor in the development of methemoglobinemia in infants. This drug-induced state is generally attributed to a deficient diaphorase activity.

Table 27-7 lists various drugs excreted in human milk and their possible effects on the nursing infant. Should a condition exist or occur that necessitates the use of one or more drugs with known or suspected effects on the nursing infant, lactation should be suppressed.

Discontinuing breastfeeding. It is rarely necessary for the mother to discontinue nursing because of drug content in breast milk. A mother who has elected to breastfeed her infant usually wants to succeed and to persevere in this psychologic and physiologic relationship. Often she is convinced that the advantages exceed any possible disadvantages or inconvenience. Breastfeeding has many positive features, such as assisting uterine involution, providing optimal nutrition (which includes a degree of antibody protection to the newborn), giving opportunity for consistent rest, and the close physical contact needed for mother/infant interaction.

Breastfeeding should be discontinued on a medical basis:

1 When the drug is so potent that minute amounts may have profound effect on the infant (radioactive products, steroids, anticoagulants, and antineoplastics)
2 When the substance has significant antigenic properties (penicillin and its cogeners)
3 When the mother exhibits evidence of decreased renal function and is taking medication that might involve the breast as a secondary means of excretion
4 When the mother has ingested a toxic substance such as a heavy metal (mercury) or benzene products
5 When the mother has a serious illness, is in recognizable negative calcium or nitrogen balance, or has a notable vitamin deficiency.

QUESTIONS

For study and review

1 What effect does alcohol have on libido and sexual response?

2 What effect on sexual response can be expected with the administration of:
   a. an adrenergic blocking drug?
   b. a parasympathetic inhibiting drug?
3 How can drug effects on the fetus be determined?
4 Interview a nurse working in a prenatal clinic, a family nurse practitioner, or an obstetrician to determine what instructions are provided to their pregnant patients concerning the use of medicines during pregnancy.
5 Interview a pregnant patient to determine what instructions she has received concerning over-the-counter drugs, smoking, and prescribed drugs.
6 What effect do the following drugs have on the nursing infant when ingested by the mother?
   a. aspirin   f. thyroid
   b. phenobarbital   g. nicotine
   c. diazepam (Valium) h. penicillin
   d. cascara
   e. oral contraceptives
7 Through library research obtain a recent article on drugs affecting sexuality, the fetus, or the nursing infant, and prepare and give a report on the information to your class.

REFERENCES

Adamsons, L., and Joelson, I.: The effects of pharmacologic agents upon fetus and newborn, Am. J. Obstet. Gyncol. **96:**437, 1966.

Adcock, E., and Greene, H.: Poliovirus antibodies in breastfed infants, Lancet **2:**662-663, 1971.

Ammann, A. J., and Steihm, E. R.: Immune globulin levels in calcium and breast milk from formula and breastfed infants, Proc. Soc. Exp. Biol. Med. **122:**1098, 1966.

Apgar, V., and others: Should you give her that drug during pregnancy? Patient Care **3:**84, 1969.

Apgar, V.: Drugs in pregnancy, J.A.M.A. **190:**840, 1964.

Apt, L., and Gaffney, W.: Congenital eye abnormalities from drugs during pregnancy. In Leopold, I. H., editor: Symposia on ocular therapy, vol. VII, St. Louis, 1974, The C. V. Mosby Co., pp. 1-22.

Arena, J. M.: Contamination of the ideal food, Nutr. Today, pp. 2-8, Winter, 1970.

Arena, J. M.: Drugs and breast feeding, Clin. Ped. **5**(8): 472, 1966.

Barnardo, D., Strothers, I., and Sharrett, M.: Breast milk, jaundice and the pill, Br. Med. J. **2:**348, 1972.

Beeson, P. B., and McDermott, W., editors: Cecil-Loeb textbook of medicine, ed. 13, Philadelphia, 1971, W. B. Saunders Co.

Bowes, W. R., Conway, E., Brackbill, Y., and Steinchneider, A.: Effects of obstetrical medication on fetus and infant, Soc. Res. Child Dev. **35**(137):1970.

Catz, C. S., and Giacoia, G. P.: Drugs and metabolites in human milk. In Galli, C., Jacini, G., and Pecile, A., editors: Dietary lipids and postnatal development, New York, 1973, Rowen Press.

Chinn, P. L.: Child health maintenance, St. Louis, 1974, The C. V. Mosby Co.

Cohlan, S. Q.: Fetal and neonatal hazards from drugs administered during pregnancy, New York J. Med. **64:**493, 1964.

Colbrinik, R., Hood, T., and Chusid, E.: The effects of narcotic addiction on the newborn infant, Pediatrics **9:**288-303, 1952.

Cushman, P.: Sexual behavior in heroin addiction and methadone maintenance, New York State J. Med. **72:**1261-1265, 1972.

Eckstein, H., and Jack, B.: Breastfeeding and anticoagulant therapy, Lancet **1:**672-673, 1970.

Erkkola, R., and Kanto, J.: Diazepam and breastfeeding, Lancet **1:**1235-1236, 1972.

Freedman, A. M., and Kaplan, H. I.: Comprehensive textbook of psychiatry, Baltimore, 1967, The Williams & Wilkins Co.

Gay, G. R., and Sheppard, C. W.: Sex in the drug culture, Med. Asp. Human Sex. **6:**28-50, 1972.

Gochfeld, M.: Pesticides and the nursing mother, Pediatrics **50:**169-170, 1972.

Greaves, G.: Sexual disturbances among chronic amphetamine users, J. Nerv. Ment. Dis. **155:**363-365, 1972.

Harris, Noel G., editor: Modern trends in psychological medicine, New York, 1948, Hoeber.

Individual differences in composition of milk, Br. Med. J. **1:**253-254, 1954.

Kaplan, H. S.: The new sex therapy, New York, 1974, Brunner/Mazel, Inc.

Knowles, J. C.: Effects on the infant of drug therapy in nursing mothers, Drug Therapy **3:**May 1973.

Lerch, C.: Maternity nursing, St. Louis, 1974, The C. V. Mosby Co.

Mellin, G. W.: Drugs in the first trimester of pregnancy and the fetal life of homo sapiens, Am. J. Obstet. Gynecol. **90:**1168-1180, 1963.

Money, J., and Anke, E.: Man and woman, boy, and girl, Baltimore, 1972, Johns Hopkins University Press.

Nelson, M. M., and Foprfar, J.: Association between drugs administered during pregnancy and congenital abnormalities of the fetus, Br. Med. J. **1:**523, 1971.

Novak, E. R., and Woodruff, J. D., editors: Gynecologic and obstetric pathology, ed. 7, Philadelphia, 1974, W. B. Saunders Co.

Rothballer, A. A.: Aggression, defense, and neurohumors, Brain Function **5:**135-170, 1972.

Schultz, H. W.: Drugs and pregnancy, Review article reprint from Pharmindex, January 1974.

Schnider, S.: A review: Fetal and neonatal effects of drugs in obstetrics, Anesth. Analg. **45:**372, 1966.

Stevenson, R. E.: The fetus and the newly born infant: Influences of the prenatal environment, St. Louis, 1973, The C. V. Mosby Co.

Sutherland, M., James, M., and Light, B.: The effect of drugs upon the developing fetus, Ped. Clin. North Am. **12:**781, 1965.

Wilson, J. G.: Present status of drugs as teratogens in man, Teratology **7:**3-16, 1974.

CHAPTER 28

Enzymes

Enzymes as a group are among the newest agents used in therapy, but it may be anticipated that their application in medicine will increase greatly in future years. Enzymes are specific structures that act as catalysts of the many chemical reactions that go on in living systems. Catalysts are substances that accelerate chemical reactions (often stimulating a thousandfold or greater the speed of reaction) without themselves being used up in the reaction. The catalytic action of enzymes can be illustrated by catalase, an enzyme present in many living cells that speeds up a reaction in which hydrogen peroxide decomposes to form water and oxygen.

$$H_2O_2 \xrightarrow{\text{Catalase}} H_2O + \tfrac{1}{2} O_2$$

Catalase permits this reaction (moles of H_2O_2 decomposing per minute) to go on many thousand times the rate that could be observed without catalase; each molecule of catalase present in solution can stimulate the decomposition of millions of molecules of hydrogen peroxide.

The role of enzymes in living organisms is an important one, because these catalysts of living origin permit the chemical reaction to go on, and this makes life possible.

One feature of enzymes of great interest to possible pharmacologic application is their specificity. Each separate enzyme catalyzes a distinct chemical reaction or reaction type, and the thousands of chemical reactions characteristic of living cells* each require their corresponding enzyme.

Because the usefulness of drugs depends to

*Examples of large groups of reaction types are: hydrolysis of peptide bonds in proteins, oxidation of aldehydes to acids, and transfer of electrons.

a large measure on their specificity or selectivity, the high specificity of enzymes in catalyzing a given reaction and in influencing no other is a promising feature. However, their potential usefulness in medicine has been limited by certain other properties. The fact that they are proteins means that they need a high degree of purification before administration; and even pure proteins derived from other species may be antigenic and cause toxic reactions of an immunologic type. Also, as proteins, most enzymes would need to be given parenterally in order to short-circuit destruction by the protein-digesting enzymes of the gastrointestinal tract. In addition, proteins cannot yet by synthesized, and the preparation of purified enzymes from natural sources is often a laborious process, yielding small amounts of ultimate product. Finally, therapeutic agents that are proteins are limited in that they do not pass into cells readily, unlike the small molecules that constitute most of the drugs considered elsewhere in this book. A further limitation is that enzymes catalyze single specific chemical reactions, and symptoms of disease are not yet understood in such simple chemical terms.

Within these limitations, however, some enzymes have become useful for certain symptomatic purposes: protein-digesting enzymes such as trypsin have been used to remove dead tissue by enzymatic digestion (chemical debridement); enzymes that digest deoxyribonucleic acid have been used to digest thick purulent exudates whose viscosity depends on large amounts of this type of nucleic acid. A beginning has also been made in the use of enzymes that can destroy specific toxic or allergic substances in the body. The detoxicating action of enzymes has promise because of the specificity of enzymes that might be employed.

Hyaluronidase, N.F., B.P.; hyaluronidase for injection, N.F. (Alidase, Diffusin, Hyazyme, Wydase)

Hyaluronic acid is a polysaccharide that constitutes an essential component of intercellular ground substance. It is present in the form of a gel in many parts of body tissues, where it serves as an intercellular cement and acts as a barrier to the diffusion of invading substances.

Hyaluronidase is a mucolytic enzyme prepared from mammalian testes. It is capable of hydrolyzing and depolymerizing hyaluronic acid. It acts as a spreading factor to facilitate absorption and distribution of infusions, local anesthetics, and drugs and to increase diffusion and absorption of local accumulations or transudates of blood.

It is especially useful to facilitate administration of fluids by hypodermoclysis particularly in infants and young children. The resulting increased rate of dispersion and absorption of the injected fluid reduces tissue tension and pain. The rate of absorption, however, should not be greater than that of an intravenous infusion. Special care must be exercised when administering the drug to children—the speed and total volume administered must be controlled to avoid overhydration. It may also be used as an adjuvant to increase absorption and dispersion of injected drugs.

Preparation, dosage, and administration. Hyaluronidase is available in a stable dried form in vials containing 150 and 1500 N.F. units in a solution for injection, 150 units in 1 ml. or 1500 units in 10 ml. A dose of 150 units is dissolved in 1 ml. of isotonic sodium chloride solution and is then added to 1000 ml. of fluid for hypodermoclysis, or it is injected into the proposed site of the clysis. For children, 15 units is added to each 100 ml. of solution. Drip rate should not exceed 2 ml. per minute.

Side effects and toxic effects. Hyaluronidase has a low level of toxicity, but caution is recommended when it is administered to patients with infections. It should not be injected into or around infected areas since it will produce spread of the infection by the same mechanism of action that causes spread of injected solutions. Patients occasionally exhibit hypersensitivity to this substance.

Streptodornase

Streptodornase is an enzyme produced by the growth of hemolytic streptococci. It promotes depolymerization of deoxyribonucleic acid and deoxyribonucleoprotein from degenerating white blood cells and injured tissue cells. Much of the stringy, slimy, viscous material in purulent exudates results from their presence. Streptodornase changes the thick purulent material to a thin, liquid material, sometimes in a very short time. Fortunately, streptodornase has no effect on nucleoprotein or the nuclei of living cells. The action of this enzyme requires the presence of the magnesium ion, but this is freely present in tissues. Activity of the enzyme is inhibited by citrate and heparin. It is most active at a pH between 7 and 8.5. Streptodornase is antigenic and may cause a sensitivity reaction.

Streptokinase

Streptokinase is an extracellular enzyme activator that is formed during the growth of various groups of hemolytic streptococci, prominent among which are the human strains of Lancefield's Group C. Streptokinase activates a factor present in human plasma known as plasminogen. Plasminogen is present in purulent, serous, and sanguineous exudates and, when activated by streptokinase, it forms an active enzyme, plasmin. Plasmin in turn promotes lysis of fibrin from a gel to a liquid and is accompanied by the formation of large polypeptides. This explains the dissolution of blood clots and fibrinous exudates. Streptokinase is therefore essentially a proteolytic enzyme active in the solution of fibrin. It exerts its maximal activity between a pH of 7.3 and 7.6.

Streptokinase-streptodornase (Varidase)

This preparation is a mixture of the two enzymes described previously. In addition to their proteolytic activity, they are capable of producing two additional reactions. One reaction is local and consists of an outpouring of white blood cells and fluid at the site of application. The second is a pyrogenic effect, especially when the enzymes are injected into a closed space with limited or delayed drainage. It is thought that the elevation of temperature is caused by the absorption of toxic products resulting from activity of the enzymes.

Uses. Streptokinase-streptodornase is used to liquefy coagulated blood, remove clots, and dissolve fibrinous material and purulent accumulations present after trauma or inflammation. The enzyme action helps antiinfective forces, such as antibiotics, promoting the healing of tissues.

Preparation, dosage, and administration. Streptokinase-streptodornase is available in the form of buccal tablets (10,000 units of streptokinase and 2500 units of streptodornase); as a powder for topical use (100,000 units of streptokinase and 25,000 units of streptodornase); as a powder for injection (20,000 units of streptokinase and 5000 units of streptodornase); and as a jelly (100,000 units of streptokinase and 25,000 units of streptodornase). The usefulness of this preparation after intramuscular or buccal administration is not fully established. It is applied topically in the form of wet dressings or as a jelly, or it is injected into cavities. Maximum effects usually occur in 12 to 24 hours. Solutions lose their potency when kept at room temperature but will keep for a week at a temperature 2° to 10° C.

Side effects and toxic effects. These enzymes are employed as supplements to, rather than as substitutes for, surgical debridement and drainage. They are not recommended for use in the presence of active hemorrhage or acute cellulitis, because they may interfere with the clotting of blood or promote the spread of a nonlocalized infection. In the absence of adequate drainage the patient may develop fever, urticaria, nausea, and vomiting when this preparation is injected into a closed cavity. The preparation should not be administered intravenously because of severe systemic adverse reactions caused by impurities in the preparation.

Trypsin, crystallized, N.F. (Tryptar, Parenzyme)

Crystallized trypsin is a purified preparation of the pancreatic enzyme obtained from mammalian pancreatic glands. It exerts a proteolytic action when brought into contact with clotted blood, exudate, and necrotic tissue. It is not harmful to living tissues because of the presence in serum of a specific trypsin inhibitor and other nonspecific inhibitory substances.

Crystallized trypsin is useful as an adjunct to surgical treatment of necrotic wounds, abscesses, empyema, sinuses, and fistulas. It is also used to liquefy hematomas and blood clots. It is sometimes employed in the treatment of bronchopulmonary conditions to reduce the viscosity of tenacious secretions that do not respond to expectorant drugs. Trypsin has received a D.E.S.I. rating of *effective* when administered as an aerosol for liquefaction of viscid sputum and *possibly effective* for intrapleural use and for topical debridement of open wounds.

It is contraindicated in cases of severe hepatic disease, for use in actively bleeding cavities, and for debridement of ulcerated carcinomas. It should be used with caution in cases of tuberculous empyema.

Preparation, dosage, and administration. Crystallized trypsin is available in the form of buccal tablets (5 mg.), as a suspension for injection (5 mg. per milliliter), as a solution for injection (5 mg. per milliliter), and as a powder in vials containing 25 mg. Crystallized trypsin is applied to surface lesions either in a dry form by means of a blower or as a freshly prepared solution in the form of wet dressings. For less accessible lesions it may be instilled or used as an irrigant. Solutions or suspensions, when given by injection, are given by deep intragluteal injection. It should never be given intravenously. It is effective within a pH range of 5 to 8. Trypsin crystallized for aerosol contains 250,000 units per vial; usual dose is 125,000 units in 3 ml. of saline daily.

Side effects and toxic effects. Pain and induration may occur at the site of intramuscular injection. Hives and urticaria occur occasionally. A severe burning sensation may be experienced on surface lesions after topical application; this can be prevented by prior application of a local anesthetic. Fever and an increased heart rate may result after injection; this can be prevented by the administration of an antihistaminic. Aerosol inhalation of trypsin may cause irritation of the eyes and nose, sore tongue, pharyngitis, and hoarseness. Toxic effects are considered negligible when the use of the enzyme is limited to local or topical administration.

Chymotrypsin, U.S.P. (Chymar, Enzeon)

Chymotrypsin is another protein-digesting enzyme that is being used to prevent and treat inflammatory reactions that cause pain, edema, and blood and lymphatic effusions associated with an episiotomy, bruises, contusions, and fractures. It is available for intramuscular injection; for systemic effects it is available in the form of buccal tablets.

Fibrinolysin (Thrombolysin)

Fibrinolysin, a proteolytic enzyme that dissolves fibrin, is prepared by activating a fraction of normal human plasma with purified streptokinase. Thus it has both profibrinolysin-activator (streptokinase) and fibrinolytic (plasmin) properties.

Fibrinolysin is administered intravenously to treat various forms of thromboembolic disease—phlebothrombosis, thrombophlebitis, pulmonary embolism, and arterial thrombosis except that involving coronary or cerebral vessels. Since the fibrinolytic process in man is highly complex, evaluation of a thrombolytic drug is very difficult. There is evidence that the drug is effective in lysing fibrin clots, recanalizing thrombi, and removing inflammatory fibrin deposits from tissues. However, this preparation should be used only under controlled conditions, in adequately equipped facilities by persons experienced in its use.

Side effects. Fibrinolysin should be considered a potentially powerful antigen and great caution should be exercised in its use, particularly with repeated administration. Side effects and toxic reactions include nausea and vomiting, chills, epigastric pain, and febrile reactions, which may occur 4 to 6 hours after administration. Hypotension, hypertension, tachycardia, and chest pain have also been reported.

Precautions and contraindications. Fibrinolysin is contraindicated in hemorrhagic disorders, severe liver dysfunction, and hypofi-brinogenemia. It must be used cautiously in patients with a history of arrhythmias. It must be used *very cautiously* after hemorrhage or extensive surgery, since bleeding from open wounds and operative sites may occur. Plasma fibrinogen and prothrombin times should be determined periodically. Anaphylactic reaction may occur and antidotes (corticosteroids, epinephrine, antihistamines) should be available.

Preparation and dosage. Preparations are not standardized and optimal dosage has not been established. The drug is available in fibrinolysin units. The manufacturer's recommended dose for adults in 50,000 to 100,000 units per hour for 1 to 6 hours daily intravenously, depending upon specific needs. Additional doses can be given daily for 3 or 4 consecutive days.

Sutilains, N.F. (Travase)

Sutilains is a sterile preparation of proteolytic enzymes isolated from culture filtrates of *Bacillus subtilis*. It is five to sixteen times greater in its action than chymotrypsin. It dissolves and aids in the removal of necrotic tissue and purulent exudate from open wounds and ulcers resulting from second and third degree burns, decubiti, peripheral vascular disease, and trauma. If dissolution does not occur in 24 to 48 hours, the drug should be discontinued.

Side effects and precautions. Side effects are mild and include transient pain, paresthesia, bleeding, and dermatitis. If bleeding or dermatitis occurs, the drug should be discontinued. Although systemic allergic reactions have not been reported, the drug is capable of causing an antibody response. This drug must be kept away from the eyes; if contact occurs, rinse the eyes with copious amounts of water.

Contraindications. Sutilains should not be applied to wounds communicating with major body cavities, wounds with exposed major nerves or nerve tissue, neoplastic ulcers, or wounds in women of child-bearing age.

Drug interactions. The use of detergents and antiseptics concomitantly should be avoided because of possible denaturation of sutilains. Compounds containing metallic ions, such as thimerosal, interfere with the action of the enzyme.

Application. The wound should be thoroughly cleansed with water or isotonic sodium chloride solution before applying a thin layer of sutilains ointment; the area should then be covered with loose wet dressings. This procedure should be repeated 3 or 4 times daily.

Preparation. Sutilains is prepared as an ointment containing 82,000 casein units of sutilains per gram of ointment base. It must be stored at a temperature between 2° and 10° C.

Bisobrin lactate (EN1661)

Bisobrin is a synthetic fibrinolytic agent under clinical investigation. Its action is long-lasting and compares favorably with that of urokinase. It acts indirectly in a manner similar to that of streptokinase.

Urokinase (Win-kinase)

Urokinase is an activator of plasminogen; it is obtained from human urine. It is under clinical investigation for treatment of pulmonary embolism. Unfortunately, its high cost limits its widespread use.

Bromelains (Ananase)

Bromelains is a mixture of proteolytic enzymes obtained from the pineapple plant. It is claimed that this oral preparation is an adjunct to the treatment of inflammation resulting from trauma, operations, and skin infections. The effectiveness of proteolytic enzymes as antiinflammatory drugs is very difficult to appraise. There is no certainty about the usefulness of this drug in the management of inflammatory conditions.

QUESTIONS

For study and review

1 Explain what is meant by the term *chemical debridement.*
2 Discuss the use and differences between the following drugs.
   a. streptokinase-streptodornase
   b. hyaluronidase
   c. fibrinolysin
   d. sutilains
3 What precautions should be taken with the storage and use of enzymatic drugs?
4 What observations are important for the nurse to make when caring for patients being treated with enzymatic agents?

REFERENCES

A. M. A. drug evaluations, ed. 2, Acton, Mass., 1973, Publishing Sciences Group, Inc.

Heimburger, N., and Trobisch, H.: Blood coagulation and fibrinolysis, Angew Chem. **10:**85, 1971.

Mitchell, J. R. A.: The search for an anti-thrombotic agent, Adv. Cardiol. **4:**233, 1970.

Modell, W., editor: Drugs of choice 1976-1977, St. Louis, 1976, The C. V. Mosby Co.

Ogston, D., and Douglas, A. S.: Anticoagulant and thrombolytic drugs, Drugs **1:**228, 1971.

Osol, A., and Pratt, R.: The United States dispensatory, ed. 27, Philadelphia, 1973, J. B. Lippincott Co.

Urokinase pulmonary embolism trial study group: Urokinase pulmonary embolism trial; phase 1 results, J.A.M.A. **214:**2163, 1970.

CHAPTER 29

Drugs that affect the eye

Anatomy and physiology of the eye
Ocular drug administration
Glaucoma
Osmotic agents
Autonomic drugs
Miotics
Carbonic anhydrase inhibitors
Mydriatics
Chemotherapy of ocular infection
Other agents

ANATOMY AND PHYSIOLOGY OF THE EYE

The eye is the receptor organ for one of the most delicate and valuable senses, vision; as such, it demands only the most thoughtful and expert care. The eyeball has three layers or coats: the protective external (corneoscleral) coat, the nutritive middle vascular (uveal) coat, and the light-sensitive inner neural receptor (retinal) layer.

The eyeball is protected in a deep depression of the skull, the orbit, and is moved in the orbit by six small extraocular muscles. The retina is connected to the brain by the optic nerve, which leaves the orbit through a bony canal in the posterior wall.

The cornea is normally transparent to light, allowing it to enter the eye. This transparency is dependent upon normal intraocular pressure; increased intraocular pressure results in loss of transparency. The cornea has no blood vessels and receives its nutrition from the aqueous humor and its oxygen supply by diffusion from the air and surrounding structures. In order to act as a lens, the cornea must have air in front of it. The corneal surface consists of a thin layer of epithelial cells, which are quite resistant to infection. However, an abraded cornea is very susceptible to infection. The cornea is also supplied with sensory fibers, and damage to the corneal epithelium will evoke pain. Seriously injured corneal tissue is replaced by scar tissue, which is usually not transparent. The sclera, which is continuous with the cornea, is nontransparent; it is the white portion of the eye.

The iris gives the eye its brown, blue, gray, green, or hazel color. It surrounds the pupil; muscles in the iris, the sphincter and dilator muscles, alter pupil size. The sphincter muscle, which encircles the pupil, is parasympathetically innervated; the dilator muscle, which runs radially from the pupil to the iris periphery, is sympathetically innervated. Contraction of the sphincter muscle, either alone or in association with relaxation of the dilator muscle, causes constriction of the pupil, or *miosis*. Contraction of the dilator muscle and relaxation of the sphincter muscle causes dilation of the pupil, or *mydriasis.*

Drugs producing miosis (miotics) do so by (1) interfering with cholinesterase activity, or (2) competing with acetylcholine for receptor sites in the sphincter muscle. Drugs producing mydriasis (mydriatics) do so by (1) interfering with the action of acetylcholine, or (2) stimulating sympathetic or adrenergic receptors. Pupil constriction normally occurs with light and when the eye is focusing on nearby objects. Pupil dilation normally occurs in dim light and when the eye is focusing on distant objects.

The lens is situated behind the iris. It is a transparent, gelatinous mass of fibers encased in an elastic capsule. The function of the lens is to ensure that the image on the retina is in sharp focus. The lens does this by changing shape (accommodation). This occurs readily in young persons but with age the lens becomes more rigid, the ability to focus close objects is lost, and the *near point* (the closest point that can be seen clearly) recedes. With age the lens may also lose its transparency and become opaque. This is known as a cataract. Unless it can be treated or removed surgically, blindness can occur.

The lens has ligaments called zonular fibers around its edge, which connect with the ciliary body. Their tension helps to change the shape of the lens. In the unaccommodated eye, the ciliary muscle is relaxed and the zonular fibers taut. For near vision the ciliary muscle fibers contract, and this relaxes the pull of the ligaments. Accommodation depends upon two factors: (1) ciliary muscle contraction, and (2) the ability of the lens to assume a more biconvex shape when tension on the ligaments is relaxed. The ciliary muscle is innervated by parasympathetic fibers. Paralysis of the ciliary muscle is termed *cycloplegia.*

Aqueous humor is formed by the ciliary body, and it bathes and feeds the lens, iris, and posterior surface of the cornea. After it is formed it flows forward between the lens and the iris into the anterior chamber. It drains out of the eye through drainage channels located near the junction of the cornea and sclera. A trabecular meshwork leads into the canal of Schlemm whereby the aqueous drains into the venous system of the eye.

PROTECTIVE MECHANISMS

Eyelashes, eyelids, blinking, and tears all serve to protect the eye. There are about 200 eyelashes for each eye. The eyelashes evoke a blink reflex whenever a foreign body touches them, momentarily closing the lids to prevent the foreign substance from entering the eye. Blinking, which is bilateral, occurs every few seconds during waking hours and serves to keep the corneal surface free of mucus and spreads the lacrimal fluid evenly over the cornea. Tears are secreted by lacrimal glands and contain lysozyme, a mucolytic enzyme with bactericidal action. Tears provide lubrication for lid movements. They wash away noxious agents, and by forming a thin film over the cornea they provide it with a good optical surface. Tear fluid is lost by evaporation and by draining into two small ducts (the lacrimal canaliculi) at the inner corners of the eyelids.

OCULAR DRUG ADMINISTRATION

Drugs used in ophthalmology in the treatment of eye disorders or for eye examinations include cholinergics, anticholinesterases, adrenergics, antiadrenergics, chemotherapeutics, anesthetics, and antiseptics.

Ocular drugs are administered by topical application of a *solution* or *ointment.* Ocular solutions are sterile, have the advantage of being easily administered, and usually do not interfere physically with vision. Their main disadvantage is the short duration of time the drug is in contact with the eye. Ocular ointments have the advantage of being quite comfortable on instillation and keeping the drug in longer contact with the eye for more prolonged effects. However, ointments form a film over the eye, which interferes with vision, and they cause a higher incidence of contact dermatitis than solutions.

Packs may also be used to apply drugs to the eye. These are cotton pledgets saturated with an ophthalmic solution and inserted into the inferior

Figure 29-1

Instillation of drops into the eye.

or superior cul-de-sac. Ocular drugs may also be administered by iontophoresis, subconjunctival injection, retrobulbar injection, and injection directly into the chambers of the eye.

Instillation of topical preparations. The patient's head is placed on a suitable rest so that his face is directed upward. He is then instructed to fix his gaze on a point above his head. Gentle traction with clean fingertips is applied to the lid bases at the bony rim of the orbit; care is taken not to apply any pressure to the eyeball itself. The dropper or ointment tube approaches the eye from below, outside the patient's field of vision, with due care to avoid contact with the eye. The drop is applied gently and is not allowed to fall more than 1 inch before it strikes the eye (Figure 29-1). Following instillation of common ophthalmic drugs, ocular massage is not necessary since the drugs have solubility characteristics that permit adequate corneal penetration.

Many of the solutions employed in ophthalmology are extremely potent and care must be taken to prevent their systemic absorption. Gentle pressure is applied for 2 minutes to the lacrimal canaliculi at the inner corner of the eyelids and is directed inward and downward against the bones of the nose. This will help to prevent the solution from entering the nasal cavity and being absorbed through the highly vascular nasal mucosa.

GLAUCOMA

Glaucoma is an eye disease characterized chiefly by abnormally elevated intraocular pressure that may result from excessive production of aqueous humor or from diminished ocular fluid outflow. Increased pressure, if sufficiently high and persistent, may lead to irreversible blindness. There are three major types of glaucoma—primary, secondary, and congenital. Primary glaucoma includes narrow-angle (acute congestive) glaucoma and wide-angle (chronic simple) glaucoma; these are determined by the angle of the anterior chamber where aqueous humor reabsorption takes place. Wide-angle glaucoma has a gradual insidious onset, and its control depends upon permanent drug therapy. Drugs are also necessary for controlling the acute attack associated with narrow-angle glaucoma, followed usually by surgery (e.g., iridectomy). Secondary glaucoma may result from previous eye disease or may follow cataract extraction; therapy of secondary glaucoma is usually with drugs for an indefinite period of time. Congenital glaucoma requires surgical treatment. Cholinergic and anticholinesterase drugs are used to treat glaucoma; selection of a drug is determined largely by the requirements of the individual patient.

OSMOTIC AGENTS

Osmotic agents are administered intravenously or orally to reduce intraocular pressure. These agents elevate the osmotic pressure of the plasma, which causes fluid from the extravascular spaces to be drawn into the blood. The effect on the eye is reduction of volume of intraocular fluid producing a decrease in intraocular pressure.

Glycerin, U.S.P. (Glycerol, Glyrol, Osmoglyn); glycerol, B.P.

Glycerin is available as 50% or 75% oral solutions and as a 0.5% ophthalmic solution. Topical application, one or two drops, is used for edema of the superficial layers of the cornea; it reduces edema and improves visualization.

Oral administration of glycerin is used to reduce intraocular pressure in patients with acute narrow-angle glaucoma prior to iridectomy. It is also used pre- and postoperatively in conditions such as congenital glaucoma, retinal detachment, cataract extraction, and keratoplasty. It may also be used in some secondary glaucomas.

Following oral administration, intraocular pressure begins to decrease within 10 minutes, reaches a maximum in 30 minutes to 2 hours, and may persist for 4 to 8 hours. Glycerin may be used with carbonic anhydrase inhibitors and miotics; these drugs may prolong the effects of glycerin.

Side effects. Glycerin has a slower onset of action and fewer side effects than mannitol or urea. Side effects include headache, nausea and vomiting, thirst, and diarrhea. Headache is the result of cerebral dehydration and may be relieved by having the patient lie down during and after oral administration of glycerin. Flavoring glycerin with lemon or lime juice, pouring it over cracked ice, and having the patient sip it through a straw may decrease the incidence of nausea and vomiting. Oral dose is 1 to 1.5 Gm. per kilogram of body weight; it may be administered at 5-hour intervals.

Precautions. Glycerin should be used cautiously in patients with cardiac, renal, or hepatic disease; the shift in body water may cause pulmonary edema or congestive heart failure. Elderly patients may be subject to dehydration. Diabetic patients receiving the drug should be carefully observed for symptoms of acidosis since the metabolism of glycerin may cause hyperglycemia and glycosuria.

Mannitol, U.S.P., B.P. (Osmitrol)

Mannitol is administered intravenously to reduce intraocular pressure. It is available in 0.5% to 25% solutions. Usual dosage is 0.5 to 2 Gm. per kilogram of body weight. The solution should be infused slowly over a period of 30 to 60 minutes. Maximal decrease in intraocular pressure occurs 30 to 60 minutes after administration and lasts about 6 hours.

Mannitol is used for the same conditions as glycerin. It should be used cautiously in patients with cardiovascular or pulmonary disease, severely ill patients, and the elderly.

Side effects. Side effects are similar to those for glycerin. In addition, the drug has caused agitation, disorientation, and convulsions. Fatalities have been reported after administration of large doses. Patients receiving mannitol should be carefully monitored for fluid and electrolyte balance, urinary output, and vital signs.

Urea, U.S.P., B.P. (Urevert, Ureaphil)

Urea is administered intravenously to reduce intraocular pressure. It is available as a powder, 40 and 90 Gm. with diluent to make a 30% solution with 10% invert sugar. Usual dosage for adults is 0.5 to 2 Gm. per kilogram of body weight of a 30% solution administered at a rate of 60 drops per minute. Dosage for children is 0.5 to 1.5 Gm. per kilogram of a 30% solution administered over a 30-minute period. Maximal decrease in intraocular pressure occurs 1 hour after injection and lasts 5 to 6 hours. It is used for the same conditions as glycerin.

Side effects. Headache, nausea and vomiting, dehydration, and massive diuresis are common side effects. Dizziness, disorientation, and agitation may also occur. Pulmonary edema, convulsions, and death have occasionally been reported.

Urea is irritating to the tissues and causes pain at the site of injection. Extravasation should be

Figure 29-2

Diagram of a section of the eyeball showing the main structures of the eye and enlargement of the canal of Schlemm showing aqueous flow.

prevented since tissue necrosis can occur. Patients should be carefully monitored for vital signs and side effects.

AUTONOMIC DRUGS

The muscles of the ciliary body receive parasympathetic innervation; those of the iris receive both parasympathetic and sympathetic innervation.

Autonomic drugs are among the most commonly used drugs in ophthalmology. These drugs are used to produce miosis, mydriasis, and cycloplegia. The mechanisms by which autonomic drugs act are discussed in Chapter 9.

MIOTICS
CHOLINERGIC DRUGS

Cholinergic drugs are chemically related to acetylcholine, the neurohormone that mediates nerve impulse transmission at all cholinergic or parasympathetic nerve sites. Applied topically to the eye, cholinergic drugs (1) cause contraction of the sphincter muscle of the iris resulting in pupil constriction (miosis); (2) cause spasms of the ciliary muscle and deepening of the anterior chamber; and (3) cause vasodilation of vessels where intraocular fluids leave the eye. The ciliary muscle effect leaves the eye in accommodation for near vision.

The cholinergic drugs are used to lower intraocular pressure in glaucoma. Contraction of the ciliary muscles and constriction of the pupil may widen the filtration angle and permit outflow of aqueous humor. Increased outflow may also result from dilation of collector channels and veins peripheral to the canal of Schlemm. Unless the elevated pressure is lowered, the result is an impaired blood supply to the optic nerve with eventual atrophy of the nerve and visual field loss.

Clinical toxicity from overdosage or unusual sensitivity to these drugs is manifested by headache, salivation, sweating, abdominal discomfort, diarrhea, asthmatic attacks, and a fall in blood pressure.

Acetylcholine chloride, U.S.P. (Miochol)

A 10% solution of acetylcholine chloride is instilled into the anterior chamber or upon the iris for rapid, intense miosis during surgery on the anterior chamber of the eye or for cataract removal, keratoplasty, peripheral iridectomy, or cyclodialysis. The rapid miosis protects the vitreous face and facilitates placement of corneal sutures by reducing the danger of imprisoning iris tissue during wound closure. Acetylcholine is promptly destroyed by cholinesterase; thus miosis may last for only 10 minutes. This fact plus its poor corneal penetration makes it of no value in the treatment of glaucoma.

Carbachol, U.S.P. (Carcholin)

The only dosage form of carbachol that is official in the United States is the solution for ophthalmic use, 0.75%, 1.5%, or 3%.

Carbachol must be combined with a wetting agent, such as benzalkonium chloride, for increased corneal penetration. Carbachol produces intense and prolonged miosis since it is resistant to destruction by cholinesterase. Its miotic action lasts 4 to 8 hours, and it is usually prescribed for use two or three times daily. Carbachol may produce a slight conjunctival hyperemia, aching of the eyes, and headache during the first few days of treatment. These symptoms subside as therapy continues. Massaging the cornea through the eyelids enhances absorption of carbachol.

Pilocarpine nitrate ophthalmic solution, U.S.P., B.P.; pilocarpine hydrochloride, U.S.P.

Pilocarpine is used in 0.5% to 6% solution. One drop in the eye will cause miosis and spasm of accommodation in 15 minutes and reaches a maximum in 30 to 60 minutes. The pupillary effect lasts for as long as 20 hours, but the fixation of the lens for near vision disappears in about 2 to 3 hours. At first intraocular pressure is increased but this is followed by a persistent fall in pressure.

Dosage of pilocarpine for wide-angle glaucoma is usually 1 to 2 drops of a 1% or 2% solution every 6 to 8 hours. For acute glaucoma pilocarpine in a 4% solution may be instilled every 10 minutes, three or more times. Excess solution must be wiped away promptly to prevent its flow into the lacrimal system and the production of systemic symptoms. Pilocarpine is also used to neutralize mydriatics used during eye examinations. Pilocarpine is widely used for treatment of early stages of wide-angle glaucoma; it is less beneficial in advanced stages. It may be used alternately with mydriatics to break adhesions be-

tween the iris and the lens. Patients may become resistant or intolerant to this drug. It is the safest and most widely used miotic.

ANTICHOLINESTERASE DRUGS

Anticholinesterase drugs inhibit the enzymatic destruction of acetylcholine (ACh) by inactivating cholinesterase. This leaves acetylcholine free to act on the effector cells of the iris sphincter and ciliary muscles causing pupil constriction and spasm of accommodation.

Physostigmine and neostigmine are short-acting "reversible" anticholinesterases; after combination with the enzyme they are gradually dissociated and inactivated. Neostigmine is not as readily absorbed as physostigmine, and higher concentrations must be used for topical treatment of glaucoma.

Isoflurophate, demecarium, and echothiophate are long-acting "irreversible" anticholinesterase drugs. They form stable complexes with cholinesterase and thus irreversibly impair the destructive function of the enzyme. Destruction of acetylcholine is then dependent upon synthesis of new enzymes. These drugs are used primarily in the management of glaucoma.

Isoflurophate, U.S.P. (diisopropyl fluorophosphate, DFP, Floropryl)

The effects of this drug are similar to those of physostigmine, but it is more powerful. It is used in a 0.01% to 0.1% concentration in peanut oil since it is rapidly hydrolyzed in water. One drop is instilled into the eye every 12 to 72 hours. It is also available as an ophthalmic ointment, 0.025%. Isoflurophate produces miosis within 20 minutes and the effect may last 2 or more weeks. Care must be taken to prevent tears or other moisture from contaminating the solution.

D.E.S.I. rating is *effective* in the management of accommodative esotropia, wide-angle glaucoma, and conditions obstructing aqueous outflow.

Physostigmine salicylate, U.S.P., B.P. (Eserine Salicylate)

Physostigmine is used in solutions as strong as 0.25%, 0.5%, and 1%, 1 or 2 drops every 4 to 6 hours. The aqueous solutions of this compound tend to oxidize on exposure to light and air and turn pink or brown. Such colored solutions should never be used. Maximum effect of topical application is reached in 30 minutes and may last as long as 2 days. Physostigmine is used in the treatment of wide-angle glaucoma. It may be applied alternately with atropine to break adhesions between the iris and lens, and it may be used after instillation of a mydriatic to shorten the period of pupil dilation and minimize the dangers of increased ocular pressure.

Physostigmine is often irritating to the eye and is rarely tolerated for prolonged periods of treatment. Conjunctivitis and allergic reactions occur frequently with this drug.

Physostigmine ointment may be prescribed for bedtime use to prevent nocturnal rise in ocular tension.

Neostigmine bromide, U.S.P. (Prostigmin)

Neostigmine is used occasionally in the treatment of wide-angle glaucoma and emergency treatment of angle-closure glaucoma. It is not as effective as physostigmine, since it does not penetrate the eye as well, but it is more stable and less irritating. It is used in 2.5 to 5% solutions, 1 or 2 drops every 4 to 6 hours.

D.E.S.I. ratings are: *effective* in the management of wide-angle glaucoma and some secondary glaucomas; *probably effective* in alternation with a mydriatic to break up adhesions of the iris, lens, and cornea.

Demecarium bromide (Humorsol)

Demecarium bromide is prepared as a 0.125% and 0.25% ophthalmic solution. It is an extremely powerful agent, and 1 drop will produce miosis within 1 hour and ciliary muscle contraction for as long as 5 to 12 days. Care must be taken to prevent general systemic absorption. One drop is instilled every 12 to 48 hours.

D.E.S.I. ratings are like those listed for isoflurophate.

Echothiophate iodide, U.S.P. (Phospholine Iodide); ecothiopate iodide, B.P.

Echothiophate is used as a 0.03%, 0.06%, and 0.125% solution. It is a very potent agent with prolonged effects similar to those of demecarium

bromide. It is extremely effective in the control of chronic wide-angle glaucoma, aphakic glaucoma, and congenital glaucoma.

Miosis occurs within 10 to 45 minutes and may persist from several days to 4 weeks. Solutions of echothiophate are relatively unstable and gradually lose their potency at room temperature; refrigeration prolongs potency. In the treatment of glaucoma, 1 drop of the 0.03% solution is usually instilled into the eye on retiring and in the morning. Frequency of administration and strength of dosage must be individually adjusted for each patient. Finger pressure should be applied at the inner canthus after instillation to minimize drainage into the nose and throat. This drug may induce cataract formation.

D.E.S.I. rating is *effective* in the management of accommodative esotropia and wide-angle glaucoma. Ratings are similar to those for isoflurophate.

Disadvantages and advantages of cholinergic and anticholinesterase drugs. There are disadvantages to the instillation of cholinergic and anticholinesterase drugs into the eye. Among these are the following:

1 Visual blurring and headache result from stimulation of accommodation.
2 Constriction of the pupil (miosis) makes it difficult to adjust quickly to changes in illumination. This may be serious in elderly persons, since their light adaptation and visual acuity are often reduced. Night time is particularly hazardous for these patients.
3 They may cause irritation, conjunctivitis, blepharitis, dermatitis, and so on.
4 Cysts of the iris, synechiae, retinal detachments, obstruction of tear drainage, and even cataracts may develop.
5 Tolerance and resistance may develop; this can occur with any of the miotics.
6 Instillation must be frequent.
7 Systemic side effects include precipitation of an asthmatic attack, nausea, fall in blood pressure, and other symptoms of parasympathetic stimulation (refer to Chapter 9).
8 Anticholinesterase drugs may cause spasm of the wink reflex, which is annoying to the patient.

The cholinergic agents are very effective in many cases of chronic glaucoma. Their side effects are less severe and occur less frequently than those caused by anticholinesterase agents.

These drugs are often effective in treating chronic glaucoma when other agents have been ineffective. Instillations are less frequent with these drugs because of their prolonged action. Another advantage is better control over the intraocular pressure and less fluctuation in pressure.

Antidotes to cholinergic drugs. Two antidotes are available for overcoming effects caused by cholinergic stimulation—atropine and pralidoxime. Pralidoxime chloride (Protopam) is effective only against anticholinesterases because it reactivates the enzyme.

CARBONIC ANHYDRASE INHIBITORS

The intraocular pressure is maintained by the production of an aqueous humor inside the eye. It has been found that one of the substances necessary for the production of this fluid is the enzyme carbonic anhydrase. In glaucoma, where the intraocular pressure is abnormally high, it is desirable to slow the production of this fluid and thus decrease the pressure. The specific drugs used to inhibit carbonic anhydrase are quite effective when taken orally. Side reactions are usually not severe and consist of lethargy, anorexia, numbness, and tingling of the face and extremities. Diureses is produced and potassium depletion can occur.

Teratogenic effects have been reported in animals from acetazolamide, ethoxzolamide, and methazolamide. They should not be used in the first trimester of pregnancy. The duration of action of a single oral therapeutic dose is 6 to 8 hours.

The commonly used preparations are as follows:

Acetazolamide, U.S.P., B.P. (Diamox)—available in 250-mg. tablets

Ethoxzolamide, U.S.P. (Cardrase)—available in 125-mg. tablets

Methazolamide, U.S.P. (Neptazane)—available in 50-mg. tablets

Dichlorphenamide, U.S.P., B.P. (Daranide)—available in 50-mg. tablets

MYDRIATICS
ANTICHOLINERGIC (PARASYMPATHETIC) DRUGS

Mydriasis (dilation of the pupil) and cycloplegia (paralysis of accommodation) are produced when *anticholinergic drugs* are applied topically to the eye. The circular smooth muscles of the iris, which constrict the pupil, are innervated by parasympathetic fibers from the oculomotor (third cranial) nerve. Anticholinergics block the neurohormonal mediator, acetylcholine. This leaves the pupil (i.e., radial fibers of the iris) under the unopposed influence of its sympathetic or adrenergic nerve supply, and pupil dilation occurs. The oculomotor nerve also supplies the ciliary muscle. Contraction of this muscle slackens the suspensory ligament of the lens and allows the lens to become more convex. Accommodation for near vision is dependent upon the ciliary muscle's ability to contract.

The mydriatics and cycloplegics are also used to treat inflammations such as uveitis and keratitis. These drugs relieve ocular pain by relaxing inflamed intraocular muscles and by putting the eye at rest.

Mydriatic agents evoke a lesser response in persons with heavily pigmented irides than in persons with lighter pigmented irides. Thus blacks tend to respond less to these drugs than whites.

The pharmacologic actions of these drugs allow for accurate measurement of refractive errors, which permits proper lens determination for eyeglasses. They are also used pre- and postoperatively in intraocular surgery.

The anticholinergic drugs used topically in the eye include atropine, scopolamine, homatropine, cyclopentolate, tropicamide, and eucatropine.

Homatropine, cyclopentolate, and tropicamide are short-acting cycloplegics. They are used for refraction in older children and adults. Instillation of a 1% pilocarpine solution may be used to counteract the mydriasis and cycloplegia of short-acting cycloplegics. Pilocarpine is not useful in counteracting the effects of atropine or scopolamine because of its short duration of action. All cycloplegics may produce flushing of the face and may induce fever.

Systemic absorption of these drugs can result in serious side effects, such as dryness of the mouth, inhibition of sweating, flushing, tachycardia, fever, delirium, and coma. Pupillary dilation from either local or systemic administration can precipitate acute glaucoma in predisposed persons, which, if unrecognized or untreated, can result in blindness.

Atropine sulfate, U.S.P., B.P.

Atropine is the most potent of all cycloplegic drugs and has a long duration of action. It is available in 0.5% to 4% aqueous solutions and in ointments containing 0.25%, 0.5%, or 1% of atropine. Atropine produces mydriasis within 30 to 40 minutes; cycloplegia is slower in onset and several applications over a period of 1 or 2 hours may be required. Residual cycloplegia may persist for 5 to 6 or more days; the mydriatic effect lasts for 10 to 12 days.

Atropine is the drug of choice for refraction of children with accommodative esotropia. It is often preferred for refraction of children under 6 years of age. It is commonly used for the initial examination of patients with convergent strabismus. It is not a desirable drug for refraction in adults because of its long duration of effect.

Atropine in a 1% solution or ointment is also used to treat inflammations of the eye such as iritis, uveitis, and keratitis. In severe cases the drug may be instilled three times a day; in mild cases administration is usually once daily. Patients should be instructed that if side effects occur and are present when the next dose of drug is to be instilled (dryness of mouth, tachycardia), the instillation should be omitted. The patient must be aware that during therapy he may be unable to focus on nearby objects and will be unusually sensitive to light. Dark glasses should be worn to decrease photophobia. The eye will be accommodated for distant vision.

Atropine is contraindicated in patients with glaucoma. Dilation of the pupil causes a narrowing of the iridocorneal angle where the canal of Schlemm is located. This restricts drainage of intraocular fluids, though secretion continues and intraocular pressure rises. This may precipitate an attack of acute glaucoma.

Since atropine is highly toxic, bottles of atropine should be stored in a safe place out of the reach of children.

Scopolamine hydrobromide, U.S.P.; hyoscine hydrobromide, B.P.

Scopolamine in aqueous solutions of 0.25%, 0.5%, and 1% has actions and side effects similar to those of atropine. Scopolamine is a more rapidly acting mydriatic and cycloplegic than atropine but its effects are of shorter duration. Instillation of a 0.5% scopolamine solution causes mydriasis in 40 to 60 minutes and cycloplegia in 30 minutes to 1 hour; effects may persist for 5 to 7 days. It is used in patients sensitive to atropine.

Homatropine hydrobromide, U.S.P., B.P.

Of the short-acting cycloplegics, homatropine has the slowest onset and most prolonged action. Mydriasis occurs in 40 to 60 minutes and cycloplegia in 30 minutes to 1 hour. These effects may last from 24 to 48 hours. For mydriasis or ophthalmoscopic examination the 1% solution is usually adequate; for cycloplegia instillation of several drops of a 2% or stronger solution at intervals of 10 to 15 minutes may be required. It is contraindicated in patients with glaucoma and those with narrow angle or shallow anterior chambers because of their susceptibility to glaucoma. It must be used cautiously in older patients.

Cyclopentolate hydrochloride, U.S.P., B.P. (Cyclogyl Hydrochloride)

Cyclopentolate is more potent than homatropine and has a shorter duration of action. Mydriasis and cycloplegia occur within 30 to 60 minutes; effects may last 6 to 24 hours. It is used solely as a mydriatic. Dosage is usually 1 drop of a 1% solution or 2 drops of 0.5% solution 5 minutes apart. In children, 3 drops 10 minutes apart may be used.

The D.E.S.I. ratings for cyclopentolate are: *effective* for mydriasis and cycloplegia for diagnostic purposes; *ineffective* for use in inflammatory conditions such as iritis, keratitis, choroiditis, and iridocyclitis, and for prevention of lenticular adhesions.

Tropicamide, U.S.P., B.P. (Mydriacyl)

Tropicamide is a rapid-acting cycloplegic and mydriatic agent with a short duration of action. Two drops of a 1% solution of tropicamide 5 minutes apart are effective within 20 to 35 minutes; there is complete recovery from the cycloplegic effect in 2 to 6 hours. Examination must be performed within 35 minutes after instillation or an additional drop must be applied.

D.E.S.I. rating is like that for cyclopentolate: *effective* for diagnostic use; *ineffective* for use in inflammatory conditions.

Eucatropine hydrochloride, U.S.P.

Eucatropine produces a more rapid and less prolonged mydriasis than that produced by most other mydriatics. Mydriasis occurs in about 30 minutes and persists for 4 to 6 hours. Eucatropine is available as a 2% or 5% solution. One or two drops are instilled and repeated in 10 to 15 minutes if necessary. It is used for diagnostic purposes and for treatment of some inflammatory conditions. It is the preferred drug for testing for angle-closure glaucoma. It is not used for measuring refractive errors as it produces only minimal cycloplegia.

ADRENERGIC DRUGS

Mydriasis and decreased congestion of conjunctival blood vessels are produced when adrenergic (sympathomimetic) drugs are applied topically to the eye. Three adrenergic drugs are used in ophthalmology—epinephrine, hydroxyamphetamine, and phenylephrine.

Adrenergic drugs applied topically to the eye elicit the following sympathetic responses:

1 Mydriasis brought about by contraction of the radial or dilator muscle of the eye
2 Constriction of conjunctival blood vessels
3 Slight relaxation of the ciliary muscle
4 Decreased formation of aqueous humor and increased outflow with a resultant drop in intraocular pressure

Exactly how these effects are produced remains uncertain but there is some evidence that alpha-adrenergic receptors are present in the outflow mechanism of the eye and, when stimulated, they increase outflow of aqueous humor. It has also been shown experimentally that vasoconstriction decreases the rate of aqueous humor formation.

Adrenergic drugs are used to treat wide-angle glaucoma and glaucoma secondary to uveitis, to produce mydriasis for ocular examination, and to relieve congestion and hyperemia. Adrenergic drugs are contraindicated in the treatment of narrow-angle glaucoma since dilation of the pupil will further restrict ocular fluid outflow and this may cause an acute attack of glaucoma. Serious systemic side effects from these drugs are unusual, but care must be taken in patients with cardiovascular disease since tachycardia and elevated blood pressure can occur with these agents.

Epinephrine hydrochloride, U.S.P.; adrenaline, B.P.

Epinephrine is available in 0.25%, 0.5%, 1%, and 2% solutions, as the bitartrate or hydrochloride salt. Dilute solutions are used at times to treat local allergies and superficial hyperemia. It is sometimes added in dilute solutions (e.g., 1:50,000) to local anesthetics since its vasoconstricting effect prevents too rapid absorption of the anesthetic. In the initial treatment of primary open-angle glaucoma it is usually combined with pilocarpine or another miotic for more effective treatment. It may also be used during cataract surgery.

Instillation of 1 drop of a 2% solution of epinephrine causes immediate vasoconstriction that lasts 2 to 3 hours; mydriasis occurs within a few minutes and lasts for several hours; fall in intraocular pressure occurs within 1 hour, reaches a maximum in 4 hours, and persists for 24 hours or longer. Frequency of instillation should be individualized and may vary from every 2 or 3 days to two times a day.

Systemic effects such as tachycardia and elevated blood pressure may occur with its use. Other side effects that can occur include eye pain, ocular irritation, and tearing. There have also been reports of epinephrine causing macular edema.

Hydroxyamphetamine hydrobromide (Paredrine)

Hydroxyamphetamine is available in a 1% solution. It is extensively used as a mydriatic; 1 or 2 drops are usually instilled into the conjunctival sac. The D.E.S.I. ratings for hydroxyamphetamine are: *effective* for production of mydriasis; *ineffective* when used with a cycloplegic to help induce a rapid and satisfactory cycloplegia.

Phenylephrine hydrochloride ophthalmic solution, U.S.P., B.P. (Neo-Synephrine)

Phenylephrine is commonly used in 0.125% solution as a decongestant in over-the-counter products. In the 2.5% solution it is used as a mydriatic for ocular examination. The 1% solution is used in conjunction with cycloplegics to decrease the amount of cycloplegic needed for refraction and to aid in rapid satisfactory cycloplegia. The 10% solution is used in intraocular surgery. The 10% solution should be used with special caution in persons with advanced arteriosclerosis and in patients with hypertension. Care must be taken to prevent systemic absorption since 1 drop of a 10% solution contains about 5 mg. of drug. This is equal to the usual subcutaneous dose and it can produce a substantial rise in blood pressure. Phenylephrine's effects are produced within 30 minutes.

CHEMOTHERAPY OF OCULAR INFECTION

The basic principles guiding the use of chemotherapy are the same in all branches of medicine. The drug of choice and the dose required should be established by adequate laboratory isolation of the offending organism; the initial culture from the infected area should be obtained before any chemotherapeutic agent is applied. However, treatment should not be withheld if the time required to make these determinations may result in increased severity of infection and if the type of infection (e.g., most cases of conjunctivitis) does not warrant the expense of laboratory analysis; these tend to be self-limiting. Prophylactic use of antibiotic agents in general is useless as well as wasteful and potentially dangerous. A large proportion of the inflammatory diseases seen in ophthalmology are caused by viruses or other agents that are not susceptible to any currently available antibiotic; obviously, the use of antibiotics in such situations is unwarranted.

ANTIBIOTICS

All known systemically administered antibiotics are available and used at indicated times to treat ocular infections. Care must be taken to use an antibiotic that will not cause local or general sensitivity and to use drugs that are unlikely to ever be used systemically, in order to avoid possible sensitization to common systemic antiinfective drugs and to discourage development of resistant strains of offending organisms.

Selection of an antibiotic for ocular infection is based on: (1) clinical experience; (2) nature and sensitivity of the organisms most commonly causing the condition; (3) the disease itself; and (4) sensitivity and response of the patient.

Most antiinfective agents do not readily penetrate the eye when given systemically. However, some systemic drugs will penetrate the inflamed eye since the blood-aqueous barrier is decreased by injury or inflammation. Topically applied antiinfectives can cause sensitivity reactions, and patients sensitized to one drug may show cross reactions to chemically related drugs. In addition, the normal flora of the eye is interfered with when antiinfective agents are applied topically, and this may encourage growth of other organisms. Eye infections require prompt treatment to help prevent spread of infection. Severe infections may damage the eye and impair vision. Solutions are preferred for treatment of eye infections, since ointment bases often tend to interfere with healing.

Some of the common ocular infections treated with antibiotics include the following:

Conjunctivitis—acute inflammation of the conjunctiva (the mucous membrane lining the back of the lids and the front of the eye except for the cornea) resulting from bacterial invasion. "Pink eye" is the acute contagious epidemic form of conjunctivitis usually caused by pneumococci. Symptoms include redness and burning of the eye, lacrimation, itching, and at times photophobia. Conjunctivitis is usually self-limiting. The eye should be protected from light.

Hordeolum (sty)—an acute localized infection of the eyelash follicles and the glands of the anterior lid margin resulting in the formation of a small abscess or cyst.

Chalazion—infection of the Meibomian (sebaceous) glands of the eyelids. A hard cyst may form from blockage of the ducts.

Blepharitis—inflammation of the margins of the eyelid resulting from bacterial infection or allergy. Symptoms are crusting, irritation of the eye, and red and edematous lid margins.

Keratitis—corneal inflammation caused by bacterial infection; herpes simplex keratitis is caused by viral infection.

Uveitis—infection of the uveal tract, or the vascular layer of the eye, which includes the iris, ciliary body, and choroid.

Penicillin

Topical application of penicillin is not recommended. Local hypersensitivity reactions are very common, and, unfortunately, the patient may develop a generalized hypersensitivity that will forever prohibit the use of penicillin.

Amphotericin B, U.S.P. (Fungizone)

Amphotericin B is an effective fungistatic drug against yeast-like fungi. Unfortunately, its toxicity is high. It is well tolerated by the eye when applied as a 0.5% ointment. It is used for fungal infections of the cornea.

Bacitracin ophthalmic ointment, U.S.P., B.P. (Baciguent); bacitracin zinc, B.P.

Bacitracin is rarely used systemically because of its nephrotoxic effects. Ophthalmic bacitracin is available as an ointment containing 500 units per gram of suitable base and as a powder containing 10,000 units for making solutions for topical use. It is particularly useful in treating superficial infections caused by gram-positive bacteria. Used in combination with neomycin and polymyxin a broader spectrum of antimicrobial activity is produced than when these drugs are used alone. D.E.S.I. rating is similar to that for neomycin. Bacitracin does not penetrate the cornea in therapeutic amounts, it is nonirritating to the eye, and it causes no systemic effects.

Since bacitracin solutions are unstable, they should be refrigerated. Solutions remain potent for about 3 weeks. Ointment preparations are stable for about 1 year at room temperature. Bacitracin is preferable to penicillin for topical use, since fewer organisms are resistant to it, allergic reactions occur less frequently, and sensitization to penicillin is avoided.

Chloramphenicol, U.S.P., B.P. (Chloromycetin)

Chloramphenicol's effectiveness against a wide variety of gram-positive and gram-negative organisms makes it an extremely useful drug for intraocular infections. It penetrates the eye much more readily than many other antibiotics. Chloramphenicol is applied topically as a 1% ointment or a 0.16%, 0.25%, or 0.5% solution. Drops may be instilled three times a day or every 3, 4, or 6 hours, and the ointment may be applied at bedtime. Prolonged or frequent use should be avoided. One case of bone marrow hypoplasia has been reported following prolonged (23 months) use of the eyedrops.

D.E.S.I. rating is *effective* for use in superficial ocular infections.

Erythromycin, U.S.P. (E-Mycin, Ilotycin)

Erythromycin is applied one or more times daily in a 0.5% ointment. It is effective against all gram-positive and many gram-negative organisms. D.E.S.I. rating is *effective* for use in superficial eye infections.

Isoniazid, U.S.P., B.P.

Isoniazid is used for tuberculous infection of the eye as a topical 10% solution or ointment; it may be given as a subconjunctival injection containing 10 to 20 mg. of the drug. Corneal penetration occurs with isoniazid. The drug is well tolerated by the eye. Resistance develops rapidly.

Neomycin sulfate, U.S.P., B.P. (Myciguent)

Neomycin is available as an ointment containing 3.5 mg. per gram of base or as a 0.5% solution. It has a broad antibacterial spectrum and a low index of allergenicity. Because of auditory and renal toxicity it is generally not used parenterally and thus is often preferred for local use. However, it is an active topical sensitizer and can cause cross-sensitivity reactions to systemically used antibiotics that are chemically related. D.E.S.I. rating is *effective* for treating superficial ocular infections involving the conjunctiva and cornea. Solutions containing neomycin and another antibiotic such as polymyxin B and gramicidin (Neosporin, Neo-Polycin) have been rated as *possibly effective* for use in superficial ocular infections.

Polymyxin B sulfate, U.S.P., B.P. (Aerosporin)

Polymyxin is used largely for its activity against gram-negative bacteria. Hypersensitivity reaction to the topical solution is practically unknown. It is applied as an ointment containing 10,000 or 20,000 units per gram and as solutions containing 10,000 or 20,000 units per milliliter. An intact corneal epithelium prevents penetration of polymyxin B into the eye, but epithelial damage from abrasion or ulceration permits effective penetration.

Tetracyclines

The tetracyclines are used topically to treat superficial infections of the eye. Generally, they are bacteriostatic rather than bactericidal; they have a broad antimicrobial spectrum. Organisms resistant to one tetracycline are usually resistant to the others. Trachoma may be treated with both topical and oral tetracycline therapy. The tetracyclines have been recommended for prophylaxis of gonorrheal ophthalmia neonatorum, since they produce a lower incidence of conjunctivitis and less irritation of the eye than does silver nitrate. Topical tetracyclines rarely cause adverse reactions.

Tetracycline hydrochloride, U.S.P. (Achromycin) is applied topically as 1% ointment or 1% suspension in oil.

Chlortetracycline hydrochloride, N.F. (Aureomycin) is applied as a 1% ointment; a sterile powder is also available for making a 0.5% solution.

Oxytetracycline hydrochloride, U.S.P. (Terramycin) is applied as a 0.5% ointment or solution.

D.E.S.I. ratings for the tetracyclines are: *effective* for treatment of superficial ocular infec-

tions caused by organisms susceptible to these antibiotics; *possibly effective* for treatment of viral ocular infections.

SULFONAMIDES
Sulfacetamide sodium, U.S.P., B.P. (Sodium Sulamyd)

Used in a 10% ointment or a 10% to 30% solution, sulfacetamide provides high local concentrations that are relatively nonirritating. The presence of purulent drainage or exudate interferes with the action of the sulfonamides, since the purulent matter contains para-amino-benzoic acid. Sulfacetamide is available only for topical use and thus is preferred over other sulfa drugs used systemically. It may cause local irritation.

D.E.S.I. ratings are: *effective* for treatment of conjunctivitis, corneal ulcer, and other superficial ocular infections caused by susceptible microorganisms, and as an adjunct in the systemic therapy of trachoma; *possibly effective* for treatment of nonpurulent blepharitis and nonpurulent conjunctivitis.

Sulfisoxazole diethanolamine (Gantrisin Diethanolamine)

Sulfisoxazole is available in a 4% ophthalmic solution and a 4% ophthalmic ointment. It is applied topically to the conjunctiva three or more times per day. D.E.S.I. ratings are similar to those for sulfacetamide.

OTHER ANTIINFECTIVES
Nitrofurazone, N.F. (Furacin)

Nitrofurazone is a highly bacteriostatic agent that has a fairly broad spectrum. Unfortunately, the rate of patient sensitization is high. Nitrofurazone is available for topical application in the eye as a 1% ointment and a 0.02% solution. The drug is well tolerated by the eye. Since its ocular penetration is insignificant, it is useful only for surface infections of the eye.

Idoxuridine, U.S.P., B.P. (Herplex, Dendrid, Stoxil)

Idoxuridine inhibits the replication of certain viruses when applied directly to the eye. The drug is too toxic for systemic use. When applied locally in the eye in a 0.1% solution, the drug is effective in the treatment of keratitis caused by the herpes simplex virus and the vaccinia virus. One drop of the drug may be applied to the conjunctiva every 1 to 2 hours (day and night) for several days. The solution should be kept refrigerated and the expiration date observed.

Idoxuridine is also available as a 0.5% ointment; it is usually applied five times a day. Its effectiveness is reported to be equal to that of the drops.

ANTISEPTICS

Many of the antiseptics that were used to treat surface infections of the eye prior to the advent of antibiotics are now obsolete. Not only were many of these drugs relatively ineffective, they also delayed healing and in some cases caused permanent damage to the eye. Antiseptic solutions are employed in ophthalmology for irrigation, dissolution of secretions, and precipitation of mucus and in certain instances in which specific antimicrobial agents cannot be used. A 2.2% boric acid solution is used as an irrigant; this concentration is thought to be isotonic with tear fluid.

Silver nitrate, U.S.P., B.P.

A solution of 1% or 2% silver nitrate is routinely employed as a prophylaxis against ophthalmia neonatorum in newborn infants. In many states this is required by law. The gonococci are particularly susceptible to silver salts. Silver nitrate is preferred to effective antibiotic agents, since these may sensitize the patient and since silver nitrate has stood the test of time. Silver nitrate ophthalmic solution, U.S.P., is available in collapsible capsules containing about 5 drops of a 1% solution. It should be rinsed from the eye immediately with water to prevent chemical conjunctivitis.

Mercury compounds

Inorganic mercuric salts such as yellow mercuric oxide ophthalmic ointment, N.F., and ammoniated mercury, U.S.P., B.P., formerly served as bacteriostatic agents. Today they are seldom used.

Benzalkonium chloride, U.S.P.

This is a cationic surface-active wetting agent that has several applications in ophthalmology. Its antiseptic properties make it useful in the preservation of other solutions and the sterilization of small instruments. It is also used in balanced salt solutions to aid in the cleansing and application of contact lenses. For topical application to the conjunctiva a 1:10,000 solution is used (1 ml. of a 0.01% solution).

Zinc sulfate, U.S.P., B.P.

An aqueous solution of 0.1% to 1% zinc sulfate is used as an astringent and mildly antiseptic eyewash in conjunctivitis caused by the Morax-Axenfeld bacillus.

Iodine tincture, U.S.P.

Iodine tincture contains 2% iodine and 2% sodium iodide in dilute alcohol. Its only ophthalmologic use is for the chemical cautery of corneal lesions produced by the herpes simplex virus.

STEROIDS

Corticosteroid therapy is indicated for all allergic reactions of the eye, nonpyogenic inflammations, and severe injury. Allergic reactions of the eye may be caused by drugs applied to the eye or by contact with substances such as weed pollen to which the individual is hypersensitive.

Ophthalmic corticosteroid therapy is not used for pyogenic (pus-producing) inflammations of the eye, since corticosteroids decrease defense mechanisms and reduce resistance to pathogenic organisms.

Eye structures are relatively delicate, and inflammation can cause functional damage, scarring, and impaired vision. Inflammation increases capillary permeability. In the eye, this results in the escape of proteins and cells from the blood vessels into the aqueous humor; this, in turn, may cause a rise in intraocular pressure.

The glucocorticoids used in ophthalmology may be applied topically, injected into the conjunctiva, or given systemically.

Corticosteroid therapy is not recommended for minor corneal abrasions. Steroids may actually increase ocular susceptibility to fungous infection. When steroids are used for various eye conditions, they should be used for a limited period of time only and the eye should be checked for increase in ocular pressure. Clinical evidence indicates that prolonged ocular steroid therapy can cause glaucoma and cataracts.

The following corticosteroids are available for topical use as solutions, suspensions, or ointments. They are available in varying strengths and in combinations with various antibiotics.

Cortisone acetate, U.S.P.
Dexamethasone, U.S.P.
Fludrocortisone acetate
Flurometholone, N.F.
Hydrocortisone, U.S.P.
Methylprednisolone, N.F.
Prednisolone, U.S.P.
Triamcinolone acetonide, U.S.P.

OTHER AGENTS
TOPICAL ANESTHESIA

Local anesthetics are used to prevent pain during surgical procedures and examinations. Unfortunately, all of the topical anesthetic drugs interfere with healing of epithelial tissue, particularly of the cornea. The practice of repeatedly applying such an anesthetic to an eye after removal of a foreign body is to be condemned.

Cocaine hydrochloride, U.S.P., B.P.

Cocaine was the first drug to be used for anesthesia of the eye (1884). One drop of cocaine produces anesthesia of the cornea in 5 to 10 minutes. Complete anesthesia lasts for approximately 10 minutes; less anesthetic effect persists for 1 or 2 hours. In addition to its anesthetic effects cocaine produces mydriasis and constriction of conjunctival vessels. Since the surface of the eye becomes dry, this may cause damage to the corneal surface. It may precipitate an acute attack of glaucoma. For these reasons, cocaine has largely been replaced by newer anesthetics.

Solutions of 1% to 4% are used for deep topical anesthesia of the eye. The drug has both anesthetizing and adrenergic effects. Local administration may produce acute cocaine poisoning with sudden severe confusion, delirium, and convulsions. Short-acting barbiturates must be given at once to prevent fatality.

Benoxinate hydrochloride (Dorsacaine)

Benoxinate is similar to proparacaine. Anesthesia occurs within 1 minute after instillation of 1 drop of a 0.4% solution and lasts about 10 to 15 minutes. A series of three instillations may extend the anesthesia to 20 minutes.

Tetracaine hydrochloride, U.S.P. (Pontocaine)

Tetracaine is used topically in a 0.5% to 2% solution for rapid, brief, superficial anesthesia. It is a widely used local ocular anesthetic. One drop of a 0.5% solution of tetracaine will produce anesthesia within 30 seconds, during which time a burning sensation may be felt by the patient. The anesthetic effect lasts for 10 to 25 minutes. Tetracaine can cause epithelial damage; therefore, it is not recommended for prolonged home use by patients.

Proparacaine hydrochloride, U.S.P. (Ophthaine, Ophthetic)

This drug is similar to tetracaine. A 0.5% solution is administered by topical instillation. Anesthesia is produced within 20 seconds and lasts for 15 minutes. It is relatively free from the burning and discomfort of other anesthetics and is often the drug of choice.

LUBRICANTS

Lubricants, or "artificial tears," are used to provide moisture and lubrication in diseases in which tear production is deficient, to lubricate artificial eyes and moisten contact lenses, and to protect the cornea during procedures on the eye. These agents are also incorporated into ophthalmic preparations to prolong the contact time of topically applied drugs.

Methylcellulose, U.S.P. (Methulose, Visculose, Isopto Tears, Lyteers, Tearisol)

Methylcellulose is used as a 0.5% to 2.5% solution. For decreased tear production 1 or 2 drops of the 0.5% solution is applied to the eye as needed; to lubricate contact lenses and artificial eyes the solution is applied directly to the lens or artificial eye. Most preparations contain benzalkonium or chlorobutanol as preservatives.

Methylcellulose is nonirritating to ocular tissue and can be used for prolonged periods without damaging the eye. However, if an excess is instilled into the eye and dries on the eyelids it may cause discomfort similar to having sand in the eyes. If this occurs, an eye wash or sterile, nonirritating irrigating solution should be used.

Polyvinyl alcohol, U.S.P. (Wetting Solution, Lens Mate, Liquifilm Tears)

Polyvinyl alcohol is a nontoxic viscous agent that is less viscous than methylcellulose and therefore must be applied more frequently when used as a substitute for tears. As artificial tears, 1 or 2 drops are applied to the eyes as needed. To moisten contact lenses the solution is applied to the lens before insertion. Preparations also contain a preservative such as benzalkonium or chlorobutanol.

DIAGNOSTIC AIDS
Fluorescein sodium, U.S.P., B.P.

Fluorescein is a nontoxic water-soluble dye that is used as a diagnostic aid. When applied to the cornea, only areas denuded of epithelium (corneal lesions or ulcers) are stained a bright green color; foreign bodies appear surrounded by a green ring. These effects permit detection of corneal epithelial defects caused by injury or infection and location of foreign bodies in the eye. Loss of conjunctiva is indicated by a yellow hue. The dye is also used in fitting contact lenses. Areas that lack fluorescein-stained tears will appear black under ultraviolet light indicating the contact lens is touching the cornea at those areas. Fluorescein is used in retinal photography to determine retinal vascular status and to identify defects in the retinal pigment epithelium. In addition, it may be used to test lacrimal patency; if after the dye is instilled into the eye it appears in the nasal secretions, the nasolacrimal drainage system is open.

Solutions of this dye are easily contaminated by *Pseudomonas aeruginosa,* which causes intense corneal ulceration. For this reason prepared solutions are never used, but strips of filter paper impregnated with the dry dye are moistened just before use. Staining of the eye disappears in 30 minutes.

Fluress

Fluress is a combination of the dye fluorescein and the local anesthetic benoxinate. It is useful for removal of foreign bodies in the eye since it provides for simultaneous staining and anesthesia. One drop of a 0.25% solution is usually used.

Silicone

Silicone fluids are being used for patients with artificial eyes to lubricate the socket, reduce irritation, and increase comfort. They prevent crusting in the lids and impart a more lifelike glistening effect to the artificial eye.

MISCELLANEOUS AGENTS
Alpha-chymotrypsin (Chymar)

This enzyme is used in selected cases to facilitate cataract extraction. It is injected behind the iris into the posterior chamber where it dissolves the filaments or zonules that hold the lens, thereby facilitating lens extraction. This effect is usually obtained in 1 to 2 minutes with 0.2 to 0.5 ml. of a freshly prepared 1:5000 solution. Chymotrypsin may cause a transient glaucoma lasting about 1 week, which can be relieved by the use of pilocarpine. It is available in ampules containing 750 units of lyophilized enzyme dissolved in 10 ml. of diluent.

Sodium chloride ointment

This 5% ointment is used to reduce the corneal edema that occurs in certain corneal dystrophies.

QUESTIONS

For study and review

1 Which of the following have a mydriatic effect only?
   a. homatropine
   b. atropine
   c. phenylephrine
   d. cyclopentolate
2 When comparing ophthalmic solutions to ointments, which of the following are true statements?

a. Antibiotics tend to be more stable in ointment form.
b. Solutions do not remain in contact with the eye as long as ointments.
c. Ointments tend to interfere more with vision than solutions.
d. Solutions cause more prolonged effects than ointments.

3 Cholinergic drugs applied to the eye have which of the following effects?
a. pupil dilation
b. vasodilator effect on eye vessels
c. ciliary muscle spasm
d. more resistance to destruction by cholinesterase than acetylcholine

4 Which of the following are cholinergic drugs?
a. pilocarpine
b. carbachol
c. physostigmine
d. isoflurophate

5 Which of the following are true about anticholinesterase drugs?
a. They inhibit the action of acetylcholine.
b. They can be termed indirect-acting drugs.
c. Synthesis of new cholinesterase is required for destruction of acetylcholine when the "irreversible" anticholinesterase drugs are used.
d. The "reversible" anticholinesterases form stable compounds with cholinesterase.

6 Which of the following are adverse reactions to drugs used to treat glaucoma?
a. Systemic absorption of a cholinergic drug resulting in toxicity and a fall in blood pressure
b. Cataract formation with the use of potent anticholinesterase drugs
c. Systemic absorption of adrenergic drugs causing tachycardia and elevated blood pressure
d. Conjunctivitis
e. Headache and ocular pain

7 Classify the drugs in Column A with their pharmacologic action listed in Column B.

Column A	Column B
physostigmine	1. cholinergic
pilocarpine	2. antiviral
isoflurophate (DFP)	3. anticholinesterase
idoxuridrine	4. gram-negative antibiotic
acetylcholine	5. carbonic anhydrase inhibitor
atropine	
polymyxin B	6. gram-positive antibiotic
bacitracin	7. parasympatholytic
phenylephrine	8. adrenergic

REFERENCES

Abrams, J. D.: The nature of glaucoma, Nurs. Times **68:**707, 1972.

Aviado, D. M.: Krantz and Carr's pharmacologic principles of medical practice, ed. 8, Baltimore, 1972, The Williams & Wilkins Co.

Bernstein, H. N.: Some iatrogenic ocular diseases from systemically administered drugs, Int. Ophthalmol. Clin. **10:**553, 1970.

Grant, M.: Toxicology of the eye, Springfield, Ill., 1973, Charles C Thomas, Publisher.

Kaufman, H. E., editor: Ocular anti-inflammatory therapy, Springfield, Ill., 1970, Charles C Thomas, Publisher.

Lemp, M. A., and Holly, F. J.: Ophthalmic polymers as ocular wetting agents, Am. J. Ophthalmol. **4:**15, 1972.

Leopold, I. H., editor: Symposia on ocular therapy, vol. 7, St. Louis, 1974, The C. V. Mosby Co.

Lieberman, T. W.: Individual responsiveness to drugs and pharmacogenetics in ophthalmology. In Leopold, I. H., editor: Symposia on ocular therapy, vol. 5, St. Louis, 1972, The C. V. Mosby Co.

Lubeck, M. J.: Effects of drugs on ocular muscles, Int. Ophthalmol. Clin. **11:**35, 1971.

Modell, W., editor: Drugs of choice 1976-1977, St. Louis, 1976, The C. V. Mosby Co.

Osol, A., and Pratt, R.: The United States dispensatory, Philadelphia, 1973, J. B. Lippincott Co.

Periera, P.: Screening for glaucoma, Nursing Times **68:**771, 1972.

Podos, S. M., Becker, B., and Kass, M. A.: Prostaglandin synthesis, inhibition and intraocular pressure, Invest. Ophthalmol. **12:**426, 1973.

Smith, M. B.: Handbook of ocular pharmacology, Acton, Mass., 1974, Publishing Sciences Group, Inc.

Spaeth, G. L.: General medications, glaucoma, and disturbances of intraocular pressure, Med. Clin. North Am. **53:**1109, 1969.

CHAPTER 30

Dermatologic agents

Preparations that soothe
Antiseptics and parasiticides
Stimulants and irritants
Keratolytics
Antipruritics
Protectives
Cleansers
Some cutaneous disorders

The skin is the largest organ of the body, but absorption from the skin is poor and uncertain. The flat cells of the outermost layer of the skin contain keratin, a substance that serves to waterproof the skin and to prevent absorption of water and other substances. Absorption is affected, however, by the presence of sweat pores and of sebaceous glands, which penetrate the epidermis from the deeper subcutaneous tissue and corium. Hair follicles, pigment cells, nerve endings, nerve networks, and blood vessels as well as collagenous and elastic fibers all contribute to the functions of the skin. Although the skin is not known for its powers of absorption, drugs that cannot penetrate the horny first layer are sometimes absorbed by way of the sebaceous glands. Absorption is increased if the skin is macerated either by water or perspiration. It is more likely to occur if the epidermis is thin, as it is in the axilla or in the skin of a child. Absorption will take place rapidly from raw or denuded surfaces.

Methyl salicylate rubbed on the skin can be found in the urine in 30 minutes. Alcohol and volatile solvents promote absorption. The nature of the vehicle affects absorption—drugs that are fat soluble can be absorbed more rapidly than water-soluble drugs, and natural fats make a better vehicle to carry the drug into the skin than do substances such as petrolatum.

A wide range of drugs are used in dermatology, some for systemic and others for local effects. It is impossible in a textbook of this kind to present more than a superficial discussion of dermatologic agents. The student, therefore, should refer to specialty texts devoted to dermatology and dermatologic therapy.

DRUGS EXCRETED BY WAY OF THE SKIN

Drugs may be excreted by the skin in small amounts. Silver, copper, arsenic, mercury, bromides, borates, phenol, salicylates, antipyrine, methylene blue, and phenolphthalein may be deposited in the skin and sweat glands, and this may explain the skin eruption sometimes noticed after their use. Many other drugs can be the cause of skin eruption.

SYMPTOMS ASSOCIATED WITH CUTANEOUS DISORDERS

Reactions or disorders of the skin are manifested by symptoms such as itching, pain, or tingling and by signs such as swelling, redness, papules, pustules, blisters, and hives.

659

A reaction of the skin that makes the patient uncomfortable or unsightly may be attributable to or related to sensitivity to drugs, allergy, infection, emotional conflict, hormonal imbalance, or degenerative disease. Many times the cause of the skin disorder is unknown and the treatment may be empiric in the hope that the right remedy will be found.

PREPARATIONS THAT SOOTHE
EMOLLIENTS

Emollients are fatty or oily substances that may be used to soften or soothe irritated skin and mucous membrane. An emollient may also serve as a vehicle for application of other medicinal substances. Olive oil and liquid petrolatum are frequently used to cleanse dry areas that would be irritated by water.

Fixed oils. These are used as emollients and include olive oil, flaxseed oil, and cottonseed oil.

Benzoinated lard. This is made by incorporating 1% benzoin with lard and then straining the preparation. The addition of the benzoin hinders the development of rancidity. The preparation is used as an ingredient of ointments.

Glycerin, U.S.P., B.P. (Glycerol). In pure form this tends to have a drying effect, but when diluted with water or rose water it is useful for application to irritated lips and skin.

Lanolin, U.S.P.; *hydrous wool fat,* B.P. Lanolin is made by combining the purified fat of sheepswool with 25% to 30% water. It is used as an ointment base. It does not become rancid, and as much as twice its weight of water can be incorporated with it. It has a somewhat unpleasant odor. It requires dilution for use in ointments, and from 20% to 100% of petrolatum may be added for this purpose.

Hydrophilic ointment, U.S.P.; *aqueous cream,* B.P. This is an ointment in which the oil in it is dispersed in the continuous water phase. It is an oil-in-water emulsion, and when medicaments are incorporated, the wetting agent in the emulsion enables the drugs to come in more direct contact with the skin and sebaceous glands. It is less greasy and more easily washed off than other ointments. Inflamed or irritated skin is often intolerant of this kind of ointment.

Petrolatum, N.F.; *soft paraffin,* B.P. (Petroleum Jelly). This is a purified, semisolid mixture of hydrocarbons derived from petroleum and used as a vehicle for medicinal agents for local application. It is an important ointment base.

Plastibase. This is a new type of ointment base that contains 95% liquid petrolatum and 5% polyethylene; it is a hydrophobic base.

Polysorb anhydrous; Aquaphor. These are absorbent ointment bases that will combine with water or aqueous solutions of drugs.

Rose water ointment, N.F. This is a pleasant smelling water-in-oil emulsion of the cold cream type. It contains spermaceti and white wax as emulsifying agents in addition to expressed almond oil, sodium borate, rose water, oil of rose, and distilled water. Nonallergic cold creams do not contain perfume, to which some patients are intolerant.

Cold cream, U.S.P. This is like rose water ointment, N.F., except that mineral oil is substituted for almond oil or persic oil.

Theobroma oil, U.S.P., B.P. (cacao or cocoa butter). This preparation is a fixed oil that is expressed from the roasted seeds of *Theobromo cacao.* It is a yellowish white solid having a faint, agreeable odor and a bland taste resembling chocolate. It is used chiefly for making suppositories and, to some extent, as a lubricant for massage and for application to sore nipples.

White ointment, U.S.P. This is a mixture of white wax and white petrolatum. It is mostly petrolatum with a little white wax added to give it stiffness. It is used as an ointment base.

Yellow ointment, N.F. This contains yellow wax and petrolatum.

Zinc oxide ointment, U.S.P. This contains 20% zinc oxide in a base of liquid petrolatum and white ointment.

Zinc ointment, U.S.P., B.P. This contains 15% zinc oxide in a base of simple ointment.

Vitamin A and D ointment. This contains vitamin A and vitamin D in a lanolin-petrolatum base.

SOLUTIONS AND LOTIONS

Soothing preparations may also be liquids that carry an insoluble powder or suspension, or they may be mild acid or alkaline solutions, such as boric acid solution, limewater, or aluminum subacetate. The bismuth salts (the subcarbonate or the subnitrate) and starch are also commonly used for their soothing effect.

Aluminum acetate solution, U.S.P. (Burow's Solution). This contains 545 ml. of aluminum subacetate solution and 15 ml. of glacial acetic acid in 1000 ml. of aqueous medium. It is diluted with 10 to 40 parts of water before application.

Aluminum subacetate solution, U.S.P. This preparation contains 145 Gm. of aluminum sulfate, 160 ml. of acetic acid, and 70 Gm. of precipitated calcium carbonate in 1000 ml. of aqueous medium. It is applied topically after dilution with 20 to 40 parts of water as a wet dressing.

Calamine lotion, U.S.P., B.P. Prepared calamine, zinc oxide, bentonite magma, glycerin, and calcium hydroxide solution are included in this lotion. It is a soothing lotion used for the dermatitis caused by poison ivy, insect bites, prickly heat, and so on. It is patted on the involved skin area.

Zinc stearate, U.S.P. This is a compound of zinc and variable proportions of stearic and palmitic acids. It contains about 14% zinc oxide and is similar to zinc oxide. It is used as a dusting powder, but caution should be observed with its use, particularly around infants, to prevent inhalation of the powder.

ANTISEPTICS AND PARASITICIDES

It is generally agreed that thorough washing of the skin with warm water and a mild soap should precede the application of antiseptics to the skin. It is impossible to sterilize the skin, but adequate soaping and washing will do much to remove bacteria and the outer, loose epithelium. Strong antiseptics may do more harm than good by producing an irritation that will decrease the natural resistance of the skin to bacterial invasion. Antiseptics that are used to lower bacterial content are presented in Chapter 22.

A number of skin conditions for which antiseptics are used are caused by staphylococci and streptococci. Invasion by these organisms is likely to occur, especially when the normal protective mechanisms of the skin are broken down.

ANTIBIOTICS

Although relatively costly, bacitracin and tyrothricin are very useful in the local treatment of infectious lesions. Bacitracin is most often used in an ointment, although it can be used to moisten wet dressings or as a dusting powder. It is odorless and nonstaining and its use seldom results in sensitization. Tyrothricin is said to be more effective in wet dressings than in a cream or an ointment. Tyrothricin does not cause local irritation and its use rarely is attended by sensitization. Neomycin has been used successfully in the treatment of a number of infections of skin and mucous membrane. It is applied topically but occasionally it irritates the skin. An ointment combining neomycin, bacitracin, and polymyxin B may be more efficacious in mixed infections than when these agents are used singly. Vioform and xeroform are helpful in skin infections; there is seldom any irritation, but temporary discoloration of the skin and linen occurs. A number of antibiotics can be given orally or parenterally for treatment of infections of the skin.

Ammoniated mercury ointment, B.P. The preparation contains 5 Gm. of ammoniated mercury in each 100 Gm. of the finished preparation along with liquid petrolatum and white ointment. In this strength local irritation seldom occurs. The preparation has no odor and does not stain. It occasionally causes sensitization, particularly when combined with salicylic acid. It may be used to treat impetigo and superficial pyodermas.

Nitrofurazone, N.F. (Furacin). This is a synthetic, bright yellow, antibacterial substance that is inhibitory to bacteria in concentrations of 1:100,000 to 1:200,000 and bactericidal in concentrations of 1:50,000 to 1:75,000. It is effective against a variety of both gram-positive and gram-negative organisms. It is least effective against *Pseudomonas aeruginosa* and *Diplococcus pneumoniae.*

Nitrofurazone is useful when applied topically in the treatment of superficial mixed infections associated with contaminated wounds, burns, ulcerations, and impetigo. It is also useful in the preparation of areas for skin grafting. Applications of nitrofurazone may produce a generalized allergic skin reaction in certain individuals. Its internal use is not recommended, although it appears to have a low level of toxicity. Any systemic untoward effects as a result of absorption from dressings seem unlikely.

Nitrofurazone is appplied locally in a 0.2% ointment-like base or as a 0.02% to 0.2% solution. It is either applied directly to the area or applied to a dressing that is then applied to the infected area. Since the base is water soluble and softens at body temperature, special reinforcement of the dressing may be required to maintain an effective contact with the area or to limit absorption into the dressing. If diluted, solutions become cloudy and should be discarded.

ANTIFUNGAL AGENTS

Salicylanilide, N.F. (Salinidol). This antifungous preparation is used externally for the treatment of ringworm of the scalp. It is available as a 5% ointment and is applied alone or along with less irritating fungistatics. The ointment is rubbed into the affected areas once or twice a day for 6 days of the week over a period of about 8 weeks.

Gentian violet, U.S.P. This is available for external application is a solution containing 1% of the dye in an alcohol-water solvent. Its principal disadvantage is that it stains clothing.

Potassium permanganate solution, U.S.P. (1:100 to 1:10,000). This solution is sometimes prescribed for foot soaks for epidermophytosis of the feet (athlete's foot). It is inexpensive and odorless but leaves brown stains on fabrics, skin, and nails.

Sulfur ointment, U.S.P.; *sulphur ointment*, B.P. Sulfur ointment contains about 10% of the precipitated sulfur in a base of liquid petrolatum and white ointment and is used in the treatment of ringworm and seborrhea. An ointment containing precipitated sulfur, salicylic acid, and resorcin may be more helpful than sulfur alone in the treatment of seborrheic dermatitis and fungous infections. It is also a scabicide.

Benzoic and salicylic acid ointment, U.S.P. (Whitfield's Ointment). This ointment contains salicylic ointment. It is used for epidermophytosis of the feet.

Nystatin, U.S.P., B.P. (Mycostatin). This drug is an antibiotic substance used to treat infections of the skin and mucous membranes caused by *Candida albicans*. Vaginal infections are treated with suppositories or tablets, each containing 100,000 units, once or twice daily. An ointment and cream are available (100,000 units per gram) for moniliasis of the skin and should be applied to the affected area once to several times a day.

Griseofulvin, U.S.P., B.P. (Fulvicin, Grifulvin). This preparation is an important addition to the treatment of superficial fungous infections, particularly those caused by the trichophyton and microsporon organisms. It is given orally in a dosage of 1 Gm. per day (in children the dosage is decreased by half). It has a fungistatic action by combining with the keratin of skin, hair, and nails. Topical therapy should be continued while the griseofulvin is ingested. It is available in 250-mg. tablets for oral administration.

Tolnaftate, U.S.P., B.P. (Tinactin). A 1% cream and a 1% solution and powder are used for the topical treatment of superficial fungous infections caused by trichophyton and related organisms. The drug is ineffective against *Candida albicans* and against gram-positive and gram-negative bacteria. Treatment twice a day for 2 to 3 weeks is usually adequate.

PEDICULICIDES—SCABICIDES

The following agents are used to kill lice or scabies caused by itch mite (7-year itch).

Gamma benzene hexachloride, U.S.P., B.P. (Gexane, Kwell). This white, crystalline powder acts both as a pediculicide and scabicide. It is toxic and its use should be supervised by a physician. One application is sufficient to remove the active parasites. The preparation does not dissolve nits and, after 1 week, a second application may be given if necessary. Repeated use should be avoided because the substance tends to cause skin irritation. It should be kept away from the eyes, since it is irritating to mucous membranes. It is applied topically as a 1% lotion or ointment. A small brush may be used to facilitate application to the scalp. All clothing and bed linen should be sterilized by boiling to prevent reinfection. Wool clothing should be dry cleaned. The patient should not bathe or wash the hair until 24 hours after the treatment. A 10% solution of acetic acid or vinegar will help to remove nits from hairy regions but should be followed by a cleansing bath.

Isobornyl thiocyanoacetate-technical (Bornate). This preparation is one of the thiocyanates that kill lice. It may be mildly irritating to the skin of certain persons, but it does not seem to act as a sensitizing agent. It should not be applied near the eyes or on mucous membranes.

An oil emulsion is used in amounts of 30 to 60 ml., depending on the amount of hair at the site of infestation. It is applied and worked into a lather, after which it is allowed to remain for 10 minutes. In a scalp treatment, the hair is then combed with a fine-tooth comb and washed with a bland soap and water. The preparation should not remain on the skin too long. More than two applications should be avoided.

Benzyl benzoate lotion, N.F., B.P. (Benylate, Albacide). Benzyl benzoate is applied in a 10% to 30% lotion or emulsion. Application is sometimes followed by a slight, transient, burning sensation. In patients with sensitive skin severe irritation sometimes develops. It should be kept away from the eyes.

The entire body should be bathed, and the lesions caused by the itch mite should be well scrubbed with soap and warm water. Then the entire body surface, except the face, should be covered with the drug in the form of the emulsion or lotion, the application being made with a swab or brush. Particular care should be given to the region of the nails. After the first application has dried, a second one should be made to the most involved areas. Sterilization of clothing and bed linen is essential. Twenty-four hours later, clean clothing is put on after a warm soaking bath. A second or third treatment should be given if the parasite has not been eradicated.

STIMULANTS AND IRRITANTS

Stimulants are those substances that produce a mild irritation and in that way promote healing and the disappearance of inflammatory exudates. Most of the irritant drugs exert a stimulating effect when applied in low concentrations. Examples of preparations that may have a stimulating effect are the tars obtained from the destructive distillation of wood and coal.

Tars, when diluted, act as antiseptics as well as irritants. Official preparations include niper tar, N.F., coal tar, U.S.P., and prepared coal tar, B.P. The tars are sometimes prescribed in the treatment of psoriasis and chronic e_zematous dermatitis. The official tars are seldom employed full strength. Coal tar is the most antiseptic but also the most irritant, and it has the most disagreeable odor. Ichthammol, N.F., derived from destructive distillation of coal, is used in the form of an ointment for eczema and seborrheic conditions of the skin.

Vulneraries are a form of tissue stimulant that are used to hasten the granulation of wounds or stimulate the growth of cells over a denuded area.

Compound benzoin tincture, U.S.P., is useful as a stimulant and protective for ulcers, bedsores, cracked nipples, and fissures of the lips, anus, and the like.

Preparations made of red blood cells also have been used to stimulate healing of indolent wounds and ulcers.

KERATOLYTICS

Keratolytics (keratin dissolvers) are drugs that soften scales and loosen the outer horny layer of the skin. Salicylic acid, U.S.P., B.P., and resorcinol, U.S.P., B.P., are drugs of choice. Their action makes possible the penetration of other medicinal substances by a cleaning of the lesions involved. Salicylic acid is particularly important for its keratolytic effect in local treatment of scalp conditions, warts, corns, fungous infections, and chronic types of dermatitis. It is used up to 20% in ointments, plasters, or collodion for this purpose.

ANTIPRURITICS

Antipruritics are drugs given to allay itching of skin and mucous membranes. There is less need for these preparations as the constitutional treatment of patients with skin disorders is better understood. Dilute solutions containing phenol as well as tars have been widely used. They may be applied as lotions, pastes, or ointments.

Dressings wet with potassium permanganate 1:4000, aluminum subacetate 1:16, boric acid, or physiologic saline solution may cool and soothe and thus prevent itching. Lotions such as calamine or calamine with phenol (phenolated calamine, U.S.P.) and cornstarch or oatmeal baths may also be employed to relieve itching.

Local anesthetics such as dibucaine and benzocaine may decrease pruritus, but their use is not recommended because of their high sensitizing and irritating effects. The application of hydrocortisone in a lotion or ointment in a strength of 0.5% to 1% has proved to be one of the best methods of relieving pruritus and decreasing inflammation. It has the additional advantage of possessing a low sensitizing index.

It may be necessary to administer sedatives that have a systemic effect. Some physicians prefer not to use barbiturates because they decrease cortical control of the scratch reflex. Tranquilizers such as meprobamate are usually effective and safe when given in small doses. Trimeprazine, one of the phenothiazine derivatives, is said to be effective for the relief of itching. Trimeprazine tartrate is administered orally. The usual dose for adults is 2.5 mg. four times a day.

In addition to the aforementioned measures to relieve itching, preparations of ergotamine are used to relieve the generalized itching associated with jaundice, cirrhosis of the liver, Hodgkin's disease, and so on. Ergotamine tartrate, U.S.P., is one of the preparations, and there are others, one of which is dihydroergotamine. This preparation is said to relieve itching in a way similar to ergotamine tartrate without producing the common undesirable side effects of that preparation (nausea, vomiting, and cardiovascular reactions).

Other preparations used to relieve itching related to allergic reactions are the antihistaminic drugs (see Index). Calamine and Benadryl, marketed under the name of Caladryl, are examples of combined drugs given to relieve itching.

PROTECTIVES

Protectives are soothing, cooling preparations that form a film on the skin. Protectives, to be useful, must not macerate the skin, must prevent drying of the tissues, and must keep out light, air, and dust. Nonabsorbable powders are usually listed as protectives, but they are not particularly useful because they stick to wet surfaces and have to be scraped off and do not stick to dry surfaces at all.

Collodion, U.S.P. Collodion is a 5% solution of pyroxylin, or guncotton, in a mixture of ether and alcohol. When collodion is applied to the skin, the ether and alcohol evaporate, leaving a transparent film that adheres to the skin and protects it.

Flexible collodion, U.S.P., B.P. This is a mixture of collodion with 2% camphor and 3% castor oil. The addition of the latter makes the resulting film elastic and more tenacious. Styptic collodion contains 20% of tannic acid and is, therefore, astringent as well as protective.

Adhesive tape. Adhesive tape is a tenacious preparation that is solid at ordinary temperature but pliable and adhesive at the temperature of the body. It consists of rubber, lead plaster, and petrolatum spread on linen or muslin. Besides its use as a general protective agent, adhesive tape is widely used to reinforce weak muscles, limit effusions, and keep dressings in place. It can cause sensitivity reactions when applied directly to the skin.

Nonabsorbable powders. These include zinc stearate, zinc oxide, certain bismuth preparations, talcum powder, and aluminum silicate. The disadvantages associated with their use have been mentioned previously.

Although it is safe to say that no substances known at present can stimulate healing at a more rapid rate than is normal under optimal conditions, preparations that act as bland protectives may help by preventing crusting and trauma. In some instances they may reduce offensive odors.

Water-soluble chlorophyll derivatives (Chloresium). A mixture of water-soluble derivatives of chlorophyll is employed topically to produce a bland, soothing effect, to deodorize, to promote tissue repair, and to relieve itching in ulcers, burns, or wounds. It is applied in solution or as an ointment. These derivatives of chlorophyll may aid in producing a clean, granulating wound base suitable for the normal repair of tissues, but they do not take the place of antiinfective agents for the treatment of infections.

Solutions containing 0.2% water-soluble chlorophyll derivatives are applied one or more times daily. A 0.5% ointment may be spread over affected areas and covered with a fine mesh gauze or dressing.

CLEANSERS

BATHS

Baths may be employed to cleanse the skin, to medicate it, or to reduce temperature. The usual method of cleansing the skin is by the use of soap and water, but this may not be tolerated in skin diseases. In some cases even water is not tolerated and inert oils must be substituted. Persons with dry skin should bathe less frequently than those with oily skin. It is possible to keep the skin clean without a daily bath. Nurses are sometimes accused of overbathing hospital patients, causing the patient's skin to become dry and itchy. An oily lotion is preferable to alcohol for the dry skin.

To render baths soothing in irritative conditions, bran, starch, or gelatin may be added in the proportion of about 1 to 2 ounces to the gallon. Oils such as Alpha-Keri, Lubath, and oilated oatmeal in a proportion of 1 ounce to the tub of water decrease the drying effect of water and thus help to relieve the itching of a sensitive, xerotic skin.

SOAPS

Ordinary soap is the sodium salt of palmitic, oleic, or stearic acids or mixtures of these. Soaps are prepared by saponifying fats or oils with the alkalies. The fats or oils used vary considerably. The oil used for castile soap is supposed to be olive oil. Some soaps are made with coconut oil to which the skin of some persons is sensitive. Soaps contain glycerin unless it has been removed from the preparation. The consistency of the soap depends upon the predominating acid and alkali used.

Although all soaps are alkaline, the presence of an excess of free alkali or acid will constitute a potential source of skin irritation. The best soaps are only slightly alkaline, and they are likely to be found among the inexpensive soaps rather than in the highly scented, highly colored, and expensive varieties.

Medicated soaps contain antiseptics and other added substances, such as cresol, thymol, and sulfur, but soaps per se are antiseptic only insofar as they favor the mechanical cleansing of the skin.

The belief that soap and water are bad for the complexion is erroneous for the most part. A clean skin helps to promote a healthy skin. The soap used in maintaining a clean skin should be mild and contain a minimum of irritating materials.

Soaps are irritating to mucous membranes, and they are used in enemas mainly because of this action. They are also used in the manufacture of pills, liniments, and tooth powders. One of the mildest soaps is shaving soap.

SOME CUTANEOUS DISORDERS

BURNS

It is said that approximately 6000 or more people die each year of burns in the United States alone. The chief cause of death is shock, a fact of considerable significance in any effective plan of treatment.

Consideration of what takes place in the damaged tissues clarifies many points of treatment. At first there is an altered capillary permeability in the local injured area. That is, the permeability is increased and a loss of plasma and weeping of the surface tissues result. If the burn is at all extensive, considerable amounts of plasma fluid may be lost in a relatively short time. This depletes the blood volume and causes a decreased cardiac output and diminished blood flow. Unless the situation is rapidly brought under control, irreparable damage may result from the rapidly developing tissue anoxia. Lack of sufficient oxygen and the accumulation of waste products from inadequate oxidation result in loss of tone in the minute blood vessels, and the increased capillary permeability then extends to tissues remote from those suffering the initial injury. Thus, a generalized edema often develops and the vicious cycle once established tends to be self-perpetuating. One of the aims in the treatment of burns is, therefore, to stop the loss of plasma insofar as it is possible and replenish that which is lost as quickly as possible.

Partial- or full-thickness burns must be thought of as open wounds with the accompanying danger of infection. The infection must be prevented or treated. The treatment, however, must be such that it will not bring any further destruction of tissue or of the small islands of remaining epithelium from which growth and regeneration can take place.

First aid treatment of burns. An important first aid treatment for minor and major burns, regardless of cause (chemical, electric, thermal), is to immediately cool the wound to remove irritants, prevent afterglow, and constrict blood vessels; this reduces the permeability of the blood vessels and checks edema formation. Cold tap water can be used to thoroughly flush the wound and to cool hot clothing. The more quickly the wound is cooled, the less tissue damage there is likely to be, and the more rapid will be the recovery. No greasy ointments, lard, butter, or dressings should be applied, since these agents will inhibit loss of heat from the burn, which will increase both discomfort and tissue damage. The burn may be left exposed to the air or cold wet compresses may be applied until the patient can be transported to a place where he can receive medical attention.

Prevention and treatment of infection. Penicillin and streptomycin are frequently used for the early treatment of burned patients other than those with a minor partial-thickness burn and an intact skin. These agents are given parenterally during the first few days and are then discontinued until debridement has been performed or until there is evidence of infection. Some physicians feel that in the treatment of burns that are not grossly contaminated it may be better to wait until there is evidence of infection, obtain a culture, and follow with the antibiotic of choice.

A booster dose of tetanus toxoid is given to the patient who has been previously immunized, and active immunization is started for those not previously immunized.

Mafenide acetate, U.S.P. (Sulfamylon). One of the most important therapeutic agents developed to combat burn infection has been the discovery of mafenide acetate, which is also known as Linberg's butter. Mafenide is a water-soluble ointment that is applied topically to the burn wound with sterile gloves following wound cleansing and debridement. The exposure method of therapy is preferred, although occasionally dressings may be applied; however, this may result in tissue maceration.

The ointment forms a protective coating over the burn. It rapidly diffuses through partial- and full-thickness burns and has proved to be one of the most effective means for preventing and retarding bacterial invasion in burn wounds. It has decreased deaths resulting from septicemia and decreased extension of the wound from infection. It has decreased the number of burn cases requiring plastic surgery or skin grafting. However, eschar separation is delayed.

Mafenide acetate is relatively nontoxic. It is rapidly broken down in the body and eliminated via the urinary tract. Since this drug is a strong carbonic anhydrase inhibitor, acidosis may occur. The patient should be carefully observed for any signs of respiratory embarrassment. If rapid or labored respirations occur, the ointment should be washed off the wound. Therapy can be interrupted for 2 to 3 days without impairing the bacterial control of the wound.

Mafenide may cause some discomfort when first applied—a burning sensation may occur that lasts from a few minutes to as long as an hour.

This is a highly stable drug. It remains active for several years and does not need to be refrigerated except in tropical countries.

Silver nitrate, U.S.P. An aqueous solution of silver nitrate, 0.5%, has been used extensively in some burn centers during the past few years. As a 0.5% solution it is a relatively safe antiseptic agent. Dressings soaked in silver nitrate, 0.5%, are applied to the burn; the dressings must be kept moist and must not be allowed to dry in order to prevent precipitation of silver salts into the wound, which would cause irritation. Concentrations of silver nitrate above 1% produce tissue necrosis; concentrations below 0.5% are not antiseptic. Silver nitrate stains anything with which it comes in contact. The brown or black tissue discoloration is usually not permanent. Silver nitrate solution, 0.5%, is a hypotonic solution, and when it is used on extensive burns or for extensive periods of time it may cause electrolyte imbalance. Blood electrolytes should be frequently determined and patients observed for symptoms of sodium or potassium depletion (change in behavior, confusion, and so on).

Silicone fluid (dimethyl polysiloxane). Silicone fluid has been used to treat hand burns. The hands are placed in plastic bags containing silicone fluid. This is a stable agent; it is inert, has a low specific gravity, and is not harmful to normal or burned skin. The bouyancy of the silicone fluid is a result of its low specific gravity. This permits the patient to move his fingers freely without great discomfort.

SUNBURN

Sunburn is an acute erythema caused by too long an exposure to the rays of the sun. In some cases, especially if a large area is involved, it may be serious, and the skin surface should be treated as in any serious burn. Exposure to the sun should be done gradually, a few minutes each day, when a general tan is desired. As would be true for any minor partial-thickness burn, when the epithelium is intact and remains so, ordinary protective demulcents or emollients are sufficient to allay irritation.

QUESTIONS

For study and review

1 What are some of the nursing problems unique to the care of patients with disorders of the skin?
2 What are some of the points for or against giving a hospital patient a daily, complete bath with soap and water?
3 What information or help would you give a patient who complains of a dry, itchy skin?
4 What constitutes a good soap? What can and cannot be expected from a soap?
5 Why is an extensive burn of the skin likely to be dangerous? What are some of the main points in treatment of burns? How are patients with burns treated in your hospital?
6 Discuss the therapeutic effectiveness and precautions to take when an extensively burned patient is treated with mafenide acetate (Sulfamylon) and with silver nitrate solution.
7 Define each of the following and give an example of each:
   a. emollients
   b. keratolytics
   c. antipruritics
8 What preparations are used in your hospital for prevention or treatment of decubitus ulcers?
9 A 1:5000 solution of potassium permanganate has been ordered for treatment of a patient with epidermophytosis. To entirely cover the feet with the solution, 10,000 ml. are required; on hand are gr. 7$\frac{1}{2}$ tablets (0.5 Gm.). How many tablets will be required to make a 1:5000 solution?

REFERENCES

A.M.A. drug evaluations, ed. 2, Acton, Mass., 1973, Publishing Sciences Group, Inc.

Aviado, D. M.: Krantz and Carr's pharmacologic principles of medical practice, ed. 8, Baltimore, 1972, The Williams & Wilkins Co.

Bromberg, B. E.: Burn wound management with biologic dressings, N.Y. State J. Med. **70:**1645, 1970.

Griffenhagen, G. B., and Hawkins, L. L., editors: Handbook of non-prescription drugs, Washington D.C., 1973, American Pharmaceutical Association.

Johns, L. A., and others: Nursing care of the thermally injured patient. In Anderson, E. H., and others, editors: Current concepts of clinical nursing, vol. IV, St. Louis, 1973, The C. V. Mosby Co.

White, M. G., and Asch, M. J.: Acid-base effects of topical mafenide acetate in the burned patient, New Eng. J. Med. **284:**1281, 1971.

CHAPTER 31

Drugs acting on gastrointestinal organs

Drugs affecting the digestive tract exert their action mainly on muscular and glandular tissues. The action may be directly on the smooth muscle and gland cells or indirectly on the autonomic nervous system. Both divisions of the autonomic system innervate the tissues of the digestive tract and discharge nerve impulses into these structures almost continuously. Under normal conditions they maintain a delicate balance of control of functions.

Drugs may bring about increased or decreased function, tone, emptying time, or peristaltic action of the stomach or bowel. In addition, drugs may be used to relieve enzyme deficiency, to counteract excess acidity or gas formation, to produce or prevent vomiting, or as diagnostic aids.

Drugs that affect the mouth

On the whole, drugs have little effect upon the mouth. Good oral hygiene that includes adequate measures for mechanically cleansing the mouth and teeth has more influence than most medicines.

FLAVORING AGENTS

Oral medications that have an unpleasant taste are usually encapsulated, but occasionally it is necessary to give a drug in liquid or powder form. Licorice syrup is particularly effective to disguise the taste of a saline substance because of its colloidal properties and because the taste lingers in the mouth. Other popular syrup flavors are raspberry and cherry.

Unpleasant-tasting drugs that are disguised in a suitable flavoring agent are further improved (psychologically, at least) by the addition of a coloring agent. A chocolate-colored medicine is often thought to have the taste of chocolate even when the flavoring agent added is something entirely different. Since the oral route of drug administration is most acceptable, consultation with the pharmacist is useful when taste problems arise.

MOUTHWASHES AND GARGLES

The efficacy of a mouthwash or gargle depends largely on the length of time it is allowed to remain in contact with the tissues of the mouth and throat. Ordinarily, these preparations cannot be used in sufficient concentration or over a period of time sufficient to ensure germicidal effects.

A 1% solution of sodium bicarbonate ($\frac{1}{2}$ teaspoonful in a glass of water) is useful to remove mucus from the mouth and throat. A 0.9% sodium chloride solution is probably as good a gargle as most mixtures used.

Chloraseptic mouthwash and *Cepacol mouthwash* are used in some institutions. Chloraseptic mouthwash provides surface anesthesia when this is indicated for oropharyngeal discomfort, as well as maintaining oral hygiene. It is to be diluted with equal parts water or sprayed full strength.

Cepacol is also available commercially. It is to be used full strength and is also produced in lozenge form.

Sodium perborate is a white, odorless, salty-tasting powder that contains not less than 9% available oxygen. It is used in 2% solution as a mouthwash and local disinfectant. Its action results from the liberation of oxygen. It may be obtained in flavored preparations that disguise the salty taste. It is a popular ingredient of tooth powder and is said to be particularly effective against Vincent's infection and pyorrhea. *Potas-*

sium permanganate (0.1%), *potassium chlorate* (1%), or *hydrogen peroxide* (25%) may also be used; they are oxidizing agents.

Other substances used in the treatment of stomatitis include boric acid, formalin, gentian violet, and zinc chloride.

Many hospital pharmacies prepare the mouthwash used in that particular institution. Nurses should inquire regarding the content of the preparation and should know whether or not the mouthwash should be diluted prior to use.

DENTIFRICES

The ordinary dentifrice contains one or more mild abrasives, a foaming agent, and flavoring materials made into a powder or paste to be used as an aid to the toothbrush in the mechanical cleansing of accessible parts of the teeth.

The following ingredients, alone or mixed, are found in a number of dentifrices:

Glycerin	Pumice (flour)
Alcohol	Stannous fluoride
Sweetening agents	Soap
Propylene glycol	Sodium borate
Precipitated calcium carbonate	Milk of magnesia

The essential requirement of a tooth powder or cleaner is that it must not injure the teeth or surrounding tissues. In the absence of a tooth paste the nurse may feel justified in having the patient use only a toothbrush and proper toothpick technique since thorough mechanical cleansing of bacterial plaques and food debris is the primary objective.

Therapeutic dentifrices. Accepted Dental Therapeutics (ADT) claims that the incidence of dental caries is low in communities with fluorine-bearing water. Approximately one part of fluoride to a million parts of water will help to control dental caries. In those communities without fluorinated water, dentists can prescribe individualized doses of sodium fluoride to children from infancy to adolescence.

The Council on Dental Therapeutics of the American Dental Association has accepted the toothpastes Crest and Colgate MFP as being effective in reducing the incidence of dental caries. Crest contains 0.4% stannous fluoride; Colgate MFP contains 0.76% sodium monofluorophosphate.

Drugs that affect the stomach

Conditions of the stomach requiring drug therapy include hyperchlorhydria, hypochlorhydria, peptic ulcer, nausea and emesis, and hypermotility. Drugs are also used for diagnostic test purposes. Some of the drugs utilized for these conditions are not unique in their treatment of gastric dysfunction but are members of other major groups of drugs, such as anticholinergic preparations and sedatives.

ANTACIDS

Antacids are chemical substances utilized in treatment of hyperchlorhydria and peptic ulcer. Although peptic ulcer is thought to be the result of several pathogenic processes, the control of hyperacidity complements other therapeutic measures.

Gastric hyperacidity causes symptoms of fullness after eating, gastric distension, eructation (belching), and what the laity call "heartburn." Antacids relieve these symptoms.

Peptic ulcer is a localized destruction in the gastrointestinal mucosa, usually in the stomach or duodenum. If the ulceration continues to be bathed in gastric juice, continued erosion may occur and lead to perforation. Neutralizing or buffering the gastric acid helps to promote healing and relieve pain and discomfort.

The major digestive substances secreted by the stomach are hydrochloric acid and pepsin. Hydrochloric acid activates the secretion of pepsin. Pepsin, in turn, begins protein digestion. Oversecretion of hydrochloric acid, however, may result in erosion, ulceration, and possible perforation of the gastric walls. Antacids are used to: (1) lower the acidity of gastric secretions by direct neutralization (example, sodium bicar-

bonate, magnesium oxide), (2) buffer the hydrochloric acid (normally pH 1 or 2) to a lower hydrogen ion concentration (sodium citrate, magnesium trisilicate), or (3) by combined absorption of the hydrogen ions of hydrochloric acid, to buffer and partially neutralize the acid (example, hydrated aluminum oxide, anion exchange resins).

Buffering hydrochloric acid to a pH of 3 or 4 is most desirable, since the proteolytic action of pepsin is then reduced and the gastric juice loses its corrosive effect. As pH approaches 7 or 8, as it does with some antacids, pepsin becomes completely inactive, the stomach empties rapidly, and a rebound of gastric secretion occurs. It is, therefore, thought to be preferable to lower gastric acidity rather than to raise pH to a state of neutral or above.

Antacids constitute one of the largest groups of drugs used in medicine and by the laity and are frequently abused drugs. Excess alkalinity can cause an uncompensated alkalosis. Nurses frequently hear requests from patients for "just a little something to settle my stomach" and must constantly be aware of their responsibility to explore the basis of that request and to instruct the patient when indicated.

When antacids are appropriately prescribed, they may be given every 1 or 2 hours throughout the 24 hours because of the continuous and often rapid gastric emptying. Many patients will prove receptive to instruction regarding this regimen and will be pleased to assume some responsibility in taking the drugs.

The following are the properties of an ideal antacid:

1 Efficiency, so that small amounts of the drug will control a relatively large amount of gastric acid
2 Absence of interference with electrolyte balance when administered in therapeutic amounts
3 Exertion of prolonged effect without secondary increase of gastric secretion
4 Palatability
5 Inexpensiveness, since administration may be prolonged
6 Will not cause constipation or diarrhea
7 Absence of release of carbon dioxide after reaction with hydrochloric acid; this may increase distention and discomfort and may lead to perforation
8 Noninterference with absorption of other drugs

Antacids may be classified as systemic or nonsystemic. Systemic antacids are soluble in gastric and intestinal secretions and are readily absorbed. Therefore they are capable of altering electrolyte balance and of producing systemic alkalosis. Alkalosis is characterized by headache, abdominal pain, nausea, and vomiting. The kidney must then bear the burden of electrolyte readjustment, and failure of the renal mechanisms would result in a more enduring metabolic alkalosis. Renal insufficiency and calcinosis have been described in patients on prolonged systemic antacid administration. Another disadvantage of systemic antacids is acid rebound, caused by increased hydrochloric acid secretion as a result of neutralization.

Nonsystemic antacids form relatively insoluble compounds that are not readily absorbed. Because they have no direct effect on the acid-base balance of the blood, they are unlikely to produce alkalosis.

SYSTEMIC ANTACIDS

Systemic antacids are found in many widely advertised proprietary preparations but are, because of aforementioned reasons, prescribed by the physician much less often than they were at one time. Their use is particularly avoided for patients who have pyloric obstruction or renal disease. However, patients sometimes experience greater relief from systemic antacids, and physicians may prescribe them in conjunction with one or more of the nonsystemic preparations. Systemic antacids are sometimes freely available on nursing units, and it is frequently a temptation to the nurse to give a patient the antacid he requests without first obtaining a physician's order. The implications of such action should be apparent.

Sodium bicarbonate, U.S.P., B.P. (baking soda); sodium citrate, U.S.P., B.P.

Sodium bicarbonate is the most common systemic antacid used medically and by the laity. Administered as a tablet or a powder, it is readily soluble and easily absorbed. It produces high pH levels (8.5) that inactivate pepsin and predispose to overneutralization and rebound secretion. Frequent use can cause systemic alkalosis. Furthermore, its reaction with hydrochloric acid liberates carbon dioxide, which may produce gastric distention, an undesirable phenomenon for patients with ulcers. It does not have a prolonged buffering effect.

$$NaHCO_3 + HCl \rightarrow NaCl + H_2CO_3 \ (H_2O \text{ and } CO_2)$$

Patients with hypertension, cardiac, or renal disease should be instructed not to use antacids containing sodium, for they can cause a substantial increase in body sodium and adverse effects on the vascular and renal systems.

Preparation, dosage, and administration. Sodium bicarbonate is a white crystalline powder that may be compressed into tablets. The usual dose is 1 to 2 Gm. (gr. 15 to 30) taken up to four times daily. It may be given with other therapeutic drugs to reduce their gastrointestinal irritability.

Sodium citrate is an absorbable systemic antacid similar to sodium bicarbonate. It differs from the latter in action in that it does not release carbon dioxide. It is seldom prescribed as an antacid in the treatment of peptic ulcer, but it is commonly found in proprietary preparations recommended to relieve gastric distress. Sodium citrate is subject to oxidation, which results in the formation of sodium bicarbonate and is therefore capable of causing alkalosis when given in large amounts.

NONSYSTEMIC ANTACIDS
Aluminum hydroxide gel, U.S.P., B.P. (Amphojel, Creamolin, Al-U-Creme, Alkagel)

Aluminum hydroxide gel is one of the more popular of the nonsystemic antacids. It is an insoluble drug that reacts with gastric acid to form aluminum chloride that, in turn, reacts with intestinal secretion to form insoluble salts.

$$Al(OH)_3 + 3 \ HCl \rightarrow AlCl_3 + 3 \ H_2O$$

The formation of aluminum chloride is responsible for both the astringent and constipating effects of the drug. The use of a mixture of aluminum hydroxide with either magnesium trisilicate or magnesium hydroxide helps to prevent constipation.

The chief action is believed to be chemical neutralization of hydrochloric acid; aluminum hydroxide has been found to buffer the gastric secretion to a pH of about 4. It is also thought to possess some adsorptive properties, but evidence regarding this is inconclusive. Onset of action is slow but it has a prolonged buffering effect.

Aluminum hydroxide interferes with absorption of phosphates from the intestine and, in the presence of a low phosphorus diet, may cause a deficiency. Aluminum hydroxide can interfere with absorption of other drugs and should not be given simultaneously with anticholinergics or barbiturates. Since aluminum hydroxide preparations contain sodium they should not be given to patients on a low sodium diet.

Preparation, dosage, and administration. Aluminum hydroxide gel is available in the form of a liquid suspension and as tablets of 300 or 600 mg. The tablets should be chewed slowly. The patient may prefer the tablet form, but the liquid preparation affords a better antacid effect. Flavoring agents are available. Aluminum hydroxide gel is given orally in doses of 4 to 8 ml. every 2 to 4 hours, although as much as 15 to 30 ml. may be given hourly. Some physicians like to have their patients take the aluminum hydroxide gel diluted in a small amount of water or milk or to drink a small amount of liquid after swallowing the antacid. Unless some fluid is taken with a small amount of the antacid it may only coat the esophagus and little or none of it may reach the stomach. It may also be administered by continuous drip through a stomach tube, in which case it is diluted and given 1 part to 2 or 3 parts of water at the rate of 15 to 20 drops per minute (1500 ml. in 24 hours).

Aluminum phosphate gel, B.P. (Phosphaljel)

The properties of this preparation are similar to those of aluminum hydroxide gel, but it does not interfere with absorption of phosphate. Larger doses of this preparation are necessary because its acid-combining power is less than half that of aluminum hydroxide gel of the same concentration.

Uses. Aluminum phosphate gel is a preparation of choice for patients with an ulcer who are unable to be maintained on a high phosphate diet or who suffer an accompanying diarrhea.

Preparation, dosage, and administration. Aluminum phosphate gel is available as a 4% suspension for oral administration. During the active phase of the ulcer 15 to 45 ml. may be given alone or with milk every 2 hours. Later, the dose may be reduced and given after each meal, at bedtime, and between meals if necessary.

Other compounds. There are a number of other aluminum compounds used as antacids, such as dihydroxyaluminum aminoacetate, N.F. (Alglyn is one of many names under which it is sold) and basic aluminum carbonate (Basaljel). They are not believed to have any marked advantage over aluminum hydroxide. "Rolaids" contains dihydroxyaluminum sodium carbonate.

Magnesium trisilicate, U.S.P., B.P.

Magnesium trisilicate is a compound of silicon dioxide and magnesium oxide with water.

$$MgO \cdot 3\ SiO_2 \cdot n\ H_2O$$

It occurs as a white, odorless, tasteless powder, insoluble in water but partially soluble in acids. It is said to compare favorably with other nonsystemic antacids and acts effectively as an adsorbent as well as providing chemical neutralization. It has a slow onset of action but prolonged buffering effect. In the stomach it has a gelatinous consistency, which explains its ability to coat and protect the crater of the ulcer. In therapeutic amounts it apparently does not affect the motility of the gastrointestinal tract.

$$2\ MgO \cdot 3\ SiO_2 \cdot n\ H_2O + 4\ HCl \rightarrow$$
$$2\ MgCl_2 + 3\ SiO_2 + (n + 2)\ H_2O$$

In the intestine the magnesium chloride reacts with the bicarbonate in the intestinal secretions to form magnesium carbonate (which is excreted) and sodium chloride (which is subject to absorption). This follows a pattern similar to that of the neutralization of the bicarbonate by the hydrochloric acid of the stomach under normal circumstances and helps to explain why electrolyte balance is not disturbed. The magnesium chloride formed after neutralization of the hydrochloride acid is also responsible for a cathartic action in the bowel. Large doses may produce diarrhea, although therapeutic doses do not seem to disturb normal motility of the gastrointestinal tract.

Uses. Magnesium trisilicate is an effective antacid for the relief of gastric hyperacidity and for pain associated with peptic ulcer. A judicious combination of magnesium trisilicate and aluminum hydroxide has resulted in an antacid preparation that is efficient, safe when given in large amounts over prolonged periods, and relatively free from constipating effects.

Preparation, dosage, and administration. Magnesium trisilicate is available in 500-mg. tablets and in powder form. The usual dose is 1 Gm. four times a day, but as much as 2 to 4 Gm. may be given hourly during the treatment of the acute phase of an ulcer. The tablets should be chewed before they are swallowed.

A combination of magnesium trisilicate and aluminum hydroxide gel is available under the trade name Gelusil (tablet and liquid form). The dosage of this preparation varies with the severity of the symptoms to be controlled; 4 to 8 ml. is an average dose, although more may be prescribed.

Mucin, aluminum hydroxide, and magnesium trisilicate (Mucotin) is an antacid mixture that provides an additional protective coating to the ulcer and the gastric mucosa because of the mucin content. The preparation is available in tablets that should be well chewed before they are swallowed. The dose recommended is two tablets every 2 hours.

Precipitated calcium carbonate, U.S.P., B.P.

Calcium carbonate (chalk) is a fine white powder that is practically insoluble in water but is somewhat soluble in water containing carbon dioxide. It is decomposed by acids, forming a salt of calcium and carbonic acid that in turn yields water and carbon dioxide.

$$CaCO_3 + 2\ HCl \rightarrow CaCl_2 + H_2CO_3\ (CO_2 + H_2O)$$

The calcium chloride will react with the sodium bicarbonate in the intestinal secretions to form calcium carbonate and sodium chloride. The sodium chloride is absorbable, but the calcium carbonate is excreted.

Uses. Calcium carbonate is used chiefly as an antacid and as a protective for patients with hy-

peracidity, gastritis, and peptic ulcer. Its effects are rapid and prolonged with a high neutralizing capacity.

Preparation, dosage, and administration. Precipitated calcium carbonate is administered orally in doses of 1 to 2 Gm. hourly when acute symptoms are to be controlled. Thereafter, the dosage may be lowered. The official dose is 1 Gm. four or more times a day.

Side effects. Calcium carbonate has a tendency to cause constipation, a disadvantage that may be avoided by alternating the administration of calcium carbonate with the use of magnesium oxide. The release of carbon dioxide may be dangerous if an ulcer is close to perforation. Large doses and prolonged administration may cause an accumulation of chalky formations in the bowel. Difference of opinion has been expressed concerning whether calcium carbonate causes a gastric rebound of acid secretion.

Some cases of hypercalcemia have occurred during chronic usage, especially in conjunction with milk and cream therapy. When large quantities are prescribed, physicians frequently measure serum calcium periodically. The nurse should be aware of symptoms of hypercalcemia, such as depression and bradycardia.

Magnesium oxide, U.S.P., B.P. (light magnesia); magnesium oxide, U.S.P. (heavy magnesium)

Magnesium oxide is a widely used nonsystemic antacid. It is a bulky white powder that is relatively insoluble in water. It reacts with hydrochloric acid to form magnesium chloride and water.

$$MgO + 2\ HCl \rightarrow MgCl_2 + H_2O$$

In the intestine magnesium chloride acts as a saline cathartic and eventually reacts with sodium to form magnesium carbonate, which is excreted, and sodium chloride, which may be absorbed. The neutralizing capacity of magnesium oxide is outstanding among the various antacids. It does not act rapidly, but its effect is prolonged since any excess remains in the stomach and serves to neutralize subsequently secreted acid. Its chief disadvantage is that it may cause diarrhea. Therefore, a frequent practice has been utilization of the laxative effect of magnesium oxide to counteract the constipating effect of certain other antacids.

Magnesium oxide is unlikely to cause alkalosis since little is absorbed, but the little that is absorbed is rapidly excreted by the kidneys and alkaline urine may result.

Preparation, dosage, and administration. The two compounds of magnesium oxide are identical in chemical composition but differ in physical properties. The former is lighter and five times more bulky than the latter. The light magnesia is more difficult to administer but affords a greater surface for reaction with the gastric content because of its greater capacity for dispersion. Recommended antacid dose is 250 mg. (250 to 500 mg., B.P.).

Magnesium carbonate, N.F., B.P.

This preparation has antacid properties almost identical with those of magnesium oxide, except that it liberates carbon dioxide upon the neutralization of hydrochloric acid. It is a bulky white powder. The official dose as an antacid is 0.5 Gm. (500 mg.) to 2 Gm. (250 to 500 mg., B.P.).

Milk of magnesia, U.S.P.; magnesium hydroxide mixture, N.F., B.P.

These preparations exhibit the characteristic antacid effect of the basic salts of magnesium. The usual antacid dose is 5 to 15 ml. In larger doses, its effect is predominantly cathartic. Maalox is a trade name for a mixture of aluminum hydroxide gel and magnesium hydroxide. It is comparable to Gelusil (aluminum hydroxide and magnesium trisilicate). The usual dosage of Maalox is 8 ml. It should be given with a little water, or a small quantity of water or milk should be swallowed after the dose.

Magaldrate, U.S.P. (Riopan)

Magaldrate is a chemical combination of aluminum and magnesium hydroxide. It is a buffer antacid that is usually not absorbed and thus unlikely to disturb the acid-base balance. In patients with impaired renal function limited absorption may cause hypermagnesemia. The chief advantage of magaldrate is its low sodium content. It is available in suspension and tablet form. Dosage for adults is 400 to 800 mg. four or more times daily. Hourly administration may be necessary to control severe symptoms.

NURSING MEASURES CONCERNING ANTACIDS

1 Patients who self-medicate with antacids for recurring gastrointestinal symptoms should be advised to seek medical care since they are treating symptoms and not the cause of the symptoms. They may be treating themselves in vain. Nurses should thoroughly question patients who routinely self-medicate with antacids.

2 Helping a patient identify the source of his gastric discomfort such as overeating, eating a wide variety of foods at one time, tension, anxiety, or other emotional stress, may enable him to avoid the causes of his discomfort and eliminate the need for antacid therapy.

3 Patients on a low-sodium diet, and patients with hypertensive, cardiac, or renal disease should be instructed to avoid antacids containing sodium, particularly if antacids are frequently used.

4 Patients taking antacid tablets that should be chewed should be instructed to thoroughly chew or pulverize the tablet. These tablets are usually hydrophobic and do not mix readily with water. The wettability of an antacid is related to its ability to provide prompt and complete action. Thus liquids are better than tablets. Chewing the tablets slowly and thoroughly helps to obtain small particle size like that present in liquid antacids, and helps to more thoroughly wet those particles for more prompt action.

5 Antacid suspensions should be well shaken before being taken.

6 Patients on medical antacid therapy should be encouraged to strictly adhere to their antacid schedule and should be given responsibility for taking their own antacids while still hospitalized.

7 Patients should be cautioned about side effects and instructed to consult their physician if these occur.

8 Evaluation of antacid therapy is important. The patient's subjective response to antacid therapy and the nurse's objective observations (e.g., frequency with which the patient takes his antacid) can help to determine effectiveness of antacid therapy.

9 The age of an antacid is important. For example, aluminum hydroxide gel becomes less reactive as it ages. Also, there is wide variation in aluminum hydroxide batches to neutralize acid, one batch being more or less effective than another. A patient not responding well to aluminum hydroxide therapy

may need a new or different supply of aluminum hydroxide.

DIGESTANTS

Digestants are drugs that promote the process of digestion in the gastrointestinal tract and constitute a type of replacement therapy in deficiency states. The most common drugs employed for this purpose are hydrochloric acid, bile salts, and gastric and pancreatic enzymes.

Hydrochloric acid

Hypochlorhydria is a term that denotes decreased secretion of hydrochloric acid in the stomach. *Achlorhydria* means an absence of hydrochloric acid, and when both acid and enzymes are absent in the gastric secretion, the condition is known as *achylia gastrica*. A deficiency of acid is said to occur in approximately 10% to 15% of the population. It is more commonly found in elderly persons. Achlorhydria is associated with gastric carcinoma, pernicious anemia, some types of gastritis, and a number of other conditions, although it is occasionally found in apparently normal individuals. Symptoms of achlorhydria are poorly defined but may consist of vague epigastric distress after meals, eructation, abdominal distention, coated tongue, nausea, and vomiting.

The hydrochloric acid of the stomach has several important functions. It is essential for the conversion of pepsinogen to active pepsin, which is important for the digestion of protein; it has a germicidal effect on numerous bacteria; it stimulates secretion of secretin in the duodenum; it neutralizes bicarbonate of the intestinal secretions and thus helps to maintain electrolyte balance; and it activates pancreatic and hepatic secretions.

Uses. This is administered to relieve symptoms that result from gastric achlorhydria.

Preparation, dosage, and administration. The following are available preparations of hydrochloric acid.

Diluted hydrochloric acid, U.S.P.; *dilute hydrochloric acid*, B.P. This preparation contains 10% hydrochloric acid, which should be further diluted in at least one-half glass of water and should be administered through a tube to avoid injury to the enamel of the teeth. The usual dose is 5 ml., although some physicians recommend doses up to 10 ml. The acid may be sipped with the meal or taken just after the meal. Even though the acid is diluted well, the taste is very sour. Food should be eaten after the last swallow of the acid or the mouth rinsed with an alkaline mouthwash.

Glutamic acid hydrochloride (Acidulin). This preparation is a combination of glutamic acid and hydrochloric acid and is available in capsules, which avoids exposure of dental enamel to the acid. The hydrochloric acid is released when the preparation comes in contact with water. The dose is 0.3 Gm., which is equivalent to 0.6 ml. of dilute hydrochloric acid. One gram doses may also be ordered. The preparation is usually administered before meals.

GASTRIC AND PANCREATIC ENZYMES
Pepsin

Pepsin is an enzyme secreted by the stomach that initiates the hydrolysis of protein. Proteolytic enzymes in the intestinal and pancreatic secretions are capable of digesting proteins completely, so that gastric pepsin is not an indispensable enzyme. Its absence occurs only as an accompaniment to achlorhydria. The absence of both pepsin and hydrochloric acid is known as gastric achylia and is most frequently observed in patients with pernicious anemia or gastric carcinoma. Pepsin is seldom used at the present time, but when it is given, the dose is 0.5 to 1 Gm. taken after meals. Pepsin contains the proteolytic enzyme obtained from fresh hog's stomach.

Pancreatin, N.F., B.P.

Pancreatin is a powdered substance obtained from the pancreas of the hog or ox. It principally contains pancreatic amylase, trypsin, and pancreatic lipase. Acid chyme entering the duodenum and vagal stimulation regulate pancreatic secretion, so replacement therapy may be necessary for patients who have had vagal fibers surgically severed, who have had surgical procedures that cause food to bypass the duodenum, who have had surgery of the jejunum, or who have pancreatitis. Some doubt has been expressed concerning the usefulness of pancreatin. The drug is available in enteric-coated capsules to avoid destruction in the stomach and is administered in 500-mg. to 1-Gm. doses. Viokase (whole hog pancreas) and Cotazym (which is *pancrelipase,* a standardized preparation of whole hog pancreas containing amylase, trypsin, and lipase) are also utilized for patients with pancreatic deficiencies. In Cotazym the lipase activity is greater than in other pancreatic enzyme preparations.

CHOLERETICS AND HYDROCHOLERETICS
Bile and bile salts

Drugs that stimulate the liver to increase bile production are known as choleretics, the most important of which are bile salts and bile acids. Hydrocholeretics are drugs stimulating the production of bile of a low specific gravity, which is desirable in disorders of the biliary tract unassociated with liver disease.

Bile is secreted by the liver into the bile duct, which drains into the duodenum. It is not an enzyme; it is composed of water, bile salts, bile pigments, cholesterol, lecithin, and inorganic salts. Of these, bile salts are most important in the digestion of fats because of their hydrotropic effect. They lower surface tension of fats and are partially responsible for the emulsification of fats before digestion and absorption in the small intestine. Bile acids stimulate the production of bile salts. Both of these substances are normally absorbed from the intestine, pass through the portal blood to the liver, are reexcreted by the liver, then pass through the bile ducts and again enter the intestine. Bile salts are essential for the absorption of fat-soluble vitamins and cholesterol.

Bile and bile salts are used for patients with various hepatic disorders to aid digestion and absorption and to increase biliary drainage. They are sometimes used for patients with prolonged drainage of the common bile duct.

Outstanding effects of parenterally administered bile salts are manifested in the circulatory and neuromuscular systems, causing hypotension, bradycardia, and skeletal muscular hyperactivity.

Dehydrocholic acid, N.F. (Decholin)

Dehydrocholic acid is a hydrocholeretic; it increases bile volume without increasing total bile acid quantity. In addition to its function in improving lipid absorption, it is frequently used to flush the biliary ducts to remove mucus, debris, and small obstructions and to prevent ascent of infections. It is used postoperatively to enhance T-tube drainage. Its hydrocholeretic effect may help outline bile ducts to determine obstructions and may improve gallbladder visualization on x-rays. It is also used to determine arm-to-tongue circulation time, in which case the drug is administered intravenously and the patient normally experiences a bitter taste within 8 to 16 seconds. Prolonged circulation times are frequently indicative of cardiac decompensation. Although dehydrocholic acid is the least toxic of the hydrocholeretic drugs, caution regarding its use in determining circulation time has been recommended. Dehydrocholic acid is not recommended for patients with complete mechanical obstruction of the biliary tract or in cases of severe hepatitis. The usual dose as a choleretic is 250 to 500 mg. two or three times daily.

Florantyrone (Zanchol)

Florantyrone is a hydrocholeretic of a synthetic nature that is closely related to dehydrocholic acid in action. It is available in 250-mg. tablets and is usually administered in doses of 750 mg. to 1 Gm. daily.

Chenodeoxycholic acid (bile acid)

Chenodeoxycholic acid is a primary bile acid under clinical investigation for the nonsurgical treatment of cholesterol gallstones. Cholesterol gallstones occur when bile contains an excess of cholesterol relative to the bile salts and phospholipid content. Since chenodeoxycholic acid is a common bile acid in humans, it alters this ratio in favor of bile salts and the phospholipid content and presumably prevents the precipitation of cholesterol. In some patients it has dissolved or reduced the size of cholesterol gallstones. Dosage varies from 0.75 to 4.5 Gm. The drug has been administered for 6 to 22 months.

Diarrhea has been reported as an adverse reaction to chenodeoxycholic acid. Some concern has been expressed about its chronic use, since it is dehydroxylated in the intestines to lithocholic acid, a known hepatotoxin in some animal species.

EMETICS

Emetics are agents given to produce vomiting, the use of which has been largely supplanted by gastric lavage. They are occasionally used as a first-aid measure when prompt evacuation of the stomach is essential.

Vomiting is a complex reflex mechanism, and drugs given to induce vomiting may act at one or more locations in the reflex arc. Vomiting can sometimes be brought about simply by tickling the back of the throat with a finger. A number of household substances can also be used to produce emesis. They include mustard water (1 level teaspoonful of dry mustard to a glass of tepid water), mild soapsuds solution, warm salt water, or plain starch in warm water. Copious amounts of warm or tepid water will usually induce vomiting. Other emetics include copper sulfate, zinc sulfate, and ipecac syrup.

Gastric lavage may be indicated at times to empty the stomach of irritating material. A glass of warm solution of sodium bicarbonate may provoke emesis and empty the stomach with much the same result as gastric lavage.

Apomorphine hydrochloride, N.F., B.P.

This drug acts by direct stimulation of the vomiting center in the medulla. The dose is 5 mg. (2 to 8 mg.), and it is administered subcutaneously or intramuscularly. Vomiting is usually produced in a few minutes. Large doses produce central depression, so that the drug should be avoided for patients who are already depressed. Tolerance does not develop to the emetic action of apomorphine. Since the drug is prepared from morphine, conformity with regulations of the Controlled Substances Act is essential.

ANTIEMETICS

Antiemetics are drugs given to produce symptomatic relief of nausea and vomiting. Control of vomiting is important and often difficult. Numerous preparations have been used, but effective treatment usually depends upon the removal of the cause. Vomiting may result from diverse phenomena, such as strong emotion, severe pain, increased intracranial pressure, and labyrinthine disturbances. Other factors include motion sickness, endocrine disturbances, the action of certain drugs, gastrointestinal pathology, reaction to roentgen treatments, and heart disease.

When there is reason to believe that the nausea and vomiting are associated with a mild disturbance of some kind, a cup of plain hot tea will often relieve a nauseated patient. Carbonated drinks are popular remedies when medication is unavailable and seem to be more effective when administered at room temperature. In patients who cannot eructate, however, they will only increase gastric distention and discomfort. Salts of bismuth, magnesium oxide, and calcium carbonate may be employed as antacids and protectives to relieve irritation and vomiting. Vomiting caused by other conditions may be relieved by central nervous system depressants, antihistaminics, and tranquilizers. Chlorpromazine is regarded as an unusually potent antiemetic acting primarily to block the chemoreceptor trigger zone. Dimenhydrinate (Dramamine), meclizine (Bonine), and several other drugs are employed effectively for motion sickness. These are discussed elsewhere (see Index). Antiemetics exert their effects on the vomiting center, the cerebral cortex, the chemoreceptor trigger zone, or the aural vestibular apparatus.

Diphenidol hydrochloride (Vontrol)

Diphenidol is a new drug recommended for the prevention and control of nausea and vomiting, the vertigo of Meniere's disease, labyrinthitis following middle or inner ear surgery, and motion sickness. It is used to control vomiting postoperatively, drug-induced vomiting, and vomiting resulting from radiation therapy. It is not recommended for control of nausea and vomiting of pregnancy since its safety during pregnancy has not been determined. Its use to control vertigo in children has not been investigated.

Diphenidol controls nausea and vomiting by

inhibiting the medullary chemoreceptor trigger zone; it controls vertigo by a specific antivertigo effect on the vestibular apparatus.

Side effects. This drug should be restricted to hospitalized or carefully supervised patients because of untoward effects that may occur, which include hallucinations, disorientation, and confusion. These usually occur within 3 days after initiation of therapy and subside within 3 days after discontinuing the drug. Other side effects include drowsiness, depression, sleep disturbances, and dry mouth. Dizziness, rash, malaise, headache, and mild transient hypotension occur rarely.

Since diphenidol has a weak peripheral anticholinergic effect it should be used cautiously in patients with glaucoma or gastrointestinal or urinary obstructions.

Preparation, dosage, and administration. Recommended oral dose for adults is 25 to 50 mg. four times a day; for children the dose is 5 mg. per kilogram of body weight daily divided into four doses. Intravenous or intramuscular dose for adults is 20 mg. Diphenidol is not recommended for infants under 6 months of age or for those weighing less than 25 pounds. Intravenous administration is not recommended for children of any age.

Diphenidol is available in 25-mg. tablets, 2-ml. ampules containing 20 mg. of diphenidol per milliliter, and as suppositories containing 25 or 50 mg. of the drug.

Trimethobenzamide hydrochloride, N.F. (Tigan)

Trimethobenzamide hydrochloride exhibits an antiemetic action similar to the phenothiazine derivatives but has a weak antihistaminic action. It is believed to depress the chemoreceptor trigger zone in the medulla rather than the vomiting center directly. It has the advantage of long duration of action and little or no sedative effect. It is recommended for the prevention or relief of nausea and vomiting caused by radiation sickness, infection, and operative procedures. It has also been used to relieve nausea and vomiting caused by a number of other conditions. It is not particularly effective for the treatment of motion sickness.

Trimethobenzamide hydrochloride is marketed in 100- and 250-mg. capsules for oral administration, in vials and ampules for intramuscular injection containing 100 mg. per milliliter, and in 200-mg. rectal suppositories. The usual adult oral dose is 100 to 250 mg. The usual adult parenteral dose is 200 mg. After oral or parenteral administration the drug is effective in 20 to 40 minutes, and action persists 3 to 4 hours or more. Dosage for children is 15 mg. per kilogram of body weight divided into three or four doses during a 24-hour period.

Incidence of adverse effects is low. Dizziness, drowsiness, diarrhea, irritation after rectal administration, and pain at the site of injection have been noted. Occasionally, the patient's nausea is intensified.

DIAGNOSTIC AIDS
AGENTS USED TO DETERMINE GASTRIC ACIDITY
Histamine

Histamine is such a potent stimulant of the gastric glands that, when injected subcutaneously or intramuscularly in doses of approximately 0.3 to 0.5 mg., its failure to stimulate secretion of hydrochloric acid is considered proof of achlorhydria. The injection may produce side effects, such as a wheal at the site of injection, headache, vertigo, superficial vasodilation, larger vessel vasoconstriction, and sometimes a drop in blood pressure.

Preparation, dosage, and administration
Histamine phosphate, U.S.P., B.P. This drug is also known as histamine diphosphate or histamine acid phosphate. When given during an augmented histamine test, it is accompanied by simultaneous administration of an antidote (usually epinephrine) so that all effects of histamine, except those on gastric secretions, are antagonized. It is given subcutaneously in doses of 0.04 mg. per kilogram of body weight, and the patient is to have had nothing by mouth since midnight. D.E.S.I. rating is *effective* for testing for gastric secretions.

Betazole hydrochloride, U.S.P. (Histalog).

This preparation, an analogue of histamine, is used more frequently than histamine phosphate because of its lower incidence of side effects. The routine administration of an antihistaminic compound is unnecessary, and augmentation of gastric secretion is equally effective. Betazole hydrochloride is to be used cautiously in patients with allergies. It is administered subcutaneously or intramuscularly in doses of 0.5 mg. per kilogram of body weight. Oral administration is under investigation. Its D.E.S.I. rating is *effective* for clinical testing of gastric secretion.

Azuresin, N.F. (Diagnex Blue)

Azuresin is a preparation utilized to detect achlorhydria without intubation. As such, it has come to replace the older quinine carbacrylic resin for tubeless gastric analysis. The blue dye in the azuresin can be displaced by the hydrogen ions of hydrochloric acid, if acid is present. The test results do not furnish exact quantitative data, but the test is a convenient screening device. However, false positive and false negative results have been reported.

Preparation, dosage, and administration. Since the patient is to have nothing by mouth after midnight in preparation, the test is usually performed in the early morning hours. Upon awakening, the patient is instructed to void, and this urine is discarded. Then 500 mg. of caffeine are administered in one glass of water in order to stimulate gastric secretions. Histamine phosphate may be substituted. One hour later, the patient is instructed to void and this urine is saved as a control specimen. Two grams of azuresin are then administered in one-fourth glass of water. Two hours after administration of the resin, the patient is again instructed to void. The concentration of dye in this last specimen is then determined by comparison of urine color to color standards. If the color indicates the presence of 0.6 mg. or more of azuresin in the urine, the patient has free gastric hydrochloric acid; if less than 0.6 mg. is present, the test is inconclusive and further evaluation is required. The patient should know that his urine will range from green to blue in color and that this condition may persist for several days.

AGENTS USED FOR ROENTGENOGRAPHIC STUDIES
Barium sulfate, U.S.P., B.P.

Barium sulfate is a fine, white, colorless, tasteless, and bulky powder free from grittiness. It is more impermeable to roentgen rays than are tissues and is therefore employed as an opaque contrast medium for radiologic examination of the gastrointestinal tract. Its property of insolubility renders it safe to use, for all soluble barium salts are exceedingly poisonous. The patient is usually first examined by means of a fluoroscope, and flat plates are later taken to determine the rate of barium passage through the digestive tract and to locate sites of abnormality.

Preparation, dosage, and administration. For examination of the stomach, the patient is to have had nothing by mouth since midnight and is given barium orally in doses of 300 Gm. (usually in 400 ml. of water). Saccharin and vanillin may be used to improve the palatability of this mixture. If the large bowel is to be examined, the patient should have nothing by mouth after midnight in addition to cathartics and/or cleansing enemas. The barium is then given in enema form. The patient should be instructed to attempt to retain the barium during the radiologic examination, a feat that sometimes proves difficult. After the examination, either cleansing enemas or cathartics should be administered, so that the remaining barium does not contribute to bowel obstruction. In both cases the patient should be informed that his stool will be very light in color after the examination.

Meglumine diatrizoate injection, U.S.P., B.P. (Gastrografin)

Diatrizoate compounds, which are utilized in varied concentrations for specific radiographic examinations, are also sometimes used for gastrointestinal examinations. A 76% oral solution of meglumine diatrizoate injection is a water-soluble, iodinated contrast agent known as Gastrografin. Because of its hypertonicity and tendency to cause distention of the bowel, it is somewhat less satisfactory than barium for radiographic examinations.

ORGANIC IODINE COMPOUNDS FOR CHOLECYSTOGRAPHY

A number of organic iodine compounds are used as diagnostic aids in examination of the liver, gallbladder, and bile ducts. These compounds are excreted by the liver into the bile and concentrated in the gallbladder. Since they cast a shadow on x-ray film, they are utilized to visualize the gallbladder outline and the presence of stones and to determine whether the organ fills and empties normally. If the gallbladder is not functioning, it does not absorb the dye and is not visualized on the film. Because an empty stomach and a clear intestinal tract are necessary for visualization of the gallbladder, patients are prepared with fat-free suppers and cathartics and may have nothing by mouth after midnight. Occasionally, after films are taken, the patient is given a fat-containing meal and additional films are taken to determine the ability of the organ to contract.

It is recommended that iodinated compounds be used cautiously, if at all, for patients with severe renal or hepatic disease. These compounds are contraindicated for patients sensitive to iodine, and their use will interfere with diagnostic radioactive isotope uptake studies.

Iodoalphionic acid (Priodax)

This compound produces fewer side effects than iodophthalein sodium. It is eventually excreted chiefly by the kidneys. Untoward effects include dysuria, nausea and vomiting, diarrhea, dryness of the mouth, and general weakness. The drug is available in 0.5-Gm. tablets for oral administration. The usual adult dose is 3 Gm. taken with several glasses of water.

Iopanoic acid, U.S.P., B.P. (Telepaque)

Iopanoic acid is a radiopaque medium used in cholecystography. It is claimed that undesirable side effects seldom occur and that it produces greater opacification of the gallbladder. When side effects do occur, they include nausea, diarrhea, and dysuria. The usual dose is 3 Gm. given orally 10 hours before the roentgenogram is to be made. The drug is available in 500-mg. tablets.

Iodipamide meglumine (Cholografin meglumine)

Iodipamide is a water-soluble organic iodine compound that is administered intravenously for cholecystography when patients are unable to ingest or absorb oral agents or when rapid visualization of the gallbladder is essential for diagnosis in emergencies and prior to surgery. It is the agent of choice for cholangiography. After injection, cholangiography can be performed in 25 minutes and cholecystography after 2 to $2\frac{1}{2}$ hours.

Drugs that affect the intestine

CATHARTICS

Cathartics are oral drugs administered to induce defecation. They may be administered for the following purposes:

1 In preparation of abdominal viscera prior to roentgen examination or surgery
2 Postoperatively
3 In cases of food and drug poisoning to promote the elimination of the offending substance from the gastrointestinal tract; saline cathartics are considered useful for this purpose
4 To keep the stool soft when it is essential to avoid the irritation or straining that accompanies the passage of a hardened stool (a rectal disorder, irritated polyps in the bowel, or cases in which straining should be avoided, as after the repair of a hernia or after a cerebral vascular accident)
5 To expel parasites and toxic anthelmintics; cathartics are routinely prescribed after certain anthelmintics for the purpose of expelling the parasites as well as the anthelmintic, which may be toxic
6 To secure a stool specimen to be examined for parasites; a saline cathartic is often preferred

The laity, however, frequently misuses cathartics, and misconceptions about the function of the bowel have long been harbored by mankind.

Almy and Steinberg state:

Drugs have been used since time immemorial for the purpose of promoting defecation. Such agents are widely self-administered by lay persons. Whatever the psychological basis, there is a durable attitude, spanning many centuries and many cultures, that associates excrement with evil and its elimination with the expiation of guilt. The practical result is that most people in our society still regard even transitory constipation as something to be directly and promptly treated with a cathartic. In the past the medical profession has abetted these tendencies by the empiric and nonspecific use of purgation in the treatment of systemic disease (even the common cold) and has been slow to disown the theory of intestinal autointoxication. As a consequence, more patients now consult the physician because of the untoward effects of chronic use of cathartics than for any condition that can be relieved by them.*

Constipation is a functional impairment of the bowel that prevents it from producing stool of normal consistency and frequency. Chronic constipation is sometimes caused by organic disease, such as benign or malignant tumors, which produces obstruction in the bowel; megacolon; hypothyroidism; anal and rectal disorders; and diseases of the liver and gallbladder. Patients who suffer from disorders of the gastrointestinal tract frequently complain of constipation. On the other hand, many persons complain of constipation when no organic disease or lesion can be found. A number of factors may operate to cause constipation in such persons.

1 Faulty diet and faulty eating habits (A diet that provides inadequate bulk and residue will contribute to the development of constipation. The gastrointestinal tract should function normally if fluids and residue are supplied in sufficient quantities to keep the stool formed but soft.)
2 Failure to respond to the normal defecation impulses and insufficient time to permit the bowel to produce an evacuation
3 Sedentary habits and insufficient exercise (Bedridden patients may be constipated because of inactivity or unnatural position for defecation.) Constipation, when not due to organic causes, is generally attributable to the above three factors.
4 The effect of drugs (The use of morphine, codeine, or ganglionic blocking agents often leads to constipation as a side effect.)

---

*From Almy, T. P., and Steinberg, H.: The choice of drugs for gastrointestinal disturbances. In Modell, W., editor: Drugs of choice 1962-1963, St. Louis, 1962, The C. V. Mosby Co., p. 339.

5 Febrile states, psychosomatic disorders, anemias, and sick headaches (Constipation can be a symptom of both functional and organic disorders.)
6 Atonic and hypertonic conditions of the musculature of the colon (These may result from habitual use of cathartics.)

RESPONSIBILITIES OF THE NURSE

As is true for all medications, the nurse must exercise caution in giving advice about cathartics. Persons who seek help because they are becoming increasingly dependent upon cathartics should be encouraged to seek the advice of a physician. Not infrequently, powerful, self-prescribed cathartics empty the whole colon, which then requires time to collect material. In the meantime, the patient may again be distressed because there has been no daily bowel movement and take another cathartic, thereby initiating a vicious cycle that may lead to dependency. Whatever the case, the patient should be helped to overcome his dependency.

Nurses should direct their efforts toward teaching the patient practices that promote normal bowel habits. In doing so, they must bear in mind that teaching in this area may be met with some resistance, so that they should attempt to achieve a nonthreatening atmosphere. The patient's bowel complaints should be listened to, and habits explored in order to determine the possible cause of the bowel disorder. Appropriate teaching can then be directed to the problem in relation to the patient's intellectual level, his socioeconomic background (which influences the type of food he eats), and his receptivity. Not infrequently, entire families have similar bowel habits and sometimes the mother is an excellent intermediary for change.

Elderly persons who have some degree of constipation cannot be treated in the same way as younger patients. They cannot be expected to change the habit patterns of a lifetime or to subject themselves to tiresome diets that disturb the peace required by the elderly person. It may be decidedly unwise to urge an elderly person to increase the roughage of his diet. He may not have the teeth or the type of bowel to make such an adjustment happily. After an examination the doctor frequently prescribes a laxative for more or less regular use, and if it produces satisfactory results (no griping or gaseous distention), there is probably little need to worry about the cathartic habit.

CONDITIONS FOR WHICH CATHARTICS MAY BE CONTRAINDICATED

There are a number of conditions for which cathartics should be given with caution, if at all.

1 Inflammatory disorders of the alimentary tract, such as appendicitis, typhoid fever, and chronic ulcerative colitis
2 Cases of undiagnosed abdominal pain; should the pain be caused by an inflamed appendix, a cathartic may bring about a rupture of the appendix by increasing intestinal peristalsis
3 After some operations such as repair of the perineum or rectum (for a time, at least)
4 Pregnancy and severe anemia; debilitated patients
5 Chronic constipation and spastic constipation
6 Bowel obstruction, hemorrhage, or intussusception

A number of ill effects may follow the use or overuse of irritant cathartics in particular; one of these is a disturbance of electrolyte balance. The small intestine contains an abundance of sodium, potassium, chloride, and bicarbonate ions that will be lost when the bowel is emptied vigorously. This can result in alkalosis or acidosis, dehydration, and potassium deficiency. Young and healthy adults may recover from the purgation without noticeable ill effect, but the same may not be true in the elderly or the debilitated patient or the patient with renal impairment.

CLASSIFICATION

Cathartics may be classified according to their source, site of action, degree of action, or method of action. The latter two classifications will be described.

Degree of action
1 Laxatives—stimulate few bowel movements, which are formed and usually unaccompanied by cramping
2 Purgatives—produce more frequent bowel movements, which are soft or liquid in nature and are frequently accompanied by cramping

Method of action
1 Irritant cathartics—increase peristalsis in the colon by irritating sensory nerve endings in the mucosa

2 Bulk cathartics—increase the volume of nonabsorbable intestinal contents, thereby distending the bowel and initiating reflex bowel activity
3 Saline cathartics—retain and increase water content of feces by virtue of osmotic qualities; may also be considered as bulk cathartics
4 Intestinal lubricants—mechanically lubricate feces in order to facilitate defecation
5 Fecal softening agents—act as dispersing wetting agents, facilitating mixture of water and fatty substances within the fecal mass; when a homogenous mixture is produced, the feces become soft

IRRITANT CATHARTICS—ANTHRACENE CATHARTICS (EMODIN CATHARTICS)

The principal members of this group are botanical drugs obtained from the bark, seed pods, leaves, and roots of a number of plants. Cascara, senna, rhubarb, and aloe yield anthraquinones in the alkaline portion of the small intestine; these are absorbed and later secreted to produce irritation in the large intestine. These compounds are partially absorbed from the intestine and may cause discoloration of the urine. They have also been found to impart a purgative effect to the milk of nursing women. The anthracene cathartics act in 6 to 12 hours and exert their main action on the large intestine, which explains their tendency to produce cramping. Aloe and rhubarb are almost obsolete irritant cathartics.

Cascara sagrada

Cascara sagrada is obtained from the bark of the *Rhamnus purshiana*, a shrub or small tree, and is one of the most extensively used cathartics. Its action is mainly on the large bowel and, although its effects are comparatively mild, it does act by irritation. It is less likely to cause griping than some of the other cathartics belonging to this group of compounds. The active ingredients reach the large bowel by way of the bloodstream, after absorption in the small bowel, as well as by passage along the alimentary tract. Bowel evacuation occurs in about 8 hours.

Preparation, dosage, and administration. Cascara is used in one of three preparations obtained by extracting the crude drug with hot water.

Cascara sagrada extract, N.F. This is a powder obtained by evaporating the water extract to dryness and adding starch; each gram represents 3 Gm. of cascara sagrada. Usual dose is 300 mg.; range of dose is 120 to 500 mg.

Cascara sagrada fluidextract, N.F.; *cascara liquid extract*, B.P. Each milliliter of this preparation represents the activity of 1 Gm. of crude drug. Alcohol is added as a preservative. Usual dose is 0.6 to 2 ml. This preparation has a very bitter taste.

Aromatic cascara fluidextract, U.S.P. This preparation is prepared using magnesium oxide as a debitterizing agent to make it more palatable. Flavoring agents, sweeteners, and alcohol are also added. Each milliliter represents 1 Gm. of cascara sagrada. The presence of magnesium oxide decreases the cathartic action requiring a higher dosage than the other preparations. Usual dose is 5 ml.; range of dose is 5 to 15 ml. For infants the dose is 1 to 2 ml.; for children, 2 to 8 ml.

Cascara tablets, N.F., B.P. These forms are available in 120-, 200-, and 300-mg. tablets. The average dose is 300 mg. (gr. 5) for adults. The dose of cascara tablets, B.P., is 120 to 250 mg.

Senna

Senna is obtained from the dried leaves of the plant, *Cassia acutifolia*, a cathartic well known to the Arabians. The dried leaves have been used to make a homemade infusion of the drug, which is decidedly potent. It produces a through bowel evacuation in 4 to 6 hours and is likely to be accompanied by griping. It resembles cascara but is more powerful. It is found in the proprietary remedies Castoria and Syrup of Figs.

Senna tea is an infusion of senna leaves made from a teaspoonful of leaves to a cup of hot water.

A powdered concentrate of senna, obtained from the pod of the plant, is said to contain the desirable laxative components but to be free of the impurities that in previous preparations have been the cause of griping. This compound is sold under the name of Senokot (tablets and granules), and the usual adult dose is two tablets or 1 teaspoon of the granules.

Preparation, dosage, and administration

Senna syrup, N.F. The usual dose is 8 ml. orally.

Senna fluidextract, N.F. The usual dose is 2 ml. orally.

OTHER IRRITANT CATHARTICS
Castor oil, U.S.P., B.P. (Oleum Ricini)

Castor oil is obtained from the seeds of the castor bean, *Ricinus communis*, a plant that grows in India but that is also cultivated in a number of places where the climate is warm. Castor oil is a bland, colorless emollient that passes through the stomach unchanged, but, like other fatty substances, it retards the emptying of the stomach and for this reason is usually given when the stomach is empty. In the intestine the oil is hydrolyzed to glycerol and a fatty acid, ricinoleic acid. This fatty acid is responsible for the irritation of the bowel, especially the small intestine. It rarely reaches the large intestine before causing irritation. Its irritating effect causes a rapid propulsion of contents from the small intestine, including any of the oil that may have escaped hydrolysis. A therapeutic dose will produce several copious semiliquid stools in 2 to 6 hours and should not be given at bedtime. Some persons have little or no griping or colic-like distress, whereas others may experience considerable abdominal cramping and exhaustion. Patients who have an irritable bowel or lesions in the bowel may be made very ill.

The fluid nature of the stool is caused by the rapid passage of the fecal content rather than by a diffusion of fluid into the bowel. Castor oil tends to empty the bowel completely; hence, no evacuation is likely to occur for a day or so after its administration. The drug is excreted into the milk of nursing mothers.

Uses. Castor oil is used much less often today than formerly. It continues to be used in the preparation of certain patients who are to have a roentgen examination of abdominal viscera. Because of its irritant action it is contraindicated for patients with ulcerative lesions of the bowel, pregnant women, or nursing mothers.

Preparation, dosage, and administration. The usual adult dose of castor oil is 15 to 60 ml. and it is given orally. Dose for children is 5 to 15 ml.

The natural oil may be unpleasant and nauseating. This may be overcome by the use of fruit juices or pharmaceutical mixtures to emulsify and disguise the oil.

Phenolphthalein tablets, N.F., B.P.

Phenolphthalein, a phenol derivative, is a synthetic substance, the cathartic action of which is similar to that of the anthracene group. It is a white powder insoluble in water but soluble in the juice of the intestine, where it exerts its relatively mild irritant action. Evacuation is produced in 6 to 8 hours, unaccompanied by griping. It acts upon both the small and large bowel, particularly the latter. When given orally, part of the drug is absorbed and resecreted into the bile and thus a prolonged cathartic action may be obtained. If the urine and feces are alkaline, they will be red in color from this drug.

Repeated doses may cause nausea, and in some susceptible individuals a skin rash may appear. In other cases a prolonged and excessive purgative effect may indicate individual idiosyncracy. The drug is odorless and tasteless and relatively pleasant to take; it is found in a number of proprietary preparations and is sold in a candy-like form and in a chewing gum. Children should not be allowed free access to these preparations, since they are likely to regard them as ordinary candy or gum and may get an overdose of the drug. Deaths have been reported from such accidents, although the dose causing toxicity is large.

Preparation, dosage, and administration. Tablets are available in 60- and 120-mg. amounts. The usual dose is 60 mg. orally.

Phenolphthalein is found in some proprietary preparations with other cathartics such as agar, liquid petrolatum, as well as with other irritant cathartics.

Bisacodyl, U.S.P., B.P. (Dulcolax)

Bisacodyl is a relatively nontoxic laxative agent that reflexly stimulates peristalsis upon contact with the mucosa of the colon. Bisacodyl has been successful in the treatment of various types of constipation. In larger doses, it is also widely used for cleansing of the bowel prior to some surgeries and proctoscopic and radiographic examinations. Bisacodyl is insoluble in

neutral or alkaline solution and should not be taken within 1 hour after antacids have been administered.

Preparation, dosage, and administration. Bisacodyl is available in tablets containing 5 mg. for oral administration and suppositories containing 10 mg. for rectal administration. The suppositories act within 15 to 60 minutes, while the tablets produce evacuation of the bowel in 6 to 12 hours. The suppositories may cause a burning sensation and proctitis. The tablets are enteric coated and should not be chewed (to avoid release of the drug in the stomach and the possibility of emesis).

BULK-FORMING CATHARTICS

Hydrophilic colloids stimulate peristalsis by increasing bulk and therefore modifying the consistency of the stool. This mechanism of cathartic action is a normal stimulus and is one of the least harmful. These drugs do not interfere with absorption of food, but they can cause fecal impaction and obstruction, so it is important to give them with adequate fluids. The effect of these cathartics may not be apparent for 12 to 24 hours, and their full effect may not be achieved until the second or third day after administration. Some physicians maintain that bran and dried fruits (such as prunes and figs) exert the same effect, and they prefer to advise these foods rather than the cathartics.

Agar, U.S.P.

Agar is a dried mucilaginous substance obtained from several varieties of algae, which is rich in indigestible cellulose. It may be obtained in the powdered, granular, or flaked form. The granular preparation is usually the one most desirable. When moistened, it swells, forming a mass of material that passes through the intestine without being affected by the digestive juices, and by its blandness and bulk it makes the stool large and soft so that it is easily moved along the colon and into the rectum.

The effect of agar is not noticed immediately. It may require a week or two to establish satisfactory evacuation, but as soon as results seem satisfactory, the dose should gradually be reduced to the smallest amount needed for a satisfactory bowel movement. Doses should then be omitted occasionally until its use is no longer necessary. This gradual reduction and cessation of dosage should constitute a principle underlying the use of all laxative cathartics to avoid undesirable reactions and habit formation.

Preparation, dosage, and administration. Agar is best taken twice daily in doses of 4 to 16 Gm. accompanied by plenty of fluid. Some find agar more palatable when it has been allowed to soak in hot water and is then added to such food as cereal, soup, or mashed potatoes or is merely taken in the soft semisolid form. When the dry agar is used, it likewise may be added to soup, cereal, potatoes, pudding, and so on. It also may be emulsified with liquid petrolatum (Petrogalar). Cascara, phenolphthalein, or milk of magnesia is sometimes added to the emulsified form.

The mineral oil and agar emulsions are widely advertised but are of little value because the agar content is so small (2% to 6%). The laxative effect of these emulsions is usually caused by the addition of some other cathartic.

Plantago seed, N.F. (psyllium seed)

Plantago seed is the dried ripe seed of the *Plantago psyllium*, *Plantago indica*, or *Plantago ovata*. The small, brown or blond seeds contain a mucilaginous material that swells in the presence of moisture to form a jelly-like indigestible mass. The main disadvantage lies in the fact that, although the seeds swell, their ends remain sharp and may be the cause of irritation in the alimentary tract. At present, only the preparations of the extracted gums are available, and these have the advantage of causing less mechanical irritation.

Preparation, dosage, and administration. The following are preparations of plantago.

Psyllium hydrophilic mucilloid (Metamucil). This compound is a white to cream-colored powder containing about 50% powdered mucilaginous portion (outer epidermis) of blond psyllium seeds and about 50% dextrose. This mixture is used in the treatment of constipation because it promotes the formation of a soft, water-retaining gelatinous residue in the lower bowel. In ad-

dition, it has a demulcent effect on inflamed mucosa. The dose is 4 to 7 Gm. one to three times daily. It should be stirred into a glass of water or other fluid, drunk while in suspension, followed by an additional glass of fluid.

Plantago ovata coating (Konsyl). This form is a cream- to brown-colored granular powder obtained from the *Plantago ovata* (blond psyllium, mucilaginous portion). The dose is 5 to 10 Gm. three times daily before meals in a glass of water or milk. It should be swallowed before it thickens.

Methylcellulose, U.S.P. (Cellothyl, Hydrolose, Methocel, Syncelose)

Methylcellulose is a synthetic hydrophilic colloid. It is a grayish white, fibrous powder that, in the presence of water, swells and produces a viscous, colloidal solution in the upper part of the alimentary tract. In the colon this solution loses water and forms a gel that increases the bulk and softness of the stool.

Preparation, dosage, and administration. Methylcellulose is available in 500-mg. tablets or as a syrup (200 mg. per milliliter). It is administered orally two to four times daily in doses of 1 to 1.5 Gm. It should be accompanied by one or two glasses of water. The dosage is gradually reduced as normal defecation reflexes establish a normal pattern for the behavior of the bowel. Tablets should not be chewed to avoid risk of esophageal obstruction.

Carboxymethylcellulose sodium, U.S.P. (Carmethose, CMC Cellulose Gum, Thylose Sodium)

Carboxymethylcellulose sodium is a synthetic, hydrophilic, colloid gum. It is similar to methylcellulose in that it forms a soft bulk in the intestine after oral ingestion. It is insoluble in gastric juices, which is not true of methylcellulose.

Preparation, dosage, and administration. Carboxymethylcellulose sodium is available in 225- and 500-mg. tablets and in 5% solution for oral administration. The usual dose is 1.5 Gm. three times daily with one or two glasses of water. Tablets should not be chewed before swallowing.

SALINE CATHARTICS

The saline cathartics are soluble salts that are only slightly absorbed from the alimentary canal. Because of their osmotic effect these salts retain and increase the water content of feces. An isotonic saline solution will inhibit absorption of water from the bowel and will therefore increase the total fluid bulk. Peristalsis will be increased and several liquid or semiliquid stools will result. A hypertonic saline solution will cause diffusion of fluid from the blood in the wall of the bowel and into the lumen of the organ until the solution has been made isotonic. This type of fluid is especially effective in relieving edema, although the action may prove exhausting to the patient. Catharsis results in 1 to 4 hours.

The intestinal membrane is not entirely impermeable to the passage of saline cathartics. Some find their way into the general circulation only to be excreted by the kidney, in which case they act as saline diuretics. Hypertonic saline solutions in the bowel may result in so much loss of fluid that little or no diuretic effect will be possible. Some ions may have a toxic effect if they accumulate in the blood in sufficient quantity. This may occur with magnesium ions if a solution is retained in the intestine for a long time or if the patient suffers from renal impairment. It may also occur when large doses of the salt are given intravenously.

Uses. The saline cathartics are the cathartics of choice for the relief of edema (cerebral, cardiac) and for securing a stool specimen for examination as well as for use with certain anthelmintics and in some cases of food and drug poisoning.

When the object is merely to empty the intestine, magnesium citrate, magnesium sulfate, sodium phosphate, or milk of magnesia is effective. Milk of magnesia (magnesium hydroxide) is the mildest of the salines and is often the cathartic of choice for children. Heavy magnesium oxide is better for adults, as a rule. Magnesium sulfate is probably the best to relieve edema, although it has a disagreeable taste. Sodium sulfate is the most disagreeable and is seldom prescribed, except in veterinary practice. The effervescent preparations are the most agreeable to take.

The sodium salts are contraindicated in cardiac patients or those on a low sodium diet. The magnesium and potassium salts are contraindicated in patients with renal disease.

Preparation, dosage, and administration. The following salts, when given for their cathartic effect, are usually given orally. Certain of them may be given rectally as an enema. The salts tend to have a rapid action, especially if administered in the morning before breakfast. Patients sometimes complain of gaseous distention after taking saline cathartics. All preparations should be accompanied by a liberal intake of water, since the salts do not readily leave the stomach and may cause vomiting unless well diluted. On the other hand, if the saline is given to reduce edema, the patient's total daily intake of fluids will probably be restricted.

When a salt such as magnesium sulfate is administered to a patient, it should not only be dissolved in an adequate amount of water but it should also be disguised in fruit juice. Grape juice is excellent unless the patient is nauseated, in which case it is better to give it in plain water (chilled) or on chipped ice since the grape juice, if vomited, will stain bedclothing.

Sodium sulfate, U.S.P., B.P. (Glauber's Salt). This compound occurs as a white powder that is readily soluble in water. It has a strong, disagreeable saline taste that may be improved with lemon juice. It is one of the least expensive of saline cathartics and is the basis of many proprietary saline cathartics such as Sal Hepatica. The usual dose is 15 Gm.

Magnesium sulfate, U.S.P., B.P. (Epsom Salt). This agent occurs as glassy, needle-like crystals or as a white powder and is readily soluble in water. It has a bitter saline taste. The usual dose for cathartic effect is 15 Gm. ($\frac{1}{2}$ ounce), although the range of dosage may be from 10 to 30 Gm.

Milk of magnesia, U.S.P.; *magnesium hydroxide mixture*, B.P. Milk of magnesia is also used as an antacid. In the stomach the magnesium hydroxide reacts with the hydrochloric acid to form magnesium chloride, which is responsible for the cathartic effect. The usual dose for adults is 15 ml. ($\frac{1}{2}$ fluidounce), although the range of dosage is 5 to 30 ml. *Magnesium hydroxide tablets*, N.F., contain 0.3 Gm. of the drug.

Magnesium oxide, U.S.P., B.P. This preparation depends on the conversion of the oxide into soluble salts of magnesium, which are responsible for the cathartic effect. The usual laxative dose is 1 to 4 Gm.

Heavy magnesium carbonate, B.P.; *light magnesium carbonate*, B.P. This cathartic is a bulky white powder that is practically insoluble in water. It is used as an antacid as well as a cathartic. Cathartic effect is dependent upon the formation of a soluble salt of magnesium. The usual dose is 2 to 8 Gm.

Magnesium citrate solution, N.F. This preparation is not very soluble, hence the need for a relatively large dose. It is not unpleasant to take because it is carbonated and flavored. The usual dose is one half to one bottle (6 to 12 ounces).

Sodium phosphate. This is a white crystalline substance readily soluble in water. Its taste is less disagreeable than that of either sodium sulfate or magnesium sulfate. The usual dose is 4 Gm.

Effervescent sodium phosphate, N.F. This preparation is made effervescent by the addition of sodium bicarbonate and citric and tartaric acids. The usual dose is 10 Gm.

A concentrated aqueous solution of sodium biphosphate and sodium phosphate is available under the name of Fleet Phospho-Soda. The usual dose as a cathartic is 4 to 15 ml. It is also marketed in a disposable enema unit.

Potassium sodium tartrate, N.F. (Rochelle Salt). The usual dose is 10 Gm. ($\frac{1}{3}$ ounce) orally. This preparation occurs as crystals or white powder, is very soluble, and has a not unpleasant taste.

Mineral waters. Mineral waters are usually artificially prepared solutions made in a factory and contain magnesium sulfate or sodium sulfate or both. Their use in the treatment of constipation is thought inadvisable.

LUBRICANT OR EMOLLIENT CATHARTICS
Mineral oil, U.S.P.; liquid paraffin, B.P.

Mineral oil (liquid petrolatum) is a mixture of liquid hydrocarbons obtained from petroleum. The oil is not digested and absorption is minimal. It softens the fecal mass and prevents excessive absorption of water. It is especially useful when it is desirable to keep feces soft and when straining at stool must be reduced, as after rectal operations, repair of hernias, or cerebrovascular or spinal cord accidents. It may be useful for patients who have a chronic type of constipation because of prolonged inactivity. Such might be the case in patients with orthopedic conditions.

Some physicians object to the use of mineral oil on the basis that it dissolves certain of the fat-soluble vitamins and bile salts and inhibits their absorption. Others maintain that only the precursor to vitamin A (carotene) is so affected and that natural vitamin A is quantitatively absorbed from the intestine in the presence of mineral oil. Another objection to its use is that in large doses it tends to seep from the rectum, which may interfere with healing of postoperative wounds in the region of the anus and perineum. Although absorption of mineral oil is very limited, it is said to give rise to a chronic inflammatory reaction in tissues where it is found after absorption. Indiscriminate use by the aged and weak should not be encouraged. Mineral oil may also produce a lipid pneumonia if drops coating the pharynx gain access to the trachea.

Preparation, dosage, and administration. Mineral oil is administered in doses that range from 15 to 30 ml. (adults) and is best given between meals or at bedtime. It should not be given immediately after meals, since it may delay the passage of food from the stomach. Most patients may have a slice of orange or glass of orange juice to relieve the oily taste in the mouth. Mineral oil is also to be found as the major ingredient of some oil retention enemas.

Olive oil, U.S.P., B.P.; corn oil, U.S.P., B.P.; cottonseed oil, U.S.P.

Olive oil and cottonseed oil are digestible oils, but if given in sufficient quantity, they may act as emollient cathartics, since part of the oil will escape hydrolysis.

When administered in doses of 30 ml., these oils act as laxatives. They may be given orally or rectally. Dose for infants is 4 to 8 ml.

FECAL MOISTENING AGENTS

With the introduction of fecal moistening agents and other less toxic synthetic drugs, there seems to be more restricted use of irritant cathartics. Fecal moistening agents are constantly being improved and have achieved a level of popular therapy.

Dioctyl sodium sulfosuccinate, N.F.

Dioctyl sodium sulfosuccinate acts in a manner similar to that of detergents and permits water and fatty substance to penetrate and to be well mixed with the fecal material. Thus, this agent promotes the formation of soft, formed stools and is a useful aid in the treatment of constipation. One or two days may be required for full effects.

It is said to have a wide margin of safety and negligible toxicity. There is some question about the advisability of giving it with mineral oil, since there is a possibility that it may promote absorption of the oil.

Uses. It is indicated for patients with rectal impaction, chronic constipation, and painful conditions of the rectum and anus and for those who should avoid straining at the time of defecation. It is particularly useful for bedridden patients, especially children.

Preparation, dosage, and administration. The following are available preparations of dioctyl sulfosuccinate.

Dioctyl sodium sulfosuccinate (Colace, Doxinate). This preparation is available in 50-, 60-, 100-, and 240-mg. capsules; in solution, 10 mg. per milliliter; and as a syrup, 4 mg. per milliliter. The usual adult dose is 50 to 100 mg. daily; 10 to 20 mg. for infants and children. Solutions of the drug are best given in fruit juice or milk.

Peri-Colace. Peri-Colace includes casantranol, which provides gentle peristaltic stimulation. Either dioctyl sodium sulfosuccinate or casantranol produces a bowel movement in 8 to 12 hours.

Dioctyl calcium sulfosuccinate, N.F. (Surfak). This drug is claimed to provide superior surfactant activity to the older chemical, dioctyl sodium. It is indicated in conditions in which cathartic therapy is undesirable but in which prevention of constipation is necessary. A wide margin of safety is claimed. The drug is administered in 240-mg. capsules; the usual dose is one capsule daily.

Dialose. Dialose is a combination of dioctyl sulfosuccinate and sodium carboxymethylcellulose. It combines the advantages of both drugs—fecal-moistening and bulk-producing agents. Dialose Plus also includes oxyphenisatin acetate, which is a peristaltic stimulant. Recommended dosages are one capsule two or three times a day, taken with a glass of water.

ANTIDIARRHEICS

Diarrhea is a symptom of a disorder of the bowel associated with rapid passage of intestinal content, frequent fluid stools, and griping. The remedies ordered to relieve diarrhea are selected on the basis of causation. The causes may be many and varied and include (1) the eating of contaminated or partially decomposed food, (2) bacterial or protozoan infection, (3) nervous disorders, (4) disturbances of gastric physiology, such as the absence of hydrochloric acid or the effects of resectional surgery of the stomach, (5) inflammatory processes of the intestine or adjacent viscera, and (6) the effects of certain drugs in the intestine (such as some of the broad-spectrum antibiotics).

The antidiarrheic drugs are less likely to be used without medical supervision than are the cathartics. Diarrhea may at times produce serious consequences in terms of dehydration, exhaustion, and loss of electrolytes, vitamins, and food materials. In view of the numerous possible causes it is evident that effective treatment depends on discovering the cause and removing it if possible. In a few instances the administration of a cathartic that brings about the emptying of the entire bowel may be the best way to relieve diarrhea by elimination of contents irritating the bowel. Since diarrhea is looked upon as a defense mechanism on the part of the bowel against irritants or toxins, the diarrhea should not be checked until the cause has been determined.

The drugs used in the treatment of diarrhea include (1) demulcents and protectives, (2) adsorbents, (3) astringents, (4) antiseptics, and (5) sedatives and antispasmodics.

DEMULCENTS AND PROTECTIVES

The demulcents are preparations that have a soothing effect on the irritated membrane of the gastrointestinal tract by coating membrane surface and thereby protecting underlying cells from irritating stimuli. The preparations used are salts of bismuth, calcium carbonate, and magnesium oxide. They are of limited efficacy and used only in mild disturbances.

ADSORBENTS

Preparations that adsorb gas or toxic substances from the stomach and bowel have been used extensively, but their value in the control of diarrhea has come to be questioned. If they are effective adsorbents, they adsorb not only undesirable substances but desirable ones such as enzymes and food nutrients as well. Hydrophilic substances such as psyllium hydrophilic mucilloid are sometimes combined with adsorbents for use as antidiarrheics. They contribute adhesiveness to the stool but do not necessarily stop the diarrhea. Adsorbents have an advantage of being inexpensive and nontoxic.

Preparation, dosage, and administration. The following are adsorbent preparations.

Activated charcoal, U.S.P. In a dry state this is one of the most effective adsorbent substances. It was formerly used to relieve flatulence and diarrhea. It is now used chiefly as a general purpose antidote for certain types of poisoning.

Kaolin, N.F.; *light kaolin*, B.P. This is a naturally occurring aluminum silicate (clay) long used by the Chinese for the relief of diarrhea. It is given suspended in water in doses of 15 to 60 Gm. every 3 or 4 hours until relief is obtained.

Kaolin mixture with pectin (Kaopectate). This mixture contains kaolin and pectin and acts as both an adsorbent and demulcent. Pectin is a coarse, yellowish powder that, when mixed with water, has a mucilaginous consistency. Ground raw apples constitute a good source of it and have been used in the treatment of diarrhea, especially diarrhea in children. Kaopectate is effective but must be given in relatively large doses, 15 to 30 ml. several times a day.

ASTRINGENTS

Astringents are substances that shrink swollen and inflamed tissues such as the intestinal mucosa of the patient suffering from diarrhea. Astringents precipitate proteins and form an insoluble substance (a protein salt) over the mucous membrane and thus protect it from irritating substances. Astringents also inhibit secretions. Tannic acid has long been used as an astringent in the treatment of diarrhea, but there is some doubt concerning its effectiveness beyond the stomach because it may combine with food substances and be destroyed by hydrolysis.

Present-day therapy is directed at the cause of the diarrhea and at the maintenance of normal extracellular fluids. For this, better agents are available.

CARMINATIVES

Carminatives are mild, irritant drugs that increase gastrointestinal motility and aid in expulsion of gas from the stomach and intestine. The active ingredients are, with few exceptions, aromatic substances such as volatile oils that possess an irritant action. Carminatives are more likely to be used in the home than in the hospital. Elderly patients may prefer them, partly because they may be accustomed to using them for the relief of mild symptoms. Whiskey or brandy in hot water or a few drops of peppermint (peppermint oil, U.S.P., or peppermint water, N.F.) in hot water are remedies commonly used in the home.

Mylicon is a drug utilized for the relief of flatulence. It is composed of simethicone (40 mg.) and relieves flatulence by its defoaming action. It acts in the stomach and intestines by changing the surface tension of gas bubbles, causing them to coalesce and enabling the patient to eliminate gas by eructating or passing flatus. The drug is available in tablet form to be chewed.

Phazyme is a phased tablet that releases pepsin, diastase, and simethicone in the stomach and pancreatin in the small intestine. It provides enzymes and gas-releasing agents to minimize gas formation and discomfort due to distention. It is administered in doses of one tablet with meals and at bedtime.

ANTISEPTICS
Sulfonamides

Several of the sulfonamide compounds that are poorly absorbed from the intestine have been used in the treatment of certain cases of bacillary dysentery. These have included sulfaguanidine and succinylsulfathiazole. However, sulfadiazine (which is absorbed from the bowel) has come to be the preparation of choice. It is also the preparation of choice for the treatment of cholera. The usual full doses of the drug are employed. The initial dose is usually 2 to 4 Gm. followed by 1 Gm. every 4 to 6 hours. Adequate fluid intake should be provided for the patient.

Salicylazosulfapyridine (Azulfidine) is employed in the treatment of secondary infections of patients who suffer from chronic ulcerative colitis. One gram is administered every 4 hours around the clock or, when the patient becomes ambulatory, 1 Gm. may be given after meals and at bedtime for a period of 1 to 2 weeks.

It has a D.E.S.I. rating of effective as adjunctive therapy in treatment of ulcerative colitis.

Antibiotics

Several of the antibiotics are bactericidal when administered orally (streptomycin, chloramphenicol, and the tetracyclines). Combinations of penicillin and streptomycin may also be given intramuscularly for certain infections of the bowel. Methicillin or vancomycin may be prescribed if *Staphylococcus aureus* is identified in the stool of patients suffering from diarrhea.

Neomycin sulfate, U.S.P., is an antibiotic that is also poorly absorbed from the gastrointestinal tract when given in oral form. It has been used as a bactericidal agent to sterilize the tract before surgery and in treatment of bacterial diarrheas. For sterilization of the intestinal tract, two tablets (0.5 Gm. each) are recommended hourly for 4 hours, then two tablets every 4 hours for four doses, The drug is contraindicated in the presence of intestinal obstruction because of the possibility of increased absorption from the diseased bowel. Caution is expressed regarding the possibility of superinfection. Chronic toxicity can result in renal damage and in damage to the eighth cranial nerve.

Kanamycin sulfate, U.S.P. (Kantrex), may also be used for similar purposes in 1- to 4-Gm. oral doses. Toxicity is low and affects the eighth cranial nerve.

Other drugs. A number of other drugs have been used for their antiseptic effect in the intestine. They include drugs such as methylene blue, gentian violet, and phenylsalicylate. Certain arsenicals, emetine, the iodohydroxyquinoline compounds, as well as certain antibiotics, are used in the treatment of amebic dysentery (see Chapter 21).

SEDATIVES AND ANTISPASMODICS

The sedatives most often used to relieve diarrhea are preparations of opium, such as paregoric and laudanum. Actually, the opium preparations do not relax the intestinal smooth muscle. They increase muscle tone so that the intestinal contents are not propelled. Codeine and morphine are sometimes used but should not be employed for chronic conditions because of the danger of producing drug dependence. Phenobarbital is used in conjunction with anticholinergic drugs, a combination that is a common base for many antispasmodic drugs.

Belladonna and its alkaloids, either natural or synthetic, are frequently employed for their antispasmodic action on the intestine. These preparations are manufactured in varied proportions and under differing trade names. Some of the more commonly used include those described in the following paragraphs.

Chardonna is a drug consisting of phenobarbital, charcoal, and extract of belladonna. It depresses cholinergic stimulating effects. It is indicated for spastic conditions of the gastrointestinal tract in doses of one tablet three times daily, to be given before meals.

Donnagel combines kaolin, pectin, atropine, and belladonna for adsorbent, demulcent, anticholinergic, and spasmolytic effects. It is specifically indicated for antidiarrheal use in doses of 1 to 2 tablespoons every 3 hours.

Donnatal is a mixture of atropine, scopolamine, and phenobarbital. It also contains belladonna alkaloids for antrispasmodic use.

Diphenoxylate hydrochloride, U.S.P., B.P., is used in combination with atropine (Lomotil) to control diarrhea in patients with irritable bowel syndrome and functional diarrhea. Dosage is variable. It is available in tablets and liquid form; each tablet or 5 ml. contains 2.5 mg. of diphenoxylate and 0.025 mg. of atropine. It is a very effective drug that acts by increasing intestinal tone and decreasing gastrointestinal motility. It is an opiatelike drug and may cause euphoria or slight sedation. It is an exempt narcotic.

Methscopolamine bromide, N.F. (Pamine) is a parasympatholytic drug that inhibits gastric secretion and also decreases gastrointestinal motility. The recommended dose is 2.5 mg. before meals and at bedtime.

QUESTIONS

For study and review

1 Differentiate between systemic and nonsystemic antacid characteristics.
2 Why is betazole hydrochloride (Histalog) preferred over histamine phosphate in diagnostic stimulation of hydrochloric acid secretion?
3 Define the mechanism of action of the Diagnex Blue test. In relation to this test, what would you consider important to tell the patient?
4 When using a salt solution for a gargle, why is it preferable to use a physiologic salt solution rather than a strong salt solution?
5 Mention some of the ways drugs may affect the stomach.
6 Name several simple emetics.
7 Name several preparations that are useful to check vomiting.
8 What are several popular misconceptions about constipation?
9 Name several conditions in which cathartics are contraindicated.
10 When a person walks into a drugstore and asks for a cathartic, why is a good druggist likely to inquire whether the person has any nausea or abdominal pain?
11 If a patient is scheduled to have a cholecystogram and a T_3 uptake on the same day, what nursing judgment would be exercised?
12 Identify and define the major modes of cathartic action, giving a drug example of each.
13 In case of food poisoning, why would castor oil be a more suitable cathartic than cascara?
14 What suggestions would you give to a person who asked you what could be done to overcome habitual constipation?
15 Evaluate the claims made for cathartics on present-day television and radio programs.
16 Identify two major objections to the use of mineral oil.

Multiple choice

Circle the answer of your choice.

17 Which of the following is a good example of a systemic antacid?
  a. calcium carbonate
  b. sodium bicarbonate
  c. lime water
  d. rhubarb and soda
18 Which of the following is a good example of a nonsystemic antacid?
  a. aluminum hydroxide
  b. calcium chloride
  c. sodium bicarbonate
  d. sodium carbonate
19 Which of the following represents the most outstanding precaution to observe when giving hydrochloric acid to a patient?
  a. dilute well with water
  b. give with meals
  c. give after meals
  d. follow administration with a drink of water
20 A potent stimulant of gastric secretions is:
  a. hydrochloric acid
  b. alcohol 7%
  c. histamine phosphate
  d. glutamic acid
21 All of the following preparations act both as an antacid and as a carthartic except:
  a. phenolphthalein
  b. magnesium hydroxide
  c. magnesium oxide
22 Kaopectate can be expected to relieve diarrhea by producing which of the following effects?
  a. cathartic and demulcent
  b. adsorbent and demulcent
  c. adsorbent and astringent
  d. carminative and sedative
23 In which of the following classifications might essence of peppermint belong?
  a. digestant
  b. antiemetic
  c. carminative
  d. antidiarrheic
24 Methylcellulose is a cathartic that acts in which of the following ways?
  a. irritation of the intestine
  b. formation of bulk
  c. stimulation of bile flow
  d. detergent action
25 Of the following cathartics which would you say is the one of choice for children?
  a. castor oil

    b. senna syrup

    c. milk of magnesia

    d. sodium sulfate

26 The physiologically least harmful of the following cathartics is:

    a. cascara sagrada

    b. milk of magnesia

    c. Dulcolax

    d. Metamucil

27 Indicate whether each of the following antacids is constipating or diarrheal.

    a. aluminum hydroxide gel

    b. magnesium trisilicate

    c. calcium carbonate

    d. milk of magnesia

28 Bile acts to aid digestion by:

    a. activating pepsin

    b. hydrolyzing protein

    c. lowering surface tension of fats

    d. flushing bile ducts

29 The active proteolytic enzyme in gastric juice is:

    a. pepsin

    b. pepsinogen

    c. trypsin

    d. amylase

30 The pharmacologic action of cascara sagrada primarily results from:

    a. central nervous system stimulation

    b. hydrophilic action

    c. antispasmodic effect

    d. mild irritating effect on the intestine

31 Which of the following statements are true?

    a. Antacids indirectly suppress peptic activity if they raise gastric pH above 4.

    b. Calcium carbonate is an antacid with a rapid onset and prolonged duration of action.

    c. The presence of an antacid in gastric contents decreases the volume of gastric juice secreted.

    d. Calcium carbonate causes acid rebound.

32 Which of the following statements are false?

    a. Aluminum hydroxide has a greater constipating potential than magnesium hydroxide.

    b. Cascara sagrada has a greater intensity of action on the intestine than castor oil

    c. The potential for harm by mineral oil used as a laxative is negligible.

    d. Sodium bicarbonate has a greater systemic alkalosis potential than aluminum hydroxide.

REFERENCES

A.M.A. drug evaluations, ed. 2, Acton, Mass., 1973, Publishing Sciences Group, Inc.

Aviado, D. M.: Krantz and Carr's pharmacologic principles of medical practice, ed. 8, Baltimore, 1972, The Williams & Wilkins Co.

Christensen, J.: The controls of gastrointestinal movements: Some old and new views, New Eng. J. Med. **285:**85, 1971.

Di Palma, J. R., editor: Drill's pharmacology in medicine, New York, 1971, McGraw-Hill Book Co.

Fordtran, J. S., and others: In vivo and in vitro evaluation of liquid antacids, New Eng. J. Med. **288:**923, 1973.

Goodman, L. S., and Gilman, A., editors: The pharmacological basis of therapeutics, ed. 5, New York, 1975, The Macmillan Co.

Goth, A.: Medical pharmacology, ed. 7, St. Louis, 1974, The C. V. Mosby Co.

Grady, G. F., and Keusch, G. T.: Pathogenesis of bacterial diarrheas, New. Eng. J. Med. **285:**831, 891, 1971.

Griffenhagen, G. B., and Hawkins, L. L., editors: Handbook of non-prescription drugs, Washington, D.C., 1973, American Pharmaceutical Association.

Grollman, A., and Grollman, E. F.: Pharmacology and therapeutics, ed. 7, Philadelphia, 1970, Lea & Febiger.

Hollander, D., and Harlan, J.: Antacids vs placebos in peptic ulcer therapy, J.A.M.A. **226:**1181, 1973.

Librach, I. M.: Peptic ulcer: Facts and figures, Nursing Mirror **134:**23, 1972.

Meyers, F. H., Jawetz, E., and Goldfien, A.: Review of medical pharmacology, ed. 4, Los Altos, Calif., 1974, Lange Medical Publications.

Modell, W., editor: Drugs of choice 1976-1977, St. Louis, 1976, The C. V. Mosby Co.

Osol, A., and Pratt, R.: The United States dispensatory, ed. 27, Philadelphia, 1973, J. B. Lippincott Co.

Redman, B. K., and Redman, R. S.: Oral care of the critically ill patient. In Bergersen, B. S., editor: Current concepts in clinical nursing, vol. 1, St. Louis, 1967, The C. V. Mosby Co.

Schiff, E. R.: Treatment of uncomplicated peptic ulcer disease, Med. Clin. North Am. **55:**305, 1971.

Thistle, J. L., and Hoffman, A. F.: Efficacy and specificity of chenodeoxycholic acid therapy for dissolving gallstones, New Eng. J. Med. **289:**655, 1973.

Turner, P., and Richens, A.: Clinical pharmacology, Edinburgh, 1973, Churchill Livingstone.

CHAPTER 32

Toxicology

General symptoms of poisoning
Source and incidence of poisoning
Poison control centers
Classification of poisons
Mechanisms of toxic actions of poisons
First-aid measures for poisoning

Treatment of poisoning

Removal of poison
Administration of suitable antidote

Toxicology is the study of poisons, their action and effects, methods for their detection, and diagnosis and treatment of poisoning. A poison can be defined as any substance that in relatively small amounts can cause death or serious bodily harm by chemical action. All drugs are potential poisons when used improperly or in excess dosage. Poisoning may be *acute* or *chronic.* In acute poisoning the effects are immediate. In chronic poisoning the effects are insidious as a result of cumulative effects of small amounts of poison absorbed over a prolonged period of time. Chronic poisoning causes chronic illness that may or may not be reversible.

GENERAL SYMPTOMS OF POISONING

When poisoning is suspected, the nurse should send for the physician. In the meantime, since time is such a precious factor, particularly in cases of acute poisoning, the nurse should learn as much about the patient as possible and apply suitable first-aid measures.

There is reason to suspect that a poison has been taken when sudden, violent symptoms occur, such as severe nausea, vomiting, diarrhea, collapse, or convulsions. It is important to find out (if possible) what poison has been taken and how much. Additional information that might prove helpful to the physician in making a diagnosis includes answers to questions or reports of observed phenomena, as follows:

1 Did the symptoms appear suddenly in an otherwise healthy individual? Did a number of persons become ill about the same time (as might happen in food poisoning)?
2 Is there anything unusual about the person, his clothing, or his surroundings? Is there evidence of burns about the lips and mouth? Are the gums discolored? Are there needle (hypodermic) pricks, pustules, or scars on the exposed and accessible surfaces of the body? (These may be seen in examination of drug addicts.) Is there any skin rash or discoloration?
3 The odor of the breath, the rate of respiration, any difficulty in respiration, and cyanosis should be noted.
4 The quality and rate of the pulse should be noted.

5 If vomitus is seen, what is its appearance and its odor? Is or was vomiting accompanied by diarrhea or abdominal pain?

6 Any abnormalities of stool and urine should be noted; change in color or the presence of blood may be significant.

7 For signs of involvement of the nervous system, the presence of excitement, muscular twitching, delirium, difficulty in speech, stupor, coma, constriction or dilation of the pupils, and elevated or subnormal temperature should be looked for.

The nurse should save all specimens of vomitus, urine, or stool in case the physician wishes to examine them and perhaps turn them over to the proper authority for analysis. This is of particular importance not only in making or confirming a diagnosis but also in the event that the case has medicolegal significance.

SOURCE AND INCIDENCE OF POISONING

Poisoning is common in the United States. About 2 million cases occur each year with about 2,000 fatalities. Most poisonings are *accidental* and caused by drug intoxication. Some poisonings are *suicide* attempts. *Criminal* poisonings are rare, since modern scientific methods permit highly accurate detection of poisons and most large cities maintain toxicologic laboratories in conjunction with law enforcement agencies. *In-dustrial* poisonings are prevalent since modern technology exposes man to numerous toxic agents in exhaust gases, radioactive substances, insecticides, and the like.

In the adult, five common drugs account for most poisonings from medicinals—barbiturates, salicylates, glutethimide, meprobamate, and phenothiazines. Scopolamine, bromides, and ethylene glycol also rank high as poisoning agents. Carbon monoxide is a chief cause of both accidental and suicidal death.

While most poisonings occur in the adult, one third of the accidental poisonings occur in children under age 5. Children are normally curious and will taste or ingest that which is easily accessible within their environment. Most of these poisonings are from medicines found within the home—aspirin, laxative tablets, barbiturates, iron pills, and tranquilizers. Other frequent causes of poisoning in children are cleaning agents, pesticides, bleaches, paint thinners, and lye. Lead and arsenic poisoning is encountered in fruit-growing areas where unwashed fruitbearing residues of insecticidal sprays are available to children and in ghetto areas where children often eat old peeling paint and plaster containing lead and arsenic. In the emergency department of a large midwestern hospital the chief cause of poisoning among children was found to be aspirin. In most cases the children had apparently mistaken the sweetened gr. 1 tablets for candy.

Table 32-1 Common poisoning agents and the symptoms and treatment of poisoning

Drug	Estimated fatal oral dose	Symptoms	Treatment
Barbiturates		Respiratory depression, hypotension, hypothermia, renal failure, coma	Respiratory assistance, renal dialysis, diuresis
Short acting	3 Gm.		
Long acting	5 Gm.		
Glutethimide	10 Gm.	Hypotension, apnea, mydriasis, flaccid paralysis	Gastric lavage, respiratory assistance, renal dialysis, diuresis
Salicylates	10 to 20 Gm.	Hyperpnea, respiratory alkalosis, metabolic acidosis occurring later, hypoprothrombinemia	Alkaline diuresis, renal dialysis, vitamin K
Phenothiazines	50 mg. per kilogram of body weight	Miosis, irritability	Supportive measures, control of convulsions
Meprobamate	12 Gm.	Respiratory depression, hypotension, coma	Respiratory assistance, renal dialysis

POISON CONTROL CENTERS

Physicians have long been concerned about the incidence of poisoning especially among young children, and as a result of such concern the first poison control center was started in Chicago in 1953 as a cooperative and integrated community activity. This idea spread to other cities in many states, and similar programs have been started, the administration of which may be the function of the local medical society, a medical school, the health department, a hospital, or a combination of these groups. Their main purpose is to serve as centers from which information about poisons can be obtained. There are now over 200 of these centers in the United States. With thousands of products on the market known only by their trade names, one of the major problems in treating the victim of a supposed poison is the proper identification of the ingredients of the product so that adequate treatment may be given or the victim and his family can be assured that the product is harmless. The collection of data that help to identify a poison is an important contribution of the center, although it has other functions. Data on all cases of poisoning are collected and centrally reported and followup visits to homes are often made to help prevent further cases of poisoning. The National Clearinghouse of Poison Centers is maintained by the National Institutes of Health for compilation of data and dissemination of information on poisons.

Poison symbols. In an attempt to reduce poisoning in children, new poison symbols are appearing for placement on containers of poisonous substances. The traditional skull and crossbones symbol seems to have lost some of its negative effectiveness, particularly for children. It was found that children associated the symbol with pirates, excitement, and adventure and that there was no national program to educate children about the intended meaning of the skull and crossbones symbol.

One new symbol is "Mr. Yuk," an ugly, green-faced, scowling, tongue-sticking-out poison warning symbol chosen by preschool children from six designs. This symbol is the official symbol of the National Poison Center Network headquartered at the Pittsburgh Poison Center. The symbol also contains the phone number of the nearest poison center. Another symbol design being used by the Poison Control Center at Denver General Hospital is "Officer UGH." The meaningful part of this symbol is the officer's hands crosswise across his mouth. Hopefully, more meaningful symbols and a national education program via televison will help to reduce the incidence of poisoning in children.

CLASSIFICATION OF POISONS

The classification of poisons is as broad as the classification of drugs since any drug is a potential poison in the tissues of the right person or when used in excess.

Poisons might be classified in various ways. They might be grouped according to chemical classifications as organic and inorganic poisons; as alkaloids, glycosides, and resins; or as acids, alkalies, heavy metals, oxidizing agents, halogenated hydrocarbons, and so on.

Another way in which they might be grouped is by locale of exposure—poisons found in the home, poisons encountered in industry, poisons encountered while camping, and so on.

Still another way in which poisons may be classified is according to the organ or tissue of the body in which the most damaging effects are produced. Some poisons injure all cells with which they have contact. Such chemical substances are sometimes called protoplasmic poisons or cytotoxins. Others have more effect on the kidney (nephrotoxins), the liver (hepatotoxins), or on the blood or blood-forming organs.

Poisons that affect chiefly the nervous system are called neurotoxins or neurotropic poisons. They must be studied separately, because different symptoms characterize each one. Symptoms of toxicity have been mentioned in connection with each of these drugs as they were presented in previous chapters. Although symptoms of this group of poisons are to some extent specific, it is also true that certain symptoms are encountered repeatedly and are associated with a large number of poisons. Drowsiness, dizziness, headache, delirium, coma, and convulsive seizures always indicate central nervous system involvement. On the other hand, one learns to associate dry mouth, dilated pupils, and difficult swallowing with overdosage of atropine or one of the atropine-like drugs; ringing in the ears, excessive perspiration, and gastric upset are associated with overdosage with salicylates.

MECHANISMS OF TOXIC ACTIONS OF POISONS

Poisons produce injurious effects in a number of ways. Many times the precise mechanism of action is not known; death may be caused by respiratory failure but exactly what happens to cause depression of the respiratory center may not be known.

It is apparent that the human body is dependent upon a constant supply of oxygen if various physiologic functions are to proceed satisfactorily. Anything that interferes with the use of oxygen by the cells or with the transportation of oxygen will produce damaging effects in cells and in some cells faster than in others. Carbon monoxide from automobile engines and unvented gas heaters is one of the most widely distributed toxic agents. It poisons by producing hypoxia and finally asphyxia. Carbon monoxide has a great affinity for hemoglobin and forms carboxyhemoglobin. Thus the production of oxyhemoglobin and the free transport of oxygen is interfered with, and oxygen deficiency soon develops in the cells. Unless exposure to the carbon monoxide is terminated quickly and before 40% of hemoglobin has been changed to carboxyhemoglobin, the anoxia may produce serious brain damage; death occurs when 60% of the hemoglobin has been changed to carboxyhemoglobin.

The cyanides act somewhat similarly in that they bring about cellular anoxia, but they do so in a different manner. They inactivate certain tissue enzymes so that cells are unable to utilize oxygen. Death may occur very rapidly.

Curare and the curariform drugs in toxic amounts bring about paralysis of the diaphragm, and again the victim dies from lack of oxygen.

Certain drugs have a direct effect on muscle tissue of the body such as that of the myocardium or the smooth muscle of the blood vessels. Death results from the failure of circulation or cardiac arrest. The nitrites, potassium salts, and digitalis drugs may exert toxic effects of this type.

Arsenic is an example of a protoplasmic poison or cytotoxin. Compounds of arsenic inhibit many enzyme systems of cells, especially those that depend on the activity of their free sulfhydryl groups. The arsenic combines with these SH groups and makes them ineffective. Hence, extensive tissue damage in the body occurs.

Methyl alcohol owes its toxic effect to an intermediate product of metabolism—formic acid. This produces a severe acidosis, lowered pH of the blood, reduced cerebral blood flow, and decreased consumption of oxygen by the brain. There is also a selective action on the retinal cells of the eye, but the exact cause of this injury is unknown.

Benzene is an example of a poison that acts by inhibiting the formation of all types of blood cells. In some instances the precursor of one type of blood cell is injured more than another. Depression of the formation of any of the blood cells can cause death.

The strong acids and alkalies denature and destroy cellular proteins. Examples of corrosive acids are hydrochloric, nitric, and sulfuric acids. Sodium, potassium, and ammonium hydroxides are examples of strong or caustic alkalies. Locally, these substances cause destruction of tissue, and death may result from hemorrhage, perforation, or shock. Corrosive poisons may also cause death by altering the pH of the blood or other body fluids, or they may produce marked degenerative changes in vital organs such as the liver or the kidney.

Many of the central nervous system depressants cause death by producing excessive depression of respiration and respiratory failure. The general anesthetics, barbiturates, chloral hydrate, and paraldehyde are examples of such drugs.

Central nervous system stimulants such as pentylenetetrazol, strychnine, and others in toxic amounts cause convulsive seizures, exhaustion, and depression of vital centers.

FIRST-AID MEASURES FOR POISONING

As mentioned previously, the duty of the nurse is to send for a physician and, pending his arrival, to ascertain if possible the cause of the symptoms and to apply suitable first-aid measures. The treatment of acute poisoning is always an emergency. Recommendations on first-aid measures for poisoning were made by the Committee on Toxicology of the American Medical Association and are presented on pp. 698-699.

Treatment of poisoning

Treatment of poisoning includes a number of general principles of action. Under many circumstances good first aid may save the patient's life and make the physician's task easier. To some extent, first aid and the later treatment may overlap. There are many things that may be done for the patient that require the direction and supervision of a physician, but the more the nurse knows about the poison and what to expect and what to have ready for use, the more help to all concerned. Occasionally, a nurse must deal with an emergency alone or under the direction of a physician contacted by telephone.

When living in or near a city it is faster and more satisfactory to bring a patient to a hospital, clinic, or physician's office than it is to wait for the physician to call at home. Professional ambulance service, the police, or fire department will frequently provide transportation, but a family car or that of a neighbor may be a faster way of solving the problem. Treatment of poisoning frequently involves (1) removal of the poison, (2) administration of a suitable antidote, (3) promotion of elimination, and (4) supportive treatment of the patient.

The order of these measures may need to be reversed, depending on the poison taken and the general condition of the patient. Sometimes the prompt removal of the poison is all the treatment that is needed.

REMOVAL OF POISON

When poisons are on the external surface of the body, in the nasal or oral cavities, or in the eye, attempts to remove them should be made by irrigating with copious amounts of plain water; this will prevent additional trauma resulting from the use of a weak base or acid. Toxic oils should be removed with organic solvents or warm, soapy water. If the poison has been swallowed recently, it is advisable to remove it from the stomach as soon as possible to decrease chances of absorption. The simplest way, provided the patient is conscious and cooperative, is to persuade him to drink an excess of tepid water and induce vomiting. Other emetics can be used, but some of them must be used with caution. Tepid water with mustard (1 teaspoon to a glass), weak salt water, starch water, or weak soap solution can do little harm, although the mustard may accentuate the discomfort of raw mucous membranes. Copper sulfate is sometimes added to water and used as an emetic, especially for arsenic poisoning, but it has been known to kill infants when the excess cupric ion was not removed. Apomorphine, gr. $1/10$, can be given hypodermically. It acts promptly but tends to be depressing and hence is not widely used. The best emetic is probably the mildest and the one most readily available.

Use of the stomach tube to remove poisons can be hazardous. This is especially true if there is (1) danger of perforating a corroded esophagus or stomach, (2) danger of aspirating the poison, or (3) danger of precipitating a convulsive seizure such as might occur in strychnine poisoning.

Use of the stomach tube is sometimes preferable to the use of emetics, because the tube has greater efficiency in emptying the stomach and because less prostration is likely to follow its use than when the patient is made to vomit. However emetics are usually the treatment of choice.

First-aid measures for poisoning

The following recommendations on first-aid measures for poisoning have been adopted by the Committee on Toxicology. These recommendations are made in response to numerous requests to the American Medical Association for general instructions for poisoning emergencies. They are intended for use in educating the public in what to do when poisoning occurs.

Emergency telephone numbers:
POISON CONTROL CENTER . . . .
PHYSICIAN . . . . FIRE DEPT . . . .
HOSPITAL . . . . . . (resuscitator) . . . .
PHARMACIST . . . . POLICE . . . . . .
RESCUE SQUADS . . . .

The aim of first-aid measures is to help prevent absorption of the poison. SPEED is essential. First-aid measures must be started at once. If possible, one person should begin treatment while another calls a physician. When this is not possible, the nature of the poison will determine whether to call a physician first or begin first-aid measures and then notify a physician. Save the poison container and material itself if any remains. If the poison is not known, save a sample of the vomitus.

MEASURES TO BE TAKEN BEFORE ARRIVAL OF PHYSICIAN
I. Swallowed poisons

Many products used in and around the home, although not labeled "Poison," may be dangerous if taken internally. For example, some medications which are beneficial when used correctly may endanger life if used improperly or in excessive amounts.

In all cases, *except those indicated below,* REMOVE POISON FROM PATIENT'S STOMACH IMMEDIATELY by inducing vomiting. This cannot be overemphasized, for it is the essence of the treatment and is often a life-saving procedure. Prevent chilling by wrapping patient in blankets if necessary. Do not give alcohol in any form.
A. Do not induce vomiting if:
　1. Patient is in coma or unconscious.
　2. Patient is in convulsions.
　3. Patient has swallowed petroleum products (kerosene, gasoline, lighter fluid).
　4. Patient has swallowed a corrosive poison (symptoms: severe pain, burning sensation in

mouth and throat, vomiting). CALL PHYSICIAN IMMEDIATELY.
　(a) Acid and acid-like corrosives: sodium acid sulfate (toilet bowl cleaners), acetic acid (glacial), sulfuric acid, nitric acid, oxalic acid, hydrofluoric acid (rust removers), iodine, silver nitrate (styptic pencil).
　(b) Alkali corrosives: sodium hydroxide-lye (drain cleaners), sodium carbonate (washing soda), ammonia water, sodium hypochlorite (household bleach).

If the patient can swallow after ingesting a *corrosive poison,* the following substances (and amounts) may be given:
　For acids: milk, water, or milk of magnesia (1 tablespoon to 1 cup of water).
　For alkalies: milk, water, any fruit juice, or vinegar.
　For patient 1-5 years old—1 to 2 cups.
　For patient 5 years and older—up to 1 quart.
B. Induce vomiting when non-corrosive substances have been swallowed:
　1. Give milk or water (for patient 1-5 years old —1 to 2 cups; for patient over 5 years—up to 1 quart).
　2. Induce vomiting by placing the blunt end of a spoon or your finger at the back of the patient's throat, or by use of this emetic—2 tablespoons of salt in a glass of warm water.

When retching and vomiting begin, place patient face down with head lower than hips. This prevents vomitus from entering the lungs and causing further damage.

II. Inhaled poisons

　1. Carry patient (do not let him walk) to fresh air immediately.
　2. Open all doors and windows.
　3. Loosen all tight clothing.
　4. Apply artificial respiration if breathing has stopped or is irregular.

5. Prevent chilling (wrap patient in blankets).
6. Keep patient as quiet as possible.
7. If patient is convulsing, keep him in bed in a semidark room; avoid jarring or noise.
8. Do not give alcohol in any form.

III. Skin contamination

1. Drench skin with water (shower, hose, faucet).
2. Apply stream of water on skin while removing clothing.
3. Cleanse skin thoroughly with water; rapidity in washing is most important in reducing extent of injury.

IV. Eye contamination

1. Hold eyelids open, wash eyes with gentle stream of running water *immediately*. Delay of few seconds greatly increases extent of injury.
2. Continue washing until physician arrives.
3. *Do not use chemicals;* they may increase extent of injury.

V. Injected poisons (scorpion and snake bites)

1. Make patient lie down as soon as possible.
2. Do not give alcohol in any form.
3. Apply tourniquet above injection site (e.g., between arm or leg and heart). The pulse in vessels below the tourniquet should not disappear, nor should the tourniquet produce a throbbing sensation. Tourniquet should be loosened for 1 minute every 15 minutes.

4. Apply ice-pack to the site of the bite.
5. Carry patient to physician or hospital; DO NOT LET HIM WALK.

VI. Chemical burns

1. Wash with large quantities of running water (except those burns caused by phosphorus).
2. Immediately cover with loosely applied clean cloth.
3. Avoid use of ointments, greases, powders, and other drugs in first-aid treatment of burns.
4. Treat shock by keeping patient flat, keeping him warm, and reassuring him until arrival of physician.

MEASURES TO PREVENT POISONING ACCIDENTS

A. Keep all drugs, poisonous substances, and household chemicals out of the reach of children.
B. Do not store nonedible products on shelves used for storing food.
C. Keep all poisonous substances in their original containers; do not transfer to unlabeled containers or to food containers such as soft drink bottles.
D. When medicines are discarded, destroy them. Do not throw them where they might be reached by children or pets.
E. When giving flavored and/or brightly colored medicine to children, *always* refer to it as medicine— *never* as candy.
F. Do not take or give medicine in the dark.
G. READ LABELS before using chemical products.

ADMINISTRATION OF SUITABLE ANTIDOTE

After the stomach has been emptied, it is necessary to administer the proper antidote. An *antidote* is any agent used to counteract the action of a poison. There are three kinds of antidotes: (1) physical or mechanical, (2) chemical, and (3) physiologic.

A *physical antidote* is one that envelops or mixes with the poison and prevents its absorption, soothes and protects the tissues, and may aid in removal of the poison.

Demulcents, emollients, emetics, cathartics, and the stomach tube are used as physical antidotes.

Milk, white of egg, boiled starch or porridge, gruels, barley water, mashed potato, and mucilage of acacia are suitable demulcents. Fixed oils such as olive cottonseed, cod liver, or liquid petrolatum may be used, but in cases where the poison is soluble in the oil, like cantharides or phosphorus, the stomach should be emptied after giving the oil.

A *chemical antidote* is one that reacts with the poison and neutralizes it. Common salt (sodium chloride) is an excellent antidote for silver nitrate. The products formed, silver chloride and sodium nitrate, are both harmless. Magnesium oxide, milk of magnesia, or baking soda are chemical antidotes for acids. In general, it should be remembered that alkalies counteract acids and vice versa. Care should be used when sodium bicarbonate is given, because if too much gas results from the reaction, the pressure may rupture the corroded stomach. For this reason, milk of magnesia or calcium carbonate may be preferable. Lemon juice, grapefruit juice, and vinegar are suitable weak acids to neutralize strong bases. Poisoning with irritant metallic salts is best treated with albumin in the form of egg white, since an insoluble albuminate is formed. The antidote for the vegetable alkaloids such as morphine, atropine, or strychnine is tannic acid or potassium permanganate. Both the tannic acid and the potassium permanganate (1:2000) may be used to wash out the patient's stomach. Tannic acid can be obtained from strong green tea; it brings about precipitation of alkaloids while potassium permanganate causes oxidation of alkaloids.

Chemical antidotes act only on such portions of the poison as have not been absorbed, and they must be given promptly. They are frequently added to the lavage solution.

A *physiologic antidote* is one that produces the opposite systemic effects from that of the poison. If a person has taken or been given too much pilocarpine, the sweating is readily counteracted by the hypodermic use of atropine (gr. $\frac{1}{60}$ to $\frac{1}{30}$). Morphine has specific antidotes (naloxone); strychnine poisoning is treated with diazepam or a barbiturate.

ANTIDOTE KIT

The following materials have been suggested to cope with poison emergencies. Others may be added (see Table 32-2). A nurse is often responsible for maintaining supplies and for seeing that all labels are clearly legible. However, the pharmacist should relabel all medications.

Activated charcoal
Alcohol
Amyl nitrite
Apomorphine tablets, 2 mg.
Aromatic spirit of ammonia
Atropine tablets (1 mg.) and parenteral form
Benadryl
Bicarbonate of sodium
Caffeine-sodium benzoate
Calcium disodium edetate (CaEDTA)
Calcium gluconate, 10%, ampules
Chloroform
Cupric sulfate, powdered
Dextrose, 50%, ampules
Dimercaprol
Epinephrine tablets, 1 mg.
Ephedrine hydrochloride, 16-mg. tablets
Limewater
Magnesia, calcined
Methylene blue, 50 ml., 1% in 1.8% sodium sulfate
Morphine sulfate tablets, 10 mg.
Nalorphine, 10 mg. in two ampules
Naloxone
Nitrite of sodium, 2%, 10-ml. ampules
Oxygen
Olive oil
Pralidoxime chloride
Penicillamine
Pentobarbital sodium, 0.5-Gm. ampules
Potassium permanganate, 1% solution, to be diluted twenty times
Thiosulfate of sodium, 30%, 10-ml. ampules
Tincture of iodine
Vasopressors
Whiskey

A hypodermic syringe and a stomach tube with a funnel should be available. The following usually can be secured at the home of the patient: boiled water, hot strong black coffee, eggs, milk, mustard, salt, starch, tea, and vinegar.

Activated charcoal, U.S.P. (Medicinal charcoal, active carbon)

Activated charcoal is a fine, black, odorless, tasteless, nongritty powder. Special treatment is required to activate the surface of charcoal to increase its absorptive power. The charcoal may be activated by treating it at high temperatures

Table 32-2 Some specific poisons, symptoms, and emergency treatment

Poison	Symptoms	Treatment
Acids (such as hydrochloric or nitric)	Parts in contact with acid are first white, later colored (brown or yellow) Pain in throat, esophagus, and stomach; dysphagia, diarrhea, shock, circulatory collapse Death may result from asphyxia from edema of glottis	Avoid stomach tube, emesis, and solutions of carbonate, such as sodium bicarbonate Give milk of magnesia, aluminum hydroxide, mild soap solution, plenty of milk or water with egg white Copious amounts of water Keep patient warm and quiet Corticosteroids to reduce fibrosis and possibility of esophageal stricture
Arsenic (found in weed killers, insecticides, sheepdip rodenticides, and so on)	Rapidity of onset of symptoms related to whether or not poison is taken with food Odor of garlic on breath and stools Faintness, nausea, difficulty in swallowing, extreme thirst, severe vomiting, gastric pain, "rice water" stools, oliguria, albuminuria, cold, clammy skin Collapse and death	Give 0.5 to 10 Gm. of activated charcoal in a glass of water followed by repeated lavage with warm or weak sodium bicarbonate solution or by an emetic (warm water, salt water, or mustard water) repeated until vomiting occurs Intravenous fluids Sedation, analgesics Dimercaprol (BAL) is the antidote of choice (see p. 705) Keep patient warm

Bromides	*Acute poisoning*
	  Deep stupor
	  Ataxia
	  Extreme muscular weakness
	  Collapse
	Chronic poisoning (bromism)
	  Bromide acne is seen on face, chest, and back
	  Salty taste in mouth
	  Foul breath
	  Gastrointestinal disturbance
	  Mental depression
	  Faulty memory
	  Pronounced apathy
	  Ataxia—slurred speech
	  Muscular weakness
	  Malnutrition
	  Anemia
		Stop the drug
		Large doses of physiologic salt solutions are given to hasten excretion of drug
		As a rule, symptoms of bromism rapidly abate if drug is withdrawn
		Diuretics are given to hasten excretion of the drug

Carbon monoxide (present in coal gas, illuminating gas, exhaust gas from motor cars, and so on)	Symptoms vary with concentration of carbon monoxide in blood Headache, dizziness, impaired hearing and vision, drowsiness, confusion, loss of consciousness Slow respiration, rapid pulse Coma, cherry-red lips and nails	Remove patient to fresh air; artificial respiration; high concentration of oxygen preferably under positive pressure Bed rest for 48 hours Keep patient warm

Continued.

Table 32-2 Some specific poisons, symptoms, and emergency treatment—cont'd

Poison	Symptoms	Treatment
Carbon tetrachloride (found in some dry-cleaning fluids and in some home fire extinguishers)	*When inhaled:* headache, nausea, vomiting, diarrhea, jaundice, oliguria, albuminuria, dark-colored urine *When swallowed:* headache, nausea, vomiting, sometimes blood in vomitus, abdominal pain, disturbance of hearing and vision, jaundice, profuse diarrhea, albuminuria, anuria	Remove patient from poisoned atmosphere; administer oxygen or oxygen with carbon dioxide Simple emetics to produce repeated vomiting if lavage not available; if possible, lavage followed by saline cathartic High-protein, high-carbohydrate, high-calcium diet General supportive measures
Chlorophenothane (dichlorodiphenyl-trichloroethane, or D.D.T.)	Headache, nausea, vomiting, diarrhea, paresthesias of lips and tongue, numbness of extremities, malaise, sore throat Coarse tremor, convulsions, respiratory failure	Induce vomiting or use gastric lavage if convulsions do not threaten Give saline cathartic, force fluids, give strong tea or coffee Avoid fats, fat solvents, and epinephrine Wash contaminated skin areas with soap and water
Cyanides	An odor of oil of bitter almonds on breath; headache, rapid breathing, dyspnea, palpitation of heart, feeling of tightness in chest, cyanosis, convulsions Death may come within few minutes	Prompt treatment sometimes successful Amyl nitrite (several pearls broken into gauze and given by inhalation), followed by 1% sodium nitrite intravenously slowly, in 10-ml. doses, to a total of 50 ml. in an hour, and this followed by slow intravenous administration of sodium thiosulfate (50 ml. of a 25% solution) Oxygen, artificial respiration, and blood transfusion may be indicated
Fluoride (found in insecticides)	Nausea, vomiting, abdominal pain, diarrhea, muscle weakness, difficult swallowing, facial paralysis, inability to speak, convulsions at times, respiratory failure and circulatory collapse	Give emetic containing soluble calcium salts (calcium lactate or gluconate) or use plenty of warm water and follow with plenty of milk Preferable to lavage promptly with 1% calcium chloride to inactivate fluoride General supportive measures
Hydrocarbons (present in kerosene, gasoline, naphtha, cleaning fluids, insecticides)	Symptoms of intoxication similar to those of alcohol; burning sensation in mouth, esophagus, and stomach Vomiting, dizziness, tremor, muscle cramps, confusion, fever Cold, clammy skin, weak pulse, thirst, unconsciousness, coma Death from respiratory failure	Emetics and lavage usually avoided unless large amounts swallowed; saline cathartics after small amounts taken Some authorities recommend large doses of mineral oil for severe poisoning, followed by lavage with 1% or 2% sodium bicarbonate solution General supportive measures
Iodine	Brown-stained lips, tongue, and mouth, which are painful Odor of iodine in vomitus Intense thirst, fainting attacks, giddiness, vomiting, burning, abdominal pain, diarrhea, shock	Give plenty of water promptly, with starch or flour or mashed potatoes Gastric lavage if possible with thin, cooked suspension of starch or 5% sodium thiosulfite solution Give drinks of milk or white of egg, with water

Table 32-2 Some specific poisons, symptoms, and emergency treatment—cont'd

Poison	Symptoms	Treatment
Lye (a severe caustic)	Severe burning pain in mouth, throat, and stomach Strong soapy taste in mouth Early violent vomiting with mucus and blood in vomitus Mucous membranes become white and swollen; lips and tongue swell; throat may become constricted Respirations difficult Skin cold and clammy Pulse rapid Violent purging Great anxiety	Emetics and lavage frequently not recommended Give large amounts of water containing weak acids, lemon, vinegar, lime juice, and so on; later give demulcents, white of egg, gruel, olive oil or salad oil Analgesics, parenteral fluids Corticosteroids
Mercury and its compounds	Burning sensation of throat Nausea and vomiting (vomitus blue if antiseptic tablets of bichloride used) Sense of constriction in throat and esophagus Ashen-gray color of mucous membranes that have been in contact with poison Bloody, profuse diarrhea, with shreds of mucous membrane in stool and vomitus Shock, albuminuria, and hematuria During acute phase, pain and prostration; late, progressive uremia	Give 0.5 to 10 Gm. of activated charcoal in a glass of water and then lavage with 5% sodium formaldehyde sulfoxylate solution followed by sodium bicarbonate solution If not feasible, give emetic of mustard water or salt water until vomiting has occurred repeatedly Give milk and egg white in water Dimercaprol indicated as specific antidote (see p. 705) Parenteral fluids Keep patient warm Recovery depends on dose taken, amount of absorption, and amount of kidney damage
Nicotine (Black Leaf 40 contains about 40% nicotine sulfate)	Burning sensation in mouth and throat, increased flow of saliva, abdominal pain, vomiting, diarrhea, headache, sweating, confusion, weakness, dilation of pupils, faintness, death from respiratory paralysis	Activated charcoal, 10 to 30 Gm. in a glass of water; lavage with 0.5% tannic acid or 1:5000 potassium permanganate Artificial respirations Wash contaminated skin with cold water
Paris green (copper arsenite and copper acetate)	Vomiting of green material followed by gastric and abdominal pain; diarrhea with dark and sometimes bloody stools; metallic taste; neuromuscular weakness Thirst, oliguria, anuria Cold, clammy skin Coma, convulsions, death	Potassium ferrocyanide, gr. 10 in water as soon as possible (forms an insoluble salt of copper), followed by lavage with sodium bicarbonate solution or a mustard-water emetic until stomach cleansed Demulcents (milk, egg white in water, gelatin) Supportive measures
Phenolic compounds (carbolic acid, cresol, Lysol, creosote)	Corrosion of mucous membranes that have come in contact with poison Severe pain, vomiting, bloody diarrhea, headache, dizziness Cold, clammy skin Oliguria, hematuria, unconsciousness, slow respiration, respiratory failure Urine dark and turns very dark on exposure to air	Of utmost importance to remove poison before absorption, prompt lavage with olive oil (a good solvent); leave some oil in stomach after lavage; give egg white and milk for demulcent effect Parenteral fluids, oxygen, carbon dioxide, analgesics Other supportive measures Phenol on skin can be removed with 50% solution of alcohol, followed by thorough rinsing with water, or wash external burns with olive oil or castor oil

Continued.

Table 32-2 Some specific poisons, symptoms, and emergency treatment—cont'd

Poison	Symptoms	Treatment
Strychnine (symptoms occur within 15 or 20 min. after drug has been taken)	Feeling of stiffness in muscles of face and neck Twitching of face and limbs Violent convulsions of whole body, at intervals varying from a few minutes to an hour Death may result from asphyxia caused by spasm of respiratory muscles or during period of relaxation from respiratory paralysis	Administer diazepam If diazepam is not available barbiturates, chloroform, paraldehyde, or tribromethanol are recommended Gastric lavage may be done with solutions of potassium permanganate 1:1000 or 2% tannic acid After convulsions have been checked, chloral hydrate or phenobarbital may be needed to prevent convulsions from returning During treatment patient should be in cool, quiet room and protected from sudden noise, jarring, or change of any kind that might precipitate another seizure
Quaternary ammonium compounds (such as Zephiran)	Burning pain in the mouth and throat, nausea and vomiting, apprehension and restlessness; muscle weakness, collapse, coma, sometimes convulsions	Induce vomiting or use gastric lavage if it can be done promptly; mild soap solution will serve as antidote for unabsorbed portions Give cathartic

with steam and carbon dioxide or with dehydrating substances like sulfuric acid, phosphoric acid, zinc chloride, or a combination of these. For medicinal purposes the charcoal must be thoroughly washed to remove inorganic matter. The surface area of 1 ml. of finely divided charcoal is estimated to be 1000 square meters.

Activated charcoal absorbs a large variety of substances both simple and complex. It is used as an adjunct in the treatment of oral poisonings caused by ingestion of heavy metals, mercuric chloride, strychnine, phenol, atropine, phenolphthalein, oxalic acid, poison mushrooms, aspirin, and most drugs. It is not effective for cyanide poisoning.

For emergency treatment, from 0.5 to 10 Gm. of the powder is stirred into a glass of water to be taken orally by the patient or to be passed through an orogastric tube. Some clinicians claim that 5 to 10 times the estimated amount of the ingested substance should be given; if the amount ingested is unknown, 15 to 30 Gm. of the charcoal may be used. The mixture should be removed from the stomach shortly afterwards by inducing vomiting or via the gastric tube.

Ipecac syrup, U.S.P.; ipecacuanha, B.P.

Ipecac is obtained from the dried roots of the ipecacuahna or acuminata plants native to Central and South America. It has a long history of use as a medicinal agent by the Indians of South America. It was introduced into Europe as a treatment for dysentery. Its chief use in the United States today is as an emetic to induce vomiting in cases of ingested noncorrosive poisons.

Ipecac probably acts both centrally and locally; it directly stimulates the vomiting center and it has an irritant effect on gastric mucosa. Usual dose for adults and children is 15 to 20 ml. followed by 200 to 300 ml. of water, milk, or fruit juice, or as much fluid as the patient can drink. Vomiting usually occurs in 15 to 30 minutes. Dose may be repeated once after 20 minutes if the first dose is not effective.

Syrup of ipecac is available without a prescription in 1-ounce bottles bearing the following instructions:

1 For emergency use to cause vomiting in poisoning. Before using call physician, Poison Control Center, or hospital emergency room immediately for advice.

2 Warning—Keep out of reach of children. Do not use if strychnine, corrosives such as alkalies (lye) and strong acids, or petroleum distillates such as kerosene, gasoline, fuel oil, coal oil, paint thinner, or cleaning fluid have been ingested.

3 Usual dosage is 1 tablespoon (15 ml.) in persons over 1 year of age.

It is recommended that syrup of ipecac be kept in every home, particularly where there are children. Ipecac syrup should not be confused with ipecac fluidextract, which is fourteen times more concentrated and which has been responsible for a number of deaths.

Ipecac syrup should not be used if the patient has ingested corrosives or caustic substances, since the vomitus may further injure the esophagus. Activated charcoal should not be given with syrup of ipecac since the charcoal will adsorb the ipecac nullifying its effects. The charcoal can be given *after* vomiting or gastric emptying has occurred.

If the patient is conscious, drug induced vomiting is usually preferable to gastric lavage, particularly in children, since aspiration of vomitus is less likely to occur. Nurses should employ the necessary measures to reduce the likelihood of aspiration of vomitus (proper positioning of patient). Induction of vomiting may be facilitated by stimulating the pharynx.

HEAVY METAL ANTAGONISTS

Dimercaprol is a highly effective antidote to arsenic, gold, or mercury poisoning; other antidotes are very useful for the treatment of some other intoxications caused by heavy metals. Most important are calcium disodium edetate and penicillamine.

Dimercaprol, U.S.P., B.P. (BAL)

$$
\begin{array}{c}
\text{H} \\
| \\
\text{HS—C—H} \\
| \\
\text{HS—C—H} \\
| \\
\text{HO—C—H} \\
| \\
\text{H}
\end{array}
$$

Dimercaprol was developed during World War II as an antidote for the arsenic-containing blister gas, Lewisite; hence, the name "BAL"

for "British Anti-Lewisite." It was used to decontaminate the skin and eyes of persons who had been in contact with the gas, but later it was found to be of value in treatment of various forms of arsenic poisoning.

Dimercaprol is a colorless liquid with a rather offensive odor. It is dispensed in 10% solution in peanut oil for intramuscular injection. One milliliter contains 100 mg. of dimercaprol.

Arsenic compounds produce their toxic effects by combining with the sulfhydryl groups of enzymes, which are necessary for normal metabolism. As a result, the processes of oxidation and reduction in the tissues are seriously hindered. BAL interferes with this combination, forms a stable combination with the arsenic, neutralizes its toxic effects, and hastens its excretion.

BAL is also indicated in the treatment of gold and mercury poisoning. Treatment should begin as soon as possible after poisoning has occurred. In mercury poisoning, if treatment does not occur within 2 hours, irreversible, extensive renal damage may occur.

Results in the treatment of poisoning from other heavy metals are disappointing or inconclusive. It may be used as an adjunct in treating lead and copper toxicity. Although the toxicity of BAL is less among patients suffering from arsenic, gold, or mercury poisoning than among persons in normal condition, doses of 300 mg. may cause nausea and vomiting, headache, a burning sensation of the mouth, throat, and eyes, a constricting sensation in the chest, muscular aching, and tingling in the extremities. This drug can also cause blood pressure elevation, capillary damage, and a condition resembling diabetic acidosis. In high doses coma and convulsions may occur. Hypersensitivity reactions are common. BAL is a potentially dangerous drug and is potentially nephrotoxic.

In the treatment of arsenic or gold poisoning, the dose is 2.5 to 5 mg. of dimercaprol per kilogram of body weight, given intramuscularly four times daily the first 2 days, reduced to two injections on the third day, and then daily for the next 10 days. In mild cases the dose may be reduced. In mercury poisoning the dosage is sometimes increased.

After intramuscular injection, maximum con-

Table 32-3 Poisonings treatable with dialysis

Ethylene glycol (contained in antifreeze preparations)
Heavy metals
Methyl alcohol
Mushroom poisoning

Dialyzable drug poisoning

Alcohol	Bromide	Paraldehyde
Ammonia	Calcium	Potassium
Amphetamines	Chloral hydrate	Quinidine
Anilines	Fluoride	Quinine
Antibiotics	Iodide	Salicylates
Barbiturates	Isoniazid	Strychnine
Boric acid	Meprobamate	Thiocyanate

centrations in the plasma occur in 2 hours; in 4 hours this is decreased to one half the maximum concentration. The drug is excreted or metabolized in 6 to 24 hours.

D.E.S.I. rating is *effective* for treatment of arsenic, gold, and mercury poisoning, and for treating acute lead poisoning when used with calcium disodium edetate.

Its use is contraindicated in hepatic insufficiency except for postarsenical jaundice.

Edetate calcium disodium, U.S.P. (Calcium Disodium Versenate, CaEDTA)

$$Na-O-\overset{\overset{\displaystyle O}{\|}}{C}-H_2C \quad CH_2-CH_2 \quad CH_2-\overset{\overset{\displaystyle O}{\|}}{C}-O-Na$$

Calcium disodium edetate (CaEDTA) is most useful in the treatment of lead poisoning. It combines with the heavy metal in the body and favors its renal excretion.

Calcium disodium edetate is available as a 20% solution for injection and in tablets containing 500 mg. It has a half-life of 20 to 60 minutes; about 50% is excreted in the urine in 1 hour and 95% in 24 hours. Thus adequate kidney function is vital during therapy.

For the treatment of lead poisoning the drug is administered by slow intravenous infusion over a period of 3 to 4 hours. One gram is added to 250 or 500 ml. of 5% dextrose in water or

to isotonic saline. Infusions may be given twice a day for 3 to 5 days. Dosage for children should be kept below 1 Gm. per 30 pounds of body weight. The drug is given in 5-day courses with a 2-day rest period between courses. Daily urinalysis should be done and dosage reduced if there is indication of renal impairment.

The drug may also be injected intramuscularly, but a local anesthetic may have to be added to the solution in order to decrease pain at the site of injection. In mild cases calcium disodium edetate may be administered orally; the usual dose for adults is 4 Gm. a day. However, the oral route is not recommended by the A.M.A. since the drug is poorly absorbed from the gastrointestinal tract. In addition, if lead is present in the gut, its absorption may be increased because the lead chelate formed is more soluble than the lead itself, and a breakdown in the lead chelate complex will release free lead. Lead should be evacuated from the gastrointestinal tract prior to treatment with CaEDTA.

Urinary excretion should be monitored during use of this drug. When the urine returns to non-toxic levels, the CaEDTA therapy should be terminated. If there is indication of renal impairment, dosage should be reduced or discontinued; if urinary excretion is not adequate, hemodialysis may be necessary.

CaEDTA is also used diagnostically in cases of suspected lead poisoning. If the 24-hour urinary excretion of lead is 500 μg. or more per liter following administration of the drug, a diagnosis of poisoning may be made before clinical symptoms and irreversible damage occur.

D.E.S.I. rating is *effective* for reduction of blood and depot lead in acute and chronic lead poisoning and lead encephalopathy; *probably effective* for the treatment of other heavy metal poisonings and in the removal of radioactive and nuclear fission products such as plutonium.

It is important not to confuse this drug with the *tri*sodium salt of ethylenediamine tetraacetic acid, the administration of which would be extremely dangerous.

Adverse effects. If more than the recommended dosage is used, renal damage may occur. particularly in children. Symptoms of acute lead poisoning, particularly cerebral symptoms, may be aggravated at the beginning of therapy. If this happens, dosage should be reduced.

Malaise, excessive thirst, paresthesias, sudden fever and shaking chills, headache, nausea and vomiting, and lacrimation may occur 4 to 8 hours after infusion of the drug.

Penicillamine, U.S.P., B.P. (Cuprimine)

Penicillamine is used to treat poisoning caused by copper and for removing copper from the body in hepatolenticular degeneration (Wilson's disease). It may also be used as a chelator of lead, iron, and mercury. It is derived from the degradation of penicillin, but it has no antibacterial activity.

The recommended dose of penicillamine is 250 mg. four times a day by mouth. Dosage for adults may be increased to 4 or 5 Gm. daily. The drug should be given on an empty stomach between meals and at bedtime to avoid interference with dietary metals. For children and infants over 6 months of age, daily dose is 250 mg. dissolved in fruit juice. Dosage must be individualized by determining the urinary excretion of copper.

Adverse effects. Rashes, blood dyscrasias, and possibly renal damage may occur following the use of penicillamine. The drug is relatively safe, however, and adverse effects do not occur frequently. Patients should be carefully observed for hypersensitivity reactions. Urinalysis and blood examinations should be performed every 3 days for the first 2 weeks of therapy and then every 10 days for the next 3 or 4 months.

Deferoxamine binds iron and promotes its excretion. As a consequence, it is useful in the treatment of iron poisoning and in diseases such as hemochromatosis in which there is a chronic accumulation of iron in the body. The complex formed when deferoxamine is combined with iron is a reddish color. Since the complex is excreted via the urinary tract, the urine of patients treated with this drug will be reddish brown. The drug seems to have little effect on hemoglobin levels.

Deferoxamine is well tolerated, and adverse effects are infrequent. Mild rash or pruritus may occur. Rapid intravenous injection may cause hypotension, tachycardia, erythema, and urticaria. Pain and tissue irritation may occur at the injection site. Patients on long-term therapy have reported allergic type reactions, blurred vision, fever, diarrhea, and leg cramps. Cataracts have been reported after prolonged deferoxamine therapy but not after short-term therapy.

Intramuscular and intravenous dose for adults and children is 1 Gm. initially followed by 0.5 Gm., which may be given every 4 to 12 hours. Total dosage should not exceed 6 Gm. in 24 hours. Intravenous dose should be given by slow infusion. The subcutaneous route should not be used since severe tissue irritation and damage may occur. In cases of acute iron poisoning several grams may be given by stomach tube followed by intravenous medication.

ORGANOPHOSPHORUS INSECTICIDE ANTIDOTES

Many organophosphorus insecticides, as well as some therapeutic agents, are highly toxic because they inactivate cholinesterase in the body. Atropine is an important antidote for poisoning caused by anticholinesterase drugs. Another antidote, pralidoxime chloride, U.S.P. (Protopam), has been developed that actually reactivates the cholinesterase enzymes in the body when they

Deferoxamine (Desferal)

are inhibited by the organophosphorus compounds, thereby removing the block at the myoneural junction. Since many widely used insecticides owe their toxicity to the fact that they combine with cholinesterase drugs, knowledge of antidotes for such poisonings is important.

Along with atropine, pralidoxime is useful for the treatment of poisoning by anticholinesterase drugs and organophosphorus pesticides.

Pralidoxime chloride is administered intravenously in a dosage of 1 Gm. perferably in 100 ml. of sodium chloride solution and infused over a period of 15 to 30 minutes or injected at a rate not exceeding 200 mg. per minute, which is repeated in 8 to 12 hours as needed. Pediatric dose is 250 mg. intravenously, which may be repeated every 8 to 12 hours. In the absence of gastrointestinal symptoms the drug may be given orally, 1 to 3 Gm. every 3 to 5 hours.

PROMOTION OF ELIMINATION

Promotion of elimination may be accomplished by the use of certain cathartics, such as saline cathartics or castor oil, or by rectal irrigation. After gastric lavage 1 ounce of 50% magnesium sulfate may be left in the stomach, followed by administration of copious amounts of water. Magnesium sulfate helps to cleanse the lower part of the bowel. In case of anuria, the artificial kidney may be life saving.

SUPPORTIVE CARE OF THE PATIENT

Sometimes the greatest need of the patient is met by giving artificial respiration. Shock is an important factor to be considered. Intravenous administration of physiologic saline or glucose solution is important to maintain adequate circulation and to replace fluid that may be lost by diarrhea or vomiting from gastrointestinal irritation. Attention to fluid needs may also help to conserve kidney and liver function, particularly in the presence of certain poisons. At times depressant drugs are indicated, at other times stimulants. Often attention must be given to keeping the patient warm and, if stuporous or comatose, to seeing that his position is changed periodically to prevent hypostatic pneumonia.

Moral support of the patient and his family is always an important aspect of nursing care.

POISONOUS FOODS

Many foods, because of their content of inherently poisonous chemicals (mushrooms and other fungi) or the presence of bacterial exotoxins, produce symptoms of poisoning when eaten. The symptoms are diverse, but intense gastrointestinal irritation is common to all of them, and they may therefore be appropriately classed as irritants. Mushroom poisoning arises through mistaking various fungi, such as poisonous mushrooms, toadstools, and truffles, for edible varieties. The toxin of some of these plants is muscarine, a deadly alkaloidal poison that causes violent vomiting, colic, thirst, dyspnea, paralysis, and death. (Atropine is the antidote.) Many of the cases of food poisoning seen especially in the warm season of the year are caused by soluble exotoxins that result from bacterial contamination of food. Foods that seem prone to cause symptoms of poisoning are corned beef, sausage, pickled or decaying fish, shellfish, ham, home-canned vegetables, salads, whipped cream, and custards. Poisoning is more likely to occur, especially from salads, whipped cream, and custards, when large amounts are made at one time and are improperly prepared and refrigerated. The treatment of food poisoning, from whatever cause, is prompt evacuation of the stomach, preferably by stomach tube. In the process of this evacuation plenty of water is used and tannic acid or strong tea is administered; a large dose of magnesium sulfate or castor oil is given to empty the bowel and prevent absorption. Morphine may be given for abdominal pain, and stimulants may be indicated if there is prostration.

QUESTIONS

For study and review

Circle the answer of your choice.
1 Which of the following conditions would lead you to suspect acute poisoning?
   a. gradual loss of weight
   b. anorexia, undue lassitude
   c. onset of sudden violent symptoms
   d. weakness, anemia, headache
2 Which of the following factors is likely to be the crucial one in the successful treatment of early and acute poisoning?

a. amount of supportive treatment
b. immediate removal of poison from the body
c. control of shock
d. administration of the right antidote

3 Which of the following kinds of antidotes are represented when sodium chloride solution is used in the treatment of silver nitrate poisoning?
a. chemical
b. physical
c. universal
d. physiologic

4 If you were working in the chemistry laboratory and splashed some hydrochloric acid in your eye, what is the first thing you would do?
a. rush to the emergency room or health center
b. search for a weak base and instill some in your eye
c. neutralize the acid with solution of sodium hydroxide
d. wash eye with copious amounts of plain water

5 BAL (British Anti-Lewisite) is a recommended antidote for poisoning from:
a. hydrocarbons
b. strong acids
c. phenolic compounds
d. certain heavy metals

6 Death from carbon monoxide is likely to be caused by:
a. changes in bone marrow
b. damage to liver and kidney
c. depression of heart
d. anoxia

7 Death from a poison like methyl alcohol is likely to result from:
a. destruction in the kidney
b. perforation, hemorrhage, or both
c. acidosis
d. depression of the respiratory center

8 Which of the following kinds of foods are least likely to be a source of bacterial contamination and food poisoning?
a. lobster salad
b. boiled dinner of cabbage, meat, and potatoes
c. chicken salad, Boston cream pie
d. ham sandwiches, iced tea

9 Which of the following statements best explains why children are often poisoned by medicines left around the house?
a. children are naturally curious about things
b. children mistake sweet-tasting tablets or pills for candy
c. children like to explore new things with their mouths
d. children like to imitate other members of the household

10 Which of the following would you do if present at the scene of a poisoning and the patient had been vomiting?
a. note odor and color of the vomitus before flushing down the toilet
b. save a specimen of vomitus and add a preservative if possible
c. save a specimen of vomitus (an early one if possible) for the doctor
d. discard emesis as fast as possible to avoid offense to the patient

REFERENCES

Arena, J. M.: The clinical diagnosis of poisoning, Pediat. Clin. North Am. **17:**477, 1970.
Arena, J. M.: Treatment of some common household poisonings, Pharmacol. Phys. **3**(9):1, 1969.
Arena, J. M.: Poisoning: Toxicology, symptoms and treatment, ed. 2, Springfield, Ill., 1970, Charles C Thomas, Publisher.
Cashman, T. M., and Shirley, H. C.: Emergency management of poisoning, Pediat. Clin. North Am. **17:**525, 1970.
Castell, D. O., and Morrison, C. C.: Common adult poisons, Res. Phys. **13:**66, 1967.
Dimijian, G. G., and Radelat, F. A.: Evaluation and treatment of the suspected drug user in the emergency room, Arch. Intern. Med. **125:**162, 1970.
Dove, A. K.: Pharmacologic principles in the treatment of poisoning, Pharmacol. Phys. **3**(7):1, 1969.
Dove, A. K.: Poisoning from common household products, Pediat. Clin. North Am. **17:**569, 1970.
Driesbach, R. H.: Handbook of poisoning: Diagnosis and treatment, ed. 8, Los Altos, Calif., 1974, Lange Medical Publications.
Joselow, M. M., Louria, D. B., and Brawder, A. A.: Mercurialism: Environmental and occupational aspects, Ann. Intern. Med. **76:**119, 1972.
Lawrence, R. A., and Haggerty, R. J.: Household agents and their potential toxicity, Mod. Treatm. **8:**511, 1971.
Leape, L. L., and others: Hazards, to health—liquid lye, New Eng. J. Med. **284:**578, 1971.
Locket, S.: Haemodialysis in the treatment of acute poisoning, Proc. Roy. Soc. Med. **63:**427, 1970.
Maher, J. F.: Nephrotoxicity of drugs and chemicals, Pharmacol. Phys. **4:**1, 1970.
Mann, J. B., and Sandberg, D. H.: Therapy of sedative overdosage, Pediat. Clin. North Am. **17:**617, 1970.
Matthew, H.: Acute poisoning: Some myths and misconceptions, Br. Med. J. **1:**519, 1971.
Matthew, H.: Gastric aspiration and lavage, Clin. Toxic. **3:**179, 1970.
Matthew, H., and Lawson, A. A. H.: Treatment of common acute poisonings, ed. 2, Edinburgh, 1972, Churchill Livingstone.
Murphy, J. V.: Intoxication following the ingestion of elemental zinc, J.A.M.A. **212:**2119, 1970.
Rodman, M. J.: Poisoning treatment and prevention, R. N. **35:**51, 1972.
Schreiner, G. E.: Dialysis of poisons and drugs—annual review, Trans. Am. Soc. Artif. Intern. Organs **16:**544, 1970.
Sjogvist, F., and Alvan, G.: Pharmacological principles in the management of accidental poisoning, Pediat. Clin. North Am. **17:**495, 1970.
Stracener, C. E., and Scherz, R. G.: Experiences with safety containers for prevention of accidental childhood poisoning, Northwest Med. **63:**334, 1970.

Index

Tensilon Chloride; *see* Edrophonium chloride
Tension
 meprobamate for, 302
 phenobarbital for, 249
 premenstrual, fluid retention in,
  chlorothiazide for, 449
Tents
 face, for administration of oxygen, 387
 oxygen, 387
Tenuate; *see* Diethylpropion hydrochloride
Tepanil; *see* Diethylpropion hydrochloride
Terbutaline sulfate as bronchodilators,
  392-393
Terpin hydrate
 and codeine elixir, 222
 as expectorant, 400-401
Terramycin; *see* Oxytetracycline
  hydrochloride
Tessalon; *see* Benzonatate
Testes
 carcinoma of
  bleomycin for, 543
  embryonal, vinblastine sulfate for, 544
  embryonal cell, mithramycin for, 543
  methotrexate for, 541
  tumors of, dactinomycin for, 543
Testicle, undescended, pituitary gonadotropic
  hormones for, 592
Testosterone
 dosage and administration of, 607
 structural formula for, 606
Testosterone cypionate, 607
Testosterone enanthate, 607
Testosterone propionate, 607
Tetanus
 chlorpromazine hydrochloride for, 288
 control of convulsive seizures in
  barbiturates for, 246
  ether for, 340
  sodium pentobarbital injection for, 251
 and gas gangrene antitoxins, 527
 paraldehyde for, 254
Tetanus antitoxin, 526-527
Tetanus immune globulin, human, 527
Tetanus toxoid, 532
 adsorbed, 532-533
Tetanus vaccine, 532
Tetany
 hypocalcemic, calcium gluconate for, 415
 due to parathyroid hormone deficiency,
  554
 uterine, magnesium sulfate for, 591
Tetracaine hydrochloride
 as local anesthetic, 357-358
 for ocular anesthesia, 656
 properties of, 359
Tetrachloroethylene for hookworm, 502-503
Tetracin; *see* Tetracycline hydrochloride
Tetracycline hydrochloride
 dosage of, 476
 structural formula for, 475
Tetracyclines, 475-477
 drug interactions with, 461, 462
 for infections of bowel, 690
 for ocular infections, 654
Tetrahydrocannabinol as active ingredient in
  cannabis drugs, 318-319
Tetraiodothyronine; *see* Thyroxine
Tetranitrol; *see* Erythrityl tetranitrate
Thalamus
 action of drugs on, 212
 anatomy and physiology of, 278
Theelin; *see* Estrone

Theobroma oil as emollient, 660
Theobromine
 as central nervous system stimulants, 267
 as diuretic, 451
Theophylline
 as bronchodilator, 393
 as central nervous system stimulants, 267
 as diuretic, structural formula and action
  of, 451
 use of, with mercurial diuretics, 445
Theophylline Ethylenediamine; *see*
  Aminophylline
Therapies, supplementary, discovery and use
  of, 12-13
Thiabendazole as anthelmintic, 503-504
Thiamine, 431-433
Thiamine hydrochloride, 431, 433
Thiamine mononitrate, 433
Thiazides
 as diuretics, 447-450
 for hypertension, 183-184
 therapy with, hypercalcemia due to, 423
 urinary excretion of, 451
Thimecil; *see* Methylthiouracil
Thimerosal as antiinfective, 516
Thioguanine for neoplastic disease, 542
Thiopental as preanesthetic agent, 335
Thiopental sodium as intravenous anesthetic,
  346-347
Thiopentone as intravenous anesthetic,
  346-347
Thiopentone sodium, dosage, administration,
  and length of action of, 247
Thiopropazate, frequency of extrapyramidal
  symptoms from, 286
Thiopropazate hydrochloride as major
  tranquilizer, 287, 292
Thioridazine, frequency of extrapyramidal
  symptoms from, 286
Thioridazine hydrochloride as major
  tranquilizer, 287, 289-290
Thiotepa for neoplastic disease, 540
Thiothixene
 as major tranquilizer, 293
 frequency of extrapyramidal symptoms
  from, 286
Thioxanthene derivatives as major
  tranquilizers, 293-294
Thorazine Hydrochloride; *see*
  Chlorpromazine hydrochloride
Threadworms, thiabendazole for, 503-504
Threshold potential, 150
Throat, infections of, lincomycin for, 486
Thrombin
 for control of capillary bleeding, 196
 for shock therapy, 194
Thromboangiitis obliterans, nicotinyl tartrate
  for, 172
Thrombocytopenia
 due to chloramphenicol, 485
 due to cytarabine, 543
 due to mechlorethamine hydrochloride,
  537
 due to para-aminosalicylic acid, 481
 due to phenylbutazone, 237
 due to sulfonamides, 471
Thrombocytopenic purpura, idiopathic,
  azathioprine for, 542
Thromboembolic phenomena, coumarin
  derivatives in prevention of, 202
Thromboembolism due to oral
  contraceptives, 603
Thrombolysin; *see* Fibrinolysin

Thrombophlebitis
 as complication of intravenous therapy,
  418
 due to diethylstilbestrol, 604
 heparin for, 200
Thrombosis
 cerebral, due to diethylstilbestrol, 604
 as complication of intravenous therapy,
  418
 due to cortisone and hydrocortisone, 569
 intravascular, drugs preventing, 198-204
 due to quinine sulfate, 495
Thylose Sodium; *see* Carboxymethylcellulose
  sodium
Thymol as antiinfective, 515
Thymolytic action of glucocorticoids, 566
Thyrocalcitonin, function of, 554
Thyroglobulin, 559
Thyroid, preparations of, 557-559
 side effects and toxic effects of, 558
 in stimulation of ovulation, 605
Thyroid gland, 554
 carcinoma of, radioiodine for, 561-562
 effect of iodine deficiency on, 557
Thyroid hormones, 554-564
 biosynthesis of, 555
 deficiency of, states produced by, 557
 drugs acting against, 559-564; *see also*
  Antithyroid drugs
 physiologic effects of, 555-557
 secretion of, regulation of, 557
Thyroid-releasing hormone (TRH), 557
Thyroid-stimulating hormone (TSH), 557
Thyroidectomy
 hypocalcemia due to, 421
 for thyrotoxicosis, 559
 use of iodide in preparation for, 560
Thyrolar; *see* Liotrix
Thyrotoxicosis, 559-564
Thyrotropic hormone (TSH), 550
Thyrotropin, 552
Thyroxine, history and chemistry of, 555
Thyroxine sodium; *see* Levothyroxine
  sodium
D-Thyroxine sodium; *see* Dextrothyroxine
  sodium
Tic douloureux, ethyl alcohol injection for,
  257-258
Tidal air, definition of, 385
Tigan; *see* Trimethobenzamide hydrochloride
Tinactin; *see* Tolnaftate
Tincture of green soap as antiinfective, 522
Tinctures, description of, 36
Tindal; *see* Acetophenazine maleate
Tinnitus due to tricyclic antidepressants, 307
Titroid; *see* Levothyroxine sodium
Tobacco smoking and nicotine, 137
Tobramycin, 479
Toclase; *see* Carbetapentane citrate
Tocopherol; *see* Vitamin E
Tofranil; *see* Imipramine hydrochloride
Tolazamide, dosage and administration of,
  582
Tolbutamide
 structural formula for, 581
 use, dosage, and administration of, 582
Tolerance
 to amphetamines, 269, 325
 to barbiturates, 248
 to caffeine, 268
 to chloral hydrate, 254
 drug, 98
 to drugs in infants and children, 84-85